ACSM's
Resource Manual for
Guidelines for Exercise Testing
and Prescription
SEVENTH EDITION

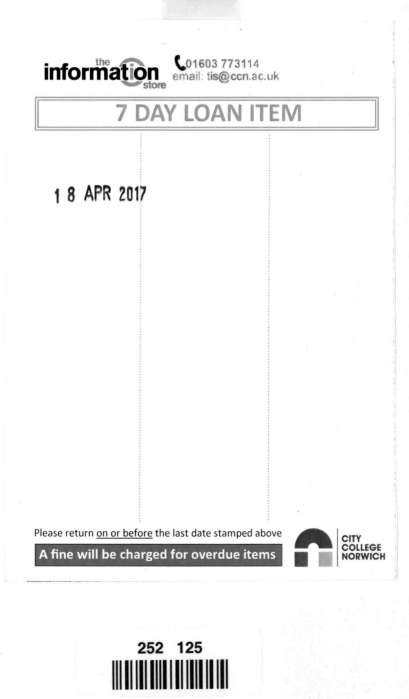

EDITORS*

SENIOR EDITOR

David P. Swain, PhD, FACSM, ACSM-CES, ACSM-PD
Professor, Human Movement Sciences Department
Old Dominion University
Norfolk, Virginia

SECTION EDITORS

Clinton A. Brawner, MS, FACSM, ACSM-CES, ACSM-RCEP
Clinical Exercise Physiologist
Henry Ford Hospital
Detroit, Michigan

Heather O. Chambliss, PhD, FACSM
Instructor, Health Promotion
University of Memphis
Memphis, Tennessee

Paul R. Nagelkirk, PhD
Assistant Professor, Exercise Science Program
Ball State University
Muncie, Indiana

Madeline Paternostro Bayles, PhD, FACSM, ACSM-CES, ACSM-PD
Associate Professor, Undergraduate Exercise Science Coordinator
Indiana University of Pennsylvania
Indiana, Pennsylvania

Ann M. Swank, PhD, FACSM
Professor, Exercise Physiology Laboratory
University of Louisville
Louisville, Kentucky

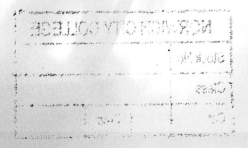

*See Appendix B for a list of editors for the previous two editions.

ACSM's
Resource Manual for
Guidelines for Exercise Testing and Prescription
SEVENTH EDITION

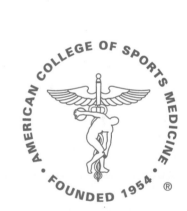

**AMERICAN COLLEGE
OF SPORTS MEDICINE**

Wolters Kluwer | Lippincott Williams & Wilkins
Health

Philadelphia · Baltimore · New York · London
Buenos Aires · Hong Kong · Sydney · Tokyo

Acquisitions Editor: Emily Lupash
Managing Editor: Meredith L. Brittain
Marketing Manager: Sarah Schuessler
Manufacturing Coordinator: Margie Orzech
Creative Director: Doug Smock
Compositor: Absolute Service, Inc.
ACSM Publication Committee Chair: Walter R. Thompson, PhD, FACSM, FAACVPR
ACSM Group Publisher: Kerry O'Rourke
Umbrella Editor: Jonathan K. Ehrman, PhD, FACSM

Seventh Edition

Copyright © 2014, 2010, 2006, 2001, 1998, 1993, 1988 American College of Sports Medicine

351 West Camden Street   Two Commerce Square / 2001 Market Street
Baltimore, MD 21201   Philadelphia, PA 19103

Printed in China

9 8 7 6 5 4 3 2 1

Library of Congress Cataloging-in-Publication Data

ACSM's resource manual for Guidelines for exercise testing and prescription / American College of Sports Medicine ; [senior editor, David P. Swain ; section editors, Clinton A. Brawner ... et al.]. — 7th ed.
    p. ; cm.
  Resource manual for Guidelines for exercise testing and prescription
  Companion to: ACSM's guidelines for exercise testing and prescription / American College of Sports Medicine. 9th ed. 2013.
  Includes bibliographical references and indexes.
  ISBN 978-1-60913-956-8
  I. Swain, David P. II. American College of Sports Medicine. III. American College of Sports Medicine. ACSM's guidelines for exercise testing and prescription. IV. Title: Resource manual for Guidelines for exercise testing and prescription.
  [DNLM: 1. Exercise Therapy—methods. 2. Exercise—physiology. 3. Exercise Test—standards. 4. Guidelines as Topic. 5. Physical Exertion—physiology. 6. Sports Medicine. WB 541]

615.8'2—dc23

2012036403

DISCLAIMER

Care has been taken to confirm the accuracy of the information present and to describe generally accepted practices. However, the authors, editors, and publisher are not responsible for errors or omissions or for any consequences from application of the information in this book and make no warranty, expressed or implied, with respect to the currency, completeness, or accuracy of the contents of the publication. Application of this information in a particular situation remains the professional responsibility of the practitioner; the clinical treatments described and recommended may not be considered absolute and universal recommendations.

The authors, editors, and publisher have exerted every effort to ensure that drug selection and dosage set forth in this text are in accordance with the current recommendations and practice at the time of publication. However, in view of ongoing research, changes in government regulations, and the constant flow of information relating to drug therapy and drug reactions, the reader is urged to check the package insert for each drug for any change in indications and dosage and for added warnings and precautions. This is particularly important when the recommended agent is a new or infrequently employed drug.

Some drugs and medical devices presented in this publication have Food and Drug Administration (FDA) clearance for limited use in restricted research settings. It is the responsibility of the health care provider to ascertain the FDA status of each drug or device planned for use in their clinical practice.

To purchase additional copies of this book, call our customer service department at (800) 638-3030 or fax orders to (301) 223-2320. International customers should call (301) 223-2300.

Visit Lippincott Williams & Wilkins on the Internet: http://www.lww.com. Lippincott Williams & Wilkins customer service representatives are available from 8:30 am to 6:00 pm, EST.

This book is dedicated to all those who strive to help others improve their health through exercise: to the scientists — such as D. Bruce Dill, Per-Olof Astrand, Martti Karvonen, Ralph Paffenbarger, and Michael Pollock — who have provided the insight; to the exercise professionals who turn knowledge into action; and to the students who will advance the cause in the future.

DPS

Preface

Exercise is critical to the health of the human organism. As humans, we are hunter-gatherers who once spent many hours in physical activity in our daily lives. Much of this activity was doubtless of a sustainable aerobic nature, whereas other activity required significant muscular power. Failure to challenge our bodies in this way results in a devolved physical condition and chronic disease.

Since August Krogh won the Nobel Prize in Physiology or Medicine in 1920 for his work on capillary blood flow in skeletal muscle, our knowledge of exercise and health has expanded enormously. In 1954, Joseph Wolffe and others founded the American College of Sports Medicine (ACSM) to bring together a group of scientists, clinicians, and other professionals dedicated to studying and promoting health through exercise.

In 1975, the ACSM published its first "*Guidelines for Graded Exercise Testing and Prescription.*" In 1978, The ACSM published its first scientifically based position stand on "The Recommended Quantity and Quality of Exercise for Developing and Maintaining Fitness in Healthy Adults" (*Med Sci Sports Exerc* 1978;10[3]:vii–x). The *Guidelines* is now in its ninth edition, and the Q&Q position stand had its fourth iteration published in 2011 (*Med Sci Sports Exerc* 2011;43[7]:1334–59). I was fortunate to have contributed as one of the authors of the 2011 position stand. Along the way, the ACSM has produced several other position stands on specific topics (resistance training, weight loss, heat illness, diabetes, etc.) to make recommendations based on available sound science.

In 1988, the ACSM developed a more comprehensive, explanatory text to accompany the "nuts and bolts" style of the *Guidelines*, and the first edition of this *Resource Manual* was published (*ACSM's Resource Manual for Guidelines for Exercise Testing and Prescription*).

As both a scientist and educator, I believe the *Resource Manual* is a tremendous asset for those wishing to translate knowledge of exercise into practice. This is the text that exercise professionals and students should turn to in order to obtain a deeper understanding of how exercise and health are interrelated and to find practical guidance in working with clients and patients.

The most important change in the seventh edition over the previous edition is an updated knowledge base using recent research, ACSM position stands (such as the 2011 Q&Q position stand), and the ninth edition of the *Guidelines*. Some reorganization was done, including the removal of the certification KSAs (knowledge, skills, and abilities) from the text. These were taken out because, although the *Resource Manual* is an excellent source book for those seeking ACSM certification, *ACSM's Certification Review* is more directly designed for certification preparation, and the placement of KSAs in the text of the *Resource Manual* interrupted the flow within the chapters.

A particularly important change is the development of Section V, Behavior Change. We professionals know that exercise is beneficial for health, and most people in the general population realize that this is true. Moreover, although there are many important details for the professional to be aware of when prescribing exercise, the basic rules aren't difficult to comprehend. I would summarize them as follows:

- Walk 30 min a day for basic health. More is better.
- Do more vigorous cardio exercise 2–3 times per week for greater benefit.
- Lift weights 2–3 times per week to develop muscular strength and maintain independence.
- To lose weight: exercise more than you eat.

The great challenge in today's world isn't getting these points across, it's motivating people to start and then adhere to a program. Material on behavior change was present in previous editions of the *Resource Manual*, and the seventh edition has expanded on that foundation, placing several chapters into a cohesive approach in working with clients.

I wish you the best in your own fitness and health, and in that of your clients.

ACKNOWLEDGMENTS

I would like to thank most the contributors and the section editors who worked tirelessly to produce this *Resource Manual*. More than 75 experts in their field contributed to the writing of the chapters in this substantial text. They are listed immediately following this preface. The *Resource Manual* is a living document produced by people with opinions.

The ACSM makes its recommendations based on the consensus opinion of experts within various fields. This process begins with the publication of peer-reviewed research in scientific journals such as *Medicine and Science in Sports and Exercise*. Individual researchers test their theories, and their reports on this research pass through a filter of other researchers in a peer-review process. Those articles that are published then enter the knowledge base in the exercise science field. Experts selected by the ACSM come together every few years to develop position stands on what the research means and what recommendations should thus be made. Using these position stands, as well as recently published studies, other experts revise the *Guidelines* in a 4–5 yr cycle. In concert with the *Guidelines*, a further set of experts — our contributors — revise this *Resource Manual*. At each step in the process, the opinions of the individuals involved are an important factor in molding the result. These opinions grow out of the scientific training that the individuals received. Does this process result in "truth"? It results in the best recommendations that our colleagues in the field can make.

The Section Editors — Paul Nagelkirk, Ann Swank, Madeline Paternostro Bayles, Clinton Brawner, and Heather Chambliss — reviewed and edited several chapters within each of their sections of the *Resource Manual*. This is a particularly demanding task and I thank them for their excellent work.

After my own review, the chapters were then reviewed by experts from the ACSM's Committee on Certification and Registry Boards, chaired by Deborah Riebe, and also reviewed by Umbrella Editor Jonathan Ehrman (Senior Editor of the sixth edition of the *Resource Manual*). The CCRB reviewers examined the chapters for content while Jon Ehrman examined them for consistency with the *Guidelines*. The entire process was assisted by staff members within the ACSM national office, Director of Publishing Kerry O'Rourke, Assistant Director of Certification Programs Traci Rush, and Certification Coordinator Kela Webster. All of these individuals were essential in the development of a text as large and comprehensive as the *Resource Manual*. I give a special thanks to Jill Livingston, who did a tremendous amount of work in preparing the references in each chapter. With thousands of references and dozens of contributors, she managed to cheerfully answer all my questions with the speed of a mouse click.

The Wolters Kluwer/Lippincott Williams & Wilkins publishing company has done an outstanding job in bringing the *Resource Manual* to publication. They have been superb partners for the publication of many of the ACSM's books and journals. Senior Acquisitions Editor Emily Lupash has been the driving force behind the LWW and ACSM connection, and Senior Product Manager Meredith Brittain deftly handled the *Resource Manual*.

I would like to add my personal thanks to some of my colleagues in ACSM: Linda Pescatello, Senior Editor of the *Guidelines*; Carol Garber, lead author of the ACSM 2011 "Quantity and Quality of Exercise" position stand; and past ACSM Presidents Barry Franklin and Ed Howley. Linda and Carol have been partners in my recent work, whereas Barry and Ed have been role models and mentors in my career. All of them have dedicated their own careers to advancing our knowledge of exercise and health.

David P. Swain, PhD, FACSM
Senior Editor

ADDITIONAL RESOURCES

ACSM's Resource Manual for Guidelines for Exercise Testing and Prescription, Seventh Edition includes additional resources for instructors that are available on the book's companion Web site at http://thepoint.lww.com/ACSMRM7e.

INSTRUCTORS

Approved adopting instructors will be given access to the following additional resources:

- Brownstone test generator
- PowerPoint presentations
- Image bank
- WebCT/Angel/Blackboard ready cartridge

In addition, purchasers of the text can access the searchable full text online by going to the *ACSM's Resource Manual for Guidelines for Exercise Testing and Prescription, Seventh Edition* Web site at http://thepoint.lww.com/ACSMRM7e. See the inside front cover of this text for more details, including the passcode you will need to gain access to the Web site.

NOTA BENE

The exercise professional should use the views and information contained in the seventh edition of *ACSM's Resource Manual for Guidelines for Exercise Testing and Prescription* as expert advice. When applying this advice in exercise testing and programmatic settings, the professional must use independent and prudent judgment. *ACSM's Resource Manual for Guidelines for Exercise Testing and Prescription* presents a framework whereby the professional may certainly — and in some cases has the obligation to — tailor to individual client or patient needs while balancing institutional or legal requirements.

Contributing Authors to the Seventh Edition*

Kent J. Adams, PhD, FACSM
California State University Monterey Bay
Seaside, California
Chapter 3: Exercise Physiology

Robert E. Alman, DEd
Indiana University of Pennsylvania
Indiana, Pennsylvania
Chapter 21: Cardiorespiratory and Health-Related
Physical Fitness Assessments

Rafael E. Bahamonde, PhD, FACSM
Indiana University-Purdue University Indianapolis
Indianapolis, Indiana
Chapter 1: Functional Anatomy

David R. Bassett, Jr, PhD
University of Tennessee
Knoxville, Tennessee
Chapter 13: Assessment of Physical Activity

Susan G. Beckham, PhD, FACSM
The Cooper Institute
Dallas, Texas
Chapter 19: Exercise Program Safety and Emergency
Procedures

Vera A. Bittner, MD, MSPH
University of Alabama at Birmingham
Birmingham, Alabama
Chapter 12: Physical Activity Status and Chronic
Diseases

**Clinton A. Brawner, MS, FACSM, ACSM-CES,
ACSM-RCEP**
Henry Ford Hospital
Detroit, Michigan
Chapter 23: Clinical Exercise Testing Procedures

Brian W. Carlin, MD
Drexel University School of Medicine
Pittsburgh, Pennsylvania
Chapter 25: Diagnostic Procedures in Patients with
Pulmonary Diseases

Ruth Ann Carpenter, MS, RD
Health Integration, LLC
Cincinnati, Ohio
Chapter 47: Methods for Delivering Physical Activity
Programs

Heather O. Chambliss, PhD, FACSM
University of Memphis
Memphis, Tennessee
Chapter 45: Principles of Behavior Change: Skill
Building to Promote Physical Activity

Dawn P. Coe, PhD, ACSM-CES
University of Tennessee
Knoxville, Tennessee
Chapter 36: Exercise Prescription in Special
Populations: Women, Pregnancy, Children, and
Older Adults

Sheri R. Colberg, PhD, FACSM, ACSM-ETT
Old Dominion University
Norfolk, Virginia
Chapter 14: Nutritional Status and Chronic Diseases
Chapter 40: Exercise Prescription for Patients with
Diabetes

Christopher B. Cooper, MD
David Geffen School of Medicine at UCLA
Los Angeles, California
Chapter 39: Exercise Prescription for Patients with
Pulmonary Disease

**Dino G. Costanzo, MA, FACSM, ACSM-RCEP,
ACSM-PD, ACSM-ETT**
The Hospital of Central Connecticut
New Britain, Connecticut
Appendix A: American College of Sports Medicine
Certifications

Adam deJong, MA
Oakland University
Rochester, Michigan
Chapter 29: Electrocardiography

Shawn M. Drake, PT, PhD, ACSM-CES
Arkansas State University
Jonesboro, Arkansas
Chapter 20: Preparation for Exercise Testing

*See Appendix C for a list of contributors for the previous two
editions.

Andrea L. Dunn, PhD, FACSM
Klein Buendel
Golden, Colorado
Chapter 9: Psychopathology

Craig A. Emter, PhD
University of Missouri-Columbia
Columbia, Missouri
Chapter 32: Adaptations to Cardiorespiratory Exercise
   Training

Maria A. Fiatarone Singh, MD, FRACP
The University of Sydney
Lidcombe NSW, Australia
Chapter 36: Exercise Prescription in Special Populations:
   Women, Pregnancy, Children, and Older Adults

Christy A. Greenleaf, PhD
University of Wisconsin
Milwaukee, Wisconsin
Chapter 45: Principles of Behavior Change:
   Skill Building to Promote Physical Activity

Trent Hargens, PhD, ACSM-CES
James Madison University
Harrisonburg, Virginia
Chapter 6: Pathophysiology and Treatment of
   Cardiovascular Disease

Chad Harris, PhD, FACSM
LaGrange College
LaGrange, Georgia
Chapter 3: Exercise Physiology

**Sam Headley, PhD, FACSM, ACSM-CES,
ACSM-RCEP**
Springfield College
Springfield, Massachusetts
Chapter 41: Exercise Prescription for Patients with
   Comorbidites and Other Chronic Diseases

David L. Herbert, JD
David L. Herbert & Associates, LLC
Canton, Ohio
Chapter 10: Legal Considerations for Exercise
   Programming

William G. Herbert, PhD, ACSM-PD
Virginia Polytechnic Institute and State University
Blacksburg, Virginia
Chapter 10: Legal Considerations for Exercise
   Programming

Jeff Herrick, PhD
George Mason University
Fairfax, Virginia
Chapter 5: Lifespan Effects of Aging and Deconditioning

Nancy Houston-Miller, BSN
Stanford School of Medicine
Stanford, California
Chapter 16: Psychosocial Status and Chronic Disease

Chun-Jung Huang, PhD
Florida Atlantic University
Boca Raton, Florida
Chapter 5: Lifespan Effects of Aging and Deconditioning

Julie M. Hughes, PhD
United States Army Research Institute of Environmental
   Medicine
Natick, MA
Chapter 42: Exercise Prescription for Patients with
   Osteoporosis

Allison Ives, MS
Temple University
Philadelphia, Pennsylvania
Chapter 44: Theoretical Foundations of Physical
   Activity Behavior Change

Megan Jablonski, MA
University of Louisville
Louisville, Kentucky
Chapter 17: Assessment of Psychosocial Status

Andrea K. Johnson, PhD
University of Tennessee
Martin, Tennessee
Chapter 5: Lifespan Effects of Aging and Deconditioning

**Anthony S. Kaleth, PhD, ACSM-HFS, ACSM-CES,
ACSM-PD, ACSM-RCEP**
Indiana University-Purdue University Indianapolis
Indianapolis, Indiana
Chapter 1: Functional Anatomy

Carol Kennedy-Armbruster, PhD, ACSM-HFS
Indiana University
Bloomington, Indiana
Chapter 34: Group Exercise Programming

Steven J. Keteyian, PhD, FACSM, ACSM-RCEP
Henry Ford Hospital
Detroit, Michigan
Chapter 23: Clinical Exercise Testing Procedures
Chapter 38: Exercise Prescription for Patients with
   Cardiovascular Disease

Duane Knudson, PhD, FASCM
Texas State University
San Marcos, Texas
Chapter 2: Biomechanics

William J. Kraemer, PhD, FACSM
University of Connecticut
Storrs, Connecticut
Chapter 31: Musculoskeletal Exercise Prescription
Chapter 33: Adaptations to Resistance Training

Maurice H. Laughlin, PhD, FACSM
University of Missouri
Columbia, Missouri
Chapter 32: Adaptations to Cardiorespiratory Exercise
    Training

Beth A. Lewis, PhD
University of Minnesota
Minneapolis, Minnesota
Chapter 44: Theoretical Foundations of Physical
    Activity Behavior Change

Hayley MacDonald, MS, ACSM-CPT
University of Connecticut
Storrs, Connecticut
Chapter 28: Exercise Assessment in Special Populations

Bess H. Marcus, PhD
University of California San Diego
La Jolla, California
Chapter 44: Theoretical Foundations of Physical
    Activity Behavior Change

Bonita L. Marks, PhD, FACSM, ACSM-CES
University of North Carolina at Chapel Hill
Chapel Hill, North Carolina
Chapter 11: General Overview of Preparticipation
    Health Screening and Risk Assessment

Scott B. Martin, PhD
University of North Texas
Denton, Texas
Chapter 45: Principles of Behavior Change:
    Skill Building to Promote Physical Activity

**Barbara S. McClanahan, EdD, PhD, ACSM-GEI,
ACSM-HFS**
University of Memphis
Memphis, Tennessee
Chapter 46: Counseling Physical Activity Behavior Change
Chapter 48: Promoting Physical Activity in the
    Community

Audrey Lynn Millar, PT, PhD, FACSM
Winston-Salem State University
Winston-Salem, North Carolina
Chapter 43: Exercise Prescription for Patients with Arthritis

Nicole Moodie, PhD
Rockhurst University
Kansas City, Missouri
Chapter 26: Diagnostic Procedures in Patients with
    Metabolic Disease

Melissa A. Napolitano, PhD
George Washington University
Washington, DC
Chapter 44: Theoretical Foundations of Physical
    Activity Behavior Change

Ildiko Nyikos, MA, ACSM-RCEP
Lakeshore Foundation
Birmingham, Alabama
Chapter 27: Occupational and Functional Assessments

Stefan M. Pasiakos, MS, ACSM-CPT
US Army Research Institute of Environmental Medicine
Natick, Massachusetts
Chapter 4: Nutrition

Susan Peacock, MEd, MS
University of Louisville
Louisville, Kentucky
Chapter 15: Assessment of Nutritional Status

Moira Petit, PhD
University of Minnesota
Minneapolis, Minnesota
Chapter 42: Exercise Prescription for Patients with
    Osteoporosis

**Wanda Koester Qualters, MS, ACSM-RCEP,
ACSM-CES**
Indiana University Health Bloomington Hospital
Bloomington, Indiana
Chapter 24: Diagnostic Procedures for
    Cardiovascular Disease

Nick Ratamess, PhD
The College of New Jersey
Ewing, New Jersey
Chapter 18: Body Composition Status and Assessment

Nancy R. Rodriguez, PhD, RD, FACSM
University of Connecticut
Storrs, Connecticut
Chapter 4: Nutrition

Jeff L. Roitman, EdD, FACSM
Rockhurst University
Kansas City, Missouri
Chapter 26: Diagnostic Procedures in Patients with
    Metabolic Disease

Lee Romer, PhD, FACSM
Brunel University London
Uxbridge, United Kingdom
Chapter 7: Pathophysiology and Treatment of
    Pulmonary Disease

Peter Ronai, MS, ACSM-RCEP, ACSM-CES
Sacred Heart University
Fairfield, Connecticut
Chapter 22: Muscular Fitness and Assessment

Alice S. Ryan, PhD, ACSM-CES
University of Maryland School of Medicine
Baltimore, Maryland
Chapter 8: Pathophysiology and Treatment of
    Metabolic Disease

Paul Salmon, PhD
University of Louisville
Louisville, Kentucky
Chapter 17: Assessment of Psychosocial Status

Patrick D. Savage, MS
Fletcher Allen Healthcare
So. Burlington, Vermont
Chapter 38: Exercise Prescription for Patients with
    Cardiovascular Disease

Matthew A. Saval, MS, ACSM-RCEP, ACSM-CES
Henry Ford Hospital
Detroit, Michigan
Chapter 37: Exercise Prescription and Medical
    Considerations

John R. Schairer, DO
Henry Ford Hospital
Detroit, Michigan
Chapter 37: Exercise Prescription and Medical
    Considerations

Lesley Scibora, DC, PhD
University of Minnesota
Minneapolis, Minnesota
Chapter 42: Exercise Prescription for Patients with
    Osteoporosis

Monica C. Serra, PhD, RD
University of Maryland School of Medicine
Baltimore VA Medical Center
Baltimore, Maryland
Chapter 8: Pathophysiology and Treatment of
    Metabolic Disease

Patricia Sevene, PhD
California State University Monterey Bay
Seaside, California
Chapter 3: Exercise Physiology

John C. Sieverdes, PhD
University of South Carolina
Columbia, South Carolina
Chapter 47: Methods for Delivering Physical Activity
    Programs

Mark A. Sloniger, PhD, FACSM
Indiana University of Pennsylvania
Indiana, Pennsylvania
Chapter 21: Cardiorespiratory and Health-Related
    Physical Fitness Assessments

Michelle Stockton, PhD
University of Memphis
Memphis, Tennessee
Chapter 46: Counseling Physical Activity Behavior
    Change
Chapter 48: Promoting Physical Activity in the
    Community

Thomas W. Storer, PhD
University of California Los Angeles
Los Angeles, California
Chapter 39: Exercise Prescription for Patients with
    Pulmonary Disease

**David P. Swain, PhD, FACSM, ACSM-CES,
ACSM-PD**
Old Dominion University
Norfolk, Virginia
Chapter 30: Cardiorespiratory Exercise Prescription

Dennis A. Tighe, MD, FACC, FACP
University of Massachusetts Medical School
Worcester, Massachusetts
Chapter 41: Exercise Prescription for Patients with
    Comorbidites and Other Chronic Diseases

Stella L. Volpe, PhD, RD, LD/N, FACSM
Drexel University
Philadelphia, Pennsylvania
Chapter 35: Weight Management

Jessica A. Whiteley, PhD
University of Massachusetts
Boston, Massachusetts
Chapter 44: Theoretical Foundations of Physical
    Activity Behavior Change

Richard E. Wood, PhD
Springfield College
Springfield, Massachusetts
Chapter 41: Exercise Prescription for Patients with
    Comorbidites and Other Chronic Diseases

Mary M. Yoke, MA, ACSM-HFS
Indiana University
Bloomington, Indiana
Chapter 34: Group Exercise Programming

Reviewers for the Seventh Edition

Sherry A. Barkley, PhD, ACSM-RCEP, ACSM-CES
Augustana College
Sioux Falls, South Dakota

Robert Berry, MS, MA, ACSM-RCEP, ACSM-CES
Baystate Medical Center
Glastonbury, Connecticut

Andy Bosak, PhD, ACSM-HFS
Armstrong Atlantic State University
Savannah, Georgia

Nikki Carosone, MS, ACSM-CPT
Plus One Fitness
Brooklyn, New York

**Brian J. Coyne, MEd, ACSM-RCEP,
ACSM/NCPAD-CIFT**
Duke University Health System
Morrisville, North Carolina

Kimberly DeLeo, BS, PTA, ACSM-CPT
Health and Exercise Connections, LLC
People First Rehabilitation
Mattapoisett, Massachusetts

Grace DeSimone, BA, ACSM-CPT, ACSM-GEI
Plus One Health Management
New York, New York

**Gregory B. Dwyer, PhD, FACSM, ACSM-RCEP,
ACSM-CES, ACSM-PD**
East Stroudsburg University
East Stroudsburg, Pennsylvania

Sabrina Fairchild, MA, ACSM-HFS
California State University, Chico
Durham, California

Yuri Feito, PhD, MPH, ACSM-RCEP, ACSM-CES
Barry University
Miami, Florida

**Diana Ferris, MS, ACSM-HFS,
ACSM/NSPAPPH-PAPHS**
Stratford, Connecticut

**Carol Ewing Garber, PhD, FACSM, ACSM-PD,
ACSM-RCEP, ACSM-ETT, ACSM-HFS**
Columbia University
New York, New York

Wanda Koester, MS, ACSM-RCEP, ACSM-CES
Indiana University Health
Bloomington, Indiana

Shel Levine, MS, MSA, ACSM-CES
Eastern Michigan University
Farmington Hills, Michigan

**Gary Liguori, PhD, FACSM, ACSM-CES,
ACSM-HFS**
University of Tennessee at Chattanooga
Chattanooga, Tennessee

**Meir Magal, PhD, FACSM, ACSM-CES,
ACSM-HFS**
North Carolina Wesleyan College
Rocky Mount, North Carolina

Peter Magyari, PhD, ACSM-HFS
University of North Florida
Jacksonville, Florida

Sharon L. McGoff, BS, JD, ACSM-HFS
Fit 4 Life Coaching, LLC
Indianapolis, Indiana

**Mark A. Patterson, MEd, ACSM-RCEP,
ACSM/ACS-CET**
Kaiser Permanente
Denver, Colorado

Deborah Riebe, PhD, FACSM, ACSM-HFS
University of Rhode Island
Kingston, Rhode Island

**Peter J. Ronai, MS, FACSM, ACSM-RCEP,
ACSM-CES, ACSM-HFS, ACSM-PD, ACSM-ETT**
Sacred Heart University
Milford, Connecticut

Brad A. Roy, PhD, FACSM, ACSM-CES
Kalispell Regional Medical Center
Kalispell, Montana

David Seigneur, MS, ACSM-CES
UPMC Mercy
Pittsburgh, Pennsylvania

Paul Sorace, MS, ACSM-CES
Hackensack University Medical Center
Bayonne, New Jersey

Thomas Spring, MS, ACSM-CES, ACSM-CPT
Beaumont Health System
Huntington Woods, Michigan

Amy-Jo Sutterluety, PhD, FACSM, ACSM-CES, ACSM-HFS
Baldwin-Wallace University
Berea, Ohio

Benjamin Thompson, PhD, ACSM-HFS
Metropolitan State College of Denver
Denver, Colorado

Hilary Welch-Petrowski, MS, ACSM-CES
Eagle Ranch Fitness Club
Eagle, Colorado

Contents

Preliminary Section: Background Materials

PAUL NAGELKIRK, PhD, *Section Editor*

Functional Anatomy

ANATOMICAL POSITION AND DEFINITIONS OF ANATOMICAL LOCATIONS AND PLANES

The anatomical position is the universally accepted reference position used to describe regions and spatial relationships of the human body and to make reference to body positions (*e.g.*, joint motions). In the anatomical position, the body is erect with the feet together and the upper limbs hanging at the sides, palms of the hands facing forward, thumbs facing away from the body, and fingers extended (*Fig. 1-1*).

Another useful tool used to describe anatomical motions are body planes, or planes of motion. There are three theoretical planes orthogonal to each other that pass through the body. The *sagittal plane* divides the body or structure into the right and left sides. The *frontal* or *coronal plane* divides the body or structure into anterior and posterior portions. The *transverse plane*

KEY TERMS

Agonist: Muscle or muscle group that is the prime mover for a joint action.

Anatomical position: The universally accepted reference position used to describe regions and spatial relationships of the human body and to make reference to body positions.

Antagonist: Muscle or muscle group that opposes the action of the prime movers (agonist).

Appendicular skeleton: All of the bones that are found in the limbs of the body.

Atrioventricular (AV) valves: Separate the atria from the ventricles. The right AV valve has three leaflets and is called the tricuspid valve. The left AV valve has two leaflets and is called the bicuspid (or mitral) valve.

Auscultation: The act of listening to sounds of the body. A practitioner can use a stethoscope to assess blood pressure, heart rate, and heart and lung sounds by auscultation.

Axial skeleton: The bones of the skeleton that form the central or supportive core, including the bones of the skull, vertebral column, ribs, and sternum.

Contractile proteins: Specialized proteins found within muscle cells that interact with one another to cause muscle force production. The major contractile proteins are actin and myosin.

Joints: The articulations between bones, typically classified according to structure as being fibrous,

cartilaginous, or synovial. Synovial joints are the most common in the body.

Motor unit: A single somatic motor neuron and the group of muscle fibers innervated by it.

Muscle fiber architecture: The orientation of the muscle fibers to the longitudinal axis of the muscle. Terms commonly used to describe muscle fiber architecture include fusiform (longitudinal) and pennate (unipennate, bipennate, and multipennate).

Planes of motion: Orthogonal planes that divide the human body and can be used to describe various body movements. The three planes of motion are commonly known as the sagittal, frontal, and transverse planes.

Regulatory proteins: Specialized proteins found within muscle cells that block the binding of the contractile proteins to one another and thus keep the muscle in a relaxed state. The regulatory proteins are troponin and tropomyosin.

Respiratory membrane: The membrane formed by the walls of the alveoli and capillaries as they come in contact with one another in the lungs. The respiratory membrane is where diffusion of oxygen and carbon dioxide occurs within the lungs.

Synergist: Muscle or muscle group that assists the agonist in performing a joint action.

Ventilation: The act of breathing in (inhalation) and out (exhalation) so that air can enter the alveoli to allow oxygen and carbon dioxide exchange.

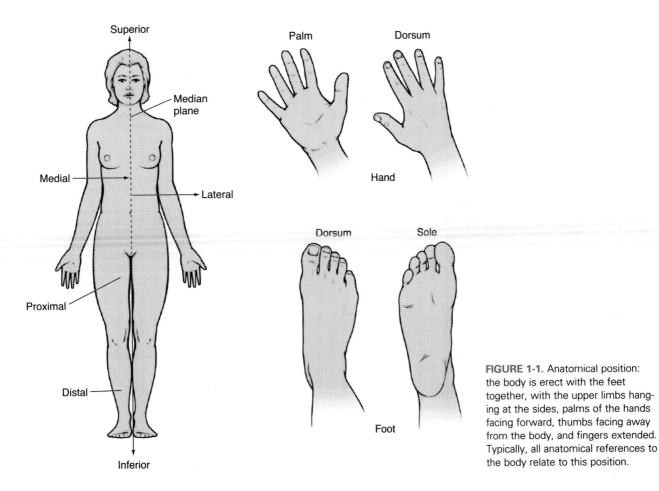

FIGURE 1-1. Anatomical position: the body is erect with the feet together, with the upper limbs hanging at the sides, palms of the hands facing forward, thumbs facing away from the body, and fingers extended. Typically, all anatomical references to the body relate to this position.

(also called the *cross-sectional* or *horizontal plane*) divides the body or structure into superior and inferior portions (*Fig. 1-2*). *Table 1-1* lists some terms commonly used to reference anatomical spatial relationships.

CARDIOVASCULAR ANATOMY

GENERAL COMPONENTS AND FUNCTIONS

The cardiovascular system is a continuous closed arrangement that includes a pump (the heart) and more than 60,000 miles of conduits (blood vessels) (24). The primary function of the cardiovascular system is to provide an environment for the transport of nutrients and removal of waste products. The cardiovascular system assists with maintaining homeostasis at rest and during exercise by performing the following specific functions (28,29,38):

1. transports oxygenated blood from the lungs to tissues and deoxygenated blood from the tissues to the lungs;
2. distributes nutrients (*e.g.*, glucose, free fatty acids, amino acids) to cells;
3. removes metabolic byproducts (*e.g.*, carbon dioxide, urea, lactate) from the periphery for elimination or reuse;
4. regulates pH to control acidosis and alkalosis;

5. transports hormones and enzymes to regulate physiological functions;
6. maintains fluid volume to prevent dehydration; and
7. maintains body temperature by absorbing and redistributing heat.

The following sections provide an overview of the basic structures and functions of the heart and blood vessels.

Heart

Location and General Landmarks

The adult heart is approximately the size of a fist and weighs between 250 and 350 g (39). The heart is positioned obliquely within the thoracic cavity in a space known as the *mediastinum* (*Fig. 1-3*). It is positioned anterior to the vertebral column and posterior to the sternum. The lungs flank the heart bilaterally and slightly overlap it.

The heart has four chambers: the two superior chambers are the *atria*, and the two inferior chambers are the *ventricles*. The external deep grooves of the heart (called *sulci*) define the boundaries of the four chambers of the heart (17,38). The coronary sulcus separates the atria from the ventricles; the interventricular sulcus separates

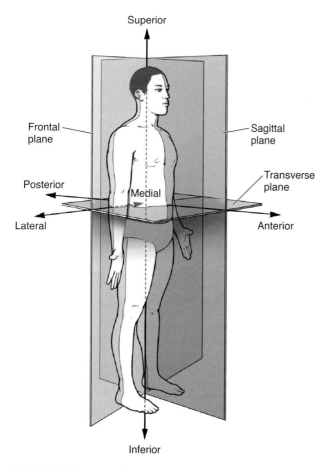

FIGURE 1-2. Anatomical planes of the body.

TABLE 1-1. Definitions of Anatomical Locations

Term	Definition
Anterior	The front of the body; ventral
Deep	Below the surface and not relatively close to the surface
Distal	Farthest point in distance from a given anatomic reference point
Inferior	Away from the head; lower
Lateral	Away from the midline of the body; to the side
Medial	Toward the midline of the body
Posterior	The back of the body; dorsal
Proximal	Closest point in distance to a given anatomic reference point
Superficial	Located close to or on the body surface
Superior	Toward the head; higher

the left ventricle (LV) and right ventricle (RV). The sulci also contain the major arteries and veins that provide circulation within the heart.

The heart has a base and an apex. The base of the heart consists mainly of the left atrium (LA), part of the right atrium (RA), and parts of the proximal portion of the large veins that enter the heart posteriorly. The base is located superiorly and near the right sternal border at the level of second and third ribs. The apex of the heart

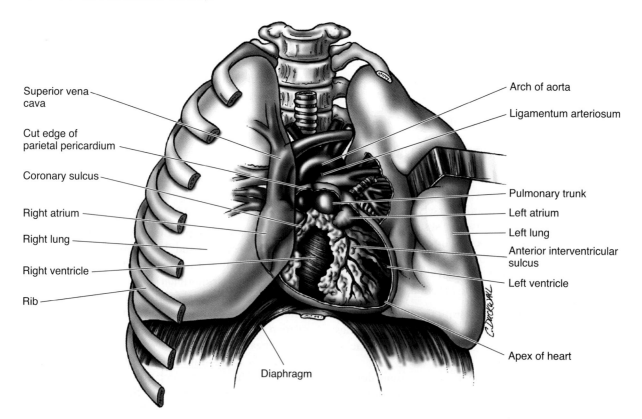

FIGURE 1-3. Anterior view of the thorax showing the position of the heart in the mediastinum.

is located inferiorly and to the left of the base at the level of the fifth intercostal space. Approximately two-thirds of the heart's mass is to the left of the midsagittal plane. Contractions of the heart can be easily discerned at the apex between the fifth and sixth ribs. This is referred to as the *point of maximal intensity* (PMI) (28).

The superior border of the heart consists of both atria and the bases of the pulmonary trunk and the aorta. The right border is formed by the RA. The left border consists of the LV and a small part of the LA. The inferior border is formed primarily by the RV and a portion of the LV at the apex. The heart is rotated to the left in the chest so that the anterior portion of the heart forms the sternocostal surface, which consists mainly of the RA and RV. The diaphragmatic surface consists mainly of the LV where it slopes and rests on the diaphragm.

Tissue Coverings and Layers of the Heart

The heart is covered by a double-walled, loose-fitting membranous sac called the *pericardium* (Fig. 1-4). The outer wall of the pericardium, the parietal pericardium, has both a fibrous (*i.e.*, tough) layer and a serous (*i.e.*, smooth) layer. The fibrous layer serves to strengthen the pericardium and anchor it within the mediastinum. The thin serous layer, called the visceral pericardium or *epicardium*, adheres to the fibrous layer of the parietal pericardium and forms a tight covering over the heart surface. Between the parietal and visceral layers is the *pericardial cavity*. The pericardial cavity contains *pericardial fluid*, which acts as a lubricant and reduces friction between the membranes during contraction. If the pericardium becomes inflamed, *pericarditis*, a condition characterized by painful adhesions, can result.

The thickest layer of tissue in the heart is the *myocardium*. The myocardium is composed of cardiac muscle. Within the myocardium is a network of crisscrossing, dense, connective tissue fibers called the *cardiac skeleton*. This cardiac skeleton provides insertion points for the fibers of the cardiac musculature, support for the valves of the heart, and some separation between the atria and ventricles.

The inner layer of the myocardium is lined with a thin layer of endothelium called the *endocardium*. The endocardium forms the innermost lining of the walls of the various heart chambers as well as the heart valves. The endocardium joins with the endothelial linings of the blood vessels as they leave and enter the heart (36).

Heart Chambers, Valves, and Blood Flow

The heart is two pumps in a single unit with four chambers or cavities: RA, LA, RV, and LV (*Fig. 1-5*). The right heart (RA and RV) and the left heart (LA and LV) make up the two pumps. The right side of the heart collects blood from the periphery and pumps it through the lungs (pulmonary circuit). The left side of the heart collects blood from the lungs and pumps it throughout the body (systemic circuit) (5,12,14,30,35).

The atria and ventricles of the heart are separated by the *interatrial septum* and the *interventricular septum*, respectively. The atria are smaller and have thinner walls than the ventricles. The LV walls and interventricular septum are two to three times thicker than the RV walls. The thicker myocardium of the LV allows the left side of the heart to pump blood against the greater resistance offered by the large vascular tree that makes up the systemic circuit. Conversely, the RV only has to pump blood a relatively short distance through the low resistance pulmonary circuit.

The heart has four valves whose function is to maintain unidirectional blood flow. The **atrioventricular (AV) valves** separate the atria from the ventricles. The *semilunar valves* separate the ventricles from the aorta and pulmonary artery trunk. The AV valves are named for the number of leaflets, or *cusps*, formed by the endocardium (*Fig. 1-6*). Whereas the right AV valve has three cusps and is called the *tricuspid valve*, the left AV valve has only two cusps and is called the *bicuspid* (or *mitral*) *valve*. The tricuspid valve controls blood flow from the RA to the RV, and the mitral valve controls blood flow from the LA to the LV. The cusps of the AV valves are attached to *chordae tendineae* (strong fibrous bands) that extend from the *papillary muscles*. The papillary muscles arise from folds and ridges of the

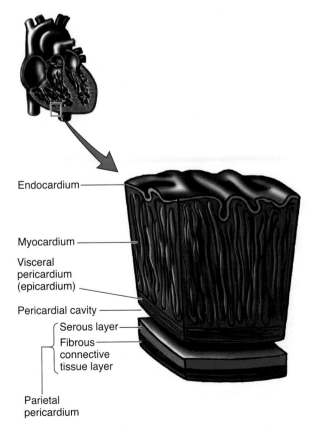

Endocardium

Myocardium

Visceral pericardium (epicardium)

Pericardial cavity

Serous layer

Fibrous connective tissue layer

Parietal pericardium

FIGURE 1-4. Endocardium, myocardium, and pericardium.

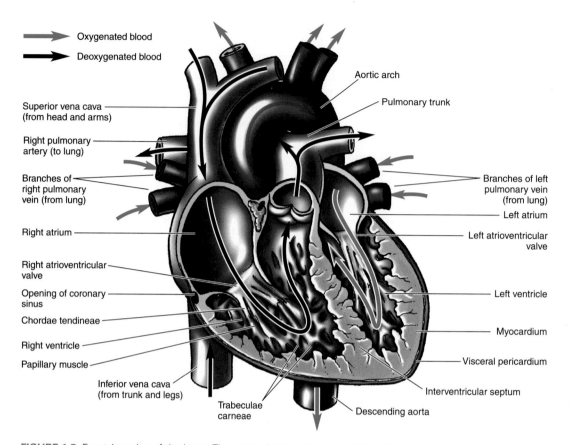

FIGURE 1-5. Frontal section of the heart. The arrows indicate the path of blood flow through the heart.

myocardium that project into the ventricular chambers. During ventricular contraction, the papillary muscles shorten and pull the chordae tendineae taut; this prevents the AV valves from swinging back into the atria, thus preventing retrograde blood flow during ventricular contraction (18).

There are two semilunar valves in the heart, each with three cusps. The *pulmonary valve* lies between the RV and the pulmonary artery. The *aortic valve* is located between the LV and the aorta. The cusps of the semilunar valves prevent the backflow of blood from the arteries to the ventricles.

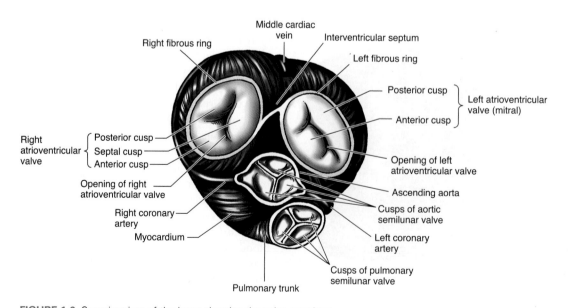

FIGURE 1-6. Superior view of the heart showing the valve openings.

Blood flow through the heart is accomplished by the following sequence of events, beginning with the return of systemic blood to the RA:

1. Venous blood flows into the RA via the superior and inferior vena cava, coronary sinus, and anterior cardiac veins; much of this blood flows into the RV through the open tricuspid valve.
2. The RA free wall (the contractile section of the RA heart wall) contracts and additional blood moves through the tricuspid valve into the RV.
3. The RV free wall contracts, the tricuspid valve closes (creating the first heart sound), the pulmonary valve opens, and blood flows through the pulmonary valve into the pulmonary artery and the branches of that system; after the ejection of blood into the pulmonary artery, pressure within the pulmonary artery closes the pulmonary valve (creating the second heart sound).
4. Blood ultimately reaches the alveolar capillaries, where gas exchange occurs.
5. Blood flows back to the LA via the pulmonary veins; much of this blood flows into the LV through the open bicuspid valve. (Step 5 occurs simultaneously with step 1.)

6. The LA free wall contracts and additional blood flows through the bicuspid valve and into the LV. (Step 6 occurs simultaneously with step 2.)
7. The LV free wall contracts, the bicuspid valve closes (creating the first heart sound), the aortic valve opens, and blood flows through the aortic valve into the aorta and its branches where it is distributed to the systemic circulation, which includes the coronary circulation; after the ejection of blood into the aorta, pressure within the aorta closes the aortic valve (creating the second heart sound). (Step 7 occurs simultaneously with step 3.) (18,19,32,39)

Heart Blood Supply

Although the interiors of the heart chambers are continuously bathed with blood, only the endocardium is directly nourished. The myocardium is too thick to permit adequate diffusion of nutrients and oxygen to the cardiac muscle cells and to the epicardium. The functional supply of blood for the heart is delivered via the *left coronary artery* (LCA) and *right coronary artery* (RCA) (*Figs. 1-7* and *1-8*). The coronary arteries arise from the *aortic sinus* at the base of the aorta just superior to the semilunar (aortic) valve cusps (*Fig. 1-9*).

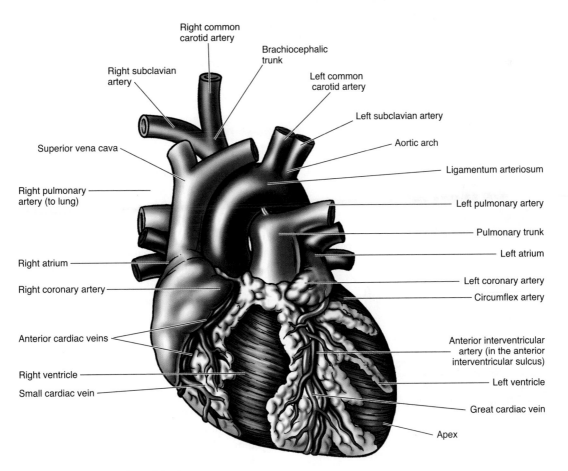

FIGURE 1-7. Anterior view of the heart.

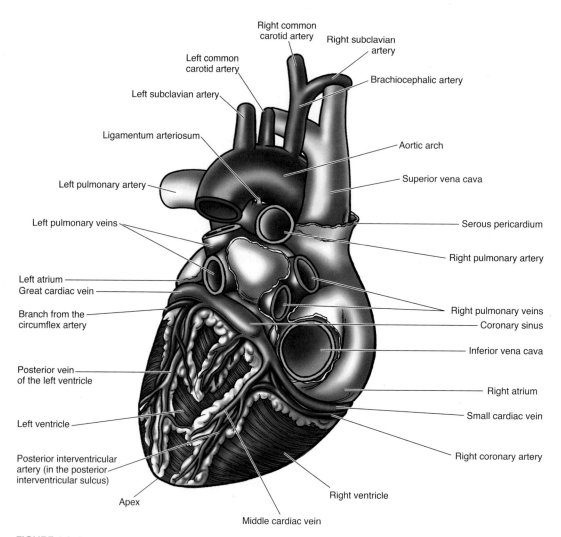

FIGURE 1-8. Posterior view of the heart.

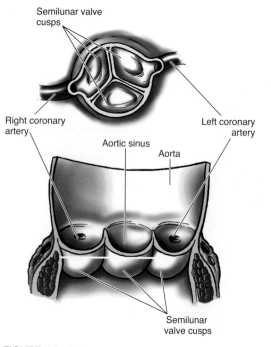

FIGURE 1-9. Origin of the coronary arteries.

The LCA angles toward the left side of the heart for about 1–2 cm before branching into the *left anterior descending* (LAD) coronary artery and the *circumflex artery* (CxA) (37). The LAD artery supplies blood to the interventricular septum and anterior walls of both ventricles. The CxA branches toward the left margin of the heart in the coronary sulcus and supplies blood to the laterodorsal walls of the LA and LV. Both the LAD artery and CxA curve around the left ventricular wall and supply small branches that interconnect (*anastomose*) with the RCA.

The RCA supplies blood to the right side of the heart as it follows the AV groove before curving to the back of the heart, giving off a *posterior interventricular artery* (*posterior descending artery*, or PDA). The RCA and PDA have numerous branches that supply blood to the anterior, posterior, and lateral surfaces of the RV and to the RA.

After blood circulates through the coronary artery system, which ends at the myocardial capillaries, it is collected by the cardiac veins. The blood then travels a path similar to that of the coronary arteries but in the opposite direction. On the posterior aspect of the heart, the cardiac veins form an enlarged vessel, the *coronary sinus*, which empties the blood into the RA. Some smaller anterior cardiac veins also empty directly into the RA.

Conduction System of the Heart

Cardiac muscle has intrinsic properties that allow it to depolarize and contract without direct neural stimulation. Cardiac cells interconnect end to end and form *intercalated discs* (29). These intercalated discs allow electrical impulses to spread from cell to cell and cause the myocardium to act as a single unit or functional *syncytium*. The components of the heart's conduction system include the *sinoatrial* (SA) *node*, the *AV node*, the *AV bundle* (*bundle of His*), the *right* and *left bundle branches*, and the *Purkinje fibers* (Fig. 1-10).

The electrical impulse, which initiates cardiac contraction, begins at the SA node, or intrinsic pacemaker, of the heart. The cells of the SA node, which lie in the wall of the RA near the opening of the superior vena cava, depolarize spontaneously about 60–80 times per minute at rest, depending on input from the autonomic nervous system (the intrinsic rate of the SA node without such influence is about 100 times per minute) (41). From the SA node, the electrical impulse spreads via internodal gaps through both atria until it reaches the AV node, which is located in the inferior part of the interatrial septum. The electrical impulse is delayed at the AV node for approximately 0.13 s to allow the atria to contract and fill the ventricles. The impulse then moves rapidly through the AV bundle (bundle of His), through the right and left bundle branches, and through the network of Purkinje fibers in the myocardium of both ventricles. The Purkinje fibers are specialized fast-conducting cells

that allow rapid conduction to the ventricles. This rapid conduction allows the ventricles to contract at approximately the same time.

The rate and forcefulness of heart contraction do not depend on intrinsic nerve stimulation; rather, they are influenced by extrinsic factors such as autonomic nervous system control and hormone activity. Sympathetic nerves and hormones (*e.g.*, norepinephrine and epinephrine) stimulate the atria and ventricles to beat faster (*chronotropic effect*) and more forcefully (*inotropic effect*). Parasympathetic nerves control the atria and slow the heart rate.

Blood Vessels

After blood flows from the heart, it enters the vascular system, which is composed of numerous blood vessels. The blood vessels (a) form a closed system to deliver blood to the tissues; (b) help promote the exchange of nutrients, metabolic wastes, hormones, and other substances with the cells; and (c) ultimately return blood back to the heart.

Arteries carry blood away from the heart (*Fig. 1-11*). Large arteries branch into smaller arteries and eventually into microscopic *arterioles*. Arterioles branch into capillaries, which allow the exchange of blood with various

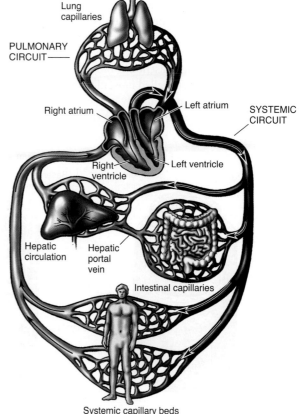

FIGURE 1-11. Schematic diagram of blood circulation.

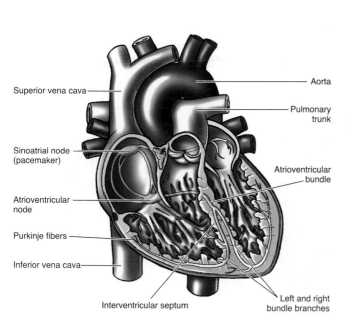

FIGURE 1-10. Electrical conduction system of the heart.

tissues (*e.g.*, the digestive system, liver, kidneys). On the venous side of the circulation, capillaries converge into microscopic *venules*, which converge to form larger vessels called *veins*. The large veins (*e.g.*, superior and inferior vena cava, pulmonary veins) return blood to the heart.

The walls of the various blood vessels vary in thickness and size because of the presence or absence of one or more layers of tissues (*Fig. 1-12*). The *tunica intima* consists of the endothelium and a thin connective tissue basement membrane. The tunica intima is the only layer common to all of the blood vessels. The internal elastic lamina separates the tunica intima from the middle layer of smooth muscle fibers and elastic fibers known as the *tunica media*. The smooth muscle fibers of the tunica media can be influenced by neural control (parasympathetic and sympathetic nerves), hormones (*e.g.*, acetylcholine, norepinephrine, epinephrine), or local factors (*e.g.*, pH, oxygen levels, carbon dioxide levels), which can cause them to vasoconstrict or vasodilate. The external elastic lamina separates the tunica media from the outermost layer of connective tissue called the *tunica adventitia* (*externa*). The adventitia helps attach vessels to surrounding tissues (38).

Arteries

Arteries can be classified as *elastic* or *muscular* according to their size and function. Large arteries such as the aorta and those of the pulmonary trunk are called elastic arteries. The tunica media of these vessels is thick and contains many elastic fibers (see *Fig. 1-12*). The elastic nature of these arteries helps maintain pressure within the vessels. Other smaller arteries distribute blood throughout the body. These arteries are called muscular arteries and their tunica media contains primarily smooth muscle fibers. Muscular arteries are less distensible than elastic arteries.

Arterioles

Arterioles are arteries very small in diameter that deliver blood to the capillaries. They have lumens smaller than 0.5 mm, and their tunica media is largely composed of smooth muscle with scattered elastic fibers (38). Arterioles play a major role in regulating blood flow to the capillaries because of their ability to vasoconstrict or vasodilate. Also, changes in arteriole diameter directly affect resistance to blood flow and thus can influence blood pressure (BP).

Capillaries

Capillaries are microscopic vessels that connect the arterioles with the venules. Capillaries form dense networks that branch throughout all tissues. The average capillary is 1 mm in length and 0.01 mm in diameter, which is just large enough for a single red blood cell (RBC) to pass through (28) (*Fig. 1-12*). Capillaries have extremely thin walls made of a single layer of endothelial cells and a basement membrane. In contrast to the other blood vessels, capillaries do not have a tunica media or tunica adventitia. This unique characteristic allows for the exchange of materials between the blood and the tissue cells.

Venules and Veins

Venules, which form from capillaries, consist mainly of tunica intima and tunica adventitia. Venules collect blood from capillaries. *Veins* receive blood from the venules and have the same three tissue layers as arteries. However, the tunica media of the veins is thinner than that found in the arteries. In general, veins are thinner and more compliant than arteries and act as blood reservoirs. The walls of some veins, such as those in the legs, contain one-way valves that help maintain venous return

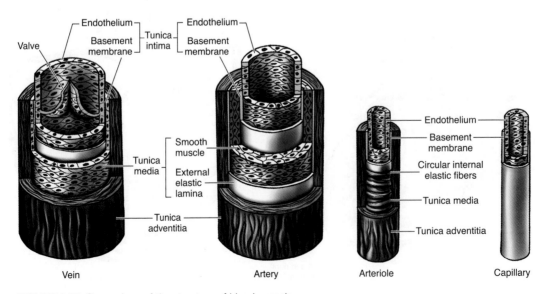

FIGURE 1-12. Comparison of the structure of blood vessels.

to the heart by preventing retrograde blood flow even under relatively low pressures (*Fig. 1-13*). The valves in the veins are made up of folds of tunica intima (endothelium) and are similar in nature to the semilunar valves of the heart. A special type of vein formed by a thin layer of endothelial cells surrounded with dense connective tissue for support is called a *venous sinus* (*e.g.*, the coronary sinus of the heart).

At rest, most (approximately 60%) of the blood volume is in systemic veins and venules. Systemic capillaries hold only about 5% of the blood volume, and systemic arteries and arterioles hold about 15%. Another 5% is within the heart itself, with the remainder in the pulmonary circulation. Blood contained in the veins and venules can be quickly redistributed to the arterial side via vasoconstriction, which is caused by smooth muscle located in the venous walls. Skeletal muscle activity such as during exercise squeezes veins (the "muscle pump"), which assists in returning venous blood to the heart.

ANATOMICAL SITES FOR BLOOD PRESSURE AND HEART RATE DETERMINATION

The measurement of arterial BP before, during, and after an exercise test or training session is routine. The systolic BP (SBP) and diastolic BP (DBP) are taken to ensure patient safety and to obtain important diagnostic

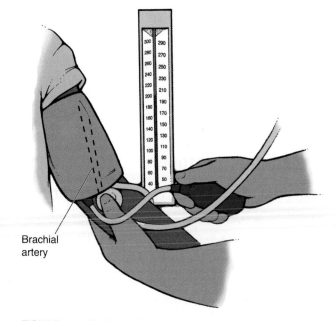

Brachial artery

FIGURE 1-14. Positions of the stethoscope head and pressure cuff.

and prognostic information. The most common method used for the determination of BP is brachial artery auscultation. The brachial artery courses through a groove formed by the bifurcation of the triceps and biceps brachii muscles on the medial (inside) aspect of the upper arm (*Fig. 1-14*).

Health fitness professionals can assess peripheral pulses to obtain an index of resting heart rate or aerobic exercise intensity. Large, superficial arteries are preferable for pulse determination because they are easily palpable. Two conventional palpation sites are the common carotid and radial arteries. The right and left common carotid arteries are located on the anterior portion of the neck in the groove formed by the larynx (Adam's apple) and the sternocleidomastoid muscles (the large muscles on the lateral aspects of the neck) just below the mandible (lower jaw). The radial artery courses deep on the lateral (thumb side) aspect of the forearm and becomes superficial near the distal head of the radius (24). Radial pulses may be difficult to obtain in individuals with large amounts of subcutaneous fat over the palpation site. Pulses may be taken at any arterial site. Other palpation sites include the temporal (temple region of skull), popliteal (behind the knee), femoral (inguinal fold of groin), and dorsal pedis (top of foot) arteries. Lower extremity pulses may provide information regarding the adequacy of peripheral blood flow.

SUMMARY

The cardiovascular system is a closed system of pumps, valves, and conduits that coordinate both anatomical and physiological functions to maintain a constant internal environment. The heart is a hollow, four-chambered

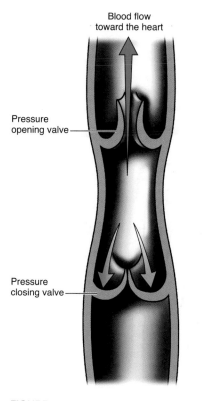

Blood flow toward the heart

Pressure opening valve

Pressure closing valve

FIGURE 1-13. Valves of a vein.

organ that pumps blood through elastic blood vessels to the lungs and systemic circulation. The compliance and elasticity of these blood vessels helps maintain BP at rest and during exercise. In times of increased cardiovascular work, the cardiovascular system functions in an even more sophisticated manner to meet those demands while it continues to maintain BP and meet tissue requirements.

PULMONARY ANATOMY

GENERAL COMPONENTS AND FUNCTIONS

This section describes the basic anatomy of the pulmonary system as it relates to function. The lungs of an average-sized person weigh about 1 kg. However, if spread out, the tissue would occupy a surface area about the size of a singles tennis court (24). The anatomy of the pulmonary system supports the basic function of exchanging carbon dioxide (CO_2), a byproduct of cellular metabolism, and oxygen (O_2), which is necessary for cellular activity (33). Other important functions include the production and metabolism of vasoactive substances and the filtration of systemic venous blood before entry into the LV. The structural components of the pulmonary system (*Fig. 1-15*) are the framework for the corresponding functions of the system (*Table 1-2*) (2,7).

TABLE 1-2. Structural Components of the Pulmonary System and Their Corresponding Function

Structural Components	Function
Respiratory center	Control of breathing
Peripheral chemoreceptors	Control of breathing
Afferent and efferent nerves	Control of breathing
Upper respiratory tract	Distribution of ventilation
Conducting airways	Distribution of ventilation
Respiratory bronchioles	Distribution of ventilation
Chest wall, respiratory muscles, and pleura	Ventilatory pump
Pulmonary arteries, capillaries, and veins	Distribution of blood flow
Functional respiratory unit	Gas exchange
Mucociliary escalator	Bronchial clearance
Alveolar macrophages	Lung clearance and defense
Lymphatic drainage	Lung clearance and defense

The pulmonary system consists of two major divisions: the upper and lower respiratory tracts. Functionally, the pulmonary system can be separated in two portions: the *conducting portion*, which is a system of interconnecting cavities and tubes (*i.e.*, the nose, mouth, pharynx, larynx,

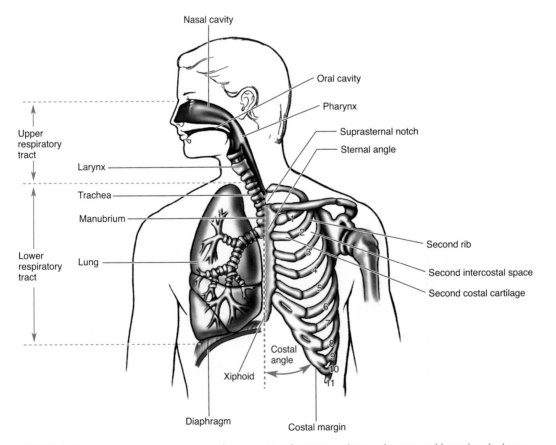

FIGURE 1-15. Pulmonary system consists of an upper respiratory tract (nose, pharynx, and larynx) and a lower respiratory tract (tracheobronchial tree and lungs).

trachea, bronchi), and the *respiratory portion*, where gas exchange occurs (*e.g.*, respiratory bronchioles, alveolar ducts, and alveoli) (*Figs. 1-15* and *1-16*).

Upper Respiratory Tract

The upper respiratory tract, which includes the nose, paranasal sinuses, pharynx, and larynx (see *Fig. 1-15*), acts as a conduction pathway for the movement of air into the lower respiratory tract. The function of these structures is to purify, warm, and humidify ambient air before it reaches the gas exchange units. During normal quiet breathing, inspired air is heated to body temperature and the relative humidity is increased to more than 90% during passage through the nose. Outside air goes into the nasal cavity via the nostrils. As air enters the nostrils, it passes through the nasal vestibule, which is lined with skin that has coarse hairs that help filter out large dust particles. Air is then moved to the upper nasal cavity. The upper nasal cavity is lined with a membrane rich in capillaries, which are responsible for warming the air. *Mucus* secreted by cells moistens the air and traps dust particles. Mucus is removed by the cilia in the pharynx where it is eliminated from the respiratory tract via swallowing or spitting. The pharynx (or throat) is a funnel-shaped tube about 13 cm long that begins at the internal nares (internal nostrils), anterior to the cervical vertebrae and posterior to the nasal and oral cavities and larynx. The pharynx is made up of skeletal muscles and is lined with mucous membrane. It serves as a passage for air and food and as a resonating chamber for speech. The pharynx is divided by the soft palate into the *nasopharynx* and the *oropharynx*. The *epiglottis*, located at the base of the tongue, protects the laryngeal opening during swallowing. The *larynx* (or voice box) contains the vocal cords, which contribute to speech and participate in coughing. It also connects the pharynx with the next respiratory organ, the trachea, which is the first organ of the lower respiratory tract.

Lower Respiratory Tract

The lower respiratory tract begins in the *trachea* (windpipe) just below the larynx and includes the bronchi, bronchioles, and alveoli (see *Figs. 1-15* and *1-16*). There are approximately 23 generations of airways. The first 16 serve as conducting airways and the last 7 are respiratory airways ending in the approximately 300 million alveoli that form the gas exchange surface.

Trachea

The trachea, or windpipe, begins at the base of the neck and extends approximately 10–12 cm to an internal ridge called the *carina* (see *Fig. 1-15*), where it divides into the right and left main bronchi. It is located anterior to the esophagus, extending from the larynx to about the fifth thoracic vertebra. The trachea consists of a series of anteriorly located horseshoe-shaped cartilaginous rings, which are closed posteriorly by a longitudinal muscle bundle. The mucous membrane of the carina is highly sensitive and is associated with the cough reflex.

Bronchi and Bronchioles

At the sternal angle, the trachea divides into *right* and *left primary bronchi*, which branch into the right and left lungs, respectively. The major bronchi contain cartilage that maintains the free passage of air as well as large numbers of mucous glands that produce secretions in response to irritation, infection, or inflammation. Once in each lung, the primary bronchi divide into smaller bronchi called *secondary (lobar) bronchi* because they go to each of the lobes of the lungs (three lobes in the right lung and two in the left lung) (*Figs. 1-16* and *1-17*). The secondary bronchi continue to branch into *tertiary (segmental) bronchi* (10 on the right and 10 on the left), then *bronchioles*, and end in *terminal bronchioles*. Beyond the terminal bronchioles are respiratory bronchioles, alveolar ducts, and alveoli (see *Figs. 1-16* and *1-17*). This branching is commonly referred as the *bronchial tree*. The structural makeup of the bronchial tree changes as it extends to its terminal branches. The C-shaped cartilage rings in the airway walls are gradually replaced by smaller plates of cartilage and then totally disappear in the bronchioles. Smooth muscle makes up more of the airway wall as the cartilage decreases. In addition, the

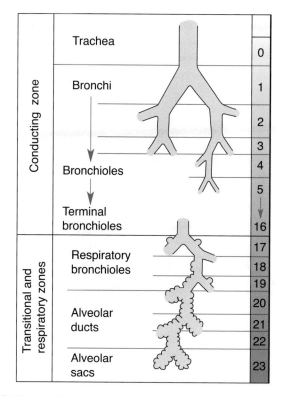

FIGURE 1-16. Branching of the airways starting from the trachea to the alveolar sacs. There are approximately 23 generations of branching in the tracheobronchial tree.

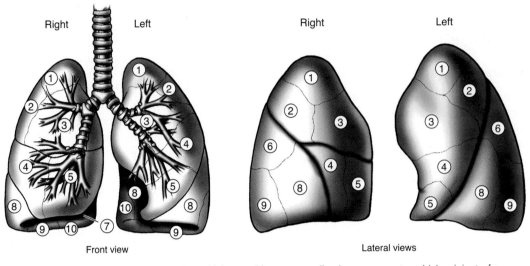

FIGURE 1-17. Structure of the tracheobronchial tree with corresponding lung segments, which originate from segmental bronchi. The right upper lobe contains segments 1–3, the right middle lobe contains segments 4 and 5, and the right lower lobe contains segments 6–10. The left upper lobe contains segments 1–5, and the left lower lobe contains segments 6–10.

inside layer of epithelium experiences structural changes as there is a transition to squamous cells in the alveoli. This transition of the epithelium is important for facilitating gas exchange.

Alveoli

The respiratory bronchioles subdivide into *alveolar ducts*, which lead to *alveolar sacs* with alveoli. Alveolar sacs are air spaces or openings shared by two or more alveoli. *Alveoli* are cup-shaped pouches lined with type I and II epithelium surrounded by a thin elastic membrane for support. The *respiratory (alveolar-capillary) membrane* consists of the alveolar epithelium, the interstitium (containing the basement membrane), and the pulmonary capillary endothelial cells (*Fig. 1-18*). Type II epithelial cells, found primarily at the junctions of alveolar walls, produce *surfactant*. A thin layer of surfactant lines the alveolus and functions to lower the surface tension in the alveolus. This helps to prevent alveolar collapse.

Respiratory Gas Exchange

Gas exchange occurs by way of two anatomical structures, the functional respiratory unit and the alveolus. As illustrated in *Figure 1-19*, a terminal bronchiole enters the center of the functional respiratory unit accompanied by a pulmonary arteriole carrying deoxygenated blood from the body tissues and muscles. The arteriole divides into a rich network of pulmonary capillaries that lie adjacent to the alveolar walls and then drain into pulmonary venules and veins.

The exchange of respiratory gases takes place by passive diffusion across the respiratory membrane. The respiratory membrane wall is very thin, about 0.5 μm

in thickness and 1/16th the diameter of a RBC. The combination of a large surface area and a thin respiratory membrane makes for rapid diffusion of the respiratory gases into and out of the blood.

Blood Supply to the Lungs

The pulmonary circulation is a low pressure system with a normal mean pressure of approximately 15 mm Hg at rest. The lungs receive blood from the pulmonary arteries, which contain systemic venous blood from the RV;

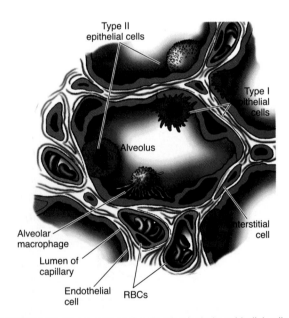

FIGURE 1-18. Major cells of the alveolus include epithelial cells (types I and II), endothelial cells of the pulmonary capillary, and alveolar macrophages. Also shown is a lumen of capillary with RBCs.

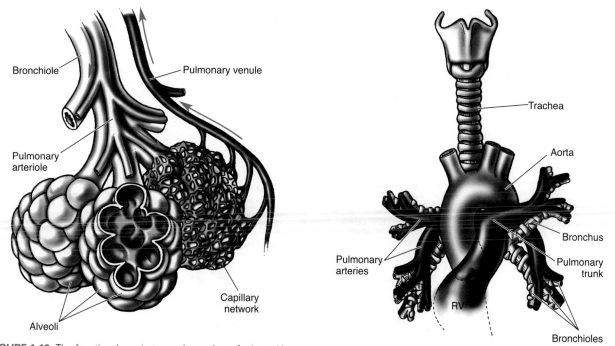

FIGURE 1-19. The functional respiratory unit consists of a bronchiole and corresponding blood supply; the pulmonary arteriole carries deoxygenated blood and the pulmonary venule carries oxygenated blood. The rich capillary network supplies the alveoli for the purpose of gas exchange.

FIGURE 1-20. Major pulmonary arteries, which originate from the right ventricle (RV). Branches of the pulmonary arteries are adjacent to the bronchi and bronchioles.

and bronchial arteries, which contain oxygenated blood from the LV (*Fig. 1-20*). The pulmonary arteries deliver blood to be oxygenated within the alveoli, and the blood within the bronchial arteries provides nourishment for the rest of the lung tissue.

Deoxygenated blood coming from the systemic circulation via the RA and RV of the heart passes through the pulmonary trunk and divides into the right and left pulmonary arteries. The pulmonary arteries divide into branches corresponding to the divisions of the bronchial tree and supply the pulmonary arterioles. In the lungs, blood releases CO_2 and gets replenished with O_2 (*respiratory gas exchange*). Oxygenated blood is then transported from the pulmonary capillaries to four pulmonary veins, which empty into the LA. The pulmonary veins also receive blood from the bronchial circulation, which accounts for a right-to-left shunt that causes blood entering the LA to be less than fully oxygenated (typically, oxygen saturation is about 98%). Oxygenated blood passes from the LA into the LV where it is pumped into the systemic circulation via the aorta and its branches.

VENTILATORY PUMP AND MECHANICS OF BREATHING

The ventilatory pump consists of the chest wall, the ventilatory muscles, and the pleural space (*Figs. 1-21 and 1-22*). These components of the ventilatory pump provide for the processes of *inhalation* (air moving into the lungs) and *exhalation* (air moving out of the lungs). Breathing involves both inhalation and exhalation so that ventilation (exchange of air) in the lungs is accomplished. Inhalation is initiated by activation of the ventilatory muscles, particularly the diaphragm. The ventilatory muscles increase the thoracic dimensions so that the pressure in the pleural space is lower than the outside atmospheric pressure. Air enters the lung until the *intrapulmonary* (inside the lung) gas pressure is equal to the atmospheric pressure. During exhalation, the ventilatory muscles relax and the thoracic dimensions decrease (*i.e.*, the ribs fall back down and the diaphragm moves upward into the thorax), thus increasing intrapulmonary pressure relative to the outside atmospheric pressure. As a result, air flows from the lungs to outside the body, thus completing the process of breathing.

Chest Wall

The chest wall includes the intercostal muscles, which are considered ventilatory muscles (see *Fig. 1-21*), and bones (the spine, ribs, and sternum). The ribs articulate with the spine so that the ribs can move upward and outward during inhalation and downward and inward during exhalation. This movement contributes to the changes in thoracic volume that are critical for driving ventilation.

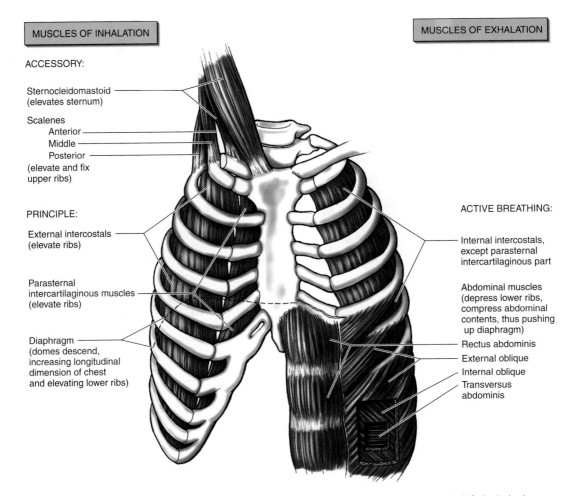

MUSCLES OF INHALATION

ACCESSORY:

Sternocleidomastoid
(elevates sternum)

Scalenes
    Anterior
    Middle
    Posterior
(elevate and fix
upper ribs)

PRINCIPLE:

External intercostals
(elevate ribs)

Parasternal
intercartilaginous muscles
(elevate ribs)

Diaphragm
(domes descend,
increasing longitudinal
dimension of chest
and elevating lower ribs)

MUSCLES OF EXHALATION

ACTIVE BREATHING:

Internal intercostals,
except parasternal
intercartilaginous part

Abdominal muscles
(depress lower ribs,
compress abdominal
contents, thus pushing
up diaphragm)

Rectus abdominis
External oblique
Internal oblique
Transversus
abdominis

FIGURE 1-21. Major muscles of ventilation. The principal muscles of inhalation, shown on the left, include the diaphragm, external intercostal muscles, and parasternal muscles. The principal muscles of exhalation, shown on the right, include the internal intercostal muscles and the abdominal muscles (rectus, transversus, and internal and external oblique muscles).

Ventilatory Muscles

The muscles of ventilation are the only skeletal muscles essential to life. The muscles of inhalation and exhalation are illustrated in *Figures 1-21* and *1-22*. The *diaphragm*, the major muscle of inhalation, is innervated by the *phrenic nerve*, which originates from the third to fifth cervical spine segments. Spinal cord transection caused by injury at or above this level compromises ventilatory muscle function and, consequently, ventilation.

The diaphragm is a domelike sheet of muscle that physically divides the abdominal and thoracic cavities. The diaphragm functions as a piston, with contraction and relaxation of the vertically oriented muscle fibers. With contraction, the diaphragm moves downward and displaces the abdominal contents so that the abdomen moves outward. Exhalation is normally passive under quiet breathing because of the elastic recoil of the lung tissue and gravity, which causes the ribs to fall back to their natural position.

However, when ventilatory requirements are increased such as during exercise, the muscles of exhalation are recruited. The major muscles of exhalation are the intercostal and the abdominal muscles (rectus abdominis, internal and external obliques, and transversus abdominis).

Pleura

The visceral and parietal pleura are thin membranes that cover the lungs and the inside of the chest wall, respectively. They converge at the lung hila (*Fig. 1-22*) (27). The pleural space, which lies between the visceral and parietal pleura, contains a small amount of fluid (*Fig. 1-22*). Because the pleural space is airtight and the chest wall and lung tissue pull against each other across the pleural space, negative pressure (relative to atmospheric pressure) is produced at rest. During inhalation, both the visceral and parietal pleura expand outward, and negative pressure develops in the pleural space.

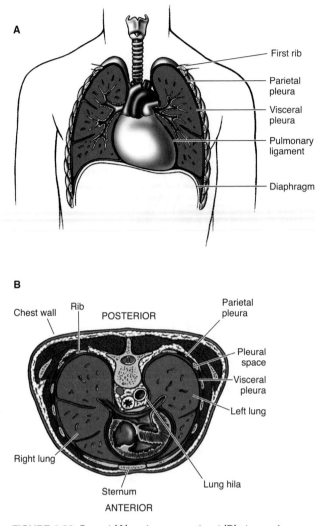

FIGURE 1-22. Frontal **(A)** and cross-sectional **(B)** views of the chest and lungs showing the pleural layers (visceral and parietal) and the pleural space. With inhalation, negative pressure develops in the pleural space. This allows air to move from the atmosphere into the tracheobronchial tree for gas exchange. The negative intrathoracic pressure also facilitates return of venous blood into the right atrium.

SUMMARY

The major function of the pulmonary system is the exchange of carbon dioxide and oxygen, which is necessary for metabolism. The pulmonary system is divided functionally into conducting zones, which filter, warm, and moisten incoming air, and respiratory zones, where gas exchange occurs. Other important functions of the pulmonary system include the production and metabolism of vasoactive substances and the filtering of particulate material before entry into the systemic circuit. The structural components of the pulmonary system are the framework for these and other important functions at rest and with physical activity.

MUSCULOSKELETAL ANATOMY

GENERAL COMPONENTS AND FUNCTIONS

One of the primary objectives of regular exercise training is the improvement of musculoskeletal fitness. The physiological adaptations of muscle to exercise training may be manifested through increased muscle force production, muscular strength and endurance, and resistance to injury. Inherent in designing effective training programs is a thorough understanding of muscle structure and function. This section provides a brief overview of the fundamentals of musculoskeletal anatomy. For in-depth study, the reader is referred to a variety of excellent sources (1,18,31,32,34).

Skeletal System (Axial Skeleton, Appendicular Skeleton, and Bone Tissue)

Beyond supporting soft tissue, protecting internal organs, and acting as an important source of nutrients and blood constituents, the bones of the skeletal system serve as rigid levers for movement. The skull, vertebral column, sternum, and ribs are considered the **axial skeleton**; the remaining bones of the upper and lower limbs are considered the **appendicular skeleton**. The major bones of the body are illustrated in *Figure 1-23*. The skeletal system consists of cartilage, periosteum, and osseous tissue. The structure of bone tissue can be explained using a typical long bone such as the humerus. The main portion of a long bone is the shaft, or *diaphysis (Fig. 1-24)*. The ends of the bone are called the *epiphyses*. The epiphyses are covered by *articular cartilage*. Cartilage is a resilient, semirigid form of connective tissue that reduces friction in synovial joints and redistributes joint loads to a wider area, thus decreasing stresses sustained by the contacting joint surfaces. The region of mature bone where the diaphysis joins the epiphyses is called the *metaphysis*. In an immature bone, this region includes the *epiphyseal plate* or *growth plate*. The *medullary cavity*, or marrow cavity, is the space inside the diaphysis. Lining the marrow cavity is the *endosteum*, which contains cells necessary for bone development. The *periosteum* is a membrane around the surface of bones that are not covered with articular cartilage. The periosteum is composed of two layers: an outer fibrous layer and an inner highly vascular layer that contains cells for the creation of new bone. The periosteum serves as an attachment point for ligaments and tendons and is critical for bone growth, repair, and nutrition.

There are two types of bone: compact and spongy. The main difference is the amount of matter and space they contain. *Compact bone* contains few spaces and forms the external layer of all bones of the body and a large portion of the diaphysis of the long bones, where it provides support for bearing weight. In contrast,

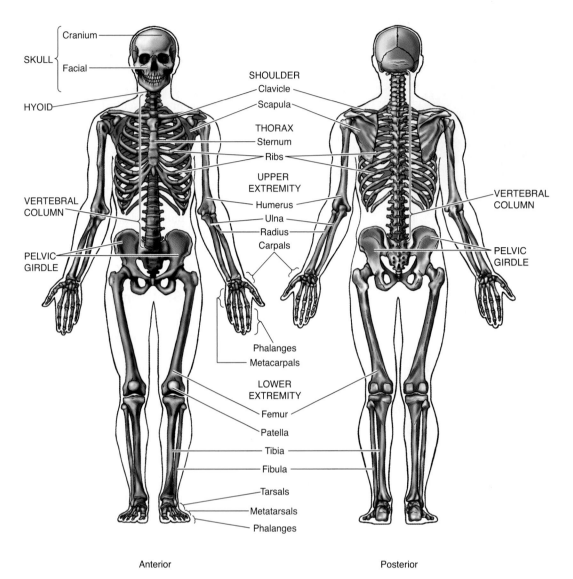

FIGURE 1-23. Divisions of the skeletal system.

spongy bone is much less dense; it consists of a three-dimensional lattice composed of beams or struts of bone called *trabeculae*. The trabeculae are oriented to provide strength and counteract the stresses normally encountered by the bone. In some bones, the space within these trabeculae is filled with *red bone marrow*, which produces blood cells.

Structure and Function of Joints in Movement

Joints are the articulations between bones. Along with bones and ligaments, they constitute the articular system. *Ligaments* are tough, fibrous connective tissues that anchor bone to bone. Joints are typically classified as (a) *fibrous*, in which bones are united by dense fibrous connective tissue; (b) *cartilaginous*, in which the bones are united by cartilage; or (c) *synovial*, in which a fibrous articular capsule and an inner synovial membrane enclose a joint cavity filled with synovial fluid. *Table 1-3* summarizes the joint classifications and provides examples in the human body.

Synovial (Diarthrodial) Joints

The most common joint in the human body is the synovial joint. *Figure 1-25* illustrates its unique capsular arrangement. There are four distinct features of a synovial joint: (a) it has a joint cavity; (b) the articulating surfaces of the bones are covered with articular cartilage; (c) it is enclosed by a fibrous joint capsule; and (d) the capsule is lined with a *synovial membrane*. The synovial membrane produces *synovial fluid*, which provides constant lubrication during movement to minimize the wear and tear effects of friction on the cartilaginous covering of the articulating bones. Synovial joints are sometimes reinforced by ligaments. These ligaments are either separate or are a thickening

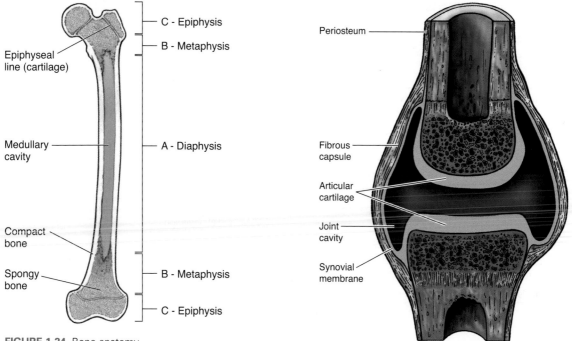

FIGURE 1-24. Bone anatomy.

FIGURE 1-25. Synovial joint.

of the outer layer of the joint capsule. Some synovial joints have other structures such as articular discs (*e.g.*, the meniscus of the knee). There are six major types of synovial joints that are classified by the shape of the articulating surface or type of movement allowed (see *Table 1-3*). *Table 1-4* summarizes the major joints of the body, joint motions, and the plane in which these motions occur (*Fig. 1-26*).

Joints are typically well perfused by numerous arterial branches and are innervated by branches of the nerves supplying the adjacent muscle and overlying skin. Proprioceptive feedback and pain are important joint sensations, which are a result of the high density of sensory fibers in the joint capsule. This feedback has obvious importance in regulating human movement and in preventing injury.

TABLE 1-3. Classifications of Joints in the Human Body	
Joint Classification	**Features and Examples**
Fibrous	
Suture	Tight union unique to the skull
Syndesmosis	Interosseous membrane between bone (*e.g.*, the union along the shafts of the radius and ulna, tibia, and fibula)
Gomphosis	Unique joint at the tooth socket
Cartilaginous	
Primary (synchondroses; hyaline cartilaginous)	Usually temporary to permit bone growth and typically fuse; some do not (*e.g.*, at the sternum and rib [costal cartilage])
Secondary (symphyses; fibrocartilaginous)	Strong, slightly movable joints (*e.g.*, intervertebral discs, pubic symphysis)
Synovial	
Plane (arthrodial)	Gliding and sliding movements (*e.g.*, acromioclavicular joint)
Hinge (ginglymus)	Uniaxial movements (*e.g.*, elbow, knee extension and flexion)
Ellipsoidal (condyloid)	Biaxial joint (*e.g.*, wrist flexion and extension, radioulnar deviation)
Saddle (sellar)	Unique joint that permits movements in all planes, including opposition (*e.g.*, the carpometacarpal joint of the thumb)
Ball and socket (enarthrodial)	Multiaxial joints that permit movements in all directions (*e.g.*, hip and shoulder joints)
Pivot (trochoidal)	Uniaxial, biaxial, and multiaxial joints that permit rotation (*e.g.*, humeroradial joint)

TABLE 1-4. Major Joint Motions and Planes of Motion

Major Joint	Type of Joint	Joint Movement(s)	Plane
Scapulothoracic	Not a true joint	Elevation–depression Upward–downward rotation Protraction–retraction	Frontal Frontal Transverse
Glenohumeral	Synovial: ball and socket	Flexion–extension Abduction–adduction Internal–external rotation Horizontal abduction–adduction Circumduction	Sagittal Frontal Transverse Transverse
Elbow	Synovial: hinge	Flexion–extension	Sagittal
Proximal radioulnar	Synovial: pivot	Pronation–supination	Transverse
Wrist	Synovial: ellipsoidal	Flexion–extension Ulnar–radial deviation	Sagittal Frontal
Metacarpophalangeal	Synovial: ellipsoidal	Flexion–extension Abduction–adduction	Sagittal Frontal
Proximal interphalangeal	Synovial: hinge	Flexion–extension	Sagittal
Distal interphalangeal	Synovial: hinge	Flexion–extension	Sagittal
Interverterbral	Cartilaginous	Flexion–extension Lateral flexion Rotation	Sagittal Frontal Transverse
Hip	Synovial: ball and socket	Flexion–extension Abduction–adduction Internal–external rotation Horizontal abduction–adduction Circumduction	Sagittal Frontal Transverse Transverse
Knee	Synovial: hinge	Flexion–extension	Sagittal
Ankle: talocrural	Synovial: hinge	Dorsiflexion–plantarflexion	Sagittal
Ankle: subtalar	Synovial: gliding	Inversion–eversion	Frontal

Joint Movements and Range of Motion

The degree of movement at a joint is typically called the *range of motion* (ROM) (13). *Active* ROM is reached by voluntary movement, and *passive* ROM is achieved by external means (*e.g.*, an examiner or device). Joint ROM is typically limited by the structure of the articulating bones, ligamentous arrangement, and soft tissue limitations.

Movement at one joint may influence the extent of movement at adjacent joints because several muscles and other soft-tissue structures cross multiple joints. For example, finger flexion decreases during wrist flexion because the muscles that flex and extend both the wrist and fingers are placed on slack and cannot generate enough tension to allow for full ROM. *Tables 1-5* and *1-6* summarize major joint movements and the muscles that produce those movements, along with example resistance exercises for the muscles.

Muscular System

There are three types of muscle tissue: skeletal, cardiac, and smooth. Skeletal muscle is attached primarily to

bones and is responsible for movement, stabilizing the body, load distribution, shock absorption, and heat generation. Skeletal muscle tissue is under voluntary control and is referred to as *striated* because of the dark and light bands that are visible under a microscope. In general, all muscle tissue has four important characteristics: (a) irritability, defined as the ability to respond to electrical or mechanical stimuli; (b) contractility, the ability to develop tension; (c) extensibility, the ability to be stretched or increase in length; and (d) elasticity, the ability to return to its original length after a stretch or compression.

Skeletal Muscle Macrostructure

The individual *muscle fibers* (muscle cells) that make up skeletal muscles are joined together by a hierarchical organization of several connective tissue membranes (*Fig. 1-27*). The outermost layer surrounding the whole muscle is the *epimysium*. Skeletal muscles are composed of multiple *fascicles*, which are bundles of muscle fibers that vary in size from 15 to 150 fibers. A layer of connective tissue called the *perimysium* surrounds each

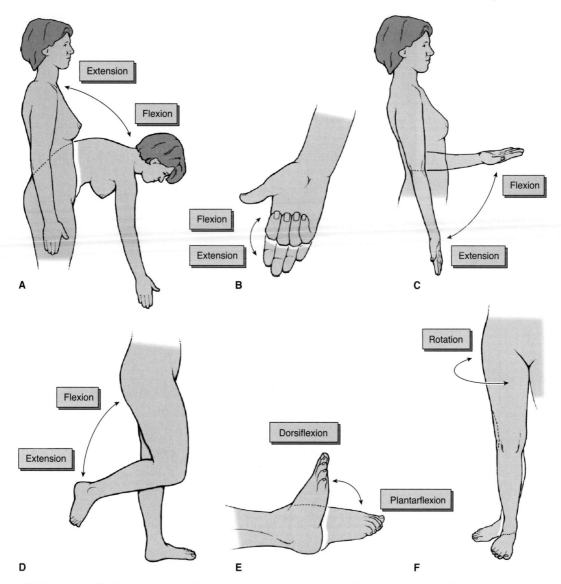

FIGURE 1-26. A–E. Flexion and extension of various parts of the body. **F.** Rotation of the lower limb at the hip joint.

individual *fasciculus*. A third connective tissue layer known as the *endomysium* envelops individual muscle fibers. Blood vessels, nerves, and lymphatic vessels pass into the muscle to reach the individual muscle fibers. An additional thin elastic membrane is found just beneath the endomysium and is called the *sarcolemma*. The sarcolemma is the true cell boundary and encloses the cellular contents of the muscle fiber, nuclei, local stores of fat, glucose (in the form of glycogen), enzymes, contractile proteins, and other specialized structures such as the mitochondria.

Skeletal muscles are anchored to the skeleton by extensions of the epimysium, perimysium, and endomysium. These connective tissues extend beyond the end of a muscle and converge to form *tendons*. In most cases, tendons are dense cords of connective tissue that attach a muscle to the periosteum of the bone. When the tendon

is flat and broad, it is called an *aponeurosis*. Tendons and aponeuroses provide the mechanical link between skeletal muscle and bone.

Skeletal muscles have different muscle fiber architecture. Fibers in a *fusiform arrangement* run in line with the pull of the muscle (*e.g.*, biceps brachii). Muscles with a *pennate arrangement* have fibers that run obliquely or at an angle to the line of pull (*Fig. 1-28*). Pennate muscles that have fibers located on only one side of the tendon are classified as *unipennate* (*e.g.*, vastus lateralis), whereas *bipennate* muscles have fibers located on both sides of a centrally positioned tendon (*e.g.*, rectus femoris), and *multipennate* are arranged with two or more fasciculi that are attached obliquely and combine to form one muscle (*e.g.*, deltoid). The muscle fiber architecture of a muscle can affect muscle force generation, velocity of shortening, and ROM. For example, muscles composed of long

TABLE 1-5. Major Movements of the Upper Extremities

Joint	Movement	Major Agonist Muscles	Examples of Resistance Exercise
Scapulothoracic	Fixation	Serratus anterior Pectoralis minor Trapezius Levator scapulae Rhomboids	Push-up Parallel bar dip Upright row Shoulder shrug Seated row
Glenohumeral	Flexion	Anterior deltoid Pectoralis major (clavicular head)	Front raises Incline bench press
	Extension	Latissimus dorsi Teres major Pectoralis major (sternocostal head)	Dumbbell pullover Chin-up Bench press
	Abduction	Middle deltoid Supraspinatus	Lateral raises, dumbbell press Low pulley lateral raise
	Adduction	Latissimus dorsi Teres major Pectoralis major	Lat pull-down Seated row Cable crossover fly
	Medial (internal) rotation	Latissimus dorsi Teres major Subscapularis Pectoralis major Anterior deltoid	Back latissimus pull-down, bent row One-arm dumbbell row Rotator cuff exercise, dumbbell press, parallel bar dip, front raise
	Lateral (external) rotation	Infraspinatus Teres minor Posterior deltoid	External rotation Back press, bent over lateral raises
Elbow	Flexion	Biceps brachii Brachialis Brachioradialis	Curls Preacher curl Hammer curl
	Extension	Triceps brachii Anconeus	Triceps dips, triceps extensions Triceps push-downs, tricep kickback
Radioulnar	Supination	Supinator Biceps brachii	Dumbbell supination
	Pronation	Pronator teres, pronator quadratus	Dumbbell pronation
Wrist	Flexion	Flexor carpi radialis and ulnaris Palmaris longus Flexor digitorum superficialis	Wrist curl
	Extension	Extensor carpi radialis longus, extensor digitorum	Reverse wrist curl brevis and ulnaris
	Adduction (ulnar deviation)	Flexor and extensor carpi ulnaris	Wrist curls, reverse wrist curl
	Abduction (radial deviation)	Extensor carpi radialis longus and brevis Flexor carpi radialis	Wrist curls, reverse wrist curl

muscle fibers tend to have fusiform arrangements and demonstrate greater ROM and velocity of shortening than pennate muscles. In contrast, pennate muscles are composed of large numbers of short fibers, providing a larger cross-sectional area capable of generating greater force production but less ROM than muscles with fusiform fiber architecture.

Muscles also can be described by the number of joints they act upon. For example, a muscle that causes movement at one joint is *uniarticular*. Muscles that cross more than one joint are referred to as *biarticular* or *multiarticular* muscles. The main advantage of biarticular and multiarticular muscles is that only one muscle is needed to generate tension in two or more joints. This is more efficient and conserves energy. In many instances, the length of the muscle stays within 100%–130% of the resting length: as one side of the muscle shortens, the other side stretches, maintaining a near constant length. This property of biarticular and multiarticular muscles enhances force production by optimizing the length–tension

TABLE 1-6. Major Movements of the Lower Extremities

Joint	Movement	Major Agonist Muscle(s)	Examples of Resistance Exercises
Intervertebral	Trunk flexion	Rectus abdominis External obliques Internal obliques	Sit-ups, crunches, leg raise Machine crunch High pulley crunch
	Trunk extension	Erector spinae	Back extension, dead lift
	Lateral flexion	Rectus abdominis External obliques Internal obliques	Roman chair side bend Dumbbell side bend Hanging leg raises
	Rotation	External obliques Internal obliques	Broomstick twist Machine trunk rotation
Hip	Flexion	Iliacus Psoas major Rectus femoris Sartorius Pectineus	Leg raise Incline leg raise Machine crunches Leg raise Cable adduction
	Extension	Gluteus maximus Hamstrings (semitendinosus, semimembranosus, long head of biceps femoris)	Squat, leg press, lunge Leg curl (standing, seated, lying)
	Abduction	Tensor fasciae latae Sartorius Gluteus medius Gluteus minimus	Cable hip abduction Standing machine abduction Floor hip abduction Seated machine abduction
	Adduction	Adductor longus, brevis, and magnus Gracilis Pectineus	Power squat Cable adduction Machine adduction
	Medial rotation	Semitendinosus Semimembranosus Gluteus medius Tensor fasciae latae Gracilis	Leg curl (standing, seated, lying) Floor hip adduction Machine abduction
	Lateral rotation	Biceps femoris Adductor longus, brevis, magnus Gluteus maximus	
Knee	Flexion	Hamstrings Gracilis Sartorius	Leg curl (standing, seated, lying)
	Extension	Quadriceps femoris (rectus femoris, vastus lateralis, medialis, and intermedius)	Lunge, squat, leg extension
Ankle: talocrural	Dorsiflexion	Tibialis anterior Extensor digitorus longus Extensor hallucis longus	Ankle dorsiflexion against resistance
	Plantarflexion	Gastrocnemius, soleus, tibialis posterior Flexor digitorum longus Flexor hallucis longus	Standing calf raise, donkey calf raise Seated calf raise
Ankle: subtalar	Eversion	Peroneus longus and brevis	Exercises against resistance
	Inversion	Tibialis anterior and posterior	Exercises against resistance

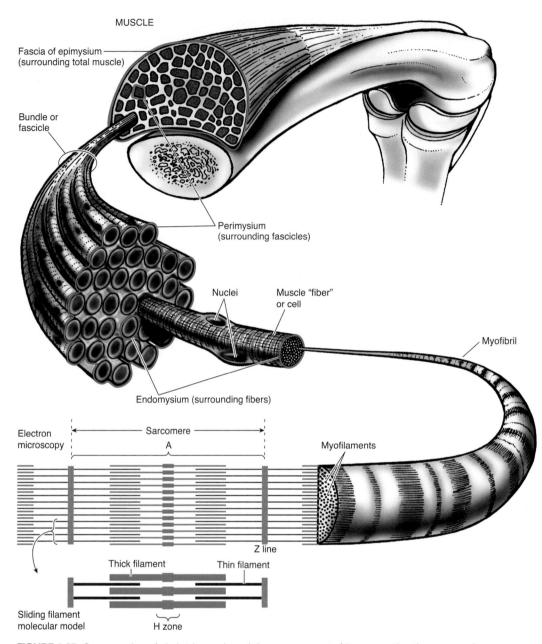

FIGURE 1-27. Cross section of skeletal muscle and the arrangement of its connective tissue wrappings.

relationship. The major superficial skeletal muscles of the body are illustrated in *Figures 1-29* and *1-30*.

Skeletal Muscle Microstructure

Skeletal muscle fibers are approximately 10–100 μm in diameter and typically many centimeters long. Each muscle fiber contains several hundred to several thousand regularly ordered, threadlike *myofibrils*. These myofibrils extend lengthwise throughout the cell and are connected to the plasma membrane by intermediate filaments. Myofibrils contain the apparatus that allows for contraction of the muscle cell, which consists primarily of two types of myofilaments: thick filaments (*myosin*) and

thin filaments (*actin*). The myosin and actin filaments are arranged longitudinally in the smallest contractile unit of skeletal muscle, the *sarcomere*. Each myofibril is composed of numerous sarcomeres joined end to end at the *Z lines*. The dark *A band* represents the region that contains both thick myosin filaments and thin actin filaments. The *H zone* is the central portion of the A band that appears only when the sarcomere is in a resting state and it is occupied only by thick filaments (see *Fig. 1-28*). A thick filament contains approximately 200 myosin molecules with the heads of the molecules protruding outwards at regular intervals. They occur in the A band where they overlap at either end with thin filaments. The thin filaments consist of the contractile protein *actin* and

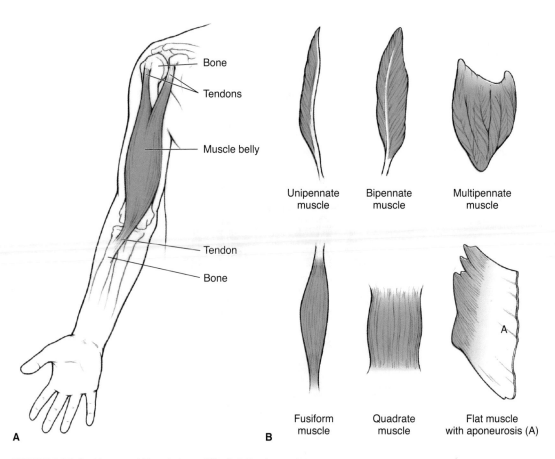

FIGURE 1-28. Architecture **(A)** and shape **(B)** of skeletal muscles.

regulatory proteins *tropomyosin* and *troponin*. One end of each actin filament is attached to a Z line, with the opposite end extending toward the center of the sarcomere, lying in the space between the myosin filaments. The actin protein has a binding site that, when exposed, serves as an attachment point for the myosin head. The site where the myosin head binds to the actin filament is known as a *crossbridge*. It is this arrangement of the myosin and actin filaments that give skeletal muscle its striated appearance.

Muscle Fiber Actions and Fiber Types

Approximately 5% of skeletal muscle weight consists of the high-energy phosphates, key minerals, and energy sources needed for force production; an additional 20% of muscle is composed of protein, principally *myosin*, *actin*, and *tropomyosin*. Water constitutes approximately 75% of muscle weight. Physical training results in a significant alteration of these constituents, depending on the specific training stimulus.

Given the wide shift in blood supply shunted to active skeletal muscle during vigorous exercise, a highly efficient vascular bed must exist throughout muscles. Likewise, the body has the ability to enhance blood supply through formation of new capillary networks stimulated by physical training that involves endurance (or aerobic) exercise.

Skeletal muscles are controlled by the central nervous system (CNS), both through higher centers and individual spinal segments, and by proprioceptive structures (*e.g.*, muscle spindles, Golgi tendon organs) inherent to the musculotendinous complex. The integration is complex yet remarkably efficient. Most evidence indicates that when stimulated to contract, muscle tissue shortens or lengthens because the myosin and actin myofilaments slide past each other without changing individual length. The contact between the actin and myosin filaments is known as *crossbridging*. *Box 1-1* summarizes the sliding-filament theory (20). This continual process of forming and releasing crossbridges permits the generation of tension. Force production continues as long as the muscle is stimulated, but the ability of the muscle to perform may be limited by intrinsic factors such as diminished production of adenosine triphosphate (ATP), decreased pH, and accumulation of metabolic byproducts (see the discussion on fatigue in *Chapter 3*).

Three common terms describing muscle contraction are *twitch*, *summation*, and *tetanus*. *Twitch* refers to a single, brief muscle contraction caused by a single action potential traveling down a motor neuron. *Summation* is the addition of individual twitch contractions to increase the intensity of the overall muscle force. Progressive stimulation frequencies increase the amount of force developed because the muscle cannot completely relax

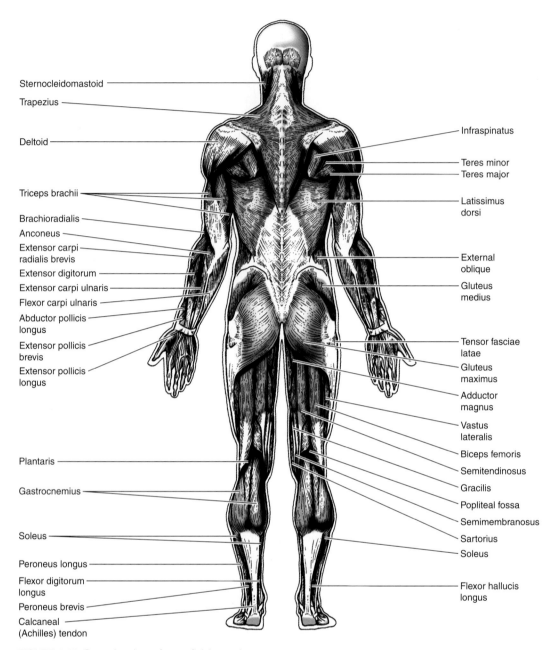

Sternocleidomastoid

Trapezius

Deltoid

Triceps brachii

Brachioradialis

Anconeus

Extensor carpi
radialis brevis

Extensor digitorum

Extensor carpi ulnaris

Flexor carpi ulnaris

Abductor pollicis
longus

Extensor pollicis
brevis

Extensor pollicis
longus

Plantaris

Gastrocnemius

Soleus

Peroneus longus

Flexor digitorum
longus

Peroneus brevis

Calcaneal
(Achilles) tendon

Infraspinatus

Teres minor
Teres major

Latissimus
dorsi

External
oblique

Gluteus
medius

Tensor fasciae
latae

Gluteus
maximus

Adductor
magnus

Vastus
lateralis

Biceps femoris

Semitendinosus

Gracilis

Popliteal fossa

Semimembranosus

Sartorius

Soleus

Flexor hallucis
longus

FIGURE 1-29. Posterior view of superficial muscles.

from the previous stimulus before the next stimulus arrives. As soon as the frequency of stimulation is high enough, full summation is achieved. This is referred to as *tetanus* and is the maximal amount of force the **motor unit** (*i.e.*, all the muscle fibers innervated by a single motor neuron) can develop. At this point, muscle fiber stimulation is of such high frequency that it is unable to return to its resting length between contractions (30).

The human body has the ability to perform a wide range of physical tasks combining varying levels of speed, power, and endurance. No single type of muscle fiber possesses the characteristics that allow optimal performance across this continuum of physical challenges.

Rather, muscle fibers possess certain characteristics that result in relative specialization. For example, motor units of specific fiber types are selectively recruited by the body for speed and power tasks of short duration, whereas others are recruited for endurance tasks of long duration and relatively low intensity. When the task requires elements of speed or power but also has an endurance component, yet another type of muscle fiber is recruited. These different fiber types, to be described more specifically later, should not be thought of as mutually exclusive. In fact, intricate recruitment and switching occurs in muscle over the performance of many tasks, and fibers designed to be optimal for one type of task can contribute to the

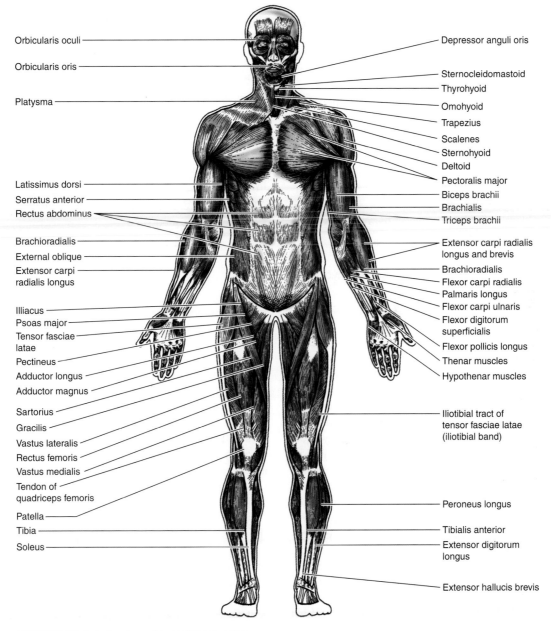

Orbicularis oculi

Orbicularis oris

Platysma

Latissimus dorsi
Serratus anterior
Rectus abdominus

Brachioradialis
External oblique
Extensor carpi
radialis longus

Illiacus
Psoas major
Tensor fasciae
latae
Pectineus
Adductor longus
Adductor magnus

Sartorius
Gracilis
Vastus lateralis
Rectus femoris
Vastus medialis
Tendon of
quadriceps femoris
Patella
Tibia
Soleus

Depressor anguli oris

Sternocleidomastoid
Thyrohyoid
Omohyoid
Trapezius
Scalenes
Sternohyoid
Deltoid
Pectoralis major
Biceps brachii
Brachialis
Triceps brachii

Extensor carpi radialis
longus and brevis
Brachioradialis
Flexor carpi radialis
Palmaris longus
Flexor carpi ulnaris
Flexor digitorum
superficialis
Flexor pollicis longus
Thenar muscles
Hypothenar muscles

Iliotibial tract of
tensor fasciae latae
(iliotibial band)

Peroneus longus

Tibialis anterior
Extensor digitorum
longus

Extensor hallucis brevis

FIGURE 1-30. Anterior view of superficial muscles.

performance of another. The net result is a functioning muscle that can respond to various tasks; and although the composition of a given muscle may lend itself to performing best in endurance activities, it can still accomplish speed and power tasks to a lesser degree.

The human body can respond adequately to most physical tasks encountered in everyday living. With muscle impairment, specific training regimens may restore normal function. Likewise, normal function can be enhanced through exercise training to accomplish physical tasks that are in excess of the demands of daily living, such as athletics (9,22).

Over the years, there has been a fair amount of controversy about the classification of muscle fiber types (3).

In addition, questions remain about whether these fiber types can change in response to an intervention such as endurance training (8,16,21,23). In either case, there is general agreement that, relative to exercise performance, two distinct fiber types — type I (slow twitch) and type II (fast twitch) — have been identified and classified by contractile and metabolic characteristics (4,13). To illustrate the variation in fiber types within humans, *Table 1-7* lists fiber type distribution in elite athletes relative to the general population.

Type I Muscle Fibers. The characteristics of type I muscle fibers, listed in *Table 1-8*, are consistent with muscle fibers that are fatigue resistant. Thus, type I fibers are selected for activities of low intensity and long duration.

BOX 1-1	Sliding-Filament Theory of Muscle Contraction and Relaxation Summary

RESTING MUSCLE

Calcium ions are bound to the SR.

Tropomyosin–troponin complex blocks attachment sites for myosin; ATP is bound to myosin heads.

MUSCLE CONTRACTION

Nerve impulse exceeding resting potential spreads across sarcolemma and down transverse tubules, causing release of calcium from the SR.

Calcium binds with troponin, which permits actin and myosin to form crossbridges.

Myosin ATPase is activated, splitting ATP; this transfer of energy causes movement of the myosin crossbridges and generates tension.

Crossbridges uncouple when ATP binds to the myosin bridge.

Coupling and uncoupling continue as long as calcium and ATP are present.

RELAXATION

When the nerve impulse ceases, calcium is taken up by the SR.

ATP binds and crossbridges uncouple; actin and myosin return to a resting state.

SR, sarcoplasmic reticulum; ATP, adenosine triphosphate.

Within whole muscle, type I motor units asynchronously contract; that is, in addition to their inherent fatigue resistance, endurance is prolonged by the constant switching that occurs to ensure unfatigued muscle as the exercise stimulus continues. Sedentary people have approximately 50% type I fibers, and this distribution is generally equal throughout the major muscle groups of the body (15). In endurance athletes, the percentage of type I fibers is greater, but this is thought to be largely a genetic predisposition, despite some evidence suggesting that prolonged exercise training can alter fiber type (*Table 1-9*) (6,10).

Essentially, those most successful at endurance activities generally have a high proportion of type I fibers, and this is most likely attributable to genetic factors enhanced through appropriate exercise training. From a metabolic perspective, type I fibers are called *aerobic* because the generation of energy for continued muscle contraction is met through the ongoing oxidation of available energy sources (*e.g.*, carbohydrates and fats). Thus, with minimal accumulation of anaerobically produced metabolites, continued muscle contraction is favored in type I fibers.

Type II Muscle Fibers. At the opposite end of the continuum, individuals who achieve the greatest success in power and high-intensity speed tasks usually have a greater proportion of type II muscle fibers distributed through the major muscle groups. Type II fibers shorten and develop tension considerably faster than type I fibers (40). Type IIx fibers are the "classic" fast-twitch fiber. Metabolically, these fibers are anaerobic fibers because they rely on energy sources intrinsic to the muscle, not the fuels used by type I fibers. When an endurance component is introduced, such as in events lasting upward of several minutes (800–1,500 m running races, for example), a second type of fast-twitch fiber, type IIa, is recruited. As noted in *Table 1-8*, type IIa fibers represent an intermediate fiber type between the type I and type IIx fibers. Metabolically, although type IIa fibers have the ability to generate a moderately large amount of force, they also have some aerobic capacity, although not as much as type I fibers. This is a logical and necessary bridge between the range of muscle fiber types and the ability to meet the various physical tasks imposed. Reference to the existence of the type IIc fiber is necessary in a complete description of human muscle fiber types. The type IIc fiber has been described as a rare and undifferentiated muscle fiber type that is most likely involved in reinnervation of impaired skeletal muscle (26).

How Muscles Produce Movement

Skeletal muscle produces force that is transferred to the tendons, which in turn pull on the bones and other structures (skin). Most muscles cross a joint, so when a muscle contracts, it pulls one of the articulating bones toward

TABLE 1-7. Muscle Fiber Composition in Selected Populations

Sport	Percentage of Type I (Slow Twitch)	Percentage of Type II (Fast Twitch)
Distance runners	60–90	10–40
Track sprinters	25–45	55–75
Weightlifters	45–55	45–55
Shot-putters	25–40	60–75
Nonathletes	47–53	47–53

Reprinted with permission from Powers SK, Howley ET. *Exercise Physiology.* Dubuque (IA): WC Brown; 1990. p. 160. The McGraw-Hill Companies, Inc.

TABLE 1-8. Structural and Functional Characteristics of Slow Twitch (I) and Fast Twitch (IIa and IIx) Muscle Fibers

Characteristics	Fiber Type		
	I	**IIa**	**IIx**
Neural Aspects			
Motor neuron size	Small	Large	Large
Motor neuron recruitment threshold	Low	High	High
Motor nerve conduction velocity	Slow	Fast	Fast
Structural Aspects			
Muscle fiber diameter	Small	Large	Large
Sarcoplasmic reticulum development	Less	More	More
Mitochondrial density	High	High	Low
Capillary density	High	Medium	Low
Myoglobin content	High	Medium	Low
Energy Substrates			
Phosphocreatine stores	Low	High	High
Glycogen stores	Low	High	High
Triglyceride stores	High	Medium	Low
Enzymatic Aspects			
Myosin-ATPase activity	Low	High	High
Glycolytic enzyme activity	Low	High	High
Oxidative enzyme activity	High	High	Low
Functional Aspects			
Twitch (contraction) time	Slow	Fast	Fast
Relaxation time	Slow	Fast	Fast
Force production	Low	High	High
Energy efficiency, "economy"	High	Low	Low
Fatigue resistance	High	Low	Low
Elasticity	Low	High	High

Reprinted with permission from Fox EL, Bowers RW, Foss ML. *The Physiological Basis of Physical Education and Athletics.* 4th ed. Dubuque (IA): WC Brown; 1989. p. 110.

TABLE 1-9. Adaptations in Skeletal Muscle Relative to Specific Training Regimens

Muscle Factor	Training			
	Slow Twitch		Fast Twitch	
	ST	**ET**	**ST**	**ET**
Percentage composition	0 or ?	0 or ?	0 or ?	0 or ?
Size	+	0 or +	+ +	0
Contractile property	0	0	0	0
Oxidative capacity	0	+ +	0	+
Anaerobic capacity	? or +	0	? or +	0
Glycogen content	0	+ +	0	+ +
Fat oxidation	0	+ +	0	+
Capillary density	?	+	?	? or +
Blood flow during work	?	? or +	?	?

ST, strength training; ET, endurance training.

0, no change; ?, unknown; +, moderate increase; + +, large increase.

Adapted with permission from Gollnick PD, Sembrowich WI. Adaptations in human skeletal muscle as a result of training. In: Amsterdam E, editor. *Exercise and Cardiovascular Health and Disease.* New York: Yorke Medical Books; 1977. p. 90; and from Katch VL, McArdle WD, Katch FI. *Essentials of Exercise Physiology.* 4th ed. Baltimore (MD): Lippincott Williams & Wilkins; 2011. 712 p.

most common type of levers in the human body and are designed for large ROM and speed of movement.

Muscle Actions. Muscle *action* is the result of neuromuscular activation that leads to the production of force and contributes to the movement or the stabilization of the musculoskeletal system (25). Muscle actions can be classified into three basic types: isometric, concentric, and eccentric. In an *isometric* (or *static*) *action*, the muscle generates force in the absence of joint movement, such as holding a dumbbell during a biceps curl without movement. An action in which the muscle length changes is often called *dynamic*. Concentric and eccentric actions are dynamic muscle actions. A *concentric action* occurs when the muscle torque being generated exceeds the torque of the resistance force and the muscle shortens in length, such as the upward phase of a biceps curl. *Eccentric actions* occur when the torque generated by the muscle is less than the torque of the resistance force being encountered. This results in the active muscle lengthening rather than shortening such as the downward phase of a biceps curl. Eccentric actions are often used when muscles have to slow down body parts or oppose external resistance forces.

Muscle Roles. Movements of the human body generally require several muscles to work together rather than a single muscle to perform all the work. Because muscles only pull and cannot push, most skeletal muscles are arranged in opposing pairs such as flexor–extensor, internal–external rotators, and so on. Muscles can be classified according to their roles during movement. When a muscle or group of muscles is responsible for the action or movement, it is called a *prime mover* or **agonist**. For example, during a biceps curl, the prime movers are the elbow flexors, which

the other. Usually, both articulating bones do not move equally; one of the articulating bones stays more stationary. The attachment that is more stationary and usually more proximal (especially in the extremities) is called the *origin*. The muscle attachment that moves the most and is usually located more distally is called the *insertion*.

Levers. Mechanically, to produce movement, the muscles, joints, and bones work as a system of levers. The bone acts as the lever, the joint functions as the center of rotation (COR), and the muscles produce the force or effort (F) to move the lever. The resistance (R), or the force that opposes the movement of the lever, could be the weight of the body part or the external resistance provided by weights. Levers are classified into three types according to the relative position of the center, axis of rotation, and the effort and resistance forces (*Fig. 1-31*). Third-class levers (*Fig. 1-31C*) are the

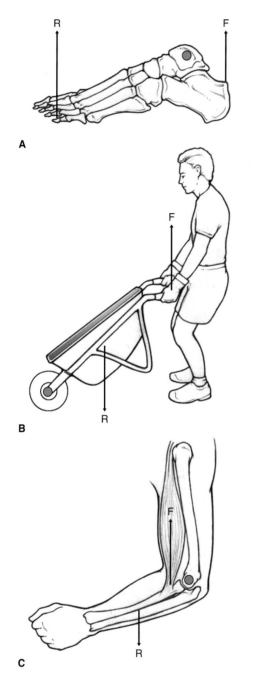

FIGURE 1-31. Examples of lever systems in the human body, where *F* is the exerted force, *R* is the reaction force, and the *green dot* (●) is the axis of rotation. Most musculoskeletal joints behave as third-class levers. **A.** First-class lever. **B.** Second-class lever. **C.** Third-class lever.

include the biceps brachii, brachialis, and brachioradialis muscles. The opposing group of muscles is called the **antagonist** (triceps brachii and anconeus). In addition, most movements also involve other muscles called **synergists**. The role of these muscles is to prevent unwanted movement, which helps the prime movers perform more efficiently. Synergist muscles can also act as fixators or stabilizers. In this role, the muscles stabilize a portion of the body against an external force. For example, the

scapular muscles (*e.g.*, rhomboids, serratus anterior, trapezius) must provide a stable base of support for the upper extremity muscles during a throwing motion.

Muscles and Exercise. Muscle actions produce force that causes joint movement during exercise. Exercise scientists and other health care professionals should have a good knowledge and understanding of which muscles are involved in the movements of the major joints. This knowledge is the basis for the development of exercise programs for use in training and rehabilitation (11). *Tables 1-5* and *1-6* give a list of common resistance training exercises and the muscles involved.

SUMMARY

Besides contributing to body shape and form, bones perform several important functions, including support, protection, movement, and storage of essential nutrients and blood cell formation. Skeletal muscle is responsible for bodily movement, body stabilization, and heat production. It is composed of varying amounts of types I, IIa, and IIx muscle fibers whose quantity and distribution are largely genetic. Physical activity patterns and sports performance characteristics develop from the varying properties of muscle fibers, the organization and integration of fiber recruitment patterns, and the levers, bones, and joints through which the muscle fibers act. Although the conversion of muscle fiber types through either disuse or training and the splitting and generation of muscle fibers are somewhat controversial, exercise training clearly results in significant metabolic adaptations of muscle fibers.

REFERENCES

1. Agur AMR, Dalley AF. *Grant's Atlas of Anatomy*. 12th ed. Philadelphia (PA): Lippincott Williams & Wilkins; 2008. 864 p.
2. Albertine KH, Williams MC, Hyde DM. Anatomy of the lungs. In: Mason RJ, editor. *Murray and Nadel's Textbook of Respiratory Medicine*. 4th ed. Oxford: Elsevier; 2005. p. 3–29.
3. Armstrong RB. Muscle fiber recruitment patterns and their metabolic correlates. In: Horton ES, Terjung RL, editors. *Exercise, Nutrition, and Energy Metabolism*. New York: Macmillan; 1988. p. 9–26.
4. Brooke MH, Kaiser KK. Muscle fiber types: how many and what kind? *Arch Neurol*. 1970;23(4):369–79.
5. Brooks GA, Fahey TD, Baldwin KM. *Exercise Physiology: Human Bioenergetics and Its Applications*. 4th ed. New York (NY): McGraw-Hill; 2005. 928 p.
6. Burke ER, Cerny F, Costill D, Fink W. Characteristics of skeletal muscle in competitive cyclists. *Med Sci Sports*. 1977;9(2):109–12.
7. Carrin B. Development and structure of the normal human lung. In: Tuner-Warwick M, editor. *Respiratory Diseases: Clinical Atlas*. London: Gower Medical Pub; 1989. p. 1–14.
8. Chi MM, Hintz CS, Coyle EF, et al. Effects of detraining on enzymes of energy metabolism in individual human muscle fibers. *Am J Physiol*. 1983;244(3):C276–87.
9. Coggan AR, Spina RJ, King DS, et al. Skeletal muscle adaptations to endurance training in 60- to 70-yr-old men and women. *J Appl Physiol*. 1992;72(5):1780–6.
10. Costill DL, Daniels J, Evans W, Fink W, Krahenbuhl G, Saltin B. Skeletal muscle enzymes and fiber composition in male and female track athletes. *J Appl Physiol*. 1976;40(2):149–54.

11. Delavier F. *Strength Training Anatomy*. 3rd ed. Champaign (IL): Human Kinetics; 2010. 192 p.

12. DeVries HA, Housh TJ. *Physiology of Exercise for Physical Education, Athletics, and Exercise Science*. 5th ed. Madison (WI): WCB Brown & Benchmark; 1994. 636 p.

13. Edstrom L, Nystrom B. Histochemical types and sizes of fibres in normal human muscles. A biopsy study. *Acta Neurol Scand.* 1969;45(3):257–69.

14. Foss ML, Keteyian SJ, Fox EL. *Fox's Physiological Basis for Exercise and Sport*. 6th ed. Boston (MA): McGraw-Hill; 1998. 620 p.

15. Fox EL, Bowers RW, Foss ML. *The Physiological Basis of Physical Education and Athletics*. 4th ed. Dubuque (IA): WC Brown; 1989. 734 p.

16. Gollnick PD, Armstrong RB, Sembrowich WL, Shepherd RE, Saltin B. Glycogen depletion pattern in human skeletal muscle fibers after heavy exercise. *J Appl Physiol.* 1973;34(5):615–8.

17. Gray H, Williams PL, Bannister LH. *Gray's Anatomy: The Anatomical Basis of Medicine and Surgery*. electronic ed. New York (NY): Churchill Livingstone; 2005.

18. Hall-Craggs ECB. *Anatomy as a Basis for Clinical Medicine*. 3rd ed. Baltimore (MD): Williams & Wilkins; 1995. 587 p.

19. Hunter GR, Harris RT. Structure and function of the muscular, neuromuscular, cardiovascular, and respiratory systems. In: Baechle TR, Earle RW, editors. *Essentials of Strength Training and Conditioning*. 3rd ed. Champaign: Human Kinetics; 2008. p. 3–21.

20. Huxley HE. The structural basis of muscular contraction. *Proc R Soc Lond B Biol Sci.* 1971;178(51):131–49.

21. Jacobs I, Esbjornsson M, Sylven C, Holm I, Jansson E. Sprint training effects on muscle myoglobin, enzymes, fiber types, and blood lactate. *Med Sci Sports Exerc.* 1987;19(4):368–74.

22. Jansson E, Kaijser L. Muscle adaptation to extreme endurance training in man. *Acta Physiol Scand.* 1977;100(3):315–24.

23. Jansson E, Sjodin B, Tesch P. Changes in muscle fibre type distribution in man after physical training. A sign of fibre type transformation? *Acta Physiol Scand.* 1978;104(2):235–7.

24. Katch VL, McArdle WD, Katch FI. *Essentials of Exercise Physiology*. 4th ed. Baltimore (MD): Lippincott Williams & Wilkins; 2011. 712 p.

25. Knudson DV, Morrison CS. *Qualitative Analysis of Human Movement*. 2nd ed. Champaign (IL): Human Kinetics; 2002. 252 p.

26. Komi PV, Karlsson J. Skeletal muscle fibre types, enzyme activities and physical performance in young males and females. *Acta Physiol Scand.* 1978;103(2):210–8.

27. Light RW. *Pleural Diseases*. 5th ed. Philadelphia (PA): Lippincott Williams & Wilkins; 2007. 427 p.

28. Marieb EN, Hoehn K, Hutchinson M. *Human Anatomy and Physiology*. 7th ed. San Francisco (CA): Pearson Benjamin Cummings; 2007. 1159 p.

29. Martini F. *Fundamentals of Anatomy and Physiology*. 6th ed. Upper Saddle River (NJ): Prentice Hall; 2003. 1264 p.

30. McArdle WD, Katch FI, Katch VL. *Exercise Physiology: Energy, Nutrition, and Human Performance*. 7th ed. Philadelphia (PA): Lippincott Williams & Wilkins; 2009.

31. Moore KL, Agur AMR, Dalley AF. *Essential Clinical Anatomy*. 4th ed. Philadelphia (PA): Lippincott Williams & Wilkins; 2010. 703 p.

32. Moore KL, Dalley AF, Agur AMR. *Clinically Oriented Anatomy*. 5th ed. Baltimore (MD): Lippincott Williams & Wilkins; 2006. 1209 p.

33. Nilsestuen J. Pulmonary physiology. In: Berghuis P, editor. *Respiration*. Redmond: SpaceLabs; 1992. p. 1–11.

34. Olson TR, Pawlina W. *A.D.A.M. Student Atlas of Anatomy*. Baltimore (MD): Williams & Wilkins; 1996. 492 p.

35. Powers SK, Howley ET. *Exercise Physiology: Theory and Application to Fitness and Performance*. 6th ed. New York (NY): McGraw-Hill Education; 2006. 624 p.

36. Shier D, Butler J, Lewis R. *Hole's Essentials of Human Anatomy and Physiology*. 10th ed. Boston (MA): McGraw-Hill; 2009.

37. Sokolow M, McIlroy M, Cheitlin M. *Clinical Cardiology*. Norwalk (CT): Appleton & Lange; 1993. 741 p.

38. Spence AP, Mason EB. *Human Anatomy and Physiology*. 4th ed. St. Paul (MN): West Pub Co; 1992. 956 p.

39. Thibodeau GA, Patton KT. *Anthony's Textbook of Anatomy & Physiology*. 16th ed. St. Louis (MO): Mosby; 1999. 1083 p.

40. Vrbova G. Influence of activity on some characteristic properties of slow and fast mammalian muscles. *Exerc Sport Sci Rev.* 1979;7:181–213.

41. Wilmore JH, Costill DL, Kenney WL. *Physiology of Sport and Exercise*. 4th ed. Champaign (IL): Human Kinetics; 2008. 574 p.

SELECTED REFERENCES FOR FURTHER READING

Aaberg E. *Muscle Mechanics*. 2nd ed. Champaign (IL): Human Kinetics; 2006. 219 p.

Calais-Germain B. *Anatomy of Movement*. Seattle (WA): Eastland Press; 2003. 316 p.

Delavier F. *Strength Training Anatomy*. 3rd ed. Champaign (IL): Human Kinetics; 2010. 192 p.

Floyd RT, Thompson CW. *Manual of Structural Kinesiology*. 17th ed. New York (NY): McGraw-Hill; 2009. 408 p.

Hamill J, Knutzen KM. *Biomechanical Basis of Human Movement*. 3rd ed. Philadelphia (PA): Lippincott Williams & Wilkins; 2008. 236 p.

Jenkins DB. *Hollinshead's Functional Anatomy of the Limbs and Back*. 9th ed. Philadelphia (PA): WB Saunders; 2009. 442 p.

Knudson DV, Morrison CS. *Qualitative Analysis of Human Movement*. 2nd ed. Champaign (IL): Human Kinetics; 2002. 252 p.

Neumann, DA. *Kinesiology of the Musculoskeletal System: Foundations for Physical Rehabilitation*. 2nd ed. St. Louis (MO): Mosby; 2010. 725 p.

Oatis, CA. *Kinesiology: The Mechanics and Pathomechanics of Human Movement*. 2nd ed. Philadelphia (PA): Lippincott Williams & Wilkins; 2008. 960 p.

INTERNET RESOURCES

- American Association of Anatomists: http://www.anatomy.org
- Anatomy on the Internet: http://www.meddean.luc.edu/lumen/MedEd/GrossAnatomy/anatomy.htm
- The Digital Anatomist Information System: http://sig.biostr.washington.edu/projects/da/
- InnerBody. Your Guide to Human Anatomy Online: http://www.innerbody.com/htm/body.html
- Muscles and Exercise Online: http://www.exrx.net/Lists/Directory.html
- NISMAT Exercise Physiology Corner: Muscle Physiology Primer: http://www.nismat.org/physcor/muscle.html
- University of California San Diego: Muscle Physiology: http://muscle.ucsd.edu/musintro/jump.shtml
- University of Michigan Muscles in Action: http://www.med.umich.edu/lrc/Hypermuscle/

2

Biomechanics

Biomechanics is the study and application of the motion of living organisms using the branch of physics known as mechanics. The study of forces and torques that cause movement is called kinetics and the description of the resulting motion is called kinematics. This chapter summarizes how professionals can use their understanding of the causes of human motion (kinetics), the effects of forces on human tissues, and kinematic measurements of human motion to modify exercise prescriptions.

KINETICS

Understanding the causes of human movement requires an understanding of several kinetic variables. This section discusses the forces and torques that create and/or modify motion; introduces Newton's laws of motion, which describe the creation and/or modification of motion; and summarizes some of the major forces that affect human movement.

KEY TERMS

Base of support: The area of the supporting surface of an object such as between and under the feet in standing or between the hands in a handstand.

Biomechanics: The study of the motion and causes of motion of living things and the application of mechanical principles.

Buoyancy: The floating force on an object immersed in a fluid.

Center of gravity: The location of a theoretical point that can be used to represent the total weight (mass) of an object.

Drag: The fluid force that acts parallel to the relative flow of fluid past an object.

Force: A push or pull that tends to modify motion or the shape of an object.

Friction: The force that acts parallel to and opposes motion between surfaces in contact.

Impulse: The effect of force acting over time.

Kinematics: The branch of mechanics that describes motion.

Kinetics: The branch of mechanics that explains the causes of motion.

Lift: The fluid force that acts at right angles to the relative flow of fluid past an object.

Mass: The quantity of matter in a body or substance.

Moment arm: The leverage of a force creating a torque or moment of force; the perpendicular distance between the line of action of the force and the axis of rotation.

Moment of force: The rotating effect of a force.

Moment of inertia: A measure of the resistance of a body to angular acceleration about a given axis.

Momentum: The quantity of motion of an object that is equal to the product of the mass and velocity of the object.

Normal reaction: The force acting at right angles between two surfaces in contact.

Stiffness: The measure of the elasticity of a material defined as the slope of the stress–strain graph in the elastic region.

Strain: A measure of the deformation of a material when acted upon by a force.

Stress: The force per unit area in a material.

Torque: Another term used to refer to a rotating effect of a force. Mechanics of materials uses *torque* to refer to torsional (twisting about a longitudinal axis) moments.

Vector: A quantity that has both magnitude (size) and direction.

FORCES AND TORQUES

For a body segment to change its state of motion, a force must be applied. A force is a linear effect that can be defined as a push, pull, or tendency to distort. Forces can be represented by vectors. Forces have four important characteristics, two of which are the vector characteristics of magnitude (size) and direction. The other two characteristics are line of action and point of application.

Forces and the vectors used to represent them can be drawn as arrows with the length representing magnitude and the arrowhead indicating direction (*Fig. 2-1*). The International System of Units (SI) of force magnitude are Newtons (N). The point of application of a force is the location at which the force acts on an object. The line of action is an imaginary line extending in both directions from the force vector (see *Fig. 2-1*). In most situations, multiple forces act on body segments, so vector addition and subtraction techniques are needed to take into account the interacting magnitudes and directions. Adding vectors together determines a resultant vector. A vector can be also broken up into equivalent parts called *components*. For example, the forces between a runner's foot and the ground are usually resolved into right-angle components (*Fig. 2-2*).

Depending on how forces are applied to an object, they may cause three kinds of motion: (a) translation or linear motion; (b) rotation or angular motion; and (c) general motion, which is a combination of translation and rotation. A force acting through the center of a mass of an object creates translation. Forces with a line of action not acting through the object's center of mass tend to create rotation and translation or general motion. The force F in *Figure 2-2* does not act through the center of gravity of the runner, so it tends to create linear and angular motion of the body.

The measure of the rotary effect of a force is called a moment of force (M), which is commonly referred to as torque. A moment can be calculated as the product of the force and its moment arm, which is the perpendicular distance from the line of action of the force to the axis

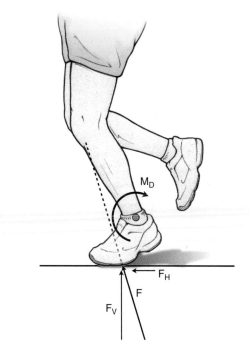

FIGURE 2-2. The ground reaction force (F) between a runner's foot in stance can be broken up into horizontal (F_H) and vertical (F_V) components. This ground reaction force acts off-center to the ankle joint axis and creates a dorsiflexing (M_D) moment of force or torque.

of rotation. The most common unit of a moment of force is Newton meters (Nm). Moments are also vector quantities that can be added to determine the net rotary effect of forces acting on an object. For instance, typical changes in the moment arm or leverage of the distal attachment of the biceps brachii at the elbow during flexion are illustrated in *Figure 2-3*.

NEWTON'S LAWS OF MOTION

Sir Isaac Newton developed three laws of motion that explain how forces create movement. The first law is the *law of inertia*, which states "a body continues in its state of rest, or uniform motion in a straight line, unless a force acts upon it." All objects have this innate property (inertia) that resists changes in state of motion. To move a motionless object, force must be applied to overcome its inertia and thus set it into motion. Likewise, the inertia of the moving object tends to keep it moving, so a force must be applied to either stop it or modify its motion.

The second law is usually called the *law of acceleration* and is represented in two dimensions by the mathematical formula $\Sigma F = ma$, where ΣF equals the sum of all forces in a given direction, m equals mass, and a equals acceleration in the same direction. This formula illustrates the relationship between kinetics and the resulting kinematics at any instant in time. The law says that "the acceleration an object experiences is proportional to the resultant force acting on the object in that

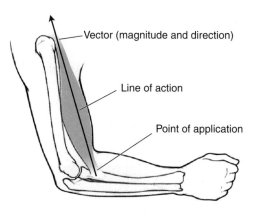

FIGURE 2-1. Vectors such as a force can be represented by an *arrow*. The four characteristics of a force are illustrated.

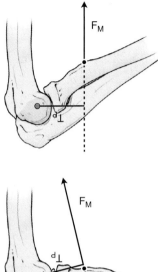

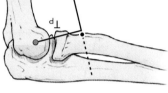

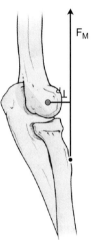

FIGURE 2-3. Schematic of the changes in the moment arm $(d_\perp)$ at the elbow for the biceps brachii. The torque or moment of force the muscle can create is affected by both changes in force and moment arm $(T = F_M \cdot d_\perp)$. The moment arm at the elbow for the long head of biceps would be affected by both shoulder and elbow joint rotation. (Note variation in the muscle angle of pull and the resulting moment arm.)

direction and is inversely proportional to the object's mass." This formula specifies the cause-and-effect relationship between forces and linear motion. Over intervals of time, Newton's second law is expressed as the impulse–momentum relationship, where the change in **momentum** of any object in a direction is equal to the net **impulse** applied ($\Delta p = \Sigma J$) in that direction.

In angular motion, the law of acceleration is written as $\Sigma M = I\alpha$, where ΣM equals the sum of the moments acting on the object, I equals the **moment of inertia** of the object, and α equals the angular acceleration of the object.

Newton's second law may be the most important because it defines the relationship between kinetics and kinematics, includes the inertia of objects (m and I), and provides for units of force. For example, a Newton of force is the linear effect that will accelerate 1 kg of mass (m) $1 \text{ m} \cdot \text{s}^{-2}$ (a). These two formulas are applied in biomechanical models to estimate the net forces and torques acting in linked segment models. This is called *inverse dynamics* because measures of kinematics (α) and body segment inertial properties (I) are used to calculate the net moments (ΣM) and forces that create the movement in the model.

Newton's third law is called the *law of action–reaction*. This says that "for every force there is an equal and opposite force." In other words, forces do not act only on one body but are an interaction between two bodies. The law can be expressed mathematically as $F_{AB} = -F_{BA}$. When objects A and B interact, object A produces an equal and opposite effect on B. In turn, the second object, B, produces an equal and opposite effect on A. Positive and negative signs in mechanics refer to the direction of vector quantities. For example, during locomotion, the foot exerts a force every time it contacts the ground; however, the ground exerts an equal and opposite force on the foot (see *Fig. 2-2*). This is an important law of kinetics that shows that forces and torques are mutual interactions between objects.

IMPORTANT FORCES IN HUMAN MOVEMENT

Forces that create human motion can be external forces between parts of the body and the environment (*i.e.*, the ground reaction forces in *Fig. 2-2*) or internal forces created by the musculoskeletal system. These forces can be classified in many ways, but the forces that are most often considered in biomechanical analyses are described in this section.

Gravity is the vertical attraction force between the earth and an object. The magnitude of this force is the body weight (BW) of the object. BW is proportional to mass from Newton's second law. Because gravitational acceleration is fairly constant on the earth ($9.81 \text{ m} \cdot \text{s}^{-2}$), a barbell with a mass of 50 kg weighs 490.5 N [$F_w = 50(9.81)$]. Skeletal muscles must skillfully balance the weight of body segments and external objects such as dumbbells to move in even the simplest exercise. Standing in the anatomical position, the weight force of the body interacts with the supporting force from the floor.

Contact between the human body and another object (*e.g.*, catching a ball, jumping, wearing ankle weights) results in external forces that are often resolved into two important components: the **normal reaction** and **friction**. Friction (F_f) is the force acting parallel to the two surfaces in contact, and it acts in the opposite direction of the motion or impending motion (*Fig. 2-4*). The force acting perpendicular to the surfaces of contact is called the normal reaction (F_N) or normal force. In dry conditions, the

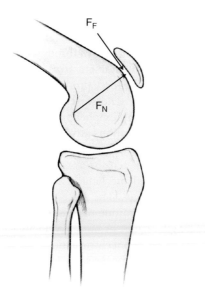

FIGURE 2-4. The contact force between two objects, such as at the patellofemoral joint, is often broken into friction (F_F) and normal reaction (F_N) components.

sizes of these two forces are related by the simple formula $F_f = F_N \cdot \mu$, where μ is the coefficient of static friction. The coefficient of static friction is a dimensionless ratio that is experimentally determined and describes the frictional properties between the two interacting surfaces. For example, tennis shoes on sports surfaces typically have coefficients of static friction ranging from 0.4 to nearly 2.0 (45). When the two surfaces start to slide past each other, the friction force decreases and a kinetic coefficient of friction must be used. Rotational friction can also be determined by how much moment of force must be applied to cause the surfaces to rotate against the other.

Some of the most important external forces in human movement are *ground reaction forces*. Ground reaction forces act between a person and the support surface on which that person moves, such as the foot of the runner shown in *Figure 2-2*. A force platform can be used to measure the changes in magnitude, direction, and point of application of the ground reaction forces during the period the foot is in contact with the platform. These ground reaction forces are resolved into three components relative to the person's direction of motion: the vertical (normal reaction) and two frictional components (anteroposterior and mediolateral). In running, the peak vertical ground reaction forces occur in midstance and are about 3 BW, and the peak anteroposterior forces are about 0.4 BW (46). If the coefficient of friction between this shoe and the platform surface was 0.8, then the maximum horizontal force that could be made before sliding would be 2.4 BW [$F_f = 0.8(3.0)$]. As such, there is little danger of slipping while running on dry surfaces. Frictional forces in wet conditions are much smaller than in similar dry conditions. A child running on a wet pool

deck might only have 0.15 BW of friction [$F_f = 0.05(3.0)$] because of the very low coefficient of friction.

Examples of internal forces are *joint reaction forces*. In linked segment biomechanical models, these forces between adjacent segments are modeled using Newton's laws of motion. In a squat exercise, for example, the downward force on an intervertebral disc from the weight of the upper body has an equal and opposite (acting upward) force from the lower body. The most common methods of inverse dynamics use Newton's laws to determine net joint reaction forces and moments of force from measurements of segment acceleration and inertial parameters. Unfortunately, the joint reaction forces are a combination of joint, muscle, and ligament forces and do not represent the true bone-on-bone forces at joints (64). Actual bone-on-bone forces and contact pressures at joint surfaces are very difficult to measure or calculate.

Important internal forces in human movement are elastic forces in muscles, tendons, and ligaments that contribute to joint reaction forces. Elastic forces often contribute to many movements and are created by the tendency of a deformed material to return to its original shape. The measure of the elasticity in a deformed material is called **stiffness** and is defined as the ratio of mechanical **stress** (σ) to **strain** (ε) in the linear (elastic) region of the curve. *Figure 2-5* shows an idealized stress/strain curve. The slope of the linear portion of the graph (σ/ε) up to the yield point gives an indication of the stiffness of the material. Stress is defined as the force per unit area of the material, and strain is usually defined as the percentage change in length. For example, the maximal muscular strength of muscle is usually reported as a stress of 25–40 N/cm^2, and the typical elongation of the Achilles tendon in a maximal voluntary contraction is a strain of

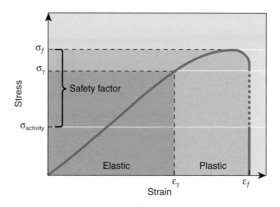

FIGURE 2-5. An idealized stress/strain curve. The elastic region is bounded by the yield point (designated by ε_y, σ_y). The plastic region is bounded by the yield point and the failure point (designated by ε_f, σ_f). The stress in musculoskeletal tissues in normal activity is much less than the yield point. The difference between the stress/strain of normal activities and the failure point is the safety factor. (Adapted with permission from Biewener AA, editor. *Biomechanics: Structures and Systems.* Oxford [UK]: Oxford University Press; 1992.)

about 5% (28). The magnitude of strain that tendons are subjected to is the major mechanical stimulus related to improvements in mechanical strength (2). Because the area of a deformed material changes, it is easier to ignore these small deformations and approximate stress–strain graphs with force–deformation graphs.

A stiff material is hard to deform (high force for small deformation) and therefore has high elasticity, tending to quickly return to its normal shape when an external force is removed. A material with low stiffness is called *compliant* because small forces can create larger deformations. Materials loaded in the elastic region of the curve return to their normal shape with minimal permanent change in shape. Stressing a material beyond the yield point and into the plastic region of the curve results in permanent change in the material's structure. Materials have an ultimate mechanical strength or failure point that represents the maximum force or stress a material can withstand before breaking. Stresses in the musculoskeletal system in normal activities are much lower than the yield point for these tissues, so there is a large safety factor (3) in most physical activities. Sometimes the mechanical strength of a material is documented as the total energy absorbed. Note that the mechanical strength of materials is different from muscular strength. This chapter refers to muscular strength as "strength" and uses "mechanical strength" to avoid confusion in terminology.

Most tissues have even more complex stress/strain curves than the one shown in *Figure 2-5*. The curves are nonlinear and the stiffness depends on the timing of force loading. This rate dependence of mechanical behavior is called *viscoelasticity*. Tissues of the musculoskeletal system have greater stiffness when they are loaded rapidly. This is a major reason why static stretching is preferred over ballistic stretching because a greater level of musculotendinous elongation can be reached using a smaller and safer amount of force. In normal and vigorous movements, however, muscles and tendons can be stretched like a spring and a large percentage of this elastic energy can be recovered in subsequent shortening (1). This storage and recovery of elastic forces is just one mechanism of the important neuromuscular strategy called the *stretch–shortening cycle*. Many powerful movements are naturally initiated with a countermovement that is stopped with an **eccentric** (*i.e.*, muscle-lengthening) action and immediately reversed to a **concentric** (*i.e.*, muscle-shortening) action in the intended direction of motion (40). For example, in the stance phase of sprinting, the plantar flexors are essentially eccentrically active in early stance, which serves to increase the force of the following concentric action in push-off.

Maybe the most important and complex internal forces affecting human movement are muscle forces. Muscles exert forces on the skeleton to create motion, stabilize posture, dampen vibration, or decrease the stress in bones created by other forces. Muscles create only tensile forces that pull on all attachments. Muscle forces also create torques about joints. The torques are always changing as the joint moves through the range of motion (ROM) because the moment arms change as joints rotate and because muscle force production is related to muscle length and velocity. Therefore, the torque a muscle group can make is a complex phenomenon that is a combination of tension variations attributable to contractile conditions and geometric moment arm changes for muscles.

The amount of tension a muscle can create depends on excitation and mechanical factors related to muscle length and velocity. The *force–velocity relationship* dictates that the magnitude of muscle force depends on the rate of length change or muscle velocity (30). The faster a muscle shortens (concentric action), the less muscle force that can be created for the same level of excitation. On the other hand, the faster the active lengthening of muscle (eccentric action), the greater the muscle force. This relationship is illustrated in *Figure 2-6*. Note that the force potentials for all three muscle actions (eccentric, isometric, concentric) are defined by the graph. Training shifts the force–velocity graph upward but cannot change the pattern of decreased or increased force potential as muscle velocity changes. The actual force or tension in eccentric muscle actions is actually much higher (150%–180% of maximal isometric values) than illustrated in *Figure 2-6* because this schematic is shortened and not to scale.

The *force–length relationship* indicates how the isometric force a muscle can create varies with its length (21,53). At intermediate lengths, muscles can produce the greatest force. Less force can be created in shortened conditions. Less active tension can also be created in lengthened conditions, but this is offset by increases in passive tension. In other words, the elastic force of stretched connective tissue and structural proteins within muscle generate tension that can be used to create subsequent motion. This passive tension is the discomfort that

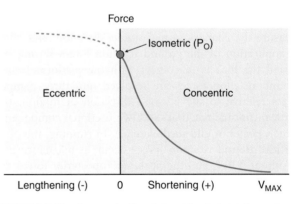

FIGURE 2-6. The force–velocity relationship of skeletal muscle illustrates skeletal muscle force potential for the rate of change of muscle length (velocity), so all three muscle actions can be visualized on the graph. (Adapted from Knudson D. *Fundamentals of Biomechanics.* New York [NY]: Kluwer; 2003, with kind permission from Springer Science+Business Media B.V.)

is felt in a vigorous stretch. Quite a bit of recent research has begun to document the complex interaction of active and passive sources of muscle tension (17,37) in muscle actions, and muscle force from passive tension can be used in some low-intensity activities that do not have to be in the extremes of the range of joint motion (47).

Clinicians and researchers often assess muscle group strength using measurements from handheld or isokinetic dynamometers. A dynamometer is a machine that measures force or torque. Isokinetic dynamometers measure torque in conditions of nearly constant joint angular velocity. Isokinetic dynamometers allow muscle group strength to be defined for all points in the ROM isometrically or at various constant speeds of shortening or lengthening. The torque-angle or moment/angle curves created by these machines illustrate the strength curves of muscle groups integrating the many mechanical factors affecting muscle force (*Fig. 2-7*). Extensive normative data are available for most joints of the body (8), and these data are usually normalized to body mass and categorized for various populations (*e.g.*, age, sex, sport). Isometric (a special case of isokinetic: angular velocity = 0 rads/s) testing is a common method of muscular strength measurement because it controls for the velocity and length dependence of muscular tension.

Dynamic measurements such as the one repetition maximum (1-RM) using various weights or resistance training machines are more commonly used field tests for estimating muscular strength because of the ease and low cost of these protocols. Another common dynamic muscular performance variable is muscular power. Peak musculoskeletal power output for various movements can be measured by combining dynamometer and kinematic measurements and has been used to establish a range of training loads that maximize power output (10,14). These studies of muscular strength and power measurements are consistent with the fitness research showing three major expressions (static, dynamic, and explosive) of muscular performance (35).

Muscles rarely work in isolation because there are multiple muscles crossing most joints with similar and/or opposing anatomical actions. Determining the contribution of individual muscles to movements is very difficult; so often, the hypothesized isolated actions of muscles made in functional anatomy are incorrect. One reason for the difference is that muscles have actions at all joints — not just the joints they cross — because of the linked segments of the human body (48,62), often referred to as the kinetic chain. The joint reaction forces acting at joints allow energy from a muscle to be transferred to segments quite distant from the segments to which the muscle attaches. Computer simulations of complex biomechanical models have begun to determine these complex actions of muscles in movements (61). Biomechanics uses various research tools to validate these observations including electromyography (EMG), movement kinematics, and direct measurements of forces in tendons. The use of EMG was one of the first technologies to show that muscular contributions to movement are more complex than hypothesized by anatomy (26). Recent EMG research has documented that many muscles have intramuscular segments (7), making them even more complicated than described in gross anatomy. The use of implanted force transducers in the tendons of animals and humans (18,39,55) and bright-mode ultrasound images of muscle and tendon length changes (36) are recent developments that help confirm the complex actions of muscles in movement. In many normal movements, muscle fibers are able to act in high-force, nearly isometric conditions because the efficient stretch and recoil of passive connective tissues within the tendon and muscle minimize the shortening velocity of the muscle fibers (37). Muscle actions most often tend to occur in short bursts (31) timed to take advantage of external forces, gravity, and biomechanical geometry (16). This coordination of muscle activation or torques has been called passive dynamics, segmental interaction, or energy that can be transferred through

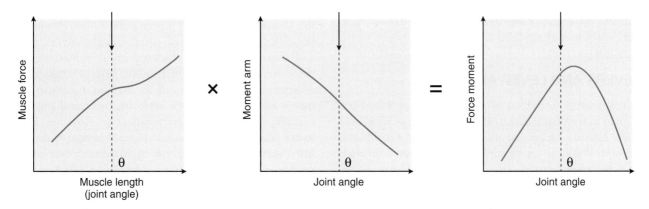

FIGURE 2-7. The joint moment/angle curve represents the strength curves of muscle groups. The shapes of these curves are a combination of muscular properties (similar to the force–length relationship) and muscle moment arms. (Adapted with permission from Zatsiorsky V, Kraemer WJ. *Science and Practice of Strength Training*. 2nd ed. Champaign [IL]: Human Kinetics; 2006.)

joints (34,43,52,64). The integration of several kinds of biomechanical research is needed to develop a good understanding of how muscles create movement.

The way muscles create movement often interacts with equipment, adding another level of complexity to helping clients. Sometimes the effects are localized, like when curve soled shoes only affect the angle and loads at the ankle joint (6). In other situations, like the use of a Smith machine for squat exercises, all sagittal plane movements are systematically altered relative to free weight squats (4). Sometimes the mechanical properties of swung equipment can be optimized for the whole biomechanical system to improve performance (11).

Other important forces affecting human movement are fluid forces. Fluid forces arise when people are submerged and move in water or air. There are three fluid forces: buoyancy, lift, and drag. Buoyancy is the supporting or flotation force of a fluid. Water exercise programs use the upward force of buoyancy to decrease the vertical loading in the joints of the lower extremities. This is an effective exercise modality for people with arthritis and people in rehabilitation programs.

When there is relative flow of a fluid past an object, the flow forces are resolved into two components: lift and drag. Lift acts at right angles to the relative flow, and drag acts in the same direction as the fluid flow and the opposite direction of the object moving through the fluid. Both of these forces increase with the square of the velocity of flow, so the resistance to body movements in water exercises increases dramatically with faster speeds of movement. There are various assistive devices that increase buoyancy, lift, and drag to adjust resistance during water exercise. For example, a life vest increases a person's buoyancy so he or she can float in an upright position. Attaching fins to the feet would increase the lift provided by kicking movements, and specialized suits can decrease drag, thereby increasing swimming speed and economy (greater speed for a given amount of energy expenditure). Cyclists or swimmers follow directly behind other competitors (draft) to decrease the drag forces of the fluid rushing past them (13). Even runners make use of this technique in the fastest races performed in a group (800 and 1,500 m).

LEVERS AND LEVER ACTIONS

Force is often described as a linear concept. However, human movement is largely determined by the rotational effect of force (*i.e.*, moment of force) around a fixed axis, or joint. Walking, for example, is accomplished through muscle contractions affecting the rotation of knee, ankle, and hip joints such that the applied force is able to overcome the resistance to movement created by the weight of the body segments. As previously described, a moment depends, in part, on the perpendicular distance between the axis and line of action. This perpendicular distance

is typically referred to as the moment arm or lever arm. A lever is a rigid bar that rotates about an axis. In the human body, the bone acts as a lever, the joint serves as the axis, and the muscles apply the force.

A **first-class lever** has an axis that is situated between the applied force and the resistance to movement. A seesaw is one example of a first-class lever. This lever arrangement is not common in the musculoskeletal system. One example would be an overhead triceps extension in which the triceps brachii pulls the olecranon process of the ulna to move a weight in the hand; the elbow joint is between the point of attachment and the resistance.

In a **second-class lever**, the applied force and resistance are on the same side of the axis with the resistance situated closer to the axis. Common examples include a wheelbarrow or nutcracker. An example related to human movement is a push-up, where the foot acts as the axis, the center of gravity serves as the resistive force, and the arms apply the movement force. There are no truly analogous examples in the human musculoskeletal system of a second-class lever.

A **third-class lever** describes an arrangement in which the applied force and resistance are situated on the same side of the axis, with the resistance being farther from the axis. A shovel is sometimes used as a third-class lever (when the hand at the end of the handle acts as the axis of rotation while the hand closer to the shovel blade applies force). This is also the most common lever found in the human musculoskeletal system. For example, during a biceps curl, the biceps brachii pulls on the radius at an attachment site close to the axis of rotation (elbow) to move a weight in the hand. This arrangement provides an advantage regarding ROM and speed of movement, particularly with light resistances. The biceps brachii may move a light weight rapidly, but must apply a much larger force than the resistive force.

KINEMATICS

Biomechanics has a long history of studies documenting the kinematics of human movements. Although most of these studies have been two-dimensional analyses, more and more research has focused on documenting the three-dimensional movements of the body. Precise three-dimensional measurement of the motion of human segments and joints has been labor intensive and involves considerable technical complexity (63). However, kinematic studies have provided useful descriptive data in many areas of human movement. Kinematic data can be used to profile the technique of athletes (19,42), help workers avoid potentially injurious work movements (33), and document normal patterns of movement such as locomotion (49,50,58).

There are several limitations in modifying client movement to match normal, skilled, or elite kinematics.

First, there are within- and between-person variabilities in movement technique. Despite the precision of kinematic measurements, there is subjectivity in determining what is considered normal or desirable given the variability of human movement. One example is the variation in running economy (mass normalized steady-state oxygen consumption for a given speed) that is fairly resistant to modifications in running technique (9,41,45). Runners naturally tend to select kinematics that maximize economy, so it is difficult to effectively modify running technique based on kinematics alone unless there is extreme deviation from normative technique. Second, kinematics measurements do not, in and of themselves, explain the causes of motion. In other words, nearly identical movements can have different muscular causes (59). For example, a physical therapist may help a patient with some muscular paralysis achieve a cosmetically normal walking pattern using other lower extremity muscles or orthotics. Therapists have been warned not to infer too much of the kinetic causes of walking from the kinematics of the patient's gait (27), and other exercise science professionals should also bear this in mind when qualitatively analyzing the kinematics of movements.

Despite the lack of explanatory power of kinematic measurements, useful information in kinematic studies can improve human movement. For example, the position and horizontal velocity of the whole-body center of mass relative to the base of support are important variables in theoretical models of stability and balance (51). The clinical value of static and dynamic measures of stance, however, is more controversial because these tests may not correlate with regaining postural control when body position is unexpectedly disturbed (50). More research on the kinematics of postural, locomotion, sport, and exercise movements may help improve the specificity of conditioning programs. This research may help inform the current emphasis on sensorimotor training in injured and athletic populations (23).

The decreasing cost and greater automation of kinematic calculations from video or position sensors may allow for the documentation of typical kinematics for more movements and with a wider variety of people (ages, skill levels, and disabilities). More examples of how kinematic data can be useful in improving human movement are summarized in the next section on the application of biomechanics in sports and exercise.

APPLICATION TO HUMAN MOVEMENT EXERCISE PRESCRIPTION

KINETICS

In prescribing exercise, professionals select the resistance and intensity of movements to match the fitness level and goals of clients. It has been hypothesized that there is an optimal window of loading that healthy people should maintain, with loading greater than this window presenting a greater risk of injury (47). The idea can be viewed as a continuum (*Fig. 2-8*) between too little loading (resulting in musculoskeletal atrophy) and too much loading (resulting in injury). Unfortunately, this window is not easily defined for several reasons. It is difficult to measure or estimate the loads in body tissues in various activities, and once known, these loads will interact with other training variables (genetics, repetition, rest, nutrition, etc.) to determine a person's response.

Prospective studies have begun to address this issue. Fuchs et al. (20) reported that drop jump training can significantly increase bone mass in young children. More research on the forces involved in typical physical training activities could then help in the development of programs that not only build aerobic and muscular fitness but also promote long-term skeletal health. Research has also begun to link the exercise resistances used by older adults in weight training to increases in bone mass (12) and the kinds of training that create the largest increases in bone mechanical strength (57).

The mechanical variables related to external forces that have been measured to examine potential injury are the magnitude of the peak force, the rate of force development, and the repetition of loading. *Figure 2-9* illustrates the difference in the vertical ground reaction force between heel–toe (rearfoot) and midfoot footstrike (46) patterns in running. The heel–toe running pattern has a passive peak or impact peak within the first 50 m of contact from the heel striking the ground. The second peak force is the active peak force that corresponds to the reversal point of the down–up motion of the body near midstance. Note how the magnitude of the active peak force is about the same in both footstrike conditions, but there is usually a higher rate of force development in the heel–toe pattern compared with the midfoot pattern.

Estimations of injury thresholds have been based on biomechanical tests of animal or cadaver tissues, test

FIGURE 2-8. The continuum of mechanical stress imposed on tissue and the likely adaptive response.

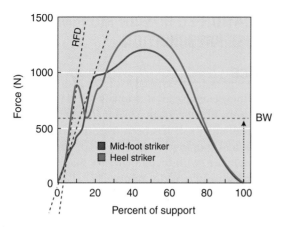

FIGURE 2-9. The vertical ground reaction force for heel and mid-foot footstrike patterns. The heel–toe (rearfoot) footstrike pattern typically had a larger rate of force development (RFD) than the midfoot pattern. BW, body weight. (Adapted with permission from Hamill J, Knutzen KM. *Biomechanical Basis of Human Movement.* Philadelphia [PA]: Lippincott Williams & Wilkins; 2003.)

dummies, and rare instances when injuries occur during biomechanical studies. Individual differences and variations in direction and pattern of application of forces make it difficult to establish reliable injury thresholds (24). Studies of the kinetics of higher risk activities, such as landings and collisions, are important not only to understand injury mechanisms but also to make changes in equipment and sport rules to decrease risk of injury to athletes (6).

During normal physical activities, the magnitude of the peak ground reaction forces usually creates stresses in lower extremity tissues within the elastic range and, therefore, does not cause acute trauma or injury. The rate of force development is an important variable because of the viscoelastic nature of tissues. The greater the rate of loading, the more stiff the tissue will be and the greater the load reached in the tissue before failure. The rate of force development is also clinically relevant because it often determines the kind of failure or fracture if loading goes beyond the elastic limit of the tissue.

Load repetition generally does not result in injury in normal physical activity in healthy individuals. It is possible, however, for long-term repeated impacts of high intensity to result in accumulation of microtrauma and the development of an overuse injury. *Overuse injuries* are usually the result of high-intensity activity over an extended period without adequate rest between training sessions. Because the long-term result of the mechanical stress of exercise can be either positive or negative, it is important for exercise professionals to be knowledgeable about symptoms of overtraining to reduce the risk of overuse injuries.

A promising area of biomechanics research involves the computer simulation of movements. In movements with simple performance criteria, computer simulations of biomechanical models can provide important information to optimize performance (25) and determine the effect of modifications in technique (32,60). A classic study

found that increasing the strength of a muscle group did not automatically improve vertical jump performance unless the coordination of the model was adjusted to take advantage of the added strength (5). In the future, the integration of biomechanics and sports medicine research may enable professionals to define general guidelines for resistances and external force loading that result in desirable hypertrophy in tissues without elevated risk of injury.

KINEMATICS

Kinematic measurements of human movement may also have some use in defining desirable exercise and sports technique. Remember that earlier in this chapter, it was noted that documenting what movement occurs (kinematics) cannot explain how the movement was created (kinetics). However, there are several ways that kinematic measurements can be used to help improve human movement.

There is some inherent value in documenting the kinematics of normal and skilled movement technique. This basic improvement in our understanding of what movements actually occur is important because many human movements are fast and difficult for professionals to see (38). Kinematic information on how movement changes with motor development (54) or learning (56) also helps the professional know what movements to look for with growth or practice. For example, kinematics measurements of walking gait (clinical gait analysis) have yielded data that are used to assist medical professionals in treating and monitoring progress for many conditions (58). For example, knowing how much trunk lateral bending occurs during normal walking helps therapists judge how much a patient has recovered. In sports, kinematic studies have improved the coaching of cricket bowling techniques and have significantly reduced intervertebral disc degeneration in athletes (15). Similar improvements in ACL injury risk in females have been achieved following training in landing technique (29). Qualitative and quantitative kinematic analysis has also been used to remediate injuries and swing mechanics in golf (22,52). The kinematic prescription of maintaining approximately normal lordosis (lumbar curvature) minimizing transverse plane twisting is likely the safest spinal alignment in golf and most activities. Coaching this spinal position in lifting and sports movements evenly loads intervertebral discs and likely reduces the risk of injury.

Two more areas in which kinematic measurements have been applied in human movement are locomotion and lifting. Walking and running speed is a kinematic variable that is often used in modifying the intensity of exercise. Speed of locomotion is also strongly related to the biomechanical variables of gait, so coaches and therapists comparing walking or running technique over time need to evaluate clients at similar speeds. Locomotion is a highly skilled activity that requires considerable kinematic control to maintain balance. Weightlifting activities are often much slower and use more stable postures. A wide **base of support** and lower **center of gravity** increase stability but tend to decrease mobility. Whereas a squatting position favors stability over mobility, the upright, forwarding-leaning stance phase of running favors mobility. Both lifting and running require balance (the control over positioning the body), but the kinematics and geometry of the postures favor different objectives (stability vs. mobility).

An object's center of gravity is a theoretical point where the weight force of the object can be considered to act. The kinematics (variation in height and horizontal distance) of the center of gravity relative to the base of support is often studied to examine the balance exhibited by performer. Running requires a skilled bounce-like motion of the center of gravity over a very small base of support in stance. In a sit-to-stand movement, the body weight is slowly shifted over the base of support where there is a transition from primarily horizontal motion to a vertical or lifting motion (*Fig. 2-10*).

Kinematics provides useful information for defining safe lifting technique. When lifting boxes from the ground, the lifter should squat with a wide base of support. Spreading the feet apart helps maintain stability and allows the load to be carried close to the body, minimizing the moment arm and resistance torques for the lower back. The lifter should also keep the trunk straight (normal lordosis)

and avoid exaggerated trunk flexion. Performing the lift slowly with the legs and without axial trunk twisting are also important mechanical factors that minimize the risk of injury (44). Unfortunately, people subconsciously tend to stoop lift (lean over), probably because small weights can be lifted with passive back muscle and ligament forces and, therefore, less metabolic cost (*Fig. 2-11B*). Repetitive

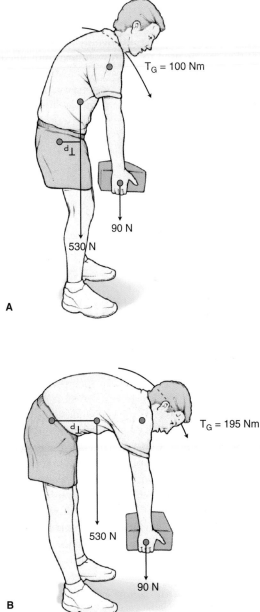

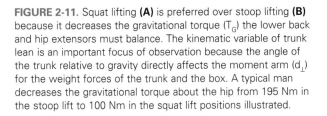

A

B

FIGURE 2-11. Squat lifting **(A)** is preferred over stoop lifting **(B)** because it decreases the gravitational torque (T_G) the lower back and hip extensors must balance. The kinematic variable of trunk lean is an important focus of observation because the angle of the trunk relative to gravity directly affects the moment arm ($d_\perp$) for the weight forces of the trunk and the box. A typical man decreases the gravitational torque about the hip from 195 Nm in the stoop lift to 100 Nm in the squat lift positions illustrated.

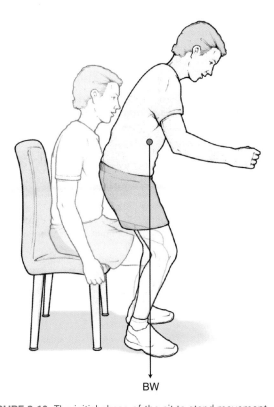

BW

FIGURE 2-10. The initial phase of the sit-to-stand movement involves trunk lean and horizontal weight shift to position the center of gravity over the new base of support (feet). The movement of the center of gravity in several directions is often used to study balance. BW, body weight.

use of this lifting technique is dangerous because of the large moment arm for the resistances and uneven spinal loading. The 30 degrees of trunk lean in the squat lift illustrated in *Figure 2-11A* decrease the moment arms for weight forces of the box and upper body by one-half (cos 60 deg = 0.5) from the stoop position, decreasing the gravitational torque loading on the lower back.

Statistical analysis of biomechanical data (including kinematics) has also been used to identify links between technique variables and performance (42). Therefore, kinematic measurements do hold promise in confirming the clinical observations of therapists and coaches, and these data may play a role in identifying key technique factors that can be used to improve human movement or reduce the risk of injury. However, kinematic data should be integrated with other studies (kinetics, EMG, training) to confirm that certain technique points are important and causative factors in performance or injury prevention.

SUMMARY

The study of biomechanics is essential to sports medicine and exercise science professionals because it forms the basis for documenting human motion (kinematics) and understanding the causes of that motion (kinetics). The key mechanical variables that explain the creation of motion are force and moment of force (torque). Newton's three laws of motion are critical to understanding how human movement is created and how it can be improved. Key forces that affect human motion are gravity, friction, normal reaction, joint reactions, ground reactions, and elastic, muscular, and fluid forces. Biomechanics also provides information to help modify exercise through studies of the kinematics of human movement. These studies precisely document the motion of the body for various movements and mover characteristics that professionals serve. Kinetic studies document the forces and moments experienced by the body during movement. The application of biomechanics in the prescription of exercise through the use of kinetic and kinematic data is being increasingly used to define desirable exercise intensities and movement amplitudes that create musculoskeletal adaptations with less risk of injury. Exercise science professionals typically use this biomechanical knowledge in the qualitative analysis of exercise technique.

REFERENCES

1. Alexander RM. Tendon elasticity and muscle function. *Comp Biochem Physiol A Mol Integr Physiol.* 2002;133(4):1001–11.
2. Arampatzis A, Peper A, Bierbaum S, Albracht K. Plasticity of human Achilles tendon mechanical and morphological properties in response to cyclic strain. *J Biomech.* 2010;43(16):3073–9.
3. Biewener AA. *Biomechanics—Structures and Systems: A Practical Approach.* Oxford (NY): IRL Press at Oxford University Press; 1992. 290 p.
4. Biscarini A, Benvenuti P, Botti F, Mastrandrea F, Zanuso S. Modelling the joint torques and loadings during squatting at the Smith machine. *J Sports Sci.* 2011;29(5):457–69.
5. Bobbert MF, Van Soest AJ. Effects of muscle strengthening on vertical jump height: a simulation study. *Med Sci Sports Exerc.* 1994; 26(8):1012–20.
6. Boyer KA, Andriacchi TP. Changes in running kinematics and kinetics in response to a rockered shoe intervention. *Clin Biomech (Bristol, Avon).* 2009;24(10):872–6.
7. Brown JM, Wickham JB, McAndrew DJ, Huang XF. Muscles within muscles: Coordination of 19 muscle segments within three shoulder muscles during isometric motor tasks. *J Electromyogr Kinesiol.* 2007;17(1):57–73.
8. Brown LE. *Isokinetics in Human Performance.* Champaign (IL): Human Kinetics; 2000. 456 p.
9. Cavanagh PR, Williams KR. Effect of stride length variation on oxygen uptake during distance running. *Med Sci Sports Exerc.* 1982; 14(1):30–5.
10. Cormie P, McCaulley GO, Triplett NT, McBride JM. Optimal loading for maximal power output during lower-body resistance exercises. *Med Sci Sports Exerc.* 2007;39(2):340–9.
11. Cross R, Nathan AM. Performance versus moment of inertia of sporting implements. *Sports Technol.* 2009;2:7–15.
12. Cussler EC, Lohman TG, Going SB, et al. Weight lifted in strength training predicts bone change in postmenopausal women. *Med Sci Sports Exerc.* 2003;35(1):10–7.
13. Delextrat A, Tricot V, Bernard T, Vercruyssen F, Hausswirth C, Brisswalter J. Drafting during swimming improves efficiency during subsequent cycling. *Med Sci Sports Exerc.* 2003;35(9):1612–9.
14. Dugan EL, Doyle TL, Humphries B, Hasson CJ, Newton RU. Determining the optimal load for jump squats: a review of methods and calculations. *J Strength Cond Res.* 2004;18(3):668–74.
15. Elliott B, Khangure M. Disk degeneration and fast bowling in cricket: an intervention study. *Med Sci Sports Exerc.* 2002; 34(11):1714–8.
16. Feldman AG, Levin MF, Mitnitski AM, Archambault P. 1998 ISEK Congress Keynote Lecture: Multi-muscle control in human movements. International Society of Electrophysiology and Kinesiology. *J Electromyogr Kinesiol.* 1998;8(6):383–90.
17. Finni T, Komi PV. Two methods for estimating tendinous tissue elongation during human movement. *J Appl Biomech.* 2002; 18(2):180–8.
18. Finni T, Komi PV, Lukkariniemi J. Achilles tendon loading during walking: application of a novel optic fiber technique. *Eur J Appl Physiol Occup Physiol.* 1998;77(3):289–91.
19. Fleisig GS, Barrentine SW, Zheng N, Escamilla RF, Andrews JR. Kinematic and kinetic comparison of baseball pitching among various levels of development. *J Biomech.* 1999;32(12):1371–5.
20. Fuchs RK, Bauer JJ, Snow CM. Jumping improves hip and lumbar spine bone mass in prepubescent children: a randomized controlled trial. *J Bone Miner Res.* 2001;16(1):148–56.
21. Gordon AM, Huxley AF, Julian FJ. The variation in isometric tension with sarcomere length in vertebrate muscle fibres. *J Physiol.* 1966;184(1):170–92.
22. Grimshaw PN, Burden AM. Case report: reduction of low back pain in a professional golfer. *Med Sci Sports Exerc.* 2000;32(10):1667–73.
23. Gruber M, Gruber SB, Taube W, Schubert M, Beck SC, Gollhofer A. Differential effects of ballistic versus sensorimotor training on rate of force development and neural activation in humans. *J Strength Cond Res.* 2007;21(1):274–82.
24. Guskiewicz KM, Mihalik JP. Biomechanics of sport concussion: quest for the elusive injury threshold. *Exerc Sport Sci Rev.* 2011; 39(1):4–11.
25. Hatze H. Biomechanical aspects of a successful motion optimization. In: Komi PV, editor. *Biomechanics VB.* Baltimore: University Park Press; 1976. p. 5–12.
26. Hellebrandt FA. Living anatomy. *Quest.* 1963;1:43–58.
27. Herbert R, Moore S, Moseley A, Schurr K, Wales A. Making inferences about muscle forces from clinical observations. *Aust J Physiother.* 1993;39(3):195–202.

28. Herzog W. Force-sharing among synergistic muscles: theoretical considerations and experimental approaches. *Exerc Sport Sci Rev.* 1996;24:173–202.

29. Hewett TE, Ford KR, Myer GD. Anterior cruciate ligament injuries in female athletes: Part 2, a meta-analysis of neuromuscular interventions aimed at injury prevention. *Am J Sports Med.* 2006; 34(3):490–8.

30. Hill AV. The heat of shortening and the dynamic constants of muscle. *Proc R Soc Lond B.* 1938;126(843):136–95.

31. Hof AL, Elzinga H, Grimmius W, Halbertsma JP. Detection of non-standard EMG profiles in walking. *Gait Posture.* 2005; 21(2):171–7.

32. Holvoet P, Lacouture P, Duboy J. Practical use of airborne simulation in a release-regrasp skill on the high bar. *J Appl Biomech.* 2002;18(4):332–44.

33. Hsiang SM, Brogmus GE, Courtney TK. Low back pain (LBP) and lifting technique—a review. *Int J Indust Ergonomics.* 1997;19(1): 59–74.

34. Hunter JP, Marshall RN, McNair PJ. Segment-interaction analysis of the stance limb in sprint running. *J Biomech.* 2004;37(9):1439–46.

35. Jackson AS, Frankiewicz RJ. Factorial expressions of muscular strength. *Res Q.* 1975;46(2):206–17.

36. Kawakami Y, Abe T, Fukunaga T. Muscle-fiber pennation angles are greater in hypertrophied than in normal muscles. *J Appl Physiol.* 1993;74(6):2740–4.

37. Kawakami Y, Fukunaga T. New insights into in vivo human skeletal muscle function. *Exerc Sport Sci Rev.* 2006;34(1):16–21.

38. Knudson DV, Morrison CS. *Qualitative Analysis of Human Movement.* 2nd ed. Champaign (IL): Human Kinetics; 2002. 252 p.

39. Komi PV, Belli A, Huttunen V, Bonnefoy R, Geyssant A, Lacour JR. Optic fibre as a transducer of tendomuscular forces. *Eur J Appl Physiol Occup Physiol.* 1996;72(3):278–80.

40. Komi PV, Nicol C. Stretch-shortening cycle of muscle function. In: Zatsiorsky VM, IOC Medical Commission, International Federation of Sports Medicine, editors. *Biomechanics in Sport: Performance Enhancement and Injury Prevention.* Malden: Blackwell Science; 2000. p. 87–102.

41. Lake MJ, Cavanagh PR. Six weeks of training does not change running mechanics or improve running economy. *Med Sci Sports Exerc.* 1996;28(7):860–9.

42. Lees A. Biochemical assessment of individual sports for improved performance. *Sports Med.* 1999;28(5):299–305.

43. Martin PE, Cavanagh PR. Segment interactions within the swing leg during unloaded and loaded running. *J Biomech.* 1990;23(6): 529–36.

44. McGill S. *Low Back Disorders: Evidence-Based Prevention and Rehabilitation.* 2nd ed. Leeds (UK): Human Kinetics; 2007. 312 p.

45. Messier SP, Cirillo KJ. Effects of a verbal and visual feedback system on running technique, perceived exertion and running economy in female novice runners. *J Sports Sci.* 1989;7(2):113–26.

46. Munro CF, Miller DI, Fuglevand AJ. Ground reaction forces in running: a reexamination. *J Biomech.* 1987;20(2):147–55.

47. Muraoka T, Muramatsu T, Takeshita D, Kanehisa H, Fukunaga T. Estimation of passive ankle joint moment during standing and walking. *J Appl Biomech.* 2005;21(1):72–84.

48. Nott CR, Zajac FE, Neptune RR, Kautz SA. All joint moments significantly contribute to trunk angular acceleration. *J Biomech.* 2010; 43(13):2648–52.

49. Novacheck TF. The biomechanics of running. *Gait Posture.* 1998; 7(1):77–95.

50. Owings TM, Pavol MJ, Foley KT, Grabiner MD. Measures of postural stability are not predictors of recovery from large postural disturbances in healthy older adults. *J Am Geriatr Soc.* 2000; 48(1):42–50.

51. Pai YC. Movement termination and stability in standing. *Exerc Sport Sci Rev.* 2003;31(1):19–25.

52. Parziale JR. Healthy swing: a golf rehabilitation model. *Am J Phys Med Rehabil.* 2002;81(7):498–501.

53. Rassier DE, MacIntosh BR, Herzog W. Length dependence of active force production in skeletal muscle. *J Appl Physiol.* 1999; 86(5):1445–57.

54. Roberton MA, Konczak J. Predicting children's overarm throw ball velocities from their developmental levels in throwing. *Res Q Exerc Sport.* 2001;72(2):91–103.

55. Roberts TJ, Marsh RL, Weyand PG, Taylor CR. Muscular force in running turkeys: the economy of minimizing work. *Science.* 1997;275(5303):1113–5.

56. Southard D. Change in throwing pattern: critical values for control parameter of velocity. *Res Q Exerc Sport.* 2002;73(4):396–407.

57. Turner CH, Robling AG. Designing exercise regimens to increase bone strength. *Exerc Sport Sci Rev.* 2003;31(1):45–50.

58. Whittle MW. *Gait Analysis: An Introduction.* 4th ed. Edinburgh (UK): Elsevier; 2007. 255 p.

59. Winter DA. Kinematic and kinetic patterns of human gait: variability and compensating effects. *Hum Mov Sci.* 1984;3(1–2):51–76.

60. Yeadon MR. The biomechanics of the human in flight. *Am J Sports Med.* 1997;25(4):575–80.

61. Zajac FE. Understanding muscle coordination of the human leg with dynamical simulations. *J Biomech.* 2002;35(8):1011–8.

62. Zajac FE, Gordon ME. Determining muscle's force and action in multi-articular movement. *Exerc Sport Sci Rev.* 1989;17:187–230.

63. Zatsiorsky VM. *Kinematics of Human Motion.* Champaign (IL): Human Kinetics; 1998. 419 p.

64. Zatsiorsky VM. *Kinetics of Human Motion.* Champaign (IL): Human Kinetics; 2002. 653 p.

SELECTED REFERENCES FOR FURTHER READING

Chaffin BD, Andersson GBJ, Martin BJ. *Occupational Biomechanics.* 4th ed. New York (NY): Wiley; 2006.

Dvir Z, editor. *Clinical Biomechanics.* New York (NY): Churchill Livingstone; 2000.

Hamill J, Knutzen K. *Biomechanical Basis of Human Movement.* 3rd ed. Baltimore (MD): Lippincott Williams & Wilkins; 2008.

Hay JG. *The Biomechanics of Sports Techniques.* 4th ed. Englewood Cliffs (NJ): Prentice-Hall; 1993.

Kirtley C. *Clinical Gait Analysis: Theory and Practice.* Edinburgh (UK): Elsevier; 2006.

Knudson D. *Fundamentals of Biomechanics.* 2nd ed. New York (NY): Springer Science; 2007.

Whiting WC, Zernicke RF. *Biomechanics of Musculoskeletal Injury.* 2nd ed. Champaign (IL): Human Kinetics; 2008.

INTERNET RESOURCES

- ACSM Biomechanics Interest Group: http://sites.google.com/site/bigacsm/
- American Society of Biomechanics: http://www.asbweb.org/
- Exploratorium: Sport Science: http://www.exploratorium.edu/explore/staff_picks/sports_science/
- Gait & Clinical Movement Analysis Society: http://www.gcmas.org/
- Hosford Muscle Tables: Skeletal Muscles of the Human Body: http://ptcentral.com/muscles
- International Society of Biomechanics: http://isbweb.org
- International Society of Biomechanics in Sports: http://www.isbs.org
- International Sports Engineering Association: http://www.sportsengineering.org/

3

Exercise Physiology

This chapter presents a review of the acute responses of the body to the exercise stressor and briefly describes some adaptations to exercise training. (*Chapters 32* and *33* discuss adaptations in more detail.) Among the topics covered are the metabolic aspects of exercise, the cardiorespiratory responses to exercise, the neuromuscular responses during exercise, the mechanisms of muscular fatigue, and the acute responses to exercise in varied environmental conditions.

KEY TERMS

Acute mountain sickness (AMS): A sickness characterized by headaches, nausea, and fatigue that is related to acute exposure to altitude.

Cardiopulmonary: The collective systems of the heart, blood vessels, and lungs that function to circulate blood in the body and exchange gases.

Cardiorespiratory: A term referring to the entire process of absorbing, circulating, and consuming oxygen in the body; "respiration" itself is the process of consuming oxygen and producing carbon dioxide within mitochondria.

Central fatigue: The progressive reduction in voluntary drive to motor neurons during exercise.

Cold stress: The loss in heat either from the core or locally that is brought on by environment, metabolism, and clothing.

Concentric: When muscle length decreases during a muscle action.

Eccentric: When muscle length increases during a muscle action.

Electron transport chain: A series of chemical reactions in the mitochondria during which electrons from the hydrogen atoms of nicotinamide adenine dinucleotide (NADH) and flavin adenine dinucleotide ($FADH_2$) are transferred to oxygen. The electrochemical energy in this process is used in production of adenosine triphosphate (ATP) from adenosine diphosphate (ADP) and inorganic phosphate (Pi).

Energy metabolism: The net effect of chemical reaction in the body resulting in ATP production.

Glycolysis: A series of chemical reactions for the conversion of glucose to pyruvate and the anaerobic production of ATP.

Heat stress: An increase in core temperature collectively brought about by the environment, metabolism, and clothing.

Hemodynamics: The mechanics of blood flow.

Hypoxic ventilatory response: The increase in ventilation seen with acute altitude exposure as a result of reduced barometric pressure and lowered arterial oxygen pressure.

Krebs cycle: A series of chemical reactions in the mitochondria in which citric acid is oxidized, resulting in the production of 3 NADH, 1 $FADH_2$, 1 guanosine triphosphate (GTP), and 2 CO_2.

Maximal oxygen consumption ($\dot{V}O_{2max}$): The maximal volume of oxygen consumed per unit time. $\dot{V}O_{2max}$ is generally established in an incremental exercise test using a large amount of muscle mass (such as treadmill running) in which a plateau of $\dot{V}O_2$ is attained ($\dot{V}O_2$ rises less than half the expected increase between the two final stages) or signs of maximal effort are attained (*e.g.*, respiratory exchange ratio >1.10).

Motor unit: A motor neuron and the muscle fibers it innervates.

Muscle fatigue: The loss of force or power output in response to voluntary effort leading to reduced performance.

Peak oxygen consumption ($\dot{V}O_{2peak}$): The greatest rate of oxygen consumption attained in a given test when indications of maximal effort were not attained or when the amount of muscle mass used was insufficient to reach a similar $\dot{V}O_2$ as that attained during treadmill exercise.

Peripheral fatigue: The loss of force and power that is independent of neural drive.

Primary pollutant: A direct source of pollution.

Secondary pollutant: A pollutant formed from the interaction of a primary pollutant with an environmental factor.

Size principle: The recruitment of motor units in order from smallest to largest according to recruitment thresholds and firing rates, resulting in a continuum of voluntary force.

FUNDAMENTALS OF EXERCISE METABOLISM

At rest, a 70-kg human has an energy expenditure of about 1.2 kcal · min^{-1}; less than 20% of resting energy expenditure is attributed to skeletal muscle. However, almost all changes that occur in the body during exercise are related to the increase in energy metabolism, largely within the contracting skeletal muscle. For example, cardiac output increases as a direct linear function of whole-body metabolism. To meet the demands on the heart, a fourfold increase in myocardial blood flow and oxygen consumption ($\dot{V}O_2$) takes place.

During intense exercise, total energy expenditure may increase 15–25 times more than resting values, resulting in a caloric expenditure of approximately 18–30 kcal · min^{-1}. Most of this increase is used to provide energy for exercising muscles. Therefore, daily caloric expenditure can be changed dramatically by simply altering the amount of physical activity performed during a day. Muscle fibers contain the metabolic machinery to produce adenosine triphosphate (ATP) by three systems: creatine phosphate (CP), glycolysis, and

aerobic oxidation of nutrients to carbon dioxide and water (oxidative phosphorylation).

The importance of the interaction of the aforementioned metabolic systems in the production of ATP during exercise should be emphasized. In reality, the energy to perform most types of exercise does not come from a single source but from a combination of anaerobic and aerobic sources (*Fig. 3-1* and *Table 3-1*). The contribution of anaerobic sources (CP system and glycolysis) to exercise energy metabolism is inversely related to the duration and positively related to the intensity of the activity. The shorter and more intense the activity, the greater the contribution of anaerobic energy production. Conversely, the longer the activity and the lower the intensity, the greater the contribution of aerobic energy production. Although proteins are used as a fuel for aerobic exercise, carbohydrates and fats are the primary energy substrates during exercise in healthy, well-fed individuals. In general, carbohydrates are used as the primary fuel at the onset of exercise and during high-intensity work (43,44,65). However, during prolonged exercise of low-to-moderate intensity (longer than 30 min), a gradual shift from carbohydrate toward an increasing reliance on fat as a substrate occurs (*Fig. 3-2*) (65,73). Although the greatest *percentage* of total energy derived from fat occurs at the lowest intensities, the greatest *quantity* of fat use (the product of percentage and intensity) occurs at about 60% of maximal aerobic capacity ($\dot{V}O_{2max}$) (1). This section of this chapter focuses on

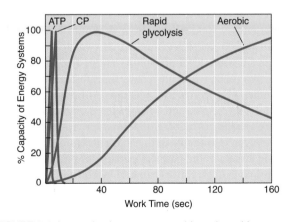

FIGURE 3-1. Interaction between anaerobic and aerobic energy sources during exercise, including adenosine triphosphate (ATP), creatine phosphate (CP), rapid glycolysis, and aerobic (oxidative phosphorylation). Note that whereas the energy to perform short-term, high-intensity exercise comes primarily from anaerobic sources, the energy for muscular contraction during prolonged exercise comes from aerobic metabolism.

TABLE 3-1. Characteristics of the Mechanisms by Which ATP Is Formed

Mechanism	Food or Chemical Fuel	Oxygen Required?	Relative ATP Yield
Anaerobic phosphocreatine	Phosphocreatine	No	Extremely limited
Glycolysis	Glycogen (glucose)	No	Extremely limited
Aerobic Krebs cycle and electron transport system	Glycogen, fats, proteins	Yes	Large

ATP, adenosine triphosphate.

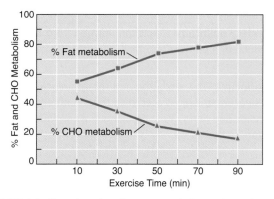

FIGURE 3-2. Alterations in substrate use during prolonged sub-maximal (<60% $\dot{V}O_{2max}$) exercise. CHO, carbohydrate. (Adapted with permission from Powers S, Byrd R, Tulley R, et al. Effects of caffeine ingestion on metabolism and performance during graded exercise. *Eur J Appl Physiol.* 1983;50:301.)

muscle bioenergetics and exercise metabolism. A detailed review of bioenergetics and exercise metabolism is provided in the suggested reading section of this chapter. A brief discussion of the energy pathways and the metabolic response to various types of exercise follows.

ENERGY FOR SHORT-TERM EXERCISE

ADENOSINE TRIPHOSPHATE

The energy released through hydrolysis of the high-energy compound ATP to form adenosine diphosphate (ADP) and inorganic phosphate (Pi) powers skeletal muscle contractions. This reaction is catalyzed by the enzyme myosin ATPase:

$$\text{(Myosin ATPase)}$$
$$\text{ATP} \rightarrow \text{ADP} + \text{Pi} + \text{energy}$$

The amount of ATP directly available in muscle at any time is small, so it must be resynthesized continuously if exercise lasts for more than a few seconds.

CREATINE PHOSPHATE

The CP system transfers high-energy phosphate from CP to rephosphorylate ATP from ADP. This reaction is catalyzed by the enzyme creatine kinase:

$$\text{(Creatine kinase)}$$
$$\text{ADP} + \text{CP} \rightarrow \text{ATP} + \text{C}$$

This system is rapid because it involves only one enzymatic step (*i.e.*, one chemical reaction); however, CP exists in finite quantities in cells, so the total amount of ATP that can be produced is limited. Oxygen is not involved in the rephosphorylation of ADP to ATP in this reaction, so the CP system is considered anaerobic (without oxygen).

Glucose
> Hexokinase

Glucose 6 – Phosphate
> Glucose 6 – Phosphate Isomerase

Fructose 6 – Phosphate
> Phosphofructokinase

Fructose 1,6 – Diphosphate
> Aldolase

Glyceraldehyde 3 – Phosphate + Dihydroxyacetone Phosphate
> Triophosphate Isomerase

Glyceraldehyde 3 – Phosphate
> Glyceraldehyde 3 – Phosphate Dehydrogenase

1,3 – Diphosphoglycerate
> Phosphoglycerate Kinase

3 – Phosphoglycerate
> Phosphoglucomutase

2 – Phosphoglycerate
> Enolase

Phosphoenolpyruvate
> Pyruvate Kinase

Pyruvate
> Lactate Dehydrogenase

Lactate

FIGURE 3-3. Enzymatic steps of glycolysis.

GLYCOLYSIS

Glycolysis is capable of producing ATP without involvement of oxygen. Glycolysis, the degradation of carbohydrate (glycogen or glucose) to pyruvate or lactate, involves a series of enzymatically catalyzed steps (*Fig. 3-3*). The net energy yield of glycolysis, without further oxidation through aerobic metabolism, is two or three ATPs through substrate-level phosphorylation. The net production is two ATPs when glucose is the substrate and three ATPs when glycogen is the substrate. Although glycolysis does not use oxygen and is considered anaerobic, pyruvate can readily participate in aerobic production of ATP when oxygen is available in the cell. Therefore, in addition to being an anaerobic pathway capable of producing ATP without oxygen, glycolysis can also be considered the first step in the aerobic degradation of carbohydrate.

ENERGY FOR LONGER DURATION EXERCISE

OXIDATIVE PHOSPHORYLATION

The final metabolic pathway for ATP production combines two complex metabolic processes: the **Krebs cycle**

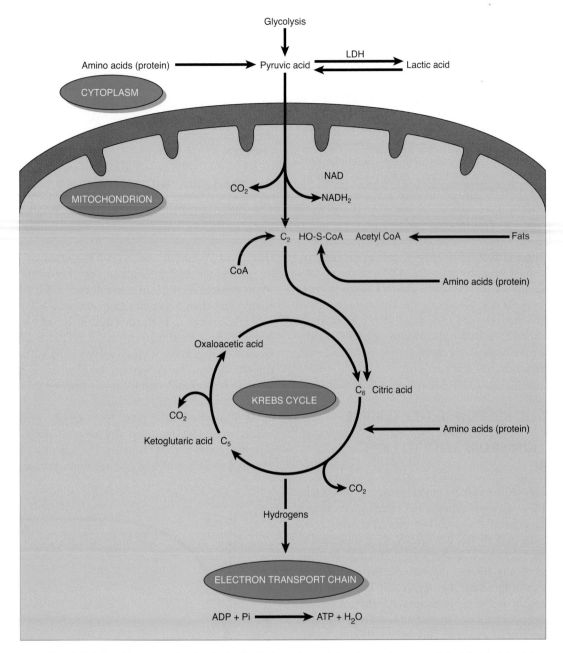

FIGURE 3-4. Relationship among the glycolysis, the Krebs cycle, and the electron transport chain. LDH, lactate dehydrogenase; NAD, nicotinamide adenine dinucleotide; CoA, coenzyme A.

and **electron transport chain**; both occur inside the mitochondria. Oxidative phosphorylation uses oxygen as the final hydrogen acceptor to form water and ATP. Unlike glycolysis, aerobic metabolism can use fat, protein, and carbohydrate as substrates to produce ATP. The interaction of these nutrients is illustrated in *Figure 3-4*.

Conceptually, the Krebs cycle can be considered a primer for oxidative phosphorylation. Entry into the Krebs cycle begins with the combination of acetyl-coenzyme A (acetyl-CoA) and oxaloacetic acid to form citric acid. The primary function of the Krebs cycle is to remove hydrogens from four of the reactants involved

in the cycle. The electrons from these hydrogens follow a chain of cytochromes (electron transport chain) in the mitochondria, and the energy released from this process is used to rephosphorylate ADP to form ATP. Oxygen is the final acceptor of hydrogen to form water, and this reaction is catalyzed by cytochrome oxidase (see *Fig. 3-4*). Complete degradation of glucose by glycolysis and oxidative phosphorylation result in a net production of 38 ATPs per glucose molecule, or 39 ATPs when the glucose molecule is derived from glycogen. These ATP values for glucose degradation may vary slightly in some sources.

FAT METABOLISM

Oxidation of fat, which provides acetyl-CoA as substrate for the Krebs cycle, is possible through aerobic metabolism. Glycolysis can also interact with the Krebs cycle in the presence of oxygen by the conversion of pyruvate to form acetyl-CoA. Fats (lipids) are present in the form of triglycerides in the body and broken down to glycerol and fatty acids by hormone-sensitive lipase, which is inhibited by insulin and activated by catecholamines (epinephrine and norepinephrine) and growth hormone. Glycerol can be metabolized through glycolysis or used to make glucose. Free fatty acids enter the blood to be ultimately used as fuel in cells via a process known as beta-oxidation. They may also be used as a precursor in the production of many substances such as cholesterol. Fatty acids must be activated using ATP and acetyl-CoA and transported via the carnitine shuttle system to enter the mitochondria for oxidation. In the mitochondrial matrix, beta-oxidation proceeds sequentially by cleaving off two carbon atoms at a time, forming acetyl-CoA, the substrate for the Krebs cycle. A 16-carbon fatty acid such as palmitate yields 129 ATPs.

METABOLIC RESPONSE TO EXERCISE

TRANSITION FROM REST TO LIGHT EXERCISE

In the transition from rest to light exercise, oxygen uptake kinetics follow a mono-exponential pattern, reaching a steady state generally within 1–4 min (*Fig. 3-5*) (69). The time required to reach a steady state increases at higher work rates and is longer in untrained individuals than in aerobically trained individuals. Because oxygen uptake does not increase instantaneously to steady state at the onset of exercise, it is implied that anaerobic energy sources contribute to meet the energy demand at the beginning of exercise. Indeed, evidence suggests that both the CP system and glycolysis contribute to the overall production of ATP at the onset of muscular work (23). As soon as a steady state is obtained, however, the ATP requirements are met by aerobic metabolism. The term *oxygen deficit* has been used to describe inadequate $\dot{V}O_2$ at the onset of exercise (see *Fig. 3-5*). Similar to short-term heavy exercise, the principal fuel used during the transition from rest to light exercise is muscle glycogen.

SHORT-TERM, HIGH-INTENSITY EXERCISE

The energy to perform short-term, high-intensity exercise (5–60 s in duration), such as weightlifting or sprinting 400 m, comes primarily from anaerobic systems (*Fig. 3-6*). Whether the ATP–CP system or glycolysis dominates the ATP production depends on the duration of the muscular effort. In general, energy for all activities lasting less than 5 s comes from the ATP–CP system. In contrast, energy to perform a 200-m sprint (30 s) would come from a combination of the ATP–CP system and anaerobic glycolysis, with glycolysis predominating. The transition from the CP system to glycolysis is not abrupt but rather a gradual shift from one pathway to another as the duration of the exercise increases.

As illustrated in *Figure 3-1*, exercise bouts lasting longer than 45 s use a combination of the CP system, glycolysis, and aerobic systems. For example, the energy required to sprint 400 m (60 s) comes primarily (about

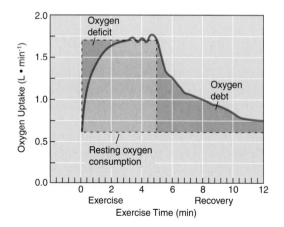

FIGURE 3-5. Oxygen uptake dynamics at onset and offset of exercise. See text for details.

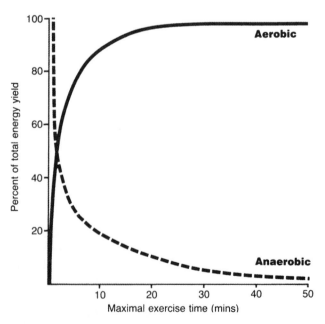

FIGURE 3-6. Relative contribution of aerobic and anaerobic metabolism during physical activity of increasing duration. In intense activities lasting 1.5–2.0 min, the ATP–CP and lactic acid energy systems generate approximately 50% of the energy, and aerobic metabolism supplies the remainder. A distance runner, on the other hand, derives essentially 98% of his or her energy from aerobic metabolism during a 50-min training run.

70%) from anaerobic sources (*i.e.*, ATP, CP, glycolysis), and the remaining ATP production is provided by aerobic metabolism. Carbohydrate (glycogen) stored in muscle is the principal fuel used during this type of exercise.

PROLONGED SUBMAXIMAL EXERCISE

Steady-state $\dot{V}O_2$ can usually be maintained during 10–60 min of submaximal continuous exercise. This rule has two exceptions. First, prolonged exercise in a hot and humid environment results in a steady drift upward of $\dot{V}O_2$ during the course of exercise (71). Second, continuous exercise at a high relative workload results in a slow rise in $\dot{V}O_2$ across time similar to that observed during exercise in a hot environment. In both cases, this drift probably occurs because of a variety of factors, such as rising body temperature and increasing blood catecholamines (38,70).

As depicted in *Figure 3-2*, both carbohydrate and fat are used as substrates during prolonged exercise. During prolonged low- and moderate-intensity exercise, there is a gradual shift from carbohydrate metabolism to the use of fat as a substrate. Explanations for this metabolic shift include the following: Fatty acids inhibit the Krebs cycle, leading to accumulation of citrate, which lowers phosphofructokinase (PFK) activity. This causes reduced uptake and oxidation of glucose. Thus, carbohydrate metabolism regulates fat metabolism during exercise and vice versa (19). The onset of exercise of low-to-moderate intensity produces a high glycolytic flux that slowly diminishes. The resulting glycolytic intermediates inhibit the carnitine transport system, thus preventing long-chain fatty acids from entering mitochondria for oxidation. Other factors that can affect the relative contribution of fat versus carbohydrate as energy substrate during prolonged exercise are nutritional status of the individual and the state of training.

PROGRESSIVE INCREMENTAL EXERCISE

Figure 3-7 illustrates the oxygen uptake during a progressive incremental exercise test. Note that oxygen

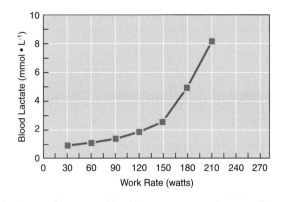

FIGURE 3-8. Changes in blood lactate concentrations as a function of work rate during incremental exercise.

uptake increases linearly with work rate until $\dot{V}O_{2max}$ is reached. After reaching a steady state, ATP used for muscular contraction during the early stages of an incremental exercise test comes primarily from aerobic metabolism. However, as the exercise intensity increases, blood levels of lactate increase (*Fig. 3-8*). Although much controversy surrounds this issue, many investigators believe that this lactate inflection point (*i.e.*, the point at which the rate of lactate appearance surpasses the rate of lactate clearance) indicates increasing reliance upon anaerobic metabolism brought about by the increased recruitment of type II or nonoxidative fast-twitch muscle fibers.

Although the precise terminology is controversial, this sudden increase in blood lactate levels — most directly termed the *lactate threshold* (LT) but referred to by some as the *anaerobic threshold* — has important implications for the prediction of performance and exercise prescription. For example, it has been shown that the LT, used in combination with other physiological variables (*i.e.*, $\dot{V}O_{2max}$), is a useful predictor of success in distance running (8). The LT may also be used as a marker of the transition from moderate- to heavy-intensity exercise and is thus useful in balancing volume and intensity in exercise prescriptions.

RECOVERY FROM EXERCISE

Oxygen uptake remains elevated above resting levels for several minutes during recovery from exercise (see *Fig. 3-5*). This elevated $\dot{V}O_2$ was previously referred to as the *oxygen debt* but is more directly termed *elevated postexercise oxygen consumption* (EPOC) (38). In general, postexercise metabolism is higher after high-intensity exercise than after light or moderate work. Furthermore, postexercise $\dot{V}O_2$ remains elevated longer after prolonged exercise than after short-term exertion. The mechanisms to explain these observations are probably linked to the fact that both high-intensity and prolonged exercise result in higher body

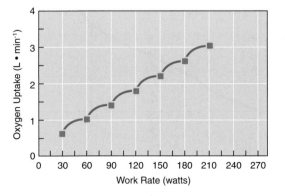

FIGURE 3-7. Changes in oxygen uptake as a function of work rate during incremental exercise.

temperatures, greater ionic disturbance, and higher plasma catecholamines than in light- or moderate-intensity short-term exercise (38).

METABOLIC OCCURRENCES DURING EXERCISE

LACTIC ACID THRESHOLD

Historically, increasing blood lactate levels during exercise were considered an indication of increased anaerobic metabolism within the contracting muscle because of a lack of oxygen. If oxygen is not available in the mitochondria to accept hydrogen released during glycolysis, pyruvate must accept hydrogen to form lactate as an end product so that glycolysis can proceed. However, the hypoxia theory is controversial. The linear increase of $\dot{V}O_2$ during incremental exercise argues against a sudden increase in anaerobic metabolism at the LT. Whether the end product of glycolysis is pyruvate or lactate also depends on other factors, including muscle fiber type and the speed of glycolytic flux. If glycolytic flux is extremely rapid, hydrogen production may exceed the transport capability of the shuttle mechanisms that move hydrogen from the cytoplasm (called *sarcoplasm* in muscle) into the mitochondria, where oxidative phosphorylation occurs. When glycolytic hydrogen production exceeds the mitochondrial transport capability, pyruvate must again accept the hydrogens to form lactate so glycolysis can continue. During exercise, epinephrine levels in the blood are elevated, which stimulates muscle *glycogenolysis* (breakdown of glycogen for fuel), increasing the rate of glycolysis. At rest and during low exercise intensities (<40% of maximal aerobic capacity), type I or slow-twitch muscle fibers are recruited predominantly. As the exercise intensity increases, more type II or fast-twitch fibers are recruited. This recruitment pattern has an important influence on lactic acid production. Conversion of pyruvate to lactate and vice versa is catalyzed by the enzyme lactate dehydrogenase (LDH), which exists in several forms (isozymes). Whereas type II muscle fibers contain an LDH isozyme that favors the formation of lactate, type I fibers contain an LDH form that promotes less conversion of pyruvate to lactate or even conversion of lactate to pyruvate. Therefore, more lactate formation occurs in type II fibers during exercise simply because of the type of LDH isozyme present, independent of oxygen availability in the muscle. Finally, type II fibers have higher activities of glycolytic enzymes than do type I fibers, indicating a greater potential of substrate flux through glycolysis.

In summary, debate over the mechanism or mechanisms responsible for muscle lactate production during exercise continues. It seems possible that any one or a combination of these possibilities may provide an explanation for muscle lactate production during exercise. The most important consequence of lactic acid production is that it immediately releases a proton (H^+), and unless this proton is buffered, a decrease in cellular pH results that may eventually disrupt enzyme function and muscle contraction and contribute to the characteristic muscle fatigue or pain that occurs with vigorous, intense exercise. However, blood lactate can also be used as a fuel by muscles and other tissues during and after exercise. Lactate concentrations increase in the blood only when the rate of lactate production begins to exceed its removal. A detailed discussion of this topic is available from other sources (41,74,75 and see Brooks et al. in the "Selected References for Further Reading").

VENTILATORY THRESHOLD

During incremental exercise, ventilation increases linearly with work rate and $\dot{V}O_2$ until the LT, at which point ventilation increases more rapidly (*Fig. 3-9*). Whereas the determination of the LT requires serial measurements of blood lactate, the ventilatory threshold (VT) can be determined noninvasively by assessment of expired gases during exercise testing, specifically pulmonary ventilation ($\dot{V}_E$), $\dot{V}O_2$, and carbon dioxide production ($\dot{V}CO_2$) (40). Oft-used methods are the modified V-slope method (determining an inflection in the relationship between $\dot{V}O_2$ and $\dot{V}CO_2$ and the ventilatory equivalents method (identifying an increase in the ventilatory equivalent for oxygen $\dot{V}_E/\dot{V}O_2$ during exercise without a corresponding increase in the ventilatory equivalent for carbon dioxide $\dot{V}_E/\dot{V}CO_2$) (40). The cause of the VT is likely multifactorial, involving central neural drive, peripheral neural feedback, hormonal responses, increasing body temperature, and decreasing blood pH.

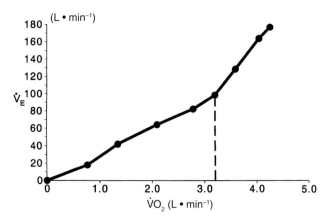

FIGURE 3-9. Relationship between intensity of exercise ($\dot{V}O_2$) and simultaneous, abrupt nonlinear increase in minute ventilation, signifying the ventilatory threshold. In this subject, the break point occurred at 3.20 L · min⁻¹, corresponding to 75% of measured $\dot{V}O_{2max}$ (4.25 L · min⁻¹).

Increased acidity of the blood from lactic acid is a likely factor that contributes to increased ventilation following chemoreceptor stimulation. A more controversial factor is the buffering of lactic acid by sodium bicarbonate in the blood, so that carbon dioxide is released in excess of that produced by muscle metabolism. These biochemical alterations are summarized by the following reaction:

$$HLa + Na\ HCO_3 \rightarrow Na\ La + H_2CO_3 \rightarrow H_2O + CO_2$$

(lactic acid) (sodium bicarbonate) (sodium lactate)
(carbonic acid)

The buffering hypothesis is controversial because chemoreceptors located at the aortic arch, carotid sinus, and medulla oblongata do not detect an increase in CO_2 during incremental exercise, but instead experience a slight decrease in CO_2 concentrations at higher intensities due to the ongoing hyperventilation.

Despite controversy regarding the mechanisms responsible for the VT (40,41,74,75), it normally coincides with the LT and obviates measurement of lactate in repeated blood samples. The close relationship between the VT and LT can be altered by glycogen depletion, suggesting that the LT does not directly cause the VT (52,67).

The VT from respiratory gas measurements is often expressed as a percentage of $\dot{V}O_{2max}$. For example, a highly trained athlete with a $\dot{V}O_{2max}$ of 4.25 L $\cdot$ min^{-1} whose break point in $\dot{V}_E$ occurs at 3.20 L $\cdot$ min^{-1} has a VT corresponding to 75% of aerobic capacity (*Fig. 3-10*). This athlete should be able to maintain exercise intensities at less than 75% of $\dot{V}O_{2max}$ without inducing a significant increase in blood lactic acid and muscle fatigue. Although the VT typically corresponds to 55% ± 8% of the $\dot{V}O_{2max}$ in healthy untrained individuals, it normally occurs at a higher percentage of the $\dot{V}O_{2max}$ (i.e., 70%–90%) in physically trained subjects (8,40).

$\dot{V}O_{2max}$ is an important predictor of performance in endurance events because it sets the upper limit for exercise intensity fueled predominantly by aerobic metabolism. In addition, several studies now suggest that the highest percentage of $\dot{V}O_{2max}$ that can be used over an extended duration without incurring significant increase in blood lactate concentration may be an even more important determinant of cardiorespiratory performance (8,40). The highest sustainable percentage of $\dot{V}O_{2max}$ in a given endurance race may be above the LT (depending on race distance). However, this percentage is more closely associated with the LT (and its marker, VT) than it is with $\dot{V}O_{2max}$ itself. Thus, LT and VT are useful for identifying training intensities.

HORMONAL RESPONSES TO EXERCISE

Several hormones are important to fuel usage during exercise. Subsequently, the response of the hormones important to metabolism change exercise intensity. Little change is seen during light exercise in catecholamines, glucagon, and growth hormone. Insulin exhibits a drop

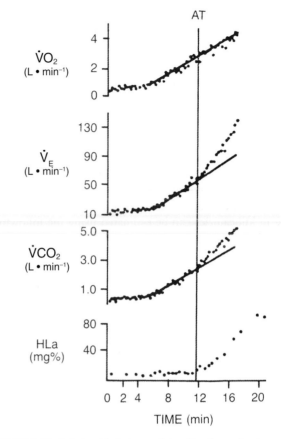

FIGURE 3-10. Relationship between intensity of exercise (oxygen consumption $\dot{V}O_2$) and simultaneous, abrupt nonlinear increases in serum lactate (HLa), carbon dioxide production ($\dot{V}CO_2$), and pulmonary ventilation ($\dot{V}_E$) occurring at the lactate and ventilatory threshold. Exercise was initiated at minute 4. (Adapted with permission from Davis JA, Vodak P, Wilmore JH, et al. Anaerobic threshold and maximal aerobic power for three modes of exercise. *J Appl Physiol*. 1976;41:544–50.)

from resting levels. The percent change in insulin concentration from rest decreases at near maximum values but still remains below that of rest. As exercise intensity increases from moderate to maximum, an increase in the response of the catecholamines, glucagon, and growth hormone is seen.

MEASUREMENT OF METABOLISM AND OXYGEN CONSUMPTION

Traditionally, whole-body metabolism is measured via direct or indirect calorimetry. The principles behind these two strategies can be explained by the following relationship:

$$Foodstuffs + O_2 \rightarrow Heat + CO_2 + H_2O$$

(indirect calorimetry)   (direct calorimetry)

Heat is liberated as a consequence of cellular respiration and muscular work. Thus, measuring the heat production of the body, calorimetry, allows an assessment of metabolism. Direct calorimetry requires that a subject be placed in an airtight chamber. As heat is released, the temperature inside the chamber increases. Typically, a circulating jacket of water used to transfer heat to the environment allows a means of determining the metabolic rate in joules or kilocalories per unit time.

Although direct calorimetry is a precise technique, construction of large chambers for measurement of metabolic rate in humans is prohibitively expensive. Also, heat produced by exercise equipment can complicate measurements using direct calorimetry. The principle of indirect calorimetry uses the measurement of $\dot{V}O_2$ to determine metabolic rate. Using this method, metabolic rate in kilocalories can be estimated using the following formula:

$$\text{Metabolic rate (kcal} \cdot \text{min}^{-1}) = \dot{V}O_2 \, (\text{L} \cdot \text{min}^{-1}) \times [4.0 + RQ]$$

where

$$RQ = \text{respiratory quotient}$$

According to the Fick equation, $\dot{V}O_2$ is equal to the volume of oxygen inhaled per unit time minus the volume exhaled per unit time:

$$\dot{V}O_2 = O_2 \text{ inhaled} - O_2 \text{ exhaled}$$
$$\dot{V}O_2 = (\dot{V}_I \cdot F_IO_2) - (V_E \cdot F_EO_2)$$

where

$$\dot{V}_I = \text{volume of inspired air per unit time}$$
$$F_IO_2 = \text{fraction of inspired oxygen}$$
$$\dot{V}_E = \text{volume of expired air per unit time}$$
$$F_EO_2 = \text{exhaled oxygen fraction}$$

The amount of O_2 taken out of the air does not equal the amount of CO_2 placed into the air (except when $RQ = 1.0$). Thus, either ventilation must be measured at both inhalation and exhalation, or a version of the Haldane transformation must be used to correct for $\dot{V}CO_2$:

$$\dot{V}O_2 = V_E \times [(1.0 - F_EO_2 - F_ECO_2)/F_IN_2] \times (F_IO_2 - F_EO_2)$$

where

$$F_ECO_2 = \text{exhaled carbon dioxide fraction}$$
$$F_IN_2 = \text{inhaled nitrogen fraction} \\ \text{(assumed to be 0.7904)}$$

The most common method of measuring $\dot{V}O_2$ uses open-circuit spirometry (*Fig. 3-11*). The exhaled ventilation is measured using a dry gas meter, turbine, or pneumotach. Gas fractions are sampled and measured by oxygen and carbon dioxide analyzers on the exhalation side. Typically, analog voltages from the gas meter and analyzers are converted to digital information and fed into a microcomputer to calculate $\dot{V}O_2$.

ENERGY COST OF ACTIVITIES

The energy cost of many types of physical activity have been established. Activities that are vigorous and involve large muscle groups usually result in more energy expended than activities that use small muscle mass or require limited exertion. Estimates of energy expenditure have been previously obtained by measuring oxygen cost of these activities in an adult population (see Ainsworth et al. (2) in the "Selected References for Further Reading").

Clinicians often use the term *metabolic equivalent* (MET) to describe exercise intensity. A single MET is equivalent to the amount of energy expended during seated rest. For simplicity, individual differences in resting energy expenditures are often overlooked, and 1 MET is considered equivalent to a $\dot{V}O_2$ of 3.5 mL $O_2 \cdot kg^{-1} \cdot min^{-1}$; hence, 1 MET represents an energy expenditure of approximately 1.2 kcal $\cdot$ min^{-1} for a 70-kg person.

SUMMARY

Exercise metabolism is a reflection of each metabolic pathway as it contributes to the increased energy demands of activity and work. Substrates for energy production include carbohydrate, fat, and protein. The mix of these substrates during exercise metabolism depends on the intensity and duration of exercise and the conditioning of the individual.

NORMAL CARDIORESPIRATORY RESPONSES TO ACUTE AEROBIC EXERCISE

The energy requirements of exercising human muscle may increase substantially in the transition from rest to maximal physical exertion. Because the available stores of ATP within muscle are limited and capable of providing energy to maintain vigorous activity for only several seconds, ATP must be constantly resynthesized to provide continuous energy production. Therefore, exercising muscle must possess a large capacity for increasing metabolic rate to produce sufficient ATP so that increased activity can continue. Energy production relies heavily on the cardiopulmonary systems for the delivery of oxygen and nutrients and for the removal of waste products to maintain the internal equilibrium of cells. Warm-up activities prior to exercise help enhance blood flow to the active tissues and increase internal temperature, which is beneficial to energy production.

The purpose of this section is to review the normal cardiorespiratory responses to acute aerobic exercise with specific reference to energy systems, hemodynamics, posture, maximal oxygen consumption ($\dot{V}O_{2max}$), the LT, dynamic versus isometric exertion, arm versus leg exercise, myocardial oxygen consumption ($M\dot{V}O_2$), and the effects of physical conditioning. This information is vital

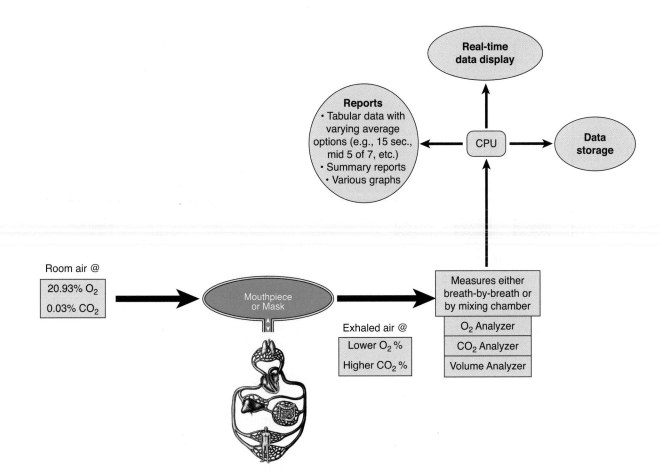

FIGURE 3-11. Open-circuit spirometry system interfaced with computer technology.

to the understanding of the role of exercise physiology in the interpretation of diagnostic and functional exercise testing and the prescription of exercise in health and disease. The responses noted generally represent those of healthy individuals. Individuals with cardiovascular, pulmonary, and/or metabolic disease may exhibit some differences in these acute cardiorespiratory responses to exercise. The magnitude of the responses may vary depending on the nature of the disease and disease severity. However, improvements in cardiorespiratory function in patients with a clinically manifest disease are possible with exercise training.

ACUTE CARDIORESPIRATORY RESPONSES TO EXERCISE

Many cardiorespiratory and hemodynamic mechanisms function collectively to support increased aerobic requirements of physical activity. The overall effect of changes in heart rate (HR), stroke volume (SV), cardiac output, blood flow, blood pressure (BP), arteriovenous oxygen difference (a-vO_2), and $\dot{V}_E$ is to oxygenate the blood and ensure that it is delivered to the active tissues.

HEART RATE

HR typically increases in a linear fashion with the work rate and oxygen uptake during dynamic exercise. The increase in HR during exercise occurs primarily at the expense of diastole (filling time), rather than systole (*Fig. 3-12*). Thus, at high exercise intensities, diastolic time may be so short as to preclude adequate ventricular filling. The magnitude of the HR response is related to age, body position, fitness, type of activity, the presence of cardiovascular disease, medications, blood volume, and environmental factors such as temperature and humidity. Maximum attainable HR decreases with age. The equation 220 − age provides an approximation of the maximum HR in healthy men and women, but the variance for any fixed age is considerable (standard deviation about ± 10 beats per minute [bpm]).

STROKE VOLUME

The SV (volume of blood ejected per heart beat) is equal to the difference between end-diastolic volume (EDV) and end-systolic volume (ESV). Whereas the former is determined by HR, filling pressure (preload),

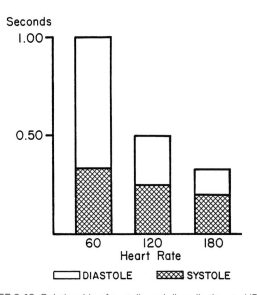

FIGURE 3-12. Relationship of systolic and diastolic time to HR. Because coronary blood flow predominates during diastole, with increased HR, as during exercise, diastolic (perfusion) time is disproportionately shortened. (Adapted with permission from Dehn MM, Mullins CB. Physiologic effects and importance of exercise in patients with coronary artery disease. *J Cardiovasc Med.* 1977;2:365–87.)

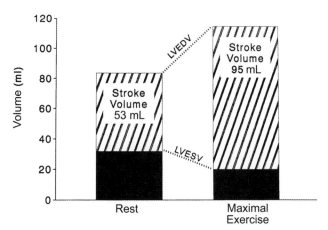

FIGURE 3-13. Changes in stroke volume from rest to maximal upright exercise are shown in young, healthy men. LVEDV, left ventricular end-diastolic volume; LVESV, left ventricular end-systolic volume. (Adapted with permission from Poliner LR, Dehmer GJ, Lewis SE, et al. Left ventricular performance in normal subjects: a comparison of the responses to exercise in the upright and supine position. *Circulation.* 1980;62:528–34.)

and ventricular compliance, the latter depends on two variables: contractility and afterload. Thus, a greater diastolic filling (preload) increases SV. In contrast, factors that resist ventricular outflow (afterload) result in a reduced SV.

SV at rest in the upright position generally varies between 60 and 100 mL · beat^{-1} among healthy adults, and maximum SV approximates 100–120 mL · beat^{-1}. During exercise in normal, healthy adults, SV increases curvilinearly with work rate until it reaches near maximum at a level equivalent to approximately 50% of aerobic capacity, increasing only slightly thereafter. Within physiological limits, enhanced venous return increases EDV, stretching cardiac muscle fibers and increasing SV via the Frank-Starling mechanism. In addition, SV can be increased by an increase in contractile state and ejection fraction (EF), which is the percentage of the EDV that leaves the ventricle during systole. EF is computed as SV/EDV.

EF is normally 65% ± 8%. Increases in SV during exercise result from both the Frank-Starling mechanism and decreased ESV (*Fig. 3-13*). The latter is attributable to increased ventricular contractility, secondary to catecholamine-mediated sympathetic stimulation. The magnitude of these changes depends on several variables, including ventricular function, body position, and the intensity of exercise. Moreover, at a higher HR, SV may actually decrease because of the disproportionate shortening in diastolic filling time (see *Fig. 3-12*).

CARDIAC OUTPUT

The product of SV and HR determines cardiac output. Cardiac output in healthy adults increases linearly with increased work rate, from a resting value of approximately 5 L · min^{-1} to a maximum of about 20 L · min^{-1} during upright exercise. However, maximum values of cardiac output depend on many factors, including age, posture, body size, presence of cardiovascular disease, and the level of physical conditioning. At exercise intensities up to 50% $\dot{V}O_{2max}$, the increase in cardiac output is facilitated by increases in HR and SV. Thereafter, the increase results almost solely from the continued increase in HR.

BLOOD FLOW

At rest, 15%–20% of the cardiac output is distributed to the skeletal muscles; the remainder goes to the visceral organs, the heart, and the brain (49). With exercise, myocardial blood flow may increase four to five times; blood supply to the brain is maintained at resting levels. As much as 85%–90% of the cardiac output is selectively delivered to working muscle and shunted away from the skin and the splanchnic, hepatic, and renal vascular beds. This redistribution of blood away from the visceral organs during exercise is caused by the sympathetic and hormonal influences on arterial smooth muscle and the resulting vasoconstriction. In active skeletal muscle, the exercise hyperemia is partly caused by local factors influenced by the increase in metabolism (*i.e.*, local autoregulation). Decreases in partial pressure of oxygen (PO_2) and increases in norepinephrine and endothelial cell shear stress in the arterial intima cause the release of *nitric oxide*, which was formerly termed *endothelial-derived relaxing factor* (EDRF). Nitric oxide exerts a vasodilatory effect on arteries and arterioles that supply the working muscles. In addition, it appears that venules paired to arterioles may release EDRFs in response to ATP release from red blood cells (RBCs). These venular EDRFs diffuse to arterioles and influence vasodilation and, therefore, blood flow (49).

BLOOD PRESSURE

There is a linear increase in systolic BP (SBP) with increasing levels of exercise, approximating 8–12 mm Hg per MET, where 1 MET = 3.5 mL $O_2 \cdot kg^{-1} \cdot min^{-1}$. Maximal values typically reach 190–220 mm Hg during aerobic incremental exercise (66). It is recommended that maximal SBP not be allowed to exceed 250 mm Hg during supervised exercise testing or training (66). Diastolic BP (DBP) may decrease slightly, remain unchanged, or increase slightly but should not exceed 115 mm Hg during supervised exercise. Pulse pressure (SBP − DBP) generally increases in direct proportion to the intensity of exercise.

Because BP is directly related to cardiac output and peripheral vascular resistance, it provides a noninvasive way to monitor the contractile performance or pumping capacity of the heart (66). Until automated devices are adequately validated, the BP response to exercise should be taken manually with a cuff and a stethoscope (85). A SBP that fails to increase or decreases with increasing workloads may signal a plateau or decrease in cardiac output, respectively. Exercise testing should be terminated in persons demonstrating exertional hypotension (SBP toward the end of a test decreasing to less than baseline standing level or SBP decreasing 10 mm Hg or more during exercise after an initial increase). This response has been shown to correlate with myocardial ischemia, left ventricular dysfunction, and an increased risk of cardiac events during follow-up (33).

ARTERIOVENOUS OXYGEN DIFFERENCE

Oxygen extraction by tissues reflects the difference between oxygen content of arterial blood (about 20 mL $O_2 \cdot dL^{-1}$ at rest) and the oxygen content of mixed venous blood (about 15 mL $O_2 \cdot dL^{-1}$), yielding a typical a-vO_2 ($CaO_2 - CvO_2$) at rest of 5 mL $O_2 \cdot dL^{-1}$. Thus, extraction at rest is approximately 25%. During exercise at maximum aerobic intensity, the mixed venous oxygen content typically decreases to 5 mL $\cdot dL^{-1}$ blood or lower, thus widening the a-vO_2 from 5 to 15 mL $\cdot dL^{-1}$ blood, corresponding to an extraction of 75%.

PULMONARY VENTILATION

$\dot{V}_E$, the volume of air exchanged per minute, generally approximates 6 L $\cdot min^{-1}$ at rest in the average sedentary adult man. At maximal exercise, however, $\dot{V}_E$ often increases 15- to 25-fold over resting values. During mild-to-moderate exercise intensities, $\dot{V}_E$ is increased primarily by increasing tidal volume, whereas increases in the ventilatory rate are more important to augment $\dot{V}_E$ during vigorous exercise. For the most part, the increase in $\dot{V}_E$ is directly proportional to the increase in oxygen consumed ($\dot{V}O_2$) and $\dot{V}CO_2$. However, at a critical exercise intensity (usually 47%–64% of the $\dot{V}O_{2max}$ in healthy untrained individuals and 70%–90% of the $\dot{V}O_{2max}$ in highly trained subjects), $\dot{V}_E$ increases disproportionately relative to $\dot{V}O_2$ paralleling the abrupt nonlinear increases in serum lactate and $\dot{V}CO_2$ (8,40). This suggests that $\dot{V}_E$ is perhaps regulated more by the requirement for carbon dioxide removal than by $\dot{V}O_2$ and that ventilation is not normally a limiting factor to aerobic capacity. However, in highly trained male athletes exercising at high intensities (>80% $\dot{V}O_{2max}$), reductions in partial pressure of arterial oxygen (PaO_2) have been documented. Furthermore, female athletes have exhibited reduction in PaO_2, and the reductions began to occur at lower exercise intensities than with the male athletes. The mechanisms leading to the hypoxemic conditions may include diffusion limitations, ventilation–perfusion inequalities, and limits to maximal flow rates (46,72). With training, the ventilatory response to submaximal exercise may be reduced by approximately 25% for a given workload. With maximal exercise, maximal minute ventilation may increase up to 25% following training.

CARDIOVASCULAR DRIFT

Steady-state upright exercise is characterized by changes in cardiovascular response despite the constant work rate. SV and mean arterial pressure progressively decrease, and HR progressively increases. Traditionally, it was thought that the increase in HR may be attributed, at least in part, to alterations in sympathetic blood flow control mechanisms, increased shunting of blood to the periphery (skin) for cooling, and decreased central blood volume (particularly in warm environments). However, it now appears that there is not a strong association between cutaneous blood flow and SV. Rather, the decrease in SV results from increased HR whereby diastolic filling time and EDV is reduced. Exercise during which dehydration occurs also contributes to cardiovascular drift, particularly if the dehydration leads to hypovolemia and hyperthermia. These conditions contribute to decreased SV and increased HR, respectively, thereby influencing the cardiovascular drift (18).

FACTORS INFLUENCING ACUTE CARDIORESPIRATORY RESPONSES TO EXERCISE

POSTURE

Posture has an effect on venous return and preload, particularly during brief bouts of physical exertion. At rest, EDV is highest when the body is recumbent. It decreases progressively as one shifts into sitting and standing postures. During exercise in the supine position, EDV remains largely unchanged. Thus, alterations in preload have little influence in increasing SV in this type of exercise. During exercise in the upright posture, EDV increases at intensities less than 50% $\dot{V}O_{2max}$. However, at higher exercise intensities, EDV and SV may decrease in some subjects (17).

DYNAMIC VERSUS STATIC EXERTION

Dynamic activity (physical exertion characterized by rhythmic, repetitive movements of large muscle groups) results in increased $\dot{V}O_2$ and HR that parallels the intensity of activity, as well as an increase in SV. There is a concomitant progressive increase in SBP with maintenance of or a slight decrease in DBP; thus, pulse pressure increases.

Blood is shunted from the viscera to working skeletal muscle, where increased oxygen extraction increases systemic a-vO_2. Thus, dynamic exercise imposes a volume load on the myocardium, which is the basis for a cardiac training effect. In contrast, isometric or static exertion involves sustained muscle contraction against a fixed load or resistance with no change in length of the involved muscle group or joint motion. The cardiovascular response to isometric exertion is apparently mediated by a neurogenic mechanism (58). Activities that involve less than 20% of the maximal voluntary contraction (MVC) of the involved muscle group evoke a modest increase in SBP, DBP, and HR. During contractions greater than 20% of the MVC, HR increases in relation to the tension exerted, and there is an abrupt and precipitous increase in SBP. The SV remains essentially unchanged, except at high levels of tension (>50% MVC), where it may decrease. The result is a moderate increase in cardiac output, which is nevertheless high for the accompanying magnitude of increased metabolism. Despite the increased cardiac output, blood flow to the noncontracting muscle does not significantly increase, probably because of mechanical vasoconstriction imposed by the contracting musculature. Vasoconstriction in other peripheral vascular beds occurs due to sympathetic drive. The combination of vasoconstriction and increased cardiac output causes a disproportionate increase in SBP, DBP, and mean BP. Thus, a significant pressure load is imposed on the heart.

TABLE 3-2. Comparison of the Relative Hemodynamic Responses to Dynamic and Static Exertion

	Dynamic (Isotonic)	Static (Isometric)
Cardiac output	+ + + +	+
Heart rate	+ +	+
Stroke volume	+ +	0
Peripheral resistance	−	+ + +
Systolic blood pressure	+ + +	+ + + +
Diastolic blood pressure	0−	+ + + +
Mean arterial pressure	0+	+ + + +
Left ventricular work	Volume load	Pressure load

+, increase; −, decrease; 0, unchanged.

A comparison of the relative hemodynamic responses to dynamic and isometric exercise is shown in *Table 3-2*.

The magnitude of the pressor response to isometric exertion depends on tension exerted relative to the greatest possible tension in the muscle group, as well as muscle mass involved (58,63). Thus, a relatively mild isometric contraction by weakened upper extremities may evoke an excessive pressor response. The increased myocardial demands are camouflaged by the relatively low aerobic requirements, so the usual warning signs of overexertion (tachycardia, sweating, and dyspnea) may be absent. In persons who have impaired coronary blood flow, a marked pressure increase may lead to threatening ventricular arrhythmias, significant ST-segment depression, angina pectoris, ventricular decompensation, and, in rare instances, sudden cardiac death (7).

ARM VERSUS LEG EXERCISE

At a fixed power output, HR, SBP, DBP, rate–pressure product (HR × SBP), $\dot{V}_E$, $\dot{V}O_2$, respiratory exchange ratio (RER), and blood lactate concentration are higher, and SV and LT (the latter expressed as a percentage of aerobic capacity) are lower during arm exercise than leg exercise (34). Because cardiac output is nearly the same in arm and leg exercise at a fixed oxygen uptake, elevated BP during arm exercise is believed to reflect increased peripheral vascular resistance. During maximal effort, physiological responses are usually greater during leg exercise than arm exercise, except when subjects are limited in their ability to perform leg work by neurological, vascular, or orthopedic impairment of the lower extremities (34,85).

The disparity in cardiorespiratory and hemodynamic response to arm exercise versus leg exercise at identical work rates appears to be attributable to several factors. Mechanical efficiency (*i.e.*, the ratio between the output of external work and caloric expenditure) is lower during arm exercise than leg exercise (34). This may reflect the involvement of smaller muscle groups and the static

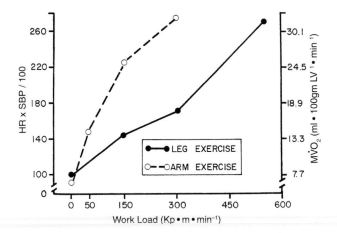

FIGURE 3-14. Mean rate–pressure product and estimated myocardial oxygen consumption ($M\dot{V}O_2$) during arm (*broken line*) and leg (*solid line*) exercise. $M\dot{V}O_2$ is estimated from its hemodynamic correlates, heart rate (HR) multiplied by systolic blood pressure (SBP). (Adapted with permission from Schwade J, Blomqvist CG, Shapiro W. A comparison of the response to arm and leg work in patients with ischemic heart disease. *Am Heart J.* 1977;94:203–8.)

effort required with arm work, which increases $\dot{V}O_2$ but does not affect the external work output. The higher rate–pressure product and estimated $M\dot{V}O_2$ at a fixed external work rate for arm work compared with leg work (*Fig. 3-14*) is believed to reflect increased sympathetic tone during arm exercise, perhaps mediated by reduced SV with compensatory tachycardia, concomitant isometric contraction, vasoconstriction in the nonexercising leg muscles, or all of these factors (78).

Peak oxygen consumption ($\dot{V}O_{2peak}$) during arm exercise in men and women generally varies between 64% and 80% of leg $\dot{V}O_{2max}$ (34). Similarly, maximal cardiac output is lower during arm exercise than leg exercise, and the maximal HR, SBP, and rate–pressure product are comparable or slightly lower during arm exercise. These factors have relevance to arm exercise training recommendations, particularly training intensity. An arm exercise prescription that assumes a maximal HR equivalent to leg exercise testing may result in an overestimation of the training HR. As a general guideline, the prescribed HR for leg training should be reduced by approximately 10 bpm for arm training (34,85).

MAXIMAL OXYGEN CONSUMPTION

The most widely recognized measure of cardiorespiratory fitness is maximal oxygen consumption, or $\dot{V}O_{2max}$. This variable is defined physiologically as the highest rate of oxygen transport and use that can be achieved at maximal physical exertion. During incremental exercise, a subject has attained $\dot{V}O_{2max}$ if he or she demonstrates a leveling off, or plateau, in $\dot{V}O_2$, in which the $\dot{V}O_2$ of the final completed stage of the protocol is no more than

that of the preceding stage. The definition of a plateau varies in the scientific literature (51), with a commonly cited definition being an increase in $\dot{V}O_2$ that is less than half of the expected increase between stages (82). In early research, the incremental exercise was typically performed in discontinuous bouts (50,82), although it is commonly performed as a single, continuous bout of incremental exercise today. In many cases, subjects fail to reach a plateau despite giving maximal effort (24,59). Several studies have followed a continuous incremental test with a verification test at a greater workload than that attained during the incremental exercise, either after a short rest (32,77) or on a separate occasion (22,47), and found no increase in $\dot{V}O_2$ during the supramaximal exercise. Therefore, it is common for a true maximal $\dot{V}O_2$ to be attained in healthy, motivated subjects during incremental exercise tests. However, the attainment of a true $\dot{V}O_{2max}$ cannot be established with certainty unless a plateau is observed or a verification test is performed. A variety of alternative criteria have been proposed to determine whether $\dot{V}O_{2max}$ was attained, such as a respiratory exchange ratio (RER = $\dot{V}CO_2/\dot{V}O_2$) of at least 1.10 and a blood lactate concentration of at least 8 mM (24). These alternative criteria are suggestive, but not conclusive.

$\dot{V}O_{2max}$ is not attained if a test is terminated due to symptoms, as may happen when testing patient populations. In such circumstances, the highest $\dot{V}O_2$ measured is termed $\dot{V}O_{2peak}$. This term is also employed despite the attainment of maximal criteria if the test protocol used a small amount of muscle mass (*e.g.*, arms only) and the subject is capable of a greater $\dot{V}O_2$ on another exercise mode (such as treadmill running). It should be noted that several modes of exercise are able to elicit high levels of $\dot{V}O_2$ when individuals are trained with that mode. Rowers, cross-country skiers, and bicyclists are all capable of attaining as high or higher $\dot{V}O_2$ values on their respective modes of exercise as they are on a treadmill (81).

Somatic $\dot{V}O_2$ may be expressed mathematically by a rearrangement of the Fick equation:

$$\dot{V}O_2 = HR \times SV \times (a\text{-}vO_2)$$

where

$$\dot{V}O_2 = \text{oxygen consumption}$$
$$(mL\ O_2 \cdot kg^{-1} \cdot min^{-1})$$

$$HR = \text{heart rate (bpm)}$$

$$SV = \text{stroke volume } (mL \cdot beat^{-1})$$

$$(a\text{-}vO_2) = \text{arteriovenous oxygen difference}$$

Thus, it is apparent that both central (*i.e.*, cardiac output) and peripheral (*i.e.*, a-vO$_2$) regulatory mechanisms affect the magnitude of body $\dot{V}O_2$.

Typical circulatory data at rest and during maximal exercise in a healthy, sedentary 30-yr-old man and a

TABLE 3-3. Hypothetical Circulatory Data at Rest and during Maximal Exercise for a Sedentary Man and a World-Class Endurance Athlete: 30-Yr-Old Subjects

Condition	Oxygen Consumption ($L \cdot min^{-1}$)	Oxygen Consumption ($mL \cdot kg^{-1} \cdot min^{-1}$)	Cardiac Output ($L \cdot min^{-1}$)	Heart Rate (bpm)	Stroke Volume ($mL \cdot beat^{-1}$)	Arteriovenous Oxygen Difference ($mL \cdot dL^{-1}$ blood)
Sedentary Man (70 kg)						
Rest	0.25	3.5	6.1	70	87	4.0
Maximal exercise	2.50	35.0	17.7	190	93	14.0
World-Class Endurance Athlete (70 kg)						
Rest	0.25	3.5	6.1	45	136	4.0
Maximal exercise	5.60	80.0	35.0	190	184	16.0

bpm, beats per minute.

similarly aged world-class endurance athlete are shown in *Table 3-3*. The absolute resting $\dot{V}O_2$ (250 mL · min^{-1}) divided by body weight (70 kg) gives the resting energy requirement, 1 MET (about 3.5 mL · kg^{-1} · min^{-1}). This expression of resting $\dot{V}O_2$ is very important in exercise physiology (14), independent of body weight and aerobic fitness. Furthermore, multiples of this value are often used to quantify respective levels of energy expenditure. For example, running at a 6-mph pace requires 10 times the resting energy expenditure; thus, the aerobic cost is 10 MET, or 35 mL O$_2$ · kg^{-1} · min^{-1}.

The tenfold maximal increase in oxygen transport and use in the sedentary individual is contrasted by a 23-fold increase in the endurance athlete, corresponding to a $\dot{V}O_{2max}$ of 35 mL · kg^{-1} · min^{-1} and 80 mL · kg^{-1} · min^{-1}, respectively. Increased aerobic capacity in trained athletes appears primarily as the result of increased maximal cardiac output rather than an increased arteriovenous extraction of oxygen. Although a-vO_2 is only slightly increased in the trained athlete, from 75% to 80%–85%, it must be noted that this percent extraction is from a much greater blood flow; thus, the skeletal muscles' capacity to extract oxygen is significantly increased. The elite athlete has double the $\dot{V}O_{2max}$ and, given the minimal change in a-vO_2, double the maximal cardiac output of the sedentary adult. Maximal HR is similar or slightly reduced with training, and thus, the greater cardiac output is due entirely to a greater maximal SV. $\dot{V}O_{2max}$ virtually defines the pumping capacity of the heart. Therefore, it is of major importance in the cardiovascular evaluation of the individual.

$\dot{V}O_{2max}$ may be expressed on an absolute or relative basis, that is, in liters per minute, reflecting total body energy output and caloric expenditure (where 1 L O$_2$ = 5 kcal), or by dividing this value by body weight in kilograms. Because large persons usually have larger absolute $\dot{V}O_2$ by virtue of larger muscle mass, the latter allows a more equitable comparison between individuals of different body mass. This variable when expressed as milliliters of oxygen per kilogram of body mass per minute is widely considered the single best index of cardiorespiratory fitness (8,85).

DETERMINATION OF THE MAXIMAL OXYGEN CONSUMPTION

$\dot{V}O_{2max}$ is usually determined during an incremental exercise test to exhaustion, while measuring expired gases as described earlier. Because it is often inconvenient to measure $\dot{V}O_{2max}$, physiologists often estimate aerobic capacity from the peak treadmill speed and grade or peak cycle ergometer work rate (also see *Chapter 23* in this *Resource Manual* and *GETP8 Chapter 5*). The conventional Bruce protocol is perhaps the most familiar and widely used treadmill protocol with normative data on $\dot{V}O_2$ so that aerobic capacity may be estimated from the workload attained (*Fig. 3-15*) (12). However, when a multistage protocol, such as the Bruce protocol, is used to predict the $\dot{V}O_{2max}$, aerobic capacity may be markedly overestimated (35). Another test methodology that may overcome some of the limitations of incremental exercise testing is ramping (68). Ramp protocols involve a nearly continuous and uniform increase in aerobic requirements that replaces the stage approach used in conventional exercise tests. With ramping, the gradual increase in demand allows for a steady increase in cardiorespiratory responses.

MYOCARDIAL OXYGEN CONSUMPTION

Determinants of $\dot{MVO}_2$ include HR, myocardial contractility, and the tension or stress developed in the ventricular wall. Wall tension reflects a combination of SBP and ventricular volume and is inversely related to myocardial wall thickness (*Fig. 3-16*). During exercise, increased HR is the major contributor to increased myocardial oxygen demand. In contrast, oxygen supply is primarily facilitated by increased coronary blood flow enabled by decreased coronary vascular resistance with only a modest increase in an already substantial myocardial oxygen difference.

Several investigators have reported excellent correlations between measured $\dot{MVO}_2$ (expressed as milliliters of oxygen per 100 g of left ventricle per minute) and HR and

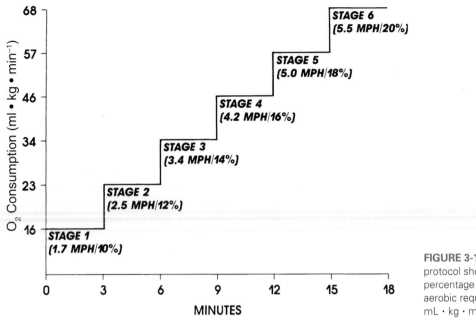

FIGURE 3-15. The standard Bruce treadmill protocol showing progressive stages (speed, percentage grade) and the corresponding aerobic requirement, expressed as mL · kg · min⁻¹.

rate–pressure product, where $\dot{M}VO_2 = (0.28 \times HR) - 14$ ($r = 0.88$) or $\dot{M}VO_2 = ([0.14 \times HR \times SBP] / 100) - 6.3$ ($r = 0.92$) (56,64). HR alone is limited in its ability to predict $\dot{M}VO_2$, especially when SBP is markedly elevated; this may occur during upper extremity work involving isometric or isodynamic efforts.

Exercise-induced angina and significant ST-segment depression (≥ 1 mm) usually occur at a reproducible rate–pressure product in an individual with ischemic heart disease. This suggests the existence of an ischemic threshold at which myocardial oxygen demand exceeds myocardial oxygen supply. The rate–pressure product

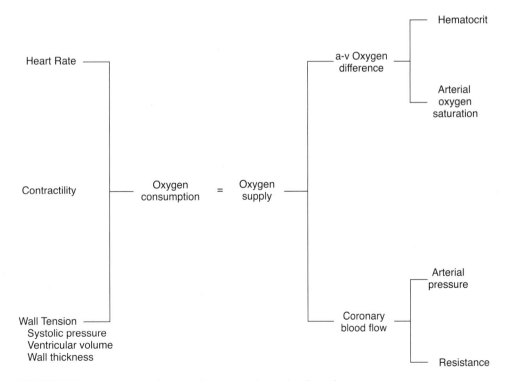

FIGURE 3-16. Determinants of myocardial oxygen demand and supply.

also provides an estimate of maximal workload that the left ventricle can perform. It has been suggested that an adequate rate–pressure product during maximal exercise is greater than 25,000 units (typically written as 250×10^2); however, this may be influenced by age, clinical status, and medications, especially β-blockers (85).

FACTORS AFFECTING THE ACUTE NEUROMUSCULAR RESPONSES TO RESISTANCE EXERCISE

Understanding the factors that affect acute resistance exercise responses is important in gaining insight into different resistance training protocols. Acute physiological changes are directly related to the configuration of external demands of resistance exercise, so resistance exercise protocols must be specific to the physiological systems targeted.

PHYSIOLOGY OF RESISTANCE EXERCISE

NEUROMUSCULAR ACTIVATION

The stimulus for muscle activation comes from a high-level central control command signal originating from the premotor cortex and the motor cortex. The signal is relayed through a lower level controller (brainstem and spinal cord) and transformed into a specific motor unit activation pattern. To perform a specific task, the required motor units meet specific demands for force production by activating associated muscle fibers (25). Various feedback loops modify force production and provide communication to other physiological systems, such as the endocrine system. The high- and low-level commands can be modified by feedback from peripheral sensory or higher central command.

MOTOR UNIT ACTIVATION

The functional unit of the neuromuscular system is the motor unit. It consists of the motor neuron and the muscle fibers it innervates. Motor units range in size from a few to several hundred muscle fibers. Muscle fibers from different motor units can be anatomically adjacent to each other; therefore, a muscle fiber may be actively generating force while the adjacent fiber moves passively with no direct neural stimulation. When maximal force is required, all available motor units are activated. Another adaptive mechanism affected by heavy resistance training is the muscle force affected by different motor unit firing rates and frequencies.

Motor unit activation is also influenced by the size principle. This principle is based on the observed relationship between motor unit twitch force and recruitment threshold. Specifically, motor units are recruited in order according to recruitment thresholds and firing rates, resulting in a continuum of voluntary force. Whereas type I motor units are the smallest and possess the lowest recruitment thresholds, type IIa and IIx motor units are larger in size and have higher activation thresholds. Therefore, as force requirements of an activity increase, the recruitment order progresses from type I to IIa to IIx motor units. Thus, most muscles contain a range of motor units (type I and II fibers), and force production can span wide levels. Maximal force production requires not only the recruitment of all motor units, including high-threshold motor units, but also recruitment at a sufficiently high firing rate. It has been hypothesized that untrained individuals cannot voluntarily recruit the highest threshold motor units or maximally activate muscles. Furthermore, electrical stimulation has been shown to be more effective in eliciting gains in untrained muscle or injury rehabilitation scenarios, suggesting further inability to activate all available motor units. Thus, training adaptation develops the ability to recruit a greater percentage of motor units when required.

Few exceptions to the size principle have been identified; however, some advanced weightlifters and other athletes may not require the order of recruitment stipulated by the size principle. It may be possible to inhibit low-threshold motor units yet activate high-threshold ones to enhance rate of force development and power production. This hypothesis emerged from observations during rapid, stereotyped movements and voluntary eccentric muscle action in humans. The central nervous system (CNS) can also limit force by engaging protective inhibitory mechanisms. For example, the Golgi tendon organs detect tension on the tendons from muscular contractions and elicit an inhibitory neuron response to limit muscular contraction. Training induced opposition of this inhibitory response may improve force production. Muscle spindles respond to stretch on the muscle. Rapid lengthening results in a contraction of the agonist muscle. This response is known as the stretch reflex and may be seen with dynamic or ballistic flexibility exercise. Thus, training may result in changes in fiber recruitment order or reduced inhibition, which assists in the performance of certain types of muscle actions.

MUSCLE FIBER TYPES

Several nomenclatures have been used to classify skeletal muscle fibers, including color (red or white), contraction speed (type I or II), oxidative or glycolytic enzyme content (fast glycolytic, fast oxidative glycolytic, or oxidative), and myosin adenosine triphosphatase (ATPase) content (type I, IIa, IIx).

It is evident that exercise-induced changes in muscle have great plasticity (36,80). This is caused partly by a complex, yet readily adaptable group of contractile and regulatory proteins. Studies have focused on the myosin molecule and examination of fiber types. Fiber typing by myosin ATPase has been the most popular classification system (36,80). The continuum of human muscle fiber types from the most oxidative (type I) to the least oxidative (type IIx) fibers are illustrated in *Chapter 33* (*Fig. 33-2*).

Three major types of polypeptide chains, including a heavy chain and two types of light chains, constitute the myosin molecule. The complexity of the system allows for different expression of isomyosin forms with different heavy- and light-chain compositions. The differential myosin expression is of interest because it is related to muscle function and adaptation. A link between the myosin ATPase fiber type distribution and myosin heavy-chain content in skeletal muscle has been investigated by examining relationships for entire biopsy samples or single fibers. The relative percentage of myosin heavy chain (MHC I, MHC IIa, MHC IIx) is highly correlated with the corresponding percentage of muscle fiber types (I, IIa, IIx) in both men and women (36).

MUSCLE SORENESS

Muscle soreness may occur after an acute resistance training session. The exact mechanisms of muscle soreness remain speculative. Soreness is typically observed after excessively intense resistance training. It is most dramatic in relatively inexperienced or novice weightlifters. However, experienced weightlifters have soreness with novel exercise or excessive progression of intensity.

Several investigations demonstrate that eccentric exercise precipitates delayed onset muscle soreness (DOMS). Eccentric contractions may damage the basic ultrastructure of the muscle cell. The focal point of the damage is the Z disk, a structural component that anchors the contractile protein actin.

The loss of structural integrity of the Z disks may be the stimulus leading to the associated symptoms. The appearance of DOMS ranges from 24 to 48 h after exercise and may last up to 10 d. Symptoms of DOMS include local muscular stiffness, tenderness, local edema, limited range of motion caused by edema, and pain, which varies from low-grade ache to severe pain. Severity and location of discomfort specifically relate to the muscles used. The reason for increased soreness associated with eccentric training is unclear. However, one bout of eccentric exercise appears to result in protection from excessive soreness from another bout for up to 5–6 wk in untrained or novice individuals. Thus, a slow progression in intensity is critical to limit soreness. It appears that excessive soreness develops from using resistance greater than the concentric one repetition maximum (1-RM).

HEMODYNAMIC RESPONSES TO ACUTE RESISTANCE EXERCISE

HEART RATE AND BLOOD PRESSURE

HR and BP increase during dynamic resistance exercise using machines, free weights, or isokinetics. Peak BP response is higher during weight training in which a concentric and an eccentric phase occur than during isokinetic exercise (31). BP and HR may increase quite dramatically, with peak BP of 320/250 mm Hg and HR of 170 bpm for a two-legged leg press at 95% of 1-RM to voluntary concentric failure with a Valsalva maneuver. HR and BP responses are also significant when the Valsalva maneuver is limited.

Peak BP and HR normally occur during the last several repetitions of a set to voluntary concentric failure. BP is higher during sets at submaximal resistance to voluntary failure than at 1-RM. In dynamic resistance exercise, BP but not HR increases during the concentric rather than the eccentric portion of a repetition. In addition, BP increases with active muscle mass, but the increase is not linear (31).

STROKE VOLUME AND CARDIAC OUTPUT

SV (determined by electrical impedance) is not significantly elevated to more than resting during the concentric phase of resistance training exercise (with or without a Valsalva maneuver). However, during the eccentric phase, SV is significantly increased to more than resting (with or without a Valsalva maneuver) and is significantly greater than during the concentric phase of a repetition (31).

During both the concentric and eccentric phases of a repetition, cardiac output may be increased. For example, cardiac output during squatting exercise may increase to approximately 20 L · min^{-1} during the eccentric phase but be only 15 L · min^{-1} during the concentric phase. However, during exercise involving smaller muscle mass (*e.g.*, knee extension), cardiac output may be elevated only during the eccentric phase. The differing response between eccentric and concentric phases may result in no overall change from rest in mean cardiac output and SV during exercise involving a small muscle mass. HR is not significantly different between the concentric and eccentric phases. Because SV is significantly greater during the eccentric than the concentric phase of a repetition, the higher cardiac output during the eccentric phase is caused by increased SV.

CALORIC COST OF RESISTANCE EXERCISE

The caloric cost of resistance exercise can be increased both during and after exercise. The caloric costs of an acute exercise session have been studied in a variety of protocols from single exercises to multiple exercise circuits. The caloric cost ranges from 14 to 75 kcal $\cdot$ kg^{-1} $\cdot$ day^{-1}. It appears that the caloric cost of resistance exercise is related to the amount of muscle mass activated, the length of the rest period, the intensity of the exercise, and the ability to tolerate higher volumes of total work (31).

SUMMARY

The acute physiological stress of the neuromuscular system during resistance exercise is related to external demands. These demands are created by acute program variables that dictate the acute resistance exercise protocol. Careful consideration of these variables affecting the demands allows optimization of the exercise prescription for resistance exercise (see *Chapter 31*).

MECHANISMS OF MUSCULAR FATIGUE

The causes of muscle fatigue have interested exercise scientists for more than a century, yet definitive fatigue agents have yet to be identified. **Muscle fatigue** is the loss of force or power output in response to voluntary effort leading to reduced performance. It is accepted that both central and peripheral factors contribute to fatigue. Whereas **central fatigue** is the progressive reduction in voluntary drive to motor neurons during exercise, **peripheral fatigue** is the loss of force and power that is independent of neural drive. The nature and extent of muscle fatigue clearly depend on the type, duration, and intensity of exercise, along with the fiber type composition of the muscle, individual fitness level, and environmental factors. For example, fatigue experienced in high-intensity, short-duration exercise depends on factors that differ from those precipitating fatigue in endurance activity. Similarly, fatigue during tasks involving heavily loaded contractions (*e.g.*, weightlifting) probably differs from that produced during relatively unloaded movement (running and swimming). This section focuses primarily on muscle fatigue resulting from two general types of activity: short-duration, high-intensity exercise and longer duration, endurance exercise.

SHORT-DURATION, HIGH-INTENSITY EXERCISE

Fatigue during short-duration, high-intensity exercise may result from impairment anywhere along the chain of command from upper brain areas to contractile proteins (*Fig. 3-17*). Although the preponderance of evidence suggests that a dysfunction within the muscle itself (peripheral mechanisms) is the most likely cause of fatigue under these circumstances, central deficits in motor drive (central mechanisms) may also occur.

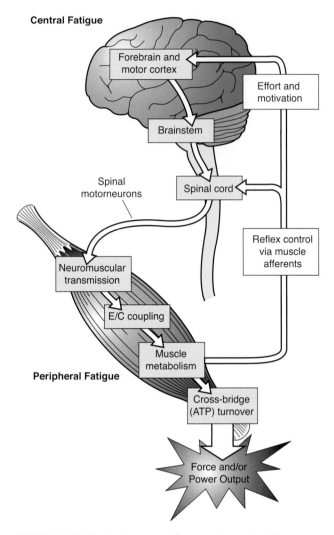

FIGURE 3-17. Chain of command for muscular contraction. Impairment along this pathway may be associated with fatigue. E/C, excitation–contraction; ATP, adenosine triphosphate.

PERIPHERAL MECHANISMS

During heavy exercise, the high level of anaerobic metabolism occurring results in decreases of ATP and CP and increases in the levels of hydrogen ion (H$^+$), Pi, ADP, and lactate. Theoretically, decreases in ATP level could contribute to fatigue because ATP supplies immediate energy for force generation in the muscles as well as provides for normal sodium–potassium pump and sarcoplasmic reticulum (SR) functioning. However, cell ATP concentration rarely decreases to less than 60%–70% of the preexercise level, even in cases of extensive fatigue (11), and it is likely that fatigue produced by other factors reduces the ATP use rate before ATP becomes limiting (21,26). Furthermore, the declines in CP concentration and tension during contractile activity follow different time courses, making a causal relationship between CP and fatigue unlikely (21).

Although the increase in ADP, Pi, and H$^+$ ions during intense contractile activity may cause fatigue by direct inhibition of ATP hydrolysis (29,30), the majority of evidence points to the effects of elevated H^+ (61). More specifically, H^+ appears to produce fatigue via the following mechanisms:

1. Inhibition of crossbridge actomyosin ATPase and ATP hydrolysis
2. Inhibition of PFK and thus the glycolytic rate
3. Competitive inhibition of Ca^{2+} binding to troponin C, reducing crossbridge activation
4. Inhibition of the SR ATPase, reducing Ca^{2+} reuptake and subsequently Ca^{2+} release (79)
5. Increase of the threshold of free Ca^{2+} required for contraction, particularly in fast-twitch fibers (29,30)

As evidenced by the preceding discussion, the primary sites of fatigue are within the muscle and do not generally involve peripheral nerves or the neuromuscular junction (NMJ). The observation that fatigued muscles generate the same tension whether stimulated directly or by the motor nerve argues against NMJ fatigue. However, there are several possible sites within the excitation–contraction coupling sequence of a muscle cell where disruptions during heavy exercise may induce fatigue. Specifically, the resting membrane potential is frequently altered, resulting in a reduced action potential (AP) amplitude and an increased AP duration that may ultimately affect Ca^{2+} release and contractile strength (11,30).

CENTRAL MECHANISMS

The possibility that specific brain mechanisms can reduce the magnitude of descending motor drive has received the least attention as a possible mediator of muscular fatigue even though willingness to maintain central motor drive (*e.g.*, willingness to maintain a maximal effort) probably contributes to fatigue in most people during activities of daily life. It has been postulated that because failure to produce the necessary force during fatigue is usually preceded by increased perceived effort, the CNS processes are at least as likely to contribute to fatigue as are those that lie within the muscle (26,30).

During fatiguing contractions, there is inhibition of central motor drive (9,30,84). Using a technique called transcranial magnetic stimulation (TMS) (42), it has been shown that the electrical stimulus reaching the muscle after magnetic stimulation of the motor cortex (motor-evoked potential) is suppressed after fatiguing exercise. Furthermore, a prolonged silent period after TMS has been demonstrated (9). These changes can result from altered voluntary drive to the motor cortex as well as intrinsic cortical processes (9,84). Therefore, the genesis of central fatigue may involve inadequate neural drive by the motor cortex at the highest levels of the brain or be influenced by peripheral conditions in the muscle via afferent feedback (3).

The influence of afferent feedback to central fatigue was demonstrated by Amann (4) using cycling time trials (TTs). Performance under nonfatigued or prefatigued conditions resulted in similar levels of peripheral fatigue markers at the end of a 5-km TT. Those results were indicative that central drive may be influenced by peripheral factors via muscle afferent input. This was further supported when group III/IV muscle afferent input was blocked during 5-km TT exercise, which resulted in exaggerated peripheral fatigue (4).

ENDURANCE EXERCISE

Numerous factors have been linked to fatigue resulting from prolonged endurance activity, including depletion of muscle and liver glycogen, decreases in blood glucose, dehydration, and increases in body temperature. Undoubtedly, each of these factors contributes to fatigue to a varying degree, the relative importance depending on environmental conditions and the nature of the activity. Mechanisms that involve various neurotransmitters and neuromodulators have also recently been proposed to explain possible CNS involvement in fatigue during prolonged exercise. This section reviews some of these factors. In particular, carbohydrate depletion, alterations in SR function, and increased brain serotonin are discussed.

GLYCOGEN DEPLETION

It has long been suggested that the rate of carbohydrate use depends on the intensity of work. This belief was based on the observation that the RER increases from rest to exercise. The early theories have been confirmed by direct measurements of glycogen use at different work intensities. The rate of body carbohydrate usage depends not only on intensity but also on the state of fitness. At a fixed workload, trained individuals have a lower RER, deplete glycogen more slowly, and can work longer than untrained individuals (8,40). High-carbohydrate diets and ingestion of carbohydrate drinks during exercise can delay fatigue by increasing the availability and oxidation of carbohydrates. These observations support the hypothesis that depletion of carbohydrate stores causes muscular fatigue during endurance activity. However, the exact mechanism is not known. Low muscle glycogen concentration may reduce NADH production and electron transport, drain intermediates of the Krebs cycle, or reduce fat oxidation, the effects of which would be to inhibit ATP production and cause fatigue (8).

It is also possible that central fatigue occurs in conjunction with carbohydrate depletion during prolonged exercise. Carbohydrate ingestion throughout exercise may attenuate the onset of negative CNS changes involving serotonin (discussed in more detail later in this section). However, the effects of carbohydrate feedings on central fatigue mechanisms and the well-established beneficial effects on the contracting muscle are difficult to distinguish. It seems apparent that future efforts should focus on the mechanisms by which glycogen depletion causes fatigue.

OTHER FACTORS

Glycogen depletion is probably not an exclusive fatigue factor during endurance exercise. Other potential candidates include disruption of important intracellular organelles, such as the mitochondria, the SR, or the myofilaments (30). The role of mitochondrial damage in fatigue is controversial (62).

The contractile proteins and, particularly, myofibril ATPase activity appear relatively resistant to change with endurance exercise (62). Ca^{2+} uptake by the SR vesicles, however, is depressed in the slow- and fast-twitch red region of the vastus lateralis, which suggests uncoupling of the transport or a leaky membrane, allowing Ca^{2+} flux back into the intracellular fluid. In addition to these functional changes, it has been demonstrated that exhaustive endurance exercise structurally damages the SR (83). The exact nature of this change and its effect on muscle function has not been elucidated.

In one study, a prolonged swim produced a significant decrease in glycogen concentration in slow type I, fast type IIa, and fast type IIx fibers of muscles, but the type IIx fibers exhibited no fatigue and no change in any of the contractile or biochemical properties measured (62). The apparent explanation is that the type IIx (fast white glycolytic) fiber is recruited less frequently during endurance activity, but glycogen use is similar to other fiber types despite fewer total contractions. It is apparent that muscle fatigue during endurance activity is somehow related to the degree of muscle use and is not entirely dependent on glycogen depletion.

In some cases, fatigue is characterized by a period of prolonged recovery during which force may be depressed for days. This low-frequency fatigue (LFF) (13) is caused by disruption of the excitation–contraction coupling process, perhaps because of excessive production of reactive oxygen species or prolonged exposure to high levels of intracellular Ca^{2+} (87).

The long recovery period after LFF may be related to the time required for repairing damaged proteins or the replacement of degraded proteins (87). Protein degradation could produce swelling and thus lead to muscle soreness. The time course of recovery from muscle soreness (i.e., days) exceeds that observed for most forms of fatigue but correlates well with recovery from LFF and reflects the time required to synthesize new muscle proteins.

Of the many proposed causes of central fatigue during prolonged exercise, the role of brain serotonin has generated the most interest. A review of the mechanisms involved in the control of brain serotonin synthesis and turnover at rest and during exercise (*Fig. 3-18*), along with its well-known influence on depression, sleepiness, mood, and pain, make it a particularly attractive candidate (10).

Concentrations of serotonin and 5-hydroxyindoleacetic acid (5-HIAA) (a major metabolite) increase in several brain regions during prolonged exercise and peak at fatigue (39,86). The administration of serotonin agonist drugs decreases, and antagonist drugs increases, run times to fatigue in the absence of any apparent peripheral markers of muscle fatigue (39).

SUMMARY

Both CNS and muscle mechanisms are likely to contribute to fatigue. After short-duration, high-intensity exercise, recovery in force production usually occurs in two components that are probably caused by separate mechanisms: (a) a rapidly reversible non–H^+-mediated perturbation, perhaps related to changes in excitation–contraction coupling and (b) a slower change that is probably mediated by H^+ and Pi. Reduction in central motor drive that occurs at the highest levels of the brain can also accompany fatigue, but this aspect is much less well studied, and the mechanisms have not been elucidated.

In prolonged endurance exercise, the depletion of skeletal muscle carbohydrate stores frequently occurs, and it appears that such glycogen depletion is an important factor in fatigue. In addition, adequate levels of muscle glycogen metabolism may be important in maintaining essential Krebs cycle intermediates. Undoubtedly, other factors are involved because muscle glycogen depletion can exist without fatigue and vice versa. Disruption of muscle protein, particularly the excitation–contraction coupling complex, has been shown to be associated with LFF. This process may be mediated by elevated levels of reactive oxygen species (free radicals) or intracellular Ca^{2+}. Increased brain serotonin metabolism has also been implicated in central fatigue under these circumstances.

ENVIRONMENTAL CONSIDERATIONS: HEAT AND COLD

The prevailing thermal environment can profoundly change the physiological response to exercise and increase the risk of an environment-related disorder. In healthy individuals, a limited core temperature range (36.1° to 37.8° C) is maintained. With this narrow temperature range, an understanding of the interrelationships between thermal environment and exercise allows better management of risk for heat or cold disorders during exercise. The physiological response to heat and cold are different, and the disorders associated with these two stressors differ fundamentally. This section presents the interaction between the environment and exercise

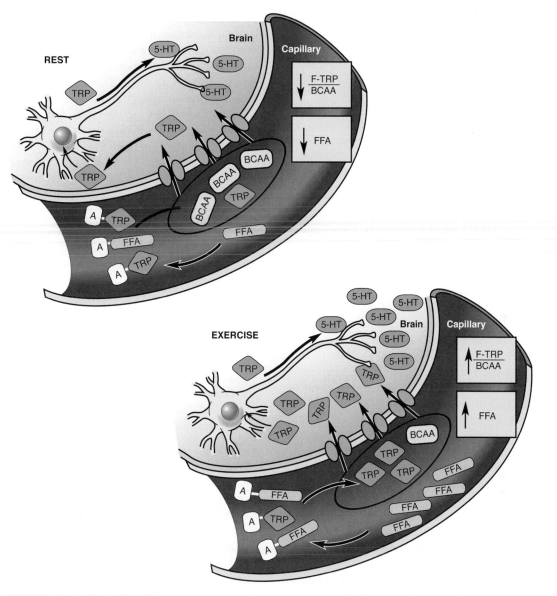

FIGURE 3-18. An illustration of the mechanisms involved in the control of brain serotonin synthesis and turnover at rest and during exercise. The well-known influence of these mechanisms on depression, sleepiness, mood, and pain make this a likely candidate for a center of fatigue. TRP, tryptophan; 5-HT, 5-hydroxytryptamine; FFA, free fatty acid; BCAA, branched chain amino acid.

and disorders that may occur. See the American College of Sports Medicine (ACSM) position stands for detailed information about environmental stressors (5,6,15).

HEAT STRESS

Heat stress is the combination of environmental conditions, metabolic rate, and clothing that increases core temperature. The traditional approach to the assessment of heat stress is to describe the balance that must be achieved between all sources of heat gain and heat loss. If a balance cannot be achieved, risk of excessive core temperature increases. A basic understanding of heat

exchange is necessary to appreciate the interactions of environment, exercise, and clothing. The risk of a serious heat-related disorder is associated with the level of heat stress, and control of risk is based on maintaining health and managing exposure to heat stress (see *Box 37-7*). Comprehensive risk reduction strategies to prevent heat-related injury and illness include (a) scheduling activities to avoid extremely hot and humid conditions, (b) individual heat acclimatization with gradual increases in work stress for at least 10–14 d, (c) monitoring of participants performing physical activity for signs and symptoms of heat strain because early recognition is key in preventing event severity, and (d) a careful monitoring of fluid replacement strategies (5,6).

HEAT BALANCE

The major source of heat gain is internal heat generated by energy metabolism. Approximately 25% of metabolic energy expenditure is actually translated to mechanical work during locomotion; the remaining 75% is released as heat in contracting muscles. As the metabolic rate increases to meet increasing demands of exercise, the rate of internal heat generation also increases. The rate of energy expenditure can be estimated using tables or equations (5). An average man (73 kg) walking on a level surface at 1.6 m · s⁻¹ (3.5 mph) has a gross metabolic rate of about 4.7 kcal · min⁻¹.

SWEAT EVAPORATIVE COOLING

The major avenue of heat loss is evaporation of sweat from the skin surface. Evaporative cooling by secreting water onto the skin surface through the eccrine sweat glands is one response to heat stress. As water absorbs heat from the skin, it changes from liquid to vapor. Surrounding air carries the vapor away. Because the heat of vaporization is quite high (590 kcal · L⁻¹), small amounts of sweat remove relatively large amounts of heat. Specifically, the evaporation of 0.5 L of sweat per hour is sufficient to remove the 280 kcal · hr⁻¹ of heat produced in the preceding walking example.

If sufficient volumes of sweat are produced quickly enough and evaporation is not impeded, thermal balance is maintained and core temperature does not increase. However, this scenario may not occur for several reasons. First, there are physiological limits to sweat evaporation. In the short term, it is not reasonable to expect a sustained sweat rate of more than 1 L · h⁻¹. In the long term (several hours), the rate of evaporation may be reduced by dehydration (6).

The physiological limit to volume of sweat produced varies by state of acclimation, by aerobic fitness, and genetically among individuals (5,6). Acclimation (also known as acclimatization) is a physiological adjustment that occurs naturally in conjunction with repeated exposure to a different environment and, in this context, exposure involving exercise. Acclimation to a heat environment increases rate of sweating, shortens onset time, and conserves sodium. Resulting benefits include reduced cardiovascular strain and lower core temperature for the same level of heat stress. Most improvement occurs over the initial 3–5 d, with smaller additional improvements over the subsequent 2–7 d (5). As a rule, 1 d of acclimation is lost for every 3 d away from exercise in heat stress, or in the case of illness, 1 d is lost per day of illness. Aerobic fitness is the single best indicator of a person's ability to tolerate heat stress.

Second, the physical limits to rate of evaporative cooling are caused by environmental conditions and clothing (5,6). The primary drive for evaporative cooling is the difference in water vapor pressures on the skin and in the air. If the difference is small, the rate of evaporative cooling decreases; if the difference is large, the evaporation rate can be sufficient to balance even high rates of metabolic heat production. Water vapor pressure on the skin is relatively constant. The vapor pressure of water in air is the primary source of differences in environmental contribution to heat stress. It is for this reason that humidity is an important factor in heat stress. Air movement also modifies the rate of evaporative cooling. If air movement is 2–3 m · s⁻¹ (4–6 mph), the maximum rate of evaporative cooling is achieved; higher speeds do not appreciably increase evaporative cooling (54).

CLOTHING

Clothing further restricts the maximum rate of evaporative cooling. Clothing between skin and the environment decreases the possibility of evaporation caused by the absorption of sweat or the prevention of vapor passage (5,54). Under some circumstances, the effect of clothing is negligible. For example, if the air is dry (low humidity) or if the metabolic rate is low, the rate of sweat evaporation through clothing is sufficient to allow adequate cooling. The resistance of clothing to sweat evaporation depends on surface area covered, nature of the fabric, number of layers, and construction of the ensemble. The following are important to minimize the effect of clothing:

- The covered surface area should be as small as is reasonable.
- The fabric should be lightweight open weave or other material that freely allows water vapor to pass through.
- Trapped air spaces from multiple layers should be minimized.
- The construction should be loose, with openings to allow easy movement of air around and through the clothing.

At the other extreme is clothing that covers most of the body; is impermeable to water vapor (*e.g.*, plastic or rubber rain clothing); and is tightly fitting around openings for arms, legs, and head. Little evaporative cooling can occur in a person wearing this type of clothing.

CONDUCTION, CONVECTION, AND RADIATION

Other factors that modify overall heat stress are conduction (transfer of heat between things in physical contact, such as a body and air), convection (transfer of heat to a moving fluid, which includes air in motion), and radiation. When the air temperature is greater than skin temperature (nominally 35° C or 95° F), heat is added by conduction and convection. Conversely, when air temperature is lower than 35° C, some heat is lost by conduction and convection. The rate of convection is enhanced by increased air movement and reduced by clothing insulation. Whereas infrared radiation from the sun and hot surfaces increase heat stress, cool surfaces accept radiation from warmer humans and reduce heat stress. Clothing insulation reduces rate of heat flow (in either direction) by radiation. Conduction, convection, and radiation combined usually account for less than 20% of heat gain or loss during exercise. An exception is during swimming, when conduction and convection are the primary sources of heat transfer.

PHYSIOLOGICAL RESPONSE

The physiological response to heat stress is reflected in body temperature, HR, and sweating. Metabolic heat increases the temperature of working muscles, and circulating blood transports heat to the central organs, causing an increase in core temperature. Additional blood flow carries excess heat to the skin. To move heat from working muscles to the skin, cardiac output increases and blood flow is shunted from the splanchnic and renal circulation.

HEAT-RELATED DISORDERS

The normal and acceptable response to heat stress includes elevated core temperature, increased HR, and water loss caused by sweating. Left unchecked, however, these responses may lead to heat-related disorders and decrements in psychomotor and cognitive performance. The disorders of particular importance during exercise are the following:

- Heat cramps
- Heat syncope
- Dehydration
- Heat exhaustion
- Heat stroke

Box 3-1 lists these disorders and describes signs, symptoms, and first aid. It is important for exercise professionals to understand these features of heat disorders. Preventive measures are described next.

BOX 3-1	Heat-Related Disorders, Including Symptoms, Signs, and First Aid

DISORDER	SYMPTOMS	SIGNS	FIRST AID
Exertional heat cramps	Painful muscle cramps, especially in abdominal or fatigued muscles	Incapacitating pain in voluntary muscles	Rest in cool environment Drink salted water (0.5% salt solution) Massage muscles
Heat syncope	Blurred vision (grayout) Fainting (brief blackout)	Brief fainting or near fainting Normal temperature	Lie on back in cool environment Drink water
Dehydration	No early symptoms Fatigue, weakness Dry mouth	Loss of work capacity Increased response time	Fluid and salt replacement
Exertional heat exhaustion	Fatigue Weakness Blurred vision Dizziness, headache	High pulse rate Profuse sweating Low blood pressure Insecure gait Pale face Collapse Body temperature normal to slightly increased	Lie flat on back in cool environment Drink water Loosen clothing
Exertional heat stroke	Chills Restlessness Irritability	Red face Euphoria Shivering Disorientation Erratic behavior Collapse Unconsciousness Convulsions Body temperature > 40° C (104° F)	Immediate, aggressive, effective cooling Transport to the hospital

HEAT CRAMPS AND SYNCOPE

Heat cramps are most likely to occur during or after sustained exercise with profuse sweating. Cramps usually appear in fatigued calf or abdominal muscles. Heat syncope may result from dehydration or excessive pooling of blood in peripheral vascular beds. The consequent hypotension may cause blackout symptoms. Recovery is relatively quick, and most people are generally aware of the occurrence. In addition to adequate hydration and maintaining salt balance, risk of syncope can be reduced by avoiding prolonged standing or rapid transition to standing.

DEHYDRATION AND HEAT EXHAUSTION

Dehydration and heat exhaustion are most likely to occur in unacclimated people and in those who do not drink enough or ignore early warning signs. In competitive sports, a 5% loss of body weight is not unusual (6). Losses greater than 1.5% should be followed by a period of recovery and rehydration. The ACSM position stand on "Exercise and Fluid Replacement" (6) provides comprehensive guidelines for fluid replacement to sustain appropriate hydration during physical activity.

HEAT STROKE

Heat stroke is a medical emergency, and the least suspicion that it may be present justifies an immediate and aggressive response to cool the body rapidly, such as packing the victim in ice. The risk of heat stroke is greatest among those who abuse alcohol or drugs, who are highly motivated and ignore symptoms of heat exhaustion, who are heat intolerant (*i.e.*, do not acclimate), or who have poor physical fitness.

HYPONATREMIA

While avoiding dehydration during exercise in the heat is critical, it is also important to avoid diluting the sodium content of the blood. Excessive drinking of fluids that are lower in sodium content than sweat such as plain water and many sports drinks dilutes the blood and results in hyponatremia. Symptoms include nausea, confusion, and fatigue, and thus it may be mistaken for heat exhaustion. In severe cases, hyponatremia is fatal. Exercisers who were thought to be experiencing heat exhaustion but were in fact in hyponatremia have been killed by "treating" them with water intake. During prolonged exercise in hot environments, sufficient water should be consumed to prevent a weight loss of 2% or more, and sufficient sodium should be consumed to maintain a serum Na^+ concentration of 135 $mEq \cdot L^{-1}$.

COLD STRESS

Cold stress is the combination of environment, metabolic rate, and clothing that results in heat loss from the core as a whole or from local areas (15,53). The physiological and/or psychological consequences of cold stress are referred to as cold strain (15). Cold-related disorders include hypothermia and varying degrees of local tissue damage (15). Again, control of cold stress is accomplished through comprehensive management of risk factors. Specifically, the ACSM recommends the use of a risk management strategy that "a) identifies/assesses the cold hazards; b) identifies/assesses contributing factors for cold-weather injuries; c) develops controls to mitigate cold stress/strain; d) implements controls into formal plans; and e) utilizes administrative oversight to ensure controls are enforced and modified." For detailed advice on these parameters, the reader should start with the ACSM position stand on "Prevention of Cold Injuries during Exercise" (15).

HEAT BALANCE

Similar to heat stress, cold stress is described as an imbalance between heat gained from metabolism and heat lost to the environment by conduction, convection, radiation, and evaporation (15). The problem, however, is net loss rather than net gain.

The sole source of heat gain during cold stress is metabolic heat released during muscular work along with basal biological processes. As exercise demands increase, the rate of heat gain from metabolism increases. If the rate of metabolic heat decreases because of fatigue or changes in demand, a disorder is more likely (15,53). Research on the effect of cold exposure on metabolism and substrate use during exercise has produced inconsistent findings (53). Future research must control the variety of factors that may exert influence on metabolism and substrate use in the cold, including duration and intensity of exercise imposed, training (fitness) status and cold acclimatization of the subjects, duration and intensity of resting preexercise cold exposure to cold conditions, duration and intensity of cold exposure during exercise, and the insulating effects of clothing (53).

HEAT LOSS

Heat is lost primarily by conduction and convection resulting from the difference between skin and ambient temperature (15). The rate of convection increases with air movement from wind (see *Box 37-12*) or motion of the body through the air (*e.g.*, while cycling or running). Sitting or lying on a cold, solid surface may cause heat loss by conduction. Periodic exercise and rest, in which heat accumulates and the person sweats under clothing, may be associated with heat loss through evaporation. Additional loss by radiant heat flow to colder surfaces is also possible.

CLOTHING

Proper clothing is the primary mechanism for achieving thermal balance during cold stress (15,53). The amount of insulation that clothing affords is described in units

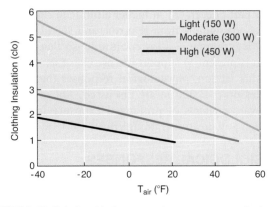

FIGURE 3-19. Relationship between air temperature and adequate clothing insulation for three levels of exercise. W, watts.

called *clo*. A wool business suit has an insulating value of approximately 1 clo. Generally, each quarter inch of clothing adds 1 clo of insulation. *Figure 3-19* illustrates the relations among air temperature, metabolic rate, and clothing in maintaining thermal balance (15). The insulating quality of clothing decreases precipitously when it becomes wet.

Sometimes clothing is sufficient to protect from hypothermia, but exposed skin is still at risk for excessive local cooling. The major method of heat loss is convection, but conduction via contact with cold objects can also occur. Adequate heating from circulating blood may not

be available because of reductions in peripheral blood flow (vasoconstriction) that naturally occur as a mechanism for heat conservation.

COLD-RELATED DISORDERS

Normal physiological response to cold stress is directed toward heat conservation, decreasing peripheral circulation, and increasing metabolic rate. These mechanisms, however, are not adequate for most cold stress, and behavioral thermal regulation is crucial for preventing cold-related disorders. Cold-related disorders can be systemic or local. *Box 3-2* is a list of some common cold-related disorders along with symptoms, signs, and steps for first aid (15).

SYSTEMIC COLD

The systemic cold disorder is hypothermia. Mild cases are marked by shivering and cold sensation in the extremities. Progression is associated with unstable cardiac function followed by CNS depression. Mild cases can be addressed by simple first aid, but moderate-to-severe hypothermia requires medical attention. As previously stated, hypothermia is best prevented by employing a comprehensive risk management strategy as detailed in the ACSM position stand (15).

BOX 3-2	Cold-Related Disorders, Including Symptoms, Signs, and First Aid		
DISORDER	**SYMPTOMS**	**SIGNS**	**FIRST AID**
Hypothermia	Chills Fatigue or drowsiness Pain in the extremities	Euphoria Slurred speech Slow, weak pulse Shivering Collapse or unconsciousness Body core temperature ≤35° C (95° F)	Move to warm area and remove wet clothing Modest external warming Drink warm fluids containing carbohydrates Transport to the hospital
Frostbite	Burning sensation at first Coldness, numbness, tingling	Skin color white or grayish yellow to reddish violet to black Blisters Response to touch depends on depth of freezing	Move to warm area and remove wet clothing External warming (*e.g.,* warm water) Drink warm fluids containing carbohydrates if conscious Treat as a burn; do not rub affected area Transport to the hospital
Frostnip	Possible itching or pain	Skin turns white	Similar to that for frostbite
Trench foot	Severe pain Tingling, itching	Edema Blisters Response to touch depends on depth of cooling	Similar to that for frostbite

LOCAL DISORDERS

Acute local disorders are associated with local tissue freezing (frostbite) or cooling (frost nip and trench foot). Frostbite can occur only when ambient temperature is less than $-1°$ C (30° F): it is marked by actual crystallization of water in tissue and subsequent destruction of cells. Because of the risk of further complications, significant cases of frostbite should be referred to medical personnel. Frostnip and trench foot are skin disorders that result from extreme cooling of the skin and underlying tissue, but without actual freezing of water in the tissue. The distinguishing characteristic between frost nip and trench foot is the presence of damp clothing that has accelerated heat loss. Predisposing factors for cold injuries and frostbite include the environmental, mechanical, physiological, and psychological domains (15).

SUMMARY

Environmental stressors such as heat and cold can significantly affect exercise and can be dangerous if uncontrolled. Adequate preventive precautions for both heat and cold are possible and should be known by exercise professionals. Situations that require medical attention are fairly common, and immediate referral of such problems is important.

EXERCISE AND THE ENVIRONMENT: ALTITUDE AND AIR POLLUTION

The condition of ambient air, which is inhaled into the lungs for respiratory gas exchange, has great importance for exercise capacity, physiological performance, and general health. This section discusses two main characteristics of ambient air: density, which changes with altitude, and contaminants, generally referred to as air pollution. It is necessary to be aware of hazards because exposure to altitude and polluted air can have profound effects on physical performance and can cause serious illnesses, even in well-trained individuals.

HIGH TERRESTRIAL ALTITUDE

Considerable evidence indicates that altitude training in preparation for competition at altitude is beneficial; therefore, many athletes spend considerable resources training at altitude. However, the value of this training for increasing performance at sea level is less certain. The lack of consensus may be attributed to differences in duration of exposure to altitude, elevations of training, initial fitness levels, and lack of a control group (28). Although continuous exposure to altitude is of little benefit, intermittent altitude exposure results in adaptations that improve sea-level performance (57,76). In particular, the "live high-train low" approach has athletes spend the greater part of each day at higher altitude to cause physiological adaptations from hypoxia, and spend a portion of the day training at a lower altitude, so that sufficient oxygen is present to support intense exercise.

In this section, physiological responses that occur at altitudes up to 3,000 m are discussed. Above 3,000 m, the negative effects of prolonged exposure to hypoxia outweigh any positive training effects (55).

PHYSIOLOGICAL RESPONSES

The amount of oxygen bound to hemoglobin in RBCs depends on the PO_2 in the inspired air (P_IO_2). P_IO_2 decreases as a result of declines in barometric pressure with increasing altitude at a constant oxygen percentage (*Table 3-4*). There is a decrease in the arterial partial pressure of oxygen (PaO_2) with the decline in P_IO_2 and, thus, in the amount of oxygen available. Acute exposure to reduced oxygen saturation triggers several compensatory mechanisms to increase oxygen transfer to tissue. After these acute reactions, acclimation occurs with more fundamental adaptations.

ACUTE PHYSIOLOGICAL RESPONSES

One of the most significant physiological compensatory reactions during acute exposure above 1,200 m (3,900 ft) is increased $\dot{V}_E$, or hypoxic ventilatory response, at rest and during exercise. Chemoreceptors in arterial blood vessels are stimulated, and signals are sent to the brain to increase ventilation. The increase in $\dot{V}_E$ is primarily associated with an increase in tidal volume, but breathing frequency also increases. Hyperventilation brings alveolar PO_2 closer to atmospheric PO_2 and substantially increases the PaO_2 when at altitude. Increased ventilation also leads to washout of carbon dioxide in the blood. Therefore, uncompensated respiratory alkalosis (higher pH) may develop. This respiratory alkalosis can cause a left shift of the oxygen–hemoglobin dissociation curve, resulting in higher arterial oxygen saturation, a second compensatory mechanism. Finally, early in exposure to altitude, reduced oxygen pressure is compensated for by small increases in cardiac output. This is primarily due

TABLE 3-4. Barometric Pressure for a Standard Atmosphere and Inspired Partial Oxygen Pressure for Five Altitudes, Accounting for the Pressure of Water Vapor in the Lungs (47 mm Hg)

Altitude (m)	Barometric Pressure (mm Hg)	Inspired Oxygen Pressure (mm Hg)
0	760	149
1,500 (4,900 ft)	627	123
2,000 (6,600 ft)	596	115
2,500 (8,200 ft)	627	107
3,000 (9,800 ft)	522	100

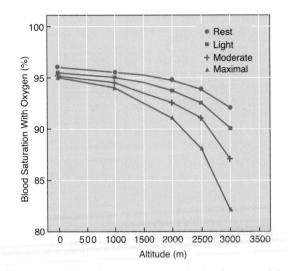

FIGURE 3-20. Effect of altitude and exercise levels on arterial oxygen saturation.

to an increased HR, which occurs because SV is constant or even slightly reduced at rest and during submaximal and maximal exercise.

Despite acute responses that compensate for lower oxygen tension at altitude, PaO_2 is decreased (*Fig. 3-20*). The magnitude of desaturation is directly related to altitude and exercise intensity. The primary pulmonary factor leading to increasing desaturation with increasing exercise intensity is limited alveolar end capillary diffusion. The result is an almost linear decrease of maximal oxygen uptake of 10% per 1,000 m (3,280 ft) altitude above 1,500 m (4,900 ft) (37). Because the oxygen uptake required by a fixed submaximal workload is not affected by altitude, the result is a higher relative exercise intensity for any given workload. Because of the nonlinear relationship between relative intensity (percentage of maximal oxygen uptake) and endurance time, the magnitude of the performance decrement at altitude is not constant but varies in proportion to the duration of the activity. Therefore, the longer the running distance, the larger the relative decrement (37).

Muscular strength and muscular endurance are not directly affected by acute exposure to altitude. However, subtle neuropsychological effects associated with acute mountain sickness (AMS) can occur at altitudes of 3,000 m within 6 h of exposure. Above 4,500 m (14,800 ft), the deterioration in most mental functions may be considerable, although variations between individuals are large (20). These neuropsychological effects may, in turn, affect muscular strength and endurance.

HIGH-ALTITUDE ILLNESS

Exposure to high altitude can lead to a number of illnesses that vary in seriousness. The speed of ascent and the absolute altitude are primary determinants of the incidence of altitude illness. Those exercising in or exposed to altitude (athletes and coaches) should anticipate the hazards and prepare through prevention and recognition of symptoms.

ACUTE MOUNTAIN SICKNESS

Acute mountain sickness (AMS) is characterized by severe headache and often accompanied by nausea, vomiting, decreased appetite, weariness, and sleep disturbances (45,60). AMS begins 6–12 h after arrival, usually peaks on the second or third day, and disappears on the fourth or fifth day. AMS normally appears above 2,500 m (8,200 ft), and the frequency of AMS increases with altitude and rate of ascent. Generally, above 3,000 m, 24 h of acclimation should be acquired for every 300-m altitude gain (45). Although AMS is self-limiting, persistence of symptoms may require medical treatment. If AMS is not at least partially resolved within 2–3 d, descent is the only effective treatment. Supplemental oxygen and pharmacological treatment (acetazolamide, furosemide, and analgesics) may be necessary for severe cases.

HIGH-ALTITUDE PULMONARY EDEMA

High-altitude pulmonary edema (HAPE) is considered a progression in the severity of AMS, associated with pulmonary edema (45). The onset may be subtle. Signs and symptoms include dyspnea, fatigue, chest pain, tachycardia, coughing, and cyanosis of the lips and extremities. As HAPE progresses, affected individuals may cough frothy or blood-tinged sputum (60). This complication can be fatal if not treated promptly. Children and young adults are at higher risk of developing HAPE than adults, and immediate medical attention is necessary. Evacuation to a lower altitude is essential. Individuals with a history of HAPE appear to be particularly susceptible to subsequent bouts upon return to high altitudes.

HIGH-ALTITUDE CEREBRAL EDEMA

High-altitude cerebral edema (HACE) may develop when the rate of ascent is too fast. The signs and symptoms of HACE include severe headache, fatigue, vomiting, nausea, ataxia, and changes of mental status (60). The incidence of HACE is low (1%), but it can be fatal if untreated. In cases of symptoms of cerebral edema, direct medical care with immediate evacuation to a low altitude and supplemental oxygen is recommended (45).

PREVENTING ALTITUDE SICKNESS

AMS can be prevented by adjusting the amount and rate of ascent. Options include an interrupted ascent with time (days) to acclimate at successive altitudes before reaching the final elevation and/or limiting daily gain in altitude to 300 m (980 ft) or less. Initially, unacclimated subjects should avoid vigorous exercise. Adequate hydration and a high-carbohydrate diet may aid prevention. Acetazolamide is the only drug for altitude sickness approved by the U.S. Food and Drug Administration (FDA). Because acetazolamide may affect exercise performance, it is contraindicated when training at high altitudes. Prophylactic administration of acetazolamide may be effective (60).

AIR POLLUTION

Air pollution can also affect exercise performance and health. Although nature contributes to pollution through ozone (O_3) from lightning, dust, sulfuric oxides from volcanic activity, and other natural pollutants, modern industrialization has exacerbated the problem. Because of the severity of pollution in many areas, organizers of sporting events and exercisers are frequently confronted with problems related to exercising in polluted air. Both large sporting events and daily activity are performed in major cities, which are generally the sites with the highest pollution levels. Also, with indoor training and sports events, the infiltration of outdoor air pollution may be significant. Furthermore, the indoor environment may actually add to the problem with indoor air pollutants emitted by the occupants, activities, and building materials.

There are two major groups or types of pollutants: primary and secondary. **Primary pollutants** are directly attributable to a source of pollution, such as carbon monoxide (CO), sulfur oxides, nitrogen oxides, hydrocarbons, and particulates (dust, smoke, and soot). **Secondary pollutants** result from an interaction of the environment (sunlight, moisture, other pollutants) with primary pollutants. These include O_3, aldehydes, sulfuric acid (H_2SO_4), and peroxyacetyl nitrate (PAN). City air commonly contains both primary and secondary pollutants.

GENERAL EFFECTOR MECHANISMS

The effect of pollutants is partly related to level of penetration. This "dosage" is determined by exposure time, concentration of pollutant in inhaled air, ventilation rate and volume, temperature and humidity of inhaled air, and route of inhalation (the nose vs. the mouth). Pollution primarily affects the respiratory tract. This tract provides a large surface area for contact by the pollutant. The mucous membranes of the nose effectively remove large particles and highly soluble gases (e.g., 99.9% of inhaled SO_2), preventing them from affecting deeper airways and lung tissue. However, smaller particles and agents with low solubility easily pass through this barrier. During exercise, when mouth breathing plays an important role, this air filtration is less efficient, and more pollutants reach the lungs, traverse the diffusion surface, and enter the blood and body tissues.

Pollutants can have several effects on the body's tissues, including the following:

- Irritation of the airways, which may lead to bronchoconstriction, hence increased airway resistance
- Reduction of alveolar diffusion capacity
- Reduction of oxygen transport capacity

Other effects of pollutants that can indirectly affect exercise performance are irritation of eyes (PAN and formaldehyde) and skin. Short-term effects of exposure to pollutants rather than long-term effects of exposure are discussed in this section.

OUTDOOR POLLUTION

Geographical distribution of outdoor pollution is strongly related to industry and population density. Automobiles, trucks, buses, aircrafts, industrial sources, and combustion of fossil fuels are major sources of CO, sulfur and nitrogen oxides, hydrocarbons, and particles. Areas with equal production of pollutants do not necessarily have equally polluted air, or smog, because climate and topography play major roles. River and mountain valleys generally have greater smog levels than hilltops and plains. High temperature and humidity typically promote photochemical smog with associated high O_3 levels. For example, in the Los Angeles area, photochemical smog, trapped by summer winds blowing toward the surrounding mountains, is a common phenomenon (48). Low temperature with a concomitant increase in fuel consumption for heating and high humidity (fog, rain) promote a different type of fog in which high sulfur oxide concentrations combined with particulate matter are converted into H_2SO_4 (acid rain) and sulfates. The most famous fog of this type is the London fog, which produced a large number of deaths in 1952 (4,000 in a 4-d period). Such fog can be persistent when temperature inversion occurs, a condition brought about by little wind and a layer of cool polluted air trapped beneath a layer of warmer air.

PREVENTION

Avoidance of exposure is the primary method for preventing acute and long-term adverse effects of outdoor pollutants. Timing and selection of optimal location for exercise and moderating intensity and duration are key factors (16). Knowledge of daily and seasonal patterns and fluctuations (*Fig. 3-21*) is important when planning an event involving high-intensity exercise. Avoiding periods and areas with heavy traffic can minimize CO exposure. Summer and early autumn afternoons can be unfavorable because of high O_3 exposure.

Information on air pollution can be acquired from local meteorological authorities, many of which provide a pollutant standards index (PSI) developed by the U.S. Environmental Protection Agency (EPA). The PSI converts measured pollutant concentration to a number on

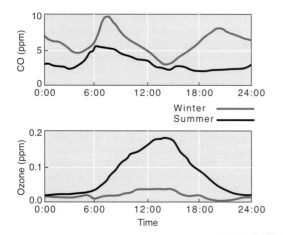

FIGURE 3-21. Daily and seasonal fluctuations in CO and ozone concentrations in the Los Angeles area. (Adapted with permission from McCafferty W. *Air Pollution and Athletic Performance*. Springfield [IL]: Charles C Thomas; 1981. 227 p.)

TABLE 3-5. National Ambient Air Quality Standards as Provided by the Environmental Protection Agency

| Pollutant | Time Period | |
	For Averaging	Standard Limit Level
Carbon monoxide	8 h	9 ppm
	1 h	35 ppm
Ozone	1 h	0.12 ppm
	8 h	0.08 ppm
Nitrogen dioxide (NO_2)	AAM	0.053 ppm
Sulfur dioxide (SO_2)	AAM	80 $\mu g \cdot m^{-3}$
	24 h	365 $\mu g \cdot m^{-3}$
Particulates (PM-2.5) ($\leq$2.5-μ diameter)	AAM	15 $\mu g \cdot m^{-3}$
	24 h	65 $\mu g \cdot m^{-3}$
Particulates (PM-10) ($\leq$10-micron diameter)	AAM	50 $\mu g \cdot m^{-3}$
	24 h	150 $\mu g \cdot m^{-3}$

AAM, annual arithmetic mean; ppm, parts per million.

For pollutants with high hourly or daily fluctuations, longer duration averages and short-term peak level limits are provided. The numbers correspond to a PSI of 100.

a scale from 0 to 500. The critical number is 100, which corresponds to the threshold established under the Clean Air Act (*Table 3-5*) (27). A PSI greater than 100 indicates pollution in an unhealthful range. PSI places maximum emphasis on acute health effects (24 h or less), rather than chronic effects, making it useful for exercise planning. It does not incorporate interactions between pollutants. *Table 3-6* has information on the PSI (27).

The important factors for controlling exposure to indoor pollution include selecting an optimal location for air intake, using low-emission building materials, regularly cleaning and use of low-dust floor coverings, clean ventilation and air conditioning systems, and sufficiently high fresh air ventilation rate.

More specifically, exercise centers and fitness facilities require higher ventilation rates than offices and living quarters. When outdoor CO_2 concentrations are 350 parts per million (ppm), an indoor CO_2 concentration limit of 1,000 ppm is considered an indicator of adequate ventilation. At that level, 80% of the users are satisfied with air quality. An indoor level of 650 ppm CO_2 is needed to increase satisfaction to 90% (27). Indoor exercise areas should maintain the lowest CO_2 concentration practically possible.

TABLE 3-6. Pollutant Standards Index and Implications for Short-Term Health Effects

Index Value	PSI Descriptor	General Health Effects	Cautionary Statements
Up to 50	Good	None for the general population	None required
51–100	Moderate	Few or none for the general population	None required
101–200	Unhealthful	Mild aggravation of symptoms among susceptible people, with irritation symptoms in the healthy population	People with existing heart or respiratory ailments should reduce physical exertion and outdoor activity; the general population should reduce vigorous outdoor activity
201–300	Very unhealthful	Significant aggravation of symptoms and decreased exercise tolerance in people with heart or lung disease; widespread symptoms in the healthy population	Elderly and people with heart or lung disease should stay indoors and reduce physical activity; general population should avoid vigorous outdoor activity
>300	Hazardous	Early onset of certain diseases in addition to significant aggravation of symptoms and decreased exercise tolerance in healthy people	Elderly and people with diseases should stay indoors and avoid physical exertion
		At PSI levels greater than 400, premature death of ill and elderly people may result	At PSI levels greater than 400, the general population should avoid outdoor activity
		Healthy people have adverse symptoms that affect normal activity	All people should remain indoors, keeping windows and doors closed, and minimize physical exertion

PSI, pollution standards index. Also see *Table 37-8.*

SUMMARY

The environmental effects of altitude and air pollution can affect exercise and athletic performance. Physiological adaptation or maladaptation (in the case of altitude sickness or exposure to air pollution) is often a factor in fitness, exercise, and training programs. Although some effects of altitude can be overcome with chronic adaptations to training at altitude, prevention of harmful effects of pollution is often a function of avoiding and minimizing exposure.

REFERENCES

1. Achten J, Gleeson M, Jeukendrup AE. Determination of the exercise intensity that elicits maximal fat oxidation. *Med Sci Sports Exerc*. 2002;34(1):92–7.
2. Ainsworth BE, Haskell WL, Whitt MC, et al. Compendium of physical activities: an update of activity codes and MET intensities. *Med Sci Sports Exerc*. 2000;32(9):S498–516.
3. Allen GM, Gandevia SC, McKenzie DK. Reliability of measurements of muscle strength and voluntary activation using twitch interpolation. *Muscle Nerve*. 1995;18(6):593–600.
4. Amann M. Central and peripheral fatigue: interaction during cycling exercise in humans. *Med Sci Sports Exerc*. 2011;43(11):2039–45.
5. American College of Sports Medicine, Armstrong LE, Casa DJ, et al. American College of Sports Medicine position stand. Exertional heat illness during training and competition. *Med Sci Sports Exerc*. 2007;39(3):556–72.
6. American College of Sports Medicine, Sawka MN, Burke LM, et al. American College of Sports Medicine position stand. Exercise and fluid replacement. *Med Sci Sports Exerc*. 2007;39(2):377–90.
7. Atkins JM, Matthews OA, Blomqvist CG, Mullins CB. Incidence of arrhythmias induced by isometric and dynamic exercise. *Br Heart J*. 1976;38(5):465–71.
8. Bassett DR Jr, Howley ET. Limiting factors for maximum oxygen uptake and determinants of endurance performance. *Med Sci Sports Exerc*. 2000;32(1):70–84.
9. Bergstrom M, Hultman E. Energy cost and fatigue during intermittent electrical stimulation of human skeletal muscle. *J Appl Physiol*. 1988;65(4):1500–5.
10. Bigland-Ritchie B, Furbush F, Woods JJ. Fatigue of intermittent submaximal voluntary contractions: central and peripheral factors. *J Appl Physiol*. 1986;61(2):421–9.
11. Bigland-Ritchie B, Rice CL, Garland SJ, Walsh ML. Task-dependent factors in fatigue of human voluntary contractions. *Adv Exp Med Biol*. 1995;384:361–80.
12. Bruce RA, Kusumi F, Hosmer D. Maximal oxygen intake and nomographic assessment of functional aerobic impairment in cardiovascular disease. *Am Heart J*. 1973;85(4):546–62.
13. Byrd SK, McCutcheon LJ, Hodgson DR, Gollnick PD. Altered sarcoplasmic reticulum function after high-intensity exercise. *J Appl Physiol*. 1989;67(5):2072–7.
14. Byrne NM, Hills AP, Hunter GR, Weinsier RL, Schutz Y. Metabolic equivalent: one size does not fit all. *J Appl Physiol*. 2005;99(3):1112–9.
15. Castellani JW, Young AJ, Ducharme MB, et al. American College of Sports Medicine position stand: prevention of cold injuries during exercise. *Med Sci Sports Exerc*. 2006;38(11):2012–29.
16. Cedaro R. Environmental factors and exercise performance: a review, II. *Air Pollution Excel*. 1992;8:161–6.
17. Concu A, Marcello C. Stroke volume response to progressive exercise in athletes engaged in different types of training. *Eur J Appl Physiol Occup Physiol*. 1993;66(1):11–7.
18. Coyle EF, Gonzalez-Alonso J. Cardiovascular drift during prolonged exercise: new perspectives. *Exerc Sport Sci Rev*. 2001;29(2):88–92.
19. Coyle EF, Jeukendrup AE, Wagenmakers AJ, Saris WH. Fatty acid oxidation is directly regulated by carbohydrate metabolism during exercise. *Am J Physiol*. 1997;273(2 Pt 1):E268–75.
20. Cudaback DD. Four-km altitude effects on performance and health. *Pub Astronom Soc Pac*. 1984;96:463–77.
21. Davis JM, Bailey SP. Possible mechanisms of central nervous system fatigue during exercise. *Med Sci Sports Exerc*. 1997;29(1):45–57.
22. Day JR, Rossiter HB, Coats EM, Skasick A, Whipp BJ. The maximally attainable VO2 during exercise in humans: the peak vs. maximum issue. *J Appl Physiol*. 2003;95(5):1901–7.
23. Di Prampero PE, Boutellier U, Pietsch P. Oxygen deficit and stores at onset of muscular exercise in humans. *J Appl Physiol*. 1983;55(1 Pt 1):146–53.
24. Duncan GE, Howley ET, Johnson BN. Applicability of VO2max criteria: discontinuous versus continuous protocols. *Med Sci Sports Exerc*. 1997;29(2):273–8.
25. Edgerton VR, Roy RR, Gregor RJ, Hager CL, Wickiewicz T. Muscle fiber activation and recruitment. In: Knuttgen HG, Vogel JA, Poortmans JR, editors. *Biochemistry of Exercise*. Champaign: Human Kinetics Publishers; 1983. p. 31–49.
26. Enoka RM, Stuart DG. Neurobiology of muscle fatigue. *J Appl Physiol*. 1992;72(5):1631–48.
27. Environmental Protection Agency Web site [Internet]. Washington (DC): Environmental Protection Agency; [cited 2008 Oct 14]. Available from: http://www.epa.gov/
28. Favier R, Spielvogel H, Desplanches D, et al. Training in hypoxia vs. training in normoxia in high-altitude natives. *J Appl Physiol*. 1995;78(6):2286–93.
29. Fitts RH. Cellular mechanisms of muscle fatigue. *Physiol Rev*. 1994;74(1):49–94.
30. Fitts RH. Cellular, molecular, and metabolic basis of muscle fatigue. In: Rowell LB, Shepherd JT, American Physiological Society, editors. *Handbook of Physiology: A Critical, Comprehensive Presentation of Physiological Knowledge and Concepts*. New York: Published for the American Physiological Society by Oxford University Press; 1996.
31. Fleck SJ. Cardiovascular responses to strength training. In: *Strength and Power in Sport*. 2nd ed. Osney Mead, United Kingdom: Blackwell Science Ltd; 2003. p. 387–408.
32. Foster C, Kuffel E, Bradley N, et al. VO2max during successive maximal efforts. *Eur J Appl Physiol*. 2007;102(1):67–72.
33. Franklin BA. Diagnostic and functional exercise testing: test selection and interpretation. *J Cardiovasc Nurs*. 1995;10(1):8–29.
34. Franklin BA. Exercise testing, training and arm ergometry. *Sports Med*. 1985;2(2):100–19.
35. Franklin BA. Pitfalls in estimating aerobic capacity from exercise time or workload. *Appl Cardiol*. 1986;14:25–6.
36. Fry AC, Allemeier CA, Staron RS. Correlation between percentage fiber type area and myosin heavy chain content in human skeletal muscle. *Eur J Appl Physiol Occup Physiol*. 1994;68(3):246–51.
37. Fulco CS, Rock PB, Cymerman A. Maximal and submaximal exercise performance at altitude. *Aviat Space Environ Med*. 1998;69(8):793–801.
38. Gaesser GA, Brooks GA. Metabolic bases of excess post-exercise oxygen consumption: a review. *Med Sci Sports Exerc*. 1984;16(1):29–43.
39. Garner SH, Sutton JR, Burse RL, McComas AJ, Cymerman A, Houston CS. Operation Everest II: neuromuscular performance under conditions of extreme simulated altitude. *J Appl Physiol*. 1990;68(3):1167–72.
40. Gaskill SE, Ruby BC, Walker AJ, Sanchez OA, Serfass RC, Leon AS. Validity and reliability of combining three methods to determine ventilatory threshold. *Med Sci Sports Exerc*. 2001;33(11):1841–8.
41. Gladden LB. Lactate metabolism: a new paradigm for the third millennium. *J Physiol*. 2004;558(Pt 1):5–30.

42. Godt RE, Nosek TM. Changes of intracellular milieu with fatigue or hypoxia depress contraction of skinned rabbit skeletal and cardiac muscle. *J Physiol.* 1989;412:155–80.

43. Gollnick PD. Metabolism of substrates: energy substrate metabolism during exercise and as modified by training. *Fed Proc.* 1985;44(2):353–7.

44. Gollnick PD, Riedy M, Quintinskie JJ, Bertocci LA. Differences in metabolic potential of skeletal muscle fibres and their significance for metabolic control. *J Exp Biol.* 1985;115:191–9.

45. Hamilton AJ, Cymmerman A, Black PM. High altitude cerebral edema. *Neurosurgery.* 1986;19(5):841–9.

46. Harms CA, McClaran SR, Nickele GA, Pegelow DF, Nelson WB, Dempsey JA. Exercise-induced arterial hypoxaemia in healthy young women. *J Physiol.* 1998;507(Pt 2):619–28.

47. Hawkins MN, Raven PB, Snell PG, Stray-Gundersen J, Levine BD. Maximal oxygen uptake as a parametric measure of cardiorespiratory capacity. *Med Sci Sports Exerc.* 2007;39(1):103–7.

48. Haymes EM, Wells CL. *Environment and Human Performance.* Champaign (IL): Human Kinetics Publishers; 1986. 164 p.

49. Hester RL, Choi J. Blood flow control during exercise: role for the venular endothelium? *Exerc Sport Sci Rev.* 2002;30(4):147–51.

50. Hill AV, Lupton H. Muscular exercise, lactic acid, and the supply and utilization of oxygen. *Q J Med.* 1923;16:135–71.

51. Howley ET, Bassett DR Jr, Welch HG. Criteria for maximal oxygen uptake: review and commentary. *Med Sci Sports Exerc.* 1995;27(9):1292–301.

52. Hughes EF, Turner SC, Brooks GA. Effects of glycogen depletion and pedaling speed on "anaerobic threshold." *J Appl Physiol.* 1982;52(6):1598–607.

53. Jett DM, Adams KJ, Stamford BA. Cold exposure and exercise metabolism. *Sports Med.* 2006;36(8):643–56.

54. Kamon E, Avellini B. Wind speed limits to work under hot environments for clothed men. *J Appl Physiol.* 1979;46(2):340–5.

55. Kayser B. Nutrition and energetics of exercise at altitude. Theory and possible practical implications. *Sports Med.* 1994;17(5):309–23.

56. Kitamura K, Jorgensen CR, Gobel FL, Taylor HL, Wang Y. Hemodynamic correlates of myocardial oxygen consumption during upright exercise. *J Appl Physiol.* 1972;32(4):516–22.

57. Levine BD, Stray-Gundersen J. A practical approach to altitude training: where to live and train for optimal performance enhancement. *Int J Sports Med.* 1992;13 Suppl 1:S209–12.

58. Lind AR, McNicol GW. Muscular factors which determine the cardiovascular responses to sustained and rhythmic exercise. *Can Med Assoc J.* 1967;96(12):706–15.

59. Lucia A, Rabadan M, Hoyos J, et al. Frequency of the VO2max plateau phenomenon in world-class cyclists. *Int J Sports Med.* 2006;27(12):984–92.

60. Malconian MK, Rock PB. Medical problems related to altitude. In: Pandolf KB, Sawka MN, Gonzalez RR, editors. *Human Performance Physiology and Environmental Medicine at Terrestrial Extremes.* Indianapolis: Benchmark Press; 1988. p. 637.

61. Metzger JM, Fitts RH. Fatigue from high- and low-frequency muscle stimulation: role of sarcolemma action potentials. *Exp Neurol.* 1986;93(2):320–33.

62. Metzger JM, Fitts RH. Role of intracellular pH in muscle fatigue. *J Appl Physiol.* 1987;62(4):1392–7.

63. Mitchell JH, Payne FC, Saltin B, Schibye B. The role of muscle mass in the cardiovascular response to static contractions. *J Physiol.* 1980;309:45–54.

64. Nelson RR, Gobel FL, Jorgensen CR, Wang K, Wang Y, Taylor HL. Hemodynamic predictors of myocardial oxygen consumption during static and dynamic exercise. *Circulation.* 1974;50(6):1179–89.

65. Newsholme EA. The control of fuel utilization by muscle during exercise and starvation. *Diabetes.* 1979;28 Suppl 1:1–7.

66. Pescatello LS, Franklin BA, Fagard R, et al. American College of Sports Medicine position stand. Exercise and hypertension. *Med Sci Sports Exerc.* 2004;36(3):533–53.

67. Podolin DA, Munger PA, Mazzeo RS. Plasma catecholamine and lactate response during graded exercise with varied glycogen conditions. *J Appl Physiol.* 1991;71(4):1427–33.

68. Porszasz J, Casaburi R, Somfay A, Woodhouse LJ, Whipp BJ. A treadmill ramp protocol using simultaneous changes in speed and grade. *Med Sci Sports Exerc.* 2003;35(9):1596–603.

69. Powers SK, Dodd S, Beadle RE. Oxygen uptake kinetics in trained athletes differing in VO2max. *Eur J Appl Physiol Occup Physiol.* 1985;54(3):306–8.

70. Powers SK, Howley ET, Cox R. A differential catecholamine response during prolonged exercise and passive heating. *Med Sci Sports Exerc.* 1982;14(6):435–9.

71. Powers SK, Howley ET, Cox R. Ventilatory and metabolic reactions to heat stress during prolonged exercise. *J Sports Med Phys Fitness.* 1982;22(1):32–6.

72. Powers SK, Martin D, Dodd S. Exercise-induced hypoxaemia in elite endurance athletes. Incidence, causes and impact on VO2max. *Sports Med.* 1993;16(1):14–22.

73. Powers SK, Riley W, Howley ET. Comparison of fat metabolism between trained men and women during prolonged aerobic work. *Res Q Exerc Sport.* 1980;51(2):427–31.

74. Richardson RS, Noyszewski EA, Leigh JS, Wagner PD. Lactate efflux from exercising human skeletal muscle: role of intracellular PO2. *J Appl Physiol.* 1998;85(2):627–34.

75. Robergs RA, Giasvand F, Parker D. Biochemistry of exercise-induced metabolic acidosis. *Am J Physiol Regul Integr Comp Physiol.* 2004;287:502–16.

76. Rodriguez FA, Casas H, Casas M, et al. Intermittent hypobaric hypoxia stimulates erythropoiesis and improves aerobic capacity. *Med Sci Sports Exerc.* 1999;31(2):264–8.

77. Rossiter HB, Kowalchuk JM, Whipp BJ. A test to establish maximum O2 uptake despite no plateau in the O2 uptake response to ramp incremental exercise. *J Appl Physiol.* 2006;100(3):764–70.

78. Schwade J, Blomqvist CG, Shapiro W. A comparison of the response to arm and leg work in patients with ischemic heart disease. *Am Heart J.* 1977;94(2):203–8.

79. Sjogaard G. Role of exercise-induced potassium fluxes underlying muscle fatigue: a brief review. *Can J Physiol Pharmacol.* 1991;69(2):238–45.

80. Staron RS, Karapondo DL, Kraemer WJ, et al. Skeletal muscle adaptations during early phase of heavy-resistance training in men and women. *J Appl Physiol.* 1994;76(3):1247–55.

81. Stromme SB, Ingjer F, Meen HD. Assessment of maximal aerobic power in specifically trained athletes. *J Appl Physiol.* 1977;42(6):833–7.

82. Taylor HL, Buskirk E, Henschel A. Maximal oxygen intake as an objective measure of cardio-respiratory performance. *J Appl Physiol.* 1955;8(1):73–80.

83. Thompson LV, Balog EM, Fitts RH. Muscle fatigue in frog semitendinosus: role of intracellular pH. *Am J Physiol.* 1992;262 (6 Pt 1):C1507–12.

84. Thompson LV, Fitts RH. Muscle fatigue in the frog semitendinosus: role of the high-energy phosphates and Pi. *Am J Physiol.* 1992;263(4 Pt 1):C803–9.

85. Thompson WR, Gordon NF, Pescatello LS, American College of Sports Medicine. *ACSM's Guidelines for Exercise Testing and Prescription.* 8th ed. Philadelphia (PA): Lippincott Williams & Wilkins; 2009. 400 p.

86. Westing SH, Cresswell AG, Thorstensson A. Muscle activation during maximal voluntary eccentric and concentric knee extension. *Eur J Appl Physiol Occup Physiol.* 1991;62(2):104–8.

87. Wilkie DR. Muscular fatigue: effects of hydrogen ions and inorganic phosphate. *Fed Proc.* 1986;45(13):2921–3.

SELECTED REFERENCES FOR FURTHER READING

Ainsworth BE, Haskell WL, Whitt MC, et al. Compendium of physical activities: an update of activity codes and MET intensities. *Med Sci Sports Exerc.* 2000;32:S498–516.

Astrand PO, Rodahl K, Dahl HA, Stromme SB. *Textbook of Work Physiology: Physiological Basis of Exercise.* Champaign (IL): Human Kinetics; 2003. 649 p.

Baechle TR, Earle RW, editors. *Essentials of Strength and Conditioning.* Champaign (IL): Human Kinetics; 2000. 658 p.

Brooks G, Fahey T, Baldwin K. *Exercise Physiology: Human Bioenergetics and Its Applications.* 4th ed. Boston (MA): McGraw Hill; 2005. 876 p.

Fleck SJ, Kraemer WJ. *Designing Resistance Training Programs.* 3rd ed. Champaign (IL): Human Kinetics; 2004. 377 p.

Gleeson M, Maughan RJ. *The Biochemical Basis of Sports Performance.* Lavallette (NJ): Oxford University Press; 2004. 257 p.

Hargreaves M, Spriet L, editors. *Exercise Metabolism.* 2nd ed. Champaign (IL): Human Kinetics; 2006. 301 p.

Hoffman J. *Physiological Aspects of Sport Training and Performance.* Champaign (IL): Human Kinetics; 2002. 343 p.

Komi PV, editor. *Strength and Power in Sport.* Malden (MA): Blackwell Science; 2003. 523 p.

Kraemer WJ, Hakkinen K, editors. *Strength Training for Sport.* Malden (MA): Blackwell Science; 2002. 186 p.

Maud PJ, Foster C, editors. *Physiological Assessment of Human Fitness.* 2nd ed. Champaign (IL): Human Kinetics; 2006. 319 p.

Nieman DC. *Exercise Testing and Prescription.* 6th ed. Boston (MA): McGraw Hill; 2007. 816 p.

Noakes T. *Lore of Running.* 4th ed. Champaign (IL): Human Kinetics; 2003. 931 p.

Plowman SA, Smith DL. *Exercise Physiology—For Health, Fitness, and Performance.* 2nd ed. San Francisco (CA): Benjamin Cummings; 2003. 636 p.

Powers SK, Howley ET. *Exercise Physiology—Theory and Application to Fitness and Performance.* 6th ed. Boston (MA): McGraw Hill; 2007. 540 p.

Saltin B, Boushel R, Secher N, Mitchell J, editors. *Exercise and Circulation in Health and Disease.* Champaign (IL): Human Kinetics; 2000. 345 p.

Shephard RJ, Astrand PO, editors. *Endurance in Sport.* Malden (MA): Blackwell Science; 1992. 638 p.

Skinner JS, editor. *Exercise Testing and Exercise Prescription for Special Cases: Theoretical Basis and Clinical Application.* 3rd ed. Philadelphia (PA): Lippincott Williams & Wilkins; 2005. 418 p.

Whiting WC, Zernicke RF. *Biomechanics of Musculoskeletal Injury.* Champaign (IL): Human Kinetics; 1998. 273 p.

INTERNET RESOURCES

- AccuWeather: http://www.accuweather.com
- American Academy of Pediatrics: http://www.aap.org
- American Association of Cardiovascular and Pulmonary Rehabilitation (AACVPR): http://www.aacvpr.org
- American Cancer Society: http://www.cancer.org
- American College of Sports Medicine: http://www.acsm.org
- American Diabetes Association: http://www.diabetes.org
- American Heart Association: http://www.americanheart.org
- American Medical Association: http://www.ama-assn.org
- Coalition for a Healthy and Active America (CHAA): http://www.chaausa.nonprofitoffice.com/
- The Cooper Institute: http://www.cooperinstitute.org
- Gatorade Sports Science Institute: http://www.gssiweb.com
- Healthy People 2010: http://www.healthypeople.gov
- International Society for Aging and Physical Activity (ISAPA): http://www.isapa.org
- National Athletic Trainers' Association: http://www.nata.org
- The National Center on Physical Activity and Disability (NCPAD): http://www.ncpad.org
- National Heart, Lung, and Blood Institute: http://www.nhlbi.nih.gov
- National Heart, Lung, and Blood Institute: *Clinical Guidelines on the Identification, Evaluation, and Treatment of Overweight and Obesity in Adults*: http://www.nhlbi.nih.gov/guidelines/obesity/ob_home.htm
- National Heart, Lung, and Blood Institute Healthy People 2010 Gateway: http://hp2010.nhlbihin.net
- The National Institute for Occupational Safety and Health (NIOSH): http://www.cdc.gov/niosh
- National Institute on Aging: http://www.nia.nih.gov
- National Institutes of Health: http://www.nih.gov
- National Osteoporosis Foundation: http://www.nof.org
- National Strength and Conditioning Association (NSCA): http://www.nsca-lift.org
- Nutrition Navigator: http://navigator.nutrition.tufts.edu/
- Sportscience: http://www.sportsci.org
- StrongWomen.com: http://www.strongwomen.com
- U.S. Department of Health and Human Services: http://www.hhs.gov/
- The Weather Channel: http://www.weather.com

4

Nutrition

A basic knowledge of nutrition principles is essential for professionals working with physically active individuals. This chapter presents fundamental information regarding the macronutrients (*i.e.*, carbohydrate, protein, fat), highlights selected vitamins and minerals with specific regard for physical activity and human performance, and provides a basis for estimating energy requirements. Incorporated throughout this chapter are nutritional considerations for athletic performance and exercise.

KEY TERMS

Acceptable macronutrient distribution range (AMDR): Represents a range of intakes for a particular macronutrient associated with reduced risk of chronic diseases while providing adequate intake of essential nutrients.

Adequate intake (AI): The recommended average daily intake level based on observed or experimentally determined approximations or estimates of nutrient intake by a group (or groups) of apparently healthy people that are assumed to be adequate — used when a recommended dietary allowance (RDA) cannot be determined.

Aerobic: Biological processes that require oxygen.

Anaerobic: Biological processes that occur in the absence of oxygen.

Antioxidants: Dietary components present in small concentrations, such as vitamins C and E, which prevent or reduce the extent of oxidative damage of cellular components such as DNA and cell membranes by scavenging free radicals.

Dietary reference intake (DRI): A set of reference values for specific nutrients that expands upon the former RDA, which includes the estimated average requirement (EAR), RDA, AI, and tolerable upper intake level (UL).

Essential amino acid (EAA): Amino acids required for maintaining proper growth and development that are not synthesized in the body and therefore must be consumed in the diet. EAAs are also referred to as indispensable amino acids.

Essential nutrient: Essential nutrient refers to any nutrient, such as essential amino acids and fatty acids, necessary for normal body functions that is not synthesized in the body and must be consumed in the diet.

Estimated average requirement (EAR): Average daily nutrient intake level estimated to meet the requirement for half of the healthy individuals of a particular sex or life stage.

Gluconeogenesis: Endogenous production of new glucose from nonglucose carbon precursors, such as amino acids, lactate, pyruvate, and glycerol, which occurs primarily in the liver and, to a lesser extent, the kidney.

Glycemic index: The rate at which ingestion of a food or food component, such as carbohydrate, increases blood glucose in comparison to a reference food, white bread in particular.

Glycogenolysis: The breakdown of liver and muscle glycogen in response to elevated glucagon and epinephrine levels to produce either glucose in the liver that is able to be circulated throughout the body or glucose in skeletal muscle made available for energy production.

Glycolysis: The breakdown of glucose into two pyruvate molecules accompanied by the formation of adenosine triphosphate. The pyruvate can be converted to lactate or enter mitochondria for aerobic metabolism.

Macronutrients: Organic energy-providing nutrients, which include carbohydrate, fat, protein, and alcohol, consumed in large quantities in the diet.

Micronutrients: Organic and inorganic nutrients including vitamins and minerals, respectively, which are consumed and/or required in much lower amounts in comparison to the macronutrients.

Nonessential amino acids (NEAAs): Often referred to as dispensable amino acids, these amino acids are synthesized in the body and therefore not essential in the diet.

Recommended dietary allowance (RDA): Average daily dietary nutrient intake level sufficient to meet the nutrient requirement of nearly all healthy individuals of a particular gender and life stage.

Tolerable upper intake level (UL): The highest average daily nutrient intake level not likely to pose any risk of adverse health effects to almost all individuals in the general population. The potential risk for adverse effects may increase as intakes exceed the UL.

NUTRITION BASICS: THE MAJOR NUTRIENTS

There are two major classes of nutrients critical to the understanding of human nutrition: macronutrients and micronutrients. Each class of nutrients has an important role in optimizing growth, development, and health status. These nutrients are also vital for physical performance regardless of an individual's training status. The macronutrients — carbohydrate, protein, and fat (and alcohol) — are organic compounds that contain carbon, hydrogen, and oxygen. Protein is unique given it also contains nitrogen as a component of its constituent amino acids. The macronutrients provide energy (i.e., kilocalories), and the respective energy contents of these nutrients are listed in *Table 4-1*. Micronutrients include vitamins and minerals and are required in much lower quantities than the macronutrients. In addition, micronutrients do not provide energy. Nonetheless, vitamins and minerals are critical to proper growth and metabolism. A list of major vitamins and minerals is provided in *Tables 4-2* and *4-3*, respectively.

The proper blend of nutrients is necessary for normal growth and development, as well as maintenance of health. The Food and Nutrition Board of the National Academy of Sciences Research Council periodically issues a set of reference values known as the dietary reference intakes (DRIs). The DRIs include the recommended dietary allowance (RDA), adequate intake (AI), tolerable upper intake level (UL), and the estimated average requirement (EAR) of each macronutrient and micronutrient necessary to meet the nutritional needs of nearly all healthy people (7). The following sections review the roles of macronutrients and selected nutrients with consideration for the level of nutrient intake necessary for healthy adults.

CARBOHYDRATE

Carbohydrate, glucose specifically, is the preferred fuel source for the body, particularly the nervous system. As an energy source, carbohydrate provides $4 \text{ kcal} \cdot \text{g}^{-1}$ (see *Table 4-1*). Classified by the number of sugar molecules they contain, carbohydrates are either simple or complex. Simple carbohydrates include monosaccharides (i.e., one sugar molecule) and disaccharides (i.e., two sugar molecules). The most common forms of monosaccharides are glucose, fructose, and galactose. The most common disaccharides are sucrose, lactose, and maltose. Sucrose is commonly referred to as table sugar and composed of glucose and fructose. It is found primarily in sugar cane, honey, and maple syrup. Lactose is composed of glucose and galactose and is the sugar most commonly found in milk. Maltose is a disaccharide composed of two glucose molecules and a byproduct of complex carbohydrate digestion. It is frequently present in various sport nutrition products.

Complex carbohydrates consist of three or more monosaccharides linked together. Depending on chain length, complex carbohydrates are oligosaccharides or polysaccharides. Oligosaccharides are between 3 and 10 monosaccharides in length and found naturally in foods such as legumes, onions, and bananas. Polysaccharides are complex carbohydrates greater than 10 monosaccharides in length. Glycogen and starch are the most common polysaccharides. Glycogen is the storage form of glucose in humans and consists of numerous branched chains of glucose molecules stored in the liver and skeletal muscle. When necessary, glycogen is easily broken down under conditions of increased glucose demand. Glycogen is the major source of energy for the exercising muscle during very high-intensity (anaerobic) exercise as well as during prolonged endurance events,

TABLE 4-1. Macronutrient and Energy Content	
Macronutrient	**Energy (kcal · g⁻¹)**
Carbohydrate	4
Protein	4
Fat	9
Alcohol	7

TABLE 4-2. Micronutrients: Vitamins

Vitamin	Major Function	Dietary Sources	Recommended Intake (Adults)
Fat Soluble			
A	Maintenance of skin, bone, teeth, growth, and vision	Carrots, broccoli, spinach, eggs, cheese, and milk	700–900 μg $\cdot$ d^{-1}
D	Maintenance and growth of bones	Milk, egg yolk, tuna, and salmon	5–15 μg $\cdot$ d$^{-1\,a}$
E	Antioxidant	Vegetable oils, whole grains, green leafy vegetables	15 mg $\cdot$ d^{-1}
K	Blood clotting	Green leafy vegetables, cabbage, and milk	90–120 μg $\cdot$ d$^{-1\,a}$
Water Soluble			
B$_1$ (thiamin)	Energy production	Breads, pasta, pork, oysters	1.1–1.2 mg $\cdot$ d^{-1}
B$_2$ (riboflavin)	Energy production	Milk, meat, cereals, pasta, dark green vegetables	1.1–1.3 mg $\cdot$ d^{-1}
B$_3$ (niacin)	Energy production	Poultry, meat, tuna, cereal, pasta, bread, nuts, legumes	14–16 mg NE $\cdot$ d^{-1}
B$_6$ (pyridoxine)	Protein and fat metabolism	Avocados, green beans, spinach, cereals, bread	1.3–1.7 mg $\cdot$ d^{-1}
B$_{12}$ (cobalamine)	Red blood cell formation	Meat, fish, milk, eggs	2.4 μg $\cdot$ d^{-1}
Folic acid	DNA synthesis, red blood cell formation	Dark green leafy vegetables, fortified cereals, wheat germ, oranges, bananas	400 μg $\cdot$ d^{-1}
Pantothenic acid	Macronutrient metabolism, hormone synthesis	Cereals, bread, nuts, eggs, dark green vegetables	5 μg $\cdot$ d$^{-1\,a}$
C (ascorbic acid)	Antioxidant, maintenance of bones, teeth, collagen	Citrus fruits, melons, strawberries, tomatoes, green peppers, potatoes	75–90 mg $\cdot$ d^{-1}
Biotin	Fatty acid synthesis, energy production	Egg yolk, green leafy vegetables	30 μg $\cdot$ d$^{-1\,a}$

NE, niacin equivalents.

[a]Adequate intakes.

TABLE 4-3. Micronutrients: Sports-Related Minerals

Mineral	Major Function	Dietary Sources	Recommended Intake (Adults)
Major Minerals			
Calcium	Growth, bone and teeth formation, nerve impulses	Dairy, dark green vegetables, sardines, clams	1,000–1,300 mg $\cdot$ d^{-1}
Sodium[b]	Body water and acid–base balance, nerve function	Abundant in most foods	1,500 mg $\cdot$ d$^{-1\,a}$
Potassium[b]	Body water and acid–base balance, nerve function	Meat, milk, fruits, vegetables, cereals, legumes	4,700 mg $\cdot$ d$^{-1\,a}$
Chloride[b]	Acid–base balance	Table salt, seafood, meats, eggs, milk	2,300 mg $\cdot$ d$^{-1\,a}$
Phosphorus	Bone and teeth formation, acid–base balance	Dairy, meat, fish, poultry, nuts, grains	700 mg $\cdot$ d^{-1}
Trace Minerals			
Iron	Component of hemoglobin and enzymes	Meats, eggs, legumes, grains, dark green vegetables	8–18 mg $\cdot$ d^{-1}
Chromium	Glucose and energy metabolism	Fats, meats, cereals	25–35 μg $\cdot$ d$^{-1\,a}$
Zinc	Component of enzymes	Milk, shellfish, wheat bran	8–11 mg $\cdot$ d^{-1}

[a]Adequate intakes.

[b]Electrolytes.

particularly at moderate to vigorous, as opposed to light, exercise intensities. Starches are the primary storage form of carbohydrates in plants. They are composed of either amylose, which consists of straight chains of glucose molecules or amylopectin, which consists of branched-chain glucose molecules. Various food sources contain starches, such as vegetables, legumes, and grains.

Fiber is another type of complex carbohydrate. The human body does not digest or absorb fiber. Fiber consumption has beneficial effects on health, including improved gastrointestinal health, glucose homeostasis, and enhanced satiety. In addition, fiber consumption may lower hypertension, improve plasma cholesterol, and reduce the risk of developing cardiovascular disease. Fiber has also been associated with reduced risk of cancer. The current DRI for fiber is 25–38 $g \cdot d^{-1}$ for adult men and women, respectively (7).

The classification of fibers depends on their solubility in water. Water-soluble and water-insoluble fibers are present in varying amounts in all plant sources. Derived from the cell walls of plants, insoluble fibers include cellulose, hemicellulose, and lignins. Vegetables such as broccoli, carrots, and green beans, celery, and potato skins are common sources of insoluble fibers. Whole wheat, wheat bran, and flaxseed lignans are other sources of insoluble fiber. Insoluble fibers increase bulk, soften stool, and shorten intestinal transit time. Soluble fibers undergo a metabolic processing via fermentation by bacteria in the large intestine. The product of this bacterial fermentation is gas and short-chain fatty acids, which can be absorbed. Soluble fibers found within plant cells include pectins, gums, and certain hemicelluloses. Dietary sources of soluble fibers include oats, apples, and beans. These soluble fibers, along with psyllium, lower blood cholesterol levels by binding cholesterol in the gut, reducing its absorption, and removing it from the body.

Carbohydrate Digestion and Absorption

Digestion and absorption of carbohydrates occur in the mouth, stomach, small intestine, and large intestine, with the assistance of several essential secretory organs. Dietary carbohydrates are ultimately broken down into monosaccharides. Sugar molecules pass across the intestine into the blood and are distributed to all tissues in the body. The rate of digestion and absorption within the intestine is not the same for all carbohydrates.

Glycemic Response and Glycemic Index

The glycemic response encompasses the rate of carbohydrate digestion and absorption, the extent carbohydrates raise blood glucose concentration, and the duration blood glucose concentration remains elevated. The glycemic response varies by type and amount of carbohydrate ingested, as well as by the other nutrients consumed with the carbohydrates. Simple sugars, starches, and refined (*i.e.*, fiber has been removed) carbohydrates typically cause a greater glycemic response as reflected by a more rapid rise in blood glucose following their consumption. Unrefined carbohydrates, which contain fiber, cause a lower glycemic response because digestion and absorption take longer. Consuming protein and fat with carbohydrates can decrease the rate of carbohydrate digestion and absorption and subsequent appearance of glucose in blood.

The glycemic index reflects the glycemic response of a specific food. Glycemic index is a ranking of how a food affects blood glucose in comparison to an equal amount of a reference carbohydrate such as white bread or glucose. The reference food is assigned a value of 100, and test foods are expressed relative to the reference value. High glycemic foods have glycemic indexes greater than or equal to 70, whereas low glycemic foods have an index less than 55. Although the glycemic index can provide information regarding food sources effects on blood glucose, the glycemic index does not predict the impact of consuming these foods as a part of a mixed meal. The role of the glycemic index with specific regard to glycogen replenishment after exercise continues to be debated (12).

Carbohydrate Metabolism

Carbohydrates produce energy in the form of adenosine triphosphate (ATP) through aerobic metabolism. Complete metabolism of one molecule of glucose yields 38 ATP. The basic formula to describe this process is

$$C_6H_{12}O_6 + 38\ ADP + 38\ Pi + 6O_2 \Rightarrow 6CO_2 + 6H_2O + 38\ ATP$$

The following sections provide a brief overview of carbohydrate metabolism and energy production.

Glycolysis

Glycolysis is a series of reactions involving highly regulated enzymes and is the first stage of glucose metabolism. Glycolysis itself is an anaerobic process but is influenced by the potential for aerobic metabolism of its end product, pyruvate. The first stage of aerobic metabolism is the conversion of pyruvate to acetyl-coenzyme A (acetyl-CoA) within the mitochondria. However, when oxygen is limited, acetyl-CoA production is limited and pyruvate is preferentially converted to lactate. Lactate is a metabolic byproduct of anaerobic glucose metabolism.

Citric Acid Cycle and Electron Transport Chain

During aerobic metabolism of glucose, acetyl-CoA produced from pyruvate within the mitochondria combines with oxaloacetate in the citric acid cycle. The citric acid cycle generates one ATP molecule for each pyruvate formed (two from one glucose molecule). This process also generates high-energy electrons transported to the final stage of aerobic glucose metabolism using reduced cofactors (nicotinamide adenine dinucleotide [NAD] and flavin adenine dinucleotide [FAD]).

The electron transport chain is the final step in aerobic glucose metabolism. It involves a chain of molecules, mostly proteins, associated with the inner mitochondrial membrane. This chain accepts high-energy electrons that are produced by glycolysis, the conversion of pyruvate to acetyl-CoA, and the citric acid cycle. Electrons are shuttled to the mitochondria and passed down the chain until they are combined with oxygen to form water. Energy is conserved during the passing of the electrons and used to generate ATP. The citric acid cycle and the electron transport chain are essential for maintaining energy-producing processes in the body. Utilization of the macronutrients for fuel is highly integrated with the citric acid cycle being the primary point of convergence (*Fig. 4-1*).

Gluconeogenesis and Glycogenolysis: The Maintenance of Blood Glucose

Some reactions of glycolysis can be reversed to produce new blood glucose in conditions where blood glucose levels are low, such as fasting or low carbohydrate intake. Gluconeogenesis is the production of new glucose and occurs primarily in the liver. The major substrates for gluconeogenesis are lactate, selected amino acids (*e.g.*, alanine), and glycerol. Gluconeogenesis is highly regulated, mostly through the action of hormones such as insulin and glucagon.

Another source of glucose for the body is glycogen stored in the liver and muscle. Liver glycogenolysis supplies blood glucose to the entire body via the bloodstream,

whereas muscle glycogen is a source of glucose exclusive to the muscle. As glycogen stores decrease, adipose tissue is degraded, providing fatty acids as an alternative fuel and glycerol for the synthesis of glucose via gluconeogenesis. During an overnight fast, gluconeogenesis and glycogenolysis work synergistically to maintain blood glucose. However, liver glycogen is depleted after approximately 30 h of fasting, and gluconeogenesis becomes the only source of new blood glucose.

Hormones and the Regulation of Blood Glucose

Insulin and glucagon are pancreatic hormones that regulate blood glucose. In response to an increase in blood glucose, insulin stimulates glucose uptake into cells and promotes glucose storage as liver glycogen. In muscle, insulin promotes glucose uptake for energy production and stimulates glycogen synthesis for energy storage in the muscle. The major role of insulin is to maintain glucose homeostasis by decreasing blood glucose levels after a meal containing carbohydrates.

In the fasted state, blood glucose levels begin to decline. Low blood glucose stimulates the release of glucagon, which stimulates gluconeogenesis and glycogenolysis in the liver to increase blood glucose. In addition to glucagon, the hormone epinephrine also promotes glucose production under conditions of increased energy demand. Overall, the role of glucagon and epinephrine are to increase blood glucose, whereas the primary action of insulin is to decrease blood glucose levels.

Recommended Carbohydrate Intake

On average, carbohydrate intake provides approximately 40%–60% of the total energy intake in the American diet. The following sections present recommendations regarding carbohydrate intake for maintaining and promoting health.

Carbohydrate Dietary Reference Intakes

Carbohydrates are not a required nutrient *per se* given the body's ability to produce glucose via gluconeogenesis. However, carbohydrates provide an important source of energy for the central nervous system as well as exercising muscle. In addition, diets high in fiber may confer health benefits. Therefore, the current DRIs suggest an RDA for total carbohydrate intake, an acceptable macronutrient distribution range (AMDR) for carbohydrates, and an AI for fiber. There is no UL for carbohydrates.

The current RDA for carbohydrates is 130 g · d^{-1} for both children and adults, which is the minimum amount of glucose required by the central nervous system. This equates to approximately 25% of the energy in a 2,000-kcal diet. The AMDR for carbohydrate intake for a healthy diet ranges from 45% to 65% of total energy. The source of carbohydrates should come from complex

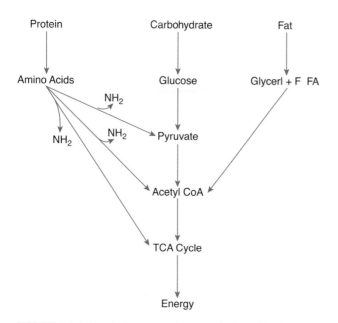

FIGURE 4-1. Integrated macronutrient metabolism. FFA, free fatty acid; CoA, coenzyme A; TCA, tricarboxylic acid.

unrefined carbohydrates with no more than 25% of the total energy derived from refined carbohydrates and less than 10% from simple sugars. The absolute intake of carbohydrate (*i.e.*, grams per day) will differ between individuals based upon total energy needs. To calculate energy intake, refer to *Table 4-4*. Once an estimated energy requirement has been determined, multiply total kilocalories by the percentage of carbohydrate intake to estimate carbohydrate kilocalories. Divide this estimate of carbohydrate kilocalories by 4 kcal · g^{-1} of carbohydrate to determine grams of carbohydrate. As previously discussed, the AI for fiber is 38 and 25 g · d^{-1} for adult men and women, respectively.

The recommendation for dietary fiber intake is the same for all athletes. Carbohydrate intakes should approximate 6–10 g · kg^{-1} for endurance athletes (2,10). To replenish and maintain adequate muscle glycogen stores for endurance performance, athletes should consume this amount of carbohydrate throughout training and competition. Depending on the athlete (*i.e.*, age, sex, height, weight, and training status), the recommended intake of carbohydrate will range from approximately 50%–65% of the total kilocalorie intake.

In conclusion, the DRIs recommend that a healthy diet contain carbohydrates in the aforementioned amounts. Americans can meet these requirements by consuming a diet high in whole grains, fruits, and vegetables. The healthy American diet should also be low in added simple sugars and refined carbohydrates such as those seen in soft drinks, bakery products, and candy.

FAT

Fat, or lipid, is the most energy-dense macronutrient. Fats provide 9 kcal · g^{-1} — more than twice the energy content of both carbohydrate and protein (see *Table 4-1*). The most recognizable forms of fats in the diet are oils, butter, high-fat dairy products, and animal products. Although a negative perception often exists with regard to consumption of fat because of its implications in the development of cardiovascular disease, some sources of dietary fats such as avocados, nuts, and certain oils confer many health benefits.

Fat is stored in the body in large amounts in adipose tissue. These fat stores represent a large energy reservoir utilized during resting conditions, certain modes of exercise, and during energy-restricted states. In addition to being a source of energy, fat serves many vital roles in the human body such as insulating and protecting vital organs. Fats are also an integral component of cell membranes and necessary for the production of steroid hormones such as testosterone and estrogen.

The primary fats in both food and in the body are in the form of triglycerides and cholesterol. Depending on their chemical structure, fats are classified as saturated or unsaturated fatty acids, which include monounsaturated and polyunsaturated fatty acids. Unsaturated fatty acids contain carbon–carbon double bonds that differ from saturated fatty acids, which contain carbons saturated with hydrogen. Unsaturated fatty acids are classified by the number of double bonds in the carbon chain, which can either be monounsaturated (one double bond) or polyunsaturated (more than one) fatty acids. Oleic acid is the most common dietary monounsaturated fatty acid and found primarily in olive and canola oil. Linoleic acid, found in corn, safflower, and soybean oils, is the most common polyunsaturated fatty acid in the diet.

Dietary fat provides the essential fatty acids (EFAs), linoleic and linolenic acids. The most common ω-3 fatty acids are α-linolenic acid, eicosapentaenoic acid (EPA), and docasahexaenoic acid (DHA), found in vegetable and fish oils. Linoleic acid, present in corn and safflower oil, and arachidonic acid, found in meat and fish, are the most common ω-6 fatty acids. These EFAs are required for growth, for healthy skin, and for producing elements

TABLE 4-4. Calculating Estimated Energy Requirements (ERR)^a

Activity Level	Determination of Physical Activity Level (PAL)			
	Boys 3–18 yr	**Girls 3–18 yr**	**Men ≥19 yr**	**Women ≥19 yr**
Sedentary	1.00	1.00	1.00	1.00
Low active	1.13	1.16	1.11	1.12
Active	1.26	1.31	1.25	1.27
Very active	1.42	1.56	1.48	1.45
Age Group	**EER Prediction Equations**^{b}			
Boys 9–18 yr	EER = 88.5 − (61.90 × Age in yr) + PAL [(26.70 × Weight in kg) + (903.0 × Height in m)] + 25			
Girls 9–18 yr	EER = 135.5 − (30.80 × Age in yr) + PAL [(10.00 × Weight in kg) + (934.0 × Height in m)] + 25			
Men ≥19 yr	ERR = 662 − (9.53 × Age in yr) + PAL [(15.91 × Weight in kg) + (539.6 × Height in m)]			
Women ≥19 yr	ERR = 354 − (6.91 × Age in yr) + PAL [(9.36 × Weight in kg) + (726.0 × Height in m)]			

^{a}Referenced from the 2005 dietary reference intakes (DRIs).

^{b}These equations are based on energy required for weight maintenance in normal-weight individuals.

of the immune system. Although the body requires only small amounts of EFA (2%–3% of total energy), obtaining sufficient amounts may require consuming a diet containing at least 10% of total energy from fat because the proportion of EFAs in the diet is small.

The position of the hydrogen atoms around the carbon–carbon double bond affects the properties of unsaturated fatty acids. Most unsaturated fatty acids have both hydrogen atoms on the same side of the double bond referred to as a *cis* configuration. Other unsaturated fatty acids with hydrogen atoms on opposing sides of the double bond are in the *trans* configuration, more commonly referred to as trans fatty acids. Naturally occurring foods do not typically contain trans fatty acids. However, unsaturated fatty acids are altered from the cis to the trans configurations and become more saturated through a process known as hydrogenation. Trans fatty acids are deleterious to health by increasing the risk of coronary artery disease (CAD) by negatively influencing blood cholesterol. Although there is no DRI for trans fatty acids, dietary intake should not exceed approximately 3% of total energy intake.

Cholesterol is a waxy, fatlike substance found in foods of animal origin. Cholesterol found in cell membranes performs several essential anatomical and physiological functions such as the formation of bile acid and steroid hormones. Plants or plant products do not contain cholesterol. The liver produces cholesterol transported in the blood by distinct particles containing both lipids and proteins (*i.e.*, lipoproteins). There are three major classes of lipoproteins: (a) low-density lipoproteins (LDLs), (b) high-density lipoproteins (HDLs), and (c) very low-density lipoproteins (VLDLs). In general, the liver produces sufficient amounts of cholesterol to meet requirements. Therefore, dietary consumption is unnecessary. However, many food sources contain cholesterol. Thus, recommendations regarding dietary cholesterol intake suggest consuming no more than 300 mg $\cdot$ d^{-1}. Although monitoring cholesterol intake is important, dietary saturated and trans fatty acids have a more substantial negative impact on blood cholesterol, a risk factor for CAD. For more information regarding cholesterol and its influence on CAD, please refer to the Adult Panel Treatment III issued by the National Cholesterol Education Program (11).

Fat Digestion and Absorption

Most fat digestion occurs in the small intestine. In the presence of fat, the small intestine releases cholecystokinin or CCK, a hormone that signals the release of bile acid from the gallbladder. Bile acids "emulsify" dietary fat in the small intestine so there is effective mixing with the fat-digesting enzymes in the small intestine, ultimately leaving triglycerides and diglycerides to monoglycerides, fatty acids, and glycerol for absorption.

The small intestine directly absorbs short- and medium-chain fatty acids along with glycerol, which then enter the bloodstream. However, the small intestine absorbs monoglycerides and long-chain fatty acids repackaged into micelles. Micelles are then repackaged into chylomicrons (*i.e.*, lipoproteins) in the intestinal cells and released into the lymphatic system and eventual into the bloodstream.

The lipoproteins, with the exception of the chylomicron, produced in the liver transport triglycerides and cholesterol through the blood. VLDLs are a major carrier of triglycerides. LDLs are principally composed of cholesterol. LDLs transport cholesterol that may be deposited in the arterial walls and contribute to atherosclerosis. The smallest group of lipoproteins, the HDLs, appears to be protective by carrying cholesterol to the liver for breakdown and excretion. Therefore, individuals with high levels of HDL, low levels of LDL, low total cholesterol, and low total cholesterol/HDL cholesterol ratio carry the lowest risk of CAD. The impact of the type of fat consumed (saturated vs. unsaturated vs. trans fatty acids) on blood lipid levels occurs through changes in the metabolism of these lipoproteins. Dietary modifications (*i.e.*, reduced total, saturated, and trans fat), along with regular exercise, have been shown to favorably influence lipoprotein profiles.

Fat and Energy Metabolism

During periods of excess energy intake, regardless of the macronutrient source, the body stores excess calories as fat in adipose tissue. Calories from dietary fat have the most efficient and direct route to storage when energy intake is higher than energy expenditure. During times of energy deficit (*e.g.*, fasting), the body can utilize dietary fat to produce energy. During endurance exercise, the body also utilizes stored fat as an energy source.

Defining Fat Intake

Fats are vital for numerous roles in the body, including energy production, structural components of cell membranes, and the production of steroid hormones. In addition, fats are necessary in the diet for the absorption of fat-soluble vitamins and the EFAs. Similar to carbohydrates and unlike protein, fats can be synthesized from endogenous nonfat precursors, which reduce their necessity in the diet. In general, American diets are composed of approximately 33% fat, more than enough to meet daily requirements for the EFAs and to allow for absorption of fat-soluble vitamins. Recommendations for a healthy diet include limiting saturated and trans fat intakes.

Fat Dietary Reference Intakes

There is no RDA for fat. However, the DRIs do include an AI and AMDR for EFAs along with an AMDR for total fat intake. Saturated fat intake should be no more than 10% of the total energy intake, and cholesterol should be less than 300 mg $\cdot$ d^{-1}. In addition, trans fat should be no more than 2.6% of the total energy intake. The AI for linoleic acid — an EFA — is 17 g $\cdot$ d^{-1} for men and 12 g $\cdot$ d^{-1} for women. The AI for α-linolenic acid is 1.6 g $\cdot$ d^{-1} for men and 1.1 g $\cdot$ d^{-1} for women. The AMDR for linoleic acid is between 5% and 10% of total energy intake, whereas the AMDR for α-linolenic acid is between 0.6% and 1.2% of total energy intake.

The AMDR for total fat intake is between 20% and 35% of the total energy intake. Diets providing fat in excess of 35% of total energy intake are likely high in calories and possibly saturated fats. On the other hand, diets providing fat intake of less than 20% of the total energy intake increase the risk of certain fat-soluble vitamin deficiencies and negative alterations in lipoprotein and blood triglyceride levels. To estimate dietary fat intake, calculate energy intake as shown in *Table 4-4*. Once an estimated energy requirement has been determined, multiply total kilocalories by the percentage of fat intake and divide it by 9 kcal $\cdot$ g^{-1} of fat.

PROTEIN

Of the macronutrients, protein is unique because of the nitrogen content of its constituent amino acids. Similar to carbohydrate, protein provides 4 kcal $\cdot$ g^{-1} (see *Table 4-1*). When proteins are oxidized for energy purposes or when dietary intake exceeds recommended amounts, CO_2 and water are produced, and the N component is (a) incorporated into urea and eliminated from the body in urine or (b) used in the synthesis of dispensable amino acids and other nitrogen-containing compounds in the body. Considered a required and vital nutrient, proteins serve structural and functional roles in the body. In addition to serving as structural components of muscle, bone, tendons, and ligaments, proteins function as enzymes critical in energy-producing reactions, hormones that regulate metabolism, transporters of other critical nutrients, and as an energy source in energy-deprived conditions. The latter function is the least desirable for this particular macronutrient.

Dietary and body proteins are composed of amino acids, which are classified as either essential (indispensable) or nonessential (dispensable). **Nonessential amino acids (NEAAs)** are amino acids made by the body, whereas **essential amino acids (EAAs)** cannot be synthesized in the body and therefore must be consumed in the diet. A list of the EAAs and NEAAs is shown in *Table 4-5*. All amino acids are needed to maintain optimal protein utilization in the body such that health, growth and development, and tissue maintenance and repair are promoted. The branched-chain amino acids (BCAA) (leucine, isoleucine, valine) are a unique class of essential amino acids used almost exclusively by skeletal muscles.

TABLE 4-5. Classification of Amino Acids

Essential (Indispensable) Amino Acids (EAAs)

Isoleucine

Leucine

Lysine

Methionine

Phenylalanine

Threonine

Tryptophan

Valine

Histidine

Nonessential (Dispensable) Amino Acids (NEAAs)

Alanine

Arginine

Aspartic acid

Asparagine

Glutamic acid

Glutamine

Glycine

Proline

Serine

Branched-Chain Amino Acids (BCAAs)

Isoleucine

Leucine

Valine

Sources of Dietary Protein and Protein Quality

Protein is abundant in meat and dairy products and found in significant levels in cereals, grains, nuts, and legumes. In addition, certain fruits (*i.e.*, apples, blueberries, and apricots) and vegetables (*i.e.*, green beans and asparagus) contain small amounts of protein. The amino acid content and the digestibility of a protein determine its quality. Proteins derived from plant foods are approximately 85% digestible; those in a mixed diet of meat products and refined carbohydrates are approximately 95% digestible. Protein quality also considers the "completeness" of the dietary protein.

Complete or high quality proteins contain all of the EAAs. Plant proteins are generally incomplete and considered to be of less quality than animal proteins. Plants do contain all of the amino acids but in lower amounts than animal proteins. One needs to eat more of a plant protein source to obtain adequate amounts of the amino acids, particularly the EAAs. In some cases, one must consume more than one source of plant protein to obtain a sufficient amount of the EAA. Grains tend to lack lysine, for example, and legumes tend to lack methionine.

Consuming both plant protein sources together allow for complementary amino acid combinations (such as soybeans and rice, wheat bread and peanut butter, pinto beans and corn tortillas) so that the diet contains sufficient amounts of EAAs. The latter point is important for individuals adhering to a vegan diet plan (15).

Protein Digestion, Absorption, and Utilization

Protein digestion begins in the stomach and is completed in the intestine. Amino acids resulting from dietary protein degradation are absorbed in the intestine. Once amino acids have been absorbed, they become available to the body. Collectively, amino acids reside in various amino acid pools, used for (a) maintenance, synthesis, or repair of body proteins; (b) synthesis of other nitrogen-containing compounds; and (c) energy production.

Protein Turnover

Protein turnover is a dynamic process that includes the synthesis and breakdown of new and existing body proteins. Amino acids derived from dietary sources and from endogenous breakdown of body proteins are used to maintain protein turnover (Fig. 4-2). The rate of protein turnover varies between proteins and is specific to their individual function. Intricate cycling of amino acids and body proteins is important for growth, maintenance, and repair of body tissues and for adaptation to different conditions.

Recommended Protein Intake and the Dietary Reference Intakes

The RDA for protein for adults is 0.8 g of protein per kilogram body mass, or approximately 0.4 g of protein per pound; the DRIs for protein range approximately from 0.7 to 1.5 g · kg^{-1} (or about 0.3–0.7 g · lb^{-1}). The DRIs

include an AMDR for dietary protein that ranges from 10% to 35% of the total kilocalories provided by the diet for optimal use of protein for various physiological challenges (e.g., aging, weight management).

To calculate protein intake using the AMDR, refer to Table 4-4 and follow the same steps previously described for carbohydrates. A diet for which protein provides 10% of the total energy intake will meet the RDA but is a relatively low-protein diet based on normal protein consumption in the United States. The upper end of the AMDR for protein provides for a higher protein diet that often raises concerns regarding kidney damage, dehydration, and increased urinary calcium excretion. These concerns do not apply to healthy individuals with normal renal function (17). The recommendations put forth by My Plate (Fig. 4-3) will help ensure the appropriate blend of protein sources necessary for a healthy diet.

Individuals should consume various proteins from both animal and plant sources. Animal sources include lean meats, poultry, fish, eggs, and low-fat dairy products, whereas vegetable sources include soy, whole grains, legumes, and vegetables.

Protein Intake for Physically Active Individuals

Protein metabolism during and following exercise is affected by sex, age, exercise intensity and duration, carbohydrate availability, type of exercise, and energy intake. The current RDA of 0.8 g · kg^{-1} of body mass does not consider the unique needs of routinely active individuals and competitive athletes. The 2005 DRIs provide a range of protein intakes (~10%–35% of total energy intake) necessary for most populations.

The noted increase in protein oxidation during endurance exercise, coupled with nitrogen balance studies,

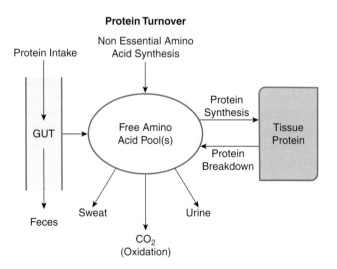

FIGURE 4-2. General representation of protein turnover.

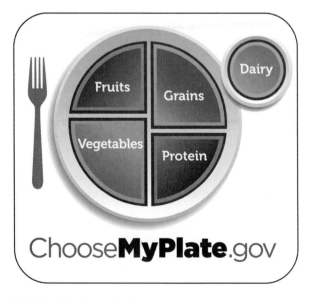

FIGURE 4-3. ChooseMyPlate.gov.

serves as the basis for recommending increased protein intakes to aid the body in recovery from habitual endurance training. Nitrogen balance studies suggested that the dietary protein intake necessary to support nitrogen balance in endurance athletes ranges from 1.2 to 1.4 g $\cdot$ kg^{-1} $\cdot$ d^{-1} (19). Resistance exercise increases protein needs to a greater extent than endurance exercise because additional amino acids and sufficient energy are needed in excess of the requirement to support muscle growth. This is particularly true at the initiation of strength training because the most significant gains in muscle size will occur in the early period. Individuals who have habitually engaged in resistance training may not require as much protein because of more efficient protein utilization (18). The recommended protein intakes for strength-trained athletes range approximately from 1.4 to 1.7 g $\cdot$ kg^{-1} $\cdot$ d^{-1}.

ALCOHOL

Alcohol (*i.e.*, ethanol) provides 7 kcal $\cdot$ g^{-1} (see *Table 4-1*). Alcohol is readily absorbed by the gastrointestinal tract by simple diffusion, with most absorption occurring in the small intestine. Rapid absorption of alcohol is responsible for its deleterious effects on mental and physical function. Body weight, sex, the type and concentration of alcohol, rate of alcohol consumption, and foods consumed with alcohol determine blood alcohol levels. The liver metabolizes most alcohol. The remainder is lost in urine or exhaled. Excess alcohol consumption can cause acute alcohol intoxication, malnutrition, and chronic diseases, particularly liver damage. However, moderate alcohol consumption (*i.e.*, one and two drinks per day for women and men, respectively), in particular consuming red wine, may confer health benefits such as improved lipoprotein profiles and reduced cardiovascular disease risk.

The effects of alcohol consumption persist for up to 48 h and compromise several factors related to athletic performance. Alcohol metabolism by the liver interferes with glycogen synthesis and glucose metabolism. Immune function, recovery from exercise or injury, and hydration status can be impaired with alcohol consumption. Therefore, athletes are discouraged from consuming alcohol during training or competition (6,10).

VITAMINS

Vitamins are vital organic compounds not synthesized by the body and are essential for optimal growth, development, and the maintenance of health. These nutrients are required, and the diet must provide small amounts on a routine basis. Vitamins are classified based upon their solubility in water or fat. Water-soluble vitamins include the B vitamins and vitamin C. There are no storage forms of water-soluble vitamins, making regular consumption important. Fat-soluble vitamins A, D, E, and K, however,

are stored in adipose tissue and thus are not required in the diet. *Table 4-2* provides a comprehensive list of the water- and fat-soluble vitamins, their primary function, dietary sources, and respective requirements for adults. The following sections provide an overview of this information with specific regard for exercise and physical performance.

Function of Vitamins

Each vitamin, be it water- or fat-soluble, has a unique role and, in some cases, works synergistically with other vitamins to contribute to health and well-being. Vitamins serve as promoters and regulators of many reactions in the body, including energy-producing reactions (thiamin, riboflavin, niacin, B$_6$, B$_{12}$, biotin, and pantothenic acid). More specifically, the B vitamins, along with biotin and pantothenic acid, act as coenzymes that bind to enzymes to promote their activity and assure proper function in the metabolism of the macronutrients. Other important roles of vitamins include aiding in the visual processes (vitamin A), blood coagulation (vitamin K), and protection of cells from oxidative damage (**antioxidants**; vitamins E and C). *Table 4-2* summarizes the major functions of these vitamins.

B Complex Vitamins

The B complex vitamins include thiamin, riboflavin, niacin, B$_6$, B$_{12}$, biotin, pantothenic acid, and folate. These vitamins have roles in energy production, red blood cell production, and amino acid metabolism.

Energy Production

Several B vitamins are essential to energy production by the body. These include thiamin, riboflavin, niacin, B$_6$, biotin, and pantothenic acid. Thiamin, riboflavin, and niacin in particular are associated with cofactors that are integral to energy-producing pathways for the macronutrients. Biotin, B$_6$, and B$_{12}$ are coenzymes for various carboxylases involved in macronutrient metabolism.

Red Blood Cell Production

Folate and B$_{12}$ are involved in red blood cell production. Deficiencies of either nutrient can lead to anemia. Given the critical role that red blood cells serve in oxygen delivery throughout the body, inadequate intake of folate or B$_{12}$ is associated with fatigue and compromised athletic performance.

Amino Acid Metabolism

Vitamin B$_6$ is required for amino acid metabolism. B$_6$ is part of several enzyme systems that are involved in nitrogen metabolism. This nutrient is essential to reactions required for protein utilization as a fuel and synthesis of nitrogen-containing compounds in the body.

Vitamin C

Vitamin C supplementation is popular, given this nutrient's roles in supporting the immune system and the healing process. Consumption of vitamin C (*i.e.*, food source or supplement) can facilitate iron absorption. Vitamin C is also a powerful antioxidant.

Fat-Soluble Vitamins

The fat-soluble vitamins (A, D, E, and K) are stored in body lipids. As a result, these nutrients can be toxic if taken in excess. *Table 4-2* describes the respective roles of these nutrients. Of the fat-soluble vitamins, only vitamin E has a role specific to exercise and human performance as an antioxidant.

Vitamin D has emerged as a nutrient of significance to healthy, physically active men, and women, as well as competitive athletes. In addition to bone health, vitamin D contributes to muscle function, the inflammatory response, and the immune system (3,13,16). The prevalence of vitamin D deficiency has increased as individuals adopt behaviors to reduce or protect themselves from exposure to sunlight. As a result, evaluation of vitamin D status is becoming more routine and supplementation strategies have been developed (13). The recommended intake of vitamin D is 600 IU for children and most adults. Dietary sources include fortified milk, fatty fish, egg yolks, margarine and some yogurts (16). Supplementation protocols vary and further research is warranted to standardize the approach to assessment of vitamin D status and interventions to manage insufficiency and deficiency of this nutrient.

Antioxidants

Vitamin E acts as an antioxidant by protecting the polyunsaturated fatty acids in cell membranes from oxidative damage (4,5). This protective action helps maintain the integrity of cell membranes. Other vitamins and minerals, such as vitamin C and selenium, also have antioxidant properties.

Dietary Sources of Vitamins

The presence of vitamins in foods is ubiquitous. Most foods contain some, if not many, of the vitamins (see *Table 4-2*). For example, grains, meat, and fish provide B vitamins. Leafy green vegetables contain large amounts of vitamins A, E, and K. Citrus fruits provide large amounts of vitamin C. Dairy products are good sources of vitamins A and D. Another source of vitamins in the diet is fortified foods. Fortification is the process of adding nutrients to foods to prevent deficiencies. Folic acid fortification, which was mandated by the U.S. Food and Drug Administration (FDA) in 1998 in an attempt to reduce serious birth defects (*i.e.*, neural tube defects), is the most recent example of nutrient fortification. The goal of the fortification program is to provide adequate nutrients for a beneficial effect without increasing the risk of vitamin toxicity.

MINERALS

Numerous metabolic reactions and physiologic processes require minerals (see *Table 4-3*). Major minerals are found in the body in amounts greater than 5 g, whereas trace minerals are needed in lesser amounts. Major minerals include calcium, phosphorus, potassium, magnesium, sulfur, sodium, and chloride. Normal body functions require common trace minerals, including iron, zinc, copper, iodine, and chromium. Mineral salts, or electrolytes, including sodium and chloride, dissolve in body water. The most noted functions of sodium, chloride, and potassium are as electrolytes involved in the regulation of water balance in the body and maintenance of electrical potentials across the membranes of excitable cells. The following sections highlight the importance and functions of calcium and iron.

Calcium

Calcium is required for healthy bones and teeth, muscle contraction, nerve transmission, and blood clotting. The role of calcium in bone formation is well known (14). Low intakes of dietary calcium result in calcium removal from the bone to maintain normal body processes. Bone turnover is compromised and bone mass is reduced if low calcium intakes persists. Routine exercise, particularly weight-bearing exercise, enhances calcium utilization and maintenance of bone mass (14,21). Although it is important for men to consume adequate calcium, women appear to be at particular risk for poor calcium intakes that may ultimately increase risk for osteoporosis later in life. The current RDA for calcium is 1,300 and 1,000 mg daily for individuals aged 13–18 and 19–30 yr, respectively. This amount of calcium, in combination with routine physical activity or exercise, will promote attainment of peak bone mass, which may reduce risk for or postpone the onset of osteoporosis later in life (20). Primary sources of calcium in the diet are dairy products, bone (*e.g.*, edible bones in sardines and canned salmon) and supplements. Dark, leafy greens and figs are among the best plant sources, but even these are limited compared to dairy and bone.

Iron

Iron is one of the most highly regarded trace minerals given its role as a component of the oxygen-carrying proteins, hemoglobin and myoglobin. Because hemoglobin carries oxygen in the body and myoglobin aids in oxygen delivery in the muscle, iron is important for aerobic metabolism and endurance exercise performance. Iron is also a constituent of several of the enzymes that constitute the electron transport chain. Therefore, iron has an essential role in energy production by the body.

Maintaining iron reserves by consistently consuming adequate amounts of iron is important for support of aerobic metabolism and energy production. Iron deficiency anemia results from compromised iron intake and reduced iron stores. Females are particularly susceptible to iron deficiency anemia. At-risk populations include female athletes, adolescent girls, athletes with low body weight, and those individuals who do not consume red meat. Iron requirements are set at 15–18 mg $\cdot$ d^{-1} for males and females, respectively (8).

The diet provides two different types of iron: heme and nonheme. Found mainly in animal products, heme iron originates mostly from hemoglobin and myoglobin. Plant products contain nonheme iron. Heme and nonheme iron are absorbed differently. Absorbed by the small intestine, heme iron is more highly bioavailable than nonheme iron. About 25% of heme iron is typically absorbed from the diet, whereas only ~17% of nonheme iron is absorbed. Dietary factors do not influence heme absorption whereas nonheme iron absorption improves with ingestion of vitamin C. Good sources of heme iron include animal products, whereas dark, leafy vegetables; beans; and raisins contain nonheme iron.

Vitamin and Mineral Supplementation

Individuals who restrict total energy intake or consume a diet with limited dietary variety are at risk of vitamin and mineral insufficiency. These individuals would benefit from a multivitamin mineral supplement that provides the recommended amounts of the micronutrients. Consumption of megadoses of vitamin or mineral supplements should be discouraged given the potential for toxicities or altered metabolism of other vitamins and minerals. Routine consumption of various nutritious foods among the basic food groups practically ensures AI of vitamins and minerals.

DIETARY GUIDELINES FOR AMERICANS

The Dietary Guidelines for Americans, 2010 are science-based directives aimed at promoting health and reducing risk for chronic diseases through diet and physical activity. Consuming a diet that meets nutritional requirements is the foundation for the dietary guidelines. Key recommendations for the general population address the following areas: adequate nutrients within calorie needs, weight management, and physical activity; and food groups to encourage fats, carbohydrates, sodium, potassium, alcoholic beverages, and food safety. In brief,

the dietary guidelines describe a healthy diet as one that emphasizes whole grains, fruits, vegetables, and fat-free or low-fat milk and milk products; includes lean meats, fish, poultry, eggs, beans, and nuts; and is low in saturated fats, trans fats, cholesterol, sodium, and added sugars. The complete recommendations contained in the report, as well as additional directives for various populations can be found at http://www.health.gov/dietaryguidelines/.

ChooseMyPlate.gov (see *Fig. 4-3*) was developed by the U.S. Department of Agriculture (USDA) to provide consumers with direction regarding portion size, food choices, and menu planning that are consistent with the Dietary Guidelines for Americans, 2010. ChooseMyPlate.gov is an interactive, user-friendly tool designed to assist people with making smart choices from each food group, finding balance between food groups, maximizing the nutrition from calories, and staying within daily calorie needs using a familiar mealtime visual, a place setting.

WATER BALANCE

Approximately two-thirds of a person's body weight is water. Water serves several functions in the body, including carrying nutrients and waste products; maintaining the integrity of proteins and glycogen; participating in metabolic reactions; providing a medium for the nutrients; maintaining blood volume, blood pressure, and body temperature; and acting as a lubricant. Although imbalances in body water can occur (*i.e.*, dehydration), the body is efficient in restoring fluid balance by regulating water intake and excretion with various mechanisms.

Fluid balance consists of water intake and water excretion. In healthy individuals, thirst controls water intake. Although thirst sensation can fall behind the body's water needs, most individuals are able to stay adequately hydrated. Sources of water to the body are liquids, foods, and metabolic water. These sources can provide approximately 1.4–3.0 L of water daily.

The kidney primarily controls water losses from the body by responding to various hormones. Water is lost from the body as excretory products (*i.e.*, urine and feces) and sweat and through ventilation. Approximately 1.4–3.0 L of cumulative water loss occurs daily. The posterior pituitary releases antidiuretic hormone (ADH) when the blood volume or blood pressure is too low, stimulating kidney reabsorption of water. Decreases in blood volume and blood pressure also elicit the release of aldosterone from the adrenal cortex, which causes sodium and water retention by the kidneys. Water balance is maintained when fluid intake from foods, liquids, and metabolism equals losses from the kidneys, skin, lungs, and feces.

Water needs are variable and dependent on the foods an individual eats, the environment (*i.e.*, heat and humidity) and activity level. The AI for total water is 3.7 and 2.7 L · d^{-1} for men and women, respectively. This recommendation is based on average intakes, because a wide range of water intakes can prevent dehydration (9).

GENERAL CONSIDERATIONS FOR ATHLETIC PERFORMANCE AND EXERCISE

Trained athletes and individuals who routinely exercise have increased energy and, therefore, macronutrient needs. These individuals should pay special attention to carbohydrate and protein intakes. Dietary carbohydrate should provide 6–8 g · kg^{-1} · d^{-1} to maintain, as well as replenish, the body's glycogen stores. Protein intake of approximately 1.2–1.7 g · kg^{-1} is needed to maintain, build, and repair tissue on a daily basis. Fat intake should be adequate to provide the EFAs and fat-soluble vitamins. In addition, dietary fat is an important energy source for weight maintenance. Active individuals should consume adequate food and fluid before, during, and after exercise to support maintenance of blood glucose levels during exercise, optimize exercise performance, and support recovery, respectively.

As long as athletes meet their energy needs to maintain body weight by consuming a varied and balanced diet, vitamin and mineral supplementation is not necessary. Micronutrient supplementation may be necessary for athletes who restrict energy intake, routinely eliminate one or more food groups from their diet, or habitually consume unbalanced diets of low micronutrient content.

Hydration status cannot be overemphasized. Athletes should be well hydrated before exercise. To balance fluid losses, effort should be made — drink adequate fluid during and after exercise (1). Consumption of sports beverages containing carbohydrates and electrolytes before, during, and after exercise can provide fuel for muscles and decrease risk of dehydration. Postexercise consumption of a beverage that contains a combination of protein and carbohydrate may enhance glycogen replacement, aid muscle repair, and promote muscle hydration better than other beverages.

SUMMARY

This chapter provides an overview of basic nutrition principles for the health fitness professional. The intent is to provide a foundation for application of essential nutrition information to the health and well-being of healthy, physically active adults. Recommendations are made with regard to appropriate food choices to balance energy intake with expenditure while acquiring **essential nutrients** from the diet. Basic nutrition concepts are consistent with the current dietary Dietary Guidelines for Americans, 2010, and where appropriate, considerations in support of exercise and athletic performance are provided.

REFERENCES

1. American College of Sports Medicine, Sawka MN, Burke LM, et al. American College of Sports Medicine position stand. Exercise and fluid replacement. *Med Sci Sports Exerc.* 2007;39(2): 377–90.
2. American Dietetic Association, Dietitians of Canada, American College of Sports Medicine, Rodriguez NR, Di Marco NM, Langley S. American College of Sports Medicine position stand. Nutrition and athletic performance. *Med Sci Sports Exerc.* 2009;41(3): 709–31.
3. Bartoszewska M, Kamboj M, Patel DR. Vitamin D, muscle function, and exercise performance. *Pediatr Clin North Am.* 2010;57(3): 849–61.
4. Bruno RS, Leonard SW, Park SI, Zhao Y, Traber MG. Human vitamin E requirements assessed with the use of apples fortified with deuterium-labeled alpha-tocopheryl acetate. *Am J Clin Nutr.* 2006;83(2):299–304.
5. Bruno RS, Traber MG. Vitamin E biokinetics, oxidative stress and cigarette smoking. *Pathophysiology.* 2006;13(3):143–9.
6. Burke L. *Practical Sports Nutrition.* Leeds (UK): Human Kinetics; 2007. 530 p.
7. *Dietary reference intakes for energy, carbohydrate, fiber, fat, fatty acids, cholesterol, protein, and amino acids* [Internet]. Washington (DC): National Academies Press; [cited July 6, 2011]. Available from: http://www.nap.edu/catalog.php?record_id=10490
8. *Dietary reference intakes for vitamin A, vitamin K, arsenic, boron, chromium, copper, iodine, iron, manganese, molybdenum, nickel, silicon, vanadium, and zinc: a report of the Panel on Micronutrients, Subcommittees on Upper Reference Levels of Nutrients and of Interpretation and Uses of Dietary Reference Intakes, and the Standing Committee on the Scientific Evaluation of Dietary Reference Intakes, Food and Nutrition Board, Institute of Medicine* [Internet]. Washington (DC): National Academy Press; [cited July 6, 2011]. Available from: http://www.nap.edu/catalog.php?record_id=10026
9. *Dietary reference intakes for water, potassium, sodium, chloride, and sulfate* [Internet]. Washington (DC): National Academies Press; [cited July 6, 2011]. Available from: http://www.nap.edu/catalog.php?record_id=10925
10. Dunford M, American Dietetic Association, Sports, Cardiovascular, and Wellness Nutritionists Dietetic Practice Group. *Sports Nutrition: A Practice Manual for Professionals.* 4th ed. Chicago (IL): American Dietetic Association; 2006. 547 p.
11. Expert Panel on Detection, Evaluation, and Treatment of High Blood Cholesterol in Adults. Executive Summary of the Third Report of The National Cholesterol Education Program (NCEP) Expert Panel on Detection, Evaluation, and Treatment of High Blood Cholesterol in Adults (Adult Treatment Panel III). *JAMA.* 2001;285(19):2486–97.
12. *GSSI Sports Science News (Web series): Using glycemic index to improve athletic performance* [Internet]. Gatorade Sports Science Institute; [cited 2008 Oct 13]. Available from: http://www.gssiweb.com/
13. Halliday TM, Peterson NJ, Thomas JJ, Kleppinger K, Hollis BW, Larson-Meyer DE. Vitamin D status relative to diet, lifestyle, injury, and illness in college athletes. *Med Sci Sports Exerc.* 2011;43(2):335–43.
14. Heaney RP, Weaver CM. Newer perspectives on calcium nutrition and bone quality. *J Am Coll Nutr.* 2005;24(6 Suppl):574S–81S.

15. Larson-Meyer DE. *Vegetarian Sports Nutrition*. Champaign (IL): Human Kinetics; 2007. 263 p.

16. Larson-Meyer DE, Willis KS. Vitamin D and athletes. *Curr Sports Med Rep*. 2010;9(4):220–6.

17. Martin WF, Armstrong LE, Rodriguez NR. Dietary protein intake and renal function. *Nutr Metab (Lond)*. 2005;2:25.

18. Phillips SM, Hartman JW, Wilkinson SB. Dietary protein to support anabolism with resistance exercise in young men. *J Am Coll Nutr*. 2005;24(2):134S–9S.

19. Rodriguez NR, Vislocky LM, Gaine PC. Dietary protein, endurance exercise, and human skeletal-muscle protein turnover. *Curr Opin Clin Nutr Metab Care*. 2007;10(1):40–5.

20. Specker B, Vukovich M. Evidence for an interaction between exercise and nutrition for improved bone health during growth. *Med Sport Sci*. 2007;51:50–63.

21. Specker BL. Evidence for an interaction between calcium intake and physical activity on changes in bone mineral density. *J Bone Miner Res*. 1996;11(10):1539–44.

SELECTED REFERENCES FOR FURTHER READING

Clark N. *Nancy Clark's Sports Nutrition Guidebook*. 4th ed. Champaign (IL): Human Kinetics; 2008.

Clinical Sports Nutrition. 3rd ed. Australia: McGraw Hill; 2006.

INTERNET RESOURCES

- Dietary Guidelines for Americans: http://www.health.gov/dietaryguidelines/
- U.S. Department of Agriculture: http://www.choosemyplate.gov

Lifespan Effects of Aging and Deconditioning

THE IMPACT OF AGING

The proportion of the population that is older than the age of 65 yr will increase worldwide from 6.9% in 2000 to 19.3% by 2050 (224). This major demographic shift means that exercise professionals need to increase their awareness of gerontology and geriatrics. Complex issues arise when attempting to distinguish the effects of aging on an individual's physiologic functions that may be caused by deconditioning and/or disease (227). More consideration is now being given to the changes in functional ability of the elderly caused by the biological aging process versus inactivity (69,77,160). Growth and development, maturation, and degeneration are the inevitable processes involved in biological aging. Health care professionals often use intervention strategies that functionally categorize individuals based solely on chronologic age. *Table 5-1* lists these chronologic stages of aging. However, caution is warranted because individual distinctions in activity level, aging, environment, and disease confound making generalizations with regard to health, fitness, and functional status. The purpose of this chapter is to identify the effects of aging and deconditioning on the systems most relevant to exercise testing and prescription.

FUNCTIONAL CAPACITY

The period from infancy through adolescence is characterized by dramatic increases in stature, body mass, and motor control. Maximal work capacity is directly related to fat-free mass (FFM), age, and sex, and indirectly related to percentage body fat in healthy children (51,87,180). However,

maximal work relative to FFM (W_{max}/FFM) is significantly related to age and sex, but not FFM. From early adulthood onward, there is a general decline in physical work capacity, which is matched with a concurrent loss in FFM. In older adults, the decline in FFM does not fully determine the observed loss in capacities for short- and long-term work (75,144). Thus, throughout the lifespan, the ability to effectively perform extended (aerobic) and short-term (anaerobic) work is notably related to FFM in addition to numerous other physiologic factors.

Aerobic capacity, assessed by maximal oxygen uptake ($\dot{V}O_{2max}$), appears to remain constant throughout childhood when expressed relative to body mass (mL · kg^{-1} · min^{-1}) (123). However, absolute aerobic capacity (L · min^{-1}) is lower in children than adults as a result of less FFM. Thus, any absolute workload will result in a greater relative work stress (% of peak load) in children compared with adults. Although children exhibit similar relative aerobic capacities as adults, during weight-bearing exercise, such as walking and running, they display significantly lower movement efficiency because of shorter stride lengths and lower ventilatory efficiency related to requirements for greater air exchange at any given level of exercise (242).

During adulthood, a steady age-related decline in $\dot{V}O_{2max}$ has been observed, with the losses averaging about 1% per year beginning at the age of 25 yr (about 5 mL O_2 · kg^{-1} · min^{-1} with each decade of aging) (27,106,204), and an accelerated decline seems to occur after the age of 50 yr (75,147). Although reduced aerobic capacity is associated with many factors, such as pulmonary and cardiovascular function and body composition (130), it has

KEY TERMS

Anaerobic capacity: The ability of the anaerobic energy systems to produce energy during short-term maximal effort exercise (86).

Deconditioning: A partial or complete reversal of physiologic adaptations to exercise resulting from a significant reduction or cessation of exercise (49,158,221).

Detraining: The process that occurs after the cessation of training in which adaptations to exercise are gradually reduced or lost (49,98,161,213,221).

Muscle atrophy: Reduction in muscle size from disuse (177).

Sarcopenia: The loss of muscle mass that results from the aging process (1,21,56,128).

TABLE 5-1. Stages of Aging

Neonatal	Birth to 3 wk
Infancy	3 wk to 1 yr
Childhood	
Early	1–6 yr
Middle	7–10 yr
Later	Prepubertal
Puberty	Girls 9–15 yr
	Boys 12–16 yr
Adolescence	Up to 6 yr after puberty
Adulthood	
Early	20–29 yr
Middle	30–44 yr
Later	45–64 yr
Senescence	
Elderly	65–74 yr
Older elderly	75–84 yr
Very old	85 yr and older

been suggested that the apparent loss of $\dot{V}O_{2max}$ is highly related to decreased levels of physical activity (224). The degree to which this decline occurs, and the time point at which the decline commences, are significantly affected by amount and intensity of physical activity. The decline in $\dot{V}O_{2max}$ parallels reduced maximum work capacity and is attributed to decreased maximal cardiac output and reduced arterial-venous oxygen difference (a-vO_2) as well as a loss of skeletal muscle mass (85,147,224). Reductions in a-vO_2 have been related to reduced levels of arterial oxygen saturation, increases in subcutaneous adipose tissue, diminished perfusion of skeletal muscle, and reductions in levels of aerobic enzymes (147,197). The decline in aerobic capacity in sedentary men and women is approximately twice that of persons who remain physically active (105,117). Exercise training has been shown to reverse the decreased energy efficiency (increased energy cost of exercise) that is associated with the aging process and that contributes to decreases in aerobic capacity (249). In addition to physical limitations resulting from sedentary lifestyles, loss of coordination, lack of familiarity of required skills, and disabling conditions such as arthritis and obesity may also play a role in limiting $\dot{V}O_{2max}$ (74,99,135,238).

Ironically, **anaerobic capacity** in children has not been well documented, although their activity patterns are exemplified by short-term anaerobic activities (10). Anaerobic power is lower in children than adults in both absolute power and relative to body mass as a consequence of differences in adenosine triphosphate (ATP), creatine phosphate (CP), muscle glycogen, ATPase, creatine kinase, phosphorylase, phosphofructokinase,

and other factors (86). Motivation and neuromuscular coordination also factor into lower anaerobic capacity in children. In adults, both sexes maintain a plateau in anaerobic capacity through about 35 yr of age, at which time it begins to decline.

By age of 65 yr, anaerobic capacity declines to essentially the level of late childhood. This decline in anaerobic performance is caused by age-related changes in the efficiency of metabolic pathways and muscle contractile and biochemical properties (*e.g.*, decreased rate of force development and enzyme activity) (179). The probable reasons for the decline in anaerobic capacity are the loss of mass in large muscles and the decrease in the size and number of glycolytic fast-twitch fibers. Intramuscular blood flow is also attenuated with aging, which contributes to a slower recovery and lactate removal rate (59,131). Even in power-trained or endurance-trained masters athletes, anaerobic power declines 50% by age of 75 yr (211). However, anaerobic training has been shown to counteract the age-related decline in muscle power and functional performance tasks (*e.g.*, 10- and 30-m walking tests at maximal speed) (37,92).

CARDIOVASCULAR SYSTEM

Heart

Although maximal cardiac output increases with growth in children, at any given level of submaximal work, cardiac output is somewhat lower in children than adults primarily because of lower stroke volume (SV) (46,54,186). Lower sympathetic stimulation of the heart in children compared with adults has been suggested as a cause for the smaller SV (19,118). However, during modest submaximal exercise, increases in SV do not seem to be related to aging. This phenomenon is a result of the Frank-Starling mechanism to compensate for a reduced number of pacemaker cells and impaired adrenergic chronotropic function (127,226). Boys exhibit greater SV and lower heart rate (HR) compared to girls in response to acute stressors such as exercise (230).

Numerous physiologic changes to the heart transpire with aging. It is imperative to differentiate between these normal biologic changes and underlying pathologies that exist in cardiovascular disease. The aging heart shows decreases in intracellular transportation and pacemaker cells as well as sensitivity to β-receptor, baroreceptor, and chemoreceptor stimulation. Furthermore, interstitial fibrosis within the myocardium and calcification of the heart's connective tissue skeleton results in collagen cross-linking and elasticity loss. The heart's function is attenuated by an increase in arterial stiffness, systolic blood pressure (SBP), and left ventricular afterload and hypertrophy. Further changes in the left ventricle result in extended diastolic relaxation (76,168).

Maximal cardiac output in a 65-yr-old person is 10%–30% less than in a young adult. Decreases in both maximal HR and maximal SV contribute to decreased maximal cardiac output of older adults. By contrast, in the period immediately after high-intensity exercise, HR recovery, return of oxygen uptake to baseline, and muscular power recovery occur faster in children than in young adults and adults (18,91,253).

Several studies over the past 25 yr have shown that resting cardiac output and SV decrease with age (183,192). Results suggest resting cardiac output decreases about 1% per year, from a mean of 6.5 L · min^{-1} in the third decade to a mean of 3.9 L · min^{-1} in the ninth decade. From 25 to 85 yr, resting SV decreases 30%, from 85 to 60 mL (192). However, in subjects who have been carefully screened for coronary artery disease, investigators have demonstrated that overall left ventricular function, using resting ejection fraction as an index, does not decline between 25 and 80 yr (183). Estimates of volume made by echocardiography and radionuclide scintigraphy demonstrate resting SV also does not decline with age. Because resting HR is also not age related, these data suggest that resting cardiac output does not decline with age in healthy individuals.

Heart Rate

In children, HR is often high at rest (80–100 bpm), apparently as a result of a low SV relative to body size (199). This low SV generally vanishes with growth and increased levels of physical activity, thus it is not age specific. In combination with an increase in the oxygen-carrying capacity of the blood secondary to hemoglobin increases that occur through the late teens, resting HR decreases to approximately 65–75 bpm by adulthood.

Resting HR is relatively unchanged throughout adulthood. However, maximal attainable HR declines proportionally with age (predicted maximum HR = 220 − age) (42). A decrease in myocardial sensitivity to catecholamines and the effect of prolonged diastolic filling appear to be responsible for this decline in maximal HR (126). In addition, as aging occurs through adulthood, a greater HR response to a given submaximal exercise intensity is observed (199). A decrease of 5–10 bpm per decade for peak HR also occurs. This age-related decline in peak HR is primarily caused by reduced sensitivity to beta-adrenergic stimulation (141,223). For those who train, this reduction in peak HR can be offset somewhat by increases in end-diastolic volume and SV, which help to reduce the negative effects on peak cardiac output. As a result, recovery HR remains higher, and recovery takes longer after maximal exercise as one ages (92).

Blood Vessels

Vascular stiffness occurs with aging and is an independent risk factor for cardiovascular disease and mortality (34,148,250). As a result, peripheral vascular resistance increases with age. The capillary-to-muscle-fiber ratio also becomes lower with age, further reducing peripheral blood flow (210). Loss of plasticity of the aorta impedes pulsatile ejection, which delays the arteries in accepting SV. In turn, this results in an increase in SBP and mean arterial pressure (13,92). Aerobic exercise training has been shown to attenuate age-related vascular stiffness (156,222), which is likely caused by the improvement of nitric oxide release (52).

PULMONARY SYSTEM

During maturation lung growth continues during the first two decades in both healthy males and females, and normal lung volumes are sustained until around 35 yr of age (195). However, after 35 yr of age, a progressive decrease occurs in both maximal expiratory flow and lung volume reserve with aging. Specifically, residual volume increases by 30%–35%, and vital capacity decreases by 40%–50% by age 70 yr (189), possibly because of a loss of elastic recoil of the lungs (199). Thoracic wall compliance decreases with age, and the ability to expand the chest cavity becomes limited, reducing pulmonary capacity during rest and exercise (13). Furthermore, during exertion, increased ventilation (L · min^{-1}) is accomplished via greater frequency of breathing rather than increased tidal volume. The overall net effect is a 20% increase in the work of ventilatory muscles (58). Despite these changes, pulmonary function does not limit exercise capacity or the ability to benefit from exercise training unless lung function is severely impaired. However, because of the increased work imposed on the ventilatory muscles, elderly individuals may report breathing discomfort (dyspnea) owing to the increased ventilatory demand caused by physical exertion, despite having normal cardiopulmonary function (109). As a result, the onset of dyspnea at lower intensities may be sufficient to reduce voluntary physical activity and further contribute to the deconditioning associated with aging.

MUSCULOSKELETAL SYSTEM

Muscle

Recent advances in laboratory technology have greatly enhanced our understanding of the number, proportion, and function of various muscle fiber types (56,212). Type I slow-twitch fibers are more resistant than type II fast-twitch fibers to atrophy until the seventh decade. Hence, the percentage of type I fibers tends to increase as a result of type II fiber disuse and subsequent degeneration. The selective loss of type II fibers may be more a function of disuse than aging *per se* given that activity patterns suggest that less muscle contraction against resistance occurs from adulthood to senescence.

The loss of skeletal muscle mass is common with the aging process and has been termed sarcopenia (56).

Declines in muscle fiber number and cross-sectional area (CSA), motor unit size and recruitment, innervation, capillarization, protein synthesis, energy production capacity, and growth factor alterations are responsible for sarcopenia (1,21,128). Sarcopenia limits muscle function with 25% of overall maximal force-generating capacity lost by the age of 65 yr and as much as 40% over a lifetime (9,196,200). Recent evidence suggests further that aging is associated with a wide variety in regard to the type of muscle force lost; specifically a 25% reduction in eccentric muscle force, 46% reduction in isometric muscle force, and 56% reduction in concentric muscle force (237). From this new evidence, it would appear that eccentric contraction muscle losses with aging are significantly less than concentric and isometric contractions and may be a target for resistance exercise prescription during early phases in an exercise program (184). Whereas the decline in muscle strength in men and women is primarily the result of muscle mass losses, neural factors are responsible for additional functional decrements (6). Specifically, an age-related decline in α-motor neurons, motor cortex activity, and motor units increases the number of denervated muscle fibers (128) and results in loss of contractile fiber participation. The dual myopathic and neuropathic etiology of sarcopenia is characterized by changes that result in functional limitations in gait, coordination, activities of daily living (2,17,149), increased risk of accidental falls (56), and onset of frailty associated with aging (71). Additionally, sarcopenia impairs thermoregulation, metabolism, and glucose sensitivity (1). There exists some agreement, however, that sarcopenia is primarily a result of diminishing stimulus secondary to sedentary lifestyles and reduced force-generating activities (42). Furthermore, changes in the architecture of muscle (pennation angle, muscle thickness, fascicle length, biochemical factors) may also impact changes in muscle function during aging (124). The evidence is unequivocal that exercise training (cardiovascular and resistance) can help to attenuate these aging processes and most likely reduces the overall net loss in muscle force capacity as a result of sarcopenia. Losses in skeletal muscle contribute significantly to the quality of life and frailty of older adults and, as such, exercise interventions that increase muscle fitness (muscle force contractility) may be required before engaging in cardiovascular activities. Given that the number of adults over 65 yr of age is expected to double over the next decade, interventions to offset sarcopenia will become critical in elderly care.

Body Composition

Approximately one-third of the population of the United States is obese and one-sixth of teenagers (age 12–19 yr) are overweight, escalating the risk of chronic disease (166). Body fat percentages are independent of sex in prepubescent children but are highly influenced by genetics as well as environmental factors. Acceptable body fat percentages for prepubescent children are between 10% and 15% (159). Sex differences begin to show during puberty and extend through adulthood with healthy ranges of approximately 10%–20% in men and 15%–25% in women, although no national standards exist for body fat percentage. Distribution of body fat is sex specific from the third to seventh decade. Women tend to exhibit greater increases in internal body fat after age 45 yr; men, however, accumulate greater subcutaneous fat. The previously discussed losses in FFM with aging have been associated with decreases in basal metabolic rate of approximately 5% per decade throughout adulthood, which in turn is a contributing factor in fat gain (31). An accumulating body of knowledge points to lifestyle changes, including decreased physical activity, as the underlying culprit in the changes in body composition (decreased FFM and increased fat mass [FM]) with aging. In elderly subjects, increased levels of body fat contribute to slower gait speed and functional limitations (217). Exercise training plays an important role in the maintenance of FFM and FM as one ages.

Bone

Bone, or *osseous tissue*, is continuously remodeling as a result of osteoblastic (formation) and osteoclastic (reabsorption) activity (42,198). Prepubescent bone maturation is greatly affected by genetics and is highly correlated to the loading factor imposed by muscle mass in accordance with Wolff's Law (243), that is, the more strain that is put on the bones, the stronger they become. Bone growth during childhood presents two primary problems because the epiphysis is not united with the bone shaft. First, overuse can result in epiphysitis during this growth period. Second, fracture may pass through the epiphyseal plate, potentially leading to abnormal growth (199). Children exposed to various weight-bearing activities exhibit positive bone growth responses (244). Peak bone mass is defined as the maximum amount of bone acquired at the end of growth (125). It is generally thought that women reach peak bone mass in their mid-to-late 20s (173). Other researchers, however, report bone mineral density (BMD) peaking at around age 35 yr (44). Men are thought to reach peak bone mass at a similar age as women. Men, however, have a higher peak bone mass mainly because of differences in endocrine status (138).

Senescence generally occurs at the beginning of the sixth decade and is characterized by predominant osteoclastic activity in which bone resorption exceeds bone formation. As a result, decreases in bone density manifested by decreases in calcium regulatory mechanisms, hormone levels, and metabolic activity occur (198). Lifestyle factors, such as physical activity level, calcium intake, and nutritional status, play a major role as well, making it difficult to determine the intrinsic contribution of aging itself on bone loss (165,198). The loss of muscle mass with aging has been associated with reductions in BMD (79). Women tend to begin losing bone mass between 30 and 35 yr of age at a rate of 0.75%–1.00% per year (198). Bone loss in men generally commences between 50 and 55 yr of age at an initial rate of 0.40% per year. This marked reduction of bone precipitates normal and pathologic fractures causing increased morbidity and mortality (97). Thus, clinical osteoporosis is a precursor to disability (165).

Joints and Flexibility

Joint flexibility, required to produce fluid and efficient motion of the body, is commonly compromised with aging. Specifically, tendons and ligaments often lose elasticity leading to decreases in joint mobility (11). This progressive loss of flexibility, resulting from several factors, including disease, deterioration of joint structures, and progressive degeneration of collagen fibers, begins during young adulthood. Increased incidence of knee and back problems from osteoarthritis has been observed beginning with middle age and progressing through old age (199). Degeneration of joints, especially the spine, is often found in elderly persons. Along with loss of strength, loss of flexibility plays a significant role in increased risk of falls and injuries. Particularly, decreased ankle flexibility has a direct link with risk of falls as a result of diminished balance and functional ability (150). The rate of deterioration accelerates beyond age 65 yr, but few specific findings are available for this age group. Exercise training and range of motion exercise help to maintain and/or increase flexibility as aging occurs.

NERVOUS SYSTEM

Infants and very young children undergo intensive learning to develop motor skills for function and performance. The central nervous system (CNS) is recognized as the predominant center for determining the outcomes of this learning. The learning process includes the integration of movement patterns that minimize physiologic cost, asymmetry, and variability of body segment coordination (112). The resulting improvement in economy of movement may decrease oxygen consumption at submaximal velocities. This improvement may also enhance reaction time, which decreases by about 15% by age 70 yr as compared with early adulthood (67).

Detrimental changes in neurotransmitters, nerve conduction velocities, and fine motor control are all indicative of normal CNS aging (193). The increased incidence of sensory deficits, particularly hearing and vision, and higher thresholds of perception for many stimuli may be related to the 35%–40% increase in falls by persons older than age 60 yr (239).

IMMUNE SYSTEM

Aging is associated with a decline in immune function (innate and adaptive immunity) known as immunosenescence, leading to increased incidence of infectious diseases (12). Innate immunity is antigen nonspecific and provides immediate defense such as the activation of natural killer (NK) cells. Adaptive immunity specifically responds to a particular foreign antigen and is mediated by T and B cells. Aging has been shown to increase NK cell number but decrease the function of these cells (154). Furthermore, elderly people exhibit a decline in the proportion and number of CD4+ T helper cells and B cells (157). Cross-sectional studies have shown the benefits of regular exercise on immune function in elderly people (121). For example, age-related decline in NK cell activity is enhanced following exercise training (202). Exercise training also improves the function of CD4+ helper T cells in elderly people (201).

Aging is also associated with a chronic inflammatory condition with elevated levels of proinflammatory cytokines such as tumor necrosis factor-α (TNF-α) and interleukin-6 (IL-6) (35,36). Research has shown the effects of physical activity on inflammatory responses. Specifically, a lower IL-6 concentration was observed in individuals who had higher self-reported physical activity levels (174). In a cross-sectional study of 1,004 elderly individuals, those who participated in moderate to high physical activity exhibited lower IL-6 levels compared with sedentary individuals (68). These data suggest that exercise training enhances immune defense with aging and may aid in the prevention of many diseases of the elderly.

RENAL FUNCTION, FLUID REGULATION, AND THERMOREGULATION

Renal function significantly declines in persons aged 50–79 yr (100) and is associated with risk factors for cardiovascular diseases (15). Aging also affects glucose tolerance with 0.7% reduction in insulin secretion per year (220). A general reduction in total cellular water occurs with aging, with a decline of 10%–50% in total body water compared with cellular water levels in early adults.

The primary maturational characteristics related to exercise in heat occur in late puberty or early adulthood. Before that time, children have a consistently lower sweat rate characterized by lower absolute and relative sweat volumes along with a higher core temperature required to start sweating. Thus, children tend to rely more on radiation and convection for heat dissipation than adults. The composition of children's sweat also differs, particularly in regard to chloride, which is lower in children than adults (72,151,185). Aging is also associated with attenuated skin blood flow, which may contribute to a reduced ability to thermoregulate. Furthermore, the effects of aging predispose older individuals to rapidly dehydrate. This may become particularly important during exercise through evaporative water loss and perspiration (119). In addition, many older adults take various medications that may further confound hydration levels, placing further limitations on thermoregulation.

Children have a greater ratio of surface area to mass than adults, which enhances convective and radiant heat transfer between skin and the environment, making tolerance to cold more difficult (120,185). However, it has been suggested that other factors that occur with aging, such as thermogenic and vasoconstrictive responses, may also limit thermoregulation to cold in children. Beyond childhood, it has been demonstrated that the ability to regulate core temperature is negatively affected by aging (225,245,251).

Summary

Growth, development, maturation, and degeneration have profound effects on the body's capability to respond to the external stresses placed on it through exercise. Lifestyle factors associated with aging make it difficult to distinguish between degeneration attributable to normal physiologic aging and alterations in habitual physical activity. Gerontologic investigations reveal that reduction of activity is predictive of lifespan and attributable at least partly to altered neurotransmission in dopamine activity (14,101). *Table 5-2* highlights selected age-related changes. The interrelationships between biologic aging and physical activity warrant further investigation.

IMPACT OF DECONDITIONING

The health/fitness professional must understand musculoskeletal adaptations to reduced physical activity so that changes in functional ability can be predicted. The appropriate exercise and/or physical activity can then be prescribed after disuse or in the rehabilitation process for a wide range of clients: weekend athletes, elite athletes, diseased, disabled, and aging populations. Deconditioning can result from detraining, bed rest, casting, use of crutches, paralysis, aging, or even exposure to microgravity during space flight (*Table 5-3*). The following section is a brief description of each of the modes of deconditioning that have yielded information regarding the effects of inactivity on the musculoskeletal system.

MODES OF DECONDITIONING

Decreased muscle activity is defined as a reduction in the intensity or amount of regularly performed activity by a muscle or muscle group. Detraining (returning to a sedentary lifestyle after formalized exercise training) does not suggest the same adaptive response as a sedentary individual would have with 1 mo of bed rest. For example, bed rest for 1 mo, which constitutes a dramatic change in the daily amount of muscle activity even for a previously sedentary individual, causes greater skeletal muscle atrophy than would the cessation of a resistance training program for the same period by an

TABLE 5-2. System Changes					
	Neonatal Infancy	**Childhood**	**Adolescence**	**Adulthood**	**Senescence**
Cardiovascular System					
Cardiac output		↑	↑	↔	↔
Stroke volume		↑	↑	↔	↓
HR$_{max}$		↑	↔	↓	↓
$\dot{V}O_{2max}$		↑	↑	↓	↓
Pulmonary System					
Vital capacity	↑	↑	↑	↓	↓
Musculoskeletal System					
Bone mineral density	↑	↑	↑	↔	↓
Fat-free body mass	↑	↑	↑	↑	↓
Anaerobic capacity		↑	↑	↑	↓
Flexibility		↑	↑	↓	↓
% Body fat		↑	↑	↑	↑
Nervous System					
Motor control	↑	↑	↑	↔	↓
Immune System					
Immune system function		↑	↑	↔	↓

↑ = increases; ↔ = no change; ↓ = decreases.

TABLE 5-3. Types of Deconditioning

Type	Noted Changes	Reference
Detraining		
	Muscle atrophy	(94)
	Decrease in muscle size	(89)
	Decrease in fiber numbers	(229)
	Capillaries undamaged	(175)
	Fiber type reverts to composition before training	(213)
Bed Rest		
	Muscle atrophy (greater than in exercising individuals)	(213)
	Considerable atrophy of fast- and slow-twitch fibers	(93)
	No change in myonuclear number per mm of fiber length	(167)
Casting		
	Decrease in strength attributed to neural factors if short term	(57)
	Severe atrophy if muscles in shortened position	(82,171)
	Neuromuscular transmission defects	(84)
Crutches		
	Reduction of strength by 20% in non–weight-bearing limb	(176)
	No changes in contralateral weight-bearing muscle	(40,176)
Paralysis		
	Reduced mitochondrial content	(40,146)
	Poor fatigue resistance	(146)
	Fast-twitch fibers greater atrophy after 6 mo	(40)
	Proportion of type IIx increases, and type IIa decreases	(40)
	Actomyosin ATPase activity not elevated	(146)
	Exercise activities generally limited to motor units above spinal cord injury	(107)
	Activities of daily living improved by strength and conditioning	(108)
	Atrophy of 50% or more after 6 mo of injury	(38,40)
Space Flight		
	Muscle atrophy	(48)
	Muscle strength decreases	(65,134)
	Greater loss in fast-twitch than slow-twitch fibers	(48)
	Bone loss to 12%	(241)
	Reduced $\dot{V}O_{2max}$	(137)
	Decreased work capacity and fatigued earlier	(48)
	Exercise counteracts harmful effects	(48)

individual who continues normal activities of daily living (90,93). Thus, the magnitude of the adaptive response to decreased activity depends on relative change in an individual's muscle use, which may be caused by injury, illness, or cessation of an exercise program.

Detraining

Detraining in athletes often occurs during the off-season or because of an injury when normal training routines are interrupted. Detraining causes a decrease in physiological variables including $\dot{V}O_{2max}$, cardiac output, and SV (50). Mitochondrial oxidative capacity also declines as a result of detraining and negatively impacts athletic performance (142).

Bed Rest

Periods of bed rest, in the clinical setting, are usually associated with some underlying disease, so differentiating musculoskeletal changes caused by inactivity versus disease process is often difficult. However, bed-resting healthy individuals has been used as an experimental model of muscle unloading to rule out disease complications and has yielded profound cardiovascular changes (decreased blood volume and SV, increased resting HR, orthostatic intolerance) along with results similar to casting or the use of crutches (24,26,60,172,190,208,248). Additionally, prolonged bed rest can result in muscle loss and weakness (4,70).

Casting

A cast characteristically places a joint in a fixed position with the objective of immobilizing injured tissue or bone. When a cast is used, the muscle activity not only decreases, but also fixes the joint position in which the muscles are held at a relatively constant length. A cast brace is specifically designed with materials that can be used in the treatment of fractures in order for an individual to return to earlier activity and early joint motion (214), which would lead to better recovery (155,170,218). Casting results in similar muscular adaptations seen during bed rest, space flight, and use of crutches. These adaptations include a decrease in muscular strength and size (4).

Crutches

The use of crutches may or may not be associated with casting. Although a lower limb in a cast often requires crutches, minor injuries (sprains and strains) may not require casting but may require nonweight bearing. Human lower limb suspension via the use of crutches has also been used as an experimental technique to study adaptations to unloading (63,89,175,182).

Paralysis

Many diseases and spinal cord injuries (SCIs) can lead to partial or total paralysis. Automobile accidents, sporting accidents (football, diving, and gymnastics), and gunshot wounds have been reported as the most common causes of SCIs (83). Although it is often difficult to distinguish how a disease process interacts with muscle disuse to produce functional changes, SCIs are unique in that affected muscles may still be innervated yet receive no input from higher nervous centers. Thus, muscles are innervated by intact motor neurons but are seldom activated except during spasm (38,41,62,94,95,146,215).

Space Flight

On a limited basis, researchers have been able to scientifically study the body's response to muscle unloading in the unique microgravity environment of outer space (4,247). Musculoskeletal changes that occur during space flight are similar to those observed during bed rest and casting. These muscular adaptations include a decrease in muscular strength and size (4). However,

with few flights and small numbers of crew members who repeat space missions, reproducibility of results has been difficult (47). Therefore, simulations of microgravity have been used and involve lower limb suspension, water immersion, and head-down tilt protocols (3,7,178). Ongoing investigations are using exercise as a means to reduce the effects of prolonged exposure to microgravity.

EFFECTS ON BONE

Exercise that promotes skeletal loading induces a compensatory adaptation in the structure and functional integrity of bone (see *Chapter 42*). The processes underlying the adaptive mechanisms of bone to loading represent a complex interaction of endocrine and musculoskeletal systems. Exercise serves as a stimulus for skeletal adaptation that includes the maintenance or addition of bone mass. Conversely, inactivity — as in bed rest because of injury or partly caused by inactivity associated with aging — reduces bone mass by adversely affecting calcium metabolism and the bone formation process.

Bone formation may be described as a dynamic lifelong process. As such, bone health has been studied in young and old subjects under conditions of short-term immobilization, prolonged bed rest, exposure to microgravity associated with space flight, and clinical conditions such as paralysis. Although results from studies are similar, comparisons across subject populations regarding bone loss and genesis are made difficult by underlying pathologies.

Depending on the length of enforced inactivity as well as underlying pathologies, recovery of lost bone or osteogenesis may be protracted. Health care practitioners need to know that extended periods of deconditioning and disuse not only result in bone loss but also compromise future bone health by increasing the patient's susceptibility to fracture and promoting early-onset osteoporosis.

The discussion that follows includes information from studies aimed at revealing the effects of inactivity, bed rest, and immobilization on bone mass and calcium metabolism in adult humans. Evidence of changes in bone mass and structural integrity has been inferred from radiologic measurements. Assays of endocrine regulators indicative of calcium absorption from the gut and deposition of calcium in bone are used in conjunction with urinary and fecal excretion of calcium to reveal the role of calcium metabolism in bone health. Several review articles offer additional detail (28,29,66,232).

Bone Mineral Density

Removing or reducing an exercise stimulus has been shown to reverse gains in lumbar spine BMD in postmenopausal women (53,104) and reduce trabecular bone mineral content in habitually active middle-aged persons (152). Bone loss was likewise observed in elderly patients (143) and male athletes (8) after a period of inactivity. Female collegiate gymnasts (209) and male ice hockey players (163) exhibit increased BMD during the competitive season compared to the off-season. A recent investigation revealed greater BMD in premenarcheal gymnasts compared with inactive control subjects (162), owing to speculation that the active subjects' more robust skeletal architecture may provide protection later in life. In support of this theory, Valdimarsson et al. (233) reported that female college soccer players had greater bone mass in the trochanter than age-matched controls nearly a decade after retiring from competition. Similarly, Nordstrom et al. (164) found a wide range of male athletes to have greater trochanter bone mass than controls at 3 and 5 yr postcompetition. Although the loss of bone mass in previously active individuals is subject to decline over time as a result of disuse, it may be only in later years that any bone accrual that results from sports participation is truly negated. Magnusson et al. (179) reported that young adult soccer players with above average BMD experienced a gradual decline in bone mass over the years, with follow-up observations at age 70 yr revealing no significant differences in bone mass between the former soccer players and control subjects. Additional study is needed to determine if highly active elderly persons present significantly different bone mass profiles than their less active counterparts.

In the absence of mechanical stress produced by weight-bearing activity, bed rest negatively affects the homeostatic mechanisms that underlie bone health. Without weight-bearing activity, calcium balance is disturbed, and, ultimately, bone mass is lost (116).

Calcium Balance

To preserve bone mass, a balance must exist between resorption of existing bone and the formation of new bone. Prolonged inactivity is known to upset this balance, resulting in excessive resorption of calcium from bone, as manifested in elevated levels of serum calcium (hypercalcemia) and a concurrent increase in urinary and fecal calcium (134). During periods of increased resorption, serum, urinary, and fecal levels of calcium fluctuate in response to hormonal regulation and decreased absorption of calcium from the intestines. Within weeks of inactivity, negative calcium balance has been observed in healthy persons subjected to bed rest (134), persons experiencing weightlessness (206), and individuals with SCIs (30).

Hormonal regulation of calcium metabolism, although altered during periods of bed rest, plays a less prominent role in the maintenance of bone mass than the influences of mechanical load. That is, reduction in mechanical load or stress appears to trigger an ordered response of bone resorption and endocrine activity, including the regulation of calcium absorption from the gut by 1,25 dihydroxyvitamin D (1,25-D) (207). Although the other prominent calcium regulator, parathyroid hormone (PTH), is unchanged or decreases slightly during periods of negative calcium balance in healthy subjects experiencing bed rest, 1,25-D decreases or does not change (134,188,234,254). Conversely, during the acute phase, individuals with SCIs who are immobilized show low PTH and 1,25-D levels (30).

Bone Mass

Site-specific losses in BMD of 1%–2% per month have been reported based on animal models, microgravity experienced by astronauts, and as a result of bed rest (20,111,133). The rate and, ultimately, the amount of bone loss may be tied to health status. Based on ultrasound calcaneal measures, healthy men lost approximately 0.017%–0.110% of bone mass per week during a 120-day bed-rest study. Persons with SCIs, however, lose as much as 33% of calcaneus bone volume within 6 mo of the injury (30). It appears that the effect of SCI on bone loss is even more pronounced in women with SCI who are postmenopausal (205).

Susceptibility to bone loss increases as a function of the proximity to mechanical load and type of bone. LeBlanc et al. (133) observed a 10% loss in BMD in the calcaneus compared with 4% at the femoral neck and spine; however, no significant reduction in bone mass occurred in the radius of the forearm after 17 wk of bed rest. During periods of unloading, trabecular bone, with its high surface-to-volume ratio, is targeted by bone-absorbing osteoclasts. Under conditions of disuse, trabecular bone loss is greatest at load-bearing sites (e.g., proximal tibia) and occurs more rapidly than cortical bone loss (133,252).

Biochemical markers of bone turnover are used extensively in bed-rest studies to assess the metabolic activity of bone. A recent study of healthy male subjects, subjected to 120 d of bed rest, showed increased bone resorption by day 7 and a decrease in bone formation by day 50 (102). Other investigators have also reported excessive bone resorption in healthy subjects during disuse (240,254), as well as in paraplegic subjects (153). However, Palle et al. (169) reported only transient changes in bone resorption early in the course of bed rest, with values returning to baseline by the fourth and final month of the study. It appears that the bone loss may be explained as a disproportionate increase in osteoclast cell activity (129). Moreover, osteoclast activity is noticeably localized in the lower body (e.g., calcaneus, tibia), ultimately compromising the structural components (e.g., matrix, collagen) of bone and increasing the risk of fracture.

An uncoupling of the bone resorption and formation process is evidenced by the fact that biochemical markers of bone formation do not increase during unloading.

Investigators have reported that biochemical markers of bone resorption remain elevated for weeks upon resumption of activity (139,231,234). Thus, individuals with a history of bone loss who subsequently undergo forced unloading are particularly vulnerable to injury caused by fracture as they regain their mobility.

Remobilization: Can Lost Bone Be Regained?

The timeline for regaining bone loss caused by disuse has been studied in animals and humans. Jaworski and Uhthoff (110) evaluated the osteogenic activity of old and young dogs after immobilization of the forelimbs for 32 wk. At 28 wk into remobilization, there was a 40% and 70% recovery of bone mass in old and young dogs, respectively. Significant deficits in bone mass were still apparent in horses who remobilized for 8 wk after 7 wk of disuse (235). In contrast, the restoration of bone architecture in young rats after 3 wk of hind-limb immobilization was nearly complete after several weeks of exercise (33). Similarly, Kaneps et al. (115) found the cancellous and cortical mechanical properties of immobilized forelimbs in dogs to be significantly less than controls at 16 wk. However, at 32 wk, including 16 wk of treadmill running, no significant difference between immobilized and control limbs was observed.

Although limited, recovery of bone mass and the associated architectural integrity in humans is protracted, with evidence that deficits can persist indefinitely. Bone mineral deficits induced by multiple space flights could still be observed in astronauts 5 yr later (228). Similarly, lumbar and femoral neck bone mass lost during 17 wk of bed rest was not regained in healthy subjects after 6 mo of normal remobilization (133). Lower extremity bone density (calcaneus and proximal tibia), however, was regained in this study sample. Although tibial bone mass may take 1.0–1.5 yr to recover after periods of non–weight-bearing associated with hip surgery (133), permanent losses in BMD were reported in the lower limbs and spines of men who suffered tibial fractures 9 yr earlier (103).

Implications and Considerations

After immobilization, the bone restoration process may be particularly difficult in certain populations (*e.g.*, elderly and those with SCIs). Depending on baseline levels and the amount of bone loss, elderly individuals may be at greater risk of fracture after immobilization. Similarly, men older than age 60 yr and postmenopausal women may be predisposed to accelerated bone loss, a condition that may exacerbate bone loss during immobilization. As such, an intervention strategy might be used that includes brief periods of assisted mobility during forced inactivity followed by remobilization at the earliest possible time. Thus, it would appear that retrieval of lost bone following periods of disuse is difficult at best even under loading conditions. However, the administration of insulin-like growth factor-1 (IGF-1) has been shown to promote osteogenesis during periods of unloading (32) and loading (140) in animal models, whereas human trials have been limited to special populations (*e.g.*, children deficient in growth hormone). Perhaps IGF-1 will be a promising intervention in the fight to regain bone mass in humans.

Considering that bone mass restoration is outpaced by increases in muscle strength, practitioners must be careful not to induce fracture by overly aggressive exercise programs. A conservative approach — including range-of-motion exercises, a gradual overload of balance and stability challenges, site-specific muscle strengthening (*Box 5-1*) as supported by clinical evaluations, and bone scans — is recommended.

| **BOX 5-1** | **Guidelines for Exercise Professionals Working with Severely Detrained or Bed Rested Individuals** |

- Emphasize strength training of back and lower limb postural muscle groups:
  — Back extensors
  — Quadriceps
  — Hip extensors
  — Ankle plantarflexors (soleus and gastrocnemius)
- Start with low-intensity training
  — To accommodate potential neuromuscular deficits
  — To minimize potential for muscle damage

- Use gradual, progressive overload
- Be aware of increased risk of bone fracture
  — Particularly in estrogen-deficient women and the elderly
  — Even after muscle strength has returned to normal
- Incorporate training for postural stability and dynamic balance

Summary

Exercise that promotes skeletal loading stimulates compensatory adaptations, resulting in structural changes and healthier bones. Inactivity, regardless of the reason, is detrimental to maintaining bone health. It is difficult to distinguish between effects of normal physiologic aging and alterations in exercise and physical activity patterns. Transient bone mass changes have been observed in athletes, persons with mobility issues, and individuals experiencing unloading for brief periods. Bone loss is greatest at distal points of loading and areas associated with postural integrity and mobility (*e.g.*, vertebra, hip). Accelerated bone loss is associated with age, menopause, space flight, SCI, and extended periods of unloading. Although hormonal regulation of calcium balance is altered during periods of inactivity, the most salient feature of bone health is the influence of mechanical loading. Recovery of lost bone is at best protracted, with evidence that deficits can persist indefinitely. Depending on baseline levels and amount of bone loss, practitioners must be careful not to rush rehabilitation because the risk of fracture is increased after immobilization.

EFFECTS ON SKELETAL MUSCLE

Morphologic Consequences

Loss of skeletal muscle as a result of aging and/or disuse is a serious consequence that reduces the independence and physical ability of older adults (80). Regardless of the mechanisms of age-related changes of skeletal muscle (see *Table* 5-3), the predominant adaptive response is skeletal muscle atrophy and a subsequent reduced capacity to generate force (41,94,128). Atrophy is the process whereby muscle CSA is reduced, almost exclusively because of reductions in the contractile proteins actin and myosin (145). Specifically, in the absence of contractile activity, proteolytic and synthetic systems are altered, resulting in an upregulation of genes that mediate the breakdown of contractile proteins (43,45), which in turn promote ubiquitination and the expression of specific atrophy genes (16,113).

For the first several weeks of disuse, atrophy is almost linearly related to duration and extent of unloading and differs among anaerobic (Type II) and aerobic (Type I) biochemical muscle properties. Generally, atrophy is most severe in the Type II muscles involved in weight bearing and postural control; extensor muscles are typically more severely affected than flexor muscles (40,89,132). Likewise, it has recently been shown that the atrophic response of thigh adductor muscles to unloading is intermediate to that of extensor and flexor muscles (25,40). Of particular concern are muscles of the thigh and calf. These are critical in normal walking and show marked atrophy in non–weight-bearing conditions, and reductions in their force generating capacity

contribute to reduced mobility and increased frailty associated with aging (40,96).

In lower mammals, fiber-type composition may influence the atrophic response to unloading; however, this has not been demonstrated in humans (41). Human skeletal muscle generally does not present the clear segmentation of fiber type found in lower mammals (187).

Fast muscle fiber subtypes, unlike slow fibers, appear to show transformation with several months of unloading or after detraining (41,90,213). Type IIx fibers in human muscle appear to serve as the default expression of the fast myosin gene, and with disuse, there appears to be a net loss of CSA of these fast-twitch fibers (128). These transformations do not markedly alter the energy demand of contraction, unlike slow to fast fiber conversions, but do significantly reduce the muscle power capacity for common activities of daily living. These combined losses in CSA and subsequent loss of power and force of both slow and fast fibers produce declines in strength that range from 30% to 35% (236).

Metabolic Consequences

The influence of unloading on metabolic characteristics of human skeletal muscle is not fully understood. However, it has been suggested that age-associated losses in VO_{2max} indirectly reduce the overall energy capacity and subsequently reduce the ability to perform mechanical work (191). Whereas homogenates of muscle biopsies show decreased concentrations of enzyme markers of aerobic oxidative capacity after unloading, anaerobic enzymes of energy supply do not seem to change (23,93). Reduced enzymes associated with aerobic capacity may reflect preferential loss of contractile protein with unloading; that is, aerobic oxidative enzyme content per fiber volume may not change, and the anaerobic enzyme content may actually increase (40,145). Also, it would appear that age-associated mitochondrial losses would severely limit the oxidative capacity of elderly adults. Indeed, it has been reported that 8% of oxidative capacity is lost every decade with aging (203). Nonetheless, fiber atrophy results in lower total mitochondrial content, so unloading compromises absolute muscular endurance (23,61,216). This also suggests that relative muscular endurance is not independently affected by atrophy associated with unloading but is partially diminished as a result of mitochondrial losses associated with sarcopenia (23). However, preferential loss of contractile protein and subsequent reduction in metabolic capacity require the remaining muscle to work against greater absolute load, which in combination would contribute to increased fatigue and decreased capacity.

Strength and Local Muscular Endurance

Unloading reduces muscular strength, regardless of the type of action or movement performed or the method of strength expression (5,22,23,26,64,81,90,132). Strength reduction is nearly linearly related to the duration of unloading and extent of muscle atrophy for the first few weeks. Atrophy accounts for a large part but not all of decreased force production, suggesting the ability to activate muscle is also compromised by unloading. This is interesting because marked force reduction during eccentric, isometric, and slow-speed concentric muscle contraction is believed to be controlled in some part by neural inhibitory mechanisms (63,246). Specifically, it would appear that motor unit activation order is partially responsible for the significantly greater losses of concentric and isometric contraction than eccentric contractions (184). Indeed, it is suggested that there is decreased agonist muscle activation coupled with increased antagonist muscle activation during concentric muscle contractions in older adults. The increased antagonist recruitment during muscle shortening may serve as a stimulus that reduces overall concentric strength (184). However, the relative decline in strength is comparable across speeds and types of muscle actions, so increased inhibition is not responsible for reduced voluntary activation, or if it is, the reduction is uniform across speeds and types of muscle actions (22,26,63,64).

The lack of shape change in the force–velocity relationship with short-term unloading may suggest that muscle fiber type composition is not altered. However, as transformation to a faster muscle occurs with long-term extreme unloading, an increased ability to maintain force as speed increases during concentric actions should be evident (88). This finding has been reported after long-term space flight (65). However, 120 d of unloading of otherwise healthy individuals did not alter relative rise time during surface electrical stimulation of the triceps surae muscle group, suggesting that myofibrillar actomyosin ATPase activity is not altered by 3 mo of disuse (122). Likewise, time to peak tension for a twitch of tibialis anterior muscle has been reported comparable between SCI patients and healthy control subjects, suggesting that long-term unloading does not markedly alter calcium kinetics (215). Comparable twitch mechanics in SCI patients and healthy controls may be interpreted to imply that fiber-type composition of muscle and, thereby, myofibrillar actomyosin ATPase activity is not altered by SCI (39,40,146). Thus, a muscle appears faster in chronic SCI patients than control subjects, yet is comparable to those of healthy individuals for myofibrillar actomyosin ATPase activity and mechanical function.

The magnitude of strength reduction is also specific to muscle group, with weight-bearing muscles most affected. For knee extensors, the decline in strength averages about 0.6% per day. In contrast, the first dorsal interosseus hand muscle is relatively resistant to adaptation after 3–5 wk of immobilization (24,78).

Muscular endurance associated with disuse has not been widely studied. However, given the reductions in mitochondrial content and reduced maximal oxygen delivery, it may be suggested that losses in the capacity to repeatedly contract over time would be significant with aging. One recent report suggests that after 4 wk of casting of the elbow flexors, endurance time was paradoxically increased in female but not male subjects. Furthermore, the electromyography (EMG) activity during the endurance test was altered in the female subjects. The EMG was associated with intermittent motor unit activity instead of the continuous activity typically observed. This suggests that motor unit activation patterns are altered after disuse, at least in women (194). The ability to maintain force over repeat contractions is not altered within 6 mo of SCI but is markedly compromised in chronic SCI patients (41,94,215).

Neuromuscular Consequences

Decreased strength with reduced use has consistently been shown to be greater than that explained by muscle atrophy (175). An exception to this concept has been reported after short-term space flight. Muscle strength decreases in proportionately similar amounts, or perhaps less than fiber size, after 5 or 11 d of unloading (about 15% vs. 20%) (65,132). This implies increased ability to recruit muscle or greater specific tension (force per unit muscle size). Neither has been reported in studies of unloading at normal gravity (26,60,93,114). Thus, neuromuscular impairment may occur after unloading.

Electromyographic studies demonstrate that maximal firing rate and maximal integrated EMG activity are decreased and periods of silent EMG activity appear during maximal voluntary contractions after unloading (114). The ability to recruit high-threshold motor units also seems to be compromised (82). The greater relative decline in strength than in size suggests that more muscle may be used to perform a given submaximal task. This has recently been reported using magnetic resonance imaging (MRI), supporting EMG analyses in which greater numbers of motor units are required to develop submaximal force (26,175,176).

The exercise professional should account for these neuromuscular adaptations to unloading in exercise prescriptions for subjects recovering from reduced muscular activity. Submaximal loads that were once easily borne require more absolute muscle involvement. In addition, individuals may not have visible muscle atrophy but may be particularly weak because of irregularities in motor control. Thus, although caution should be taken when training an older person following disuse, recent studies indicate that significant gains in strength, rate of contraction, and muscle size are accrued after several months of training following periods of disuse (219). It may be beneficial for exercise professionals to focus on movement focused skills independent of external resistance in the early phases of a resistance training program.

Indeed, once the movement appears coordinated then it may be beneficial to incorporate either static or dynamic resistance to build overall strength.

Vulnerability of Muscle Damage

Unloading lower limb skeletal muscle for 5 wk has demonstrated increased vulnerability to eccentric exercise-induced dysfunction and muscle injury (176). MRI obtained 3 d after eccentric exercise demonstrated muscle damage over the unloaded CSA, but none was evident in the contralateral weight-bearing limb. These results have practical importance to the exercise professional. Dysfunction and injury during reloading may prolong recovery. In the previous study, 10 d after the eccentric exercise, strength remained reduced by 20% (before unloading). Low-intensity exercise should be used with care during renewal of walking to minimize muscle dysfunction and injury. Further, during early phases of a resistance training program, it may be more advantageous to train motor skills prior to adding a resistance stimulus.

Increased vulnerability to exercise-induced muscle injury has also been reported in elderly individuals (145). Whether this is caused by aging, low physical activity or both is not known, but when starting an exercise program for an elderly person, it is important to be cautious.

Possible Countermeasures

Few data exist regarding the efficacy of various countermeasures designed to prevent muscle atrophy and dysfunction or to enhance recovery during disuse. Endurance activity enhances fatigue resistance of skeletal muscle during unloading. Electrical stimulation of tibialis anterior muscle for 45 min to 2 h · d^{-1} in complete SCI patients evoked a marked increase in ability to maintain force during contraction. This response is partly attributed to increased muscle fiber aerobic–oxidative enzyme content (146,215). Resistance-like exercise (high-force intermittent stimulation) in patients with SCI, as well as ladder climbing in hind- limb-suspended rats, has been shown to increase muscle size (62), the former to near preinjury levels. One report using only four subjects suggests that wearing a Penguin antigravity suit for 10 h a day and performing resistance exercise for 15 min each hour can prevent muscle atrophy associated with bed rest (167). A more practical approach to offsetting the muscle-wasting effects of disuse comes from the work of Rittweger et al., who found that subjects who engaged in flywheel resistive exercise lost significantly less power and recovered power significantly faster than control subjects (181).

Although neuromuscular dysfunction cannot be attributed solely to disuse in elderly patients, it is clear that resistance exercise induces gains in strength, muscle mass, and functional mobility while reducing frailty (55,73,229). Thus, resistance exercise is an effective countermeasure to the loss of muscle associated with disuse, ultimately reducing disability and supporting independent, healthy aging (136).

SUMMARY

Muscle atrophy, regardless of the method of unloading (decreased training, bed rest, space flight), results in decreased strength, poor motor control, and possible dysfunction and muscle injury. Therefore, individuals need to engage in activities that increase strength and are weight bearing. For older adults, resistance training may ultimately support independence and promote a high quality of life. Older adults that have maintained a lifestyle of physical activity may further benefit by offsetting the muscle losses associated with both natural aging and physical inactivity. In closing, maintaining muscle mass with a program of resistance training is essential for healthy aging in adults.

REFERENCES

1. *ACSM Current Content: Exercise and the older adult* [Internet]. Indianapolis (IN): American College of Sports Medicine; [cited 2011 Feb 14]. Available from: http://www.acsm.org/AM/Template.cfm?Section=Current_Comments1&Template=/CM/ContentDisplay.cfm&ContentID=8636
2. *ACSM Current Content: The Physiology of Aging* [Internet]. Indianapolis (IN): American College of Sports Medicine; [cited 2011 Feb 14]. Available from: http://www.acsm.org/AM/Template.cfm?Section=Current_Comments1&Template=/CM/ContentDisplay.cfm&ContentID=8623
3. Adams GR. Human unilateral lower limb suspension as a model for spaceflight effects on skeletal muscle. *J Appl Physiol.* 2002;93(4):1563–5; author reply 1565–6.
4. Adams GR, Caiozzo VJ, Baldwin KM. Skeletal muscle unweighting: spaceflight and ground-based models. *J Appl Physiol.* 2003;95(6):2185–201.
5. Adams GR, Hather BM, Dudley GA. Effect of short-term unweighting on human skeletal muscle strength and size. *Aviat Space Environ Med.* 1994;65(12):1116–21.
6. Akima H, Kano Y, Enomoto Y, et al. Muscle function in 164 men and women aged 20–84 yr. *Med Sci Sports Exerc.* 2001;33(2):220–6.
7. Akima H, Kuno S, Suzuki Y, Gunji A, Fukunaga T. Effects of 20 days of bed rest on physiological cross-sectional area of human thigh and leg muscles evaluated by magnetic resonance imaging. *J Gravit Physiol.* 1997;4(1):S15–21.
8. Alfredson H, Nordstrom P, Lorentzon R. Prolonged progressive calcaneal bone loss despite early weightbearing rehabilitation in patients surgically treated for Achilles tendinosis. *Calcif Tissue Int.* 1998;62(2):166–71.
9. Aoyagi Y, Shephard RJ. Aging and muscle function. *Sports Med.* 1992;14(6):376–96.
10. Armstrong N, Welsman JR, Williams CA, Kirby BJ. Longitudinal changes in young people's short-term power output. *Med Sci Sports Exerc.* 2000;32(6):1140–5.
11. Arnesen SM, Lawson MA. Age-related changes in focal adhesions lead to altered cell behavior in tendon fibroblasts. *Mech Ageing Dev.* 2006;127(9):726–32.

12. Aw D, Silva AB, Palmer DB. Immunosenescence: emerging challenges for an ageing population. *Immunology*. 2007;120(4):435–46.

13. Babb TG. Mechanical ventilatory constraints in aging, lung disease, and obesity: perspectives and brief review. *Med Sci Sports Exerc*. 1999;31(1 Suppl):S12–22.

14. Backman L, Lindenberger U, Li SC, Nyberg L. Linking cognitive aging to alterations in dopamine neurotransmitter functioning: recent data and future avenues. *Neurosci Biobehav Rev*. 2010;34(5):670–7.

15. Baggio B, Budakovic A, Perissinotto E, et al. Atherosclerotic risk factors and renal function in the elderly: the role of hyperfibrinogenaemia and smoking. Results from the Italian Longitudinal Study on Ageing (ILSA). *Nephrol Dial Transplant*. 2005;20(1):114–23.

16. Bajotto G, Shimomura Y. Determinants of disuse-induced skeletal muscle atrophy: exercise and nutrition countermeasures to prevent protein loss. *J Nutr Sci Vitaminol (Tokyo)*. 2006;52(4):233–47.

17. Bales CW, Ritchie CS. Sarcopenia, weight loss, and nutritional frailty in the elderly. *Annu Rev Nutr*. 2002;22:309–23.

18. Baraldi E, Cooper DM, Zanconato S, Armon Y. Heart rate recovery from 1 minute of exercise in children and adults. *Pediatr Res*. 1991;29(6):575–9.

19. Barontini M, Lazzari JO, Levin G, Armando I, Basso SJ. Age-related changes in sympathetic activity: biochemical measurements and target organ responses. *Arch Gerontol Geriatr*. 1997;25(2):175–86.

20. Barou O, Valentin D, Vico L, et al. High-resolution three-dimensional micro-computed tomography detects bone loss and changes in trabecular architecture early: comparison with DEXA and bone histomorphometry in a rat model of disuse osteoporosis. *Invest Radiol*. 2002;37(1):40–6.

21. Bemben MG, Mccalip GA. Strength and power relationships as a function of age. *J Strength Cond Res*. 1999;13(4):330–8.

22. Berg HE, Dudley GA, Haggmark T, Ohlsen H, Tesch PA. Effects of lower limb unloading on skeletal muscle mass and function in humans. *J Appl Physiol*. 1991;70(4):1882–5.

23. Berg HE, Dudley GA, Hather B, Tesch PA. Work capacity and metabolic and morphologic characteristics of the human quadriceps muscle in response to unloading. *Clin Physiol*. 1993;13(4):337–47.

24. Berg HE, Eiken O, Miklavcic L, Mekjavic IB. Hip, thigh and calf muscle atrophy and bone loss after 5-week bedrest inactivity. *Eur J Appl Physiol*. 2007;99(3):283–9.

25. Berg HE, Larsson L, Tesch PA. Lower limb skeletal muscle function after 6 wk of bed rest. *J Appl Physiol*. 1997;82(1):182–8.

26. Berg HE, Tesch PA. Changes in muscle function in response to 10 days of lower limb unloading in humans. *Acta Physiol Scand*. 1996;157(1):63–70.

27. Betik AC, Hepple RT. Determinants of VO2 max decline with aging: an integrated perspective. *Appl Physiol Nutr Metab*. 2008;33(1):130–40.

28. Bikle DD, Halloran BP. The response of bone to unloading. *J Bone Miner Metab*. 1999;17(4):233–44.

29. Bloomfield SA. Changes in musculoskeletal structure and function with prolonged bed rest. *Med Sci Sports Exerc*. 1997;29(2):197–206.

30. Bloomfield SA, Mysiw WJ, Jackson RD. Bone mass and endocrine adaptations to training in spinal cord injured individuals. *Bone*. 1996;19(1):61–8.

31. Bosy-Westphal A, Eichhorn C, Kutzner D, Illner K, Heller M, Muller MJ. The age-related decline in resting energy expenditure in humans is due to the loss of fat-free mass and to alterations in its metabolically active components. *J Nutr*. 2003;133(7):2356–62.

32. Boudignon BM, Bikle DD, Kurimoto P, et al. Insulin-like growth factor I stimulates recovery of bone lost after a period of skeletal unloading. *J Appl Physiol*. 2007;103(1):125–31.

33. Bourrin S, Palle S, Genty C, Alexandre C. Physical exercise during remobilization restores a normal bone trabecular network after tail suspension-induced osteopenia in young rats. *J Bone Miner Res*. 1995;10(5):820–8.

34. Boutouyrie P, Tropeano AI, Asmar R, et al. Aortic stiffness is an independent predictor of primary coronary events in hypertensive patients: a longitudinal study. *Hypertension*. 2002;39(1):10–5.

35. Bruunsgaard H, Pedersen BK. Age-related inflammatory cytokines and disease. *Immunol Allergy Clin North Am*. 2003;23(1):15–39.

36. Bruunsgaard H, Pedersen M, Pedersen BK. Aging and proinflammatory cytokines. *Curr Opin Hematol*. 2001;8(3):131–6.

37. Caserotti P, Aagaard P, Puggaard L. Changes in power and force generation during coupled eccentric-concentric versus concentric muscle contraction with training and aging. *Eur J Appl Physiol*. 2008;103(2):151–61.

38. Castro MJ, Apple DF Jr, Hillegass EA, Dudley GA. Influence of complete spinal cord injury on skeletal muscle cross-sectional area within the first 6 months of injury. *Eur J Appl Physiol Occup Physiol*. 1999;80(4):373–8.

39. Castro MJ, Apple DF Jr, Melton-Rogers S, Dudley GA. Muscle fiber type-specific myofibrillar Ca(2+) ATPase activity after spinal cord injury. *Muscle Nerve*. 2000;23(1):119–21.

40. Castro MJ, Apple DF Jr, Rogers S, Dudley GA. Influence of complete spinal cord injury on skeletal muscle mechanics within the first 6 months of injury. *Eur J Appl Physiol*. 2000;81(1–2):128–31.

41. Castro MJ, Apple DF Jr, Staron RS, Campos GE, Dudley GA. Influence of complete spinal cord injury on skeletal muscle within 6 mo of injury. *J Appl Physiol*. 1999;86(1):350–8.

42. Christiansen JL, Grzybowski JM, Spreadbury D. *Biology of Aging: An Introduction to the Biomedical Aspects of Aging*. New York (NY): McGraw-Hill, Primis Custom Pub; 1999.

43. Clarke BA, Drujan D, Willis MS, et al. The E3 Ligase MuRF1 degrades myosin heavy chain protein in dexamethasone-treated skeletal muscle. *Cell Metab*. 2007;6(5):376–85.

44. Cohen AJ, Roe FJ. Review of risk factors for osteoporosis with particular reference to a possible aetiological role of dietary salt. *Food Chem Toxicol*. 2000;38(2–3):237–53.

45. Cohen S, Brault JJ, Gygi SP, et al. During muscle atrophy, thick, but not thin, filament components are degraded by MuRF1-dependent ubiquitylation. *J Cell Biol*. 2009;185(6):1083–95.

46. Collis T, Devereux RB, Roman MJ, et al. Relations of stroke volume and cardiac output to body composition: the strong heart study. *Circulation*. 2001;103(6):820–5.

47. Convertino VA. Insight into mechanisms of reduced orthostatic performance after exposure to microgravity: comparison of ground-based and space flight data. *J Gravit Physiol*. 1998;5(1):P85–8.

48. Convertino VA. Planning strategies for development of effective exercise and nutrition countermeasures for long-duration space flight. *Nutrition*. 2002;18(10):880–8.

49. Coupe M, Fortrat JO, Larina I, Gauquelin-Koch G, Gharib C, Custaud MA. Cardiovascular deconditioning: from autonomic nervous system to microvascular dysfunctions. *Respir Physiol Neurobiol*. 2009;169 Suppl 1:S10–2.

50. Coyle EF, Martin WH,3rd, Sinacore DR, Joyner MJ, Hagberg JM, Holloszy JO. Time course of loss of adaptations after stopping prolonged intense endurance training. *J Appl Physiol*. 1984;57(6):1857–64.

51. Crawford K, Fleishman K, Abt JP, et al. Less body fat improves physical and physiological performance in army soldiers. *Mil Med*. 2011;176(1):35–43.

52. d'Alessio P. Aging and the endothelium. *Exp Gerontol*. 2004;39(2):165–71.

53. Dalsky GP, Stocke KS, Ehsani AA, Slatopolsky E, Lee WC, Birge SJ Jr. Weight-bearing exercise training and lumbar bone mineral content in postmenopausal women. *Ann Intern Med*. 1988;108(6):824–8.

54. de Simone G, Devereux RB, Daniels SR, et al. Stroke volume and cardiac output in normotensive children and adults. Assessment of relations with body size and impact of overweight. *Circulation*. 1997;95(7):1837–43.

55. De Vos NJ, Singh NA, Ross DA, Stavrinos TM, Orr R, Singh MAF. Optimal load for increasing muscle power during explosive resistance training in older adults. *J Gerontol A Biol Sci Med Sci.* 2005;60(5):638–47.

56. Deschenes MR. Effects of aging on muscle fibre type and size. *Sports Med.* 2004;34(12):809–24.

57. Deschenes MR, Giles JA, McCoy RW, Volek JS, Gomez AL, Kraemer WJ. Neural factors account for strength decrements observed after short-term muscle unloading. *Am J Physiol Regul Integr Comp Physiol.* 2002;282(2):R578–83.

58. DeVries HA, Adams GM. Comparison of exercise responses in old and young men. I. The cardiac effort-total body effort relationship. *J Gerontol.* 1972;27(3):344–8.

59. Donato AJ, Uberoi A, Wray DW, Nishiyama S, Lawrenson L, Richardson RS. Differential effects of aging on limb blood flow in humans. *Am J Physiol Heart Circ Physiol.* 2006;290(1): H272–8.

60. Duchateau J. Bed rest induces neural and contractile adaptations in triceps surae. *Med Sci Sports Exerc.* 1995;27(12):1581–9.

61. Duchateau J, Hainaut K. Effects of immobilization on contractile properties, recruitment and firing rates of human motor units. *J Physiol.* 1990;422:55–65.

62. Dudley GA, Castro MJ, Rogers S, Apple DF Jr. A simple means of increasing muscle size after spinal cord injury: a pilot study. *Eur J Appl Physiol Occup Physiol.* 1999;80(4):394–6.

63. Dudley GA, Duvoisin MR, Adams GR, Meyer RA, Belew AH, Buchanan P. Adaptations to unilateral lower limb suspension in humans. *Aviat Space Environ Med.* 1992;63(8):678–83.

64. Dudley GA, Duvoisin MR, Convertino VA, Buchanan P. Alterations of the in vivo torque-velocity relationship of human skeletal muscle following 30 days exposure to simulated microgravity. *Aviat Space Environ Med.* 1989;60(7):659–63.

65. Edgerton VR, Zhou MY, Ohira Y, et al. Human fiber size and enzymatic properties after 5 and 11 days of spaceflight. *J Appl Physiol.* 1995;78(5):1733–9.

66. Ehrlich PJ, Lanyon LE. Mechanical strain and bone cell function: a review. *Osteoporos Int.* 2002;13(9):688–700.

67. Elia EA. Exercise and the elderly. *Clin Sports Med.* 1991;10(1): 141–55.

68. Elosua R, Bartali B, Ordovas JM, et al. Association between physical activity, physical performance, and inflammatory biomarkers in an elderly population: the InCHIANTI study. *J Gerontol A Biol Sci Med Sci.* 2005;60(6):760–7.

69. Erickson KI, Prakash RS, Voss MW, et al. Aerobic fitness is associated with hippocampal volume in elderly humans. *Hippocampus.* 2009;19(10):1030–9.

70. Evans WJ. Skeletal muscle loss: cachexia, sarcopenia, and inactivity. *Am J Clin Nutr.* 2010;91(4):1123S–7S.

71. Evans WJ, Paolisso G, Abbatecola AM, et al. Frailty and muscle metabolism dysregulation in the elderly. *Biogerontology.* 2010;11(5):527–36.

72. Falk B, Bar-Or O, Smolander J, Frost G. Response to rest and exercise in the cold: effects of age and aerobic fitness. *J Appl Physiol.* 1994;76(1):72–8.

73. Fiatarone MA, Marks EC, Ryan ND, Meredith CN, Lipsitz LA, Evans WJ. High-intensity strength training in nonagenarians. Effects on skeletal muscle. *JAMA.* 1990;263(22):3029–34.

74. Fitzgerald PL. Exercise for the elderly. *Med Clin North Am.* 1985;69(1):189–96.

75. Fleg JL, Morrell CH, Bos AG, et al. Accelerated longitudinal decline of aerobic capacity in healthy older adults. *Circulation.* 2005;112(5):674–82.

76. Franklin SS. Hypertension in older people: part 1. *J Clin Hypertens (Greenwich).* 2006;8(6):444–9.

77. Freedman VA, Martin LG. Contribution of chronic conditions to aggregate changes in old-age functioning. *Am J Public Health.* 2000;90(11):1755–60.

78. Fuglevand AJ, Bilodeau M, Enoka RM. Short-term immobilization has a minimal effect on the strength and fatigability of a human hand muscle. *J Appl Physiol.* 1995;78(3):847–55.

79. Gentil P, Lima RM, Jaco de Oliveira R, Pereira RW, Reis VM. Association between femoral neck bone mineral density and lower limb fat-free mass in postmenopausal women. *J Clin Densitom.* 2007;10(2):174–8.

80. Glass D, Roubenoff R. Recent advances in the biology and therapy of muscle wasting. *Ann N Y Acad Sci.* 2010;1211:25–36.

81. Gogia PP, Schneider VS, LeBlanc AD, Krebs J, Kasson C, Pientok C. Bed rest effect on extremity muscle torque in healthy men. *Arch Phys Med Rehabil.* 1988;69(12):1030–2.

82. Goldspink DF, Morton AJ, Loughna P, Goldspink G. The effect of hypokinesia and hypodynamia on protein turnover and the growth of four skeletal muscles of the rat. *Pflugers Arch.* 1986;407(3):333–40.

83. Gordon T, Mao J. Muscle atrophy and procedures for training after spinal cord injury. *Phys Ther.* 1994;74(1):50–60.

84. Grana EA, Chiou-Tan F, Jaweed MM. Endplate dysfunction in healthy muscle following a period of disuse. *Muscle Nerve.* 1996; 19(8):989–93.

85. Granath A, Jonsson B, Strandell T. Circulation in healthy old men, studied by right heart catheterization at rest and during exercise in supine and sitting position. *Acta Med Scand.* 1964;176:425–46.

86. Green S. A definition and systems view of anaerobic capacity. *Eur J Appl Physiol Occup Physiol.* 1994;69(2):168–73.

87. Gulmans VA, de Meer K, Binkhorst RA, Helders PJ, Saris WH. Reference values for maximum work capacity in relation to body composition in healthy Dutch children. *Eur Respir J.* 1997; 10(1):94–7.

88. Harris RT, Dudley GA. Factors limiting force during slow, shortening actions of the quadriceps femoris muscle group in vivo. *Acta Physiol Scand.* 1994;152(1):63–71.

89. Hather BM, Adams GR, Tesch PA, Dudley GA. Skeletal muscle responses to lower limb suspension in humans. *J Appl Physiol.* 1992;72(4):1493–8.

90. Hather BM, Tesch PA, Buchanan P, Dudley GA. Influence of eccentric actions on skeletal muscle adaptations to resistance training. *Acta Physiol Scand.* 1991;143(2):177–85.

91. Hebestreit H, Mimura K, Bar-Or O. Recovery of muscle power after high-intensity short-term exercise: comparing boys and men. *J Appl Physiol.* 1993;74(6):2875–80.

92. Henwood TR, Riek S, Taaffe DR. Strength versus muscle power-specific resistance training in community-dwelling older adults. *J Gerontol A Biol Sci Med Sci.* 2008;63(1):83–91.

93. Hikida RS, Gollnick PD, Dudley GA, Convertino VA, Buchanan P. Structural and metabolic characteristics of human skeletal muscle following 30 days of simulated microgravity. *Aviat Space Environ Med.* 1989;60(7):664–70.

94. Hillegass EA, Dudley GA. Surface electrical stimulation of skeletal muscle after spinal cord injury. *Spinal Cord.* 1999;37(4):251–7.

95. Ho CH, Wuermser LA, Priebe MM, Chiodo AE, Scelza WM, Kirshblum SC. Spinal cord injury medicine. 1. Epidemiology and classification. *Arch Phys Med Rehabil.* 2007;88(3 Suppl 1):S49–54.

96. Hodges P, Holm AK, Hansson T, Holm S. Rapid atrophy of the lumbar multifidus follows experimental disc or nerve root injury. *Spine (Phila Pa 1976).* 2006;31(25):2926–33.

97. Hofbauer LC, Brueck CC, Shanahan CM, Schoppet M, Dobnig H. Vascular calcification and osteoporosis—from clinical observation towards molecular understanding. *Osteoporos Int.* 2007;18(3): 251–9.

98. Houston ME, Froese EA, Valeriote SP, Green HJ, Ranney DA. Muscle performance, morphology and metabolic capacity during strength training and detraining: a one leg model. *Eur J Appl Physiol Occup Physiol.* 1983;51(1):25–35.

99. Ike RW, Lampman RM, Castor CW. Arthritis and aerobic exercise: a review. *Physician Sportsmed.* 1989;17(2):128–39.

100. Imai E, Horio M, Yamagata K, et al. Slower decline of glomerular filtration rate in the Japanese general population: a longitudinal 10-year follow-up study. *Hypertens Res.* 2008;31(3):433–41.

101. Ingram DK. Age-related decline in physical activity: generalization to nonhumans. *Med Sci Sports Exerc.* 2000;32(9):1623–9.

102. Inoue M, Tanaka H, Moriwake T, Oka M, Sekiguchi C, Seino Y. Altered biochemical markers of bone turnover in humans during 120 days of bed rest. *Bone.* 2000;26(3):281–6.

103. Ito M, Matsumoto T, Enomoto H, Tsurusaki K, Hayashi K. Effect of nonweight bearing on tibial bone density measured by QCT in patients with hip surgery. *J Bone Miner Metab.* 1999;17(1):45–50.

104. Iwamoto J, Takeda T, Ichimura S. Effect of exercise training and detraining on bone mineral density in postmenopausal women with osteoporosis. *J Orthop Sci.* 2001;6(2):128–32.

105. Jackson AS, Sui X, Hebert JR, Church TS, Blair SN. Role of lifestyle and aging on the longitudinal change in cardiorespiratory fitness. *Arch Intern Med.* 2009;169(19):1781–7.

106. Jackson AS, Wier LT, Ayers GW, Beard EF, Stuteville JE, Blair SN. Changes in aerobic power of women, ages 20–64 yr. *Med Sci Sports Exerc.* 1996;28(7):884–91.

107. Jacobs PL, Mahoney ET. Peak exercise capacity of electrically induced ambulation in persons with paraplegia. *Med Sci Sports Exerc.* 2002;34(10):1551–6.

108. Jacobs PL, Nash MS, Rusinowski JW. Circuit training provides cardiorespiratory and strength benefits in persons with paraplegia. *Med Sci Sports Exerc.* 2001;33(5):711–7.

109. Janssens JP. Aging of the respiratory system: impact on pulmonary function tests and adaptation to exertion. *Clin Chest Med.* 2005;26(3):469–84, vi–vii.

110. Jaworski ZF, Uhthoff HK. Reversibility of nontraumatic disuse osteoporosis during its active phase. *Bone.* 1986;7(6):431–9.

111. Jee WS, Wronski TJ, Morey ER, Kimmel DB. Effects of spaceflight on trabecular bone in rats. *Am J Physiol.* 1983;244(3):R310–4.

112. Jeng SF, Liao HF, Lai JS, Hou JW. Optimization of walking in children. *Med Sci Sports Exerc.* 1997;29(3):370–6.

113. Judge AR, Koncarevic A, Hunter RB, Liou HC, Jackman RW, Kandarian SC. Role for IkappaBalpha, but not c-Rel, in skeletal muscle atrophy. *Am J Physiol Cell Physiol.* 2007;292(1):C372–82.

114. Kandarian SC, Boushel RC, Schulte LM. Elevated interstitial fluid volume in rat soleus muscles by hindlimb unweighting. *J Appl Physiol.* 1991;71(3):910–4.

115. Kaneps AJ, Stover SM, Lane NE. Changes in canine cortical and cancellous bone mechanical properties following immobilization and remobilization with exercise. *Bone.* 1997;21(5):419–23.

116. Karlsson MK. Does exercise during growth prevent fractures in later life? *Med Sport Sci.* 2007;51:121–36.

117. Kasch FW, Boyer JL, Van Camp SP, Verity LS, Wallace JP. The effect of physical activity and inactivity on aerobic power in older men (a longitudinal study). *Physician Sportsmed.* 1990;18(4):73–83.

118. Kaye D, Esler M. Sympathetic neuronal regulation of the heart in aging and heart failure. *Cardiovasc Res.* 2005;66(2):256–64.

119. Kenney WL. Control of heat-induced cutaneous vasodilatation in relation to age. *Eur J Appl Physiol Occup Physiol.* 1988;57(1):120–5.

120. Kenney WL, Tankersley CG, Newswanger DL, Hyde DE, Puhl SM, Turner NL. Age and hypohydration independently influence the peripheral vascular response to heat stress. *J Appl Physiol.* 1990;68(5):1902–8.

121. Kohut ML, Cooper MM, Nickolaus MS, Russell DR, Cunnick JE. Exercise and psychosocial factors modulate immunity to influenza vaccine in elderly individuals. *J Gerontol A Biol Sci Med Sci.* 2002;57(9):M557–62.

122. Koryak Y. Contractile properties of the human triceps surae muscle during simulated weightlessness. *Eur J Appl Physiol Occup Physiol.* 1995;70(4):344–50.

123. Krahenbuhl GS, Skinner JS, Kohrt WM. Developmental aspects of maximal aerobic power in children. *Exerc Sport Sci Rev.* 1985;13:503–38.

124. Kubo K, Kanehisa H, Azuma K, et al. Muscle architectural characteristics in women aged 20–79 years. *Med Sci Sports Exerc.* 2003;35(1):39–44.

125. Lafage-Proust MH, Combe C, Barthe N, Aparicio M. Bone mass and dynamic parathyroid function according to bone histology in nondialyzed uremic patients after long-term protein and phosphorus restriction. *J Clin Endocrinol Metab.* 1999;84(2):512–9.

126. Lakatta EG. Age-associated cardiovascular changes in health: impact on cardiovascular disease in older persons. *Heart Fail Rev.* 2002;7(1):29–49.

127. Lakatta EG. Cardiovascular regulatory mechanisms in advanced age. *Physiol Rev.* 1993;73(2):413–67.

128. Lang T, Streeper T, Cawthon P, Baldwin K, Taaffe DR, Harris TB. Sarcopenia: etiology, clinical consequences, intervention, and assessment. *Osteoporos Int.* 2010;21(4):543–59.

129. Laugier P, Novikov V, Elmann-Larsen B, Berger G. Quantitative ultrasound imaging of the calcaneus: precision and variations during a 120-Day bed rest. *Calcif Tissue Int.* 2000;66(1):16–21.

130. Laukkanen JA, Laaksonen D, Lakka TA, et al. Determinants of cardiorespiratory fitness in men aged 42 to 60 years with and without cardiovascular disease. *Am J Cardiol.* 2009;103(11):1598–604.

131. Lawrenson L, Poole JG, Kim J, Brown C, Patel P, Richardson RS. Vascular and metabolic response to isolated small muscle mass exercise: effect of age. *Am J Physiol Heart Circ Physiol.* 2003;285(3): H1023–31.

132. LeBlanc A, Gogia P, Schneider V, Krebs J, Schonfeld E, Evans H. Calf muscle area and strength changes after five weeks of horizontal bed rest. *Am J Sports Med.* 1988;16(6):624–9.

133. Leblanc AD, Schneider VS, Evans HJ, Engelbretson DA, Krebs JM. Bone mineral loss and recovery after 17 weeks of bed rest. *J Bone Miner Res.* 1990;5(8):843–50.

134. LeBlanc A, Schneider V, Spector E, et al. Calcium absorption, endogenous excretion, and endocrine changes during and after long-term bed rest. *Bone.* 1995;16(4 Suppl):301S–4S.

135. Lelieveld OT, van Brussel M, Takken T, van Weert E, van Leeuwen MA, Armbrust W. Aerobic and anaerobic exercise capacity in adolescents with juvenile idiopathic arthritis. *Arthritis Rheum.* 2007;57(6):898–904.

136. Leveille SG, Guralnik JM, Ferrucci L, Langlois JA. Aging successfully until death in old age: opportunities for increasing active life expectancy. *Am J Epidemiol.* 1999;149(7):654–64.

137. Levine BD, Lane LD, Watenpaugh DE, Gaffney FA, Buckey JC, Blomqvist CG. Maximal exercise performance after adaptation to microgravity. *J Appl Physiol.* 1996;81(2):686–94.

138. Loomba-Albrecht LA, Styne DM. Effect of puberty on body composition. *Curr Opin Endocrinol Diabetes Obes.* 2009;16(1):10–5.

139. Lueken SA, Arnaud SB, Taylor AK, Baylink DJ. Changes in markers of bone formation and resorption in a bed rest model of weightlessness. *J Bone Miner Res.* 1993;8(12):1433–8.

140. Machwate M, Zerath E, Holy X, Pastoureau P, Marie PJ. Insulin-like growth factor-I increases trabecular bone formation and osteoblastic cell proliferation in unloaded rats. *Endocrinology.* 1994;134(3):1031–8.

141. Madden KM, Levy WC, Stratton JR. Normal aging impairs upregulation of the beta-adrenergic but not the alpha-adrenergic response: aging and adrenergic upregulation. *J Cardiovasc Pharmacol.* 2006;48(4):153–9.

142. Madsen K, Pedersen PK, Djurhuus MS, Klitgaard NA. Effects of detraining on endurance capacity and metabolic changes during prolonged exhaustive exercise. *J Appl Physiol.* 1993;75(4):1444–51.

143. Magnusson HI, Linden C, Obrant KJ, Johnell O, Karlsson MK. Bone mass changes in weight-loaded and unloaded skeletal regions following a fracture of the hip. *Calcif Tissue Int.* 2001;69(2):78–83.

144. Makrides L, Heigenhauser GJ, McCartney N, Jones NL. Maximal short term exercise capacity in healthy subjects aged 15–70 years. *Clin Sci (Lond).* 1985;69(2):197–205.

145. Manfredi TG, Fielding RA, O'Reilly KP, Meredith CN, Lee HY, Evans WJ. Plasma creatine kinase activity and exercise-induced muscle damage in older men. *Med Sci Sports Exerc.* 1991;23(9): 1028–34.

146. Martin TP, Stein RB, Hoeppner PH, Reid DC. Influence of electrical stimulation on the morphological and metabolic properties of paralyzed muscle. *J Appl Physiol.* 1992;72(4):1401–6.

147. McGavock JM, Hastings JL, Snell PG, et al. A forty-year follow-up of the Dallas Bed Rest and Training study: the effect of age on the cardiovascular response to exercise in men. *J Gerontol A Biol Sci Med Sci.* 2009;64(2):293–9.

148. Meaume S, Benetos A, Henry OF, Rudnichi A, Safar ME. Aortic pulse wave velocity predicts cardiovascular mortality in subjects >70 years of age. *Arterioscler Thromb Vasc Biol.* 2001;21(12):2046–50.

149. Melton LJ,3rd, Khosla S, Crowson CS, O'Connor MK, O'Fallon WM, Riggs BL. Epidemiology of sarcopenia. *J Am Geriatr Soc.* 2000;48(6):625–30.

150. Menz HB, Morris ME, Lord SR. Foot and ankle characteristics associated with impaired balance and functional ability in older people. *J Gerontol A Biol Sci Med Sci.* 2005;60(12):1546–52.

151. Meyer F, Bar-Or O, MacDougall D, Heigenhauser GJ. Drink composition and the electrolyte balance of children exercising in the heat. *Med Sci Sports Exerc.* 1995;27(6):882–7.

152. Michel BA, Lane NE, Bloch DA, Jones HH, Fries JF. Effect of changes in weight-bearing exercise on lumbar bone mass after age fifty. *Ann Med.* 1991;23(4):397–401.

153. Minaire P, Neunier P, Edouard C, Bernard J, Courpron P, Bourret J. Quantitative histological data on disuse osteoporosis: comparison with biological data. *Calcif Tissue Res.* 1974;17(1):57–73.

154. Mocchegiani E, Malavolta M. NK and NKT cell functions in immunosenescence. *Aging Cell.* 2004;3(4):177–84.

155. Mohtadi N. Injured limbs recover better with early mobilization and functional bracing than with cast immobilization. *J Bone Joint Surg Am.* 2005;87(5):1167.

156. Moreau KL, Donato AJ, Seals DR, DeSouza CA, Tanaka H. Regular exercise, hormone replacement therapy and the age-related decline in carotid arterial compliance in healthy women. *Cardiovasc Res.* 2003;57(3):861–8.

157. Moro-Garcia MA, Alonso-Arias R, Lopez-Vazquez A, et al. Relationship between functional ability in older people, immune system status, and intensity of response to CMV. *Age (Dordr).* 2012;34(2):479–495.

158. Mujika I, Padilla S. Muscular characteristics of detraining in humans. *Med Sci Sports Exerc.* 2001;33(8):1297–303.

159. Muller MJ, Grund A, Krause H, Siewers M, Bosy-Westphal A, Rieckert H. Determinants of fat mass in prepubertal children. *Br J Nutr.* 2002;88(5):545–54.

160. Murphy MP, Partridge L. Toward a control theory analysis of aging. *Annu Rev Biochem.* 2008;77:777–98.

161. Narici MV, Roi GS, Landoni L, Minetti AE, Cerretelli P. Changes in force, cross-sectional area and neural activation during strength training and detraining of the human quadriceps. *Eur J Appl Physiol Occup Physiol.* 1989;59(4):310–9.

162. Nickols-Richardson SM, Modlesky CM, O'Connor PJ, Lewis RD. Premenarcheal gymnasts possess higher bone mineral density than controls. *Med Sci Sports Exerc.* 2000;32(1):63–9.

163. Nordstrom A, Olsson T, Nordstrom P. Bone gained from physical activity and lost through detraining: a longitudinal study in young males. *Osteoporos Int.* 2005;16(7):835–41.

164. Nordstrom A, Olsson T, Nordstrom P. Sustained benefits from previous physical activity on bone mineral density in males. *J Clin Endocrinol Metab.* 2006;91(7):2600–4.

165. O'Flaherty EJ. Modeling normal aging bone loss, with consideration of bone loss in osteoporosis. *Toxicol Sci.* 2000;55(1):171–88.

166. Ogden CL, Yanovski SZ, Carroll MD, Flegal KM. The epidemiology of obesity. *Gastroenterology.* 2007;132(6):2087–102.

167. Ohira Y, Yoshinaga T, Ohara M, et al. Myonuclear domain and myosin phenotype in human soleus after bed rest with or without loading. *J Appl Physiol.* 1999;87(5):1776–85.

168. Ong KL, Cheung BM, Man YB, Lau CP, Lam KS. Prevalence, awareness, treatment, and control of hypertension among United States adults 1999–2004. *Hypertension.* 2007;49(1):69–75.

169. Palle S, Vico L, Bourrin S, Alexandre C. Bone tissue response to four-month antiorthostatic bedrest: a bone histomorphometric study. *Calcif Tissue Int.* 1992;51(3):189–94.

170. Pathare NC, Stevens JE, Walter GA, et al. Deficit in human muscle strength with cast immobilization: contribution of inorganic phosphate. *Eur J Appl Physiol.* 2006;98(1):71–8.

171. Pattullo MC, Cotter MA, Cameron NE, Barry JA. Effects of lengthened immobilization on functional and histochemical properties of rabbit tibialis anterior muscle. *Exp Physiol.* 1992;77(3):433–42.

172. Pawelczyk JA, Zuckerman JH, Blomqvist CG, Levine BD. Regulation of muscle sympathetic nerve activity after bed rest deconditioning. *Am J Physiol Heart Circ Physiol.* 2001;280(5):H2230–9.

173. Picone R. The female athlete triad. In: Brzycki M, editor. *The Female Athlete: Train for Success.* Terre Haute: Wish Publishing; 2004. p. 105–130.

174. Pischon T, Hankinson SE, Hotamisligil GS, Rifai N, Rimm EB. Leisure-time physical activity and reduced plasma levels of obesity-related inflammatory markers. *Obes Res.* 2003;11(9):1055–64.

175. Ploutz-Snyder LL, Tesch PA, Crittenden DJ, Dudley GA. Effect of unweighting on skeletal muscle use during exercise. *J Appl Physiol.* 1995;79(1):168–75.

176. Ploutz-Snyder LL, Tesch PA, Hather BM, Dudley GA. Vulnerability to dysfunction and muscle injury after unloading. *Arch Phys Med Rehabil.* 1996;77(8):773–7.

177. Powers SK, Kavazis AN, McClung JM. Oxidative stress and disuse muscle atrophy. *J Appl Physiol.* 2007;102(6):2389–97.

178. Prisk GK. Microgravity and the lung. *J Appl Physiol.* 2000;89(1): 385–96.

179. Reaburn P, Dascombe B. Anaerobic performance in masters athletes. *Eur Rev Aging Clin Activ.* 2009;6(1):39–53.

180. Ridgway CL, Brage S, Anderssen S, Sardinha LB, Andersen LB, Ekelund U. Fat-free mass mediates the association between birth weight and aerobic fitness in youth. *Int J Pediatr Obes.* 2011; 6(2-2):e590–6.

181. Rittweger J, Felsenberg D, Maganaris C, Ferretti JL. Vertical jump performance after 90 days bed rest with and without flywheel resistive exercise, including a 180 days follow-up. *Eur J Appl Physiol.* 2007;100(4):427–36.

182. Rittweger J, Winwood K, Seynnes O, et al. Bone loss from the human distal tibia epiphysis during 24 days of unilateral lower limb suspension. *J Physiol.* 2006;577(Pt 1):331–7.

183. Rodeheffer RJ, Gerstenblith G, Becker LC, Fleg JL, Weisfeldt ML, Lakatta EG. Exercise cardiac output is maintained with advancing age in healthy human subjects: cardiac dilatation and increased stroke volume compensate for a diminished heart rate. *Circulation.* 1984;69(2):203–13.

184. Roig M, Macintyre DL, Eng JJ, Narici MV, Maganaris CN, Reid WD. Preservation of eccentric strength in older adults: Evidence, mechanisms and implications for training and rehabilitation. *Exp Gerontol.* 2010;45(6):400–9.

185. Rowland T. Thermoregulation during exercise in the heat in children: old concepts revisited. *J Appl Physiol.* 2008;105(2):718–24.

186. Rowland T, Popowski B, Ferrone L. Cardiac responses to maximal upright cycle exercise in healthy boys and men. *Med Sci Sports Exerc.* 1997;29(9):1146–51.

187. Roy RR, Baldwin KM, Edgerton VR. The plasticity of skeletal muscle: effects of neuromuscular activity. *Exerc Sport Sci Rev.* 1991;19:269–312.

188. Ruml LA, Dubois SK, Roberts ML, Pak CY. Prevention of hypercalciuria and stone-forming propensity during prolonged bedrest by alendronate. *J Bone Miner Res.* 1995;10(4):655–62.

189. Schneider EL. *Handbook of the Biology of Aging*. 3rd ed. San Diego (CA): Academic Press; 1990.

190. Schneider SM. Bed rest and orthostatic-hypotensive intolerance. In: Greenleaf JE, editor. *Deconditioning and Reconditioning*. Boca Raton: CRC Press; 2004. p. 137–156.

191. Schrack JA, Simonsick EM, Ferrucci L. The energetic pathway to mobility loss: an emerging new framework for longitudinal studies on aging. *J Am Geriatr Soc*. 2010;58 Suppl 2:S329–36.

192. Schulman SP, Lakatta EG, Fleg JL, Lakatta L, Becker LC, Gerstenblith G. Age-related decline in left ventricular filling at rest and exercise. *Am J Physiol*. 1992;263(6 Pt 2):H1932–8.

193. Schut LJ. Motor system changes in the aging brain: what is normal and what is not. *Geriatrics*. 1998;53 Suppl 1:S16–9.

194. Semmler JG, Kutzscher DV, Enoka RM. Gender differences in the fatigability of human skeletal muscle. *J Neurophysiol*. 1999;82(6):3590–3.

195. Sharma G, Goodwin J. Effect of aging on respiratory system physiology and immunology. *Clin Interv Aging*. 2006;1(3):253–60.

196. Shephard RF. *Body Composition in Biological Anthropology*. Cambridge (NY): Cambridge University Press; 1991. 345 p.

197. Shephard RJ. Age and physical work capacity. *Exp Aging Res*. 1999;25(4):331–43.

198. Shephard RJ. *Aging, Physical Activity, and Health*. Champaign (IL): Human Kinetics; 1997. 488 p.

199. Shephard RJ. Physiologic changes over the years. In: Durstine JL, editor. *ACSM's Resource Manual for Guidelines for Exercise Testing and Prescription*. 2nd ed. Philadelphia: Lea & Febiger; 1993. p. 397–408.

200. Shephard RJ, Montelpare W, Plyley M, McCracken D, Goode RC. Handgrip dynamometry, Cybex measurements and lean mass as markers of the ageing of muscle function. *Br J Sports Med*. 1991;25(4):204–8.

201. Shimizu K, Kimura F, Akimoto T, et al. Effect of moderate exercise training on T-helper cell subpopulations in elderly people. *Exerc Immunol Rev*. 2008;14:24–37.

202. Shinkai S, Konishi M, Shephard RJ. Aging, exercise, training, and the immune system. *Exerc Immunol Rev*. 1997;3:68–95.

203. Short KR, Bigelow ML, Kahl J, et al. Decline in skeletal muscle mitochondrial function with aging in humans. *Proc Natl Acad Sci U S A*. 2005;102(15):5618–23.

204. Shvartz E, Reibold RC. Aerobic fitness norms for males and females aged 6 to 75 years: a review. *Aviat Space Environ Med*. 1990;61(1):3–11.

205. Slade JM, Bickel CS, Modlesky CM, Majumdar S, Dudley GA. Trabecular bone is more deteriorated in spinal cord injured versus estrogen-free postmenopausal women. *Osteoporos Int*. 2005;16(3):263–72.

206. Smith SM, Wastney ME, Morukov BV, et al. Calcium metabolism before, during, and after a 3-mo spaceflight: kinetic and biochemical changes. *Am J Physiol*. 1999;277(1 Pt 2):R1–10.

207. Smith SM, Wastney ME, O'Brien KO, et al. Bone markers, calcium metabolism, and calcium kinetics during extended-duration space flight on the mir space station. *J Bone Miner Res*. 2005;20(2):208–18.

208. Smorawinski J, Nazar K, Kaciuba-Uscilko H, et al. Effects of 3-day bed rest on physiological responses to graded exercise in athletes and sedentary men. *J Appl Physiol*. 2001;91(1):249–57.

209. Snow CM, Williams DP, LaRiviere J, Fuchs RK, Robinson TL. Bone gains and losses follow seasonal training and detraining in gymnasts. *Calcif Tissue Int*. 2001;69(1):7–12.

210. Spina RJ. Cardiovascular adaptations to endurance exercise training in older men and women. *Exerc Sport Sci Rev*. 1999;27:317–32.

211. Spirduso WW, Francis KL, MacRae PG. *Physical Dimensions of Aging*. 2nd ed. Champaign (IL): Human Kinetics; 2005. 374 p.

212. Staron RS. The classification of human skeletal muscle fiber types. *J Strength Cond Res*. 1997;11:67.

213. Staron RS, Leonardi MJ, Karapondo DL, et al. Strength and skeletal muscle adaptations in heavy-resistance-trained women after detraining and retraining. *J Appl Physiol*. 1991;70(2):631–40.

214. *Stedman's Medical Dictionary for the Health Professions and Nursing*. 5th ed. Philadelphia (PA): Lippincott Williams & Wilkins; 2005. 2000 p.

215. Stein RB, Gordon T, Jefferson J, et al. Optimal stimulation of paralyzed muscle after human spinal cord injury. *J Appl Physiol*. 1992;72(4):1393–400.

216. Stein TP, Wade CE. Metabolic consequences of muscle disuse atrophy. *J Nutr*. 2005;135(7):1824S–8S.

217. Sternfeld B, Ngo L, Satariano WA, Tager IB. Associations of body composition with physical performance and self-reported functional limitation in elderly men and women. *Am J Epidemiol*. 2002;156(2):110–21.

218. Stevens JE, Walter GA, Okereke E, et al. Muscle adaptations with immobilization and rehabilitation after ankle fracture. *Med Sci Sports Exerc*. 2004;36(10):1695–701.

219. Suetta C, Aagaard P, Magnusson SP, et al. Muscle size, neuromuscular activation, and rapid force characteristics in elderly men and women: effects of unilateral long-term disuse due to hip-osteoarthritis. *J Appl Physiol*. 2007;102(3):942–8.

220. Szoke E, Shrayyef MZ, Messing S, et al. Effect of aging on glucose homeostasis: accelerated deterioration of beta-cell function in individuals with impaired glucose tolerance. *Diabetes Care*. 2008;31(3):539–43.

221. Taaffe DR, Henwood TR, Nalls MA, Walker DG, Lang TF, Harris TB. Alterations in muscle attenuation following detraining and retraining in resistance-trained older adults. *Gerontology*. 2009;55(2):217–23.

222. Tanaka H, Dinenno FA, Monahan KD, Clevenger CM, DeSouza CA, Seals DR. Aging, habitual exercise, and dynamic arterial compliance. *Circulation*. 2000;102(11):1270–5.

223. Tanaka H, Monahan KD, Seals DR. Age-predicted maximal heart rate revisited. *J Am Coll Cardiol*. 2001;37(1):153–6.

224. Tanaka H, Seals DR. Endurance exercise performance in Masters athletes: age-associated changes and underlying physiological mechanisms. *J Physiol*. 2008;586(1):55–63.

225. Tankersley CG, Smolander J, Kenney WL, Fortney SM. Sweating and skin blood flow during exercise: effects of age and maximal oxygen uptake. *J Appl Physiol*. 1991;71(1):236–42.

226. Tate CA, Hyek MF, Taffet GE. Mechanisms for the responses of cardiac muscle to physical activity in old age. *Med Sci Sports Exerc*. 1994;26(5):561–7.

227. Thompson WR, Gordon NF, Pescatello LS, American College of Sports Medicine. *ACSM's Guidelines for Exercise Testing and Prescription*. 8th ed. Philadelphia (PA): Lippincott Williams & Wilkins; 2009.

228. Tilton FE, Degioanni JJ, Schneider VS. Long-term follow-up of Skylab bone demineralization. *Aviat Space Environ Med*. 1980;51(11):1209–13.

229. Tseng BS, Marsh DR, Hamilton MT, Booth FW. Strength and aerobic training attenuate muscle wasting and improve resistance to the development of disability with aging. *J Gerontol A Biol Sci Med Sci*. 1995;50 Spec No:113–9.

230. Turley KR, Wilmore JH. Cardiovascular responses to submaximal exercise in 7- to 9-yr-old boys and girls. *Med Sci Sports Exerc*. 1997;29(6):824–32.

231. Uebelhart D, Bernard J, Hartmann DJ, et al. Modifications of bone and connective tissue after orthostatic bedrest. *Osteoporos Int*. 2000;11(1):59–67.

232. Uebelhart D, Demiaux-Domenech B, Roth M, Chantraine A. Bone metabolism in spinal cord injured individuals and in others who have prolonged immobilisation. A review. *Paraplegia*. 1995;33(11):669–73.

233. Valdimarsson O, Alborg HG, Duppe H, Nyquist F, Karlsson M. Reduced training is associated with increased loss of BMD. *J Bone Miner Res*. 2005;20(6):906–12.

234. van der Wiel HE, Lips P, Nauta J, Netelenbos JC, Hazenberg GJ. Biochemical parameters of bone turnover during ten days of bed rest and subsequent mobilization. *Bone Miner.* 1991;13(2):123–9.

235. van Harreveld PD, Lillich JD, Kawcak CE, Turner AS, Norrdin RW. Effects of immobilization followed by remobilization on mineral density, histomorphometric features, and formation of the bones of the metacarpophalangeal joint in horses. *Am J Vet Res.* 2002;63(2):276–81.

236. Vandervoort AA. Aging of the human neuromuscular system. *Muscle Nerve.* 2002;25(1):17–25.

237. Vandervoort AA. Potential benefits of warm-up for neuromuscular performance of older athletes. *Exerc Sport Sci Rev.* 2009;37(2):60–5.

238. Vanhecke TE, Franklin BA, Miller WM, deJong AT, Coleman CJ, McCullough PA. Cardiorespiratory fitness and sedentary lifestyle in the morbidly obese. *Clin Cardiol.* 2009;32(3):121–4.

239. Verghese J, Holtzer R, Lipton RB, Wang C. Quantitative gait markers and incident fall risk in older adults. *J Gerontol A Biol Sci Med Sci.* 2009;64(8):896–901.

240. Vico L, Chappard D, Alexandre C, et al. Effects of a 120 day period of bed-rest on bone mass and bone cell activities in man: attempts at countermeasure. *Bone Miner.* 1987;2(5):383–94.

241. Vico L, Collet P, Guignandon A, et al. Effects of long-term microgravity exposure on cancellous and cortical weight-bearing bones of cosmonauts. *Lancet.* 2000;355(9215):1607–11.

242. Walker JL, Murray TD, Jackson AS, Morrow JR Jr, Michaud TJ. The energy cost of horizontal walking and running in adolescents. *Med Sci Sports Exerc.* 1999;31(2):311–22.

243. Wang J, Horlick M, Thornton JC, Levine LS, Heymsfield SB, Pierson RN Jr. Correlations between skeletal muscle mass and bone mass in children 6–18 years: influences of sex, ethnicity, and pubertal status. *Growth Dev Aging.* 1999;63(3):99–109.

244. Wang Q, Alen M, Nicholson P, et al. Weight-bearing, muscle loading and bone mineral accrual in pubertal girls—a 2-year longitudinal study. *Bone.* 2007;40(5):1196–202.

245. Weinert D, Waterhouse J. The circadian rhythm of core temperature: effects of physical activity and aging. *Physiol Behav.* 2007;90(2–3):246–56.

246. Westing SH, Seger JY, Thorstensson A. Effects of electrical stimulation on eccentric and concentric torque-velocity relationships during knee extension in man. *Acta Physiol Scand.* 1990;140(1):17–22.

247. Widrick JJ, Romatowski JG, Norenberg KM, et al. Functional properties of slow and fast gastrocnemius muscle fibers after a 17-day spaceflight. *J Appl Physiol.* 2001;90(6):2203–11.

248. Wilson TE, Shibasaki M, Cui J, Levine BD, Crandall CG. Effects of 14 days of head-down tilt bed rest on cutaneous vasoconstrictor responses in humans. *J Appl Physiol.* 2003;94(6):2113–8.

249. Woo JS, Derleth C, Stratton JR, Levy WC. The influence of age, gender, and training on exercise efficiency. *J Am Coll Cardiol.* 2006;47(5):1049–57.

250. Yildiz O. Vascular smooth muscle and endothelial functions in aging. *Ann N Y Acad Sci.* 2007;1100:353–60.

251. Young AJ. Effects of aging on human cold tolerance. *Exp Aging Res.* 1991;17(3):205–13.

252. Young DR, Niklowitz WJ, Brown RJ, Jee WS. Immobilization-associated osteoporosis in primates. *Bone.* 1986;7(2):109–17.

253. Zanconato S, Cooper DM, Armon Y. Oxygen cost and oxygen uptake dynamics and recovery with 1 min of exercise in children and adults. *J Appl Physiol.* 1991;71(3):993–8.

254. Zerwekh JE, Ruml LA, Gottschalk F, Pak CY. The effects of twelve weeks of bed rest on bone histology, biochemical markers of bone turnover, and calcium homeostasis in eleven normal subjects. *J Bone Miner Res.* 1998;13(10):1594–601.

SELECTED REFERENCES FOR FURTHER READING

Cox H. *Annual Editions: Aging 11/12.* New York (NY): McGraw-Hill; 2012. 192 p.

Rikli R, Jones CJ. *Senior Fitness Test Manual.* Champaign (IL): Human Kinetics; 2001. 176 p.

Signorile J. *Bending the Aging Curve: The Complete Exercise Guide for Older Adults.* Champaign (IL): Human Kinetics; 2011. 328 p.

INTERNET RESOURCES

- ISAPA: International Society for Aging and Physical Activity: http://www.isapa.org
- National Institute on Aging: http://www.nia.nih.gov
- NCPAD: National Center on Physical Activity and Disability: http://www.ncpad.org
- Tufts University Health & Nutrition Newsletter: http://healthletter.tufts.edu
- WebMD: http://www.webmd.com

Pathophysiology and Treatment of Cardiovascular Disease

The World Health Organization estimates that cardiovascular disease (CVD) kills 17.1 million people worldwide each year, with an estimated 82% of those deaths occurring in low- and middle-income countries. In the United States, CVD kills more people than cancer, pulmonary diseases, accidents and diabetes mellitus combined, and was the underlying cause of 33.6% of all deaths in 2007. Approximately 2,200 Americans die each day from CVD, an average of one death every 39 s. An estimated 82,600,000 American adults have one or more types of CVD, which will generate over $286 billion in direct and indirect health care costs. This includes $167 billion in expenditures (direct costs, which include cost of physicians, prescribed medications, home health care, etc.) and $119 billion in lost productivity resulting from premature mortality (indirect costs) (47).

This chapter will discuss the outcomes and manifestations of specific CVDs, the physiologic process of atherosclerosis, and treatments of CVDs, including pharmacologic, surgical, and lifestyle interventions. Furthermore, the role of cardiovascular risk factors in CVD will be presented as well as the goals of risk factor modification strategies.

ATHEROSCLEROSIS

Our understanding of atherosclerosis has evolved over the past several decades, and the disease is no longer viewed as a passive deposition of cholesterol in the arterial wall causing progressive arterial stenosis and ultimately creating an occlusive thrombus. Today, we recognize that atherosclerosis is an active process involving molecular signals that produce altered cellular behavior as well as endothelial dysfunction and a subsequent inflammatory response (35). Although lipid deposition is a fundamental part of the atherosclerotic process, interactions among blood-borne molecules and intrinsic cells of the arterial wall are now recognized as important contributors to the pathogenesis of this disease.

Although atherosclerosis is often considered in chronologic phases, the disease is far more complex than this simplistic perspective suggests. Initiation of the process typically occurs in childhood. The lesion progresses to form a fatty streak, typically during young adulthood through middle age. Ultimately, the lesion matures to form a complex fibrous plaque that may produce symptoms or complications such as myocardial infarction (MI), sudden cardiac death, or stroke, typically as a result of an occlusive thrombus. The rate at which an individual lesion progresses through these stages may vary greatly over time and is related to the presence of classic and emerging risk factors.

Initiation of the atherosclerotic process begins with injury of the endothelial lining of the arterial wall, stemming from several possible causes including carbon monoxide or other tobacco-related irritants, hypertension, low-density lipoprotein cholesterol (LDL-C), and homocysteine. For reasons that are still unclear, normal endothelial function is not restored by the inherent

---

KEY TERMS

Myocardial infarction: The death of myocardial tissue resulting from prolonged ischemia.

Angina pectoris: Chest pain or discomfort that is caused by myocardial ischemia.

Cardiovascular disease: Class of diseases that affect the heart or circulatory system.

Ischemia: A lack of blood flow relative to tissue needs.

Morbidity: The rate of incidence of a particular disease.

Mortality: The number of deaths in a given time or place.

Peripheral arterial disease: Condition in which blood flow through noncoronary arterial beds is impaired.

Sudden cardiac death: An unexpected death that results from the abrupt loss of heart function and that occurs within 1 h of the onset of symptoms.

Thrombus: A blood clot that may cause a vascular obstruction.

repair mechanisms (29). Platelets adhere to the damaged arterial wall, aggregate, and become activated, secreting growth factors and vasoconstrictive substances such as thromboxane A2.

LDL-C passes through the endothelial monolayer at the site of injury and undergoes the process of oxidation. Oxidized phospholipids such as LDL-C can elicit the expression of vascular adhesion molecules on the surface of the endothelial cells, promoting the adhesion of peripheral blood monocytes to the area of injury. Furthermore, constituents of oxidized LDL-C can stimulate the expression of chemoattractant cytokines, such as MCP-1, which encourage migration of monocytes into the subendothelial space (35). Activated platelets induce an inflammatory reaction in cells of the vascular wall (45), which induces endothelial activation and secretion of chemoattractants, further promoting monocyte recruitment (9,22,50,59). Upon moving into the arterial wall, monocytes are transformed into macrophages and collect the subintimal LDL-C, further augmenting the oxidative and subsequent inflammatory processes. At this point of development, the lesion consists primarily of foam cells (*i.e.*, engorged macrophages), as well as T- and B-lymphocytes and mast cells (19). It is referred to as a *fatty streak*, reflecting its appearance and composition (*Fig. 6-1*).

Lipid accumulation during this phase may be slowed or reversed through the cardioprotective effects of high-density lipoprotein cholesterol (HDL-C). HDL-C uses the reverse cholesterol transport mechanism to remove cholesterol from engorged macrophages and carry it out of the subendothelial space to be excreted (55). In addition, HDL holds antioxidant enzymes that may mitigate inflammation as well as the endothelial expression of vascular adhesion molecules that augment atherosclerotic progression (1,35).

With continued maturation, a fatty streak progresses to a more fibrous plaque (*Fig. 6-2*). Specific cells in and around the lesion are affected by signaling mechanisms

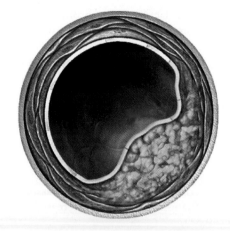

FIGURE 6-2. Disease progression of atherosclerosis: fibrous plaque. (Asset provided by Anatomical Chart Co.)

from platelets, monocytes, and endothelial cells that result in growth and proliferation (39). Fibroblasts and smooth muscle cells (SMCs) migrate to the intima from the media layer of the blood vessel (37). SMCs create the primary components of the complex extracellular matrix, including collagens, elastin, and glycosaminoglycans. In the intima, expression of these molecules gives rise to the characteristic structure of atherosclerotic plaque, including a rigid fibrous cap (34,52). Beneath this cap lies one or more lipid cores, which typically contain macrophage foam cells, inflammatory molecules, SMCs, calcium, dead cells, and acellular debris.

It was previously believed that atherosclerotic lesions would progress to occlusive stenoses that ultimately resulted in an ischemic event. It is now understood that compensatory arterial enlargement (*i.e.*, remodeling) allows for considerable atherosclerotic development without substantial lumenal occlusion (51) and that most adverse cardiovascular events are the result of plaque erosion or rupture with subsequent thrombus development (*Fig. 6-3*). Physical disruption of the lesion exposes

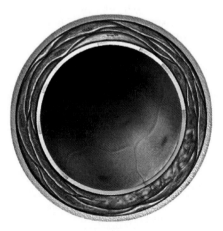

FIGURE 6-1. Disease progression of atherosclerosis: fatty streak. (Asset provided by Anatomical Chart Co.)

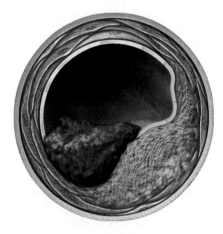

FIGURE 6-3. Disease progression of atherosclerosis: complicated lesion with blood clot. (Asset provided by Anatomical Chart Co.)

blood coagulation factors to prothrombotic stimuli that reside in the core of the plaque. The ensuing blood clot may dissolve, may become large enough to occlude the artery at the site of rupture, may become dislodged from the arterial wall and substantially occlude a downstream artery, or may be incorporated into the rapidly growing lesion. Plaques that are most vulnerable to rupture tend to have a large lipid core with reduced collagen content, a thin fibrous cap, and pronounced outward remodeling of the arterial wall (53). Atherothrombotic events also depend on the thrombogenic properties of the blood (36), and the risk of ischemic events is associated with elevated coagulation activity and decreased fibrinolytic capacity (49,57).

OUTCOMES AND MANIFESTATIONS OF CARDIOVASCULAR DISEASE AND THE UNIQUE PATHOPHYSIOLOGIES RESPECTIVE TO EACH CONDITION

HYPERTENSION

Hypertension is defined as having systolic blood pressure (SBP) 140 mm Hg or diastolic blood pressure (DBP) 90 mm Hg or higher, or taking antihypertensive medication. The most commonly diagnosed CVD — hypertension — affects an estimated one of every three American adults, or approximately 76,400,000 people older than the age of 20 yr (47). Age-adjusted prevalence of hypertension is greater in men than in women, and African Americans have higher prevalence than other ethnic groups (47). The number of deaths from hypertension rose 56.4% from 1994 to 2004 (25). Elevated BP increases risk of heart failure (HF) (27), end-stage renal disease (38), MI (13), and stroke (13), and is associated with reduced overall life expectancy (15).

In general, hypertension causes a constriction of peripheral arteries, increasing the workload of the heart. In a relatively small number of diagnosed cases of hypertension, the elevated BP is caused by another abnormality such as renal disorders or congenital narrowing of particular arteries. However, 90%–95% of all cases of high BP are "essential" or "primary" hypertension. That is, the elevated BP is not the result of a separate disorder but is a disorder unto itself associated with various risk factors (such as obesity and inactivity).

CORONARY HEART DISEASE

Coronary heart disease (CHD) is the manifestation of advanced atherosclerotic progression in one or more coronary arteries. CHD is the single largest killer of American men and women, causing one of every six deaths in the United States in 2007 (47). It has been projected that direct medical costs of CHD will exceed $106 billion by the year 2030, a 198% increase from 2010 ($35.7 billion) (21). Indirect costs, resulting from lost productivity, are expected to increase more than 50% during that same period, exceeding $112 billion. Common sequelae of CHD include angina pectoris, MI, and sudden cardiac death.

Angina pectoris is referred pain resulting from myocardial ischemia. The pain is often described as substernal pressure, heaviness, or burning that is sometimes accompanied by dyspnea. Chronic stable angina pectoris is typically elicited by physical or emotional stress and is relieved by rest or nitrate medication. Unstable angina pectoris does not share the predictability of chronic stable angina and may present itself with no provocation. Unstable angina may result from coronary vasospasm or transient occlusion and is relieved by spontaneous arterial relaxation and/or thrombolysis. Vasospastic or Prinzmetal angina is caused by focal coronary artery vasospasm, typically at the site of, or adjacent to, a fixed stenosis. Animal experiments suggest that coronary vasospasm is caused primarily by vascular smooth muscle hypercontraction and not by local endothelial dysfunction. The molecular mechanism(s) of this smooth muscle cell abnormality remains unclear.

HEART FAILURE

HF is a chronic, degenerative condition in which the ability of one or both ventricles to fill with (diastolic failure) or eject (systolic failure) blood is impaired (see *Table 6-1* for disease classification). Primarily a condition of the elderly, incidence of HF is increasing, and more Medicare dollars are spent for the diagnosis and treatment of HF than for any other diagnosis (40). Total medical costs of HF in 2010 (direct and indirect) were approximately $34.4 billion (21). Principal manifestations of HF include dyspnea, fatigue, exercise intolerance, and fluid retention. HF may be caused by any number of conditions that damage the heart, including cardiomyopathies, CHD, or established risk factors for CVD such as smoking, obesity, hypertension, high cholesterol, and diabetes mellitus (27). Most patients

TABLE 6-1. Classification of Heart Failure (27)

Stage	Definition
A	At high risk for HF but without structural heart disease or symptoms of HF
B	Structural heart disease but without signs or symptoms of HF
C	Structural heart disease with prior or current symptoms of HF
D	Refractory HF requiring specialized interventions

HF, heart failure.

experience symptoms that result from an impairment of left ventricular myocardial function and exhibit both systolic and diastolic abnormalities (27). Ventricular dysfunction in HF typically progresses, resulting in a change in the structure of the ventricle such that it becomes more spherical. This "cardiac remodeling" increases hemodynamic stress on the chamber walls and may increase regurgitant blood flow through the mitral valve, further exacerbating the remodeling process. Activation of neurohormonal systems also contributes to cardiac remodeling. Patients with HF have elevated catecholamines, cytokines, aldosterone, and angiotensin II. These hormonal changes may increase hemodynamic stress and have direct toxic effects on cardiac myocytes, as well as stimulate myocardial fibrosis, resulting in the further alteration of cardiac geometry and depressed function of the heart (27).

STROKE

Stroke is one of the leading causes of death and long-term disability in America (47). It is described as the loss of brain function subsequent to the interruption of blood flow. This may occur because of hemorrhage or obstruction, typically by an occlusive thrombus or embolism. Depending on the hemisphere of the brain that is affected, stroke patients may experience hemiplegia, altered coordination, vertigo, memory loss, problems with speech or vision, and behavioral changes.

Approximately 87% of all strokes are ischemic in nature rather than hemorrhagic (47), and transient ischemic attacks (TIAs) are particularly predictive of a stroke. The risk of stroke is 3%–17% within the first 90 d after a TIA; approximately 15% of all strokes are preceded by a TIA (18). In addition, approximately 12%–13% of persons who experience a TIA will die within 1 yr (47). The pathogenic mechanism of TIA is similar to ischemic stroke, but the transient attack is defined by neurologic symptoms that last less than 24 h (16). Patients with TIA and stroke have a high prevalence of asymptomatic coronary disease (11,12,48), so strategies for the prevention of ischemic stroke include modifying cardiovascular risk factors, such as dyslipidemia, hypertension, obesity, smoking, and physical inactivity (16). Furthermore, individuals with atrial fibrillation, women who are pregnant or within 6 wk postpartum, and postmenopausal women are at greater risk of stroke than their age- and sex-matched counterparts (3,30,60).

PERIPHERAL ARTERIAL DISEASE

Peripheral arterial disease (PAD) refers to a series of disorders in which blood flow through noncoronary arterial beds is impaired (see *Table 6-2* for disease classification). This condition most commonly affects the

TABLE 6-2. Fontaine's Classification of Peripheral Arterial Disease

Stage	Clinical Finding
I	Asymptomatic
IIa	Mild claudication
IIb	Moderate-to-severe claudication
III	Ischemic rest pain
IV	Ulceration or gangrene

femoral, popliteal, tibial, iliac, abdominal aorta, renal, and mesenteric arteries. PAD affects an estimated 8 million Americans, including 12%–20% of Americans aged 65 yr and older (23). Despite the prevalence and significant morbidity and mortality associated with PAD, only 25% of those diagnosed are undergoing treatment (2).

PAD is primarily caused by atherosclerosis and related thrombotic processes that may occlude the affected vessel and produce ischemia in downstream muscle tissue. Risk factors for PAD include age, obesity, sedentary lifestyle, dyslipidemia, hyperhomocysteinemia, hypertension, and especially smoking and diabetes mellitus. The classic manifestation of PAD is intermittent claudication: leg pain (*e.g.*, cramping, burning) that predictably follows physical exertion and is relieved by rest. It should be noted, however, that only approximately 10% of PAD patients report having intermittent claudication, approximately 50% report some variety of leg symptoms, and 40% do not report leg pain (8,23). PAD is associated with increased risk of other cardiovascular complications, such as MI and stroke, and, left untreated, may lead to gangrene and amputation. Treatment of PAD includes risk factor modification, weight-bearing exercise (such as walking), pharmacologic intervention, and possibly surgical revascularization.

SURGICAL TREATMENTS FOR CARDIOVASCULAR DISEASE

In situations in which primary prevention strategies have been unsuccessful in decreasing or reversing the progression of CVD, surgical intervention may be necessary to restore perfusion to the affected tissues. Revascularization techniques have advanced over the years and physicians now have a large arsenal of procedures, including some minimally invasive methods that require little or no convalescence.

Catheter-based interventions utilize a thin, flexible tube that is threaded through an artery from the groin or arm and into the occluded arteries. The catheter may then be used to perform a percutaneous coronary intervention such as an angioplasty, in which a small balloon is positioned over a lesion and expanded to

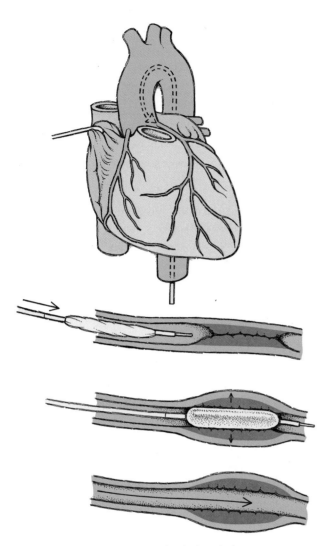

FIGURE 6-4. Percutaneous transluminal angioplasty. (Acknowledgment: Neil O. Hardy, Westpoint, CT.)

compress the plaque against the vessel wall (*Fig. 6-4*). One of the primary drawbacks of the balloon procedure is the risk of restenosis (33). To prevent restenosis, the angioplasty procedure commonly includes the use of a stent, a small metal tube that provides support to the opened vessel. Stents may be bare metal or drug coated, or carries time-released medicine (drug-eluting stent). A catheter may also be used to perform an atherectomy. A laser or rotating burr is used to break the lesion and thus remove the plaque from the artery. In some cases, a stent or balloon angioplasty is performed after the atherectomy.

The location or number of arterial blockages may necessitate the more invasive coronary artery bypass graft (CABG). A blood vessel (usually a saphenous vein, internal mammary artery, or radial artery) is surgically grafted to a coronary artery, bypassing an area that is narrowed as a result of advanced atherosclerosis. The conventional CABG procedure involves opening the chest with a sternum-splitting incision, stopping the heart, and using a cardiopulmonary bypass pump to sustain circulation. Surgical advances have led to techniques in which a CABG can be completed without separating the sternum and/or without the use of a bypass pump, leading to shorter recovery times and improved operative mortality rates. Currently, this primarily occurs only in very high-risk patients who are not acceptable candidates for traditional CABG (10,58).

CARDIOVASCULAR RISK FACTORS: ROLE IN DISEASE PROGRESSION, GOALS FOR RISK FACTOR MODIFICATION

Although it is not possible to control for all CVD risk factors such as age and family history, adopting a lifestyle that focuses on each of the controllable risk factors — and using medications in many cases — may positively affect cardiovascular morbidity and mortality. The American College of Sports Medicine positive risk factors for CVD that may be modified through lifestyle choices are cigarette smoking, sedentary lifestyle, obesity, hypertension, dyslipidemia, and impaired fasting glucose. A recent study of a large cohort of healthy men estimated that more than 60% of all primary coronary events could be prevented with a healthy lifestyle (7), further supporting the well-established benefits of risk factor modification.

SMOKING

Cigarette smoke contains several thousand chemicals and at least 40 known carcinogens. Several constituents of smoke contribute to the initiation and progression of atherosclerosis. Absorbed through active smoking or through passive exposure, cigarette smoke damages endothelial cells, leads to acute increases in BP, and increases platelet aggregation.

The smoking risk factor threshold is defined as a current smoking habit or having quit within the previous 6 mo or exposure to environmental tobacco smoke. Complete smoking cessation is the goal of this risk factor modification. Furthermore, patients should be urged to completely avoid exposure to environmental tobacco smoke.

HYPERTENSION

High BP (SBP ≥140 mm Hg and/or diastolic pressure ≥90 mm Hg, *or* on antihypertensive medication) contributes to nearly all CVDs, as well as to renal failure, aneurysm, and eye damage.

It is recommended that all patients with elevated BP initiate or maintain lifestyle modifications, including weight control, increased physical activity, and a diet that is low in sodium and saturated fat (*Table 6-3*).

TABLE 6-3. Lifestyle Modifications to Manage Hypertension[a,b] (8)

Modification	Recommendation	Approximate SBP Reduction
Weight reduction	Maintain normal body weight (BMI 18.5–24.9 kg · m^{-2}).	5–20 mm Hg/10 kg weight loss
Adopt DASH eating plan	Consume a diet rich in fruits, vegetables, and low fat dairy products with a reduced content of saturated and total fat.	8–14 mm Hg
Dietary sodium reduction	Reduce dietary sodium intake to no more than 100 mmol · d^{-1} (2.4 g sodium or 6 g sodium chloride).	2–8 mm Hg
Physical activity	Engage in regular aerobic physical activity such as brisk walking (at least 30 min · d^{-1}, most days of the week).	4–9 mm Hg
Moderation of alcohol consumption	Limit consumption to no more than 2 drinks (e.g., 1 oz or 30 mL ethanol; 24 oz beer, 10 oz wine; or 3 oz 80-proof whiskey) per day in most men and to no more than 1 drink per day in women and lighter weight persons.	2–4 mm Hg

SBP, systolic blood pressure; BMI, body mass index; DASH, Dietary Approaches to Stop Hypertension.

[a]For overall cardiovascular risk reduction, stop smoking.

[b]The effects of implementing these modifications are dose and time dependent and could be greater for some individuals.

BP–lowering medication is necessary for optimal control for many patients. The goal of BP control is to reduce BP to <140/90 or <130/80 mm Hg if the patient has diabetes or chronic kidney disease. The Seventh Report of the Joint National Committee on Prevention, Detection, Evaluation and Treatment of High Blood Pressure (JNC 7) (6) points out that the risk of CVD doubles with each increment of 20/10 mm Hg higher than 115/75 mm Hg and first introduced the classification of *prehypertensive*, which is defined as having slightly elevated BP (SBP 120–139 mm Hg, DBP 80–89 mm Hg). The JNC 7 report recommends health-promoting lifestyle modifications even for patients whose BP does not reach the threshold of hypertension.

DYSLIPIDEMIA

As previously discussed, cholesterol plays a significant role in atherogenesis. LDL-C plays a primary role in the initiation and progression of lesion development. Conversely, high serum concentration of HDL-C may slow or reverse atherosclerosis and is considered a negative risk factor. The most recent recommendations of the NCEP indicate that the goal of lipid management techniques is to keep LDL-C concentrations <100 mg · dL^{-1} if triglycerides are ≥200 mg · dL^{-1}, and all non-HDL-C should be <130 mg · dL^{-1} (56). All individuals should be encouraged to reduce dietary intake of saturated fats, *trans*-fatty acids, and cholesterol, and to increase consumption of plant sterols, viscous fiber, and ω-3 fatty acids. Promotion of weight management and regular physical activity should accompany these dietary recommendations. For many patients, LDL-lowering medication is necessary. For patients with CHD, statin medications are considered mandatory, even if LDL-C is <100 mg · dL^{-1}.

SEDENTARY LIFESTYLE

The positive effects of regular exercise on CVD are diverse and well documented in the scientific literature. All individuals are encouraged to accumulate a minimum of 30 min of moderate-intensity aerobic activity on at least 5 d · wk^{-1} or half this duration of vigorous-intensity aerobic activity (17,20). Double these levels of moderate and vigorous physical activity are recognized as more effective. In addition, combinations of moderate and vigorous intensity activity can be done to meet the recommendations (17,20). This is in addition to routine daily lifestyle activity of light intensity. Resistance training should be done 2 or more days per week. A medical and physical activity history should be assessed before participation in an exercise program, and high-risk patients should be advised to participate in medically supervised programs.

OBESITY

Obesity, defined as having a body mass index (BMI) ≥30 kg · m^{-2} or waist girth >102 cm for men and >88 cm for women, is a major independent risk factor for numerous hypokinetic diseases, including CVD. Furthermore, excess body fat is closely related to the presence of other CVD risk factors. It is estimated that as much as 75% of hypertension may be attributed to obesity, although the mechanism for this relationship is not fully understood (32). Increased total body weight has a strong effect on lipoprotein metabolism and is a determinant of decreased HDL-C and elevated triglycerides and LDL-C. Obesity also contributes to glucose intolerance and may be responsible for ≥50% of the variance in insulin sensitivity (32). It should also be noted that fat distribution patterns are likely to mediate the effect of obesity on CVD risk. Abdominal fat, in particular, is highly correlated with insulin resistance and, thus, complications of CVD. The goal for weight management is to maintain a BMI of 18.5–24.9 kg · m^{-2} with a waist circumference (measured horizontally at the iliac crest) <40 in for men and <35 in for women. Weight maintenance and reduction should be accomplished with a healthy balance of regular exercise and caloric intake.

IMPAIRED FASTING GLUCOSE

Chronic hyperglycemia, a hallmark of diabetes mellitus, is associated with accelerated atherosclerosis (44) and may bring about neurologic and cardiovascular complications. Transgenic mouse models and human autopsy studies suggest that diabetes-induced hyperglycemia, independent from dyslipidemia that is common among this patient population, results in accelerated lesion formation (26,41,42,46). Elevations in blood glucose concentrations also promote monocyte recruitment and adherence to the endothelial monolayer by stimulating expression of endothelial adhesion molecules (4,7). Diabetes and elevated glucose concentrations are related to advanced atherosclerotic plaques and clinical outcomes, but it is unclear if these effects are direct or simply secondary to the accelerated lesion initiation (28). The goal of glucose control management strategies is to maintain glycosylated hemoglobin (HbA1C) levels of <7%. Patients should initiate lifestyle changes and, as warranted, pharmacologic interventions.

PHARMACOLOGIC TREATMENT OF CARDIOVASCULAR DISEASE

Blood coagulation activity is elevated around a complicated atherosclerotic lesion and is responsible for most acute cardiovascular events. Thus, pharmacologic treatment of CVD often includes drugs that prevent the development of an occlusive thrombus. Antiplatelet medications, such as aspirin and clopidogrel, interfere with platelet activation and/or aggregation, thus interfering with one of the initial steps of the coagulation process. Aspirin is recommended not only for treatment but also for the prevention of heart disease in those at risk, provided that there are no hemorrhagic problems at present. Other common anticoagulant agents, such as warfarin and heparin, interfere with the coagulation cascade either by preventing hepatic synthesis of vitamin K-dependent clotting factors or stimulating coagulation enzyme inhibitors.

Other common medications used in the treatment of CVD focus on controlling one or more risk factors. One of the key components of strategies for primary and secondary prevention of CVD is the control of hypertension. As such, several medications are available for the maintenance of healthy BP, including diuretics, β-blockers, calcium channel blockers, angiotensin-converting enzyme (ACE) inhibitors, and angiotensin receptor blockers (ARBs).

β-Blockers (*e.g.*, atenolol, propanolol, metaprolol) bind to β-adrenergic receptors, inhibiting the action of endogenous catecholamines. These drugs reduce the sympathetic effects of catecholamines on the heart and blood vessels resulting in reduced heart rates and BP and decreasing myocardial oxygen demand.

Voltage-gated calcium channels, when stimulated in the heart and blood vessels, allow the influx of calcium into the cells resulting in vasoconstriction and increased myocardial contractility. Calcium channel blockers (*e.g.*, diltiazem, verapamil) inhibit stimulation of these voltage-regulated gates and promote vasodilation, decreased peripheral resistance, and cardiac output. However, calcium antagonists have negative inotropic effects and must be used with caution, if at all, in patients with CVD.

A diuretic (*e.g.*, furosemide, thiazides, amiloride, spironolactone) is a medication that controls BP by modulating the rate of urine excretion and, thus, plasma volume. The various classes of diuretic accomplish this in slightly different ways such as inhibiting reabsorption of sodium in the kidney (promoting osmotic diuresis) or inhibiting vasopressin (antidiuretic hormone) or aldosterone. Although diuretics are often not tolerated as well as some of the newer classes of antihypertensive medications, recent evidence suggests diuretic therapy may be more effective at reducing BP and preventing various forms of CVD (43).

The ACE catalyzes the conversion of angiotensin I to angiotensin II, which is a potent vasoconstrictor. ACE inhibitors (*e.g.*, enalapril, ramipril, lisinopril) block this reaction and the ensuing increase in BP related to vessel constriction is stopped. ACE inhibitors may also impart secondary cardiovascular benefits. Angiotensin II stimulates expression of pro-inflammatory cytokines as well as vascular adhesion molecules on the surface of endothelial cells (5,31). Thus, ACE inhibitors may slow the rate of atherosclerotic initiation and progression. Furthermore, ACE inhibition may enhance the ability to dissolve fibrin blood clots, reducing risk of complications related to occlusive thrombi (61).

The effect of angiotensin II on BP may also be minimized through the use of ARBs. Blockade of the angiotensin II receptor causes vasodilation and reduced secretion of aldosterone and vasopressin, ultimately reducing BP and myocardial workload. ARBs (*e.g.*, irbesartan, losartan, valsartan) are typically used in the treatment of hypertension and HF.

Control of blood cholesterol is another key focus of CVD treatment and prevention. Several medications are available that affect concentrations of total cholesterol, LDL-C, and/or HDL-C. Statins (*e.g.,* simvastatin, lovastatin, atorvastatin) are the most popular cholesterol-lowering medication. They are very effective at lowering LDL-C and may increase HDL-C and lower triglyceride concentration. Statins inhibit hepatic synthesis of cholesterol and increase the number of LDL receptors on hepatocytes, enhancing the elimination of LDL from the blood. Side effects of statins include skeletal muscle and liver damage, and routine blood tests are performed to monitor these concerns. In rare cases, statins may cause rhabdomyolysis — a severe myopathy that can result in renal failure. Resins (*e.g.,* cholestyramine) bind to bile acids in the intestine, preventing their reabsorption and thereby increasing their excretion. The increased bile acid excretion promotes increased cholesterol metabolism. Resins decrease total cholesterol and LDL-C. Fibrates (*e.g.,* gemfibrozil, fenofibrate) produce moderate decreases in blood concentrations of LDL-C and increases in HDL-C but are extremely effective at lowering triglyceride (54). Some gastrointestinal side effects have been reported, and fibrates may interact with anticoagulant medication. Nicotinic acid (niacin) increases serum levels of HDL-C substantially and also lowers total cholesterol, LDL-C, very-low-density lipoprotein (VLDL), and triglycerides. The mechanism of the antihyperlipidemic action of nicotinic acid is not well understood, but it is thought that the effect is mediated, in part, via decreases in the release of free fatty acids from adipose tissue and the rate of production of hepatic VLDL.

Other medications and nutritional supplements are commonly used in the treatment of CVD. Vasodilators such as nitroglycerin are used in tablet, spray, or transdermal patch form and relieve ischemia-related pain by dilating blood vessels. Antioxidant vitamins, such as vitamins E, C, and β-carotene, are thought to reduce the risk of CVD by preventing the oxidation of LDL-C. The lack of data from well-designed clinical trials makes it premature to recommend dietary supplements to prevent CVD, but all patients should be encouraged to consume a diet rich in food sources of antioxidant and other cardioprotective nutrients, such as ω-3 fatty acids.

PATHOPHYSIOLOGY OF THE HEALING MYOCARDIUM

Each year, an estimated 785,000 Americans will experience a new MI, and 470,000 more will have a recurrent attack (47). The healing process that follows an MI includes a series of changes in ventricular function, tissue composition, and regional deformation, as well as several possible complications.

In the first 4–6 h following an MI, the myocardium experiences acute ischemia. The infarcted tissue loses the ability to generate force and is changed to a passive, viscoelastic body. The loss of systolic power is the primary functional change in this phase. Several hours later, inflammation and necrosis become the dominant pathologic processes. This phase of healing typically lasts approximately 7 d, although signs of necrosis may persist for several months (14). The infarcted area may expand, growing thinner and occupying greater endothelial surface area. This remodeling process, in which the chamber dilates and weakens, may exacerbate increases in ventricular wall stress. The healing infarct soon transitions to a phase in which collagen deposition rapidly increases, leading to increased myocardial stiffness, impaired filling, and potentially impaired systolic function. Eventually, systolic function improves because of a decline in stiffness despite continued increases in collagen content. The infarct "scar" shrinks in this final stage of healing to occupy a smaller percentage of the ventricular wall. Chamber dilation decreases and wall-motion abnormalities partially resolve. Although the myocardium experiences dramatic improvements in structure and function, the tissue may never stabilize to the point that the healing process could be considered complete (24) (*Box 6-1*).

| **BOX 6-1** | **Potential Ways of Healing Infarct May Impair Left Ventricular Function (22)** |

- Infarct may fail or rupture.
- Infarct bulging or stretching wastes energy generated by healthy myocardium.
- Infarct stiffness may limit diastolic function of healthy myocardium.
- Infarct expansion and cavity dilation may increase wall stress throughout the chamber.
- Coupling to the infarct may limit deformation of the adjacent myocardium.
- Material properties of the infarct determine pattern of ventricular remodeling and hypertrophy.

REFERENCES

1. Barter PJ, Nicholls S, Rye KA, Anantharamaiah GM, Navab M, Fogelman AM. Antiinflammatory properties of HDL. *Circ Res*. 2004;95(8):764–72.

2. Becker GJ, McClenny TE, Kovacs ME, Raabe RD, Katzen BT. The importance of increasing public and physician awareness of peripheral arterial disease. *J Vasc Interv Radiol*. 2002;13(1):7–11.

3. Bonita R. Epidemiology of stroke. *Lancet*. 1992;339(8789):342–4.

4. Booth G, Stalker TJ, Lefer AM, Scalia R. Mechanisms of amelioration of glucose-induced endothelial dysfunction following inhibition of protein kinase C in vivo. *Diabetes*. 2002;51(5):1556–64.

5. Chen XL, Tummala PE, Olbrych MT, Alexander RW, Medford RM. Angiotensin II induces monocyte chemoattractant protein-1 gene expression in rat vascular smooth muscle cells. *Circ Res*. 1998;83(9):952–9.

6. Chobanian AV, Bakris GL, Black HR, et al, National Heart, Lung, and Blood Institute Joint National Committee on Prevention, Detection, Evaluation, and Treatment of High Blood Pressure, National High Blood Pressure Education Program Coordinating Committee. The Seventh Report of the Joint National Committee on Prevention, Detection, Evaluation, and Treatment of High Blood Pressure: the JNC 7 report. *JAMA*. 2003;289(19):2560–72.

7. Cipolletta C, Ryan KE, Hanna EV, Trimble ER. Activation of peripheral blood CD14+ monocytes occurs in diabetes. *Diabetes*. 2005;54(9):2779–86.

8. Criqui MH, Fronek A, Klauber MR, Barrett-Connor E, Gabriel S. The sensitivity, specificity, and predictive value of traditional clinical evaluation of peripheral arterial disease: results from noninvasive testing in a defined population. *Circulation*. 1985;71(3):516–22.

9. Danese S, de la Motte C, Reyes BM, Sans M, Levine AD, Fiocchi C. Cutting edge: T cells trigger CD40-dependent platelet activation and granular RANTES release: a novel pathway for immune response amplification. *J Immunol*. 2004;172(4):2011–5.

10. Detter C, Reichenspurner H, Boehm DH, et al. Minimally invasive direct coronary artery bypass grafting (MIDCAB) and off-pump coronary artery bypass grafting (OPCAB): two techniques for beating heart surgery. *Heart Surg Forum*. 2002;5(2):157–62.

11. Di Pasquale G, Andreoli A, Pinelli G, et al. Cerebral ischemia and asymptomatic coronary artery disease: a prospective study of 83 patients. *Stroke*. 1986;17(6):1098–101.

12. Di Pasquale G, Pinelli G, Grazi P, et al. Incidence of silent myocardial ischaemia in patients with cerebral ischaemia. *Eur Heart J*. 1988;9 Suppl N:104–7.

13. Fields LE, Burt VL, Cutler JA, Hughes J, Roccella EJ, Sorlie P. The burden of adult hypertension in the United States 1999 to 2000: a rising tide. *Hypertension*. 2004;44(4):398–404.

14. Fishbein MC, Maclean D, Maroko PR. The histopathologic evolution of myocardial infarction. *Chest*. 1978;73(6):843–9.

15. Franco OH, Peeters A, Bonneux L, de Laet C. Blood pressure in adulthood and life expectancy with cardiovascular disease in men and women: life course analysis. *Hypertension*. 2005;46(2):280–6.

16. Furie KL, Kasner SE, Adams RJ, et al. Guidelines for the prevention of stroke in patients with stroke or transient ischemic attack: a guideline for healthcare professionals from the American Heart Association/American Stroke Association. *Stroke*. 2011;42(1):227–76.

17. Garber CE, Blissmer B, Deschenes MR, et al. Quantity and quality of exercise for developing and maintaining cardiorespiratory, musculoskeletal, and neuromotor fitness in apparently healthy adults: guidance for prescribing exercise. *Med Sci Sports Exerc*. 2011;43(7):1334–59.

18. Hankey GJ. Long-term outcome after ischaemic stroke/transient ischaemic attack. *Cerebrovasc Dis*. 2003;16 Suppl 1:14–9.

19. Hansson GK, Libby P, Schonbeck U, Yan ZQ. Innate and adaptive immunity in the pathogenesis of atherosclerosis. *Circ Res*. 2002;91(4):281–91.

20. Haskell WL, Lee IM, Pate RR, et al. Physical activity and public health: updated recommendation for adults from the American College of Sports Medicine and the American Heart Association. *Med Sci Sports Exerc*. 2007;39(8):1423–34.

21. Heidenreich PA, Trogdon JG, Khavjou OA, et al. Forecasting the future of cardiovascular disease in the United States: a policy statement from the American Heart Association. *Circulation*. 2011;123(8):933–44.

22. Henn V, Slupsky JR, Grafe M, et al. CD40 ligand on activated platelets triggers an inflammatory reaction of endothelial cells. *Nature*. 1998;391(6667):591–4.

23. Hirsch AT, Criqui MH, Treat-Jacobson D, et al. Peripheral arterial disease detection, awareness, and treatment in primary care. *JAMA*. 2001;286(11):1317–24.

24. Holmes JW, Borg TK, Covell JW. Structure and mechanics of healing myocardial infarcts. *Annu Rev Biomed Eng*. 2005;7:223–53.

25. *Incidence and Prevalence: 2006 Chart Book on Cardiovascular and Lung Diseases* [Internet]. Bethesda (MD): National Institutes of Health; National Heart, Lung, and Blood Institute; [cited 2011 Feb 14]. Available from: http://www.nhlbi.nih.gov/resources/docs/06a_ip_chtbk.pdf

26. Jarvisalo MJ, Putto-Laurila A, Jartti L, et al. Carotid artery intima-media thickness in children with type 1 diabetes. *Diabetes*. 2002;51(2):493–8.

27. Jessup M, Abraham WT, Casey DE, et al. 2009 focused update: ACCF/AHA Guidelines for the Diagnosis and Management of Heart Failure in Adults: a report of the American College of Cardiology Foundation/American Heart Association Task Force on Practice Guidelines: developed in collaboration with the International Society for Heart and Lung Transplantation. *Circulation*. 2009;119(14):1977–2016.

28. Kanter JE, Johansson F, LeBoeuf RC, Bornfeldt KE. Do glucose and lipids exert independent effects on atherosclerotic lesion initiation or progression to advanced plaques? *Circ Res*. 2007;100(6):769–81.

29. Karra R, Vemullapalli S, Dong C, et al. Molecular evidence for arterial repair in atherosclerosis. *Proc Natl Acad Sci U S A*. 2005;102(46):16789–94.

30. Kittner SJ, Stern BJ, Feeser BR, et al. Pregnancy and the risk of stroke. *N Engl J Med*. 1996;335(11):768–74.

31. Kranzhofer R, Schmidt J, Pfeiffer CA, Hagl S, Libby P, Kubler W. Angiotensin induces inflammatory activation of human vascular smooth muscle cells. *Arterioscler Thromb Vasc Biol*. 1999;19(7):1623–9.

32. Krauss RM, Winston M, Fletcher BJ, Grundy SM. Obesity: impact on cardiovascular disease. *Circulation*. 1998;98(14):1472–6.

33. Kushner FG, Hand M, Smith SC Jr, et al. 2009 Focused Updates: ACC/AHA Guidelines for the Management of Patients With ST-Elevation Myocardial Infarction (updating the 2004 Guideline and 2007 Focused Update) and ACC/AHA/SCAI Guidelines on Percutaneous Coronary Intervention (updating the 2005 Guideline and 2007 Focused Update): a report of the American College of Cardiology Foundation/American Heart Association Task Force on Practice Guidelines. *Circulation*. 2009;120(22):2271–306.

34. Lafont A, Libby P. The smooth muscle cell: sinner or saint in restenosis and the acute coronary syndromes? *J Am Coll Cardiol*. 1998;32(1):283–5.

35. Libby P, Ridker PM. Inflammation and atherothrombosis. From population biology and bench research to clinical practice. *J Am Coll Cardiol*. 2006;48(9 Suppl).

36. Libby P, Theroux P. Pathophysiology of coronary artery disease. *Circulation*. 2005;111(25):3481–8.

37. Libby P, Warner SJ, Salomon RN, Birinyi LK. Production of platelet-derived growth factor-like mitogen by smooth-muscle cells from human atheroma. *N Engl J Med.* 1988;318(23):1493–8.

38. Martinez-Maldonado M. Hypertension in end-stage renal disease. *Kidney Int Suppl.* 1998;68:S67–72.

39. Massberg S, Vogt F, Dickfeld T, Brand K, Page S, Gawaz M. Activated platelets trigger an inflammatory response and enhance migration of aortic smooth muscle cells. *Thromb Res.* 2003;110(4):187–94.

40. Massie BM, Shah NB. Evolving trends in the epidemiologic factors of heart failure: rationale for preventive strategies and comprehensive disease management. *Am Heart J.* 1997;133(6):703–12.

41. McGill HC Jr, McMahan CA, Malcom GT, Oalmann MC, Strong JP. Relation of glycohemoglobin and adiposity to atherosclerosis in youth. Pathobiological Determinants of Atherosclerosis in Youth (PDAY) Research Group. *Arterioscler Thromb Vasc Biol.* 1995;15(4):431–40.

42. McGill HC Jr, McMahan CA, Zieske AW, Malcom GT, Tracy RE, Strong JP. Effects of nonlipid risk factors on atherosclerosis in youth with a favorable lipoprotein profile. *Circulation.* 2001; 103(11):1546–50.

43. Moser M. Current recommendations for the treatment of hypertension: are they still valid? *J Hypertens Suppl.* 2002;20(1):S3–10.

44. Nathan DM, Cleary PA, Backlund JY, et al, Diabetes Control and Complications Trial/Epidemiology of Diabetes Interventions and Complications (DCCT/EDIC) Study Research Group. Intensive diabetes treatment and cardiovascular disease in patients with type 1 diabetes. *N Engl J Med.* 2005;353(25):2643–53.

45. Pitsilos S, Hunt J, Mohler ER, et al. Platelet factor 4 localization in carotid atherosclerotic plaques: correlation with clinical parameters. *Thromb Haemost.* 2003;90(6):1112–20.

46. Renard CB, Kramer F, Johansson F, et al. Diabetes and diabetes-associated lipid abnormalities have distinct effects on initiation and progression of atherosclerotic lesions. *J Clin Invest.* 2004;114(5): 659–68.

47. Roger VL, Go AS, Lloyd-Jones DM, et al. Heart disease and stroke statistics—2012 update: a report from the American Heart Association. *Circulation.* 2012;125(1):e2–e220.

48. Rokey R, Rolak LA, Harati Y, Kutka N, Verani MS. Coronary artery disease in patients with cerebrovascular disease: a prospective study. *Ann Neurol.* 1984;16(1):50–3.

49. Salomaa V, Stinson V, Kark JD, Folsom AR, Davis CE, Wu KK. Association of fibrinolytic parameters with early atherosclerosis. The ARIC Study. Atherosclerosis Risk in Communities Study. *Circulation.* 1995;91(2):284–90.

50. Schober A, Manka D, von Hundelshausen P, et al. Deposition of platelet RANTES triggering monocyte recruitment requires P-selectin and is involved in neointima formation after arterial injury. *Circulation.* 2002;106(12):1523–9.

51. Schoenhagen P, Ziada KM, Kapadia SR, Crowe TD, Nissen SE, Tuzcu EM. Extent and direction of arterial remodeling in stable versus unstable coronary syndromes: an intravascular ultrasound study. *Circulation.* 2000;101(6):598–603.

52. Schwartz SM, Virmani R, Rosenfeld ME. The good smooth muscle cells in atherosclerosis. *Curr Atheroscler Rep.* 2000;2(5):422–9.

53. Shah PK. Insights into the molecular mechanisms of plaque rupture and thrombosis. *Indian Heart J.* 2005;57(1):21–30.

54. Staels B, Dallongeville J, Auwerx J, Schoonjans K, Leitersdorf E, Fruchart JC. Mechanism of action of fibrates on lipid and lipoprotein metabolism. *Circulation.* 1998;98(19):2088–93.

55. Tall AR, Jiang X, Luo Y, Silver D. 1999 George Lyman Duff memorial lecture: lipid transfer proteins, HDL metabolism, and atherogenesis. *Arterioscler Thromb Vasc Biol.* 2000;20(5):1185–8.

56. *Third report of the National Cholesterol Education Program (NCEP) Expert Panel on Detection, Evaluation, and Treatment of High Blood Cholesterol in Adults (adult treatment panel III) manuscript version* [Internet]. Bethesda (MD): The Program; [cited 2011 Feb 1]. Available from: http://www.nhlbi.nih.gov/guidelines/cholesterol/atp3_rpt.htm

57. Thompson SG, Kienast J, Pyke SD, Haverkate F, van de Loo JC. Hemostatic factors and the risk of myocardial infarction or sudden death in patients with angina pectoris. European Concerted Action on Thrombosis and Disabilities Angina Pectoris Study Group. *N Engl J Med.* 1995;332(10):635–41.

58. Verma S, Fedak PW, Weisel RD, et al. Off-pump coronary artery bypass surgery: fundamentals for the clinical cardiologist. *Circulation.* 2004;109(10):1206–11.

59. von Hundelshausen P, Weber KS, Huo Y, et al. RANTES deposition by platelets triggers monocyte arrest on inflamed and atherosclerotic endothelium. *Circulation.* 2001;103(13):1772–7.

60. Wolf PA, Abbott RD, Kannel WB. Atrial fibrillation as an independent risk factor for stroke: the Framingham Study. *Stroke.* 1991; 22(8):983–8.

61. Wright RA, Flapan AD, Alberti KG, Ludlam CA, Fox KA. Effects of captopril therapy on endogenous fibrinolysis in men with recent, uncomplicated myocardial infarction. *J Am Coll Cardiol.* 1994; 24(1):67–73.

SELECTED REFERENCES FOR FURTHER READING

Libby P, Ridker P. Inflammation and atherothrombosis: from population biology and bench research to clinical practice. *Am Coll Cardiol.* 2007;48:A33–46.

Sanz J, Moreno PR, Fuster V. The year in atherothrombosis. *J Am Coll Cardiol.* 2007;49:1740–9.

INTERNET RESOURCES

- American Heart Association: http://www.americanheart.org
- Centers for Disease Control — Heart Disease: http://www.cdc.gov/heartdisease/
- Mayo Clinic — Coronary Artery Disease: http://www.mayoclinic.com/health/coronary-artery-disease/DS00064
- National Heart, Lung, Blood Institute: http://www.nhlbi.nih.gov/

Pathophysiology and Treatment of Pulmonary Disease

Successful implementation of an exercise program in individuals with pulmonary disease can be a challenging task. The low exercise capacity extending from the type and severity of pulmonary disease affects the ability to perform any type of physical activity, including activities of daily living. Additionally, the severity of the physiologic aberration can be further amplified by physical activity. Dyspnea and fatigue initiate the perpetuating process of anxiety, activity avoidance, and progressive disability.

A basic understanding of disease pathophysiology, particularly in the context of the physiology of exercise, improves the efficacy and success of any exercise program for these patients. The design of the exercise program can be enhanced by recognizing disease features that can be used to individualize the program and optimize the individual exercise response. Through this knowledge base, elements key to the evaluation or assessment of the exercise response become more apparent, providing further direction to modifications that will enhance program design. Acquiring this knowledge base can be a large and complicated task, particularly if the diseases are approached in an individual manner.

This task can be simplified by grouping diseases based on physiologic similarities. Four groups of diseases can be defined and named for their primary limitation: obstructive pulmonary disease, restrictive pulmonary disease, pulmonary vasculature disease, and disturbances in ventilatory control. The physiologic pattern associated with each category can be generally applied to all the diseases in the respective category.

This chapter provides an overview of the key pathophysiologic principles important to exercising individuals with chronic pulmonary disease. A categorical approach is used to convey these concepts. The more prevalent diseases are used to exemplify these concepts. *Chapter 25* reviews assessment and limitations associated with pulmonary disease.

OBSTRUCTIVE PULMONARY DISEASE

Increased airway resistance is a major physiologic limitation in obstructive pulmonary disease. Generally, a reduced cross-sectional airway diameter attributable to

KEY TERMS

Asthma: A chronic inflammatory disease of the airways characterized by airflow obstruction that is often reversible and usually associated with airway hyperresponsiveness.

Bronchiectasis: A pulmonary disease characterized by irreversible dilation of the distal bronchi, commonly associated with bacterial infection.

Chronic bronchitis: Chronic inflammation of the conducting airways associated with the inhalation of noxious particles or gases (usually tobacco smoke).

Chronic obstructive pulmonary disease (COPD): A disease state characterized by airway obstruction because of chronic bronchitis and emphysema.

Emphysema: An element of COPD that primarily destroys the elastic-connective tissue structure

of the lung resulting in enlargement of distal airspaces.

Interstitial lung diseases (ILDs): A group of restrictive pulmonary diseases involving pathology primarily confined to the lung parenchyma.

Obstructive pulmonary disease: A category of diseases of the pulmonary system characterized by increased airway resistance.

Pulmonary hypertension: A pathophysiological condition characterized by elevated pulmonary arterial pressure at rest and usually associated with pulmonary vascular disease.

Restrictive pulmonary disease: A category of pulmonary diseases in which the underlying pathologic process interferes with normal lung expansion.

structural or dynamic changes in the airway accounts for the increase in airway resistance. Structural airway abnormalities are chronic, specified by disease processes, and usually related to disease severity. Dynamic changes are variable and precipitated by acute stimuli such as physical activity, stress, or acute illness. Clinically, airway resistance can be attributed to both processes, particularly in exercising individuals. Regardless of the causation, the common endpoint for high airway resistance is air trapping and lung hyperinflation (102).

CHRONIC OBSTRUCTIVE PULMONARY DISEASE

Chronic obstructive pulmonary disease (COPD) is characterized by progressive airflow obstruction that is not fully reversible, and is associated with an abnormal inflammatory response of the lung to inhaled tobacco smoke and other noxious particles (54). It is a leading but underrecognized cause of morbidity and mortality and a major health care cost. Epidemiological studies from various countries estimate that up to about one-quarter of adults aged 40 yr or older may have airflow obstruction consistent with COPD (21,60,84). It is now the fourth leading cause of death, accounting for 4.8% of all deaths worldwide, and is projected to become the third leading cause of death by 2020 (80). In recent years, the number of deaths from COPD was greater among women than men (62). In the European Union, direct health care expenditure in 2000 was estimated at €38.7 billion (79). In the United States, the projected annual cost of health care in 2010 was $29.5 billion (95).

The pathologic features of COPD are chronic bronchitis and emphysema (130). Chronic bronchitis is the inflammation and eventual scarring of the airways. It is defined as the presence of cough and sputum production for at least 3 mo in each of two consecutive years (54,130). Emphysema, on the other hand, is the permanent enlargement of airspaces distal to the terminal bronchioles accompanied by destruction of alveolar walls. COPD is characterized by a specific pattern of inflammation involving increased numbers of macrophages, neutrophils and cytotoxic T-lymphocytes (predominately CD8+), and the release of multiple inflammatory mediators. These mediators attract inflammatory cells from the circulation (chemotactic factors), amplify the inflammatory response (proinflammatory cytokines), and induce structural changes (growth factors) (14). An imbalance between proteases that destroy the elastic and connective tissue in the lung and antiproteases that protect against this process is thought to be responsible for generating emphysema. An inherited deficiency of the most well-known antiprotease, α_1-antitrypsin, is a significant risk factor for early development of emphysema, although this deficiency explains <3% of all cases (3). From a practical perspective, it is usually difficult to separate chronic bronchitis and emphysema, and these conditions frequently coexist.

Various factors interact to cause exercise intolerance in patients with COPD (81,103). Progressive narrowing of small airways in chronic bronchitis causes an increase in airway resistance. Degradation of alveolar and parenchymal elastin in emphysema causes marked reductions in elastic recoil and airway tethering. Both processes impede expiration and result in lung hyperinflation. Static hyperinflation is caused by the lungs exerting less inward recoil to counter the outward recoil of the chest wall, resulting in equilibrium of recoil forces at an elevated resting volume. Dynamic hyperinflation, which can occur independently or in addition to static hyperinflation, results from air trapping within the lungs after each breath because of an imbalance between the volumes inhaled and exhaled. The increase in airway resistance resulting from airway narrowing and more collapsible airways in COPD increases the time needed to exhale a given volume of air. This effect is exacerbated during exercise as the increased demand for ventilation may not allow sufficient time for exhalation of tidal volume to return to the relaxation volume. Lung hyperinflation decreases the capacity of the inspiratory muscles to generate pressure and increases the elastic work of breathing. Increased inward recoil of the chest wall in combination with dynamic airway collapse often results in air trapping, and a significant amount of work may be required to overcome the intrinsic load during inspiration. In severe COPD, the mechanical inefficiency and respiratory muscle load during maximal exercise may lead to hypoventilation. The resultant hypercapnia and hypoxemia lead to decreased systemic oxygen delivery and reduced pH, both of which stimulate ventilatory drive and compromise peripheral skeletal muscle function, thereby contributing to the sensations of dyspnea and limb discomfort.

The severity of COPD influences treatment selection and exercise prescription. Multiple classification schemas have been proposed to describe disease severity. The Global Initiative for Chronic Obstructive Lung Disease (GOLD) guidelines (54) recommend spirometric classification (*Table 7-1*). A post-bronchodilator $FEV_{1.0}/FVC$ ratio <0.70 indicates airflow obstruction that is not fully reversible. Because lung volumes are affected by normal healthy aging, however, using a fixed ratio may result in over diagnosis of COPD in the elderly and under diagnosis in adults younger than 45 yr (122). To minimize the potential misclassification, values for $FEV_{1.0}$ can be compared with age-related, post-bronchodilator reference values (see *Table 7-1*). This latter recommendation is consistent with American Thoracic Society/European Respiratory Society (ATS/ERS) guidelines (28).

A limitation of spirometric classification is that it does not represent the complex clinical consequences of COPD. Accordingly, the BODE index was developed

TABLE 7-1. Global Initiative for Chronic Obstructive Lung Disease: Guidelines for Diagnosis and Staging of Chronic Obstructive Pulmonary Disease

Stage[a]	Severity	FEV$_{1.0}$[b]	Symptoms[c]
I	Mild	≥80% predicted	Intermittent
II	Moderate	50%–79% predicted	Persistent
III	Severe	30%–49% predicted	Exacerbations
IV	Very severe	<30% or <50% predicted with chronic ventilatory failure	Ventilatory failure

FEV$_{1.0}$, forced expiratory volume in 1 s.

[a]For stages I through IV, the FEV$_{1.0}$/FVC ratio needs to be <70%.

[b]FEV$_{1.0}$ values are based on postbronchodilator measurements.

[c]Symptoms are useful in clinical management, but may not correlate with FEV$_{1.0}$.

Adapted from Global Initiative for Chronic Obstructive Lung Disease (GOLD). *Global Strategy for the Diagnosis, Management, and Prevention of Chronic Obstructive Pulmonary Disease.* 2010.

as a way to assess the systemic as well as the pulmonary manifestations of COPD (27). The BODE index is a multidimensional scale that assigns points based on the results of four measures: body mass index (B), a marker/indicator of nutritional status; airflow obstruction (O), measured as a percentage of the predicted FEV$_{1.0}$ (94); dyspnea (D), assessed with the modified Medical Research Council scale (82); and exercise capacity (E), measured as the best of two 6-min walk tests performed at least 30 min apart (7). The variables are graded 0–3 (0 or 1 for body mass index) and summed to give a total score between 0 and 10 (*Table 7-2*). The BODE index is much better at predicting mortality than spirometry data alone (27), with higher scores indicating a greater risk of death. In addition, the BODE index captures the beneficial effects induced by pulmonary rehabilitation (32).

COPD lung damage is irreversible, but a patient's quality of life can be improved with appropriate treatment.

TABLE 7-2. Assignment of Points for the BODE Index

	0 Point	1 Point	2 Points	3 Points
FEV$_{1.0}$ (% predicted)	≥65	50–64	36–49	≤35
6 min walk distance (m)	≥350	250–349	150–249	≤149
Dyspnea (MMRC scale)	0–1	2	3	4
BMI (kg · m^{-2})	>21	≤21		

BODE: body-mass index, airflow obstruction, dyspnea, and exercise capacity; FEV$_{1.0}$, forced expiratory volume in 1 s; MMRC scale, Modified Medical Research Council scale; BMI, body mass index.

Adapted from Celli BR, Cote CG, Marin JM, et al. The body-mass index, airflow obstruction, dyspnea, and exercise capacity index in chronic obstructive pulmonary disease. *N Engl J Med.* 2004;350:1005–12.

Smoking cessation is an important goal to slow the progression of COPD (6). Before starting an exercise program, it is important to maximize pulmonary function by pharmacotherapy (99). The principal bronchodilator treatments are β$_2$-adrenoreceptor agonists (formoterol, salmeterol, albuterol), anticholinergics (ipratropium, oxitropium, tiotropium), and methylxanthines (aminophylline, theophylline) (54). All categories of bronchodilators have been shown to increase exercise tolerance in COPD, without necessarily producing significant changes in FEV$_{1.0}$ (1). The beneficial effect of bronchodilators may be mediated by reduced airway resistance, increased airflow, and enhanced lung emptying. Such changes would be expected to decrease dynamic hyperinflation, thereby leading to a reduction in dyspnea (115). Combining bronchodilators may improve efficacy and decrease the risk of side effects compared with increasing the dose of a single bronchodilator (119). Regular treatment with long-acting bronchodilators is often more effective and convenient than short-acting bronchodilators (54). Oral medication with phosphodiesterase-4 inhibitors (roflumilast) reduces inflammation and has recently been shown to improve FEV$_{1.0}$ when added to long-acting bronchodilators (22,46). Inhaled glucocorticosteroids should be added to the treatment of symptomatic patients with an FEV$_{1.0}$ <50% of predicted (*i.e.*, GOLD stage III and IV) and repeated exacerbations (54). Chronic treatment with oral glucocorticosteroids has no proven benefit in COPD and is associated with a high risk of serious adverse side effects (54).

After pharmacotherapy, the need for oxygen therapy should be assessed. Hypoxemia is determined by the diffusion capacity of the lungs, the ability of the lung to match alveolar ventilation to the appropriate metabolic rate, and the ability to direct pulmonary blood flow to those alveoli that are adequately ventilated. As COPD progresses, derangements in all three of these components contribute significantly to the hypoxemia and hypercapnia observed during exercise and contribute substantially to exercise limitations in this patient population. Long-term oxygen therapy (15 h or more per day) should be initiated if the arterial oxygen tension is ≤55 mm Hg or oxyhemoglobin saturation is ≤88% while breathing room air (54). These same guidelines apply when considering supplemental oxygen during exercise (99,130). Interestingly, supplemental oxygen often increases exercise tolerance in nonhypoxemic patients — patients who would not normally meet the criteria for supplemental oxygen (18). The improvement in exercise tolerance with oxygen therapy may be caused, in part, by a reduction in ventilatory drive consequent to a reduction in the carotid bodies' responses to hypoxemia and hydrogen ions. This, in turn, allows more time to exhale between breaths and reduces dynamic hyperinflation, resulting in reduced exertional dyspnea (26). In hypoxemic patients, exercise tolerance may also be improved through an increase in cardiac function or an increase in oxygen delivery to the working muscles (83).

ASTHMA

Asthma is a chronic inflammatory disorder of the airways that is characterized by airway hyperresponsiveness, airflow obstruction that is often reversible, and pulmonary symptoms, including recurrent episodes of wheezing, dyspnea, chest tightness, and coughing (45,53). It affects approximately 300 million people worldwide (87). The global prevalence ranges from 1% to 18% of the population (87). It is the twenty-fifth leading cause of disability-adjusted life years lost annually, accounting for 1% of the total global disease burden (87). It accounts for about 1 in every 250 deaths worldwide (87). The social and economic consequences are considerable, both in terms of direct medical costs (such as hospital admissions and medication costs) and indirect nonmedical costs (such as time lost from work and premature death) (87).

The relationship between COPD and asthma has long been debated (114). One perspective considers chronic bronchitis, emphysema, and asthma as mutually exclusive diseases, sometimes manifesting overlapping features (*Fig. 7-1*). More recent versions of this diagram have modified the boundaries based on proportional classification of the COPD subgroups (86,129). An alternative perspective, which was proposed in 1961 and debated recently (13,74), claims that asthma, chronic bronchitis, and emphysema should not be considered as separate diseases but as different expressions of one disease entity. This perspective, which later became termed the *Dutch hypothesis* (113), seems to be driven by the high degree of variability seen in the manner in which these three diseases manifest clinically. For now, the general consensus is that COPD refers to chronic bronchitis and emphysema alone. Partially reversible airflow obstruction is the primary physiologic abnormality of COPD. The reversible component to the airflow obstruction seen in COPD may sometimes be linked to the coexistence of asthma.

A consistent feature of asthma is airway inflammation. Activation of several inflammatory cells (such as mast cells, eosinophils, neutrophils, CD4+ T-lymphocytes, natural killer cells) leads to the release of various chemical mediators (such as chemokines, cysteinyl leukotrienes, cytokines, histamine, nitric oxide, prostaglandin D_2), which contribute to the persistence of inflammation (14). Chronic airway inflammation inevitably leads to morphologic changes to both the airway smooth muscle and the pulmonary epithelium, often described as airway remodeling (12,52,61). Increased deposition of collagen and proteoglycans under the basement membrane and other layers of the airway wall results in fibrosis. Airway smooth muscle increases in mass by hypertrophy and hyperplasia, and bronchial blood vessels increase in size and number (angiogenesis). These structural changes result in thickening of the airway wall that may result in relatively irreversible narrowing of the airways. Mucous gland enlargement and goblet cell differentiation result in mucous hypersecretion, which predisposes the individual to distal airway plugging. This development, in combination with an increased surface tension through disruption of surfactant function, leads to atelectasis (closure of peripheral lung units). Atelectasis results in a reduced functional lung volume and hypoxia through a mismatch between ventilation and perfusion.

Risk factors that trigger airway inflammation are important to recognize and avoid if possible (53). Allergens (such as house dust mites, furred animals, cockroaches, pollens, fungi, molds, and yeasts) increase the risk of airway inflammation. Occupational asthma has been associated with more than 300 substances including plastic resin, wood dust, certain metals, and plant–animal biologic products (73). Latex sensitivity is increasingly prevalent in health care workers and must be taken into consideration in the rehabilitation environment. Outdoor air pollutants (such as particulates, tobacco smoke, sulphur dioxide, nitrogen oxide, and ozone) and indoor air pollutants (such as carbon monoxide, nitric oxide, and nitrogen dioxide) are known to trigger airway inflammation. Drugs (such as aspirin and β-blockers) are also common risk factors in susceptible individuals. Exercise is a cause of bronchoconstriction in approximately 90% of people with asthma, and for some it is the only cause. Water loss and cooling of the airways by increased ventilation during exercise are likely involved in the pathogenesis of exercise-induced bronchoconstriction (5,23). There is mounting evidence that obesity is an independent risk factor for asthma. How obesity influences the development of asthma is unclear, but mechanical factors, altered inflammation, and immune responses relating to the obese state may be involved (39).

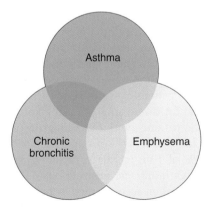

FIGURE 7-1. The interrelationship between asthma, chronic bronchitis, and emphysema depicted as a Venn diagram. (Adapted from American Thoracic Society. Standards for the diagnosis and care of patients with chronic obstructive pulmonary disease. *Am J Respir Crit Care Med.* 1995;152:S77–121.)

A diagnosis of asthma is often made by using a combination of an individual's medical history, symptoms, and pulmonary function. An increase in $FEV_{1.0}$ of at least 12% (or 200 mL) 15 min after inhalation of a short-acting β_2-agonist (e.g., 200–400 µg albuterol) or a more sustained improvement over days or weeks after the introduction of effective controller treatment (e.g., inhaled glucocorticosteroids) indicates reversible airflow obstruction consistent with asthma (53,110). In addition, asthma is suspected if peak expiratory flow (PEF) increases by at least 20% (or 60 L · min^{-1}) after inhalation of a bronchodilator or if there is a day-to-day variation in PEF of at least 20% (or 10% with twice daily readings) (53). In individuals with symptoms consistent with asthma but with normal baseline lung function, airway responsiveness to direct airway challenges (e.g., methacholine, histamine) and/or indirect challenges (e.g., mannitol, exercise) may help establish a diagnosis of asthma (4). Direct test results are usually expressed as the concentration of the challenge agent that gives rise to a specific (often 20%) decline in $FEV_{1.0}$. Generally, indirect tests are considered more specific for asthma whereas direct tests are more sensitive (31). Noninvasive markers of airway inflammation, such as hypertonic saline-induced sputum for eosinophilic or neutrophilic inflammation, may be useful. Exhaled nitric oxide and carbon monoxide have been suggested as noninvasive markers of airway inflammation, but these measures are nonspecific for asthma (15,137). Skin tests with allergens or measurement of specific immunoglobulin E (IgE) in serum can be used to detect the presence of allergies and help to identify risk factors that cause asthma symptoms. However, a positive test does not necessarily mean that the disease is allergic or that it is causally involved in asthma.

Exercise-induced bronchoconstriction should be suspected in individuals with symptoms of wheezing, dyspnea, or cough after exercise. A firm diagnosis is based on a decline in $FEV_{1.0}$ from baseline of at least 10% within 30 min after exercise (33,42). Running for 6–8 min at an intensity >80% of predicted maximum heart rate is usually recommended, but rapid incremental protocols (8–12 min) may also be diagnostic (33,42). Inhalation of dry, cold air during exercise markedly increases the test's sensitivity while maintaining a high degree of specificity (33,42). Other measures of indirect bronchial responsiveness include eucapnic voluntary hyperpnea and inhalation of hypertonic saline or mannitol (23).

Differential diagnoses of asthma require some consideration. Cough-variant asthma is a condition in which cough is the predominant or sole symptom. It must be distinguished from eosinophilic bronchitis in which patients have cough and sputum eosinophils but normal lung function (38). Postviral hyperreactive airways syndrome has an asthma-like presentation that occurs after a viral illness. So-called cardiac asthma refers to the wheezing associated with left ventricular failure. It is caused by airway compression that is a consequence of pulmonary edema causing signs and symptoms that mimic asthma. Gastroesophageal reflux disease (GERD) — that is, the backflow of stomach contents into the esophagus — is a common cause of cough and is nearly three times as prevalent in patients with asthma compared with the general population (67). Acid in the distal esophagus can, via a vagally mediated reflex, provoke bronchoconstriction and airway hypersensitivity. It is diagnosed by symptom disappearance with antireflux treatment, which involves dietary and lifestyle changes, acid suppression therapy (H_2-receptor antagonist or proton pump inhibitor), and prokinetic therapy. Exercise can potentially induce gastroesophageal reflux in susceptible individuals through an increase in the thoracoabdominal pressure gradient (8). Rigorous exercise does not need to be avoided in individuals manifesting GERD, but measures should be implemented to minimize the severity of reflux. Nonpharmacologic interventions include maintaining head elevation at a minimum of 30 degrees while exercising, and avoiding stomach overdistention with food or fluids before exercise.

A common differential diagnosis or coexisting factor to asthma is vocal cord dysfunction (VCD). VCD is characterized by abnormal adduction of the vocal cords, usually during inhalation, resulting in variable airway obstruction and symptoms mimicking asthma. VCD may arise from an alteration in the autonomic balance between the glottis and central control areas, with potential aggravation from direct laryngeal insult, laryngeal hyperresponsiveness, and psychological factors (9). Many people with VCD are wrongly diagnosed with asthma and suffer morbidity from unnecessary treatment such as high-dose glucocorticosteroid and bronchodilator use. The true population figures for exercise-induced VCD are unclear, but the estimated incidence in people with refractory asthma may be as much as 30% with VCD as the single cause of dyspnea in about one-third and coexisting asthma in two-thirds of these individuals (98). It is typically a condition of younger women, and rhinosinus conditions and GERD are often associated with this entity. The current gold standard for diagnosis rests with visualization of the vocal cords by laryngoscopy while the patient is symptomatic (51). Spirometry may be useful for diagnosing VCD in about one-fifth of asymptomatic patients, with flattening/truncation of the inspiratory loop (i.e., ratio of expiratory to inspiratory flows at 50% of FVC <1.0) confirming the presence of a variable extrathoracic obstruction (110). Exercise-induced VCD is often accompanied by inspiratory stridor over the larynx and inspiratory flow oscillations ("sawtooth" pattern) during the exercise (64). This contrasts with exercise-induced bronchoconstriction, in which wheezing is heard over the thorax and airflow obstruction usually occurs after exercise and during expiration.

BOX 7-1	Classification of Asthma Severity by Clinical Features before Treatment

INTERMITTENT

Symptoms <1 per week
Brief exacerbations
Nocturnal symptoms ≤2 per month
   $FEV_{1.0}$ or PEF ≥80% predicted
   PEF or $FEV_{1.0}$ variability <20%

MILD PERSISTENT

Symptoms >1 per week but <1 per day
Exacerbations may affect activity and sleep
Nocturnal symptoms >2 per month
   $FEV_{1.0}$ or PEF 60%–80% predicted
   PEF or $FEV_{1.0}$ variability <20%–30%

MODERATE PERSISTENT

Symptoms daily
Exacerbations may affect activity and sleep

Nocturnal symptoms >1 per week
Daily use of inhaled short-acting β_2-agonist
   $FEV_{1.0}$ or PEF 60%–80% predicted
   PEF or $FEV_{1.0}$ variability >30%

SEVERE PERSISTENT

Symptoms daily
Frequent exacerbations
Frequent nocturnal asthma symptoms
Limitation of physical activities
   $FEV_{1.0}$ or PEF ≤60% predicted
   PEF or $FEV_{1.0}$ variability >30%

$FEV_{1.0}$, forced expiratory volume in 1 s; PEF, peak expiratory flow.

Adapted from Global Initiative for Asthma (GINA). *Global Strategy for Asthma Management and Prevention.* 2010.

Treatment of VCD typically involves speech therapy, breathing techniques, pharmacologic management of associated factors (asthma, rhinosinus conditions, and GERD), and psychological counseling.

Traditionally, asthma severity has been classified into four categories based on the level of symptoms, airflow obstruction, and lung function variability (*Box 7-1*). Although such classification schema may be useful at the initial assessment of an individual, they cannot guide treatment decisions or predict an individual's response to treatment. For these reasons, the most recent guidelines recommend a classification system by level of control (45,53) (see *Table 39-3*). In clinical practice, these classifications should be used in conjunction with an assessment of the patient's clinical condition and the potential risks and benefits of changing treatment.

An individual's current level of asthma control and treatment can be used to guide treatment selection (45,53). Interruption of the inflammatory pathways is pivotal to asthma treatment. Inflammatory control is achieved primarily through inhaled glucocorticosteroids, although uncontrolled asthma may also require extra controller options, such as a long-acting β_2-agonist (formoterol, salmeterol), a leukotriene modifier (montelukast, pranlukast, zafirlukast, zileuton), or sustained release theophylline. Inhaled short-acting β_2-agonists (fenoterol, metaproterenol, pirbuterol, albuterol, terbutaline) are effective relief treatments that should be used as needed. Alternative reliever treatments include inhaled anticholinergics (ipratropium bromide, oxitropium bromide), short-acting oral β_2-agonists, some long-acting β_2-agonists, and short-acting theophylline

(aminophylline). In individuals with allergic asthma who are uncontrolled on high-dose glucocorticosteroids, anti-IgE treatment with omalizumab injections has been shown to reduce symptoms, decrease the need for reliever medications, and produce fewer exacerbations.

For people with exercise-induced bronchoconstriction, inhalation of a short-acting β_2-agonist 10–15 min before exercise provides full protection for 2–3 h (24). Long-acting β_2-agonists have the same protective effect for up to 10–12 h, but the onset of protection is treatment dependent. Specifically, formoterol has an onset of protection as rapid as short-acting β_2-agonists, whereas salmeterol is active against exercise-induced bronchoconstriction from 30 min after inhalation (24). Inhalation of a cromone (disodium cromoglycate or nedocromil sodium) 15 min before exercise offers partial protection against exercise-induced bronchoconstriction for 1–2 h, whereas combining these drugs prolongs the protection to 4 h (24). Inhaled glucocorticosteroids, methylxanthines, and leukotriene modifiers also offer partial protection against exercise-induced bronchoconstriction (24). The World Anti-doping Agency (WADA) regulations for use of asthma drugs in sports currently prohibit the administration of oral glucocorticosteroids and oral β_2-agonists. Also prohibited are inhaled β_2-agonists, except albuterol (maximum 1,600 µg over 24 h) and salmeterol (when taken in accordance with the manufacturers' recommended therapeutic regimen). If inhaled β_2-agonists other than albuterol and salmeterol are used by athletes in international competition, a Therapeutic Use Exemption is required (http://www .wada-ama.org). Several nonpharmacologic interventions aimed at reducing the severity of exercise-induced bronchoconstriction have been proposed. A warm-up can be effective in decreasing the severity and duration of exercise-induced bronchoconstriction triggered by a subsequent exercise bout (90). Incorporating a cooldown after exercise also appears to be beneficial. Dietary modifications, such as antioxidant or fish oil supplementation and salt restriction, may also be useful in decreasing the severity of exercise-induced bronchoconstriction (93,112,133). Prophylactic measures that may minimize the deleterious effect of dry, cold air on airway function include nasal breathing during low-intensity activities, covering the mouth and nose with a scarf or mask, avoiding exercise during the early morning or evening, and exercising indoors when possible.

Side effects associated with β_2-agonist therapy, such as tachycardia, palpitations, dysrhythmias, and tremors, require consideration in the context of exercise. Many of the β_2-agonist preparations are not entirely selective for bronchial tissue in that β_1-adrenergic receptors in the heart can also be stimulated (20). Levalbuterol was developed as a selective β_2-agonist, having less direct effect on β_1-receptors in the heart, thereby minimizing cardiac stimulation. Another consideration is that regular use of short- and long-acting β_2-agonists may reduce the protection against asthma via desensitization and downregulation of the β_2-receptor, a phenomenon known as tachyphylaxis (124). Based on evidence that long-term β_2-agonist use may increase the risk of asthma-related death, current guidelines recommend that long-acting β_2-agonists should only be used in combination with an appropriate dose of inhaled glucocorticosteroid (30,53). Although recent meta-analyses have shown small increases in the number of deaths in patients receiving long-acting β_2-agonists in combination with inhaled corticosteroids (125), such finding need to be balanced against the benefits of improved asthma control that these medications bring when combined with glucocorticosteroids (30,53).

BRONCHIECTASIS

Bronchiectasis is a condition characterized by irreversible airway dilation, usually arising from recurrent or chronic bronchial infection (55,72). Airway inflammation and inadequate host defense mechanisms are the dominant features of the disease. The cause of bronchiectasis is unknown in most cases. However, genetic disorders such as cystic fibrosis are most likely in younger patients, whereas pulmonary tuberculosis, whooping cough, and measles are common causes in developing countries. The prevalence and economic burden of bronchiectasis are substantial. In the United States, the average age-adjusted hospitalization rate from 1993 to 2006 was 16.5 per 100,000 people and the median cost for inpatient care was $7,827 (126).

The clinical features of bronchiectasis usually include chronic cough that produces purulent sputum with or without blood (hemoptysis), dyspnea, rhinosinusitis, fatigue, and lung crackles that are often bibasal (55,72). Differentiating between a diagnosis of bronchiectasis and chronic bronchitis can be challenging because both entities are characterized by daily sputum production and dyspnea. Furthermore, many patients with COPD have associated bronchiectasis (108). High-resolution computed tomography (CT) scanning of the chest is the gold standard for diagnosis of bronchiectasis (89). Spirometry usually reveals moderate airflow obstruction, although a restrictive defect may also be noted in patients with advanced disease and extensive parenchymal destruction. Airway hyperresponsiveness to bronchial provocation is also a common finding and may represent coexistent asthma.

The aims of treatment are to inhibit or abolish the underlying host deficiency, relieve bronchoconstriction, control airway inflammation, and improve clearance of secretions (29,88,107). Regular treatment with systemic antibiotics may produce small benefits in reducing sputum volume and purulence, reducing colonizing microbes in sputum, improving exacerbations and symptoms, and reducing airway inflammation (43). In patients with airflow obstruction or hyperresponsiveness, therapy with bronchodilators may be useful. Inhaled glucocorticosteroids may provide some benefit by reducing the volume of sputum and improving health-related quality of life, but the evidence is insufficient to justify regular use (70). Indomethacin, on the other hand, has been shown to reduce sputum volume and improve dyspnea (111). Inhaled mucolytic drugs alter the properties of sputum to make it easier to clear. One such drug, bromhexine, has been shown to reduce sputum production as well as the difficulty associated with sputum clearance (104). Another inhaled drug, recombinant human deoxyribonuclease (rhDNase), is contraindicated in patients with noncystic fibrosis bronchiectasis but does assist sputum clearance and improve spirometry in patients with bronchiectasis associated with cystic fibrosis (101). Agents that increase the osmolarity of lung mucus, such as hypertonic saline and dry-powder mannitol, have been shown to improve airway clearance (35,135). In patients who have a reduction in $FEV_{1.0}$ after inhaling mannitol, premedication with a standard dose of either formoterol or sodium cromoglycate can inhibit this reduction (19).

Chest physiotherapy is often used to enhance airway clearance. Various manual and mechanical interventions have been used, including chest wall percussion and vibration, postural and autogenic drainage, mechanically assisted cough, forced expiration ("huffing"), positive expiratory pressure, and airway oscillation (78). Although such interventions are considered to be mainstays in the treatment of bronchiectasis, only a small number of studies have evaluated their long-term effectiveness. A recent randomized crossover study (96) found a significant improvement in cough, sputum production, and exercise capacity after 3 mo of twice daily chest physiotherapy using an oscillating positive expiratory pressure device in patients with bronchiectasis. These results suggest that regular chest physiotherapy may have small but significant benefits in this population. Theoretically, chest physiotherapy before exercise may improve exercise quality if mucous plugging impedes the distal lung unit from participation in gas exchange and promotes air trapping. Exercise training does not appear to increase the clearance of sputum but may be effective in improving exercise tolerance (97).

RESTRICTIVE PULMONARY DISEASE

The restrictive pulmonary disease category encompasses many diseases. The overall incidence for these diseases is low compared with that for obstructive pulmonary disease. The pathologic process involved with each disease interferes with the ability for normal lung expansion. The restricted lung expansion extends from alterations in the lung parenchyma or because of disease of the pleura, the chest wall, or the neuromuscular system.

INTERSTITIAL LUNG DISEASE

Interstitial lung disease (ILD), also called diffuse parenchymal lung disease, is a heterogeneous group of disorders primarily confined to the lung parenchyma (*Fig. 7-2*) (41). Under normal conditions, the lung interstitium is a potential space that exists between the basement membrane of the alveolar epithelium and capillary endothelium. The matrix or stroma contains collagen and noncollagenous proteins along with a sporadic number of macrophages, fibroblasts, and myofibroblasts. With ILD, the interstitial stroma consists of a higher percentage of protein material, and the cellularity is often increased. Further magnifying the problem, the pathology is often not limited to the interstitium, and there is involvement of the alveoli and terminal bronchi. The lungs become stiff and noncompliant, lending to the restrictive physiology and diffusion abnormality often seen with this disease. Different etiologies are encountered for each ILD (*Box 7-2*).

Three primary pathologic features are fundamental to the classification of ILD: infiltration, inflammation, and infection. Diseases classified as infiltrating show deposition of a dominant substance within the interstitium,

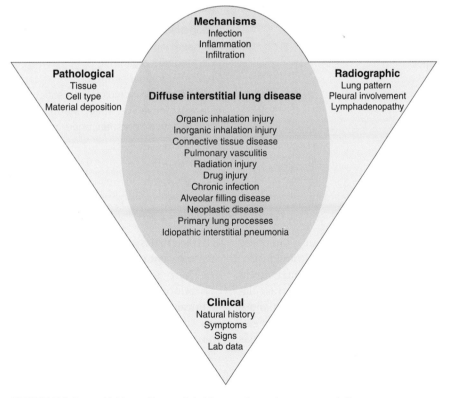

FIGURE 7-2. Interstitial lung disease (*circle*) comprises a large group of diseases. The etiology for these diseases (*lower circle*) can be linked to three basic mechanisms of injury (*upper circle*). Multiple factors are used to characterize each of these diseases. These factors can be simplified by grouping into pathologic, radiographic, and clinical differences (*corners of triangle*). This figure is used to illustrate the complexity of features to consider when diagnosing diseases within this category and the high degree of overlap seen in the characteristics that describe each disease.

BOX 7-2	Interstitial Lung Diseases Outlined by Pathogenesis

ORGANIC INHALATION

Farmer's lung
Bird fancier's lung

INORGANIC INHALATION

Asbestosis
Silicosis
Pneumoconiosis
Berylliosis

CONNECTIVE TISSUE DISEASE

Rheumatoid arthritis
Scleroderma
Sjögren syndrome
Systemic lupus erythematosus
Polymyositis/dermatomyositis

PULMONARY VASCULITIS

Wegener granulomatosis
Microscopic polyangiitis
Churg-Strauss syndrome

PHYSICAL AGENTS

Radiation
Oxygen
Mechanical ventilation

DRUGS

Amiodarone
Methotrexate
Bleomycin
Paraquat
Cocaine

CHRONIC INFECTION

Virus
Fungus
Mycobacterial disease
Parasites

ALVEOLAR FILLING DISEASE

Alveolar proteinosis
Amyloidosis
Microlithiasis

NEOPLASTIC DISEASE

Pulmonary lymphoma
Bronchoalveolar cell carcinoma
Lymphangitic carcinomatosis

PRIMARY LUNG PROCESSES

Sarcoidosis
Langerhans cell histiocytosis
Amyloidosis
Lymphangioleiomyomatosis

IDIOPATHIC INTERSTITIAL PNEUMONIA

Idiopathic pulmonary fibrosis
Nonspecific interstitial pneumonia
Cryptogenic organizing pneumonia
Acute interstitial pneumonia
Respiratory bronchiolitis interstitial lung disease
Desquamative interstitial pneumonia
Lymphocytic interstitial pneumonia

---

such as an amyloid or tumor. Cardiogenic pulmonary edema is arbitrarily included as an infiltrating process because water is displaced into the interstitium by hydrostatic forces within the pulmonary vasculature. Diseases classified as inflammatory include those processes that have inflammatory mediators propagating the pathogenesis. Idiopathic interstitial pneumonias and noncardiogenic pulmonary edema (acute respiratory distress syndrome) are assigned to this category. The infectious classification includes processes whereby microorganisms are known to be involved. This classification schema — used here to simplify the approach to ILD — not only helps with disease organization but also has clinical utility by simplifying the differential diagnosis for this large and diverse group of diseases. In actuality, most diseases within this group manifest overlapping

characteristics and mechanisms of injury, which leads to the inherent complexity of this disease group.

There is no diagnostic "gold standard" for ILD. Therefore, current ILD guidelines emphasize an integrated clinical, radiological, histopathological, and physiological approach to diagnosis (16,116). Symptoms common to ILD include exertional dyspnea, nonproductive cough, exercise intolerance, and generalized fatigue. An accurate diagnosis can often be made using high-resolution CT. Lung biopsy may improve the diagnostic accuracy, particularly in individuals with idiopathic interstitial pneumonias for which a correct diagnosis can profoundly influence treatment decisions and dictate different prognoses. Spirometry typically reveals a restrictive pattern, defined as a reduction in total lung capacity (TLC) below the fifth percentile of the predicted value and a normal $FEV_{1.0}$/FVC ratio (110). Pulmonary fibrosis may enhance expiratory flow by increasing lung elastic recoil at high lung volumes, whereas airway resistance may be decreased because of abnormally high radial traction on the airway walls by the surrounding parenchyma. Some ILDs are characterized by both pulmonary restriction and pulmonary obstruction. The diseases typically associated with both processes include sarcoidosis, hypersensitivity pneumonitis, and pulmonary Langerhans cell histiocytosis. Individuals who smoke and develop a restrictive pulmonary disorder often have COPD as a comorbid condition.

Gas exchange is often disrupted in patients with ILD. The diffusing capacity of the lung for carbon monoxide in ILD is often low at rest. This abnormality reflects impaired gas diffusion through the alveolar-capillary membrane. This diffusion abnormality usually does not translate into clinically significant hypoxemia until the disease is advanced. During exercise, the arterial oxygen tension tends to fall dramatically even in the early stages of the disease process (2,63). The exercise-induced hypoxemia primarily extends from a mismatch between ventilation and blood flow within the lung. This ventilation-perfusion mismatching occurs because of an increase in dead-space ventilation. Increased dead-space ventilation extends from a disproportionate rise in the ventilatory rate during exercise, leading to rapid shallow breathing. A reduced capillary bed surface area accentuates the dead-space ventilation. This surface area reduction can occur either in the form of pathological disruption of the capillary bed or impairment in capillary bed recruitment through the secondary development of pulmonary hypertension. Even though the diffusing capacity is abnormal, hypoxemia does not usually result from a diffusion defect because of the high oxygen diffusion rates. Only with a high level of exercise or with alveolar proteinosis can a diffusion defect account for the hypoxia.

There have been only a small number of well-conducted therapeutic clinical studies in ILD. Nevertheless, current ILD guidelines do provide strong recommendations for some aspects of treatment (16,116). The choice of treatment depends on several factors including the cause of the disease and the overall health status of the patient. Corticosteroids are often used to reduce inflammation in ILD. Sometimes, immune-suppressing drugs such as prednisone or cyclophosphamide are also given. Patients with ILD have an increased risk of developing lung cancer and smoking has a multiplicative effect on cancer risk. Therefore, patients with ILD who smoke should be offered specialist support for smoking cessation. Long-term oxygen therapy is recommended for the treatment of patients with ILD who are hypoxemic at rest. Ambulatory oxygen is recommended for patients who are hypoxemic during exercise if a clear beneficial effect on exercise capacity or dyspnea is evident.

Selected comorbidities such as gastroesophageal reflux and pulmonary hypertension may contribute to pulmonary deterioration in ILD; these medical comorbidities should be considered in the treatment of patients with ILD. Recent randomized controlled studies in patients with ILD have shown that exercise training elicits improvements in symptoms, functional exercise capacity, and quality of life (47,66,100). Thus, pulmonary rehabilitation is recommended for most patients with ILD.

OTHER RESTRICTIVE PULMONARY DISEASES

The restrictive pulmonary diseases extrinsic to the lung parenchyma can be viewed either as intrapleural or extrapleural. Intrapleural processes can be viewed by physical properties creating the abnormal pleural characteristics. Pneumothorax occurs when there is a collection of air within the pleural space. When liquid accumulates within the pleural space, it is referred to as a *pleural effusion*. There are many causes of pleural effusions, including renal disease, liver disease, heart failure, pneumonia, and malignancy. Infiltration of a solid substance into the pleural space occurs with certain fibrotic processes and malignancy. The last group of restrictive pulmonary diseases includes extrapleural processes that affect the normal function of the thoracic cage or the respiratory muscles. Thoracic deformities, such as kyphoscoliosis or ankylosing spondylitis, and morbid obesity can interfere with the expansion of the thoracic cage. Neuromuscular disorders such as poliomyelitis, Guillain-Barré syndrome, amyotrophic lateral sclerosis, myasthenia gravis, muscular dystrophies, or spinal cord injury can cause respiratory muscle weakness. Reduced chest wall compliance and respiratory muscle weakness constrain the ventilatory response to exercise by limiting the increase in tidal volume.

PULMONARY VASCULATURE DISORDERS

The healthy pulmonary vasculature is a low-pressure system with a low resistance to flow. **Pulmonary hypertension** is a rare condition characterized by increased pulmonary vascular resistance and ultimately in right-heart failure (48,91). Pulmonary hypertension has a multifactorial pathophysiology consisting of vasoconstriction, vascular remodeling, and thrombosis all contributing to the increased pulmonary vascular resistance. Pulmonary arterial hypertension (PAH) is distinguished from other forms of pulmonary hypertension, which can occur as a consequence of left-heart disease, pulmonary diseases/hypoxia (such as COPD, ILD, hypoventilation disorders, or residence at high altitude), thromboembolic disease, or disorders directly affecting the pulmonary vasculature (such as sarcoidosis) (*Box 7-3*). PAH is

BOX 7-3	**World Health Organization Classification of Pulmonary Hypertension**

1. Pulmonary arterial hypertension
2. Pulmonary venous hypertension
3. Hypoxia-associated pulmonary hypertension
4. Thromboembolic pulmonary hypertension
5. Pulmonary hypertension with unclear/ multifactorial mechanisms

Adapted from Simonneau G, Galie N, Rubin L, et al. Clinical classification of pulmonary hypertension. *J Am Coll Cardiol.* 2004;43 Suppl 1:S5–12.

classified into subgroups. Idiopathic PAH — that is, PAH with no obvious cause — is most prevalent in women and accounts for about 40% of patients with PAH. Familial PAH involves genetic transmission of PAH and accounts for about 6%–10% of patients with PAH. Associated PAH is pulmonary hypertension associated with various risk factors or conditions, including connective tissue diseases (such as scleroderma or lupus erythematosus), congenital heart disease, portal hypertension, HIV infection, and drugs/toxins (such as appetite suppressants, cocaine, or amphetamines). Other subgroups include PAH associated with significant venous or capillary involvement and persistent pulmonary hypertension of the newborn. The prevalence of PAH in the adult population is about 15–50 cases per million (109).

Dyspnea, especially when exercising, is the primary symptom of pulmonary hypertension (131). Other symptoms that can develop as the condition progresses include fatigue, angina, syncope, edema, tachycardia, palpitations, and cough. Dyspnea can be attributed to an increased ventilatory response to exercise, resulting from a mismatch between ventilation and perfusion that leads to an elevated ratio of dead-space volume to tidal volume. A second mechanism for the increased ventilatory response to exercise is increased hydrogen ion and carbon dioxide production resulting from early lactic acidosis. A third mechanism is arterial hypoxemia owing to a reduced functional capillary bed and an abnormally rapid transit time of red blood cells through the pulmonary capillary bed, shortening the time available for diffusion equilibrium. Another important cause of arterial hypoxemia is a right-to-left shunt through a patent foramen ovale (132), which is a congenital communication between the right and left atria. In patients with a patent foramen ovale and abnormally high pulmonary vascular resistance, exercise-induced increases in venous return cause right atrial pressure to rise. When right atrial exceeds left atrial pressure, venous return can flow from the right to the left atrium, diverting deoxygenated,

acidotic, and carbon dioxide–rich blood to the systemic arterial circulation. This stimulates arterial chemoreceptors so that ventilation is increased in proportion to the shunted hydrogen ion and carbon dioxide load. Fatigue associated with pulmonary hypertension may also limit exercise tolerance. The fatigue may be attributed to blunted cardiac output during exercise because pulmonary vasoconstriction reduces the delivery of blood to the left atrium. In addition, the reduction in oxygen delivery consequent to arterial hypoxemia results in an increased rate of anaerobic glycolysis, early lactic acidosis, and impaired contractility of working muscles.

Pulmonary hypertension is defined as a mean pulmonary artery pressure ≥ 25 mm Hg at rest as assessed by right heart catheterization. The definition for PAH adds the criterion that pulmonary capillary wedge pressure must be ≤ 15 mm Hg. A definition of pulmonary hypertension based on measurements of pulmonary artery pressure during exercise is no longer supported by current guidelines (11,48,91). Severity of pulmonary hypertension is determined using the WHO functional classification, which is an adaptation of the New York Heart Association (NYHA) classification for congestive heart failure (*Box 7-4*). Establishment of the correct diagnosis and the specific classification can influence the treatment a patient receives.

Treatments for pulmonary hypertension include supportive therapy (chronic oxygen supplementation, anticoagulants, and diuretics) and a combination of disease-targeted therapies (calcium channel blockers, prostanoids, endothelin-receptor antagonists, and phosphodiesterase type 5 inhibitors) (10,48,91). Such treatments have been shown to improve symptoms, exercise tolerance, quality of life, and possibly survival. Surgical treatments for severely ill patients include the creation

BOX 7-4	**World Health Organization Functional Classification of Pulmonary Hypertension**

Class I   Asymptomatic. No physical limitations

Class II Slight limitation of physical activity. Comfortable at rest. Symptomatic with ordinary exercise

Class III Marked limitation of physical activity. Comfortable at rest. Symptomatic with less than ordinary exercise

Class IV Unable to perform any physical activity without symptoms. Symptomatic at rest. Signs of right heart failure

Adapted from Barst RJ, McGoon M, Torbicki A, et al. Diagnosis and differential assessment of pulmonary arterial hypertension. *J Am Coll Cardiol.* 2004;43:S40–7.

of a right-to-left interatrial shunt (atrial septostomy), removal of clot formation from the pulmonary arteries (thromboendarterectomy), and lung or combined heart and lung transplantation (40,48,91). Exercise in patients with pulmonary hypertension is controversial (10). Theoretically, an increase in cardiac output resulting in elevation of pulmonary arterial pressure and pulmonary vascular resistance may predispose to right ventricular decompensation and circulatory collapse. Results from two recent studies, however, suggest that closely monitored intensive exercise training is safe and can improve exercise capacity, peak oxygen consumption, quality of life, and functional status in patients with severe pulmonary hypertension (59,92). Current guidelines recommend low-intensity aerobic exercise as the mainstay of therapy (48,91). Patients should be monitored for exercise-induced hypertension or hypotension, and exercise should be stopped if the patient develops severe dyspnea, dizziness, or chest pain (37). Any activities that could increase intrathoracic pressure such as high-intensity aerobic exercise or weightlifting without controlled breathing should be avoided as they may precipitate circulatory collapse (37).

DISTURBANCES IN VENTILATORY CONTROL

HYPERVENTILATION DISORDERS

Hyperventilation, characterized as a reduced partial pressure of carbon dioxide in arterial blood (hypocapnia), is the result of alveolar ventilation that is excessive in relation to metabolically produced carbon dioxide. To compensate for metabolic acidosis and minimize the fall in arterial blood and central chemoreceptor pH that would otherwise occur, ventilation is increased until the partial pressure of arterial carbon dioxide is reduced to a new lower set point. Examples of metabolically induced hyperventilation include excessive ingestion of acid (ethanol, methanol, aspirin), poorly controlled diabetes mellitus (diabetic ketoacidosis), hypoglycemia, chronic renal failure, renal tubular acidosis, or the result of using carbonic anhydrase inhibitor drugs (acetazolamide). The consequence of metabolic acidosis before exercise is a marked elevation in the ventilatory requirement to perform a given work rate. Consequently, the sensation of dyspnea is high, and, in patients with other pulmonary diseases, ventilation may encroach on the breathing reserve, resulting in premature curtailment of exercise (127).

Chronic "idiopathic" hyperventilation is defined as sustained hypocapnia at rest and during exercise with no other apparent pathologies (49,68,69). The etiology of idiopathic hyperventilation is controversial (49). Behavioral factors, such as stress and anxiety, are often assumed to be involved, but these factors may be absent or secondary to hyperventilation. Psychosomatic disorders have also been implicated because many such individuals have a high incidence of depression and phobias. An increase in progesterone during the luteal phase of the menstrual cycle, and particularly during pregnancy, results in hyperventilation through the combined effect of progesterone and estrogen on the central and peripheral chemoreceptors. This effect of sex hormones on ventilation may explain why the incidence of idiopathic hyperventilation is higher in women. Regardless of etiology, many individuals with idiopathic hyperventilation are compromised in activities of daily living and quality of life because of symptoms such as chest pain, dyspnea, light-headedness, and paresthesia.

HYPOVENTILATION DISORDERS

Hypoventilation is characterized by an elevated partial pressure of carbon dioxide in arterial blood (hypercapnia). It overlaps with other pulmonary disease categories, particularly when the disease is severe. For example, severe COPD may elicit hypoventilation because of decreased responsiveness to hypoxia and hypercapnia, increased ventilation-perfusion mismatch leading to increased dead-space ventilation, and abnormal respiratory muscle function owing to fatigue and muscular disadvantage from hyperinflation. Patients with hypoventilation can develop clinically significant hypoxemia, which aggravates the clinical manifestations of hypoventilation. Two hypoventilation disorders — obesity hypoventilation syndrome and obstructive sleep apnea–hypopnea syndrome — require consideration.

Obesity hypoventilation syndrome is defined as obesity (body mass index >30 kg $\cdot$ m^{-2}) in combination with awake hypercapnia (arterial partial pressure of carbon dioxide >45 mm Hg) without any other known causes of hypoventilation (105). Historically, the disorder was referred to as Pickwickian syndrome. The mechanisms responsible for obesity hypoventilation syndrome are not clearly defined, but may result from complex relationships between disordered ventilatory mechanics, abnormalities in central ventilatory control, sleep-disordered breathing, and neurohormonal impairments (34). Many individuals with the disorder also have obstructive sleep apnea–hypopnea syndrome, which is the frequent complete (apnea) or partial (hypopnea) cessation of airflow during sleep resulting in hypercapnia and arterial hypoxemia. Significant contributing factors in obese individuals include excess fat deposition around the upper airway and reduced traction on the trachea owing to reduced operating lung volumes (36). The symptoms of both disorders include extreme daytime drowsiness (hypersomnolence), fatigue, mood disorders, and nocturnal or morning headaches. Left untreated, individuals may be at increased risk of pulmonary hypertension, right ventricular hypertrophy (cor pulmonale), cardiac ischemia, arrhythmias, and stroke.

Patients with hypoventilation disorders can be treated successfully using noninvasive positive-pressure ventilation via a nasal mask (34,105). Bilevel intermittent positive airway pressure (BiPAP) is used to treat obesity hypoventilation syndrome, whereas nocturnal continuous positive airway pressure (CPAP) is used to treat obstructive sleep apnea–hypopnea syndrome. Such interventions are effective means of maintaining upper airway patency, eliminating apneas and hypopneas, correcting daytime hypercapnia, and alleviating symptoms. Weight loss and exercise may be effective treatments for reversing the pulmonary complications of obesity (106,118). Multiple factors associated with obesity may have considerable impact on exercise. Obese individuals require extra energy to move heavy legs during cycling or a large body mass while walking. The extra O_2 needed to perform external work results in a greater than normal cardiopulmonary response. The added mass on the chest wall and the increased pressure in the abdomen increases the load on the inspiratory muscles. The increased abdominal pressure may impair diaphragmatic excursion during inspiration, reducing the vital capacity. Expiratory reserve volume (ERV) is reduced in obese individuals because of a decrease in functional residual capacity (FRC). The reductions in ERV and FRC can result in atelectasis and hypoxemia at rest. Arterial oxygenation usually improves during exercise because lung inflations re-expand the atelectatic lung units. The pulmonary complications that are associated with obesity are accentuated in the supine position. Therefore, exercise in a recumbent position should be minimized in these individuals.

PULMONARY REHABILITATION

Pulmonary rehabilitation is defined as an evidence-based, multidisciplinary, and comprehensive intervention for patients with chronic pulmonary disease who are symptomatic and often have decreased daily life activities (99). The components of pulmonary rehabilitation are outlined in *Box 7-5* and should be prescribed depending on the individual needs of the patient.

The goal of pulmonary rehabilitation is not to improve lung function, but rather to reverse the systemic consequences of the disease (99,134). For example, peripheral muscle weakness is common in patients with chronic pulmonary disease and, at the level of the muscle, this weakness is associated with reduced capillarization, a shift from type I to type IIa fibers, reduced oxidative enzyme activities, and increased concentrations of glycolytic enzymes (71). The consequences of such alterations are twofold. First, metabolic acidosis is encountered at low work rates, resulting in an increased drive to breathe and dynamic hyperinflation that increases the work

---

| BOX 7-5 | Components of Pulmonary Rehabilitation Program |

PATIENT ASSESSMENT

Pulmonary function
Symptoms (dyspnea and fatigue)
Activity levels
Exercise capacity
Weight and body composition
Respiratory and limb muscle function
Quality of life

EXERCISE TRAINING

Endurance and strength training of lower and upper extremities
Flexibility and balance training
Respiratory muscle training

NUTRITIONAL INTERVENTION

Calorie supplementation
Fat loss through exercise

EDUCATION AND SELF-MANAGEMENT

Knowledge of disease
Breathing techniques

Energy conservation and pacing techniques
Secretion clearance techniques
Prevention of exacerbations
Treatment (medication, oxygen, and surgery)
Bronchial hygiene
Irritant avoidance
Leisure, travel, and sexuality
End-of-life planning

PHARMACOLOGIC INTERVENTION (ANABOLIC STEROIDS, GROWTH HORMONE)

Psychosocial support
Smoking cessation
Stress management
Relaxation training
Patient and family support groups

Adapted from Nici L, Donner C, Wouters E, et al. American Thoracic Society/European Respiratory Society statement on pulmonary rehabilitation. *Am J Respir Crit Care Med.* 2006;173:1390–413.

BOX 7-6	**Benefits of Pulmonary Rehabilitation**

- Improved quality of life
- Improved psychological well-being (cognitive functioning, anxiety, depression, self-esteem)
- Improved symptoms (dyspnea)
- Increased functional status
- Increased participation in everyday activities
- Reduced health care costs

Adapted from Ries AL, Bauldoff GS, Carlin BW, et al. Pulmonary rehabilitation. Joint ACCP/AACVPR evidence-based clinical practice guidelines. *Chest.* 2007;131:4S–42S.

of breathing. Second, the peripheral muscles are more susceptible to fatigue, resulting in task failure and early exercise termination. The exercise training component of pulmonary rehabilitation aims at reversing these systemic consequences. The benefits resulting from pulmonary rehabilitation are shown in *Box 7-6*.

Patients with COPD make up the largest proportion of those referred for pulmonary rehabilitation, and most of the research has been conducted in this area (76). Treatable comorbidities, however, are common to all chronic pulmonary diseases, and treatment strategies have been applied to an increasingly wide range of pulmonary conditions, including asthma (117), bronchiectasis (97), cystic fibrosis (17), ILD (65), and pulmonary hypertension (37). Pulmonary rehabilitation has also been successfully used in the preparation and selection of patients for surgical treatments such as lung transplantation and lung volume reduction surgery (121). Furthermore, rehabilitation after surgery is beneficial because the improved lung function after the surgery facilitates exercise at higher intensity.

EXERCISE TRAINING

Exercise training is the cornerstone of pulmonary rehabilitation and, when optimally delivered, produces the greatest improvements in exercise tolerance (99,120,134). The optimal duration of the exercise program has not been clearly defined. Physiologic changes can occur within just a few weeks but longer training programs produce larger and more sustained effects. Patients should perform at least three supervised sessions per week, although two supervised sessions per week in combination with one or more unsupervised sessions at home may be acceptable. The benefits of exercise training tend to decline gradually over time. Health-related benefits, however, appear better preserved than exercise tolerance and may still be identified up to 2 yr after the intervention. The role of maintenance programs after the initial training is uncertain, but

evidence to date suggests only a modest effect of such programs on long-term benefits. Guidelines for the general prescription of exercise training are outlined in *Chapter 30* and for those with pulmonary disease in *Chapter 39*.

ADJUNCTIVE THERAPIES

As indicated in previous sections, bronchodilator and oxygen therapy in the acute setting can improve exercise tolerance in patients with airflow limitation. More recent evidence suggests that both strategies may enhance the effects of pulmonary rehabilitation, probably by enabling patients to exercise at higher intensities for longer durations (25,120).

Another adjunctive therapy that may benefit selected patients with pulmonary disease is noninvasive positive-pressure ventilation (99,120). Noninvasive ventilation during an acute bout of exercise can reduce dyspnea and increase exercise tolerance, potentially by reducing the load on the respiratory muscles (75,136). More recent evidence suggests that exercise training with noninvasive ventilation in patients with severe disease can improve exercise tolerance through increasing training intensity and duration. An alternative way to reduce the load on the ventilatory muscles is to breathe a low-density gas mixture such as 79% helium, 21% oxygen (heliox). Heliox has been shown to be beneficial in reducing dynamic hyperinflation, relieving symptoms, and improving exercise tolerance in patients with chronic pulmonary disease (44,77,85). In addition, breathing a combined mixture of heliox and hyperoxia has additive effects on improving exercise tolerance (44,77,85).

Ventilatory muscle training is another treatment strategy that may benefit patients with pulmonary disease. If the training load is properly controlled, ventilatory muscle training alone or combined with aerobic training has been shown in patients with COPD to improve ventilatory muscle function, reduce exertional dyspnea, and increase exercise tolerance (50). Less clear, however, is whether there is an additive effect of ventilatory muscle training and aerobic training on physiological function (57). Additional breathing techniques that may be effective in alleviating symptoms of dyspnea in patients with COPD include forward leaning and active expiration against pursed lips (56). Diaphragmatic breathing — that is, the conscious expansion of the abdominal wall during diaphragmatic inhalation — is not recommended because it increases the work of breathing and reduces the mechanical efficiency of breathing (58).

An adjunctive therapy that may be beneficial in patients who are bedbound or suffering from extreme peripheral muscle weakness is neuromuscular electrical stimulation (123,128). Transcutaneous stimulation of the nerve roots supplying the limb locomotor muscles has been shown to improve muscle strength and endurance, symptoms, and exercise tolerance in patients with moderate-to-severe pulmonary disease. The advantages of the technique are that it is safe, well tolerated, and relatively inexpensive; it can be implemented at home; and it may help to prevent functional decline during exacerbations.

SUMMARY

Exercise in patients with chronic pulmonary disease can be performed regardless of the illness severity. Pulmonary rehabilitation principles should be used as the framework for the exercise prescription, but disease-specific principles should also be incorporated. Disease-specific principles can be easily identified with a basic understanding of lung pathophysiology as it relates to pattern recognition for each of the disease categories. These principles also facilitate identification of the proper therapeutic interventions. Incorporating modifications based on the patient's response to exercise can further individualize the exercise program.

REFERENCES

1. Aguilaniu B. Impact of bronchodilator therapy on exercise tolerance in COPD. *Int J Chron Obstruct Pulmon Dis.* 2010;5:57–71.
2. Agusti AG, Roca J, Gea J, Wagner PD, Xaubet A, Rodriguez-Roisin R. Mechanisms of gas-exchange impairment in idiopathic pulmonary fibrosis. *Am Rev Respir Dis.* 1991;143(2):219–25.
3. American Thoracic Society, European Respiratory Society. American Thoracic Society/European Respiratory Society statement: standards for the diagnosis and management of individuals with alpha-1 antitrypsin deficiency. *Am J Respir Crit Care Med.* 2003;168(7):818–900.
4. Anderson SD, Brannan JD. Bronchial provocation testing: the future. *Curr Opin Allergy Clin Immunol.* 2011;11(1):46–52.
5. Anderson SD, Kippelen P. Exercise-induced bronchoconstriction: pathogenesis. *Curr Allergy Asthma Rep.* 2005;5(2):116–22.
6. Anthonisen NR, Connett JE, Kiley JP, et al. Effects of smoking intervention and the use of an inhaled anticholinergic bronchodilator on the rate of decline of FEV1. The Lung Health Study. *JAMA.* 1994;272(19):1497–505.
7. ATS Committee on Proficiency Standards for Clinical Pulmonary Function Laboratories. ATS statement: guidelines for the six-minute walk test. *Am J Respir Crit Care Med.* 2002;166(1):111–7.
8. Ayazi S, Demeester SR, Hsieh CC, et al. Thoraco-abdominal pressure gradients during the phases of respiration contribute to gastroesophageal reflux disease. *Dig Dis Sci.* 2011;56(6):1718–22.
9. Ayres JG, Gabbott PL. Vocal cord dysfunction and laryngeal hyperresponsiveness: a function of altered autonomic balance? *Thorax.* 2002;57(4):284–5.
10. Badesch DB, Abman SH, Simonneau G, Rubin LJ, McLaughlin VV. Medical therapy for pulmonary arterial hypertension: updated ACCP evidence-based clinical practice guidelines. *Chest.* 2007;131(6):1917–28.
11. Badesch DB, Champion HC, Sanchez MA, et al. Diagnosis and assessment of pulmonary arterial hypertension. *J Am Coll Cardiol.* 2009;54(1 Suppl):S55–66.
12. Bai TR. Evidence for airway remodeling in chronic asthma. *Curr Opin Allergy Clin Immunol.* 2010;10(1):82–6.
13. Barnes PJ. Against the Dutch hypothesis: asthma and chronic obstructive pulmonary disease are distinct diseases. *Am J Respir Crit Care Med.* 2006;174(3):240–3; discussion 243–4.
14. Barnes PJ. Immunology of asthma and chronic obstructive pulmonary disease. *Nat Rev Immunol.* 2008;8(3):183–92.
15. Barnes PJ, Dweik RA, Gelb AF, et al. Exhaled nitric oxide in pulmonary diseases: a comprehensive review. *Chest.* 2010;138(3):682–92.
16. Bradley B, Branley HM, Egan JJ, et al. British Thoracic Society Interstitial Lung Disease Guideline Group, British Thoracic Society Standards of Care Committee, Thoracic Society of Australia, New Zealand Thoracic Society, Irish Thoracic Society. Interstitial lung disease guideline: the British Thoracic Society in collaboration with the Thoracic Society of Australia and New Zealand and the Irish Thoracic Society. *Thorax.* 2008;63 Suppl 5:v1–58.
17. Bradley J, Moran F. Physical training for cystic fibrosis. *Cochrane Database Syst Rev.* 2008;(1):CD002768.
18. Bradley JM, Lasserson T, Elborn S, Macmahon J, O'neill B. A systematic review of randomized controlled trials examining the short-term benefit of ambulatory oxygen in COPD. *Chest.* 2007;131(1):278–85.
19. Briffa PJ, Anderson SD, Burton DL, Young IH. Sodium cromoglycate and eformoterol attenuate sensitivity and reactivity to inhaled mannitol in subjects with bronchiectasis. *Respirology.* 2011;16(1):161–6.
20. Broadley KJ. Beta-adrenoceptor responses of the airways: for better or worse? *Eur J Pharmacol.* 2006;533(1–3):15–27.
21. Buist AS, McBurnie MA, Vollmer WM, et al. International variation in the prevalence of COPD (the BOLD Study): a population-based prevalence study. *Lancet.* 2007;370(9589):741–50.
22. Calverley PM, Rabe KF, Goehring UM, et al. Roflumilast in symptomatic chronic obstructive pulmonary disease: two randomised clinical trials. *Lancet.* 2009;374(9691):685–94.
23. Carlsen KH, Anderson SD, Bjermer L, et al. Exercise-induced asthma, respiratory and allergic disorders in elite athletes: epidemiology, mechanisms and diagnosis: part I of the report from the Joint Task Force of the European Respiratory Society (ERS) and the European Academy of Allergy and Clinical Immunology (EAACI) in cooperation with GA2LEN. *Allergy.* 2008;63(4):387–403.
24. Carlsen KH, Anderson SD, Bjermer L, et al. Treatment of exercise-induced asthma, respiratory and allergic disorders in sports and the relationship to doping: Part II of the report from the Joint Task Force of European Respiratory Society (ERS) and European Academy of Allergy and Clinical Immunology (EAACI) in cooperation with GA(2)LEN. *Allergy.* 2008;63(5):492–505.
25. Casaburi R, Kukafka D, Cooper CB, Witek TJ Jr, Kesten S. Improvement in exercise tolerance with the combination of tiotropium and pulmonary rehabilitation in patients with COPD. *Chest.* 2005;127(3):809–17.
26. Casaburi R, Porszasz J. Reduction of hyperinflation by pharmacologic and other interventions. *Proc Am Thorac Soc.* 2006;3(2):185–9.
27. Celli BR, Cote CG, Marin JM, et al. The body-mass index, airflow obstruction, dyspnea, and exercise capacity index in chronic obstructive pulmonary disease. *N Engl J Med.* 2004;350(10):1005–12.
28. Celli BR, MacNee W, ATS/ERS Task Force. Standards for the diagnosis and treatment of patients with COPD: a summary of the ATS/ERS position paper. *Eur Respir J.* 2004;23(6):932–46.
29. Chang AB, Bell SC, Byrnes CA, et al. Chronic suppurative lung disease and bronchiectasis in children and adults in Australia and New Zealand. *Med J Aust.* 2010;193(6):356–65.
30. Chowdhury BA, Dal Pan G. The FDA and safe use of long-acting beta-agonists in the treatment of asthma. *N Engl J Med.* 2010;362(13):1169–71.
31. Cockcroft DW. Direct challenge tests: Airway hyperresponsiveness in asthma: its measurement and clinical significance. *Chest.* 2010;138(2 Suppl):18S–24S.
32. Cote CG, Celli BR. Pulmonary rehabilitation and the BODE index in COPD. *Eur Respir J.* 2005;26(4):630–6.
33. Crapo RO, Casaburi R, Coates AL, et al. Guidelines for methacholine and exercise challenge testing-1999. This official statement of

the American Thoracic Society was adopted by the ATS Board of Directors, July 1999. *Am J Respir Crit Care Med.* 2000;161(1):309–29.

34. Crummy F, Piper AJ, Naughton MT. Obesity and the lung: 2. Obesity and sleep-disordered breathing. *Thorax.* 2008;63(8):738–46.

35. Daviskas E, Anderson SD, Eberl S, Young IH. Effect of increasing doses of mannitol on mucus clearance in patients with bronchiectasis. *Eur Respir J.* 2008;31(4):765–72.

36. Dempsey JA, Veasey SC, Morgan BJ, O'Donnell CP. Pathophysiology of sleep apnea. *Physiol Rev.* 2010;90(1):47–112.

37. Desai SA, Channick RN. Exercise in patients with pulmonary arterial hypertension. *J Cardiopulm Rehabil Prev.* 2008;28(1):12–6.

38. Dicpinigaitis PV. Chronic cough due to asthma: ACCP evidence-based clinical practice guidelines. *Chest.* 2006;129(1 Suppl):75S–9S.

39. Dixon AE, Holguin F, Sood A, et al. An official American Thoracic Society Workshop report: obesity and asthma. *Proc Am Thorac Soc.* 2010;7(5):325–35.

40. Doyle RL, McCrory D, Channick RN, Simonneau G, Conte J, American College of Chest Physicians. Surgical treatments/interventions for pulmonary arterial hypertension: ACCP evidence-based clinical practice guidelines. *Chest.* 2004;126(1 Suppl):63S–71S.

41. Du Bois RM, Richeldi L, European Respiratory Society. *Interstitial Lung Diseases.* Sheffield (UK): European Respiratory Society; 2009. 395 p.

42. ERS Task Force, Palange P, Ward SA, et al. Recommendations on the use of exercise testing in clinical practice. *Eur Respir J.* 2007;29(1):185–209.

43. Evans DJ, Bara AI, Greenstone M. Prolonged antibiotics for purulent bronchiectasis in children and adults. *Cochrane Database Syst Rev.* 2007;(2):CD001392.

44. Eves ND, Petersen SR, Haykowsky MJ, Wong EY, Jones RL. Helium-hyperoxia, exercise, and respiratory mechanics in chronic obstructive pulmonary disease. *Am J Respir Crit Care Med.* 2006;174(7):763–71.

45. *Expert Panel Report 3: Guidelines for the Diagnosis and Management of Asthma* [Internet]. Bethesda (MD): National Heart, Lung, and Blood Institute, National Asthma Education and Prevention Program; [cited 2011 Mar 15]. Available from: http://www.nhlbi .nih.gov/guidelines/asthma/asthgdln.pdf

46. Fabbri LM, Calverley PM, Izquierdo-Alonso JL, et al. Roflumilast in moderate-to-severe chronic obstructive pulmonary disease treated with longacting bronchodilators: two randomised clinical trials. *Lancet.* 2009;374(9691):695–703.

47. Ferreira A, Garvey C, Connors GL, et al. Pulmonary rehabilitation in interstitial lung disease: benefits and predictors of response. *Chest.* 2009;135(2):442–7.

48. Galie N, Hoeper MM, Humbert M, et al. Guidelines for the diagnosis and treatment of pulmonary hypertension: the Task Force for the Diagnosis and Treatment of Pulmonary Hypertension of the European Society of Cardiology (ESC) and the European Respiratory Society (ERS), endorsed by the International Society of Heart and Lung Transplantation (ISHLT). *Eur Heart J.* 2009;30(20):2493–537.

49. Gardner WN. The pathophysiology of hyperventilation disorders. *Chest.* 1996;109(2):516–34.

50. Geddes EL, Reid WD, Crowe J, O'Brien K, Brooks D. Inspiratory muscle training in adults with chronic obstructive pulmonary disease: a systematic review. *Respir Med.* 2005;99(11):1440–58.

51. Gimenez LM, Zafra H. Vocal cord dysfunction: an update. *Ann Allergy Asthma Immunol.* 2011;106(4):267–74.

52. Girodet PO, Ozier A, Bara I, Tunon de Lara JM, Marthan R, Berger P. Airway remodeling in asthma: New mechanisms and potential for pharmacological intervention. *Pharmacol Ther.* 2011;130(3):325–37.

53. *Global Strategy for Asthma Management and Prevention* [Internet]. GINA: Global Initiative for Asthma; [cited 2008 Oct 8]. Available from: http://www.ginasthma.org/Guidelineitem .asp??l1=2&l2=1&intId=1561

54. *Global Strategy for the Diagnosis, Management, and Prevention of COPD* [Internet]. Global Initiative for Chronic Obstructive Lung Disease (Gold); [cited 2011 Apr 6]. Available from: http://www .goldcopd.org/

55. Goeminne P, Dupont L. Non-cystic fibrosis bronchiectasis: diagnosis and management in 21st century. *Postgrad Med J.* 2010;86(1018):493–501.

56. Gosselink R. Breathing techniques in patients with chronic obstructive pulmonary disease (COPD). *Chron Respir Dis.* 2004;1(3):163–72.

57. Gosselink R, De Vos J, van den Heuvel SP, Segers J, Decramer M, Kwakkel G. Impact of inspiratory muscle training in patients with COPD: what is the evidence? *Eur Respir J.* 2011;37(2):416–25.

58. Gosselink RA, Wagenaar RC, Rijswijk H, Sargeant AJ, Decramer ML. Diaphragmatic breathing reduces efficiency of breathing in patients with chronic obstructive pulmonary disease. *Am J Respir Crit Care Med.* 1995;151(4):1136–42.

59. Grunig E, Ehlken N, Ghofrani A, et al. Effect of exercise and respiratory training on clinical progression and survival in patients with severe chronic pulmonary hypertension. *Respiration.* 2011;81(5):394–401.

60. Halbert RJ, Natoli JL, Gano A, Badamgarav E, Buist AS, Mannino DM. Global burden of COPD: systematic review and meta-analysis. *Eur Respir J.* 2006;28(3):523–32.

61. Halwani R, Al-Muhsen S, Hamid Q. Airway remodeling in asthma. *Curr Opin Pharmacol.* 2010;10(3):236–45.

62. Han MK, Postma D, Mannino DM, et al. Gender and chronic obstructive pulmonary disease: why it matters. *Am J Respir Crit Care Med.* 2007;176(12):1179–84.

63. Hansen JE, Wasserman K. Pathophysiology of activity limitation in patients with interstitial lung disease. *Chest.* 1996;109(6):1566–76.

64. Haverkamp H, Miller J, Rodman J, et al. Extrathoracic obstruction and hypoxemia occurring during exercise in a competitive female cyclist. *Chest.* 2003;124(4):1602–5.

65. Holland A, Hill C. Physical training for interstitial lung disease. *Cochrane Database Syst Rev.* 2008;(4):CD006322.

66. Holland AE, Hill CJ, Conron M, Munro P, McDonald CF. Short term improvement in exercise capacity and symptoms following exercise training in interstitial lung disease. *Thorax.* 2008;63(6):549–54.

67. Irwin RS. Chronic cough due to gastroesophageal reflux disease: ACCP evidence-based clinical practice guidelines. *Chest.* 2006;129(1 Suppl):80S–94S.

68. Jack S, Rossiter HB, Pearson MG, Ward SA, Warburton CJ, Whipp BJ. Ventilatory responses to inhaled carbon dioxide, hypoxia, and exercise in idiopathic hyperventilation. *Am J Respir Crit Care Med.* 2004;170(2):118–25.

69. Jack S, Rossiter HB, Warburton CJ, Whipp BJ. Behavioral influences and physiological indices of ventilatory control in subjects with idiopathic hyperventilation. *Behav Modif.* 2003;27(5):637–52.

70. Kapur N, Bell S, Kolbe J, Chang AB. Inhaled steroids for bronchiectasis. *Cochrane Database Syst Rev.* 2009;(1):CD000996.

71. Kim HC, Mofarrahi M, Hussain SN. Skeletal muscle dysfunction in patients with chronic obstructive pulmonary disease. *Int J Chron Obstruct Pulmon Dis.* 2008;3(4):637–58.

72. King PT. The pathophysiology of bronchiectasis. *Int J Chron Obstruct Pulmon Dis.* 2009;4:411–9.

73. Kogevinas M, Zock JP, Jarvis D, et al. Exposure to substances in the workplace and new-onset asthma: an international prospective population-based study (ECRHS-II). *Lancet.* 2007;370(9584):336–41.

74. Kraft M. Asthma and chronic obstructive pulmonary disease exhibit common origins in any country! *Am J Respir Crit Care Med.* 2006;174(3):238–40; discussion 243–4.

75. Kyroussis D, Polkey MI, Hamnegard CH, Mills GH, Green M, Moxham J. Respiratory muscle activity in patients with COPD walking to exhaustion with and without pressure support. *Eur Respir J*. 2000;15(4):649–55.

76. Lacasse Y, Goldstein R, Lasserson TJ, Martin S. Pulmonary rehabilitation for chronic obstructive pulmonary disease. *Cochrane Database Syst Rev*. 2006;(4):CD003793.

77. Laude EA, Duffy NC, Baveystock C, et al. The effect of helium and oxygen on exercise performance in chronic obstructive pulmonary disease: a randomized crossover trial. *Am J Respir Crit Care Med*. 2006;173(8):865–70.

78. Lester MK, Flume PA. Airway-clearance therapy guidelines and implementation. *Respir Care*. 2009;54(6):733–50; discussion 751–3.

79. Loddenkemper R, Gibson GJ, Sibille Y, European Respiratory Society, European Lung Foundation. *European Lung White Book: The First Comprehensive Survey on Respiratory Health in Europe*. Lausanne (Switzerland): European Respiratory Society: European Lung Foundation; 2003. 182 p.

80. Lopez AD, Shibuya K, Rao C, et al. Chronic obstructive pulmonary disease: current burden and future projections. *Eur Respir J*. 2006;27(2):397–412.

81. Loring SH, Garcia-Jacques M, Malhotra A. Pulmonary characteristics in COPD and mechanisms of increased work of breathing. *J Appl Physiol*. 2009;107(1):309–14.

82. Mahler DA, Wells CK. Evaluation of clinical methods for rating dyspnea. *Chest*. 1988;93(3):580–6.

83. Maltais F, Simon M, Jobin J, et al. Effects of oxygen on lower limb blood flow and O2 uptake during exercise in COPD. *Med Sci Sports Exerc*. 2001;33(6):916–22.

84. Mannino DM, Buist AS. Global burden of COPD: risk factors, prevalence, and future trends. *Lancet*. 2007;370(9589):765–73.

85. Marciniuk DD, Butcher SJ, Reid JK, et al. The effects of helium-hyperoxia on 6-min walking distance in COPD: a randomized, controlled trial. *Chest*. 2007;131(6):1659–65.

86. Marsh SE, Travers J, Weatherall M, et al. Proportional classifications of COPD phenotypes. *Thorax*. 2008;63(9):761–7.

87. Masoli M, Fabian D, Holt S, Beasley R, Global Initiative for Asthma (GINA) Program. The global burden of asthma: executive summary of the GINA Dissemination Committee report. *Allergy*. 2004;59(5):469–78.

88. McCool FD, Rosen MJ. Nonpharmacologic airway clearance therapies: ACCP evidence-based clinical practice guidelines. *Chest*. 2006;129(1 Suppl):250S–9S.

89. McGuinness G, Naidich DP. CT of airways disease and bronchiectasis. *Radiol Clin North Am*. 2002;40(1):1–19.

90. McKenzie DC, McLuckie SL, Stirling DR. The protective effects of continuous and interval exercise in athletes with exercise-induced asthma. *Med Sci Sports Exerc*. 1994;26(8):951–6.

91. McLaughlin VV, Archer SL, Badesch DB, et al. ACCF/AHA 2009 expert consensus document on pulmonary hypertension a report of the American College of Cardiology Foundation Task Force on Expert Consensus Documents and the American Heart Association developed in collaboration with the American College of Chest Physicians; American Thoracic Society, Inc.; and the Pulmonary Hypertension Association. *J Am Coll Cardiol*. 2009;53(17):1573–619.

92. Mereles D, Ehlken N, Kreuscher S, et al. Exercise and respiratory training improve exercise capacity and quality of life in patients with severe chronic pulmonary hypertension. *Circulation*. 2006;114(14):1482–9.

93. Mickleborough TD, Lindley MR, Montgomery GS. Effect of fish oil-derived omega-3 polyunsaturated fatty acid supplementation on exercise-induced bronchoconstriction and immune function in athletes. *Phys Sportsmed*. 2008;36(1):11–7.

94. Miller MR, Hankinson J, Brusasco V, et al. Standardisation of spirometry. *Eur Respir J*. 2005;26(2):319–38.

95. *Morbidity and Mortality: 2009 Chart Book on Cardiovascular, Lung and Blood Diseases* [Internet]. Bethesda (MD): National Heart, Lung and Blood Institute, National Institutes of Health; [cited 2011 May 10]. Available from: http://www.nhlbi.nih.gov/resources/docs/cht-book.htm

96. Murray MP, Pentland JL, Hill AT. A randomised crossover trial of chest physiotherapy in non-cystic fibrosis bronchiectasis. *Eur Respir J*. 2009;34(5):1086–92.

97. Newall C, Stockley RA, Hill SL. Exercise training and inspiratory muscle training in patients with bronchiectasis. *Thorax*. 2005;60(11):943–8.

98. Newman KB, Mason UG,3rd Schmaling KB. Clinical features of vocal cord dysfunction. *Am J Respir Crit Care Med*. 1995;152 (4 Pt 1):1382–6.

99. Nici L, Donner C, Wouters E, et al. American Thoracic Society/European Respiratory Society statement on pulmonary rehabilitation. *Am J Respir Crit Care Med*. 2006;173(12):1390–413.

100. Nishiyama O, Kondoh Y, Kimura T, et al. Effects of pulmonary rehabilitation in patients with idiopathic pulmonary fibrosis. *Respirology*. 2008;13(3):394–9.

101. O'Donnell AE, Barker AF, Ilowite JS, Fick RB. Treatment of idiopathic bronchiectasis with aerosolized recombinant human DNase I. rhDNase Study Group. *Chest*. 1998;113(5):1329–34.

102. O'Donnell DE. Hyperinflation, dyspnea, and exercise intolerance in chronic obstructive pulmonary disease. *Proc Am Thorac Soc*. 2006;3(2):180–4.

103. O'Donnell DE, Laveneziana P. Physiology and consequences of lung hyperinflation in COPD. *European Respiratory Review*. 2006;15(100):61–7.

104. Olivieri D, Ciaccia A, Marangio E, Marsico S, Todisco T, Del Vita M. Role of bromhexine in exacerbations of bronchiectasis. Double-blind randomized multicenter study versus placebo. *Respiration*. 1991;58(3–4):117–21.

105. Olson AL, Zwillich C. The obesity hypoventilation syndrome. *Am J Med*. 2005;118(9):948–56.

106. Parameswaran K, Todd DC, Soth M. Altered respiratory physiology in obesity. *Can Respir J*. 2006;13(4):203–10.

107. Pasteur MC, Bilton D, Hill AT. British Thoracic Society guideline for non-CF bronchiectasis. *Thorax*. 2010;65 Suppl 1:i1–58.

108. Patel IS, Vlahos I, Wilkinson TM, et al. Bronchiectasis, exacerbation indices, and inflammation in chronic obstructive pulmonary disease. *Am J Respir Crit Care Med*. 2004;170(4):400–7.

109. Peacock AJ, Murphy NF, McMurray JJ, Caballero L, Stewart S. An epidemiological study of pulmonary arterial hypertension. *Eur Respir J*. 2007;30(1):104–9.

110. Pellegrino R, Viegi G, Brusasco V, et al. Interpretative strategies for lung function tests. *Eur Respir J*. 2005;26(5):948–68.

111. Pizzutto SJ, Upham JW, Yerkovich ST, Chang AB. Inhaled non-steroid anti-inflammatories for children and adults with bronchiectasis. *Cochrane Database Syst Rev*. 2010;(4):CD007525.

112. Pogson Z, McKeever T. Dietary sodium manipulation and asthma. *Cochrane Database Syst Rev*. 2011;(3):CD000436.

113. Postma DS, Boezen HM. Rationale for the Dutch hypothesis. Allergy and airway hyperresponsiveness as genetic factors and their interaction with environment in the development of asthma and COPD. *Chest*. 2004;126(2 Suppl):96S–104S; discussion 159S–161S.

114. Postma DS, Kerkhof M, Boezen HM, Koppelman GH. Asthma and COPD: Common genes, common environments? *Am J Respir Crit Care Med*. 2011;183(12):1588–94.

115. Raghavan N, Webb K, Amornputtisathaporn N, O'Donnell DE. Recent advances in pharmacotherapy for dyspnea in COPD. *Curr Opin Pharmacol*. 2011;11(3):204–10.

116. Raghu G, Collard HR, Egan JJ, et al. An official ATS/ERS/JRS/ALAT statement: Idiopathic pulmonary fibrosis: Evidence-based guidelines for diagnosis and management. *Am J Respir Crit Care Med*. 2011;183(6):788–824.

117. Ram FS, Robinson SM, Black PN, Picot J. Physical training for asthma. *Cochrane Database Syst Rev.* 2005;(4):CD001116.

118. Randerath WJ, Verbraecken J, Andreas S, et al. Non-CPAP therapies in obstructive sleep apnoea. *Eur Respir J.* 2011;37(5):1000–28.

119. Rennard SI, Stoner JA. Challenges and opportunities for combination therapy in chronic obstructive pulmonary disease. *Proc Am Thorac Soc.* 2005;2(4):391–3; discussion 394–5.

120. Ries AL, Bauldoff GS, Carlin BW, et al. Pulmonary rehabilitation: Joint ACCP/AACVPR evidence-based clinical practice guidelines. *Chest.* 2007;131(5 Suppl):4S–42S.

121. Ries AL, Make BJ, Lee SM, et al. The effects of pulmonary rehabilitation in the national emphysema treatment trial. *Chest.* 2005;128(6):3799–809.

122. Roberts SD, Farber MO, Knox KS, et al. FEV1/FVC ratio of 70% misclassifies patients with obstruction at the extremes of age. *Chest.* 2006;130(1):200–6.

123. Roig M, Reid WD. Electrical stimulation and peripheral muscle function in COPD: a systematic review. *Respir Med.* 2009;103(4):485–95.

124. Salpeter SR, Ormiston TM, Salpeter EE. Meta-analysis: respiratory tolerance to regular beta2-agonist use in patients with asthma. *Ann Intern Med.* 2004;140(10):802–13.

125. Salpeter SR, Wall AJ, Buckley NS. Long-acting beta-agonists with and without inhaled corticosteroids and catastrophic asthma events. *Am J Med.* 2010;123(4):322–8.e2.

126. Seitz AE, Olivier KN, Steiner CA, Montes de Oca R, Holland SM, Prevots DR. Trends and burden of bronchiectasis-associated hospitalizations in the United States, 1993–2006. *Chest.* 2010;138(4):944–9.

127. Shea SA, Andres LP, Shannon DC, Banzett RB. Ventilatory responses to exercise in humans lacking ventilatory chemosensitivity. *J Physiol.* 1993;468:623–40.

128. Sillen MJ, Speksnijder CM, Eterman RM, et al. Effects of neuromuscular electrical stimulation of muscles of ambulation in patients with chronic heart failure or COPD: a systematic review of the English-language literature. *Chest.* 2009;136(1):44–61.

129. Soriano JB, Davis KJ, Coleman B, Visick G, Mannino D, Pride NB. The proportional Venn diagram of obstructive lung disease: two approximations from the United States and the United Kingdom. *Chest.* 2003;124(2):474–81.

130. Standards for the diagnosis and care of patients with chronic obstructive pulmonary disease. American Thoracic Society. *Am J Respir Crit Care Med.* 1995;152(5 Pt 2):S77–121.

131. Sun XG, Hansen JE, Oudiz RJ, Wasserman K. Exercise pathophysiology in patients with primary pulmonary hypertension. *Circulation.* 2001;104(4):429–35.

132. Sun XG, Hansen JE, Oudiz RJ, Wasserman K. Gas exchange detection of exercise-induced right-to-left shunt in patients with primary pulmonary hypertension. *Circulation.* 2002;105(1):54–60.

133. Tecklenburg SL, Mickleborough TD, Fly AD, Bai Y, Stager JM. Ascorbic acid supplementation attenuates exercise-induced bronchoconstriction in patients with asthma. *Respir Med.* 2007;101(8):1770–8.

134. Troosters T, Casaburi R, Gosselink R, Decramer M. Pulmonary rehabilitation in chronic obstructive pulmonary disease. *Am J Respir Crit Care Med.* 2005;172(1):19–38.

135. Wills P, Greenstone M. Inhaled hyperosmolar agents for bronchiectasis. *Cochrane Database Syst Rev.* 2006;(2):CD002996.

136. Wrigge H, Golisch W, Zinserling J, Sydow M, Almeling G, Burchardi H. Proportional assist versus pressure support ventilation: effects on breathing pattern and respiratory work of patients with chronic obstructive pulmonary disease. *Intensive Care Med.* 1999;25(8):790–8.

137. Zhang J, Yao X, Yu R, et al. Exhaled carbon monoxide in asthmatics: a meta-analysis. *Respir Res.* 2010;11:50.

SELECTED REFERENCES FOR FURTHER READING

American Association of Cardiovascular and Pulmonary Rehabilitation. *Guidelines for Pulmonary Rehabilitation Programs.* 4th ed. Champaign (IL): Human Kinetics; 2011. 184 p.

Durstine JL, Moore GE, Painter P, Roberts S, editors. *ACSM's Exercise Management for Persons with Chronic Diseases and Disabilities.* 3rd ed. Champaign (IL): Human Kinetics; 2009. 407 p.

Lumb AB. *Nunn's Applied Respiratory Physiology.* 7th ed. Philadelphia: Elsevier; 2010. 568 p.

West JB. *Pulmonary Pathophysiology: The Essentials.* 7th ed. Philadelphia: Lippincott Williams & Wilkins; 2007. 224 p.

INTERNET RESOURCES

- American Thoracic Society Best of the Web Reviews: http://www.thoracic.org/clinical/best-of-the-web/reviews.php
- American Thoracic Society/European Respiratory Society COPD Guidelines: http://www.ersnet.org/lrPresentations/copd/files/main/index.html
- American Thoracic Society statements: http://www.thoracic.org/statements
- eMedicine: http://www.emedicine.com/med/PULMONOLOGY.htm
- Global Initiative for Asthma (GINA): http://www.ginasthma.org
- Global Initiative for Obstructive Lung Disease (GOLD): http://www.goldcopd.org
- MedlinePlus: http://www.nlm.nih.gov/medlineplus/lungsandbreathing.html
- National Asthma Education and Prevention Program (Expert Panel Report 3: Guidelines for the Diagnosis and Management of Asthma): http://www.nhlbi.nih.gov/guidelines/asthma/asthgdln.htm
- Pulmonary Hypertension Association (PHA): http://www.phassociation.org

Pathophysiology and Treatment of Metabolic Disease

Diabetes mellitus (henceforth referred to as *diabetes*, but not to be confused with other diseases that produce polyuria, such as diabetes insipidus) contributes to elevated rates of morbidity and mortality by increasing the risk of cardiovascular disease (CVD), kidney failure, and other chronic metabolic conditions. Diabetes is a complex heterogeneous disease that requires the management of serum glucose levels, lipid parameters, blood pressure, and thrombotic factors. Intensive lifestyle modification of increased physical activity and adaptation of a heart healthy diet is usually a first-line of therapy for individuals with Type 2 diabetes. Regular exercise reduces body weight and fat mass, improves insulin sensitivity, blood pressure control and lipid profiles, and reduces cardiovascular risk. This chapter will define the types of diabetes, describe risk factors for diabetes, provide information on the metabolic syndrome, and focus on the effects of regular exercise and physical activity on glucose metabolism and the metabolic syndrome. The importance of exercise and physical activity on risk factors for diabetes such as central obesity, insulin resistance, hypertension, hypertriglyceridemia, and associated metabolic abnormalities will be further elucidated. Finally, the role of oral antidiabetic drugs in maintaining normal glycemia as diabetes progresses will be discussed.

DESCRIPTION OF NORMAL GLUCOSE METABOLISM, TYPE 1, AND TYPE 2 DIABETES

The 2010 statement of the American Diabetes Association (ADA) outlines the diagnosis and classification of diabetes mellitus (3). Four criteria are used for the diagnosis of diabetes (*Table 8-1*) (3). The criteria for hemoglobin A1C (HbA1C) levels, fasting plasma glucose (FPG), and the 2-h plasma glucose during a 75-g oral glucose tolerance test (OGTT) must be confirmed on a subsequent day unless unequivocal symptoms of hyperglycemia are present. The criteria have changed in recent years by the advice of experts from several groups including the International Expert Committee with members of the ADA, the International Diabetes Federation (IDF) and the European Association for the Study of Diabetes. These groups now recommend the use of the HbA1C test to diagnose diabetes with the specific value of $\geq 6.5\%$. The ADA recommends screening for diabetes in asymptomatic people at any age who are overweight or obese by the body mass index (BMI) criteria (≥ 25 kg $\cdot$ m^{-2}) and also have at least one additional risk factor for diabetes (3). Some of these risk factors include lack of physical activity, first-degree

KEY TERMS

Diabetes mellitus: A metabolic disease marked by high levels of glucose resulting from defects of insulin secretion, insulin action, or both.

Exercise: Physical activity that is planned, structured, and repetitive for the purpose of improving or maintaining one or more components of physical fitness.

Gestational diabetes: Carbohydrate intolerance of variable severity with onset or first recognition during pregnancy.

Physical Activity: Bodily movement produced by contraction of skeletal muscle that increases energy expenditure above basal level.

Prediabetes: A condition of insulin resistance and hyperglycemia that is not severe enough to meet the criteria for diagnosis of diabetes.

Type 1 diabetes mellitus: An autoimmune disease that causes pancreatic beta cell destruction and the inability of the body to produce insulin.

Type 2 diabetes mellitus: A metabolic disorder that results from the inability of the body to respond appropriately to insulin and, as the need for insulin rises, the pancreas gradually loses its ability to produce it.

TABLE 8-1. Criteria for the Diagnosis of Diabetes

1.	Hemoglobin A1C ≥6.5%. The test should be performed in a laboratory using a method that is certified by NGSP and is standardized to the DCCT assay.
	or
2.	FPG ≥126 mg · dL^{-1} (7.0 mmol · L^{-1}). Fasting is defined as no caloric intake for at least 8 h.
	or
3.	A 2-h plasma glucose ≥200 mg · dL^{-1} (11.1 mmol · L^{-1}) during an OGTT. The test should be performed according to the World Health Organization, using a glucose load containing the equivalent of 75-g anhydrous glucose dissolved in water.
	or
4.	A patient with classic symptoms of hyperglycemia or hyperglycemic crisis, a random plasma glucose ≥200 mg · dL^{-1} (11.1 mmol · L^{-1}). The classic symptoms of diabetes include polyuria, polydipsia, and unexplained weight loss.

NGSP, National Glycohemoglobin Standardization Program; DCCT, Diabetes Control and Complications Trial; FPG, fasting plasma glucose; OGTT, oral glucose tolerance test.

relative with diabetes, high risk because of race or ethnicity (African American, Latino, Native American), hypertension, and history of CVD. The ADA further recommends that individuals without these additional risk factors should be tested for diabetes beginning at 45 yr of age and repeated at least every 3 yr if results are normal.

A normal FPG concentration is defined as <100 mg · dL^{-1} (5.6 mmol · L^{-1}). Hyperglycemia that does not meet the criteria for Type 2 diabetes is classified as impaired fasting glucose (IFG), defined as FPG of 100–125 mg · dL^{-1} (5.6–6.9 mmol · L^{-1}). Similarly, impaired glucose tolerance (IGT) is defined as a 2-h OGTT plasma glucose of 140–199 mg · dL^{-1} (7.8–11.0 mmol · L^{-1}), whereas a value ≥200 mg · dL^{-1} is diagnostic for diabetes. These categories of IFG and IGT are referred to as "prediabetes," because both of these conditions are risk factors for the development of diabetes and CVD.

Type 1 diabetes, an immune-mediated disease, is characterized by β-cell destruction that usually leads to absolute insulin deficiency. Serologic markers of pancreatic destruction such as islet cell autoantibodies, insulin autoantibodies, glutamic acid decarboxylase (GAD$_{65}$), and human leukocyte antigens may be present upon diagnosis and support the autoimmune nature of this disease (2). The rate of β-cell destruction varies widely and is typically slow in infants and fast in adults (2). This type of diabetes accounts for only 5%–10% of all cases of diabetes and is characterized by islet cell autoantibodies, autoantibodies to insulin, autoantibodies to GAD$_{65}$, and autoantibodies to the tyrosine phosphatases IA-2 and IA-2β, any of which are present in 85%–90% of individuals when hyperglycemia is

discovered (2). Children and adolescents may present with ketoacidosis, whereas others may have modest fasting hyperglycemia that can quickly change to severe hyperglycemia and/or ketoacidosis. Adults with Type 1 diabetes may not present with ketoacidosis for many years because they maintain some β-cell function. Ketoacidosis occurs when a high level of ketones (β-hydroxybutyrate, acetoacetate) are produced as a byproduct of incomplete fatty acid metabolism. In Type 1 diabetes, the combination of deficient insulin and increased counterregulatory hormones (*e.g.*, catecholamines, cortisol, glucagon) results in excessive ketone production and metabolic acidosis (2). Type 1 diabetes is more common in children and adolescents but can occur at all ages, even among the elderly. Type 1 diabetes has many genetic predispositions and likely environmental influences. Patients are rarely obese, but obesity is possible in Type 1 diabetes. Patients with Type 1 diabetes are also at risk to develop other autoimmune disorders, such as Grave disease, Hashimoto thyroiditis, Addison disease, vitiligo, celiac sprue, autoimmune hepatitis, myasthenia gravis, and pernicious anemia. Other forms of Type 1 diabetes that are more rare have no known etiology (idiopathic diabetes). The idiopathic type is strongly inherited and patients are mainly of African or Asian descent.

Type 2 diabetes is characterized predominantly by insulin resistance with relative insulin deficiency and can progress to an insulin secretory defect with insulin resistance. *Insulin resistance* is defined as a reduction in glucose disposal rate elicited by a given insulin concentration (31). This type of diabetes occurs in ~90%–95% of cases of diabetes. Specific etiologies are not known and there are many different causes of Type 2 diabetes, but autoimmune destruction of the β-cell does not occur. Many individuals with Type 2 diabetes go undiagnosed because hyperglycemia develops gradually and there are no classic symptoms. Most patients with Type 2 diabetes are obese and/or have central obesity and are at risk for the development of microvascular and macrovascular complications. Type 2 diabetes can occur in children and adolescents, likely because of obesity and reduced physical activity.

Given the rise in overweight and obesity in women, the recommendations for screening in pregnancy have changed. The International Association of Diabetes and Pregnancy Study Groups (IADPSG) convened in 2008–2009 and revised the recommendations for diagnosing gestational diabetes mellitus (GDM). GDM has been defined for many years as any degree of carbohydrate intolerance of variable severity with onset or first recognition during pregnancy (2). It is recommended that all women who do not have known diabetes get screened for GDM at 24–28 wk of gestation by undergoing a 75-g OGTT. For those women with risk factors, they should be screened at their first prenatal visit. The IADPSG also developed specific cut points for fasting, 1-h and 2-h plasma glucose levels. The group acknowledges that more women will be diagnosed with GDM than previously. Further recommendations of the ADA include (a) women with GDM be screened for diabetes 6–12 wk postpartum and (b) those with a history of GDM have lifelong screening for the development of diabetes or prediabetes at least every 3 yr. Significant differences exist between the guidelines from the United States and the United Kingdom with respect to the screening, diagnosis, and management of GDM (101). Risk factors for GDM include marked obesity, personal history of GDM or delivery of a previous large-for-gestational-age infant, glycosuria, polycystic ovary syndrome, or a strong family history of diabetes (2). Central adiposity by high waist-to-hip ratio (121) as well as African American race and Latino ethnicity (7) are also associated with the development of GDM. Women with a history of GDM are at an increased risk for the development of Type 2 diabetes mellitus (3,53,55,75).

The ADA has also classified other specific types of diabetes. Maturity-onset diabetes of the young (MODY), for example, is characterized by genetic defects in β-cell function whereby hyperglycemia occurs at an early age (generally before 25 yr) and impaired insulin secretion but no problems with insulin action. Other etiologies include genetic defects in insulin action, injury to the pancreas such as pancreatitis, infection, etc., and endocrinopathies where hormones antagonize insulin action. Diabetes can also be caused by infections and drug- or chemical-induced diabetes. Immune-mediated diabetes and other genetic syndromes associated with diabetes can occur. More detail is provided for these types of diabetes elsewhere (2).

DEVELOPMENT, RISK FACTORS AND COMORBIDITIES FOR DIABETES

Obese individuals, particularly those with visceral fat accumulation, are more likely to develop Type 2 diabetes. Increased body fat mass is associated with higher levels of inflammatory adipocyte cytokines (adipokines). Inflammation not only plays an important role in atherosclerosis but also in the development of diabetes and its microvascular complications. Factors that augment inflammation in patients with Type 2 diabetes include increased oxidative stress, hyperglycemia, and the formation of advanced glycation end products (85,88,119). In the Strong Heart Study, elevated A1C, 2-h glucose, fasting insulin, albuminuria, and obesity were significant predictors of the conversion from prediabetes to diabetes in approximately 1,700 individuals over an 8-yr follow-up (113). Moreover, conversion from normal glucose tolerance was associated with lower age, elevated fasting insulin, and lower physical activity. Thus, modifiable

risk factors such as obesity and physical activity are important to these categorical conversions. Prospective studies indicate an association between physical activity and the development of Type 2 diabetes (64,70,71). In a population-based prospective study that directly measured fitness by a maximal exercise test, men in the low-fitness group had a 1.9-fold higher risk for IGT and a 3.7-fold higher risk for the development of Type 2 diabetes compared to men in the high-fitness group (115). These associations persist even after adjustment for age, parental history of diabetes, alcohol consumption, and cigarette smoking (115). Thus, it appears that physical fitness may be a major factor to reduce the development of Type 2 diabetes.

Risk factors for diabetes include age ≥45 yr; BMI ≥25 kg · m^{-2}; habitual physical inactivity; having a first-degree relative with diabetes; being a member of a high-risk ethnic population such as African American, Latino, Native American, Asian American, or Pacific Islander; delivering a baby weighing >9 lb or having a past diagnosis of GDM; and having polycystic ovary syndrome (3). Additional risk factors include hypertension (≥140/90 mm Hg), low high-density lipoprotein (HDL) cholesterol (<35 mg · dL^{-1} or 0.90 mmol · L^{-1}), high triglyceride level (>250 mg · dL^{-1} or 2.82 mmol · L^{-1}), previous diagnosis of IGT or IFG, other clinical conditions associated with insulin resistance, and a history of vascular disease (3). The National Heart, Lung, and Blood Institute (NHLBI) also classified central obesity (waist circumference as a surrogate for visceral fat) with BMI level as a risk factor for Type 2 diabetes (12). For example, men with a waist circumference of ≥40 in and women whose waist is ≥35 in with BMI in the overweight category (25.0–29.9 kg · m^{-2}) are at a high risk. This increases to extremely high risk at BMI levels of morbid obesity (≥40 kg · m^{-2}) (12). A sedentary lifestyle is an important and modifiable risk factor for Type 2 diabetes with a 30%–50% risk reduction associated with a physically active, compared to a sedentary, lifestyle (104).

Insulin resistance, a primary defect in patients with Type 2 diabetes, affects all of the normal metabolic actions of insulin including glucose transport, hexokinase activity, glycogen synthesis, and glucose oxidation. Skeletal muscle is the primary site of glucose disposal under insulin-stimulated conditions. In response to insulin binding, insulin receptors on skeletal muscle cells undergo autophosphorylation on tyrosine residues, leading to activation of the receptor tyrosine kinase and subsequent tyrosine phosphorylation of insulin receptor substrate-1 (IRS-1) (46). IRS-1, in turn, associates with the regulatory subunit of phosphatidylinositol 3 kinase, which is necessary for mediating insulin's metabolic effects, including glucose transporter 4 (GLUT4) translocation, glucose disposal, and increasing the activity of glycogen synthase and hexokinase (46). Impaired glucose clearance from the circulation by skeletal muscle and adipose tissue and, to a lesser degree, an increase in the production of glucose by hepatocytes and portal adipocytes are key aspects of the metabolic dysfunction that are associated with insulin resistance and impaired insulin secretion. Patients with diabetes often have multiple comorbid CVD risk factors including dyslipidemia and hypertension.

DEVELOPMENT AND RISK FACTORS FOR OTHER METABOLIC CONDITIONS

METABOLIC SYNDROME

Syndrome X was first introduced by Reaven (91) as a disorder characterized by IGT, dyslipidemia, and hypertension, which were associated with increased risk of Type 2 diabetes and CVD. The primary underlying mechanism for the syndrome was attributed to insulin resistance at the level of the skeletal muscle. In 2001,

the Third Report of the National Cholesterol Education Program (NCEP) Expert Panel on Detection, Evaluation, and Treatment of High Blood Cholesterol in Adults (Adult Treatment Panel III [ATP III]) (26) called attention to the importance of the metabolic syndrome. The World Health Organization (WHO) also selected criteria to define the metabolic syndrome (1). The IDF, which reflects the ATP III and WHO definitions, also created their definition of the metabolic syndrome (42). Most recently, the American Heart Association (AHA) and the NHLBI issued an executive summary that modified the definitions. These definitions of the metabolic syndrome are presented in *Table 8-2* (32). The modifications of earlier definitions include allowing for lower thresholds of the waist circumference for ethnic groups or individuals prone to insulin resistance; counting triglycerides, HDL-cholesterol (HDL-C) levels and blood pressure as abnormal if a person is receiving drug treatment for these factors; counting glucose as elevated if ≥ 100 mg $\cdot$ dL^{-1};

TABLE 8-2. Adult Treatment Panel III (ATP III) (26), World Health Organization (WHO) (1), International Diabetes Federation (42), American Heart Association and National Heart, Lung, and Blood Institute (32) Criteria for the Metabolic Syndrome

	ATP III (3 or more criteria below)	WHO Insulin Resistance (Impaired glucose tolerance, impaired fasting glucose or Type 2 diabetes, +2 or more criteria subsequently)	International Diabetes Federation (Central obesity plus any two of remaining four criteria)	American Heart Association and National Heart, Lung, and Blood Institute
Central obesity/obesity	Abdominal obesity: waist circumference >102 cm in men and >88 cm in women	Abdominal obesity: waist-to-hip ratio >0.90 in men and >0.85 in women and/or BMI >30 kg $\cdot$ m^{-2}	Waist circumference $\geq$94 cm for Europid men and $\geq$80 cm for Europid women, with ethnicity specific values for other groups	Elevated waist circumference: $\geq$102 cm in men and $\geq$88 cm in women
Lipid	Hypertriglyceridemia: $\geq$150 mg $\cdot$ dL^{-1}	Hypertriglyceridemia: $\geq$150 mg $\cdot$ dL^{-1}	Hypertriglyceridemia: $\geq$150 mg $\cdot$ dL^{-1}	Hypertriglyceridemia: $\geq$150 mg $\cdot$ dL^{-1} or drug treatment for elevated TG
Lipid	Low HDL-C: <40 mg $\cdot$ dL^{-1} in men and <50 mg $\cdot$ dL^{-1} in women	Low HDL-C: <35 mg $\cdot$ dL^{-1} in men and <39 mg $\cdot$ dL^{-1} in women	Low HDL-C: <40 mg $\cdot$ dL^{-1} in men and <50 mg $\cdot$ dL^{-1} in women or specific treatment for this lipid abnormality	Low HDL-C: <40 mg $\cdot$ dL^{-1} in men and <50 mg $\cdot$ dL^{-1} in women or drug treatment for elevated HDL-C
Blood pressure	High blood pressure: $\geq$130/85 mm Hg	High blood pressure: $\geq$140/90 mm Hg and/or antihypertensive medication	High blood pressure: $\geq$130/85 mm Hg or treatment of previously diagnosed hypertension	High blood pressure: $\geq$130 mm Hg systolic BP or $\geq$85 mm Hg diastolic BP or drug treatment for hypertension
Glucose	High fasting glucose: $\geq$110 mg $\cdot$ dL^{-1}	Impaired glucose regulation or Type 2 diabetes Insulin resistance (under hyperinsulinemic euglycemic conditions, glucose uptake below lowest quartile for background population under investigation)	High fasting glucose: $\geq$100 mg $\cdot$ dL^{-1} or previously diagnosed Type 2 diabetes	High fasting glucose: $\geq$100 mg $\cdot$ dL^{-1} or drug treatment for elevated glucose
Microalbuminuria		Urine albumin excretion rate: $\geq$20 μg $\cdot$ min^{-1} or albumin:creatinine ratio $\geq$30 mg $\cdot$ g^{-1}		

BMI, body mass index; TG, triglycerides; HDL-C, high-density lipoprotein cholesterol; BP, blood pressure.

and clarifying that either elevated systolic or diastolic pressure defines elevated blood pressure. The group also states that the "most important underlying risk factors are abdominal obesity and insulin resistance" — conditions that are modifiable by behavior and lifestyle (32).

The ATP III discusses the presence of prothrombotic and proinflammatory states as part of the metabolic syndrome. These components associated with the metabolic syndrome include inflammation (29,67,74,78,87), intimal-medial wall thickness of the carotid arteries (74) and coagulation markers (29,87). Participants in National Health and Nutrition Examination Survey (NHANES III) with the metabolic syndrome according to ATP III criteria had elevated C-reactive protein (CRP) concentrations, and higher fibrinogen concentrations and white blood cell (WBC) counts than those adults without the metabolic syndrome (29). Furthermore, physically active individuals with the metabolic syndrome had lower levels of CRP, WBC counts, and fibrinogen levels as well as other adipokines including serum amyloid-A, interleukin-6, and tumor necrosis factor-α (TNF-α) levels than sedentary individuals with the metabolic syndrome (87). Consistent with this, lean mass, visceral fat area and plasma soluble TNF receptor 1 concentration (sTNFR1) are independently related to the severity of metabolic syndrome (i.e., the number of components) in postmenopausal women (120). These studies suggest that inflammation is a risk factor for the presence of the metabolic syndrome.

Several teams investigated the WHO and ATP III definitions of the metabolic syndrome in different populations to see if they concur and if they differ in relation to mortality (41,72,98,112). In a study of over 1,500 patients with Type 2 diabetes, 78% fulfilled the ATP III criteria and 81% met the WHO criteria indicating a good agreement between the two definitions of the metabolic syndrome (72). In the Cardiovascular Health Study, there was an 80% concordance in classifying the participants (98). In a sample of approximately 400 obese adults, the prevalence of the metabolic syndrome was higher in those defined by WHO than the ATP III criteria (112). Of approximately 2,800 participants in the San Antonio Heart Study, one-fourth met both WHO and ATP III criteria for the metabolic syndrome with an additional one-fourth of adults meeting only one of the criteria (41). Furthermore, both definitions were predictive of all-cause and cardiovascular mortality, but the ATP III definition was slightly more predictive in lower risk adults in the San Antonio Heart Study (41). Finally, the metabolic syndrome defined by ATP III and not by WHO was an independent predictor of coronary or cerebrovascular events (98) suggesting that the ATP III criteria may be especially useful in this regard. In a review of prospective studies between 1998 and 2004, Ford et al. (30)

concluded that the population-attributable fraction for the metabolic syndrome is approximately 6%–7% for all-cause mortality, 12%–17% for CVD, and 30%–52% for diabetes. Using the most recent AHA and NHLBI definition of metabolic syndrome, Ho et al. (37) followed more than 30,000 men for 13.6 yr and reported that all of the metabolic syndrome parameters were significantly associated with both all-cause and cardiovascular mortality. Furthermore, they found that hypertension was the most potent predictor of all-cause and cardiovascular mortality even after adjustment for age and metabolic syndrome variables. Likewise, central obesity and hypertriglyceridemia increased all-cause and cardiovascular mortality even after adjustment for other risk factors. Physical activity should also be considered in the examination of metabolic syndrome and mortality. A study of more than 10,000 middle-aged men and women with an 11-yr follow-up indicated that coronary heart disease risk associated with the metabolic syndrome was significantly lower in physically active individuals (10). Moreover, physically active men and women with the metabolic syndrome had a lower CVD risk than inactive people with the metabolic syndrome, suggesting a protective effect of physical activity.

A report of the ADA and the European Association for the Study of Diabetes provides a critical view of the definition, pathogenesis, and utility of the metabolic syndrome (49). This review concludes that clinicians should evaluate and treat all CVD risk factors without regard to whether the patient meets the criteria for diagnosis of the metabolic syndrome. Another published review provides an examination of the mechanisms underlying the metabolic syndrome and the management of the metabolic syndrome (22).

A sedentary lifestyle is associated with metabolic risk in men and women older than the age of 60 yr (5). Using the accelerometry data from the 2003–2006 NHANES, Bankoski et al. (5) found that people with the metabolic syndrome spent a greater percentage of time being sedentary, had lower intensity during sedentary time, and had longer sedentary bouts than those individuals without the metabolic syndrome. Leisure time physical activity level assessed by self-report is inversely associated with the metabolic syndrome in a population of 58-yr-old men (6). These studies would indicate that reducing sedentary behavior and increasing leisure activities could be important in controlling the metabolic syndrome.

There is also evidence to suggest that a low cardiorespiratory fitness is associated with increased clustering of metabolic abnormalities of the metabolic syndrome (117). Additionally, a follow-up of healthy men and women with the metabolic syndrome showed that a low cardiorespiratory fitness was a risk factor for premature mortality (51). In another study (27), the age and smoking-adjusted prevalence of the metabolic syndrome in women was highest (19%) in those with the lowest cardiorespiratory fitness, and decreased across quintiles of increasing fitness levels. The significance of cardiorespiratory fitness in the metabolic syndrome is that fitness levels attenuate the effect of the metabolic syndrome on all-cause and CVD mortality (52).

Several studies have examined the amount of physical activity associated with a reduction in the prevalence of the metabolic syndrome. Men who engage in >1 h · wk^{-1} but <3 h · wk^{-1} of moderate-intensity leisure-time physical activity are 60% more likely to have the metabolic syndrome (using a modified definition of the WHO) than those who participate in ≥3 h · wk^{-1} (61). In young adults from the Bogalusa Heart study, the White and African American women who were moderately active compared to physical inactive women had significantly less risk of having three components of the metabolic syndrome (33). Finally, leisure-time physical activity levels determined by questionnaire are inversely associated with the prevalence of the metabolic syndrome in White, African American, and Native American women (45).

ROLE OF EXERCISE/PHYSICAL ACTIVITY AND BODY WEIGHT ON DIABETES

TYPE 2 DIABETES

Significant progress has been made towards an understanding of the molecular basis underlying the beneficial effects of exercise training in stimulating the entry of glucose into tissue responsive to insulin action (46,122). Accordingly, it is well accepted that regular physical exercise offers an effective therapeutic intervention to improve insulin action in skeletal muscle and adipose tissue in insulin-resistant individuals. Chronic exercise results in numerous physiologic and cellular adaptations that favor sustained improvement in insulin action (*Fig. 8-1*) (46,122).

The link between physical inactivity and insulin resistance was first noted in migrant populations who experienced dramatic increases in the incidence of Type 2 diabetes after exposure to a more Westernized environment that was quite different from their traditional lifestyles. Japanese migrants living in Hawaii had an elevated risk of diabetes compared to their

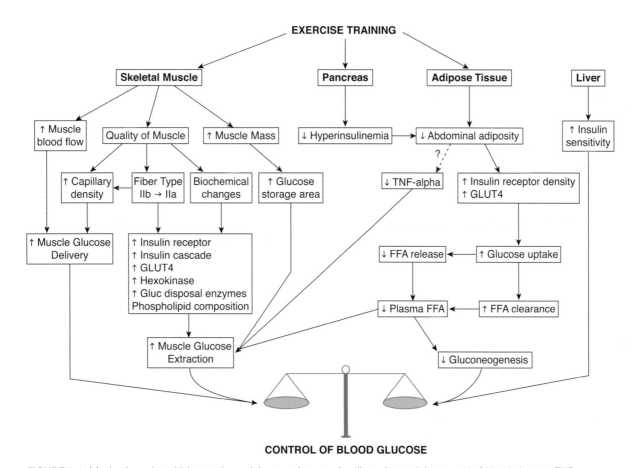

FIGURE 8-1. Mechanisms by which exercise training may improve insulin action and the control of blood glucose. TNF-α, tumor necrosis factor-α; GLUT4, glucose transporter 4; FFA, free fatty acid. (Reprinted with permission from Ivy JL, Zderic TW, Fogt DL. Prevention and treatment of non-insulin-dependent diabetes mellitus. *Exerc Sport Sci Rev.* 1999;27:1–35.)

counterparts living in Hiroshima (54). Likewise, Pima Indians in rural Mexico living a traditional Pima Indian lifestyle have markedly lower rates of diabetes compared to the Arizona Pimas consuming a westernized diet and maintaining a sedentary lifestyle (90). The difference in the prevalence of diabetes in these populations despite the similarity in genetic background can directly be attributed to changes in lifestyle behavior, in particular the level of habitual physical activity. A further illustration of this point is the finding that hunter–gatherer societies exhibit only a 1%–2% prevalence of diabetes compared to a much higher prevalence in industrialized nations (21,76).

Additional evidence to support the hypothesis that physical inactivity plays a significant role in the increased incidence of diabetes is provided by observational and retrospective studies (35,68,70,71). Data from the University of Pennsylvania Alumni study document a 6% lower risk of diabetes for each 500 kcal $\cdot$ wk^{-1} of self-reported leisure-time physical activity (35). In the Physician Health Studies (70,71) the risk of diabetes was ~35% less for females who reported vigorous exercise at least once per week, whereas men who exercised vigorously five or more times per week showed a 42% reduction in the age-adjusted risk of diabetes compared to those who exercised less than once per week, suggesting a dose-response relationship between increased physical activity and diabetes risk.

Prospective studies also document the beneficial effects that physical activity (38,39,116) and fitness (62,65) play in reducing the incidence of diabetes. The Nurses Health Study showed that brisk walking for at least 2.5 h $\cdot$ wk^{-1} was associated with a 25% reduction in diabetes over an 8-yr follow-up period (39). Data from the Women Health Study demonstrated that participants who reported walking 2–3 h $\cdot$ wk^{-1} were 34% less likely to develop diabetes than women who reported no exercise (116). Furthermore, participants enrolled in The Women Health Initiative Observational Study stratified to the lowest quartile of total energy and walking energy expenditure had a 22% and 18% higher risk of developing diabetes compared to women in the highest quartiles of energy expenditures (38). Higher levels of fitness are associated with a reduced risk of developing Type 2 diabetes in women (108). Thus, there is strong evidence of a graded inverse association between levels of self-reported physical activity and incident diabetes over long follow-up periods. Middle-aged Finnish men in the lowest quartile of cardiorespiratory fitness ($\dot{V}O_{2max}$ <25.8 mL $\cdot$ kg^{-1} $\cdot$ min^{-1}) were more than four times as likely to develop diabetes as men in the highest two quartiles of fitness ($\dot{V}O_{2max}$ >31.1 mL $\cdot$ kg^{-1} $\cdot$ min^{-1}) (65). At the Cooper Institute for Aerobics Research, a 6-yr longitudinal study demonstrated that men in the lowest fitness group (the least fit 20% of the cohort) at the time of enrollment had a

greater risk for IFG and diabetes compared with those in the highest fitness groups (the most fit 40% of the cohort) (114). These studies support the hypothesis that a sedentary lifestyle and low cardiorespiratory fitness play a significant role in the progression from normal glucose tolerance to Type 2 diabetes.

Randomized clinical trials in high-risk populations with impaired glycemic control also provide evidence to support the hypothesis that implementation of a lifestyle behavior that incorporates an increase in leisure-time physical activity can prevent or postpone the development of Type 2 diabetes (56,84,89,110). Chinese men encouraged to increase their daily physical activity (30 min of mild-intensity activity, 20 min of moderate-intensity activity, 10 min of strenuous activity, or 5 min of very strenuous exercise) were 46% less likely to develop diabetes than a control group over a 6-yr period (84). During a mean follow-up of 3–4 yr in the Finnish and U.S. Diabetes Prevention studies, the progression to frank diabetes was 60% lower for men and women with IGT assigned to an intense lifestyle intervention that included regular physical activity (~150 min $\cdot$ wk^{-1} of moderate to vigorous intensity activities), modest weight loss, and healthier dietary habits compared to glucose intolerant men and women in the control group (56,110). In another randomized controlled trial with a 30-mo follow-up, there was a significant reduction in incidence of diabetes in Asian Indians with IGT who underwent either lifestyle modification or oral medication, but the combination did not further reduce risk for diabetes (89). Thus, there remains little doubt that incorporating physical activity into the lifestyle of high-risk individuals is a critical modification to reduce the worsening of glucose metabolism.

Intervention studies demonstrate that structured and supervised training regimens that utilize either aerobic or resistive training have positive effects on insulin sensitivity and glucose homeostasis in individuals with IGT and Type 2 diabetes. Chronic training leads to improvements in glucose tolerance, the insulin response to glucose, and insulin sensitivity of up to 30% (with insulin sensitivity measured via euglycemic-hyperinsulinemic or hyperglycemic clamps) (17,18,40,48,93–95). Exercise training reduces the HbA1C concentration in patients with Type 2 diabetes (9), indicating improved glycemic control. In a randomized clinical trial, an exercise program consisting of two times per week aerobic and resistive training improved physical fitness and reduced HbA1C levels, systolic and diastolic blood pressure, low-density lipoprotein (LDL) cholesterol, and waist circumference compared to a counseling control group (4). In a small sample of individuals with Type 2 diabetes, aerobic training alone and a combined exercise program of aerobic and resistive training reduced HbA1C after only 16 wk (73). In a randomized clinical trial of 39- to 70-yr-old men and women with Type 2 diabetes,

6-mo community-based programs of aerobic, resistive, and aerobic + resistive training also reduced HbA1C, with the greatest effect observed in the combined group (100). A meta-analysis of 14 randomized clinical trials indicates a 0.74 percentage point reduction in HbA1C after moderate-intensity exercise training in patients with Type 2 diabetes compared to no change in a control group (9). High-intensity resistance training interventions were also very effective in reducing HbA1C in patients with Type 2 diabetes with absolute change of up to 1.2% (11,20). A review of the literature of yoga-based programs indicated that yoga may improve risk profiles of individuals with Type 2 diabetes, but considering the limitations of many of the 25 studies that were reviewed, no firm conclusions can be drawn on the effectiveness of this type of physical activity (43). Recommendations for physical activity in Type 2 diabetes are provided in a consensus statement of the American College of Sports Medicine (ACSM) and the ADA (14).

In summary, there is an extensive body of observational and experimental evidence supporting the hypothesis that an active lifestyle prevents the dysregulation in glucose homeostasis and substantially delays the progression from a state of impaired glycemic control to frank diabetes.

TYPE 1 DIABETES

Patients with Type 1 diabetes should be encouraged to perform regular exercise similar to healthy individuals and those with Type 2 diabetes because of the long-term benefits of physical activity in improving known risk factors for atherosclerosis and CVD. Physical activity has been linked in prospective epidemiological studies to reduced cardiovascular mortality in Type 1 diabetes (77). During a 6-yr follow-up period, patients with Type 1 diabetes in the lowest quintile of reported baseline physical activity had a sixfold and fourfold higher mortality rate in men and women, respectively, compared to the quintile with the highest physical activity level even after controlling for potential confounding variables such as age, BMI, insulin dose, cigarette smoking, and alcohol drinking (77). Children and adolescents with Type 1 diabetes may show signs of atherosclerosis, but those who exercise more than 60 min · d^{-1} have higher arterial flow-mediated dilation (109), suggesting benefits to endothelial function by physical activity. Because diabetes is associated with an increased risk of macrovascular disease, the benefit of exercise is hypothesized to derive from its antiatherogenic effects on lipid and lipoprotein metabolism (59,123). In fact, a randomized controlled clinical trial in patients with Type 1 diabetes showed that 12–16 wk of aerobic exercise training at 60%–80% $\dot{V}O_{2peak}$ produced favorable changes in lipid, lipoprotein and apolipoprotein levels. The amount of aerobic activity was inversely associated with triglyceride levels and

directly associated with the apolipoprotein AI (*APOA1*)/apolipoprotein B (*APOB*) ratio even after controlling for adiposity and glycemic control (59). Expected, $\dot{V}O_{2max}$ improves with exercise training in children with Type 1 diabetes (19,99). Although HbA1C levels did not improve, daily doses of injectable insulin were reduced with training (19). In another randomized trial, 6 mo of exercise training improved HbA1C levels and reduced insulin requirements in children, adolescents, and young adults (96). The ADA concluded in 2004 that exercise training studies fail to show an independent effect of physical activity on improving glycemic control as measured by HbA1C in patients with Type 1 diabetes (123). In a more recent meta-analysis of exercise interventions of adults with Type 1 diabetes, HbA1C levels were reduced by 0.33% units between treatment and controls (15). In summary, the benefits of exercise training in individuals with Type 1 diabetes include a reduction in CVD risk factors and, thus, patients are encouraged to perform regular aerobic exercise.

PHARMACOLOGICAL AND MEDICAL TREATMENT OF DIABETES

TYPE 2 DIABETES

The pathogenesis of Type 2 diabetes involves peripheral and hepatic insulin resistance and impaired or abnormal insulin and glucagon secretion from the pancreas. Hyperglycemia gradually develops as a result of the decrease in insulin sensitivity and abnormal metabolic adaptations (*e.g.*, decrease in glucose uptake in peripheral tissue and increase glucose output from the liver) (46,122). Diabetes is a complex chronic disease that requires adequate management of hyperglycemia and other comorbid physiologic dysfunctions such as dyslipidemia, high blood pressure, and elevated thrombotic factors — conditions that are highly associated with insulin resistance. Therefore, achieving metabolic control via tight monitoring of fasting and postprandial glucose and HbA1C is clinically important to decrease the risk of CVD in patients with diabetes (3).

The United Kingdom Prospective Diabetes Study (UKPDS), a randomized multicenter clinical trial, provided the knowledge and standard for clinical practice with the primary goal of maintaining HbA1C concentrations between 6.5% and 7.0% (3,23,44). The maintenance of HbA1C to near normoglycemia with intensified treatment in the form of oral antidiabetic agents, insulin, or combination therapy significantly reduced the development of microvascular and macrovascular complications associated with diabetes (13,57). Because of the beneficial effects of improved insulin sensitivity, improved glucose tolerance, and reduction in the risk of cardiovascular complications, the first-line of therapy for newly diagnosed patients with Type 2 diabetes is the implementation of an intensive lifestyle modification of increased physical activity and adaptation of a heart healthy diet (3,13). A common recommendation is to eventually reduce body weight by 5%–10% because most patients that present with diabetes are overweight or obese. Weight loss of ~10% improves insulin sensitivity and, in overweight individuals with Type 2 diabetes, has been shown to reduce fasting blood glucose (FBG) by 2–3 mmol · L^{-1} and HbA1C by 1 or more percentage points (86,103). Unfortunately, long-term compliance with such programs tends to be poor. The UKPDS demonstrate that only 25% of the patients were able to maintain the optimal HbA1C levels of <7% after 9 yr without an oral agent or insulin (44). Glycemic control frequently deteriorates with conventional therapies as diabetes progresses, despite the initial drop in HbA1C. Therefore, the need may arise to use oral antidiabetic agents in combination therapy to aggressively maintain glycemic control to as near normal as possible. However, the use of oral agents in this aggressive manner can only maintain adequate HbA1C levels for an estimated period of ~10 yr, after which many patients may require insulin therapy (13).

There are currently five groups of oral antidiabetic drugs according to their principal mode of action: (a) those that increase insulin secretion (insulin secretagogues); (b) those that enhance the activity of other insulin secretagogues; (c) those that delay the rate of carbohydrates digestion and absorption (α-glucosidase inhibitors); (d) those that affect signaling pathways of hepatic gluconeogenesis; and (e) those with direct effects on insulin responsive tissue (insulin sensitizers).

Insulin secretagogues, such as sulfonylureas and glinides, lower circulating blood glucose by enhancing pancreatic insulin secretion (13,57). However, because the hypoglycemic effect of this class of drugs is attributable to increased insulin secretion, its effectiveness is highly dependent on adequate β-cell function. Fasting glucose levels decrease with these drugs by 2–4 mmol · L^{-1} with an accompanying decrease in HbA1C of 1–2 percentage points (13,57).

The class of drugs known as dipeptidyl peptidase-4 (DPP-4) inhibitors prolong and enhance the activity of the insulin secretagogue, incretin. The main two molecules that fulfill criteria for being an incretin — glucagon-like peptide-1 (GLP-1) and gastric inhibitory peptide (GIP) — are intestinal hormones that amplify the postprandial secretion of insulin but are rapidly degraded by the enzyme DPP-4. Unlike GIP, which has not been thoroughly examined in humans, GLP-1 improves glucose-dependent insulin secretion, suppresses glucagon secretion, delays gastric emptying, and promotes satiety (13,36). DPP-4 inhibitors decrease HbA1C by 0.5–1.0 percentage points (81). They also improve FPG and postprandial glucose, with low risk of hypoglycemia.

α-Glucosidase inhibitors, such as acarbose, miglitol, and voglibose, reduce the rate of digestion of carbohydrates in the proximal small intestine, primarily lowering postprandial glucose concentrations as they inhibit intestinal α-glucosidase enzymes. The chance of causing hypoglycemia is very minimal in this class of drugs because of their mode of action. α-Glucosidase inhibitors generally reduce HbA1C by 0.5–1.0 percentage points depending on the dosage on the drug. These inhibitors typically reduce postprandial glucose concentrations by 1–4 mmol · L^{-1}, thereby resulting in a significant reduction in the incremental area under the postprandial glucose curve (13,57).

Although the action of bile acid sequestrants, such as colesevelam, on lipid metabolism has been extensively explored, their action on glucose metabolism has not been well delineated. It appears that bile acid sequestrants bind to bile acids in the intestines, modulating the signaling pathways of enzymes involved in hepatic glucose production (105,106). In addition to lowering LDL-cholesterol 15%–26% and modestly increasing HDL-C 4%–8%, they decrease HbA1C 0.5–1.0 percentage points.

The insulin sensitizers are attractive oral agents for therapy in patients with Type 2 diabetes because peripheral insulin resistance is a primary defect in these individuals. Biguanides, such as metformin, are the therapy of choice for overweight and obese individuals with Type 2 diabetes. Biguanides improve insulin action in hepatic tissue, adipose tissue (28), and, to a lesser extent, skeletal muscle (34,47). However, because metformin does not increase insulin release, the presence of insulin is crucial for its effectiveness. The principal modes of action are to decrease hepatic glucose output by reducing gluconeogenesis, decrease hepatic extraction of gluconeogenic substrates, decrease hepatic glycogenolysis, and enhance insulin stimulated glucose uptake in adipose tissue and to a lesser extent skeletal muscle (13,57). Metformin, the only biguanide currently available for clinical use, typical reduce fasting glucose by 2–4 mmol · L^{-1} with corresponding decreases in HbA1C of 1–2 percentage points. Thiazolidinediones (TZDs), such as pioglitazone, are also insulin sensitizers that improve whole-body insulin sensitivity via multiple actions on gene regulation (13,57). TZD treatments effectively control glycemia by altering cellular mechanisms in tissues such as muscle, adipose tissue, and liver thereby improving insulin action. The metabolic effects observed in skeletal muscle tissue include increases in glucose uptake, glycolysis, glucose oxidation, and inconsistent changes in glycogenesis. The metabolic effects observed in adipose tissue include an increase in glucose uptake, fatty acid uptake, lipogenesis, and preadipocyte differentiation. The metabolic effects observed in the liver include a decrease in gluconeogenesis, glycogenolysis, and an increase in lipogenesis and glucose uptake. TZD agents reduce HbA1C 0.5–1.5 percentage points.

In addition to the oral medications, there are two commonly used classes of injectable antidiabetic drugs also used in the treatment of diabetes: GLP-1 analogues and amylinomimetic agents. Both classes are peptide analogs, mimicking the action of human hormones involved in glucose metabolism.

The GLP-1 analogues have glucoregulatory effects similar to those of GLP-1 but have a low affinity for DDP-4. They often are not considered first-choice drugs, but instead are used as combination therapy in patients with Type 2 diabetes who are not adequately controlled with oral medications. Two common injectable GLP-1 receptor agonists are exenatide and liraglutide. Exenatide treatment typically result in a 0.5–1.0 percentage points decrease in HbA1C, 1.4 mmol · L^{-1} decrease in FPG, and a 2–3 kg decline in body mass, whereas liraglutide results in a 1–2 percentage point decline in HbA1C and a 1–3 kg body mass loss (13,66,111).

Amylinomimetic agents, such as pramlintide, are synthetic versions of the human hormone called amylin, which modulates gastric emptying, prevents the postprandial rise in plasma glucagon, and causes early satiety (102). Provided through subcutaneous injections, amylinomimetic agents decrease HbA1C 0.5–1.0 percentage points and body mass by ~2 kg.

Insulin is usually the last line of treatment and is reserved for those patients who fail to respond adequately to a combination of orals and injectable antidiabetic agents, whose glycemic control continues to deteriorate despite adequate drug combinations, and for whom safety and efficacy considerations favors its use as the drug of choice, such as in cases of pregnancy or severe hepatic and renal impairments (3,13,57). Inability to achieve adequate glycemic control with combinations of oral and injectable therapies probably indicate that the natural history of the disease has progressed to a state of severe β-cell failure and a switch to insulin therapy is usually recommended (57). An insulin pump can be used to manage some patients with Type 2 diabetes and gestational diabetes. Management of GDM focuses on similar interventions that are commonly recommended in Type 2 diabetes; however, insulin therapy can be initiated when glucose control is not achieved and reduces serious perinatal complications (16). Insulin administered by syringe is injected into subcutaneous tissue using a rotation of sites, including the abdomen (fastest absorption rate), upper arms, lateral thigh, and buttocks. Continuous Subcutaneous Insulin Infusion (CSII) is subcutaneously delivered only in the abdominal area. Insulin administered by syringe can be rapid-acting (peak action: 0.5–1.0 h), short-acting (peak action: 2–3 h), intermediate-acting (peak action: 4–10 h), or long-acting (peak action: sustained for 20–24 h). A mixed dose of different types of insulin produces a more normal glucose response and is used most commonly. Usually, rapid-acting insulin is used with CSII.

In summary, irrespective of the treatment modality, any intervention is likely to improve the probability that a patient will experience better long-term glycemic control. This is especially true if the diagnosis of diabetes is detected early when the metabolic abnormalities usually associated with this chronic disease are less severe. As our knowledge of the pathogenesis of this complicated disease continues to grow, it is certain that this information will facilitate the development of new therapeutic agents that will more effectively attain and maintain normal glycemic control while minimizing the risk of hypoglycemia.

TYPE 1 DIABETES

Type 1 diabetes mellitus is associated with long-term complications of the eyes, kidneys, and peripheral and autonomic nervous system (3). In addition, Type 1 diabetes is associated with a 10-fold increase in CVD as compared with aged-matched nondiabetic individuals (60). Because hyperglycemia appears to play a significant role in the pathophysiology of these complications, the need to achieve glycemic control to near-normal blood glucose and HbA1C concentrations as safely as possible without inducing hypoglycemia with insulin therapy is crucial for long-term clinical benefits (3). The Diabetes Control and Complication Trial (DCCT) was designed to assess whether intensive insulin therapy (at least three insulin injections per day or continuous infusion of insulin with an external pump with at least four blood measurement of glucose per day) would reduce the risk of macrovascular and microvascular complications compared to conventional therapy (one or two insulin injections per day with one urine or blood glucose test per day). The desired goal for the intensive therapy was to maintain blood glucose and HbA1C to as close to normal range as possible, whereas conventional therapy had no glucose goal except to prevent symptoms of hyperglycemia and hypoglycemia (24). At the end of the 6.5 yr of the DCCT, mean HbA1C was 7.2% in the intensive therapy group versus 9% in the conventional therapy group. Subsequently, intensive insulin therapy reduced the risk of development and progression of microvascular and neuropathic complications by 35% and 76% (20), respectively, and decreased the progression of intima-media thickness, a sensitive marker for coronary and cerebral vascular disease in patients with Type 1 diabetes (80,92). The DCCT/Epidemiology of Diabetes Interventions and Complications Research Group also demonstrated that intensive therapy to maintain near-normal HbA1C concentrations has beneficial effects on long-term complications associated with Type 1 diabetes (79,80,92). The risk of progressive nephropathy remained lower in the intensive versus the conventional treatment group 4 yr after the completion of the DCCT trials (92), whereas progressive retinopathy remained lower 10 yr following completion (118). Seventeen-year follow-up showed reduced risk of cardiovascular events by 42%, and the risk of severe clinical events such as non-fatal myocardial infarction, stroke, or death from CVD was reduced by 57% in the intensive treatment group (79). In summary, intensive therapy implemented early to achieve glycemic control to as near normal as possible is beneficial in patients with Type 1 diabetes to reduce the short- and long-term macrovascular and microvascular complications associated with this disease (3).

SUMMARY

The clinical importance of physical activity in diabetes is underscored by studies that indicate that a low level of physical fitness is associated with increased risk of all-cause and CVD mortality (25,63,97,115). Men who improve their physical fitness reduce their mortality risk by approximately 44% (8). In addition, both avoiding obesity and beginning moderately vigorous sports activity are separately associated with lower death rates from all causes and from CVD and reductions in the incidence of coronary events in middle-aged and older men and postmenopausal women (50,58,69,82,83). Maintaining a healthy body weight, not smoking, exercising moderately or vigorously 30 min $\cdot$ d^{-1}, and eating a healthy diet results in more than an 80% reduction in the incidence of coronary events (107). Therefore, increased physical activity is an effective treatment that yields significant health benefits in diabetes and other metabolic conditions.

REFERENCES

1. Alberti KG, Zimmet PZ. Definition, diagnosis and classification of diabetes mellitus and its complications. Part 1: diagnosis and classification of diabetes mellitus provisional report of a WHO consultation. *Diabet Med.* 1998;15(7):539–53.
2. American Diabetes Association. Diagnosis and classification of diabetes mellitus. *Diabetes Care.* 2011;34 Suppl 1:S62–9.
3. American Diabetes Association. Standards of medical care in diabetes—2011. *Diabetes Care.* 2011;34 Suppl 1:S11–61.
4. Balducci S, Zanuso S, Nicolucci A, et al. Effect of an intensive exercise intervention strategy on modifiable cardiovascular risk factors in subjects with type 2 diabetes mellitus: a randomized controlled trial: the Italian Diabetes and Exercise Study (IDES). *Arch Intern Med.* 2010;170(20):1794–803.
5. Bankoski A, Harris TB, McClain JJ, et al. Sedentary activity associated with metabolic syndrome independent of physical activity. *Diabetes Care.* 2011;34(2):497–503.
6. Behre CJ, Bergstrom G, Schmidt CB. Increasing leisure time physical activity is associated with less prevalence of the metabolic syndrome in healthy middle-aged men. *Angiology.* 2011;62(6):509–12.
7. Berkowitz GS, Lapinski RH, Wein R, Lee D. Race/ethnicity and other risk factors for gestational diabetes. *Am J Epidemiol.* 1992;135(9):965–73.
8. Blair SN, Kohl HW,3rd, Barlow CE, Paffenbarger RS Jr, Gibbons LW, Macera CA. Changes in physical fitness and all-cause mortality. A prospective study of healthy and unhealthy men. *JAMA.* 1995;273(14):1093–8.

9. Boule NG, Haddad E, Kenny GP, Wells GA, Sigal RJ. Effects of exercise on glycemic control and body mass in type 2 diabetes mellitus: a meta-analysis of controlled clinical trials. *JAMA.* 2001;286(10):1218–27.
10. Broekhuizen LN, Boekholdt SM, Arsenault BJ, et al. Physical activity, metabolic syndrome, and coronary risk: the EPIC-Norfolk prospective population study. *Eur J Cardiovasc Prev Rehabil.* 2011;18(2):209–17.
11. Castaneda C, Layne JE, Munoz-Orians L, et al. A randomized controlled trial of resistance exercise training to improve glycemic control in older adults with type 2 diabetes. *Diabetes Care.* 2002;25(12):2335–41.
12. *Clinical Guidelines on the Identification, Evaluation, and Treatment of Overweight and Obesity in Adults* [Internet]. Bethesda (MD): National Institutes of Health; National Heart, Lung, and Blood Institute; [cited 2011 Jan 19]. Available from: http://www.nhlbi.nih.gov/guidelines/obesity/ob_home.htm
13. Cohen A, Horton ES. Progress in the treatment of type 2 diabetes: new pharmacologic approaches to improve glycemic control. *Curr Med Res Opin.* 2007;23(4):905–17.
14. Colberg SR, Sigal RJ, Fernhall B, et al. Exercise and type 2 diabetes: the American College of Sports Medicine and the American Diabetes Association: joint position statement. *Diabetes Care.* 2010;33(12):e147–67.
15. Conn VS, Hafdahl AR, Lemaster JW, Ruppar TM, Cochran JE, Nielsen PJ. Meta-analysis of health behavior change interventions in type 1 diabetes. *Am J Health Behav.* 2008;32(3):315–29.
16. Crowther CA, Hiller JE, Moss JR, et al. Effect of treatment of gestational diabetes mellitus on pregnancy outcomes. *N Engl J Med.* 2005;352(24):2477–86.
17. Dengel DR, Hagberg JM, Pratley RE, Rogus EM, Goldberg AP. Improvements in blood pressure, glucose metabolism, and lipoprotein lipids after aerobic exercise plus weight loss in obese, hypertensive middle-aged men. *Metabolism.* 1998;47(9):1075–82.
18. Dengel DR, Pratley RE, Hagberg JM, Rogus EM, Goldberg AP. Distinct effects of aerobic exercise training and weight loss on glucose homeostasis in obese sedentary men. *J Appl Physiol.* 1996;81(1):318–25.
19. D'hooge R, Hellinckx T, Van Laethem C, et al. Influence of combined aerobic and resistance training on metabolic control, cardiovascular fitness and quality of life in adolescents with type 1 diabetes: a randomized controlled trial. *Clin Rehabil.* 2011;25(4):349–59.
20. Dunstan DW, Daly RM, Owen N, et al. High-intensity resistance training improves glycemic control in older patients with type 2 diabetes. *Diabetes Care.* 2002;25(10):1729–36.
21. Eaton SB, Konner M, Shostak M. Stone agers in the fast lane: chronic degenerative diseases in evolutionary perspective. *Am J Med.* 1988;84(4):739–49.
22. Eckel RH, Grundy SM, Zimmet PZ. The metabolic syndrome. *Lancet.* 2005;365(9468):1415–28.
23. Effect of intensive blood-glucose control with metformin on complications in overweight patients with type 2 diabetes (UKPDS 34). UK Prospective Diabetes Study (UKPDS) Group. *Lancet.* 1998;352(9131):854–65.
24. The effect of intensive treatment of diabetes on the development and progression of long-term complications in insulin-dependent diabetes mellitus. The Diabetes Control and Complications Trial Research Group. *N Engl J Med.* 1993;329(14):977–86.
25. Ekelund LG, Haskell WL, Johnson JL, Whaley FS, Criqui MH, Sheps DS. Physical fitness as a predictor of cardiovascular mortality in asymptomatic North American men. The Lipid Research Clinics Mortality Follow-up Study. *N Engl J Med.* 1988;319(21):1379–84.
26. Expert Panel on Detection, Evaluation, and Treatment of High Blood Cholesterol in Adults. Executive Summary of the Third Report of the National Cholesterol Education Program (NCEP) Expert Panel on Detection, Evaluation, and Treatment of High Blood Cholesterol in Adults (Adult Treatment Panel III). *JAMA.* 2001;285(19):2486–97.

27. Farrell SW, Cheng YJ, Blair SN. Prevalence of the metabolic syndrome across cardiorespiratory fitness levels in women. *Obes Res.* 2004;12(5):824–30.

28. Fischer M, Timper K, Radimerski T, et al. Metformin induces glucose uptake in human preadipocyte-derived adipocytes from various fat depots. *Diabetes Obes Metab.* 2010;12(4):356–9.

29. Ford ES. The metabolic syndrome and C-reactive protein, fibrinogen, and leukocyte count: findings from the Third National Health and Nutrition Examination Survey. *Atherosclerosis.* 2003;168(2):351–8.

30. Ford ES. Risks for all-cause mortality, cardiovascular disease, and diabetes associated with the metabolic syndrome: a summary of the evidence. *Diabetes Care.* 2005;28(7):1769–78.

31. Godsland IF, Stevenson JC. Insulin resistance: syndrome or tendency? *Lancet.* 1995;346(8967):100–3.

32. Grundy SM, Cleeman JI, Daniels SR, et al. Diagnosis and management of the metabolic syndrome: an American Heart Association/National Heart, Lung, and Blood Institute Scientific Statement. *Circulation.* 2005;112(17):2735–52.

33. Gustat J, Srinivasan SR, Elkasabany A, Berenson GS. Relation of self-rated measures of physical activity to multiple risk factors of insulin resistance syndrome in young adults: the Bogalusa Heart Study. *J Clin Epidemiol.* 2002;55(10):997–1006.

34. Hallsten K, Virtanen KA, Lonnqvist F, et al. Rosiglitazone but not metformin enhances insulin- and exercise-stimulated skeletal muscle glucose uptake in patients with newly diagnosed type 2 diabetes. *Diabetes.* 2002;51(12):3479–85.

35. Helmrich SP, Ragland DR, Leung RW, Paffenbarger RS Jr. Physical activity and reduced occurrence of non-insulin-dependent diabetes mellitus. *N Engl J Med.* 1991;325(3):147–52.

36. Hinnen D, Nielsen LL, Waninger A, Kushner P. Incretin mimetics and DPP-IV inhibitors: new paradigms for the treatment of type 2 diabetes. *J Am Board Fam Med.* 2006;19(6):612–20.

37. Ho JS, Cannaday JJ, Barlow CE, Mitchell TL, Cooper KH, FitzGerald SJ. Relation of the number of metabolic syndrome risk factors with all-cause and cardiovascular mortality. *Am J Cardiol.* 2008;102(6):689–92.

38. Hsia J, Wu L, Allen C, Oberman A, et al. Physical activity and diabetes risk in postmenopausal women. *Am J Prev Med.* 2005;28(1):19–25.

39. Hu FB, Sigal RJ, Rich-Edwards JW, et al. Walking compared with vigorous physical activity and risk of type 2 diabetes in women: a prospective study. *JAMA.* 1999;282(15):1433–9.

40. Hughes VA, Fiatarone MA, Fielding RA, et al. Exercise increases muscle GLUT-4 levels and insulin action in subjects with impaired glucose tolerance. *Am J Physiol.* 1993;264(6 Pt 1):E855–62.

41. Hunt KJ, Resendez RG, Williams K, Haffner SM, Stern MP, San Antonio Heart Study. National Cholesterol Education Program versus World Health Organization metabolic syndrome in relation to all-cause and cardiovascular mortality in the San Antonio Heart Study. *Circulation.* 2004;110(10):1251–7.

42. *The IDF consensus worldwide definition of the metabolic syndrome* [Internet]. Brussels (Belgium): International Diabetes Federation; [cited 2008 Apr 3]. Available from: http://www.idf.org/webdata/docs/MetS_def_update2006.pdf

43. Innes KE, Vincent HK. The influence of yoga-based programs on risk profiles in adults with type 2 diabetes mellitus: a systematic review. *Evid Based Complement Alternat Med.* 2007;4(4):469–86.

44. Intensive blood-glucose control with sulphonylureas or insulin compared with conventional treatment and risk of complications in patients with type 2 diabetes (UKPDS 33). UK Prospective Diabetes Study (UKPDS) Group. *Lancet.* 1998;352(9131):837–53.

45. Irwin ML, Ainsworth BE, Mayer-Davis EJ, Addy CL, Pate RR, Durstine JL. Physical activity and the metabolic syndrome in a tri-ethnic sample of women. *Obes Res.* 2002;10(10):1030–7.

46. Ivy JL, Zderic TW, Fogt DL. Prevention and treatment of non-insulin-dependent diabetes mellitus. *Exerc Sport Sci Rev.* 1999;27:1–35.

47. Johnson AB, Webster JM, Sum CF, et al. The impact of metformin therapy on hepatic glucose production and skeletal muscle glycogen synthase activity in overweight type II diabetic patients. *Metabolism.* 1993;42(9):1217–22.

48. Joseph LJ, Farrell PA, Davey SL, Evans WJ, Campbell WW. Effect of resistance training with or without chromium picolinate supplementation on glucose metabolism in older men and women. *Metabolism.* 1999;48(5):546–53.

49. Kahn R, Buse J, Ferrannini E, Stern M, American Diabetes Association, European Association for the Study of Diabetes. The metabolic syndrome: time for a critical appraisal: joint statement from the American Diabetes Association and the European Association for the Study of Diabetes. *Diabetes Care.* 2005;28(9):2289–304.

50. Kanaya AM, Vittinghoff E, Shlipak MG, et al. Association of total and central obesity with mortality in postmenopausal women with coronary heart disease. *Am J Epidemiol.* 2003;158(12):1161–70.

51. Katzmarzyk PT, Church TS, Blair SN. Cardiorespiratory fitness attenuates the effects of the metabolic syndrome on all-cause and cardiovascular disease mortality in men. *Arch Intern Med.* 2004;164(10):1092–7.

52. Katzmarzyk PT, Church TS, Janssen I, Ross R, Blair SN. Metabolic syndrome, obesity, and mortality: impact of cardiorespiratory fitness. *Diabetes Care.* 2005;28(2):391–7.

53. Kaufmann RC, Schleyhan FT, Huffman DG, Amankwah KS. Gestational diabetes diagnostic criteria: long-term maternal follow-up. *Am J Obstet Gynecol.* 1995;172(2 Pt 1):621–5.

54. Kawate R, Yamakido M, Nishimoto Y, Bennett PH, Hamman RF, Knowler WC. Diabetes mellitus and its vascular complications in Japanese migrants on the Island of Hawaii. *Diabetes Care.* 1979;2(2):161–70.

55. Kim C, Newton KM, Knopp RH. Gestational diabetes and the incidence of type 2 diabetes: a systematic review. *Diabetes Care.* 2002;25(10):1862–8.

56. Knowler WC, Barrett-Connor E, Fowler SE, et al. Reduction in the incidence of type 2 diabetes with lifestyle intervention or metformin. *N Engl J Med.* 2002;346(6):393–403.

57. Krentz AJ, Bailey CJ. Oral antidiabetic agents: current role in type 2 diabetes mellitus. *Drugs.* 2005;65(3):385–411.

58. Kushi LH, Fee RM, Folsom AR, Mink PJ, Anderson KE, Sellers TA. Physical activity and mortality in postmenopausal women. *JAMA.* 1997;277(16):1287–92.

59. Laaksonen DE, Atalay M, Niskanen LK, et al. Aerobic exercise and the lipid profile in type 1 diabetic men: a randomized controlled trial. *Med Sci Sports Exerc.* 2000;32(9):1541–8.

60. Laing SP, Swerdlow AJ, Slater SD, et al. Mortality from heart disease in a cohort of 23,000 patients with insulin-treated diabetes. *Diabetologia.* 2003;46(6):760–5.

61. Lakka TA, Laaksonen DE, Lakka HM, et al. Sedentary lifestyle, poor cardiorespiratory fitness, and the metabolic syndrome. *Med Sci Sports Exerc.* 2003;35(8):1279–86.

62. LaMonte MJ, Blair SN, Church TS. Physical activity and diabetes prevention. *J Appl Physiol.* 2005;99(3):1205–13.

63. Lie H, Mundal R, Erikssen J. Coronary risk factors and incidence of coronary death in relation to physical fitness. Seven-year follow-up study of middle-aged and elderly men. *Eur Heart J.* 1985;6(2):147–57.

64. Lipton RB, Liao Y, Cao G, Cooper RS, McGee D. Determinants of incident non-insulin-dependent diabetes mellitus among blacks and whites in a national sample. The NHANES I Epidemiologic Follow-up Study. *Am J Epidemiol.* 1993;138(10):826–39.

65. Lynch J, Helmrich SP, Lakka TA, et al. Moderately intense physical activities and high levels of cardiorespiratory fitness reduce the risk of non-insulin-dependent diabetes mellitus in middle-aged men. *Arch Intern Med.* 1996;156(12):1307–14.

66. Madsbad S. Exenatide and liraglutide: different approaches to develop GLP-1 receptor agonists (incretin mimetics)—preclinical and clinical results. *Best Pract Res Clin Endocrinol Metab.* 2009;23(4):463–77.

67. Malik S, Wong ND, Franklin S, Pio J, Fairchild C, Chen R. Cardiovascular disease in U.S. patients with metabolic syndrome, diabetes, and elevated C-reactive protein. *Diabetes Care.* 2005;28(3):690–3.

68. Manson JE, Greenland P, LaCroix AZ, et al. Walking compared with vigorous exercise for the prevention of cardiovascular events in women. *N Engl J Med.* 2002;347(10):716–25.

69. Manson JE, Hu FB, Rich-Edwards JW, et al. A prospective study of walking as compared with vigorous exercise in the prevention of coronary heart disease in women. *N Engl J Med.* 1999;341(9):650–8.

70. Manson JE, Nathan DM, Krolewski AS, Stampfer MJ, Willett WC, Hennekens CH. A prospective study of exercise and incidence of diabetes among US male physicians. *JAMA.* 1992;268(1):63–7.

71. Manson JE, Rimm EB, Stampfer MJ, et al. Physical activity and incidence of non-insulin-dependent diabetes mellitus in women. *Lancet.* 1991;338(8770):774–8.

72. Marchesini G, Forlani G, Cerrelli F, et al. WHO and ATPIII proposals for the definition of the metabolic syndrome in patients with Type 2 diabetes. *Diabet Med.* 2004;21(4):383–7.

73. Marcus RL, Smith S, Morrell G, et al. Comparison of combined aerobic and high-force eccentric resistance exercise with aerobic exercise only for people with type 2 diabetes mellitus. *Phys Ther.* 2008;88(11):1345–54.

74. McNeill AM, Rosamond WD, Girman CJ, et al. Prevalence of coronary heart disease and carotid arterial thickening in patients with the metabolic syndrome (The ARIC Study). *Am J Cardiol.* 2004;94(10):1249–54.

75. Metzger BE, Cho NH, Roston SM, Radvany R. Prepregnancy weight and antepartum insulin secretion predict glucose tolerance five years after gestational diabetes mellitus. *Diabetes Care.* 1993; 16(12):1598–605.

76. Mokdad AH, Ford ES, Bowman BA, et al. Prevalence of obesity, diabetes, and obesity-related health risk factors, 2001. *JAMA.* 2003; 289(1):76–9.

77. Moy CS, Songer TJ, LaPorte RE, et al. Insulin-dependent diabetes mellitus, physical activity, and death. *Am J Epidemiol.* 1993; 137(1):74–81.

78. Nakanishi N, Shiraishi T, Wada M. C-reactive protein concentration is more strongly related to metabolic syndrome in women than in men: the Minoh Study. *Circ J.* 2005;69(4):386–91.

79. Nathan DM, Cleary PA, Backlund JY, et al. Intensive diabetes treatment and cardiovascular disease in patients with type 1 diabetes. *N Engl J Med.* 2005;353(25):2643–53.

80. Nathan DM, Lachin J, Cleary P, et al. Intensive diabetes therapy and carotid intima-media thickness in type 1 diabetes mellitus. *N Engl J Med.* 2003;348(23):2294–303.

81. Neumiller JJ, Wood L, Campbell RK. Dipeptidyl peptidase-4 inhibitors for the treatment of type 2 diabetes mellitus. *Pharmacotherapy.* 2010;30(5):463–84.

82. Paffenbarger RS Jr, Blair SN, Lee IM. A history of physical activity, cardiovascular health and longevity: the scientific contributions of Jeremy N Morris, DSc, DPH, FRCP. *Int J Epidemiol.* 2001;30(5):1184–92.

83. Paffenbarger RS Jr, Hyde RT, Wing AL, Lee IM, Jung DL, Kampert JB. The association of changes in physical-activity level and other lifestyle characteristics with mortality among men. *N Engl J Med.* 1993;328(8):538–45.

84. Pan XR, Li GW, Hu YH, et al. Effects of diet and exercise in preventing NIDDM in people with impaired glucose tolerance. The Da Qing IGT and Diabetes Study. *Diabetes Care.* 1997;20(4):537–44.

85. Pennathur S, Heinecke JW. Mechanisms of oxidative stress in diabetes: implications for the pathogenesis of vascular disease and antioxidant therapy. *Front Biosci.* 2004;9:565–74.

86. Petersen KF, Dufour S, Befroy D, Lehrke M, Hendler RE, Shulman GI. Reversal of nonalcoholic hepatic steatosis, hepatic insulin resistance, and hyperglycemia by moderate weight reduction in patients with type 2 diabetes. *Diabetes.* 2005;54(3):603–8.

87. Pitsavos C, Panagiotakos DB, Chrysohoou C, Kavouras S, Stefanadis C. The associations between physical activity, inflammation, and coagulation markers, in people with metabolic syndrome: the ATTICA study. *Eur J Cardiovasc Prev Rehabil.* 2005;12(2):151–8.

88. Pradhan AD, Ridker PM. Do atherosclerosis and type 2 diabetes share a common inflammatory basis? *Eur Heart J.* 2002;23(11):831–4.

89. Ramachandran A, Snehalatha C, Mary S, et al. The Indian Diabetes Prevention Programme shows that lifestyle modification and metformin prevent type 2 diabetes in Asian Indian subjects with impaired glucose tolerance (IDPP-1). *Diabetologia.* 2006;49(2):289–97.

90. Ravussin E, Valencia ME, Esparza J, Bennett PH, Schulz LO. Effects of a traditional lifestyle on obesity in Pima Indians. *Diabetes Care.* 1994;17(9):1067–74.

91. Reaven GM. Banting lecture 1988. Role of insulin resistance in human disease. *Diabetes.* 1988;37(12):1595–607.

92. Retinopathy and nephropathy in patients with type 1 diabetes four years after a trial of intensive therapy. The Diabetes Control and Complications Trial/Epidemiology of Diabetes Interventions and Complications Research Group. *N Engl J Med.* 2000;342(6):381–9.

93. Ryan AS, Hurlbut DE, Lott ME, et al. Insulin action after resistive training in insulin resistant older men and women. *J Am Geriatr Soc.* 2001;49(3):247–53.

94. Ryan AS, Nicklas BJ, Berman DM. Aerobic exercise is necessary to improve glucose utilization with moderate weight loss in women. *Obesity (Silver Spring).* 2006;14(6):1064–72.

95. Ryan AS, Pratley RE, Goldberg AP, Elahi D. Resistive training increases insulin action in postmenopausal women. *J Gerontol A Biol Sci Med Sci.* 1996;51(5):M199–205.

96. Salem MA, Aboelasrar MA, Elbarbary NS, Elhilaly RA, Refaat YM. Is exercise a therapeutic tool for improvement of cardiovascular risk factors in adolescents with type 1 diabetes mellitus? A randomised controlled trial. *Diabetol Metab Syndr.* 2010;2(1):47.

97. Sandvik L, Erikssen J, Thaulow E, Erikssen G, Mundal R, Rodahl K. Physical fitness as a predictor of mortality among healthy, middle-aged Norwegian men. *N Engl J Med.* 1993;328(8):533–7.

98. Scuteri A, Najjar SS, Morrell CH, Lakatta EG, Cardiovascular Health Study. The metabolic syndrome in older individuals: prevalence and prediction of cardiovascular events: the Cardiovascular Health Study. *Diabetes Care.* 2005;28(4):882–7.

99. Seeger JP, Thijssen DH, Noordam K, Cranen ME, Hopman MT, Nijhuis-van der Sanden MW. Exercise training improves physical fitness and vascular function in children with type 1 diabetes. *Diabetes Obes Metab.* 2011;13(4):382–4.

100. Sigal RJ, Kenny GP, Boule NG, et al. Effects of aerobic training, resistance training, or both on glycemic control in type 2 diabetes: a randomized trial. *Ann Intern Med.* 2007;147(6):357–69.

101. Simmons D, McElduff A, McIntyre HD, Elrishi M. Gestational diabetes mellitus: NICE for the U.S.? A comparison of the American Diabetes Association and the American College of Obstetricians and Gynecologists guidelines with the U.K. National Institute for Health and Clinical Excellence guidelines. *Diabetes Care.* 2010;33(1):34–7.

102. Singh-Franco D, Perez A, Harrington C. The effect of pramlintide acetate on glycemic control and weight in patients with type 2 diabetes mellitus and in obese patients without diabetes: a systematic review and meta-analysis. *Diabetes Obes Metab.* 2011;13(2):169–80.

103. Sjoberg N, Brinkworth GD, Wycherley TP, Noakes M, Saint DA. Moderate weight loss improves heart rate variability in overweight and obese adults with type 2 diabetes. *J Appl Physiol.* 2011;110(4):1060–4.

104. Skerrett PJ, Manson JE. Reduction in risk of coronary heart disease and diabetes. In: Ruderman N, Devlin JT, Schneider SH, Kriska AM, American Diabetes Association, editors. *Handbook of Exercise in Diabetes.* 2nd ed. Alexandria: American Diabetes Association; 2002. p. 155–81.

105. Sonnett TE, Levien TL, Neumiller JJ, Gates BJ, Setter SM. Colesevelam hydrochloride for the treatment of type 2 diabetes mellitus. *Clin Ther.* 2009;31(2):245–59.

106. Staels B, Handelsman Y, Fonseca V. Bile acid sequestrants for lipid and glucose control. *Curr Diab Rep.* 2010;10(1):70–7.

107. Stampfer MJ, Hu FB, Manson JE, Rimm EB, Willett WC. Primary prevention of coronary heart disease in women through diet and lifestyle. *N Engl J Med.* 2000;343(1):16–22.

108. Sui X, Hooker SP, Lee IM, et al. A prospective study of cardiorespiratory fitness and risk of type 2 diabetes in women. *Diabetes Care.* 2008;31(3):550–5.

109. Trigona B, Aggoun Y, Maggio A, et al. Preclinical noninvasive markers of atherosclerosis in children and adolescents with type 1 diabetes are influenced by physical activity. *J Pediatr.* 2010;157(4):533–9.

110. Tuomilehto J, Lindstrom J, Eriksson JG, et al. Prevention of type 2 diabetes mellitus by changes in lifestyle among subjects with impaired glucose tolerance. *N Engl J Med.* 2001;344(18): 1343–50.

111. Tzefos M, Olin JL. Glucagon-like peptide-1 analog and insulin combination therapy in the management of adults with type 2 diabetes mellitus. *Ann Pharmacother.* 2010;44(7–8):1294–300.

112. Vidal J, Morinigo R, Codoceo VH, Casamitjana R, Pellitero S, Gomis R. The importance of diagnostic criteria in the association between the metabolic syndrome and cardiovascular disease in obese subjects. *Int J Obes (Lond).* 2005;29(6):668–74.

113. Wang H, Shara NM, Calhoun D, Umans JG, Lee ET, Howard BV. Incidence rates and predictors of diabetes in those with prediabetes: the Strong Heart Study. *Diabetes Metab Res Rev.* 2010;26(5):378–85.

114. Wei M, Gibbons LW, Mitchell TL, Kampert JB, Lee CD, Blair SN. The association between cardiorespiratory fitness and impaired fasting glucose and type 2 diabetes mellitus in men. *Ann Intern Med.* 1999;130(2):89–96.

115. Wei M, Kampert JB, Barlow CE, et al. Relationship between low cardiorespiratory fitness and mortality in normal-weight, overweight, and obese men. *JAMA.* 1999;282(16):1547–53.

116. Weinstein AR, Sesso HD, Lee IM, et al. Relationship of physical activity vs body mass index with type 2 diabetes in women. *JAMA.* 2004;292(10):1188–94.

117. Whaley MH, Kampert JB, Kohl HW,3rd, Blair SN. Physical fitness and clustering of risk factors associated with the metabolic syndrome. *Med Sci Sports Exerc.* 1999;31(2):287–93.

118. White NH, Sun W, Cleary PA, et al. Prolonged effect of intensive therapy on the risk of retinopathy complications in patients with type 1 diabetes mellitus: 10 years after the Diabetes Control and Complications Trial. *Arch Ophthalmol.* 2008;126(12):1707–15.

119. Yan SF, Ramasamy R, Naka Y, Schmidt AM. Glycation, inflammation, and RAGE: a scaffold for the macrovascular complications of diabetes and beyond. *Circ Res.* 2003;93(12):1159–69.

120. You T, Ryan AS, Nicklas BJ. The metabolic syndrome in obese postmenopausal women: relationship to body composition, visceral fat, and inflammation. *J Clin Endocrinol Metab.* 2004;89(11): 5517–22.

121. Zhang S, Folsom AR, Flack JM, Liu K. Body fat distribution before pregnancy and gestational diabetes: findings from coronary artery risk development in young adults (CARDIA) study. *BMJ.* 1995;311(7013):1139–40.

122. Zierath JR. Invited review: Exercise training-induced changes in insulin signaling in skeletal muscle. *J Appl Physiol.* 2002;93(2):773–81.

123. Zinman B, Ruderman N, Campaigne BN, Devlin JT, Schneider SH, American Diabetes Association. Physical activity/exercise and diabetes. *Diabetes Care.* 2004;27 Suppl 1:S58–62.

SELECTED REFERENCES FOR FURTHER READING

American College of Sports Medicine. *ACSM's Exercise Management for Persons with Chronic Diseases and Disabilities.* 3rd ed. Champaign (IL): Human Kinetics; 2009. 440 p.

The American College of Sports Medicine and the American Diabetes Association. Exercise and Type 2 Diabetes: Joint Position Statement. *Diabetes Care.* 2010;33(12):e147–67.

American Diabetes Association. Clinical Practice Recommendations 2011. *Diabetes Care.* 2011;34(Suppl 1).

INTERNET RESOURCES

- Academy of Nutrition and Dietetics: http://www.eatright.org
- American Association of Diabetes Educators: http://www.diabeteseducator.org
- American Diabetes Association: http://www.diabetes.org/
- National Heart, Lung and Blood Institute: http://www.nhlbi.nih.gov/guidelines/obesity/obesity2/index.htm

DEFINING MENTAL ILLNESS

Disturbances in psychological functioning are commonly encountered by exercise professionals who work with a variety of patients. Some disorders are more prevalent in certain clinical populations, such as those with chronic disease (32). Developing an understanding of mental disorders is important because of their effects on exercise participation and on overall health and well-being. Population studies consistently show that persons with mental disorders are less likely to be physically active and have greater rates of early mortality (21,25,26). Furthermore, there is consistent evidence of bidirectional influences of mental illness and physical diseases. For example, depressed persons are more likely to develop cardiovascular disease (CVD) and diabetes. Similarly, if individuals have CVD and/or diabetes and also have depressive symptoms, they are more likely to have worse outcomes compared with those with chronic disease without depressive symptoms (11,12,24).

Mental health and mental illness are considered part of a continuum of mental functioning. Mental health involves being able to engage in useful work, joining in productive relationships with others, and being able to cope with change and adversity. Disruptions in mental health are likely to occur in nearly half of all people in the United States at least once in their lifetime (17). These disruptions can be transient or chronic and can range from

KEY TERMS

Anorexia nervosa: An eating disorder that either restricts calories or has recurrent episodes of binge eating or purging and leads to a significantly low weight and fear of gaining weight.

Binge-eating disorder: An eating disorder that involves lack of control and eating large portions of food at least once a week for 3 mo and is not associated with inappropriate compensatory behaviors that occur during anorexia or bulimia nervosa.

Bipolar disorder: A disorder of mood that involves alternating periods of symptoms of depression (see Major depressive disorder) and at least one manic episode characterized by an abnormally and persistently elevated mood or irritability. There are many subtypes of bipolar disorder.

Bulimia nervosa: An eating disorder that involves recurrent binge-eating episodes and compensatory behaviors like purging, misuse of laxatives, and/or excessive exercise to prevent weight gain.

Generalized anxiety disorder (GAD): Excessive worry about two or more aspects of daily living that occur more days than not for 6 mo or more. There are many types of anxiety disorders but GAD is most prevalent.

Major depressive disorder (MDD): A mood disorder that is characterized by depressed mood or loss of interest or pleasure most of the day, nearly every day, for at least 2 wk; weight loss or weight gain; insomnia or hypersomnia; psychomotor retardation or agitation; fatigue; feelings of worthlessness or guilt; inability to think; and recurrent thoughts of death. There are many subtypes of depressive disorders.

Mental illness: A diagnosable disorder that involves alterations in thinking, mood or behavior that are associated with impaired functioning.

Substance dependence: A type of disorder that results in significant impairment with at least three of the following symptoms in a 12-mo period: tolerance, withdrawal, taking the substance in larger amounts over a longer period, unsuccessful efforts to quit or cut down, spending a great deal of time to obtain substances, giving up activities in favor of using substances, or continued use despite knowledge that use is problematic. A wide variety of substances are included in substance dependence, and substance dependence can lead to substance abuse.

Adapted from the American Psychiatric Association, American Psychiatric Association, Task Force on DSM-IV. *Diagnostic and Statistical Manual of Mental Disorders: DSM-IV.* 4th ed. Washington (DC): American Psychiatric Association; 1994. 886 p.

mild to severe. Some may require referral to treatment by a specialist or to a support group, or they may resolve over time (36). In this chapter, the most common mental health problems that are likely to be encountered by the exercise professional will be discussed. Terminology established by the most recent Surgeon General's Report on Mental Health that differentiates *mental health problems* and *mental illness* will be used. Also, criteria for diagnosis for mental disorders established by the fourth edition of the American Psychiatric Association in the *Diagnostic and Statistical Manual of Mental Disorders (DSM-IV)* are the basis for describing symptoms (1). Discussion will be limited to disorders described in *DSM-IV*. *DSM-V* is scheduled for publication in May of 2013.

Mental illness refers to diagnosable mental disorders and involves alterations in thinking, mood, or behavior or some combination of these, and these alterations are associated with impaired functioning. **Mental health** problems are those signs and symptoms that are not of a sufficient level of severity and duration that they can be diagnosed, although some of these mental health problems can also lead to impairments in functioning or later diagnosable illness (18,27,36). Each type of mental health problem or mental disorder including signs and symptoms, methods of assessment, effective treatments, and considerations for referral will be described. It is important that exercise professionals understand that effective treatments for most mental illnesses and mental health problems are available, and that they are able to recognize symptoms of mental health problems to refer individuals to appropriate treatment resources. Often, the delay or failure of receiving treatment results in worsening of symptoms and greater functional impairment (37).

RECOGNIZING STRESS: SYMPTOMS, ASSESSMENT, TREATMENT, AND REFERRAL

Psychological stress is something everyone experiences to varying degrees. The causes of stress may be specific life events, such as the death of a loved one or the loss of a job, or acute or chronic illness. Stress also can be caused by less identifiable triggers, such as daily hassles, difficult work, or maladaptive coping strategies. Symptoms of stress often overlap those of depression and anxiety disorders (*Box 9-1*).

Physical symptoms of acute stress include autonomic nervous system activation, such as elevated heart rate and blood pressure. Prolonged stress may impair the immune system, resulting in susceptibility to illness. In addition, persons experiencing high levels of stress often report higher pain ratings and feelings of anger and irritability. They may be at increased risk for injury. High levels of stress may negatively influence health behaviors, including smoking, exercise, diet, and medication (8).

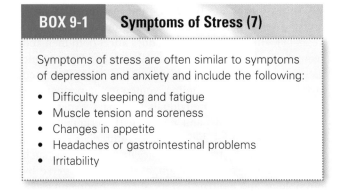

BOX 9-1   **Symptoms of Stress (7)**

Symptoms of stress are often similar to symptoms of depression and anxiety and include the following:

- Difficulty sleeping and fatigue
- Muscle tension and soreness
- Changes in appetite
- Headaches or gastrointestinal problems
- Irritability

Formal assessment of stress typically involves the administration of questionnaires to measure an individual's experience and appraisal of stressful life events. A reliable and valid questionnaire that is commonly used to measure an individual's perception of stress is the Perceived Stress Scale, which is publicly available in the original 14-item scale or validated, shorter versions of 4 or 10 items (7,8). This instrument quantifies the degree to which individuals appraise their lives as unpredictable, uncontrollable, and overloaded.

Interventions for stress often include social support networks, including family and friends, self-help groups (*e.g.*, general group therapy, relaxation, or meditation), or support groups for specific issues such as trauma or grief. In addition, assisting individuals with resilience training can enable them to identify solutions and reduce the risk of developing other serious mental or physical disorders (6,35). More formal interventions including psychotherapy or biofeedback training may be needed to help individuals develop appropriate coping strategies.

Exercise professionals should be able to recognize when stress is negatively affecting a patient's daily functioning or is causing health problems. Many people find relief from stress by participating in exercise, and exercise professionals can work with their patients to determine the most appropriate types of activities for meeting fitness goals and reducing stress.

RECOGNIZING DEPRESSION: SYMPTOMS, ASSESSMENT, TREATMENT, AND REFERRAL

The burden of depressive disorders is significant. According to the Global Burden of Disease Study conducted by the World Health Organization, major depression ranks second behind ischemic heart disease regarding the years that individuals live with disability, and by 2030, depression is predicted to lead ischemic heart disease (38). The projected lifetime risk of having any mood disorder by the age of 75 yr in the United States is 31.4% (17).

Depression occurs twice as often in women as men, and the sex differences are seen beginning in the teen years (1). However, depression does affect both men and women of all age groups, ethnicities, and socioeconomic categories (1). Certain populations may be at increased risk for depression, including women in the perinatal or menopausal periods, individuals who have experienced a stressful life event, and people with certain medical conditions, such as heart disease and diabetes (25). Depression can be triggered by negative life events, such as the loss of a spouse or a job, or it can be triggered by physiologic and biologic factors, such as having an acute or chronic disease. Family and genetic factors, biologic factors, and cognitive factors may all play a causal role in the development of depressive disorders (30). Depressive disorders are diagnosed according to clinical criteria such as the *DSM-IV* (1) (*Box 9-2*).

There are many subtypes of depression that also include bipolar disorder, which is characterized by periods of both depression and mania. Symptoms of mania include extreme elation or irritability, increased energy and decreased need for sleep, grandiose ideas, inflated self-esteem, distractibility, physical agitation, and poor judgment or inappropriate behavior (1).

Questionnaires such as the Beck Depression Inventory (BDI) (2,3), the Center for Epidemiological Studies Depression Scale (CES-D) (29), and, more recently, the Patient Health Questionnaire for depression (PHQ-8) (19) are commonly used to assess symptoms of depression. Self-report instruments assess the frequency and/or severity of symptomatology and commonly include items relating to emotional, cognitive, and/or physical symptoms of depression. Although questionnaires can give a good indication of presence of depressive symptoms, depressive disorders should only be diagnosed by a physician using criteria set forth by resources such as *DSM-IV* (1). Consultation with a mental health counselor, psychiatrist, psychologist, or physician is important to rule out any other potential causes of symptoms, such as medication or illness, and to develop an appropriate treatment plan.

Effective treatments for depression are available, but many individuals do not seek treatment or receive inadequate treatment, and it is estimated there is a 4-yr delay in seeking treatment for any type of mood disorder in the United States (37). Treatment of depression depends on type and severity of symptoms and patient preference. Effective treatments include classes of antidepressant medications, such as selective serotonin reuptake inhibitors (SSRIs), tricyclic antidepressants (TCAs), and monoamine oxidase inhibitors (MAOIs) (28). Antidepressant pharmacotherapy takes several weeks before symptoms begin to decrease, and often, the dosage must be adjusted for optimal therapeutic effect. Psychotherapy has also been found to be effective in managing depression and may include cognitive behavioral therapy (CBT) and interpersonal psychotherapy. Psychotherapy may be used alone or in combination with antidepressant medication to treat depression. In cases of mild depression, new guidelines from the American Psychiatric Association suggest exercise may be a good treatment alternative as long as symptoms are carefully monitored (28). In cases of severe depression or when depression persists despite treatment, electroconvulsive therapy (ECT) may be used and has been found to be effective (28). Regardless of the treatment modality, it is important that patients are regularly assessed throughout the course of treatment to ensure remission of depressive symptoms. For individuals who do not respond to the initial course of treatment, it may be necessary to use a combination of treatments, change medication dose, or switch treatment modalities. This process often requires long-term follow-up and continued treatment (28).

Exercise professionals working with individuals who are receiving antidepressant treatment should be aware of the type of medication and any potential somatic or cardiac effects. For example, TCAs have been found to cause cardiac arrhythmias in some patients (28). Although most antidepressant medications should not affect response to exercise, some medication side effects, such as weight change, sedation, or insomnia, may be relevant to exercise participation. In addition, regarding the possibility of using exercise as a first treatment for mild cases of depression, exercise is also recommended by practice guidelines to promote good overall health and should be encouraged as an adjunctive treatment for individuals who have depressive disorders (28).

Patients should inform their mental health providers about their exercise participation. If untreated depression is suspected, individuals can be referred to several community resources that are able to provide diagnostic and treatment services (*Box 9-3*).

BOX 9-2	**Symptoms of Major Depressive Disorder (MDD) (1)**

Symptoms of depression include the following:

- Persistent feelings of sadness or irritability
- Loss of interest in previously enjoyed activities
- Feelings of guilt, worthlessness, or helplessness
- Fatigue or decreased energy
- Difficulty thinking or concentrating
- Sleep disturbances, including insomnia or oversleeping
- Changes in appetite and/or weight gain or loss
- Psychomotor agitation or retardation
- Thoughts of death or suicide

BOX 9-3	Treatment Resources of Mental Health

First-line resources for local mental health services include the following:

- Mental health practitioners, including psychiatrists, psychologists, social workers, or mental health counselors
- Family practice/internal medicine physicians
- Community mental health centers
- Hospital psychiatry departments and outpatient clinics
- Family service, social agencies, religious organizations, and clergy

BOX 9-4	Symptoms of Anxiety (1)

Common symptoms of anxiety disorders include the following:

- Intense worry, fear, or dread
- Difficulty sleeping
- Sympathetic nervous system activation with physical symptoms, such as dry mouth, increased heart rate, sweating, trembling, agitation, or gastrointestinal distress

An exercise professional may encounter someone who expresses such hopelessness or depression to the degree that suicide risk is suspected. It may be necessary to directly inquire if a person is thinking about suicide. Simply asking, "You seem pretty down. Have you had any recent thoughts of harming yourself?" may help determine a person's intent (20). People will usually respond honestly, which allows the opportunity to gauge the seriousness of such thoughts. Immediate action is needed if a person communicates planned harmful or suicidal intentions. If the person is not under the care of mental health provider, he or she can be referred to a local suicide or crisis center or be taken directly to a hospital emergency room. It is important to make sure that the person is accompanied to the treatment center and that the person is not left alone until professional help is available. The National Hopeline Network (1-800-SUICIDE) is a 24-h hotline that connects individuals to trained counselors at a local crisis center.

RECOGNIZING ANXIETY: SYMPTOMS, ASSESSMENT, TREATMENT, AND REFERRAL

The most prevalent of the mental disorders are anxiety disorders with estimated projected lifetime prevalence in the United States of 36% (17). As with depression, women are twice as likely as men to suffer from anxiety disorders. In contrast to the feelings of fear that people experience during a stressful event, anxiety disorders are characterized by chronic symptoms that may worsen if left untreated (*Box 9-4*). Some of the most common types of anxiety disorders include generalized anxiety disorder, obsessive-compulsive disorder, specific phobias, posttraumatic stress disorder, and social anxiety disorder. The disorders are diagnosed according to *DSM-IV* symptom profile (1).

Generalized anxiety disorder (GAD) is characterized by chronic, exaggerated worry that occurs more days than not for at least 6 mo. A person with anxiety has at least three of the following six symptoms: (a) restlessness or feeling keyed up, (b) difficulty concentrating, (c) being irritable, (d) easy to fatigue, (e) muscle tension, and (f) sleep disturbances such as difficulty falling or staying asleep. Diagnosis of the disorder requires that symptoms are not due to a physiological cause such as overtraining, substance use, or hyperthyroidism; do not occur only during a mood disorder; and cause an impairment in daily areas of functioning (1).

Specific phobias are specific and intense fears that occur by the presence or anticipation of specific objects or situations (*e.g.*, excessive fear of heights, animals, or blood). When a person is exposed to the object or situation, it is highly likely to induce a panic attack, and symptoms can include excessive sweating, heart pounding, shaking, shortness of breath, and/or nausea. Diagnosis is made by ruling out other types of anxiety disorders (1).

Obsessive-compulsive disorder (OCD) involves the experience of disturbing and irrational thoughts (obsessions) and the need to engage in repeated behaviors or rituals (compulsions) to prevent or relieve the anxiety. Individuals with OCD usually recognize that their thoughts and behaviors are senseless, but they are controlled by the troubling thoughts and the urgent need to engage in rituals. Rituals often involve counting, checking, or washing and may significantly interfere with daily functioning (1).

Posttraumatic stress disorder (PTSD) develops after experiencing or witnessing an intense, terrifying event, such as a violent attack, serious accident, natural disaster, or abuse, and involves extreme fear or helplessness. Symptoms include repeated disturbing thoughts of the trauma, nightmares, sleep disturbances, or feeling as if the event is recurring. A person with PTSD tries to avoid thoughts or feelings of the trauma, often has disinterest in activities that were once important, a restricted range of affect, and low expectations for a normal life. These individuals also have a heightened sense of hypervigilance and often have sleep difficulties, irritability and startle easily. This disorder causes significant impairment in daily functioning (1).

Social anxiety disorder is also known as social phobia. This disorder is characterized by intense anxiety and self-consciousness during normal social situations. Individuals with this disorder have a persistent, excessive fear of being watched and evaluated by others and worry of being embarrassed or humiliated. Social anxiety disorder can be specific to certain situations, such as speaking or eating in public, or be generalized to any social setting (1).

In addition to these different types of anxiety disorders, there are additional subtypes of anxiety disorders just as there are with depressive disorders (1). Questionnaires are commonly used to assess symptoms of anxiety including self-report instruments, such as the State/Trait Anxiety Inventory (STAI), which assess the frequency and/or intensity of symptoms in emotional, cognitive, and/or physical domains (34). Self-report questionnaires can give a good indication of the presence and severity of symptoms of anxiety, but they cannot provide a diagnosis of the type of anxiety disorder (*i.e.*, social phobia, GAD, etc.). Thus, the presence of anxiety disorders can only be determined by trained professionals using standard diagnostic criteria (1). Referral to a mental health counselor, psychologist, psychiatrist, or physician is important to develop an appropriate treatment plan, which may include psychotherapy and/or medication.

Common medications for anxiety include antidepressants, benzodiazepines, and β-blockers. SSRI antidepressant medications are often prescribed for panic disorder, OCD, PTSD, and social phobia; however, SSRIs often take several weeks to achieve full therapeutic effect and thus are not useful for immediate anxiety symptom relief. Benzodiazepines quickly reduce anxiety symptoms and are commonly used in the treatment of panic disorder, social phobia, and GAD. However, people develop tolerance to benzodiazepines and may become dependent on them; symptom rebound may occur when medication is discontinued. β-Blockers, typically used to treat heart conditions, may be used to minimize physical symptoms when an anxiety-provoking event is anticipated (10).

Targeted psychotherapy is often indicated for anxiety disorders (15). CBT, in particular, has been found to be useful for treatment of panic disorder and social phobia. Exposure therapy, a type of behavioral therapy, is often used to treat specific phobias, OCD, and PTSD. This technique involves exposing individuals to the feared object or situation in a safe environment so that individuals can practice controlling their anxiety and responding in more appropriate and productive ways (23). Relaxation training including breathing exercises and biofeedback may also be used as a component of anxiety treatment (16). Treatment plans for an anxiety disorder should also include evaluation and treatment of comorbid mental disorders because depression, substance abuse, or other anxiety disorders often co-occur with one another (1).

If a person exhibits symptoms of anxiety, he or she can be referred to the same community mental health resources that treat depression. In addition, self-help groups can be useful for individuals who share the same concerns and are seeking to resolve problems related to daily functioning.

As with antidepressant medications, exercise professionals working with individuals receiving antianxiety medication should be aware of the type of medication and any potential side effects. Some types of medication may affect the sympathetic nervous system response to exercise so that heart rate or blood pressure may not increase as expected (9). As with depressive symptoms, research suggests that exercise may be useful in reducing symptoms of stress and anxiety (14). Although individuals with panic disorder may avoid participating in exercise for fear of inducing a panic attack, the attacks are not more likely to occur during physical activity than during other daily activities (5). By understanding a person's individual concerns, exercise professionals can work to create a safe and comfortable environment by minimizing potential exposure to anxiety-inducing situations.

RECOGNIZING EATING DISORDERS: SYMPTOMS, ASSESSMENT, TREATMENT, AND REFERRAL

Disordered eating comprises a spectrum of behavioral, cognitive, and emotional symptoms involving disturbances in eating and body image. Eating disorders are diagnosed according to standard criteria and include the disorders of anorexia nervosa, bulimia nervosa, and binge-eating disorders (1). Eating disorders are more common in women than in men, and disorders often develop in adolescence or young adulthood. Because eating disorders can cause significant health problems including early death, recognition and treatment is critical. Symptoms of eating disorders are presented in *Box 9-5*.

BOX 9-5	**Symptoms of Eating Disorders (1)**

Symptoms of eating disorders include the following:
- Extreme eating patterns, including restriction and overeating
- Body weight loss or gain
- Purging behaviors, including vomiting, laxative use, or excessive exercise
- Unusual eating behaviors, including preferences or phobias of certain foods and obsessive rituals
- Excessive weighing or avoidance of weighing
- Distorted body image, low self-esteem, or feelings of guilt and self-disgust

Anorexia nervosa is characterized by an insufficient calorie intake to sustain a normal weight for age and height. Individuals who have this disorder have intense fear of becoming fat and a distorted body image. Sometimes there are also disturbances in menstrual cycles in women. Health complications of this disorder include osteoporosis and muscle atrophy, electrolyte imbalances, cardiac arrhythmias, and sometimes early death (22).

Bulimia nervosa involves episodes of binge eating and compensatory behaviors like purging, misuse of laxatives, or excessive exercise to prevent weight gain. Individuals with this disorder are often of normal body weight but may express intense body dissatisfaction and desire to lose weight. Health consequences of bulimia nervosa include gastrointestinal disturbances, electrolyte imbalances, esophageal ruptures, pancreatitis, and erosion of tooth enamel (33).

Binge-eating disorder involves recurrent binge-eating episodes where the individual lacks control over how much he or she is eating. This behavior occurs at least once per week for 3 mo and, unlike bulimia nervosa, does not involve compensatory behaviors to prevent weight gain. The episodes often involve rapid eating, feeling uncomfortably full, eating when not hungry, eating alone, and feelings of guilt or disgust (4).

Symptoms of eating disorders are often readily recognizable to outside observers. However, determining the severity is often difficult because individuals with these disorders often hide their behaviors and resist intervention. Professional assessment of eating disorders involves multiple components: (a) medical evaluation to assess body weight and health problems, (b) psychological evaluation to assess the severity of the eating disorder and presence of comorbid mental disorders, and (c) nutritional consultation to evaluate current eating habits.

Treatment is a multifaceted process that often involves a team of health care professionals, including mental health counselors, physicians, psychologists, and nutritionists. Eating disorders like anorexia nervosa are sometimes treated in an inpatient setting so that weight can be stabilized and medical conditions can be treated. Psychotherapy is an important component of treatment to reduce inappropriate eating behaviors and explore psychological issues such as body image, self-esteem, and interpersonal relationships. Nutritionists and exercise professionals can play an important role on the intervention team to regulate energy balance through appropriate caloric intake and energy expenditure. Finally, SSRI medications may be helpful in the treatment of some eating disorders (13).

Exercise professionals can play an important role by recognizing symptoms of eating disorders and referring individuals to treatment when appropriate. When working with patients who have eating disorders, care should be taken to monitor energy balance and to modify exercise prescriptions to accommodate any medical problems. Furthermore, the exercise professional should use sensitivity when weighing or conducting body composition measurements and communicate appropriate messages to protect body image and self-esteem.

RECOGNIZING SUBSTANCE-USE DISORDERS: SYMPTOMS, ASSESSMENT, TREATMENT, AND REFERRAL

Substance-use disorders include any disorders related to problems associated with the use of alcohol, drugs of abuse, prescribed or over-the-counter medications, and toxins such as inhalants. Substance-use disorders include substance dependence and substance abuse (1).

Substance dependence is characterized by a use pattern that leads to impairment or distress three or more times in any year-long period. Specific symptoms of substance dependence include tolerance to the substance, such as a need for a greater amount to achieve an effect, and also withdrawal symptoms in the absence of the substance. Additional symptoms include an inability to control use of the substance, such as trying to quit but being unable to do so; neglect of daily obligations; and continued use despite psychological or health problems (1).

Substance abuse refers to a condition in which repeated substance use results in significant adverse effects that produce distress or impairment in functioning. Use of the substance interferes with role obligations, creates hazardous situations, and can result in legal, interpersonal, or social problems (1).

Professional assessment of substance-use disorders is critical to ensure the safety of the individual and to implement appropriate treatment. Substance abuse commonly occurs with other mental disorders, such as depression, and treatment may involve a combination of individual therapy, group therapy, and/or medication (31). Local hospitals and substance-abuse centers can provide medical and psychological evaluation and treatment in inpatient or outpatient settings.

Exercise professionals are most likely to recognize symptoms of substance use during acute intoxication or when the patient reports questionable behaviors, such as recurrent overindulgent behaviors or blackouts (39). Often, individuals with drug or alcohol problems may deny a problem and resist treatment; however, they may be open to receiving referrals if the information is presented in a professional and caring manner.

SUMMARY

Mental disorders are common problems affecting people of all ages and backgrounds. Mental health problems can be effectively managed, and individuals can achieve significant improvements in psychological functioning, physical health, and quality of life. In most cases, exercise is a useful adjunctive therapy in the treatment of mental disorders and results in both physical and mental health benefits for clients. Exercise might also be a more acceptable first-line treatment for mild severity depressive symptoms and is likely to be effective in preventing symptoms of stress, anxiety, and depression (26,28). Exercise professionals should be able to recognize symptoms of mental disorders and refer patients to appropriate community resources for treatment.

REFERENCES

1. American Psychiatric Association, American Psychiatric Association, Task Force on DSM-IV. *Diagnostic and Statistical Manual of Mental Disorders: DSM-IV.* 4th ed. Washington (DC): American Psychiatric Association; 1994. 886 p.

2. Beck AT, Steer RA, Garbin MG. Psychometric properties of the Beck Depression Inventory: twenty-five years of evaluation. *Clin Psychol Rev.* 1988;8(1):77–100.

3. Beck AT, Ward CH, Mendelson M, Mock J, Erbaugh J. An inventory for measuring depression. *Arch Gen Psychiatry.* 1961;4:561–71.

4. Brownley KA, Berkman ND, Sedway JA, Lohr KN, Bulik CM. Binge eating disorder treatment: a systematic review of randomized controlled trials. *Int J Eat Disord.* 2007;40(4):337–48.

5. Cameron OG, Hudson CJ. Influence of exercise on anxiety level in patients with anxiety disorders. *Psychosomatics.* 1986;27(10):720–3.

6. Cicchetti D. Resilience under conditions of extreme stress: a multilevel perspective. *World Psychiatry.* 2010;9(3):145–54.

7. Cohen S, Kamarck T, Mermelstein R. A global measure of perceived stress. *J Health Soc Behav.* 1983;24(4):385–96.

8. Cohen S, Kessler RC, Underwood Gordon L. *Measuring Stress: A Guide for Health and Social Scientists.* New York (NY): Oxford University Press; 1995. 236 p.

9. Davidson JR. Pharmacologic treatment of acute and chronic stress following trauma: 2006. *J Clin Psychiatry.* 2006;67 Suppl 2:34–9.

10. Den Boer JA, van Vliet IM, Westenberg HG. Recent developments in the psychopharmacology of social phobia. *Eur Arch Psychiatry Clin Neurosci.* 1995;244(6):309–16.

11. Evans DL, Charney DS, Lewis L, et al. Mood disorders in the medically ill: scientific review and recommendations. *Biol Psychiatry.* 2005;58(3):175–89.

12. Fenton WS, Stover ES. Mood disorders: cardiovascular and diabetes comorbidity. *Curr Opin Psychiatry.* 2006;19(4):421–7.

13. Hainer V, Kabrnova K, Aldhoon B, Kunesova M, Wagenknecht M. Serotonin and norepinephrine reuptake inhibition and eating behavior. *Ann N Y Acad Sci.* 2006;1083:252–69.

14. Herring MP, O'Connor PJ, Dishman RK. The effect of exercise training on anxiety symptoms among patients: a systematic review. *Arch Intern Med.* 2010;170(4):321–31.

15. Hunot V, Churchill R, Silva de Lima M, Teixeira V. Psychological therapies for generalised anxiety disorder. *Cochrane Database Syst Rev.* 2007;(1):CD001848.

16. Jorm AF, Christensen H, Griffiths KM, Parslow RA, Rodgers B, Blewitt KA. Effectiveness of complementary and self-help treatments for anxiety disorders. *Med J Aust.* 2004;181(7 Suppl):S29–46.

17. Kessler RC, Angermeyer M, Anthony JC, et al. Lifetime prevalence and age-of-onset distributions of mental disorders in the World Health Organization's World Mental Health Survey Initiative. *World Psychiatry.* 2007;6(3):168–76.

18. Klein DN, Shankman SA, Lewinsohn PM, Seeley JR. Subthreshold depressive disorder in adolescents: predictors of escalation to full-syndrome depressive disorders. *J Am Acad Child Adolesc Psychiatry.* 2009;48(7):703–10.

19. Kroenke K, Strine TW, Spitzer RL, Williams JB, Berry JT, Mokdad AH. The PHQ-8 as a measure of current depression in the general population. *J Affect Disord.* 2009;114(1–3):163–73.

20. Meyer RE, Salzman C, Youngstrom EA, et al. Suicidality and risk of suicide—definition, drug safety concerns, and a necessary target for drug development: a consensus statement. *J Clin Psychiatry.* 2010;71(8):e1–21.

21. *Morbidity and Mortality in People with Serious Mental Illness* [Internet]. Alexandria, VA: National Association of State Mental Health Program Directors; 2006 [cited 2011 Apr 8]. 87 p. Available from: http://www.nasmhpd.org/general_files/publications/med_directors_pubs/Technical%20Report%20on%20Morbidity%20and%20Mortaility%20-%20Final%2011–06.pdf

22. Morris J, Twaddle S. Anorexia nervosa. *BMJ.* 2007;334(7599):894–8.

23. Norton PJ, Price EC. A meta-analytic review of adult cognitive-behavioral treatment outcome across the anxiety disorders. *J Nerv Ment Dis.* 2007;195(6):521–31.

24. Pan A, Lucas M, Sun Q, et al. Bidirectional association between depression and type 2 diabetes mellitus in women. *Arch Intern Med.* 2010;170(21):1884–91.

25. Pan A, Lucas M, Sun Q, et al. Increased mortality risk in women with depression and diabetes mellitus. *Arch Gen Psychiatry.* 2011;68(1):42–50.

26. Physical Activity Guidelines Advisory Committee. *Physical Activity Guidelines Advisory Committee Report, 2008* [Internet]. Washington, DC: U.S. Department of Health and Human Services; 2008 [cited 2011 Apr 28]. 683 p. Available from: http://www.health.gov/paguidelines/committeereport.aspx

27. Pickles A, Rowe R, Simonoff E, Foley D, Rutter M, Silberg J. Child psychiatric symptoms and psychosocial impairment: relationship and prognostic significance. *Br J Psychiatry.* 2001;179:230–5.

28. *Practice Guidelines for the Treatment of Patients with Major Depressive Disorder* [Internet]. 3rd ed. Arlington (VA): American Psychiatric Association; 2010 [cited 2011 Apr 6]. 152 p. Available from: http://www.psych.org/guidelines/mdd2010

29. Radloff LS. The CES-D Scale: a self-report depressive scale for research in the general population. *J Appl Psychol Meas.* 1977;1:385–401.

30. Reinherz HZ, Paradis AD, Giaconia RM, Stashwick CK, Fitzmaurice G. Childhood and adolescent predictors of major depression in the transition to adulthood. *Am J Psychiatry.* 2003;160(12):2141–7.

31. Riggs PD, Mikulich-Gilbertson SK, Davies RD, Lohman M, Klein C, Stover SK. A randomized controlled trial of fluoxetine and cognitive behavioral therapy in adolescents with major depression, behavior problems, and substance use disorders. *Arch Pediatr Adolesc Med.* 2007;161(11):1026–34.

32. Scott KM, Bruffaerts R, Tsang A, et al. Depression-anxiety relationships with chronic physical conditions: results from the World Mental Health surveys. *J Affect Disord.* 2007;103(1–3):113–20.

33. Shapiro JR, Berkman ND, Brownley KA, Sedway JA, Lohr KN, Bulik CM. Bulimia nervosa treatment: a systematic review of randomized controlled trials. *Int J Eat Disord.* 2007;40(4):321–36.

34. Spielberger CD, Gorsuch RL, Lushene RE. *STAI Manual for the State-Trait Anxiety Inventory ("Self-Evaluation Questionnaire").* Palo Alto (CA): Consulting Psychologists Press; 1970. 24 p.

35. Timmermans M, van Lier PA, Koot HM. The role of stressful events in the development of behavioural and emotional problems from early childhood to late adolescence. *Psychol Med.* 2010;40(10):1659–68.

36. United States Public Health Service, Office of the Surgeon General, Center for Mental Health Services (U.S.), National Institute of Mental Health (U.S.). *Mental Health: A Report of the Surgeon General.* Rockville, MD: U.S. Department of Health and Human Services, U.S. Public Health Service; For sale by the Supt. of Docs; 1999. 487 p.

37. Wang PS, Angermeyer M, Borges G, et al. Delay and failure in treatment seeking after first onset of mental disorders in the World Health Organization's World Mental Health Survey Initiative. *World Psychiatry.* 2007;6(3):177–85.

38. World Health Organization. *The Global Burden of Disease Update, 2004*. Geneva (Switzerland): World Health Organization; 2008. 146 p.

39. Zeigler DW, Wang CC, Yoast RA, et al. The neurocognitive effects of alcohol on adolescents and college students. *Prev Med.* 2005;40(1):23–32.

SELECTED REFERENCES FOR FURTHER READING

Brownell KD, Fairburn CG. *Eating Disorders and Obesity: A Comprehensive Handbook*. New York (NY): Guilford Press; 1995. 583 p.

Davis M, Eshelman ER, McKay M. *The Relaxation & Stress Reduction Workbook*. 5th ed. Oakland (CA): New Harbinger Publications, Inc.; 2000. 294 p.

Morey B, Mueser KT. *The Family Intervention Guide to Mental Illness: Recognizing Symptoms and Getting Treatment*. Oakland (CA): New Harbinger Publications, Inc.; 2007. 227 p.

Sapolsky RM. *Why Zebras Don't Get Ulcers*. 3rd ed. New York (NY): Henry Holt and Company; 2004. 560 p.

Thakore J, editor. *Physical Consequences of Depression*. Petersfield (United Kingdom): Wrightson Biomedical Publishing Ltd.; 2001. 239 p.

Wood JC. *Getting Help: The Complete & Authoritative Guide to Self-Assessment & Treatment of Mental Health Problems*. Oakland (CA): New Harbinger Publications, Inc.; 2007. 287 p.

INTERNET RESOURCES

- Anxiety and Depression Association of America: http://www.adaa.org (information about anxiety disorders, effective treatments, and referral)
- Depression and Bipolar Support Alliance: http://www.dbsalliance.org (information on depression and local treatment resources, screening)
- Mental Health America: http://www.depression-screening.org/depression_screen.cfm (site to assess symptoms of depression and resources for effective treatments)
- Mind Garden: http://www.mindgarden.com/ (publisher of psychological assessments and instruments)
- National Association of Anorexia Nervosa and Associated Disorders: http://www.anad.org (information about anorexia and bulimia treatment services)
- National Eating Disorders Association: http://edap.org (information about eating disorders, effective treatments, and referral)
- National Institute on Alcohol Abuse and Alcoholism: http://www.niaaa.nih.gov (information on alcohol abuse and alcoholism)
- National Institute on Drug Abuse: http://www.nida.nih.gov (information on substance abuse and dependence)
- National Institute of Mental Health: http://www.nimh.nih.gov (information about all disorders, effective treatments, referral)
- Substance Abuse Treatment Facility Locator: http://dasis3.samhsa.gov (information about local substance-abuse treatment services)

Legal Considerations for Exercise Programming

Legal considerations associated with fitness evaluations and exercise tests, physical activity counseling, activity prescription, giving exercise recommendations, and leading/supervising fitness programs for apparently healthy adults or individuals with stable chronic diseases seemingly are becoming more important and complex as time passes. One area of critical concern to personal trainers, health fitness specialists, and clinical exercise specialists is the professional–client relationship and the activities performed within the confines of that relationship. Other considerations with special significance, when evaluated from a legal perspective, include the physical setting — areas in which program activities are conducted — the specific purpose for which exercise services are performed, the equipment used, the techniques applied with clients, and the instruction and supervision provided to those individuals.

The law impacts exercise professionals in each of these domains, as well as in others. Furthermore, expectations are substantially affected by the exercise environment — recreational, commercial, or clinical — by the type of client being served, and by the nature of the services being provided. Regardless of the situation, sensitivity to legal issues, adherence to current professional guidelines, and the rigorous application of risk management principles may enhance not only the quality of provided service but client satisfaction as well. Moreover, the use of risk management techniques may reduce the service-related injuries, the likelihood of personal injury litigation, and the extent of damage to the provider in the event of claim and lawsuit.

Laws that affect these matters vary considerably from state to state. Nonetheless, certain legal principles have broad application to preexercise screening, exercise testing, exercise program planning, activity supervision, and emergency response considerations. All exercise program personnel should know these principles and endeavor to develop practices aimed at reducing the risks of claims and lawsuits. Such conduct, fortunately, also improves the delivery of service.

In carefully screened and supervised adult populations, the risks of serious cardiovascular accidents in exercise programs are very low. Even for those with some signs of disease who undergo clinical tests, the cardiovascular complication rate appears to be no greater than 7 in 10,000 participants, and for aerobic exercise sessions performed by patients with heart disease, these rates are less than 1 in 20,000 (9,31). Recent survey findings indicate that facility readiness, staff training, and practice for serious adverse events in the health and fitness industry are abysmal despite the fact that more and more such facilities accept older patients and those with controlled chronic diseases (13,27,28). More than 75% of these facilities reported that they had summoned emergency medical services at least once in 5 yr. This suggests a high potential for personal injury lawsuits

KEY TERMS

Assumption of risk (waiver): An agreement by a client, provided before beginning participation, to give up, relinquish, and waive the participant's rights to legal remedy (damages) in the event of injury, even when such injury arises as a result of a provider's ordinary negligence.

Informed consent: A process that entails conveying information to a client so that the client achieves an understanding about the options to choose to participate in a procedure, test, service, or program.

Negligence: A failure to conform one's conduct to a generally accepted standard or duty.

Risk management: An initial and ongoing process to identify relevant risks associated with the delivery of a service and then, through the application of various techniques, to eliminate, reduce, or transfer those risks through the implementation of operational strategies to the program activities designed to benefit clients and program.

(13,27,28). Until the 1990s, only a small fraction of all personal injury cases resulted in claims against exercise professionals. In recent years, however, there has been a definite increase in exercise-related claims processed through the legal system, especially claims against health/fitness facilities (25,26). Those dealing with emergency response deficiencies in the industry also appear to be on the increase (18). Although tort reform proposals may help stem this trend, the future portends an ever-increasing risk of claims and lawsuits for health care professionals generally; exercise professionals are not likely to escape the same problem.

TERMINOLOGY AND CONCEPTS

Generally, legal claims against exercise professionals center on alleged violations of either contract or tort law. These two broad concepts, along with written and statutory laws, define and govern most legal relationships between individuals, including the interrelationship of exercise professionals with clients.

CONTRACT LAW

The law of contracts defines and governs the undertakings that may be specified among individuals. A contract is simply a promise or performance bargained for and given in exchange for another promise or performance, all of which is supported by adequate consideration (i.e., something of value).

In examining exercise testing procedures and recommendations for structured physical activity provided to clients, it is important for professionals to understand how the law of contracts affects their relationships with clients. Examples are numerous and include clients receiving physical fitness information; recommendations given on intensity, duration, and modalities for exercise training; or even instructions on techniques for exercise participation. Likewise, the professional may perform exercise testing in exchange for payment or some other consideration of value. This contractual relationship also encompasses any related activities that occur before and after exercise testing, such as health screening before testing, as well as first aid and emergency care that may arise out of the provision of provider services. If client expectations during this relationship are not fulfilled, a lawsuit for breach of contract may be instituted. Such potential suits allege nonfulfillment of certain promises or a breach of alleged warranties that the law sometimes imposes on many contractual relationships. Apart from professional–client relationships, contract law also has implications for interprofessional relations, such as those dealing with equipment companies, independent service contractors, and employees.

INFORMED CONSENT

Aside from breach of contract claims arising from a lack of promise fulfillment, claims against exercise professionals can be based on a type of breach of contract for failure to obtain adequate informed consent from exercise participants. Although claims based on lack of informed consent, founded upon contract principles, are somewhat archaic today, suits based on such failures are still put forth in some jurisdictions. More frequently today, however, such claims are brought forth in connection with negligence actions rather than breach-of-contract suits. Before an exercise professional administers a specific exercise procedure with a client, the individual must give informed consent to participate in the procedure. Informed consent is intended to ensure that the client entered into the procedure with adequate knowledge of the relevant material risks, any alternative procedures that might satisfy certain of the objectives, and the benefits associated with that activity. This consent can be expressed (written) or implied by law simply as a function of how the two parties to the procedure conducted themselves. See *Figure 3-1* of *GETP9* for a sample of informed consent document.

To give valid consent to a procedure, the person must be of legal age, not be mentally incapacitated, know and fully understand the importance and relevance of the material risks and benefits, and give consent voluntarily and not under any mistake of fact or duress (19). Written consent is certainly preferable to any oral or implied form of consent, and of great importance, it expressly demonstrates the process if questions arise later whether that was the case.

In many states, adequate information must be provided to ensure that the participant knows and understands the risks and circumstances associated with a procedure before informed consent can be given. In such states, a so-called subjective test is used to determine whether that person understood and comprehended the risks and procedures associated with the matter at hand. Other states have adopted a less rigid rule and provide an objective test to determine consent to a procedure or treatment. Under this test, the determination centers on whether the participant, as a reasonable and ordinary person, understood the facts and circumstances associated with the procedure so as to give voluntary consent. Although some states do not require the use of informed consent for nonsurgical procedures or when a test is performed for non–health care related purposes, adherence to the process is a desired approach and an apparent part or expectation associated with the applicable standard of care for the exercise profession. Examples of informed consent documents for exercise testing and training programs are available elsewhere (1,2,19,29).

In lawsuits arising out of the informed consent process, an injured party commonly claims that a professional was negligent in the explanation of the procedure, including the risks, and that the participant would not, in absence of the professional's negligence, have undergone the procedure that resulted in some harm or injury to the client. These cases are often decided upon the testimony of expert witnesses who express opinions on the issue of whether the professional engaged in substandard conduct in securing the informed consent. These cases can involve claims related to contract law, warranties, negligence, and malpractice. Lawsuits arising from alleged deficiencies in the informed consent process related to testing, exercise prescription, or physical activity supervision have become more commonplace. The law is moving toward a broadening requirement for disclosure of risk to participants. Some courts have even gone so far as to require the disclosure of all possible risks, as opposed to those that are simply material (12). Such a requirement imposes unusual burdens on programs and raises substantial medicolegal concerns (14). These concerns require individual analysis and response by individual legal counsel.

One element of the informed consent process relates to confidentiality and disclosure of personal and sensitive information that may be gathered from the client in the course of evaluating his or her health status or delivering services. Provision should be made in the informed consent or other documentation to secure the written authorization from clients to disclose specific test results, exercise progress reports, and so on to health care professionals who have a need to know, such as a primary care physician. Written authorization may also be secured from clients if there is intent to use data in reporting group statistics for program evaluation or research purposes, even when such information is only to be presented in ways not identifiable with the client. Many states and the federal government have promulgated privacy statutes that may affect the release of personally identifiable material regarding a program participant that requires the creation and adoption of privacy policies as well as consents or authorizations for the disclosure of information.

The Health Information Portability and Accountability Act (HIPAA) is a federal privacy law that became effective in early 2003 (11). The HIPAA law was enacted for several purposes, including the promotion of access for consumers to health insurance, protecting the privacy of health care data, and to standardize and promote efficiency of billing and insurance claims processing in the health care industry. Its provisions for protecting the rights of individual consumers define what providers and others must do to safeguard patients' personal medical and health information. The rule assures patient's access to his or her own health information and, at the same time, eliminates inappropriate uses. It applies to health care providers, medical claims clearinghouses, and health insurance carriers. Health and fitness and

rehabilitative exercise professionals who interact with physicians, nurses, medical technicians, and billing clerks and who access a patient's medical records in conjunction with delivery of their services are affected by the HIPAA requirements. Just a few of the several important provisions include (a) individual patients must be provided with copies of the HIPAA privacy rule, (b) patients' prior written authorization must be obtained before information disclosure or use by any third party, and (c) the purposes for which the information is to be used and the time limits of the authorization must be provided to the patient.

Most states have enacted laws to clarify and complement the HIPAA provisions, and these vary among jurisdictions. There are many examples of information routinely collected and maintained by health and fitness and exercise rehabilitation professionals, the uses and disclosure of which are affected by HIPAA. These include not only data collected in the exercise service setting, such as clinical exercise test results, blood pressure, and electrocardiographic records, but also untoward outcome events. With equal certainty, the rule affects the release of information to an exercise professional by health care professionals when the former seeks data needed for safeguarding patients in the process of delivering exercise services (e.g., medical history and laboratory data for preexercise screening or results of clinical exercise tests). The extent to which the HIPAA provisions apply to exercise professionals should be determined through consultation with risk managers and local legal counsel. Nonetheless, all should review and understand the rule, the content of which may be accessed on the Internet at the Health Resources and Services Administration's (U.S. Department of Health and Human Services [USDHHS]) Web site. The HIPAA provisions may be subject to revision or updating, as may the target Web site reference for related U.S. government information. At the time of this writing, the Web site containing this information may be found at http://www.hhs.gov/ocr/hipaa/. The application of these laws to a program and rights to release information depends on a variety of factors that only individual counsel can properly address.

TORT LAW

A tort is simply a civil wrong. Most tort claims affecting exercise professionals are based on allegations of negligence or malpractice causing personal injury or death.

NEGLIGENCE

Although negligence has no precise definition in law, it is regarded as failure to conform one's conduct to a generally accepted standard or duty. A legal cause of action based on claims of negligence may be established given proof of certain facts, specifically, that one person failed to provide due care to protect another to whom the former owed some duty or responsibility and that such failure proximately caused some injury to the latter person (19). Thus, the validity of negligence claims is typically established through a specific process that examines certain facts and establishes whether

- a defendant owed a particular duty or had specific responsibilities to some person who has asserted a claim of negligence,
- one or more failures (breaches) occurred in the performance of that duty compared with a particular set of behaviors that were expected (due care, standard of care), or
- the injury or damage in question was attributable to an established act or a failure to perform (*i.e.*, a negligent act or omission was the proximate cause of the injury or damage).

When negligence claims are asserted, the critical question centers on whether an exercise professional provided service in accordance with the so-called standard of care. After a duty is established, the nature and scope of expected performance are usually determined by one or more expert witnesses' references to published standards and guidelines from peer professional associations. Although standards of care are discussed in a different section of this chapter, ultimately, the most effective shield against claims of negligence may be the daily pattern of delivering services to clients and documenting fulfillment so as to show compliance with the most rigorous published guidelines that are relevant to the established activity.

MALPRACTICE

Malpractice is a specific type of negligence action involving claims against defined professionals. Malpractice actions generally involve claims against professionals who have been provided with public authority to practice (arising from specific state statutes) for alleged breaches of professional duties and responsibilities toward patients or other persons to whom they owed a particular standard of care or duty (19). Historically, malpractice claims have been confined to actions against physicians and lawyers. By statute or case law, however, some states have expanded this group to include nurses, physical therapists, dentists, psychologists, and other health professionals. In 1995, Louisiana became the first state to pass legislation to license and regulate exercise practitioners who work under the authority of physicians with patients in cardiopulmonary rehabilitation treatment programs (20–22). The Louisiana State Board of Medical Examiners now provides regulatory management for this practitioner group. Other states in recent

years such as Georgia, Maryland, Massachusetts, and California have also examined legislative proposals with various provisions to publicly regulate health and fitness and clinical exercise professionals, but no statutes have yet been enacted in jurisdictions beyond Louisiana. To date, no published reports have addressed the effect of this relatively new public regulation on cardiac rehabilitation professionals in Louisiana. The more obvious possibilities of the effect include the level of autonomy in practice, changes in provisions of liability insurance, costs of such insurance, and exposure to claims of malpractice. The advantages and disadvantages of licensure for exercise practitioners have been debated for many years. The issues are complex and involve divergent perspectives from different stakeholders (*e.g.*, those who have the goal of improving quality of service and safety for patients). Imposing added regulatory costs in an era of scarce public resources, intensifying competition with established licensed professions, raising the costs of credentialing and liability insurance for practitioners, and increasing negligence-type claims and suits are byproducts of licensure and are not in the best interests of the profession. It remains to be seen whether the advent of licensure for exercise physiologists in Louisiana has generally succeeded in areas originally of greatest concern to the advocates.

DEFENSES TO NEGLIGENCE OR MALPRACTICE ACTIONS

The proper conduct of the informed consent process can sometimes be used as defense against legal claims based on either tort or contract principles. In such cases, defense counsel may seek to characterize consent as an assumption of risk by the plaintiff. Assumption of risk to a procedure, however, is often difficult to establish without an explicit written statement or clear conduct that demonstrates such an assumption. In addition, an assumption of risk never relieves the exercise professional of the duty to perform in a competent and professional manner. Even when a valid informed consent with assumption of risk is obtained from a client, this doesn't preclude a spouse, children, or heirs from independently filing suits against the exercise professional for loss of consortium-type claims or wrongful death actions in some jurisdictions, even when the participant could not have asserted these claims because of his or her own assumption of risk (5,21). In some jurisdictions, it may be advisable or even necessary to obtain consent from a participant, a spouse, and, perhaps, in a limited number of states, to make it binding on any children or the executor, administrators, and heirs to an estate. Certainly, such consents should be binding on estates if certain of these negligence and malpractice claims from some such parties are to be successfully avoided; again, this may depend on the jurisdiction (21,22). Thus, exercise professionals need to secure individual advice from legal counsel and, if applicable, their institutional risk managers to determine the legally sufficient elements of informed consent that must be presented to clients in their settings and the extent to which "loss of consortium" issues should be addressed.

Informed consent often is confused with so-called releases. Releases are statements sometimes written into consent-type documents that contain exculpatory language — that is, wording that relieves the provider of legal responsibility in the event of an injury or death caused by any error, omission, or even negligence. Release documents, sometimes called prospective waivers of liability or responsibility, are disfavored in some states. Moreover, in a medical setting, the use of such releases, with certain limited exceptions, has been declared invalid and against public policy. In nonmedical settings, however, particularly with certain ultrahazardous activities, such as auto racing, skydiving, and even exercise-related activities, the use of such releases may be valid in some jurisdictions, under certain circumstances, if they are properly drafted and administered. In fact, when they are well defined and properly written, such documents may have substantial benefit to programs. In recent years, there has been a definite trend toward the increased use of waivers and judicial "approval" of such documents in health and fitness and recreational exercise settings to reduce providers' exposure to damage and loss arising from negligence actions. However, improperly developed waivers can fail to protect providers. Consequently, a qualified attorney should be consulted to determine his or her applicability and to prepare these documents. Materials are available to assist in the drafting and application of waivers (6). Although waivers may provide protection against simple or ordinary negligence, they are unlikely to protect against gross negligence. Negligence is a failure to perform at an accepted standard, and gross negligence is to do so willfully. As an example, if a client is injured using equipment that had a frayed cable, the staff might be negligent in having failed to perform appropriate maintenance; the negligence would be gross if the staff knew that the cable was frayed prior to the accident.

Several other defenses to claims of negligence or malpractice are also available. In some states, for example, proof of negligence committed by the participant, referred to in law as *contributory negligence*, can preclude any recovery of damages from a defendant. In many states, however, this rule has been modified by adoption of a so-called system of comparative negligence. Under this rule, negligence of the injured party is compared with negligence of all defendants in the case. Then, if the negligence of the injured party is found to be less than that of all defendants in the case (or in some states, of any defendant in the case), the plaintiff is allowed to recover, albeit in an amount reduced by the contribution of negligence by the injured party (6).

Liability insurance is an effective mechanism to protect against financial loss in the event of claims and lawsuits. Such insurance policies pay for the defense of any covered claims and lawsuits and provide indemnification from any judgment or settlement that is not excluded from the terms of coverage, up to the limits of coverage defined by the provisions of the policy. Proper professional liability insurance, which covers the activities and personnel in question, is readily available through individual purchase or many professional associations as a fee-based option for qualified members (7). In some cases, these liability policies may include special categories, provisions, and pricing for members who hold special credentials (*e.g.*, certification). The extent of liability policy coverage considered sufficient for a given exercise professional depends on individual judgment, exposure incurred in the delivery of service, and the advice of insurance professionals. The decision on the purchase of insurance also should be affected by whether the professional is self-employed, employed by an organization that extends coverage to the professionals who engage only in services on behalf of the organization, or function in both contexts at the same time.

STANDARDS OF PRACTICE

Standards of practice (or care) express how contemporary services should be delivered to give reasonable assurance that desired outcomes will be achieved in a safe manner. In most professions, such standards are developed and periodically revised by consensus among professionals or national associations of providers. Standards documents address what are considered to be benchmark methods, procedures, processes, and protocols that are applied in almost all settings regardless of location, resources, or training of the provider.

In reality, the prevailing or applicable national standard of practice is influenced by a variety of sources, including published statements from professional associations, research findings, government policies, state and national government regulations, litigation, prevailing professional practices in the field, and other factors. In recent years, the promulgation of standards for fitness and health care has increased dramatically. These circumstances mandate that professionals stay abreast of new pronouncements and regulations. Without knowledge of the most relevant and current standards and incorporation of these tenets into the operating protocols and records of service fulfillment, individual practitioners become vulnerable to damage and loss in the event of legal challenges arising from personal injury or wrongful death lawsuits.

In negligence actions, courts rely heavily on interpretations of standards from expert witnesses to determine what should or what should not have been done in particular cases. The use of these standards in certain cases dealing with exercise testing and exercise leadership has already occurred (26).

In recent years, there has been a tendency for certain health care and fitness-related professionals to favor couching their pronouncements on how care should be delivered in the framework of "guidelines," as opposed to "standards" documents. The latter term implies an immutable requirement for practice and implies no flexibility or exceptions in individual applications. A guideline should be interpreted to mean a highly recommended method, procedure, or way of providing service that is advocated by leaders of the field or their consensus. The motivation for the guidelines approach is that although it may have clarity and specificity, it is also written to express the importance of individual practitioners being able to apply sound judgment in how they implement practice parameters for a particular situation or client without incurring increased risk of claim and lawsuit in the event of an untoward outcome. Although a profession-wide shift toward practice parameters that are defined as guidelines or recommendations rather than standards may have a solid rationale from a professional perspective, the extent to which this may add a margin of provider protection in the event of negligence-type lawsuits is difficult to predict. In the past, the absence of definitive standards of practice may have led to an increased legal vulnerability for defendants. This has been because in the absence of clear and uniform standards from the profession, the opinions of individual expert witnesses brought by the plaintiff can have increased sway in the legal determination of what care was expected for a particular client who suffered a personal injury in a given situation.

Many organizations have published documents that influence the legal standard of care in the health, fitness, exercise, and rehabilitation fields. Some of the most important are those of the American College of Sports Medicine (ACSM) (3,29), Agency for Healthcare Policy and Research, American Association of Cardiovascular and Pulmonary Rehabilitation (AACVPR) (10,30,32), American College of Cardiology, American Heart Association (AHA) (3,4,8,23,34), American Medical Association, International Health Racquet, and Sportsclub Association, and the National Strength and Conditioning Association (33) (also see the most current electronic "Internet Resources" from these organizations). Documents from these organizations vary in their scope and applicability. Professionals should carefully examine their own services, uses of technologies and procedures, and types of clients they serve before deciding which standards and guidelines are most applicable to their own programs or situations. At least one such statement has been rejected as a legal standard of care by a federal court in New York because of a disclaimer

provision contained at the beginning of the publication, which provided that the statement should not be used to establish a legal standard of care (17).

Published guidelines may be incomplete or not entirely uniform. In the event of injury or death of a participant, such deficits may create confusion rather than define the professional behavior expected in a specific setting. In the area of exercise testing, standards of the ACSM, AACVPR, and AHA are inconsistent regarding the need for significant involvement of a physician during graded exercise testing (2,8,23,29,34).

On the matter of exercise prescription, one AHA publication (34) explicitly identifies a nurse as an individual who may "assess physical activity habits, prescribe exercise, and monitor responses in healthy persons and cardiac patients." Another contemporary AHA source (23) acknowledges that exercise by patients with heart disease may be appropriately supervised by physicians, nurses, or exercise physiologists, as long as supervisors are trained and their duties are consistent with state statutes governing the practice of medicine and certain other allied health care professions. If deficiencies or disparities in the published guidelines have implications for safety and legal exposure in a particular situation, the development of low-risk protocols and procedures may be a matter of critical importance that requires the advice of local counsel.

Health care professions are in the midst of a movement that may eventually see written standards and guidelines covering nearly every major dimension of care. Fitness and rehabilitation professionals are in similar circumstances and must keep up to date with consensus publications that affect services. To reduce medicolegal risks, it is prudent to adopt the most stringent standards possible. Fulfillment is equally important: Practitioners should not only update program operating manuals to verify adoption of current standards but also document day-to-day client records of service delivery to show what was done and how it was done.

In fact, documentation is vital to many aspects of risk management, not just verification of adherence to standards. Documentation should include contemporaneous recording of critical response levels that arise in exercise testing or training (*e.g.*, important symptoms, estimations of effort, and activity demand, along with signs suggesting myocardial ischemia or poor ventricular response) and annotations about how these occurrences are referred to appropriate health care providers in a timely way. It also encompasses notations on program incidents, especially care delivered in emergencies (perhaps the most important setting in which to demonstrate, after the fact, what and when the essential steps were performed). Follow-up should always be performed and program records maintained to verify the outcome of the situation whenever emergency and nonemergency incidents occur.

In 1998, the AHA and ACSM released a joint position statement recommending certain basic policies and procedures for preexercise screening and emergency readiness in all health/fitness facilities, even in hotels offering only unsupervised access (3). These recommendations of AHA/ACSM were expanded and updated in 2002 to delineate emergency response capabilities that include automated external defibrillation (AED) (4). Every health club and recreational fitness center should evaluate the key features of their organizations and clients, finding how best to structure written policies, procedures, and fulfillment relative to these important safety functions so as to adhere to this new recommendation (3). From a risk management point of view, the adequacy of any policy or procedure is a function of its being committed to written form, kept up to date relative to changing professional guidelines, and linked to ongoing evidence of fulfillment (13,24). Regarding emergency readiness, fulfillment may be partially shown by keeping dated records of regular emergency drills. Another dimension of documenting fulfillment may be achieved by maintaining records that show the names of staff members who practiced in emergency drills and notations on staff performance and any improvements made in the emergency drills. These formal drills prepare staff members for rapid and effective response when a genuine emergency arises. If a legal challenge should ever occur, this record of fulfillment may be quite helpful in establishing that a particular standard of care was adopted and routinely followed (15).

Forms may also be developed for staff members to use routinely in ensuring standardization in operational areas in which injury or legal risks are considered significant. Examples of these situations include forms for preexercise screening and consultation, instruction of new clients in exercise routines, specific cautions for avoidance of injury to patients, and staff inspection of equipment and facilities. Effective forms demonstrate how a facility has linked an important standard to a critical area of service. Use of such forms, along with routine annotation of patient records, shows consistency of fulfillment.

UNAUTHORIZED PRACTICE OF MEDICINE AND ALLIED HEALTH PROFESSIONAL STATUTES

In recent years, the growing prominence of exercise testing and other health and fitness services increasingly places exercise professionals in collaborative roles with licensed health care providers. This evolution has stimulated a variety of initiatives to clarify roles and responsibilities, promote professionalism, and increase professional opportunities. Competency credentials of the ACSM (*e.g.*, ACSM Certified Clinical Exercise Specialist®, ACSM Certified Health Fitness Specialist[SM], ACSM Registered Clinical Exercise Physiologist®), the AACVPR's core competency position statement for cardiac rehabilitation

specialists, and efforts to establish licensure are illustrations of initiatives that affect the positioning of specialists and greater role delineation (10,20).

Providing exercise services with some degree of independence in collaboration with licensed providers can create legally precarious circumstances for some exercise professionals. A prime example of confusion in this area is reflected in questions that often arise about the competency and legal authority needed to provide emergency cardiac care in community- or clinic-based settings in exercise settings where the purpose of the exercise services may be defined as treatment for diagnosed or suspected cardiovascular or other major chronic diseases. The standard for emergency response in this situation is clear and universal. It calls for a defibrillator; a crash cart with artificial airways, suction pump, and emergency drugs; and the competency of an on-site provider who can administer the AHA's advanced cardiac life support (ACLS) skills when needed (1,8,30). This provider, however, must understand that he or she cannot assume such duties unless the physician in charge has given written standing orders to that effect or the individual also has legal authorization under state statutes to accept such standing orders or to otherwise carry out the activity. This is almost never the case for unlicensed exercise professionals who provide exercise services within the health care setting, such as a hospital-based exercise testing or cardiac rehabilitation program, with or without current ACLS training. Thus, there is no legal authority for an exercise professional to evaluate the need for or perform defibrillation on a patient in these circumstances, *unless* he or she has independently completed training and licensure requirements to perform these procedures in the jurisdiction.

Recent advances in technology and new state and federal statutes are changing public expectations regarding use of AEDs. This evolution may soon alter the standard of care for emergency service in the health and fitness setting (16). It is expected, because of the ongoing development of published statements from professional organizations (17,29) and continuing litigation as to AED issues (24), that the use of AEDs is fast reaching the point that it has become the standard of care owed by health/fitness facilities toward their patrons. This time may have already come (29).

The continuing evolution of health care reform further confuses the roles of health care providers. This may often be problematic for exercise professionals working in diagnostic exercise laboratories or rehabilitation centers. A significant part of this evolution has been aimed at reducing costs by using paraprofessionals in increasingly important clinical roles. In fact, various states have undertaken efforts to expand nursing practice and other provider practice laws beyond mere observation, reporting, and recording of a patient's signs and symptoms. Various physician assistant and similar paraprofessional

BOX 10-1	**Tips for Exercise Professionals**

Some tips for exercise professionals regarding legal matters include the following:

1. Know and apply in practice the most rigorous and current peer-developed guidelines applicable to your services, clients, and organization or environment.
2. Maintain credentials relevant to your service (*e.g.*, personal certification or public licensure) and professional liability insurance coverage.
3. Use appropriate informed consent for all services in which such consent is relevant (consult with qualified attorney and risk manager).
4. Instruct clients in techniques of participation and limitations relevant to their health and physical capabilities, observe their related participation, correct problems, and follow up to verify that they manage their own participation safely and effectively.
5. Document fulfillment of your service in a manner consistent with standard of care and your written program policies and procedures.
6. Communicate critical information in a timely way to authorized parties.
7. Develop emergency response plans, rehearse for emergencies, document and upgrade procedures based on rehearsal experiences, and institute automated external defibrillation programs as applicable.
8. Report incidents and follow up to continuously improve emergency readiness and performance.
9. Maintain equipment and inspect facilities on a frequent and regular basis.

practice laws provide expanded treatment authority to nonphysicians.

Until health care reform is complete, however, some nonphysicians will continue to be engaged in certain practices that might be characterized as the practice of medicine or some other statutorily defined and controlled allied health profession. In such situations, the unlicensed provider runs the risk of engaging in unauthorized practices that could lead to both criminal and civil sanctions. Many states have defined the practice of medicine broadly so that persons engaged in exercise testing and prescription activities could, under some circumstances, fall within the range of such statutes.

As previously indicated in this chapter, published standards are not always definitive in expressing the roles and responsibilities for exercise professionals, particularly regarding the delivery of services for patients with documented diseases or even those with no outward signs of disease (*e.g.*, silent myocardial ischemia). Thus, without the presence or assistance of a licensed physician or other allied health professional for certain aspects of the provision of exercise services, claims as to the unauthorized practice of medicine or some other provider practice could be put forth. Under some of these state statutes, such practices are often classified as crimes, usually misdemeanors, punishable by imprisonment for less than 1 yr, a fine, or both. In some jurisdictions, felony classification for such offenses has been established with greater potential punishment.

In addition, a person found to have engaged in the unauthorized practice of medicine or some other allied health profession faces (after the fact) the legal expectation that he or she should have provided an elevated standard of care in the event of injury to or death of a participant.

Under this rule, the actions of an exercise professional would be compared with the presumed standard of care of a physician or other allied health professional acting under the same or similar circumstances. In the event that the actions do not meet this standard (which the nonphysician or allied health professional cannot meet because of inadequacies of knowledge, skill, authorization, and experience), liability may result (*Box 10-1*).

SUMMARY

More and more individuals are becoming exposed to organized exercise programs. Exercise professionals and fitness facility operators should note that middle-aged and older adults represent one of the fastest growing segments of their membership. These individuals tend to have more chronic disease risk factors, medical considerations affecting exercise participation, and likely a higher occurrence of undiagnosed diseases than any other group that might enter their programs. Therefore, the actual number of untoward events in exercise programs, avoidable or otherwise, will inevitably increase. Increased numbers of these occurrences will result in negligence claims that will ultimately find resolution in court. The probabilities of such traumatic actions are low, particularly for individuals and organizations that operate programs in a manner commensurate with accepted professional standards. Awareness of the areas of special legal vulnerability and adoption of legally sensitive practices, however, will keep the risks of litigation low and lead to safer and more efficacious programs. Professionals are advised to keep current concerning developments in this ever-changing medicolegal field (19).

REFERENCES

1. American Association of Cardiovascular and Pulmonary Rehabilitation. *Guidelines for Cardiac Rehabilitation and Secondary Prevention Programs.* 4th ed. Champaign (IL): Human Kinetics; 2004. 280 p.

2. American Association of Cardiovascular and Pulmonary Rehabilitation. *Guidelines for Pulmonary Rehabilitation Programs.* 4th ed. Champaign (IL): Human Kinetics; 2011. 184 p.

3. Balady GJ, Chaitman B, Driscoll D, et al. Recommendations for cardiovascular screening, staffing, and emergency policies at health/fitness facilities. *Circulation.* 1998;97(22):2283–93.

4. Balady GJ, Chaitman B, Foster C, et al. Automated external defibrillators in health/fitness facilities: supplement to the AHA/ACSM recommendations for cardiovascular screening, staffing, and emergency policies at health/fitness facilities. *Circulation.* 2002;105(9):1147–50.

5. Child sues for "loss of consortium." *Lawyers Alert.* 1984;3:249.

6. Cotten D, Cotten MB. *Legal Aspects of Waivers in Sport, Recreation & Fitness Activities.* Canton (OH): PRC Pub; 1997. 206 p.

7. Eickhoff-Shemek J. Distinguishing "general" and "professional" liability insurance. *ACSM's Health & Fitness Journal.* 2003;7(1):28–30.

8. Field JM, Hazinski MF, Sayre MR, et al. Part 1: executive summary: 2010 American Heart Association guidelines for cardiopulmonary resuscitation and emergency cardiovascular care. *Circulation.* 2010;122(18 Suppl 3):S640–56.

9. Foster C, Porcari JP. The risks of exercise training. *J Cardiopulm Rehabil.* 2001;21(6):347–52.

10. Hamm LF, Sanderson BK, Ades PA, et al. Core competencies for cardiac rehabilitation/secondary prevention professionals: 2010 update: position statement of the American Association of Cardiovascular and Pulmonary Rehabilitation. *J Cardiopulm Rehabil Prev.* 2011;31(1):2–10.

11. Health Insurance Portability and Accountability Act, 104 USC (1988) (August 21, 1996).

12. *Hedgecorth v United States,* 618 F Supp 627, No. 83-0770, 1985 U.S. Dist. LEXIS 18014 (ED Mo 1985)

13. Herbert DL. Health clubs may not be meeting standards of care. *Exerc Stand Malpract.* 2002;15(12).

14. Herbert DL. Informed consent documents for stress testing to comport with Hedgecorth v. United States. *Exerc Stand Malpract.* 1987;1(81).

15. Herbert DL. Plan to save lives: create and rehearse an emergency response plan. *ACSM's Health Fit J.* 1997;1(5):34–5.

16. Herbert DL. Standards of care for health and fitness facilities are ever evolving: will automated external defibrillators be required? *ACSM' Health Fit J.* 2000;4(2):18–20.

17. Herbert DL. U.S. District Court in New York rules: ACSM health and fitness facility standards and guidelines are not legal standards. *Exerc Stand Malpract.* 2011;12.

18. Herbert DL. Working out the risks: inadequate response to emergencies by fitness center employees has led to lawsuits. Widespread use of defibrillators could avert tragedies and reduce claims. *Best's Review.* 2000;99.

19. Herbert DL, Herbert WG. *Legal Aspects of Preventive, Rehabilitative, and Recreational Exercise Programs.* 4th ed. Canton (OH): PRC Pub; 2002. 508 p.

20. Herbert WG. Licensure of clinical exercise physiologists: impressions concerning the new law in Louisiana. *Exerc Stand Malpract.* 1995;9(5):65,68–70.

21. Herbert WG, Herbert DL. Exercise testing in adults: legal and procedural considerations for the physical educator and exercise specialist. *JOPER.* 1975;46(6):17–9.

22. Koeberle BE. *Legal Aspects of Personal Fitness Training.* Canton, (OH): Professional Reports Corporation; 1990. 186 p.

23. Leon AS, Franklin BA, Costa F, et al. Cardiac rehabilitation and secondary prevention of coronary heart disease: an American Heart Association scientific statement from the Council on Clinical Cardiology (Subcommittee on Exercise, Cardiac Rehabilitation, and Prevention) and the Council on Nutrition, Physical Activity, and Metabolism (Subcommittee on Physical Activity), in collaboration with the American Association of Cardiovascular and Pulmonary Rehabilitation. *Circulation.* 2005;111(3):369–76.

24. Lives, liabilities and lawsuits on the line: defibrillators are becoming part of the "standard of care" for recreation facilities. *Recreation Management* [Internet]. [cited 2011 May 10]. Available from: http://www.recmanagement.com/issue-content-search.php?q=herbert&s=0&e=10&user_e=10

25. *Mandel v Canyon Ranch, Inc., et al.,* No. 3122777 (Ariz. Super Ct., Pima County 1998).

26. *Mathis v New York Health Club,* 261 AD2d 345, 690 NYS2d 433, 1999 U.S. Dist. LEXIS 5800 (NY App. Div. May 27, 1999).

27. McInnis K, Herbert W, Herbert D, Herbert J, Ribisl P, Franklin B. Low compliance with national standards for cardiovascular emergency preparedness at health clubs. *Chest.* 2001;120(1):283–8.

28. McInnis KJ, Hayakawa S, Balady GJ. Cardiovascular screening and emergency procedures at health clubs and fitness centers. *Am J Cardiol.* 1997;80(3):380–3.

29. Peterson JA, Tharrett SJ, American College of Sports Medicine. *ACSM's health/fitness Facility Standards and Guidelines.* 4th ed. Champaign (IL): Human Kinetics; 2011. 211 p.

30. Ries AL, Bauldoff GS, Carlin BW, et al. Pulmonary rehabilitation: Joint ACCP/AACVPR evidence-based clinical practice guidelines. *Chest.* 2007;131(5 Suppl):4S–42S.

31. Rochmis P, Blackburn H. Exercise tests. A survey of procedures, safety, and litigation experience in approximately 170,000 tests. *JAMA.* 1971;217(8):1061–6.

32. Sanderson BK, Southard D, Oldridge N, Writing Group. AACVPR consensus statement. Outcomes evaluation in cardiac rehabilitation/secondary prevention programs: improving patient care and program effectiveness. *J Cardiopulm Rehabil.* 2004;24(2):68–79.

33. *Strength and Conditioning Professional Standards and Guidelines* [Internet]. Colorado Springs (CO): National Strength and Conditioning Association; 2001 [cited 2011 May 10]. 48 p. Available from: http://www.nsca-lift.org/Publications/SCStandards.pdf

34. Thompson PD, Franklin BA, Balady GJ, et al. Exercise and acute cardiovascular events placing the risks into perspective: a scientific statement from the American Heart Association Council on Nutrition, Physical Activity, and Metabolism and the Council on Clinical Cardiology. *Circulation.* 2007;115(17):2358–68.

SELECTED REFERENCES FOR FURTHER READING

Herbert DL, Herbert WG. *Legal Aspects of Preventive, Rehabilitative, and Recreational Exercise Programs.* 4th ed. Canton (OH): PRC Pub; 2002. 508 p.

Koeberle BE. *Legal Aspects of Personal Fitness Training.* Canton (OH): Professional Reports Corporation; 1990. 186 p.

McInnis K, Herbert W, Herbert D, Herbert J, Ribisl R, Franklin B. Low compliance with national standards for cardiovascular emergency preparedness at health clubs. *Chest.* 2001;120(1):283–8.

INTERNET RESOURCES

- Agency for Healthcare Research and Quality: http://www.ahrq.gov
- American Association of Cardiovascular and Pulmonary Rehabilitation: http://www.aacvpr.org
- American College of Cardiology: http://www.cardiosource.org/acc
- American Heart Association: http://www.my.americanheart.org/professional/index.jsp
- American Medical Association: http://www.ama-assn.org
- International Health, Racquet and Sportsclub Association: http://www.ihrsa.org
- National Strength and Conditioning Association: http://www.nsca-lift.org

Health Appraisal, Risk Assessment, and Safety of Exercise

ANN M. SWANK, PhD, FACSM, *Section Editor*

General Overview of Preparticipation Health Screening and Risk Assessment

A physically active lifestyle reduces the risk of several major chronic diseases. Regular physical activity has been shown to be beneficial in the primary prevention of cardiovascular disease (CVD), stroke, diabetes, obesity, osteoporosis, anxiety, depression, and some cancers (16,28). Given the high prevalence of a sedentary lifestyle and obesity (8,11), there is little doubt that considerable public health benefit would accrue if inactive individuals became more active.

JOB TASK ANALYSIS, DOMAIN I

ACSM Certified Clinical Exercise Specialist® (CES): Patient Clinical Assessment, 20%

ACSM Registered Clinical Exercise Physiologist® (RCEP): Clinical Assessment, 16%

ACSM Certified Personal Trainer℠ (CPT): Initial Client Consultation and Assessment, 26%

ACSM Certified Health Fitness Specialist℠ (HFS): Health and Fitness Assessment, 25%

ACSM Certified Group Exercise Instructor℠ (GEI): Participant and Program Assessment, 10%

The many health-related benefits, as well as the responsible physiologic mechanisms, of a physically active lifestyle are well documented. However, it is essential to realize that to be most effective, regular exercise must be combined with other positive lifestyle interventions, such as proper nutrition, healthy sleep habits, cessation of smoking, etc., and, when applicable, with appropriate medical therapy. Furthermore, although exercise is safe for most individuals, it is prudent to take certain precautions to optimize the benefit-to-risk ratio. The two most common risks associated with starting a new physical activity program or performing an exercise test are sudden cardiac events and orthopedic injury. The risks associated with physical activity and exercise testing are detailed in Chapter 1 of *ACSM's Guidelines for Exercise Testing and Prescription, Ninth Edition (GETP9)*.

To ensure an optimal benefit-to-risk ratio, exercise professionals should incorporate some form of health appraisal before performing fitness testing or initiating an exercise program. Although Chapter 2 of the *GETP9* provides a thorough description of proper preparticipation health screening and risk assessment, the intent of this chapter is to provide a general overview of the process as well as address medical conditions

KEY TERMS

Medical screening examination: A thorough medical examination performed by a health care professional, often a physician, to assess readiness of starting a physical activity program; often, the need of obtaining a medical screening examination is identified during the preparticipation health screening and risk assessment (see *GETP9*, Chapter 3).

Physical Activity Readiness Questionnaire (PAR-Q): A widely used and simple prescreening health assessment questionnaire developed by the British

Columbia Ministry of Health for assessing readiness of starting a physical activity program (see *GETP9*, *Fig. 2-1*).

Preparticipation health screening and risk assessments: Standardized tools for identifying existing medical conditions with the goal of assessing the risks associated with starting a new exercise program or performing an exercise test (see *GETP9*, *Figs. 2-1* and *2-2*).

that demand special consideration. The purpose of the prepartication health screening is to provide pertinent health information that may be relevant to the safety of the individual during exercise testing and training. Furthermore, it is important to identify additional factors that require special consideration when developing and designing appropriate exercise prescription and programming that will optimize adherence, minimize risks, and maximize benefits. The purposes of the prepartication health screen include the following:

- Identification and exclusion of individuals with medical contraindications to exercise testing (see *GETP9*, Chapter 3)
- Identification of individuals who should undergo a medical evaluation and exercise testing before starting an exercise program because of increased risk for disease because of symptoms or risk factors (see *GETP9*, *Tables 2-2* and *2-3*)
- Identification of persons with clinically significant disease who should participate in medically supervised exercise programs
- Identification of individuals with other special needs

The precise nature and extent of the appraisal should be determined by the age, sex, and perceived health status characteristics of the participants, as well as the personnel and equipment resources. Most prospective participants in exercise programs conducted in nonmedical settings are sedentary individuals who consider themselves "generally healthy" and whose goals are to improve their fitness and well-being, reduce weight, and reduce risk of chronic disease. The routine recommendation for all individuals to undergo exercise testing prior to beginning an exercise program has been revised. It is now acknowledged that unless there are specific medical concerns, asymptomatic individuals do not need to consult with a physician or health care provider for a prepartication evaluation when embarking upon a low-to-moderate intensity exercise program (16). Symptomatic individuals or those with chronic disease should consult with a qualified health professional prior to substantially increasing their level of physical activity. The primary safety goal of a prepartication health appraisal is to identify individuals who should receive further medical evaluation to determine whether there are contraindications to exercise testing or training or whether referral to a medically supervised exercise program is necessary. Health appraisals can range from a short questionnaire to interviews and sophisticated computerized evaluations. Many appraisals include common screening measurements including height, weight, circumferences, percent body fat, blood pressure (BP), and blood testing (serum lipids and glucose). Specifics of these screening items are addressed in detail in Chapter 3 (*Tables 3-1–3-4*) and Chapter 4 (*Tables 4-1–4-6*) of the *GETP9*. The most common

method of prescreening health assessment is the use of standardized forms, and several standardized forms are available that can be used to risk stratify individuals. Standardized forms should be viewed as a minimal standard for entry into a new exercise program. In general, these forms are aimed at identifying individuals at moderate-to-high risk who should receive medical referral before beginning or increasing their level of physical activity. Two reputable standardized forms are the Physical Activity Readiness Questionnaire (PAR-Q) and the American Heart Association/American College of Sports Medicine (AHA/ACSM) Health/Fitness Facility Prepartication Screening Questionnaire. The PAR-Q has been used and tested extensively (26) and is designed to be used when a person wants to begin a program of light-to-moderate physical activity. One of the benefits of the PAR-Q is simplicity, so much so that in some circumstances in which there is no alternative, the PAR-Q can be self-administered by the participant. The **AHA/ACSM Health/Fitness Facility Prepartication Screening Questionnaire** is designed to be completed when the participant registers at a health/fitness facility or program (5) (see *GETP9*, *Fig. 2-2*). This form is more complex than the PAR-Q and uses history, symptoms, and risk factors (including age) to assess the need for physician evaluation before beginning a new exercise program. This form was specifically designed for prescreening in health/fitness facilities. It can be completed in a few minutes, identifies moderate- and high-risk individuals, documents the results of the screening, educates the consumer and staff, and encourages appropriate use of the health care system. The use of the PAR-Q and AHA/ACSM Health/Fitness Facility Prepartication Screening Questionnaire is explained in detail, and sample forms are provided in Chapter 2 of *GETP9*. Both of these forms have limitations and should only be interpreted by qualified staff, who should always document the results. However, it needs to be emphasized that many sedentary individuals can safely begin a light- to moderate-intensity physical activity program without the need for extensive medical screening.

No form or set of guidelines for prepartication screening can cover all situations. Furthermore, the use of the PAR-Q can only identify those who are at high risk; it does not differentiate between those at low and moderate risk. In addition, most forms do not make recommendations based on intensity of the proposed exercise program. The ACSM's recommendations for medical examinations and exercise testing before participation in a new exercise program both stratify individuals into categories of low, moderate, and high risk and combine this with proposed exercise intensity to assess need of medical evaluation before the start of a new exercise program.

Although a variety of risks are associated with exercise participation, the most important is the precipitation of major cardiac events, such as a myocardial infarction or sudden cardiac death. Several studies demonstrate that the transiently increased risk of cardiac arrest occurring during vigorous exercise results largely from the presence of preexisting cardiac abnormalities, particularly CVD (5,23). The importance of identifying individuals at high risk of CVD or demonstrating symptoms associated with CVD is critical for ensuring safe participation in a physical activity program. Thus, it is of great importance for exercise professionals to have a good understanding of the medical history, signs, and symptoms that require evaluation by a physician before a moderate to higher risk/symptomatic individual starts a new physical activity program. Risks for exercise include any heart conditions, such as heart attack, cardiac catheterization, abnormal rhythms, valve disease, or congenital conditions. As described in *GETP9, Table 2-3*, the common CVD risk factors are all deserving of attention and include age, impaired fasting glucose, sedentary lifestyle, obesity, high cholesterol, smoking, hypertension, and family history of CVD. Important signs and symptoms (see *GETP9, Table 2-2*) include any form of chest discomfort or unreasonable shortness of breath with exertion, dizziness, fainting, blackouts, or cramping or burning in the legs, ankle edema, palpitations or tachycardia, and dyspnea when in a horizontal position (orthopnea) or that wakes someone who was sleeping (paroxysmal nocturnal dyspnea). Limitations attributable to bone or joint issues or previous injuries should also be addressed. This is a brief overview of the medical history, signs, and symptoms that should raise concern in the exercise professional and are usually associated with referral for physician clearance. Both the ACSM (*GETP9*) and the AHA (16) provide guidance on when a medical referral is recommended. It should also be noted that detection of elevated BP, cholesterol, or glucose should also trigger a medical referral (7,9,10,15,19,20,32). After an individual has been provided with medical clearance to participate in an exercise program (as a recommended follow-up to preparticipation screening or a more comprehensive health appraisal), it is important for the exercise professional to determine whether there are any additional health-related factors that require special consideration.

OVERVIEW OF THE MEDICAL SCREENING EXAMINATION

A medical screening examination to evaluate the risk of starting a new physical activity program can range in complexity from a simple clinical examination to extensive diagnostic testing, depending on the age, medical history, risk factors, and symptoms of the individual. At a minimum, the medical screening examination should include a detailed medical history and thorough physical examination. In obtaining the medical history, every effort should be made to acquire specific information about previous medical diagnoses, particularly those pertaining to cardiac and vascular disease, as well as the associated risk factors such as hypertension, diabetes, high cholesterol, tobacco use, and family history. Particular attention should also be given to reviewing past skeletal and muscular injuries and current physical limitations caused by either acute injury or chronic conditions such as arthritis or osteoporosis. A review of the individual's medications is an important part of the medical history to identify medical problems that may have been missed during the interview and also to identify any medications that may alter the exercise prescription. Although a review of symptoms should be a standard part of the examination, any symptoms of chest discomfort or shortness of breath associated with exertion should be explored in detail.

If dictated by preliminary screening, a standard physical examination should be performed. These are performed for those at moderate risk who wish to participate in vigorous exercise or anyone at high risk wishing to perform any intensity exercise. There should be particular importance placed on the assessment of the cardiovascular and pulmonary systems as well as the musculoskeletal system. BP and heart rate (HR) should be measured, and an auscultatory examination of the heart and lungs should be performed. Weight and height should be measured to classify the individual as normal weight, overweight, or obese, but also to assess the potential impact of excess weight on joint health. Joint mobility should be checked as well as range of motion (ROM) and strength. A neurologic examination that includes a balance test should be administered. Examining the feet, looking for open wounds, is particularly important in elderly individuals and those with diabetes.

Based on the information obtained during the history and examination combined with the participant's exercise goals and in accordance with standards of care, the examining physician may elect to order or perform more advanced diagnostic or screening tests. These include exercise stress tests with or without nuclear imaging (technetium or thallium), radiographs, magnetic resonance imaging (MRI), or even cardiac catheterization if symptoms warrant. For more detailed information about the medical screening, refer to Chapter 3 of the *GETP9*.

COMMON RISK-STRATIFICATION SCHEMA AND THEIR USES

The use of national guidelines to stratify risk of adverse health events, usually cardiac, can be very useful. Common sources of risk-stratification schema include the National Cholesterol Education Program Expert Panel on Detection, Evaluation, and Treatment of High Blood Cholesterol in Adults (10,15); the Seventh Report of the Joint National Committee on Prevention, Detection, Evaluation, and Treatment of High Blood Pressure (7,9,20); and the combined updated recommendations issued by the ACSM and AHA (16).

MEDICAL CONDITIONS THAT COMPLICATE THE EXERCISE PRESCRIPTION

There are several issues that warrant special consideration when assessing the need for further screening before a patient begins a physical activity program. There are varieties of conditions that may affect the exercise prescription; a few of the more common ones are discussed here. However, a safe strategy when a complicating medical condition is present is to assure that the individual's health care professional is aware of the individual's desire to become physically active and that the professional has approved this change in behavior.

CARDIOVASCULAR DISEASE

It is well documented that regular exercise has powerful benefits for both preventing and treating CVD. However, it is also well known that an acute bout of exercise, particularly in sedentary individuals, can precipitate a cardiac event in those with preexisting CVD. Thus, exercise prescription in individuals with CVD must be done with both physician approval and input (16). Often, individuals with CVD need to start their program under medically supervised conditions, and some individuals may never progress to unsupervised exercise. Although a good strategy for all sedentary individuals starting a new exercise program, it is especially important for individuals with CVD to start slowly and progress gradually in exercise intensity and duration. The recommended physical activity goal for patients with coronary and other vascular diseases is to progress to daily aerobic exercise sessions (i.e., 7 d a week, with 5 being the minimum frequency) and incorporate a moderate intensity, with each session lasting between 30 and 60 min in duration. Furthermore, it is suggested that this standard aerobic program be supplemented with additional lifestyle activities as well as twice-a-week resistance training (19,27). All individuals with CVD who wish to start an exercise program must be taught the warning signs of acute cardiac events such as chest pain, unreasonable shortness of breath, and tingling in jaw or left hand. For more detailed discussions related to exercise for individuals with CVD, see Chapter 9 of *GETP9*, Chapters 24 and 38 of this *Resource Manual*, recommendations cited in *Circulation* (16,27,28) and *Stroke* (14), as well

as Web sites for the AHA (http://www.americanheart.org) and the American Association of Cardiovascular and Pulmonary Rehabilitation (AACVPR) (http://www.aacvpr.org).

HYPERTENSION

As noted earlier in this chapter, hypertension is listed as a positive risk factor for heart disease. Hypertension is an insidious disorder wherein during the initial stages there are often no signs or symptoms, lending to its ominous nickname "the silent killer." It is pervasive, with more than 1 billion people worldwide, including 50 million Americans, diagnosed as hypertensive (7,9,20). Hypertension is often present as an underlying disease process within diabetes, chronic obstructive pulmonary disease (COPD), renal failure, and ischemic stroke (7,9,14,20). Therefore, when considering exercise testing procedures and designing exercise prescriptions for hypertensive patients, it is usually necessary to account for the impact of multiple disease processes. For more detailed discussions related to exercise for individuals with hypertension, see Chapter 10 in *GETP9*; the ACSM position stand on exercise and hypertension (22); recommendations cited in the *Journal of the American Medical Association* (*JAMA*) (9), *Circulation* (16,19,27), and *Stroke* (14); the American Society of Hypertension's Web site (http://www.ash-us.org); and the AHA and AACVPR Web sites mentioned previously.

CHRONIC OBSTRUCTIVE PULMONARY DISEASE

COPD is a general term used to describe long-term illnesses of the respiratory system, including such diseases as asthma, chronic bronchitis, and emphysema. It has a long preclinical development period such that physiological changes progress unnoticed until relatively major symptoms occur due to more extensive lung damage (24,25). There is no longer an "at risk" stage of development as there is insufficient evidence that those exhibiting symptoms (*e.g.*, chronic cough with sputum) actually progress to a more severe COPD stage. Rather, there are simply four objectively defined risk stages: Stage I, mild (forced expiratory volume in one second [$FEV_{1.0}$] ≥80% of predicted); Stage II, moderate ($FEV_{1.0}$ 50%–80% of predicted); Stage III, severe ($FEV_{1.0}$ 30%–50% of predicted); and Stage IV, very severe ($FEV_{1.0}$ ≤30% of predicted) (13,24,25). (See also *GETP9, Table 3-5* for revised spirometric information and classification schemas for identifying and managing pulmonary conditions.)

Evidence-based research has demonstrated that a multidisciplinary individualized approach to pulmonary rehabilitation is effective in reducing symptoms, enhancing quality of life, and, in some instances, potentially reversing the disease process (24,25). It is also recommended that pulmonary rehabilitation is beneficial for those with chronic pulmonary illnesses who do not fall within the category of COPD. In addition to the standard pulmonary therapies offered by physicians, nurses, psychologists, and respiratory, physical, and occupational therapists, exercise specialists must also be involved. Regular exercise is an important component of the rehabilitative process. Because short-term programs have limited long-term efficacy, it is recommended that pulmonary rehabilitation programs extend at least 12 wk or more for sustainable health benefits. A 6-mo pulmonary rehabilitation program incorporating 2 mo of inpatient therapy coupled with 4 mo of outpatient therapy produced statistically significant and clinically relevant improvements in exercise capacity (24,25).

Although exercise training can help improve endurance and feelings of dyspnea (24,25), supplemental oxygen may still be needed during the rehabilitative exercise sessions, especially for those with severe exercise-induced hypoxemia. Furthermore, in order to realize endurance gains, the use of supplemental oxygen use may be beneficial during high-intensity exercise even in those patients without exercise-induced hypoxemia. For monitoring dyspnea severity, in addition to using the standard dyspnea 1–4 rating scale used during exercise (*Fig. 5-4* in *GETP9*), the Modified Medical Research Council Questionnaire for Assessing the Severity of Breathlessness created by the British Medical Research Council (MRC) is an excellent adjunct health prescreening tool (13). It consists of five short questions assessing which activity patterns bring on breathlessness, with the activity pattern ranging from simple activities of daily living to strenuous exercise. The MRC questionnaire has a demonstrated relationship with other health risk assessments as well as mortality predictive value (6,21). The Pulmonary Rehabilitation Executive Summary issued in 2007 via a joint proclamation by the American College of Chest Physicians (ACCP)/AACVPR offered the following updated exercise recommendations (24,25). A mandatory recommendation was the inclusion of exercise training the specific musculature responsible for ambulation in pulmonary rehabilitation sessions (24,25). Specific exercise modality recommendations were not mentioned but the therapy should include both lower and upper body exercise. Higher intensity, lower extremity exercise training is encouraged over lower intensity due to demonstrated greater physiological benefits. Unsupported endurance training of the upper body is also encouraged. Strength training for both the lower and upper body is also encouraged in order to increase/maintain muscle mass and corresponding strength. However, as with all aspects of therapy, the exercise plan must be individualized. Therefore, if a patient cannot tolerate higher intensity exercise, lower intensity exercise is still beneficial. Patient education is key for self-management of COPD,

and teaching patients how to manage their exercise program when an exercise therapist is not available is recommended. Lastly, research has shown insufficient efficacy for the routine use of inspiratory muscle training, but patients with severe COPD may benefit from use of noninvasive ventilation procedures as an adjunctive therapy to exercise (24,25).

As with most chronic diseases, it is important to have permission from the individual's health care professional before starting a program. In summary, it is likely that health care professionals will be involved in a patient's pulmonary rehabilitation program and perhaps more so during initial stages for individuals who have been sedentary for an extended period of time. Previously sedentary patients will benefit from starting slowly and progressing gradually in exercise intensity and duration. One important safety consideration when working with anyone with a breathing disorder is making sure the individual always has enough "rescue" medication available when exercising, particularly individuals with asthma. For more detailed discussion related to exercise for individuals with COPD, see Chapter 10 of *GETP9*; Chapters 25 and 39 of this *Resource Manual*; and two Web sites — the Global Initiative for Chronic Obstructive Lung Disease (http://www.goldcopd.com) and the American Lung Association (http://www.lungusa.org).

DIABETES

Diabetes is a strong and independent contributor to the risk of developing CVD. This excessive risk includes CVD, peripheral arterial disease, and congestive heart failure. Diabetes is a metabolic disease that requires specific diet and exercise therapy alone or in combination with prescribed medications. Regular physical activity greatly reduces both the risk of developing diabetes and the medical complications associated with diabetes. Approximately 150 min of moderate-to-vigorous aerobic exercise per week coupled with resistance training (two to three times a week) is recommended, allowing no more than 2 consecutive days of no activity weekly (4). However, given the large CVD risk associated with having diabetes, the prescription of exercise for individuals with the disorder must be done with great thought and care (4,5). Additional long-term complications such as retinopathy and autonomic/peripheral neuropathy must also be considered. Vigorous exercise may exacerbate retinal detachment. Peripheral neuropathy results in decreased pain sensation and can contribute to increased risk of skin tissue breakdown and subsequent infection. Due to decreased cardiac responsiveness, autonomic neuropathy can decrease the ability of patients with diabetes to thermoregulate and adjust to postural changes (4). Given these known risks, it is important for patients with diabetes desiring to begin an exercise program to confer with their health care provider(s) for individualized exercise testing and training recommendations (2). If a patient plans to participate in low-intensity physical activity, then it may not be necessary for him or her to undergo an exercise stress test. Not only has evidence-based research failed to demonstrate a need for an exercise stress test prior to low-level physical activity participation, it has been suggested that requiring a preexercise stress test can actually demotivate a patient from beginning a walking program. However, if more vigorous exercise is planned or if the exercise will exceed the routine demands of everyday living of sedentary and/or older adults with diabetes, then a standard CVD preexercise assessment is recommended (2). It is important to not only assess risk based on medical history, symptoms, physical limitations, macrovascular and microvascular complications, and exercise stress test results, but also to evaluate glycemic control measures as glucose-related medication requirements are likely to change with participation in an exercise program.

Many individuals with diabetes are at risk for foot ulceration most often attributable to peripheral neuropathy or peripheral vascular disease. For these individuals, it may be advisable to limit their physical activity to non–weight-bearing exercises, such as swimming or bicycling. Also, some acute issues related to blood glucose must be addressed when an individual with diabetes who is treated with insulin or a secretagogue starts a new exercise program. For example, for these individuals, blood glucose should be checked before and after each exercise session. Those with blood glucose levels <100 mg $\cdot$ dL^{-1} should consume 20–30 g of carbohydrate before exercising, whereas those >300 mg $\cdot$ dL^{-1} should preclude exercise until blood glucose control is restored. Those taking other antidiabetic medications may benefit from blood glucose assessment when beginning an exercise program but can reduce the frequency of monitoring if their blood glucose values are stable. Furthermore, hypoglycemia may occur hours after the exercise session if the individual is on exogenous insulin. For more details related to exercise and diabetes, see the position stand by the ACSM (2), Chapter 10 of *GETP9*, Chapters 26 and 40 of this *Resource Manual*, or the American Diabetes Association's (ADA) recommendations (4,32) (http://www.diabetes.org).

OLDER ADULTS

Regular exercise contributes to successful aging. Just as with younger adults, older adults (65 yr of age and older) should engage in regular physical activity most days of the week and avoid becoming sedentary. Evidence-based research suggests that an active lifestyle in older adulthood affords physiological, psychological, and cognitive benefits. An older adult's exercise plan should include not only aerobic exercise, muscular strength training, and flexibility exercise but also balance and mobility

training to decrease risk of falling. For those without medical conditions, the exercise prescription recommendations are similar to that of younger adults. As with all exercise programs, special considerations must be taken into account for individuals with chronic diseases, medical limitations, or previously sedentary behavior. Therefore, the need for medical clearance and preexercise testing will be determined in part by the mode and intensity of exercise desired, as well as the specific medical conditions presented (3,16,30).

Several physiologic changes occur with aging, and they affect how older individuals respond to acute exercise and training. Maximal HR, left ventricular (LV) function, and cardiac output decrease with age, and there is general loss of muscle mass. For more details regarding the physiologic response to aging, refer to Chapter 5 in this *Resource Manual*. The musculoskeletal changes are further complicated by compromised balance and mobility in older individuals. Given the concerns of comorbidities, the referral of older individuals to their primary care physicians for clearance may be the prudent course of action. Although healthy older adults may begin a low-to-moderate intensity exercise program in an unsupervised setting, others may indeed need to begin in medically supervised exercise programs and then potentially graduate to unsupervised sessions (3). Older individuals who have been sedentary for an extended period will need to have an extended buildup period, in terms of both intensity and duration, as they begin a new exercise program. This buildup period could take a few weeks but as much as a few months. Furthermore, given the high prevalence of functional limitations in this population, low-impact simple activities such as walking or stationary biking are recommended. Additional information about exercise testing and prescription for older adults is provided in Chapter 10 of *GETP9*; Chapters 5, 28, and 36 of this *Resource Manual*; and the ACSM position stand (3). Furthermore, the National Institute on Aging (NIA), a division of the National Institutes of Health (NIH), and the American Association of Retired People (AARP) Web sites provide excellent public resources for exercise in elderly individuals (http://nihseniorhealth.com; http://www.aarp.org/health/fitness).

ARTHRITIS

Regular exercise can reduce joint pain and stiffness and increase flexibility, muscle strength, cardiac fitness, and endurance in individuals with arthritis. It also helps with weight reduction and contributes to an improved sense of well-being. Exercise is considered by many health professionals to be one part of a comprehensive arthritis treatment plan. Individuals with arthritis should discuss exercise options with their physicians and other health care providers. A physician may refer the patient to a physical therapist or other exercise professional who can help design an appropriate exercise program and teach patients about pain relief methods, proper body mechanics, and joint protection. There are many types of arthritis. Experienced physicians, physical therapists, and occupational therapists can recommend exercises that are particularly helpful for specific types of arthritis. Physicians and therapists also know specific exercises for particularly painful joints. There may be exercises that are off limits for people with a particular type of arthritis or when the joints are swollen and inflamed. Many people with arthritis begin with easy, ROM exercises and low-impact aerobics. People with arthritis can participate in a variety of, but not all, exercise programs. The three types of exercise often cited as best for people with arthritis are ROM exercises, resistance training, and aerobic exercises. Weight control can be important to people who have arthritis because extra weight puts extra pressure on the joints. Some studies show that aerobic exercise can reduce inflammation in some joints. For more details related to exercise and arthritis, refer to Chapter 10 of *GETP9*, Chapter 43 in this *Resource Manual*, and the Arthritis Foundation's Web site (http://www.arthritis.org).

OSTEOPOROSIS

Aerobic weight-bearing exercise and resistance training have an important role in both the prevention and treatment of osteoporosis (1,12,17,18,29,31). It is well known that the best way to build bone is by increasing the magnitude of strain in several different directions on the skeleton, thereby imposing sufficient overload to facilitate skeletal adaptations (18). Although this may be optimal for bone mass improvement, and especially relevant for the treatment of osteopenia, it is generally not optimal for the clinical management of osteoporosis. In fact, some research has shown that most middle-aged and older adults exercise within their "comfort zone" (not an overload zone), which will assist in the maintenance of bone mass but will not stimulate the growth of new bone (12). The diagnosis and management of osteoporosis has its own set of safety concerns, and the start of any new exercise in an individual with osteoporosis should not be undertaken without physician approval, licensed physical therapist, or certified/registered clinical exercise physiologist consultation (29). Particular attention must be given to individuals with a previous history of falls or impaired balance. Certain movements (*e.g.*, twisting of the spine, high-impact aerobics, bending from the waist) should be avoided in individuals with osteoporosis (29). A primary concern in individuals with osteoporosis is avoiding fractures, and preventing falls is essential to this goal. Thus, when working with individuals with osteoporosis, helping prevent opportunities to fall should always be a top priority. For more detailed information, refer to Chapter 10 of *GETP9*, Chapter 42

in this *Resource Manual*, the ACSM position stand (17), *WHO Global Report on Falls Prevention in Older Age* (31), and the National Osteoporosis Foundation Web site (http://www.nor.org).

SPECIAL SAFETY CONSIDERATIONS FOR RESISTANCE TRAINING

Numerous investigations in healthy adults, low-risk patients with cardiac disease, and those with other medical conditions have reported few orthopedic complications or cardiovascular events associated with light-to-moderate resistance training (1,23,29). The revised 2009 ACSM position stand on resistance training for healthy adults incorporates the vast array of resistance training paradigms available for more advanced training. It does not, however, address the safety of resistance testing and training in moderate-risk to higher risk populations such as patients with cardiac disease or those with other medical conditions. Contraindications to resistance training are similar to those used to assess readiness to start an aerobic exercise program. Contraindications to resistance training include unstable angina; uncontrolled hypertension; uncontrolled dysrhythmias; recent history of congestive heart failure, which has not been evaluated and effectively treated; severe stenotic or regurgitant valvular disease; and hypertrophic cardiomyopathy. Because patients with myocardial ischemia or poor LV function may develop wall-motion abnormalities or serious ventricular arrhythmias during resistance training exertion, moderate-to-good LV function and cardiorespiratory fitness (>5 metabolic equivalents) without anginal symptoms or ischemic ST-segment depression have been suggested as additional prerequisites for participation in traditional resistance training programs, with cardiac medications maintained as clinically indicated.

Low-to-moderate risk patients with cardiac disease who wish to initiate mild-to-moderate resistance training should first participate in a traditional aerobic exercise program for a minimum of 5 wk (*GETP9*, Chapter 9). This period permits sufficient surveillance of the patient in a supervised setting and allows the cardiorespiratory and musculoskeletal adaptations that may reduce the potential for complications to occur (1).

A preliminary orientation should establish appropriate weight loads and instruct the participant on proper lifting techniques, ROM for each exercise, correct breathing patterns to avoid straining, and the Valsalva maneuver. Because systolic BP measurements taken by the standard cuff method immediately after resistance exercise may significantly underestimate true physiologic responses, such measurement is usually not recommended. For more details related to resistance training and health, see Chapters 7 and 9 in *GETP9*, Chapter 31 in this *Resource Manual*, Pollock et al. (23), and the ACSM's 2009 position stand on resistance training in adults (1).

SUMMARY

The purpose of preparticipation health screening is to provide information relevant to the safety of fitness testing or beginning exercise training to identify known diseases and risk factors for CVD so that appropriate lifestyle interventions can be initiated. Furthermore, it is important to identify additional factors that require special consideration when developing appropriate exercise prescription and programming that will optimize adherence, minimize risks, and maximize benefits. The precise nature and extent of the appraisal should be determined by the age, sex, and perceived health status characteristics of the participants, as well as the available economic, personnel, and equipment resources. The primary safety goal of a preparticipation health appraisal is to identify individuals who should receive further medical evaluation to determine whether there are contraindications to exercise testing or training or whether referral to a medically supervised exercise program is necessary.

REFERENCES

1. American College of Sports Medicine. American College of Sports Medicine position stand. Progression models in resistance training for healthy adults. *Med Sci Sports Exerc*. 2009;41(3):687–708.
2. American College of Sports Medicine, American Diabetes Association. Exercise and type 2 diabetes: American College of Sports Medicine and the American Diabetes Association: joint position statement. *Med Sci Sports Exerc*. 2010;42(12):2282–303.
3. American College of Sports Medicine, Chodzko-Zajko WJ, Proctor DN, et al. American College of Sports Medicine position stand. Exercise and physical activity for older adults. *Med Sci Sports Exerc*. 2009;41(7):1510–30.
4. American Diabetes Association. Standards of medical care in diabetes—2009. *Diabetes Care*. 2009;32 Suppl 1:S13–61.
5. Balady GJ, Chaitman B, Driscoll D, et al. Recommendations for cardiovascular screening, staffing, and emergency policies at health/fitness facilities. *Circulation*. 1998;97(22):2283–93.
6. Bestall JC, Paul EA, Garrod R, Garnham R, Jones PW, Wedzicha JA. Usefulness of the Medical Research Council (MRC) dyspnoea scale as a measure of disability in patients with chronic obstructive pulmonary disease. *Thorax*. 1999;54(7):581–6.
7. *Cardiovascular Risk Reduction Guidelines in Adults: Cholesterol Guideline Update (ATP IV) Hypertension Guideline Update (JNC 8) Obesity Guideline Update (Obesity 2) Integrated Cardiovascular Risk Reduction Guideline: Timeline for Release of Updated Guidelines* [Internet]. Bethesda (MD): National Heart, Lung and Blood Institute; National Institutes of Health; 2011 [cited 2011 Jul 7]. Available from: http://www.nhlbi.nih.gov/guidelines/cvd_adult/background.htm
8. Centers for Disease Control and Prevention. Prevalence of no leisure-time physical activity—35 States and the District of Columbia, 1988-2002. *MMWR Morb Mortal Wkly Rep*. 2004;53(4):82–6.
9. Chobanian AV, Bakris GL, Black HR, et al. The Seventh Report of the Joint National Committee on Prevention, Detection, Evaluation, and Treatment of High Blood Pressure: the JNC 7 report. *JAMA*. 2003;289(19):2560–72.
10. Expert Panel on Detection, Evaluation, and Treatment of High Blood Cholesterol in Adults. Executive Summary of the Third Report of the National Cholesterol Education Program (NCEP) Expert Panel on Detection, Evaluation, and Treatment of High Blood Cholesterol in Adults (Adult Treatment Panel III). *JAMA*. 2001;285(19):2486–97.
11. Flegal KM, Carroll MD, Ogden CL, Curtin LR. Prevalence and trends in obesity among US adults, 1999-2008. *JAMA*. 2010;303(3):235–41.
12. Frost HM. Why do marathon runners have less bone than weight lifters? A vital-biomechanical view and explanation. *Bone*. 1997;20(3):183–9.
13. *Global Strategy for the Diagnosis, Management, and Prevention of COPD* [Internet]. Bethesda (MD): Global Initiative for Chronic Obstructive Lung Disease; 2011 [cited 2011 Apr 6]. 90 p. Available from: http://www.goldcopd.org/
14. Goldstein LB, Bushnell CD, Adams RJ, et al. Guidelines for the primary prevention of stroke: a guideline for healthcare professionals from the American Heart Association/American Stroke Association. *Stroke*. 2011;42(2):517–84.
15. Grundy SM, Cleeman JI, Merz CN, et al. Implications of recent clinical trials for the National Cholesterol Education Program Adult Treatment Panel III guidelines. *Circulation*. 2004;110(2):227–39.
16. Haskell WL, Lee IM, Pate RR, et al. Physical activity and public health: updated recommendation for adults from the American College of Sports Medicine and the American Heart Association. *Circulation*. 2007;116(9):1081–93.
17. Kohrt WM, Bloomfield SA, Little KD, Nelson ME, Yingling VR, American College of Sports Medicine. American College of Sports Medicine position stand: physical activity and bone health. *Med Sci Sports Exerc*. 2004;36(11):1985–96.
18. Manske SL, Lorincz CR, Zernicke RF. Bone health: part 2, physical activity. *Sports Health*. 2009;1(4):341–6.
19. Mosca L, Benjamin EJ, Berra K, et al. Effectiveness-based guidelines for the prevention of cardiovascular disease in women—2011 update: a guideline from the American Heart Association. *Circulation*. 2011;123(11):1243–62.
20. *NICE Guidelines. Hypertension: Clinical Management of Primary Hypertension in Adults* [Internet]. London, United Kingdom: NHS; National Institute for Health and Clinical Excellence; 2011 [cited 2011 Jul 8]. 39 p. Available from: http://www.nice.org.uk/nicemedia/live/12167/53225/53225.pdf
21. Nishimura K, Izumi T, Tsukino M, Oga T. Dyspnea is a better predictor of 5-year survival than airway obstruction in patients with COPD. *Chest*. 2002;121(5):1434–40.
22. Pescatello LS, Franklin BA, Fagard R, et al. American College of Sports Medicine position stand. Exercise and hypertension. *Med Sci Sports Exerc*. 2004;36(3):533–53.
23. Pollock ML, Franklin BA, Balady GJ, et al. AHA Science Advisory. Resistance exercise in individuals with and without cardiovascular disease: benefits, rationale, safety, and prescription: an advisory from the Committee on Exercise, Rehabilitation, and Prevention, Council on Clinical Cardiology, American Heart Association; Position paper endorsed by the American College of Sports Medicine. *Circulation*. 2000;101(7):828–33.
24. Ries AL, Bauldoff GS, Carlin BW, et al. Joint American College of Chest Physicians/American Association of Cardiovascular and Pulmonary Rehabilitation Evidence-Based Clinical Practice Guidelines. *Chest*. 2007;131(5 Suppl):S1–3.
25. Ries AL, Bauldoff GS, Carlin BW, et al. Pulmonary Rehabilitation: Joint ACCP/AACVPR Evidence-Based Clinical Practice Guidelines. *Chest*. 2007;131(5 Suppl):4S–42S.
26. Shephard RJ, Thomas S, Weller I. The Canadian Home Fitness Test. 1991 update. *Sports Med*. 1991;11(6):358–66.
27. Smith SC Jr, Allen J, Blair SN, et al. AHA/ACC guidelines for secondary prevention for patients with coronary and other atherosclerotic vascular disease: 2006 update: endorsed by the National

Heart, Lung, and Blood Institute. *Circulation*. 2006;113(19): 2363–72.

28. *The Surgeon General's Vision for a Healthy and Fit Nation 2010* [Internet]. Rockville (MD): U.S. Department of Health and Human Services; 2010 [cited 2011 Jul 8]. 21 p. Available from: http://www .surgeongeneral.gov/library/obesityvision/obesityvision2010.pdf

29. Swank AM. *Resistance Training for Special Populations: Quick Reference Guide*. Clifton Park (NY): Delmar Pub; 2009. 538 p.

30. U.S. Department of Health and Human Services. Active older adults. In: *2008 Physical Activity Guidelines for Americans: Be Active, Healthy, and Happy!* Washington: U.S. Department of Health and Human Services; 2008. p. 29–34.

31. *WHO Global Report on Falls Prevention in Older Age* [Internet]. Geneva, Switzerland: World Health Organization; 2007 [cited 2011 Jul 8]. 53 p. Available from: http://whqlibdoc.who.int/publications/ 2008/9789241563536_eng.pdf

32. Zinman B, Ruderman N, Campaigne BN, Devlin JT, Schneider SH, American Diabetes Association. Physical activity/exercise and diabetes. *Diabetes Care*. 2004;27 Suppl 1:S58–62.

SELECTED REFERENCES FOR FURTHER READING

American Association of Cardiovascular and Pulmonary Rehabilitation. *AAVCPR Cardiac Rehab Resource Manual*. Champaign (IL): Human Kinetics; 2006.

American Association of Cardiovascular and Pulmonary Rehabilitation. *Guidelines for Cardiac Rehabilitation and Secondly Prevention Programs*. 4th ed. Champaign (IL): Human Kinetics; 2004.

National Strength and Conditioning Association. *Essentials of Strength Training and Conditioning*. 3rd ed. Champaign (IL): Human Kinetics; 2008.

INTERNET RESOURCES

- American Association of Cardiovascular and Pulmonary Rehabilitation: http://www.aacvpr.org
- American Association of Retired People (AARP): http://www.aarp .org/health/fitness
- American Diabetes Association: http://www.diabetes.org
- American Heart Association: http://www.americanheart.org
- American Lung Association: http://www.lungusa.org
- American Society of Hypertension: http://www.ash-us.org
- Arthritis Foundation: http://www.arthritis.org
- Global Initiative for Chronic Obstructive Lung Disease: http:// www.goldcopd.com
- National Institute of Aging (NIA): http://nihseniorhealth.com
- National Osteoporosis Foundation: http://www.nor.org
- World Health Organization, Aging and Falls Prevention: http:// www.who.int/ageing/projects/falls_prevention_older_age/en/ index.html

Physical Activity Status and Chronic Diseases

The purpose of this chapter is to examine the relationship between physical activity and physical fitness and chronic disease with particular emphasis on risk for all-cause and cardiovascular mortality, cardiovascular disease, stroke, Type 2 diabetes mellitus, hypertension, and cancer. Available data that relate changes in physical activity level or physical fitness to health outcomes will also be examined.

It has been recognized since antiquity that regular physical activity is necessary for human well-being and that, in turn, physical inactivity is a major modifiable risk factor for premature mortality and development of chronic disease (19,21,63,100,126). Given the high prevalence of physical inactivity observed in many developed and developing nations, the burden of physical inactivity on public health is substantial (18,28,106,134,135).

A recent report from the World Health Organization estimates that close to 60% of the world population is inactive or insufficiently active and that this physical inactivity causes 21%–25% of breast and colon cancer, 27% of diabetes, and 30% of the worldwide ischemic heart disease burden (135).

In October 2008, the U.S. Federal Government released "The Physical Activity Guidelines for Americans" (1). This document, for the first time, provides a national government-sanctioned recommendation for physical activity for all ages. These guidelines were developed with the broader view that links physical inactivity to the development of many chronic diseases. There are also specific guidelines for those with disabilities, children, and pregnant/postpartum women. The Surgeon General's Report on Physical Activity and Health serves

KEY TERMS

Confidence interval (CI): A range around a relative risk estimate that refers to the probability that the range includes the true value of the relative risk estimate.

Dose-response relationship: A relationship between two variables in which any increase or change in one variable is associated with a corresponding change in the other variable. A dose-response relationship does not have to be linear, but it can follow several patterns (*e.g.*, curvilinear, quadratic).

Epidemiology: The study of the distribution and determinants of disease or injury in large populations.

Intervention study: A study in which participants are assigned to undergo an intervention to test the strength of that intervention on previously selected outcome variables, such as cardiorespiratory fitness, serum levels of lipids or lipoproteins, parameters of insulin action, bone mineral density, muscle strength and endurance, or the like. The best intervention studies are those that randomly assign participants to treatment assignment, one of which is a null intervention assignment or control group, which

are carried out in parallel. These are referred to as *randomized controlled clinical trials* (RCTs) and carry the highest level of evidence relating an activity or intervention to prespecified outcomes.

Physical activity: Any bodily movement produced by the contraction of skeletal muscles that substantially increases energy expenditure.

Physical fitness: An attained set of attributes (*e.g.*, cardiorespiratory capacity and endurance; flexibility; body composition; skeletal muscle strength and endurance) that relates to the ability to perform physical activity.

Physical inactivity: A behavioral state of not achieving, on a regular basis, a certain minimal common standard of physical activity.

Relative risk (RR): The risk of disease or injury in one group compared with another group. The two groups usually differ in terms of one or more key factors (*e.g.*, physical activity levels). RR is usually expressed as a risk ratio comparing incidence or prevalence rates among two groups.

as a valuable resource of the body of literature available before 1996 (126). A report of the Institute of Medicine that briefly reviews physical activity and chronic disease is available (109), summarizing some of the new data available before October 2006.

IS PHYSICAL ACTIVITY OR PHYSICAL FITNESS THE APPROPRIATE PREDICTOR FOR HEALTH OUTCOMES?

A question of interest to epidemiologists, public health officials, and clinicians is whether physical activity or physical fitness best predicts the risk of chronic disease. Physical fitness as assessed by measurement of maximal oxygen uptake has a strong inherited or familial component in that between 30% and 50% of the variation in cardiorespiratory fitness levels among untrained sedentary individuals can be explained by genetic and shared lifestyle factors (20). Although physical fitness can be accurately and precisely measured, such measurements are equipment-intensive and expensive and generally not feasible in large population based studies. Physical activity can also be measured directly through doubly labeled water techniques or use of accelerometers, but such measurements are cumbersome and costly and motion sensors are only suitable for certain activities (132). Most large epidemiological investigations thus rely on physical activity assessments by self-report, which are low in cost and generally well received by participants (13). These self-report instruments include diaries, logs of specific activities, and questionnaires of varying detail and participant burden. Such self-report instruments are, however, subject to inaccurate recall and report bias and several tend to underestimate very low intensity activities (13,70,72). Although both physical fitness and physical activity show a strong dose-response relationship with health outcomes, this relationship is steeper for physical fitness than for physical activity (15,138).

To date, there are no randomized intervention study in healthy populations that have assessed the link between changes in physical activity and subsequent mortality or cardiovascular events. The length of time required for such trials make them impractical. However, several exercise training trials in populations with established risk factors or cardiovascular illness have been conducted in recent years and will be reviewed later in this chapter. Several smaller trials with intermediate endpoints (*e.g.*, cardiorespiratory fitness and metabolic measures) in sedentary but otherwise healthy populations have been published that suggest that even relatively modest changes in physical activity can have substantial benefits (24,116). Public health interventions designed to increase physical activity levels thus have a firm scientific basis. Future studies should assess the optimal intensity, frequency, and type of activity (*e.g.*, aerobic exercise vs. resistance training vs. both) for specific intermediate health outcomes (*e.g.*, improvements in glucose metabolism, insulin sensitivity, lipid metabolism, blood pressure control, and in the inflammatory state) as well as subsequent clinical events and mortality.

THE SCIENTIFIC EVIDENCE

Epidemiology is the study of the distribution and determinants of disease or injury in large populations, and physical activity epidemiologists place a particular emphasis on physical inactivity and poor physical fitness as risk factors for disease and injury. The studies described in this chapter use mainly observational prospective designs in which a group of people is evaluated for a given set of baseline characteristics (*e.g.*, age, sex, physical activity, physical fitness, obesity) and followed over time to describe the incidence of disease, injury, or mortality. In most studies, the incidence of chronic disease in two or more groups that differ from one another in their level of physical activity or fitness are compared using a ratio called the relative risk (RR). The confidence in the point estimate of the RR (*i.e.*, the precision) is generally expressed as a 90% or 95% confidence interval (CI) around the RR. If the 95% CI crosses the value of 1 (*i.e.*, a ratio of equal risk in the two populations being compared), the RR is not statistically significant. For an in-depth description of the study designs used in epidemiology with reference to research in exercise science, readers are referred to the reviews of Heath (54) and Paffenbarger (99) and the book edited by Lee (76).

Modern physical activity epidemiology arguably began with the classic studies of occupational physical activity and subsequent incidence of coronary heart disease (CHD) conducted by Jeremy Morris et al. in the 1950s (100). These early studies demonstrated that men in physically demanding occupations (bus conductors and postmen) had lower incident CHD rates than men in less demanding occupations (bus drivers and office workers) (92). A comprehensive review of the physical activity or physical fitness literature that has accumulated over the last 60 yr is beyond the scope of this chapter. Rather, this chapter will cite relevant reviews or meta-analyses and illustrate study methodology and outcomes with selected studies for each outcome as appropriate.

PHYSICAL ACTIVITY OR PHYSICAL FITNESS AND ALL-CAUSE MORTALITY

Among the major causes of mortality in the United States are heart disease (26.3%), cancer (22.9%), stroke (6.2%), and diabetes mellitus (3.0%) (36). Thus, discussions of physical activity or physical fitness and all-cause mortality largely reflect the relationship between physical activity or physical fitness and these major chronic diseases. Readers are referred to several excellent reviews and meta-analyses of the topic (29,67,78,80,83,97,140). Several key studies are used here to illustrate the relationships between physical activity and physical fitness, respectively, and all-cause mortality.

The Harvard Alumni Study is a prospective observational study of approximately 17,000 men who attended Harvard University between 1916 and 1950. The results of a 16-yr follow-up of physical activity levels and all-cause mortality revealed an inverse dose-response relationship between physical activity levels and all-cause mortality (*Fig. 12-1*, bottom panel) (101). Greater levels of physical activity were associated with a lower risk of death from all causes, and men who expended $\geq$2,000 kcal $\cdot$ week^{-1} (8,372 kJ $\cdot$ week^{-1}) of energy in physical activity had a 27% lower risk of mortality compared with men expending <2,000 kcal $\cdot$ week^{-1}. Although this study was limited to young men, similarly strong associations between physical activity level and mortality have been found for middle-aged and older women and men as summarized in several recent meta-analyses (29,67,83,97,140). The greatest reduction in mortality is seen between sedentary subjects and those who are mildly or moderately active, whereas further increases in physical activity level are associated with additional but smaller incremental benefit.

The Aerobics Center Longitudinal Study (ACLS) is a prospective observational study that assessed physical fitness and health outcomes among men and women receiving a preventive medical examination, including a graded exercise treadmill test, at the Cooper Clinic in Dallas, Texas. The results depicted in *Figure 12-1* are from an analysis of approximately 10,000 men and 3,000 women followed for 8 yr for all-cause mortality in relation to initial level (quintiles) of cardiorespiratory fitness (*Fig. 12-1*, top panel) (17). A strong inverse relationship between cardiorespiratory fitness and all-cause mortality was observed in both sexes. Men and women in the lowest fitness quintile were 3.44 (95% CI: 2.05–5.77) and 4.65 (95% CI: 2.22–9.75) times more likely to die of any cause compared with men and women in the highest quintile, respectively. The greatest decrease in the risk of mortality was observed between the first and second quintiles.

In the St. James Women Take Heart Project, more than 5,000 asymptomatic women without known CHD were followed for 8 yr after undergoing treadmill exercise testing at baseline (50). Exercise capacity was strongly predictive of mortality with a 17% decline in risk of death for every 1 metabolic equivalent (MET) greater exercise capacity. The prognostic value of exercise capacity was independent of the Framingham Risk Score. Among asymptomatic women in the Lipid Research Clinics Study, exercise capacity was a similarly powerful predictor of mortality over 20 yr of follow-up (91).

The prospective relationship between cardiorespiratory fitness and mortality also holds for individuals with cardiovascular disease as demonstrated in an

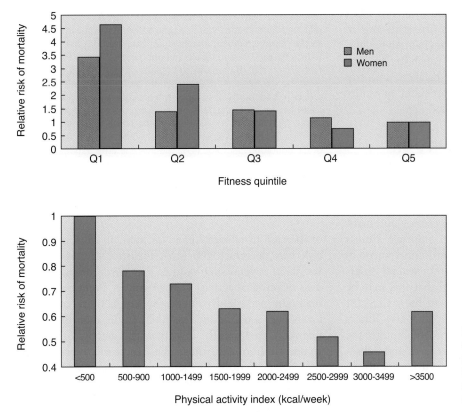

FIGURE 12-1. Relative risks of all-cause mortality across levels of cardiorespiratory fitness in the Aerobics Center Longitudinal Study (17) (*top panel*) and physical activity in the Harvard Alumni Study (101) (*bottom panel*).

8.5-yr follow-up study from the Lipid Research Clinics Study (32). The RRs of all-cause mortality for physical fitness (per two standard deviation lower treadmill time) in healthy men and men with cardiovascular disease were 1.8 (95% CI: 1.2–2.6) and 2.9 (95% CI: 1.7–4.9), respectively. An analysis from the ACLS, shows that the relationship between cardiorespiratory fitness (high-fit vs. low-fit) and all-cause mortality is similar for normotensive men (RR = 0.50 [95% CI: 0.37–0.68]), hypertensive men (RR = 0.42 [95% CI: 0.27–0.66]) and individuals with white-coat hypertension (RR = 0.44 [95% CI: 0.29–0.68]) (25). Similar results were also seen for cardiovascular disease mortality in all three groups (25). Another analysis from the ACLS cohort examined the relationship between cardiorespiratory fitness and mortality in men with Type 2 diabetes (n = 1,263) (129). Compared with men in the low-fit group, men in the high-fit group had an RR of all-cause mortality of 0.48 (95% CI: 0.34–0.67) after adjustment for age, examination year, and traditional lifestyle and conventional risk factors. Thus, there is consistent evidence that physically fit men with existing chronic conditions such as cardiovascular disease, hypertension, or Type 2 diabetes have a lower risk of mortality compared with men who are unfit. More research is required to confirm these findings in women and different ethnic groups.

Kodama et al. recently summarized data from 33 studies of cardiorespiratory fitness and mortality and reported that a 1 MET level difference in maximal aerobic capacity was associated with a 13% decrement in all-cause mortality, a risk decrease comparable to that associated with a 5 mm Hg lower systolic blood pressure (67). For older individuals, maximal cardiorespiratory fitness testing on a treadmill may be difficult. A recent meta-analysis suggests that other measures of physical capability such as walking speed, chair rising, standing balance, and grip strength are also associated with subsequent mortality and can thus be used for prognostication (29).

CHANGES IN PHYSICAL ACTIVITY OR FITNESS AND ALL-CAUSE MORTALITY

The studies cited earlier show associations between physical activity and physical fitness level at a single time and all-cause mortality, but we cannot automatically infer that physical training to improve fitness level would also be associated with an improvement in mortality. There is indirect evidence from several observational data sets, however, to suggest that this may be the case (12,16,34,47,69,82,102,128). In the ACLS, for example, almost 10,000 men participated in two fitness evaluations, allowing the investigators to explore the relationship between change in fitness level and subsequent mortality (16). Men who improved from unfit to fit had a 44% reduction in mortality compared to men who were unfit at both examinations. For every minute

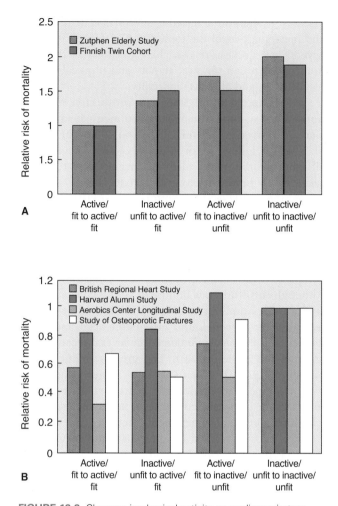

FIGURE 12-2. Changes in physical activity or cardiorespiratory fitness and relative risks of all-cause mortality. **A** presents the results of two studies that used the active/fit to active/fit group as the reference group; results in left bars are from the Zutphen Elderly Study (12), and results in right bars are from a Finnish twin cohort (69). **B** presents the results of four studies that used the inactive/unfit to inactive/unfit group as the reference group; results from left to right bars are from the British Regional Heart Study (128), results in red are from the Harvard Alumni Study (102), results in pink are from the Aerobics Center Longitudinal Study (16), and results in white are from the Study of Osteoporotic Fractures (47). The average time between successive measurements of physical activity and cardiorespiratory fitness ranged from approximately 6 yr to 11–15 yr.

of increase in maximal exercise time, all-cause mortality risk was decreased 8% (16). *Figure 12-2* presents the results of several such studies that used comparable fitness or physical activity change groups. Participants who maintain persistently high physical activity or fitness levels over a period are less likely to die than those who maintain consistently low physical activity or fitness levels. Additionally, those who increase their level of physical activity or fitness over time have a decreased risk of mortality compared with those who were consistently physically inactive or unfit. Among individuals who were active/fit initially, but then decreased their activity or fitness level, prognosis was worse than among those who maintained their activity or fitness level, but still better than among those who were persistently inactive/unfit. This finding suggests that there is a beneficial "legacy effect" of physical activity and fitness that persists over time, similar to what has been reported with some pharmacological interventions for metabolic risk factors (*e.g.*, cholesterol lowering treatment, glucose lowering treatment).

As suggested earlier, when differences in prognosis are charted for successive quintiles, the greatest decrease in mortality is found between the least fit and the next higher quintile. Not surprisingly, even modest walking regimens are associated with measurable benefit (51). Improvements in fitness level that would reclassify an individual from the lowest quintile for fitness to the next higher quintile can be achieved by participating in a program similar to the American College of Sports Medicine (ACSM)/American Heart Association (AHA) recommendations for physical activity for health (*i.e.*, a minimum of 30 min of moderate-intensity aerobic physical activity on 5 d each week or 20 min of vigorous-intensity aerobic activity on 3 d each week [53]) or the more recently issued National Physical Activity Guidelines (1).

PHYSICAL ACTIVITY AND CORONARY HEART DISEASE

Over the last 60 yr, a large body of evidence linking physical inactivity to the risk of incident and recurrent CHD has accumulated, and the relationship between physical activity and CHD is believed to be causal. In cross-sectional studies, active individuals have better CHD risk factor profiles than their sedentary counterparts. Physical activity levels predict incident risk factors in longitudinal observational studies, and exercise training interventions clearly demonstrate that several classic risk factors for CHD can be favorably altered by exercise, including blood pressure, blood cholesterol, blood glucose and inflammatory markers. Therefore, it is likely that a significant proportion of the benefit of physical activity on CHD outcomes is mediated through these classic CHD risk factors. However, an inverse association between physical activity and CHD persists even after adjustment for traditional CHD risk factors, suggesting an additional direct impact of physical activity on CHD risk (90).

A 1990 meta-analysis of studies investigating the relationship between physical activity and CHD estimated a summary RR of 1.4 (95% CI: 1.0–1.8) based on four studies comparing sedentary versus active occupations and a summary RR of 1.6 (95% CI: 1.3–1.8) based on five studies comparing low versus high leisure time physical activity (10). The corresponding analysis for CHD death produced a summary (five studies) RR of 1.9 (95% CI: 1.6–2.2) comparing sedentary and active occupations

and a summary (two studies) RR of 1.9 (95% CI: 1.0–3.4) for low versus high leisure time physical activity (10). A more recent analysis supports the notion that the relationship between physical activity and CHD follows a dose-response pattern (68). This dose-response relationship, however, has yet to be proven rigorously in a prospective randomized clinical trial.

Exercise capacity as determined by exercise treadmill testing in the clinical setting also predicts future CHD events among individuals with stable CHD or prior myocardial infarction (7,38). Exercise capacity can also be assessed in the clinical setting by questionnaires such as the Duke Activity Status Index (DASI) (56). This index, validated against exercise capacity achieved by Bruce treadmill protocol exercise testing, proved to be a powerful prognostic indicator among women with suspected ischemia enrolled in the Women's Ischemia Syndrome Evaluation Study (115). Women with an exercise capacity ≥10 METs had a 95% 5-yr survival rate free of death or myocardial infarction compared to a rate of 85% among women with estimated exercise capacity of ≤4.7 METs. In this cohort, 67% of all deaths or myocardial infarctions occurred in women whose DASI METs were ≤4.7.

The most direct evidence that exercise training affects cardiac mortality comes from the randomized clinical trials of cardiac rehabilitation among individuals with prevalent CHD. In a meta-analysis of 48 such trials that enrolled predominantly individuals with prior myocardial infarctions, Taylor and colleagues reported a 20% decrease in all-cause mortality and a 24% decrease in cardiac mortality in the active intervention group (120). This benefit was seen with exercise only trials as well as trials of more comprehensive cardiac rehabilitation. An updated analysis recently reported statistically significant reductions in cardiovascular and total mortality of 13% and 26%, respectively, in studies with 12 or more months follow-up and a reduction in hospital admissions by 31% in shorter term studies (55).

Given this strong scientific foundation, recommendations for physical activity as an integral part of a healthy lifestyle have been included in clinical guidelines and performance measures for primary and secondary prevention of CHD (5,31,93,95,104,108,117,122).

PHYSICAL ACTIVITY AND STROKE

Selected prospective studies of physical activity/fitness and risk of stroke are summarized in *Table 12-1* (2,3,11,35,44,52,59,64,74,77,79,81,111–113,127). As reviewed in a meta-analysis by Lee et al., these studies support a link between moderate and high physical activity and reduced risk of stroke (75), stronger for total and ischemic stroke compared to hemorrhagic stroke. The dose-response relationship between physical activity and stroke is less well documented than that between physical activity and CHD. One study

TABLE 12-1. Results of Selected Prospective Longitudinal Studies of Physical Inactivity or Physical Fitness and Risk of Stroke

Population	Sample Size	Stroke Classification	Activity/Fitness Classification	RR (95% CI)
Finnish women (112)	3,688	Incident stroke (ICD 430–437)	None vs. some LTPA	1.30 (0.73–2.16)[a]
Finnish men (112)	3,978	Incident stroke (ICD 430–437)	None vs. some LTPA	1.00 (0.65–1.62)[a]
Swedish men (52)	7,495	Total stroke mortality	PA score 1 vs. scores 2–4	1.20 (0.80–1.80)
		Subarachnoid hemorrhage mortality	PA score 1 vs. scores 2–4	1.80 (0.60–5.50)
		Intracerebral hemorrhage mortality	PA score 1 vs. scores 2–4	1.10 (0.40–3.70)
		Cerebral infarction mortality	PA score 1 vs. scores 2–4	1.20 (0.70–2.00)
		Unspecified stroke mortality	PA score 1 vs. scores 2–4	1.20 (0.60–2.20)
Seventh-day Adventist men (81)	9,484	Stroke mortality	Low vs. moderate PA	1.28 (1.00–1.64)
			Low vs. high PA	1.06 (0.74–1.54)
British men (127)	7,630	Incident stroke (ICD 430–438)	None vs. occasional PA	1.25 (0.59–2.50)
			None vs. light PA	1.67 (0.77–5.00)
			None vs. moderate PA	1.67 (0.67–5.00)
			None vs. moderately vigorous PA	1.67 (0.63–5.00)
			None vs. vigorous PA	5.00 (0.67– >10.00)
Asian American men (2)	7,530	Incident hemorrhagic stroke	Middle vs. high tertile PA	2.20 (0.80–6.40)
			Low vs. high tertile PA	3.70 (1.30–10.40)
		Incident thromboembolic stroke	*Nonsmokers*	
			Middle vs. high tertile PA	1.70 (1.00–2.80)
			Low vs. high tertile PA	1.80 (1.10–3.10)
			Smokers	
			Middle vs. high tertile PA	0.60 (0.40–1.00)
			Low vs. high tertile PA	1.20 (0.80–1.80)
Framingham Study men (64)	1,228	Incident stroke	Tertile 1 vs. tertile 2 PA	2.44 (1.45–4.17)
			Tertile 1 vs. tertile 3 PA	1.89 (1.19–2.94)
Framingham Study women (64)	1,676	Incident stroke	Tertile 1 vs. tertile 2 PA	1.03 (0.68–1.56)
			Tertile 1 vs. tertile 3 PA	0.83 (0.51–1.33)
U.S. white women (44)	1,473	Incident stroke	Moderate vs. high LTPA	1.80 (0.52–6.22)
			Low vs. high LTPA	3.13 (0.95–10.32)
		Incident nonhemorrhagic stroke	Moderate vs. high LTPA	1.54 (0.44–5.42)
			Low vs. high LTPA	2.89 (0.87–9.55)
U.S. white men (44)	1,285	Incident stroke	Moderate vs. high LTPA	1.17 (0.61–2.27)
			Low vs. high PA	1.24 (0.63–2.41)
		Incident nonhemorrhagic stroke	Moderate vs. high LTPA	1.16 (0.58–2.32)
			Low vs. high LTPA	1.10 (0.54–2.23)
U.S. black men and women (44)	771	Incident stroke	Moderate vs. high LTPA	1.33 (0.63–2.79)
			Low vs. high PA	1.33 (0.67–2.63)
		Incident nonhemorrhagic stroke	Moderate vs. high LTPA	1.34 (0.61–2.94)
			Low vs. high LTPA	1.43 (0.70–2.94)
Swedish men (111)	7,142	Stroke mortality	Sedentary vs. moderate/high PA	1.12 (0.61–2.04)
Dutch men (11)	802	Stroke mortality (ICD 430–438)	Low vs. middle tertile PA	1.54 (0.80–3.03)
			Low vs. upper tertile PA	1.82 (0.79–4.17)

TABLE 12-1. Results of Selected Prospective Longitudinal Studies of Physical Inactivity or Physical Fitness and Risk of Stroke (*Continued*)

Population	Sample Size	Stroke Classification	Activity/Fitness Classification	RR (95% CI)
Harvard University alumni (79)	11,130	Incident stroke	<4,184 vs. 4,184–8,367 kJ · wk⁻¹ PA	1.32 (1.02–1.69)
			<4,184 vs. 8,368–12,548 kJ · wk⁻¹ PA	1.85 (1.32–2.63)
			<4,184 vs. 12,549–16,736 kJ · wk⁻¹ PA	1.28 (0.87–1.89)
			<4,184 vs. ≥16,736 kJ · wk⁻¹ PA	1.22 (0.88–1.72)
Reykjavik men (3)	4,484	Incident stroke (ICD 430–434,436)	None vs. some PA after age 40 yr	1.45 (0.99–2.13)
		Incident ischemic stroke	None vs. some PA after age 40 yr	1.61 (1.03–2.50)
ARIC study men and women (35)	14,575	Incident ischemic stroke	Low vs. high quartile LTPA	1.12 (0.73–1.75)
U.S. male physicians (77)	21,823	Incident stroke	None vs. vigorous PA 1 time · wk⁻¹	1.27 (0.97–1.64)
			None vs. vigorous PA 2–4 times · wk⁻¹	1.25 (1.01–1.54)
			None vs. vigorous PA 5 times · wk⁻¹	1.27 (0.97–1.64)
		Incident ischemic stroke	None vs. vigorous PA 1 time · wk⁻¹	1.18 (0.88–1.56)
			None vs. vigorous PA 2–4 times · wk⁻¹	1.19 (0.93–1.49)
			None vs. vigorous PA 5 times · wk⁻¹	1.15 (0.86–1.52)
		Incident hemorrhagic stroke	None vs. vigorous PA 1 time · wk⁻¹	1.69 (0.85–3.33)
			None vs. vigorous PA 2–4 times · wk⁻¹	1.45 (0.86–2.44)
			None vs. vigorous PA 5 times · wk⁻¹	1.82 (0.89–3.70)
U.S. female nurses (59)	72,488	Incident stroke	Quintile 1 vs. 2 PA	1.02 (0.78–1.33)
			Quintile 1 vs. 3 PA	1.22 (0.91–1.64)
			Quintile 1 vs. 4 PA	1.35 (0.99–1.85)
			Quintile 1 vs. 5 PA	1.52 (1.10–2.13)
		Incident ischemic stroke	Quintile 1 vs. 2 PA	1.15 (0.81–1.61)
			Quintile 1 vs. 3 PA	1.20 (0.84–1.72)
			Quintile 1 vs. 4 PA	1.32 (0.90–1.92)
			Quintile 1 vs. 5 PA	1.92 (1.25–3.03)
		Incident hemorrhagic stroke	Quintile 1 vs. 2 PA	1.09 (0.62–1.89)
			Quintile 1 vs. 3 PA	1.12 (0.63–2.00)
			Quintile 1 vs. 4 PA	1.45 (0.76–2.78)
			Quintile 1 vs. 5 PA	0.98 (0.55–1.72)
U.S. men (74)	16,877	Stroke mortality (ICD 430–438)	Low vs. moderate aerobic fitness	2.70 (1.20–5.88)
			Low vs. high aerobic fitness	3.13 (1.22–8.33)
U.S. women (113)	39,315	Incident stroke	<200 kcal · wk⁻¹	Referent
			200–599 kcal · wk⁻¹	1.11 (0.87–1.41)
			600–1,499 kcal · wk⁻¹	0.86 (0.67–1.10)
			≥1,500 kcal · wk⁻¹	0.83 (0.63–1.08)

RR, relative risk; CI, confidence interval; ICD, International Classification of Diseases; LTPA, leisure-time physical activity; PA, physical activity; ARIC, Atherosclerosis Risk in Communities.

ᵃ95% confidence interval calculated from 90% confidence interval reported in study.

has examined an objective measure of cardiorespiratory fitness in relation to the risk of stroke mortality (74). A sample of 16,878 men from the ACLS was followed prospectively for 10 yr to evaluate the relationship between baseline cardiorespiratory fitness level and stroke mortality. Men in the low-fitness category had 2.70 (95% CI: 1.20–5.88) and 3.13 (95% CI: 1.22–8.33) times the risk of developing a stroke during the follow-up period compared with men in the moderate- and high-fit categories, respectively (74). Physical fitness may thus be a stronger correlate of stroke risk than habitual activity level.

As for CHD prevention, the protective effect of physical activity may be partly mediated through its role in reducing blood pressure and controlling other risk factors for cardiovascular disease including body weight, diabetes, lipid parameters, and measures of coagulation and thrombolysis (45). The AHA/American Stroke Association Primary Prevention Guidelines for Stroke thus view physical inactivity as an important modifiable risk factor for stroke (Class I, Level of Evidence B) and recommend increased physical activity as outlined by the Centers for Disease Control and Prevention and the National Institutes of Health of regular exercise (30 min of moderate-intensity activity daily) as part of a healthy lifestyle (Class IIa, Level of Evidence B) (45). Detailed recommendations for exercise among stroke survivors are also available (46).

PHYSICAL ACTIVITY AND HYPERTENSION

Hypertension is a highly prevalent condition in developed and developing nations. In the United States, one in three adults has hypertension and prehypertension, and the prevalence of hypertension has increased among children and adolescents in recent years (110). Following publications by Paffenbarger in 1983 and Blair in 1984 (14,103) several population-based studies have reproduced their findings of an inverse relationship between physical activity/fitness and incident hypertension. Regular leisure time physical activity was found to be inversely associated with incident hypertension among young adults (22) and middle-aged individuals (105). Regular leisure time physical activity tends to be protective in men and women and in Whites and African Americans, although there is some variability among subgroup analyses. The protective effect of regular activity is independent of body weight in both sexes (60). Similar to what was described earlier for CHD, changes in physical activity relate to changes in risk of incident hypertension (137).

Exercise training lowers resting blood pressure in individuals with normal blood pressure and those with hypertension and in individuals with and without prevalent cardiovascular disease. Whelton and colleagues summarized 54 trials of aerobic exercise training with 2,419 participants in a meta-analysis and reported a significant reduction in mean systolic blood pressure (-3.84 mm Hg [95% CI: -4.97 to -2.72 mm Hg]) and mean diastolic blood pressure (-2.58 mm Hg [95% CI: -3.35 to -1.81 mm Hg]) (133). Similar reductions in systolic blood pressure have been observed among participants in clinical trials of cardiac rehabilitation (120). Blood pressure reductions of similar magnitude can also be achieved with moderate-intensity resistance training (30). In sedentary populations, even low level activity such as walking 30–60 min · wk^{-1} has measurable benefit (61). An "optimal" dose (frequency, intensity and duration) of exercise for blood pressure lowering has not been defined.

PHYSICAL ACTIVITY, TYPE 2 DIABETES, AND THE METABOLIC SYNDROME

More than 25 million individuals in the United States have diabetes mellitus (mostly Type 2 diabetes) and 35% of U.S. adults have prediabetes (94). Diabetes is the seventh leading cause of death in the United States and a major contributor to CHD and stroke (94). Like many of the chronic diseases associated with modern living, Type 2 diabetes mellitus is a multifactorial disease with no established single cause. Risk factors that predispose individuals to develop the disease include obesity, physical inactivity, older age, a family history of diabetes, history of gestational diabetes, race or ethnicity, and certain medications (94). Whereas older age, a family history of diabetes, race or ethnicity, and a history of gestational diabetes are nonmodifiable risk factors, physical inactivity and obesity are modifiable risk factors, that is, risk factors over which individuals have control. There is consistent evidence that a physically active lifestyle provides protection against the development of Type 2 diabetes, and several studies document that individuals with higher cardiorespiratory fitness level are at lower risk of developing diabetes mellitus than their unfit counterparts (9,23). Selected examples of such studies in women and men are described subsequently.

Using 8-yr follow-up data from the Nurses' Health study, Hu et al. (58) examined the relationship between total physical activity expressed in quintiles of MET score and incidence of Type 2 diabetes and compared the benefits of walking versus more vigorous activity on diabetes risk. After multivariate adjustment, the RRs of developing Type 2 diabetes across quintiles of physical activity (least to most) were 1.00, 0.77, 0.75, 0.62, and 0.54 (p for trend < 0.001). The benefits of physical activity and the dose response remained statistically significant after further adjustment for body mass index. In the subset of women who did not participate in any vigorous activities, the investigators documented significant risk reductions across quintiles of walking with RRs of 1.00, 0.91, 0.73, 0.69, and 0.58, respectively (p for trend < 0.001), that also remained significant after further adjustment for body mass index. Faster usual walking pace was independently associated with decreased risk. Equivalent energy expenditures from walking and vigorous activity resulted in comparable reductions of diabetes risk. Similar benefits of walking were also reported from the Women's Health Study and the Iowa Women's Health Study (39,130), thus supporting current physical activity guidelines that recommend moderate-intensity activity on most days of the week (1). Among younger women, observational data suggest that low physical activity levels prior to pregnancy and during early pregnancy are highly predictive of the development of gestational diabetes mellitus (124).

Strong associations between physical activity and decreased risk of incident Type 2 diabetes have also been observed in male cohorts. In the Physicians' Health Study, men who exercised vigorously at least once a week had a 36% lower incidence of Type 2 diabetes over 5 yr of follow-up (95% CI, 49% to 18%; $p < .001$) compared to their sedentary counterparts, and there was a dose-response relationship across strata of exercise frequency (86). In the Health Professionals' Follow-up Study, 10-yr risk of Type 2 diabetes was reduced across increasing quintiles of MET-hours per week (RRs 1.00, 0.78, 0.65, 0.58, and 0.51, p for trend < 0.001) after taking into account age, smoking, alcohol use, and other covariates (57). Hours of television watching in this cohort were inversely associated with diabetes risk, with an almost threefold increase in risk among men who watched more than 40 h $\cdot$ wk^{-1} versus those who watched less than 2 h $\cdot$ wk^{-1}. A recent meta-analysis linking television watching and health outcomes concluded that every 2 h of TV viewing per day were associated with an excess of 176 cases of Type 2 diabetes per 100,000 individuals per year (49).

Similarly strong relationships between physical activity level and health outcomes have also been shown in populations with prevalent Type 2 diabetes. In the National Health and Interview Survey, for example, individuals who walked at least 2 h $\cdot$ wk^{-1} had a 39% lower mortality rate (95% CI: 52% to 22%) and a 34% (95% CI: 55% to 4%) lower cardiovascular mortality rate compared to sedentary individuals during 8 yr of follow-up (48). The protective effect was present across age, race, and sex subgroups and independent of diabetes duration, comorbid conditions or other physical limitations. A dose response was present in that all-cause and cardiovascular mortality rates were lowest in individuals walking 3–4 h $\cdot$ wk^{-1} and those who reported more vigorous activities (48).

In addition to the epidemiologic evidence, intervention studies have highlighted the importance of physical activity alone or as a component of a multifactorial intervention in the prevention of Type 2 diabetes in high-risk individuals (65,98,125) and the importance of exercise in the management of Type 2 diabetes (85,121). The Finnish Diabetes Prevention Study (DPS) was a trial that randomized 522 middle-aged, overweight adults with impaired glucose tolerance to either a control group or a lifestyle intervention that was aimed at reducing body weight, improving diet, and increasing physical activity (125). After an average of 3.2 yr of follow-up, the risk of developing Type 2 diabetes was 58% lower in the lifestyle intervention group compared with the control group. Similarly, the U.S. Diabetes Prevention Program (DPP) was an intervention that randomized 3,234 participants into one of three groups: (a) placebo

control, (b) metformin therapy (850 mg twice daily), or (c) lifestyle-modification program. The lifestyle program in this study reduced the risk of developing Type 2 diabetes by 58% compared with the control group over an average of 2.8 yr of follow-up and was significantly more effective than pharmacologic therapy with metformin (31% reduction in incidence) (65).

A meta-analysis of 14 randomized controlled exercise trials among individuals with diabetes showed significant improvements in glycemic control, visceral adiposity, exercise capacity, and plasma triglyceride levels (121). Cardiovascular outcomes and mortality were not assessed in these studies. The Look AHEAD (Action for Health in Diabetes) trial is a multicenter randomized clinical trial that compares an intensive lifestyle intervention with diabetes support and education in 5,145 overweight or obese individuals with Type 2 diabetes. Improvements in risk factors and exercise capacity in the intensive lifestyle intervention group have been documented after 1 yr and 4 yr of follow-up (84,85). The trial is ongoing and expected to be completed by December of 2014.

Current recommendations for exercise in the prevention and management of diabetes are summarized in the 2010 Joint Position Statement by the ACSM and the American Diabetes Association (27) and a 2009 scientific statement by the AHA (87).

PHYSICAL ACTIVITY AND CANCER

Malignant neoplasms are the second most common cause of death in the United States with more than 500,000 deaths annually and approximately 10 million individuals with a history of cancer (36,66). Risk factors for specific cancers vary widely. Physical inactivity is increasingly recognized as an important contributor to the risk of cancer, especially breast and colon cancer (36). The mechanisms by which physical activity could decrease cancer risk are complex and still not well understood (36,40,123). Physical activity's role in helping to maintain a healthy weight may be particularly important because overweight and obesity are associated with higher circulating levels of sex hormones and insulin, which are known to stimulate cell and tumor growth (36). Modulation of immune function, reduction of oxidative damage and improved DNA repair may also play a role (36,40,123).

A large body of evidence links a sedentary lifestyle to an increased risk of colon cancer. Wolin and colleagues reviewed 52 observational studies and compared most active with least active individuals across studies (139). Greater activity in this analysis was associated with a 24% reduction in the risk of developing colon cancer with similar reductions for men and women. Associations with colon cancer risk have been observed for both leisure time and occupational activity measures (123). A relationship between physical activity and rectal cancer has not been consistently observed. Whether physical activity differentially affects cancers of the ascending, transverse, or descending colon is an area for future investigation. Investigators have hypothesized that a lower risk of colon cancer may be conferred by a decreased transit time for fecal matter through the colon of physically active individuals, leading to decreased exposure of the susceptible regions of the intestinal wall to carcinogens.

Monninkhof and colleagues reviewed 19 cohort studies and 29 case-control studies designed to assess the association between physical activity and breast cancer (89). The authors found a strong and consistent reduction in risk of at least 20% for postmenopausal breast cancer among more active individuals, whereas evidence for reduction in premenopausal breast cancer was less conclusive. A dose-response relationship between amount of physical activity and change in breast cancer risk was apparent in about half the studies included in the systematic review. The observed association between physical activity and breast cancer risk was independent of body mass index. Studies have investigated different types of activities and different timing of these activities (adolescence and young adulthood, mildlife and post-menopausal), but the results are inconclusive. A recent report from the Nurses' Health study suggested that an activity increase after menopause among women who were sedentary during the perimenopausal transition was beneficial, reinforcing current physical activity recommendations (33).

MUSCULOSKELETAL FITNESS AND HEALTH OUTCOMES

All of the studies of the relationship between physical activity/fitness and mortality or incidence of chronic diseases described thus far in this chapter have been concerned with the effects of aerobic physical activities and cardiorespiratory fitness. There are increasing data, however, that musculoskeletal fitness is also an important determinant of health and prognosis (43,136). Musculoskeletal fitness includes aspects of bone health, joint flexibility, and muscular strength and endurance. As shown in *Table 12-2*, higher levels of muscular strength have been associated with lower all-cause mortality in middle-aged and older populations (4,6,37,41, 42,62,71,88,96,107,114). Although some studies suggest that this relationship may differ in men and women, more research is clearly needed in this area. An analysis from the ACLS suggests that muscular fitness as assessed by sit-ups, leg press, and bench press performance predicts mortality even after adjustment for cardiorespiratory fitness (37). Resistance training of 30 min or more per week has been associated with a 23% lower 12-yr risk of CHD in men enrolled in the Health Professionals' Follow-up Study (119). Resistance training

TABLE 12-2. Selected Prospective Longitudinal Studies of Musculoskeletal Fitness and Mortality

Population	Sample Size	Age Range (yr)	Follow-up Length (yr)	Indicators of Musculoskeletal Fitness	Results
American men and women (37)	9,105	20–82	14	Sit-ups, bench press, and leg press	Mortality rates were lower in men and women with moderate and high muscular fitness compared with those with low fitness
Canadian men and women (62)	8,116	20–69	13	Grip strength, sit-ups, push-ups, trunk flexibility	Sit-ups (men and women) and grip strength (men) inversely related to mortality
American men (88)	1,071	Not reported	17.5	Grip strength	Grip strength related to mortality in total sample and in men ≥60 yr old in particular
Australian men and women (6)	1,464	70–84	6	Grip strength	Grip strength inversely related to mortality in combined sample of men and women
Japanese American men (107)	6,040	45–68	30	Grip strength	Grip strength inversely related to mortality within several body mass index categories
Danish men and women (114)	406	75	5	Knee extension and body extension strength	Knee extension strength inversely related to mortality in women only
Japanese men and women (41)	7,286	40–85	6.1	Grip strength, sit-ups, side step, vertical jump, trunk flexion	Grip strength, side step, and vertical jump inversely related to mortality in men only
Finnish men and women (71)	463	75–80	4.0–4.8	Grip strength and knee extension strength	Grip strength and knee extension strength inversely related to mortality in combined sample of men and women
British men and women (42)	800	>65	24	Grip strength	Grip strength inversely related to mortality in men but not in women

was independently predictive even when participant baseline characteristics and other forms of exercise were taken into account. Resistance training also improves many markers of the metabolic syndrome including body composition, blood glucose levels, insulin sensitivity, and blood pressure (43,118,136). Resistance training can also be incorporated safely into activity regimens for patients with established cardiovascular disorders, such as CHD and heart failure, and has been shown to improve functional status in these populations (136). Further research is needed to define dose-response characteristics and minimum thresholds of resistance training for specific health outcomes for healthy individuals and those with established cardiovascular disorders.

SUMMARY

There is abundant evidence in observational data sets that physical activity and physical fitness levels are inversely associated with the risk of premature mortality and many chronic diseases, including CHD, stroke, hypertension, Type 2 diabetes, and some cancers (particularly of the colon and breast). Dose-response relationships have been observed in many studies that have used multiple physical activity or physical fitness categories. Importantly, however, much of the benefit from physical activity can be achieved with moderate intensity activities such as walking, which are often more acceptable to sedentary individuals and can be safely performed even at advanced ages. Exercise training studies demonstrate metabolic improvements and decreased incidence of conditions such as Type 2 diabetes mellitus and have shown mortality reductions among individuals with prevalent CHD.

Physical activity interventions for primary and secondary prevention are cost-effective (26,73,131). Assessment of physical activity during routine clinical encounters, counseling to increase physical activity, and referral to exercise training programs as appropriate are now recommended in many guidelines and have been incorporated into performance measures (5,31,45,93,95,104,108,117). The reader is also referred to selected Internet resources listed at the end of this section. Awareness of physical inactivity as a risk factor for disease in the U.S. population remains low. Knowledge that increasing an individual's physical activity level results in a reduction in disease risk should be highlighted in public health campaigns designed to increase physical activity levels of the population. Equally, if not more, important are the many efforts under way to create communities with exercise-friendly environments such as walking trails and bicycle paths (8).

REFERENCES

1. *2008 Physical Activity Guidelines for Americans* [Internet]. Washington (DC): U.S. Department of Health and Human Services; [cited 2011 Sep 2]. Available from: http://www.health .gov/paguidelines/pdf/paguide.pdf

2. Abbott RD, Rodriguez BL, Burchfiel CM, Curb JD. Physical activity in older middle-aged men and reduced risk of stroke: the Honolulu Heart Program. *Am J Epidemiol.* 1994;139(9):881–93.

3. Agnarsson U, Thorgeirsson G, Sigvaldason H, Sigfusson N. Effects of leisure-time physical activity and ventilatory function on risk for stroke in men: the Reykjavik Study. *Ann Intern Med.* 1999;130(12):987–90.

4. Albanes D, Blair A, Taylor PR. Physical activity and risk of cancer in the NHANES I population. *Am J Public Health.* 1989;79(6): 744–50.

5. American Association of Cardiovascular and Pulmonary Rehabilitation, American College of Cardiology Foundation, American Heart Association Task Force on Performance Measures (Writing Committee to Develop Clinical Performance Measures for Cardiac Rehabilitation), et al. AACVPR/ACCF/AHA 2010 Update: Performance Measures on Cardiac Rehabilitation for Referral to Cardiac Rehabilitation/Secondary Prevention Services Endorsed by the American College of Chest Physicians, the American College of Sports Medicine, the American Physical Therapy Association, the Canadian Association of Cardiac Rehabilitation, the Clinical Exercise Physiology Association, the European Association for Cardiovascular Prevention and Rehabilitation, the Inter-American Heart Foundation, the National Association of Clinical Nurse Specialists, the Preventive Cardiovascular Nurses Association, and the Society of Thoracic Surgeons. *J Am Coll Cardiol.* 2010;56(14):1159–67.

6. Anstey KJ, Luszcz MA, Sanchez L. A reevaluation of the common factor theory of shared variance among age, sensory function, and cognitive function in older adults. *J Gerontol B Psychol Sci Soc Sci.* 2001;56(1):P3–11.

7. Arena R, Myers J, Williams MA, et al. Assessment of functional capacity in clinical and research settings: a scientific statement from the American Heart Association Committee on Exercise, Rehabilitation, and Prevention of the Council on Clinical Cardiology and the Council on Cardiovascular Nursing. *Circulation.* 2007;116(3):329–43.

8. Artinian NT, Fletcher GF, Mozaffarian D, et al. Interventions to promote physical activity and dietary lifestyle changes for cardiovascular risk factor reduction in adults: a scientific statement from the American Heart Association. *Circulation.* 2010;122(4):406–41.

9. Bassuk SS, Manson JE. Epidemiological evidence for the role of physical activity in reducing risk of type 2 diabetes and cardiovascular disease. *J Appl Physiol.* 2005;99(3):1193–204.

10. Berlin JA, Colditz GA. A meta-analysis of physical activity in the prevention of coronary heart disease. *Am J Epidemiol.* 1990;132(4): 612–28.

11. Bijnen FC, Caspersen CJ, Feskens EJ, Saris WH, Mosterd WL, Kromhout D. Physical activity and 10-year mortality from cardiovascular diseases and all causes: the Zutphen elderly study. *Arch Intern Med.* 1998;158(14):1499–505.

12. Bijnen FC, Feskens EJ, Caspersen CJ, Nagelkerke N, Mosterd WL, Kromhout D. Baseline and previous physical activity in relation to mortality in elderly men: the Zutphen elderly study. *Am J Epidemiol.* 1999;150(12):1289–96.

13. Blair SN, Cheng Y, Holder JS. Is physical activity or physical fitness more important in defining health benefits? *Med Sci Sports Exerc.* 2001;33(6 Suppl):S379–99; discussion S419–20.

14. Blair SN, Goodyear NN, Gibbons LW, Cooper KH. Physical fitness and incidence of hypertension in healthy normotensive men and women. *JAMA.* 1984;252(4):487–90.

15. Blair SN, Jackson AS. Physical fitness and activity as separate heart disease risk factors: a meta-analysis. *Med Sci Sports Exerc.* 2001;33(5):762–4.

16. Blair SN, Kohl HW 3rd, Barlow CE, Paffenbarger RS Jr, Gibbons LW, Macera CA. Changes in physical fitness and all-cause mortality. A prospective study of healthy and unhealthy men. *JAMA.* 1995;273(14):1093–8.

17. Blair SN, Kohl HW 3rd, Paffenbarger RS Jr, Clark DG, Cooper KH, Gibbons LW. Physical fitness and all-cause mortality. A prospective study of healthy men and women. *JAMA*. 1989;262(17):2395–401.

18. Booth FW, Chakravarthy MV. Physical activity and dietary intervention for chronic diseases: a quick fix after all? *J Appl Physiol*. 2006;100(5):1439–40.

19. Booth FW, Lees SJ. Fundamental questions about genes, inactivity, and chronic diseases. *Physiol Genomics*. 2007;28(2):146–57.

20. Bouchard C, Daw EW, Rice T, et al. Familial resemblance for VO2max in the sedentary state: the HERITAGE family study. *Med Sci Sports Exerc*. 1998;30(2):252–8.

21. Bouchard C, Shephard RJ. *Physical Activity, Fitness, and Health: International Proceedings and Consensus Statement*. Champaign (IL): Human Kinetics; 1994. 1055 p.

22. Carnethon MR, Evans NS, Church TS, et al. Joint associations of physical activity and aerobic fitness on the development of incident hypertension: coronary artery risk development in young adults. *Hypertension*. 2010;56(1):49–55.

23. Caspersen CJ, Fulton JE. Epidemiology of walking and type 2 diabetes. *Med Sci Sports Exerc*. 2008;40(7 Suppl):S519–28.

24. Church TS, Earnest CP, Skinner JS, Blair SN. Effects of different doses of physical activity on cardiorespiratory fitness among sedentary, overweight or obese postmenopausal women with elevated blood pressure: a randomized controlled trial. *JAMA*. 2007;297(19):2081–91.

25. Church TS, Kampert JB, Gibbons LW, Barlow CE, Blair SN. Usefulness of cardiorespiratory fitness as a predictor of all-cause and cardiovascular disease mortality in men with systemic hypertension. *Am J Cardiol*. 2001;88(6):651–6.

26. Clark AM, Hartling L, Vandermeer B, McAlister FA. Meta-analysis: secondary prevention programs for patients with coronary artery disease. *Ann Intern Med*. 2005;143(9):659–72.

27. Colberg SR, Sigal RJ, Fernhall B, et al. Exercise and type 2 diabetes: the American College of Sports Medicine and the American Diabetes Association: joint position statement. *Diabetes Care*. 2010;33(12):e147–67.

28. Colditz GA. Economic costs of obesity and inactivity. *Med Sci Sports Exerc*. 1999;31(11 Suppl):S663–7.

29. Cooper R, Kuh D, Hardy R, Mortality Review Group, FALCon and HALCyon Study Teams. Objectively measured physical capability levels and mortality: systematic review and meta-analysis. *BMJ*. 2010;341:c4467.

30. Cornelissen VA, Fagard RH. Effect of resistance training on resting blood pressure: a meta-analysis of randomized controlled trials. *J Hypertens*. 2005;23(2):251–9.

31. Drozda J Jr, Messer JV, Spertus J, et al. ACCF/AHA/AMA-PCPI 2011 Performance Measures for Adults With Coronary Artery Disease and Hypertension: a report of the American College of Cardiology Foundation/American Heart Association Task Force on Performance Measures and the American Medical Association-Physician Consortium for Performance Improvement. *Circulation*. 2011;124(2):248–70.

32. Ekelund LG, Haskell WL, Johnson JL, Whaley FS, Criqui MH, Sheps DS. Physical fitness as a predictor of cardiovascular mortality in asymptomatic North American men. The Lipid Research Clinics Mortality Follow-up Study. *N Engl J Med*. 1988;319(21):1379–84.

33. Eliassen AH, Hankinson SE, Rosner B, Holmes MD, Willett WC. Physical activity and risk of breast cancer among postmenopausal women. *Arch Intern Med*. 2010;170(19):1758–64.

34. Erikssen G, Liestol K, Bjornholt J, Thaulow E, Sandvik L, Erikssen J. Changes in physical fitness and changes in mortality. *Lancet*. 1998;352(9130):759–62.

35. Evenson KR, Rosamond WD, Cai J, et al. Physical activity and ischemic stroke risk. The atherosclerosis risk in communities study. *Stroke*. 1999;30(7):1333–9.

36. Eyre H, Kahn R, Robertson RM, et al. Preventing cancer, cardiovascular disease, and diabetes: a common agenda for the American Cancer Society, the American Diabetes Association, and the American Heart Association. *Circulation*. 2004;109(25):3244–55.

37. FitzGerald SJ, Barlow CE, Kampert JB, Morrow JR Jr, Jackson AW, Blair SN. Muscular fitness and all-cause mortality: prospective observations. *J Phys Activ Health*. 2004;1(1):7–18.

38. Fletcher GF, Balady GJ, Amsterdam EA, et al. Exercise standards for testing and training: a statement for healthcare professionals from the American Heart Association. *Circulation*. 2001;104(14):1694–740.

39. Folsom AR, Kushi LH, Hong CP. Physical activity and incident diabetes mellitus in postmenopausal women. *Am J Public Health*. 2000;90(1):134–8.

40. Friedenreich CM, Orenstein MR. Physical activity and cancer prevention: etiologic evidence and biological mechanisms. *J Nutr*. 2002;132(11 Suppl):3456S–64S.

41. Fujita Y, Nakamura Y, Hiraoka J, et al. Physical-strength tests and mortality among visitors to health-promotion centers in Japan. *J Clin Epidemiol*. 1995;48(11):1349–59.

42. Gale CR, Martyn CN, Cooper C, Sayer AA. Grip strength, body composition, and mortality. *Int J Epidemiol*. 2007;36(1):228–35.

43. Garber CE, Blissmer B, Deschenes MR, et al. Quantity and quality of exercise for developing and maintaining cardiorespiratory, musculoskeletal, and neuromotor fitness in apparently healthy adults: guidance for prescribing exercise. *Med Sci Sports Exerc*. 2011;43(7):1334–59.

44. Gillum RF, Mussolino ME, Ingram DD. Physical activity and stroke incidence in women and men. The NHANES I Epidemiologic Follow-up Study. *Am J Epidemiol*. 1996;143(9):860–9.

45. Goldstein LB, Bushnell CD, Adams RJ, et al. Guidelines for the primary prevention of stroke: a guideline for healthcare professionals from the American Heart Association/American Stroke Association. *Stroke*. 2011;42(2):517–84.

46. Gordon NF, Gulanick M, Costa F, et al. Physical activity and exercise recommendations for stroke survivors: an American Heart Association scientific statement from the Council on Clinical Cardiology, Subcommittee on Exercise, Cardiac Rehabilitation, and Prevention; the Council on Cardiovascular Nursing; the Council on Nutrition, Physical Activity, and Metabolism; and the Stroke Council. *Circulation*. 2004;109(16):2031–41.

47. Gregg EW, Cauley JA, Stone K, et al. Relationship of changes in physical activity and mortality among older women. *JAMA*. 2003;289(18):2379–86.

48. Gregg EW, Gerzoff RB, Caspersen CJ, Williamson DF, Narayan KM. Relationship of walking to mortality among US adults with diabetes. *Arch Intern Med*. 2003;163(12):1440–7.

49. Grontved A, Hu FB. Television viewing and risk of type 2 diabetes, cardiovascular disease, and all-cause mortality: a meta-analysis. *JAMA*. 2011;305(23):2448–55.

50. Gulati M, Pandey DK, Arnsdorf MF, et al. Exercise capacity and the risk of death in women: the St James Women Take Heart Project. *Circulation*. 2003;108(13):1554–9.

51. Hamer M, Chida Y. Walking and primary prevention: a meta-analysis of prospective cohort studies. *Br J Sports Med*. 2008;42(4):238–43.

52. Harmsen P, Rosengren A, Tsipogianni A, Wilhelmsen L. Risk factors for stroke in middle-aged men in Goteborg, Sweden. *Stroke*. 1990;21(2):223–9.

53. Haskell WL, Lee IM, Pate RR, et al. Physical activity and public health: updated recommendation for adults from the American College of Sports Medicine and the American Heart Association. *Med Sci Sports Exerc*. 2007;39(8):1423–34.

54. Heath GW. Epidemiologic research: a primer for the clinical exercise physiologist. *Clin Exerc Physiol*. 2000;2(2):60–7.

55. Heran BS, Chen JM, Ebrahim S, et al. Exercise-based cardiac rehabilitation for coronary heart disease. *Cochrane Database Syst Rev*. 2011;(7):CD001800.

56. Hlatky MA, Boineau RE, Higginbotham MB, et al. A brief self-administered questionnaire to determine functional capacity (the Duke Activity Status Index). *Am J Cardiol.* 1989;64(10):651–4.

57. Hu FB, Leitzmann MF, Stampfer MJ, Colditz GA, Willett WC, Rimm EB. Physical activity and television watching in relation to risk for type 2 diabetes mellitus in men. *Arch Intern Med.* 2001;161(12):1542–8.

58. Hu FB, Sigal RJ, Rich-Edwards JW, et al. Walking compared with vigorous physical activity and risk of type 2 diabetes in women: a prospective study. *JAMA.* 1999;282(15):1433–9.

59. Hu FB, Stampfer MJ, Colditz GA, et al. Physical activity and risk of stroke in women. *JAMA.* 2000;283(22):2961–7.

60. Hu G, Barengo NC, Tuomilehto J, Lakka TA, Nissinen A, Jousilahti P. Relationship of physical activity and body mass index to the risk of hypertension: a prospective study in Finland. *Hypertension.* 2004;43(1):25–30.

61. Ishikawa-Takata K, Ohta T, Tanaka H. How much exercise is required to reduce blood pressure in essential hypertensives: a dose-response study. *Am J Hypertens.* 2003;16(8):629–33.

62. Katzmarzyk PT, Craig CL. Musculoskeletal fitness and risk of mortality. *Med Sci Sports Exerc.* 2002;34(5):740–4.

63. Kesaniemi YK, Danforth E Jr, Jensen MD, Kopelman PG, Lefebvre P, Reeder BA. Dose-response issues concerning physical activity and health: an evidence-based symposium. *Med Sci Sports Exerc.* 2001;33(6 Suppl):S351–8.

64. Kiely DK, Wolf PA, Cupples LA, Beiser AS, Kannel WB. Physical activity and stroke risk: the Framingham Study. *Am J Epidemiol.* 1994;140(7):608–20.

65. Knowler WC, Barrett-Connor E, Fowler SE, et al. Reduction in the incidence of type 2 diabetes with lifestyle intervention or metformin. *N Engl J Med.* 2002;346(6):393–403.

66. Kochanek KD, Xu J, Murphy SL, Miniño AM, Kung H. Deaths: preliminary data for 2009. *Natl Vital Stat Rep.* 2011;59(4):1–51.

67. Kodama S, Saito K, Tanaka S, et al. Cardiorespiratory fitness as a quantitative predictor of all-cause mortality and cardiovascular events in healthy men and women: a meta-analysis. *JAMA.* 2009;301(19):2024–35.

68. Kohl HW 3rd. Physical activity and cardiovascular disease: evidence for a dose response. *Med Sci Sports Exerc.* 2001;33(6 Suppl):S472–83; discussion S493–4.

69. Kujala UM, Kaprio J, Koskenvuo M. Modifiable risk factors as predictors of all-cause mortality: the roles of genetics and childhood environment. *Am J Epidemiol.* 2002;156(11):985–93.

70. Lamonte MJ, Ainsworth BE. Quantifying energy expenditure and physical activity in the context of dose response. *Med Sci Sports Exerc.* 2001;33(6 Suppl):S370–8; discussion S419–20.

71. Laukkanen P, Heikkinen E, Kauppinen M. Muscle strength and mobility as predictors of survival in 75-84-year-old people. *Age Ageing.* 1995;24(6):468–73.

72. Le Grande MR, Elliott PC, Worcester MU, Murphy BM, Goble AJ. An evaluation of self-report physical activity instruments used in studies involving cardiac patients. *J Cardiopulm Rehabil Prev.* 2008;28(6):358–69.

73. Lee AJ, Strickler GK, Shepard DS. The economics of cardiac rehabilitation and lifestyle modification: a review of literature. *J Cardiopulm Rehabil Prev.* 2007;27(3):135–42.

74. Lee CD, Blair SN. Cardiorespiratory fitness and stroke mortality in men. *Med Sci Sports Exerc.* 2002;34(4):592–5.

75. Lee CD, Folsom AR, Blair SN. Physical activity and stroke risk: a meta-analysis. *Stroke.* 2003;34(10):2475–81.

76. Lee I. *Epidemiologic Methods in Physical Activity Studies.* Oxford (NY): Oxford University Press; 2009. 328 p.

77. Lee IM, Hennekens CH, Berger K, Buring JE, Manson JE. Exercise and risk of stroke in male physicians. *Stroke.* 1999;30(1):1–6.

78. Lee IM, Paffenbarger RS Jr. Do physical activity and physical fitness avert premature mortality? *Exerc Sport Sci Rev.* 1996;24:135–71.

79. Lee IM, Paffenbarger RS Jr. Physical activity and stroke incidence: the Harvard Alumni Health Study. *Stroke.* 1998;29(10):2049–54.

80. Lee IM, Skerrett PJ. Physical activity and all-cause mortality: what is the dose-response relation? *Med Sci Sports Exerc.* 2001;33(6):S459–71.

81. Lindsted KD, Tonstad S, Kuzma JW. Self-report of physical activity and patterns of mortality in Seventh-Day Adventist men. *J Clin Epidemiol.* 1991;44(4–5):355–64.

82. Lissner L, Bengtsson C, Bjorkelund C, Wedel H. Physical activity levels and changes in relation to longevity. A prospective study of Swedish women. *Am J Epidemiol.* 1996;143(1):54–62.

83. Lollgen H, Bockenhoff A, Knapp G. Physical activity and all-cause mortality: an updated meta-analysis with different intensity categories. *Int J Sports Med.* 2009;30(3):213–24.

84. Look AHEAD Research Group, Pi-Sunyer X, Blackburn G, et al. Reduction in weight and cardiovascular disease risk factors in individuals with type 2 diabetes: one-year results of the Look AHEAD trial. *Diabetes Care.* 2007;30(6):1374–83.

85. Look AHEAD Research Group, Wing RR. Long-term effects of a lifestyle intervention on weight and cardiovascular risk factors in individuals with type 2 diabetes mellitus: four-year results of the Look AHEAD trial. *Arch Intern Med.* 2010;170(17):1566–75.

86. Manson JE, Nathan DM, Krolewski AS, Stampfer MJ, Willett WC, Hennekens CH. A prospective study of exercise and incidence of diabetes among US male physicians. *JAMA.* 1992;268(1):63–7.

87. Marwick TH, Hordern MD, Miller T, et al. Exercise training for type 2 diabetes mellitus: impact on cardiovascular risk: a scientific statement from the American Heart Association. *Circulation.* 2009;119(25):3244–62.

88. Metter EJ, Talbot LA, Schrager M, Conwit R. Skeletal muscle strength as a predictor of all-cause mortality in healthy men. *J Gerontol A Biol Sci Med Sci.* 2002;57(10):B359–65.

89. Monninkhof EM, Elias SG, Vlems FA, et al. Physical activity and breast cancer: a systematic review. *Epidemiology.* 2007;18(1):137–57.

90. Mora S, Cook N, Buring JE, Ridker PM, Lee IM. Physical activity and reduced risk of cardiovascular events: potential mediating mechanisms. *Circulation.* 2007;116(19):2110–8.

91. Mora S, Redberg RF, Cui Y, et al. Ability of exercise testing to predict cardiovascular and all-cause death in asymptomatic women: a 20-year follow-up of the lipid research clinics prevalence study. *JAMA.* 2003;290(12):1600–7.

92. Morris JN, Heady JA, Raffle PA, Roberts CG, Parks JW. Coronary heart-disease and physical activity of work. *Lancet.* 1953;265(6796):1111–20.

93. Mosca L, Benjamin EJ, Berra K, et al. Effectiveness-based guidelines for the prevention of cardiovascular disease in women—2011 update: a guideline from the American Heart Association. *Circulation.* 2011;123(11):1243–62.

94. *National diabetes fact sheet, 2011: National estimates and general information on diabetes and prediabetes in the United States* [Internet]. Atlanta (GA): U.S. Department of Health and Human Services, Centers for Disease Control and Prevention; [cited 2011 Mar 10]. Available from: http://www.cdc.gov/diabetes/pubs/factsheet11.htm

95. Nelson ME, Rejeski WJ, Blair SN, et al. Physical activity and public health in older adults: recommendation from the American College of Sports Medicine and the American Heart Association. *Circulation.* 2007;116(9):1094–105.

96. Newman AB, Kupelian V, Visser M, et al. Strength, but not muscle mass, is associated with mortality in the health, aging and body composition study cohort. *J Gerontol A Biol Sci Med Sci.* 2006;61(1):72–7.

97. Nocon M, Hiemann T, Muller-Riemenschneider F, Thalau F, Roll S, Willich SN. Association of physical activity with all-cause and cardiovascular mortality: a systematic review and meta-analysis. *Eur J Cardiovasc Prev Rehabil.* 2008;15(3):239–46.

98. Orozco LJ, Buchleitner AM, Gimenez-Perez G, Roqué I Figuls M, Richter B, Mauricio D. Exercise or exercise and diet for preventing type 2 diabetes mellitus. *Cochrane Database Syst Rev.* 2008;(3):CD003054.

99. Paffenbarger RS Jr. Contributions of epidemiology to exercise science and cardiovascular health. *Med Sci Sports Exerc.* 1988;20(5):426–38.

100. Paffenbarger RS Jr, Blair SN, Lee IM. A history of physical activity, cardiovascular health and longevity: the scientific contributions of Jeremy N Morris, DSc, DPH, FRCP. *Int J Epidemiol.* 2001;30(5):1184–92.

101. Paffenbarger RS Jr, Hyde RT, Wing AL, Hsieh CC. Physical activity, all-cause mortality, and longevity of college alumni. *N Engl J Med.* 1986;314(10):605–13.

102. Paffenbarger RS Jr, Hyde RT, Wing AL, Lee IM, Jung DL, Kampert JB. The association of changes in physical-activity level and other lifestyle characteristics with mortality among men. *N Engl J Med.* 1993;328(8):538–45.

103. Paffenbarger RS Jr, Wing AL, Hyde RT, Jung DL. Physical activity and incidence of hypertension in college alumni. *Am J Epidemiol.* 1983;117(3):245–57.

104. Pearson TA, Blair SN, Daniels SR, et al. AHA Guidelines for Primary Prevention of Cardiovascular Disease and Stroke: 2002 Update: Consensus Panel Guide to Comprehensive Risk Reduction for Adult Patients Without Coronary or Other Atherosclerotic Vascular Diseases. American Heart Association Science Advisory and Coordinating Committee. *Circulation.* 2002;106(3):388–91.

105. Pereira MA, Folsom AR, McGovern PG, et al. Physical activity and incident hypertension in black and white adults: the Atherosclerosis Risk in Communities Study. *Prev Med.* 1999;28(3):304–12.

106. Powell KE, Blair SN. The public health burdens of sedentary living habits: theoretical but realistic estimates. *Med Sci Sports Exerc.* 1994;26(7):851–6.

107. Rantanen T, Masaki K, Foley D, Izmirlian G, White L, Guralnik JM. Grip strength changes over 27 yr in Japanese-American men. *J Appl Physiol.* 1998;85(6):2047–53.

108. Redberg RF, Benjamin EJ, Bittner V, et al. ACCF/AHA 2009 performance measures for primary prevention of cardiovascular disease in adults: a report of the American College of Cardiology Foundation/American Heart Association Task Force on Performance Measures (Writing Committee to Develop Performance Measures for Primary Prevention of Cardiovascular Disease) developed in collaboration with the American Academy of Family Physicians; American Association of Cardiovascular and Pulmonary Rehabilitation; and Preventive Cardiovascular Nurses Association: endorsed by the American College of Preventive Medicine, American College of Sports Medicine, and Society for Women's Health Research. *J Am Coll Cardiol.* 2009;54(14):1364–405.

109. Report of the Institute of Medicine, the National Academy of Sciences. *Adequacy of Evidence for Physical Activity Guidelines Development* [Internet]. Washington (DC): National Academies Press; [cited 2011 Sep 2]. Available from: http://www.nap.edu/catalog/11819.html

110. Roger VL, Go AS, Lloyd-Jones DM, et al. Heart disease and stroke statistics—2012 update: a report from the American Heart Association. *Circulation.* 2012;125(1):e2–e220.

111. Rosengren A, Wilhelmsen L. Physical activity protects against coronary death and deaths from all causes in middle-aged men. Evidence from a 20-year follow-up of the primary prevention study in Goteborg. *Ann Epidemiol.* 1997;7(1):69–75.

112. Salonen JT, Puska P, Tuomilehto J. Physical activity and risk of myocardial infarction, cerebral stroke and death: a longitudinal study in Eastern Finland. *Am J Epidemiol.* 1982;115(4):526–37.

113. Sattelmair JR, Kurth T, Buring JE, Lee IM. Physical activity and risk of stroke in women. *Stroke.* 2010;41(6):1243–50.

114. Schroll M, Avlund K, Davidsen M. Predictors of five-year functional ability in a longitudinal survey of men and women aged 75 to 80. The 1914-population in Glostrup, Denmark. *Aging (Milano).* 1997;9(1–2):143–52.

115. Shaw LJ, Olson MB, Kip K, et al. The value of estimated functional capacity in estimating outcome: results from the NHBLI-Sponsored Women's Ischemia Syndrome Evaluation (WISE) Study. *J Am Coll Cardiol.* 2006;47(3 Suppl):S36–43.

116. Slentz CA, Houmard JA, Kraus WE. Modest exercise prevents the progressive disease associated with physical inactivity. *Exerc Sport Sci Rev.* 2007;35(1):18–23.

117. Smith SC Jr, Allen J, Blair SN, et al. AHA/ACC guidelines for secondary prevention for patients with coronary and other atherosclerotic vascular disease: 2006 update: endorsed by the National Heart, Lung, and Blood Institute. *Circulation.* 2006;113(19):2363–72.

118. Strasser B, Siebert U, Schobersberger W. Resistance training in the treatment of the metabolic syndrome: a systematic review and meta-analysis of the effect of resistance training on metabolic clustering in patients with abnormal glucose metabolism. *Sports Med.* 2010;40(5):397–415.

119. Tanasescu M, Leitzmann MF, Rimm EB, Willett WC, Stampfer MJ, Hu FB. Exercise type and intensity in relation to coronary heart disease in men. *JAMA.* 2002;288(16):1994–2000.

120. Taylor RS, Brown A, Ebrahim S, et al. Exercise-based rehabilitation for patients with coronary heart disease: systematic review and meta-analysis of randomized controlled trials. *Am J Med.* 2004;116(10):682–92.

121. Thomas DE, Elliott EJ, Naughton GA. Exercise for type 2 diabetes mellitus. *Cochrane Database Syst Rev.* 2006;(3):CD002968.

122. Thompson PD, Buchner D, Pina IL, et al. Exercise and physical activity in the prevention and treatment of atherosclerotic cardiovascular disease: a statement from the Council on Clinical Cardiology (Subcommittee on Exercise, Rehabilitation, and Prevention) and the Council on Nutrition, Physical Activity, and Metabolism (Subcommittee on Physical Activity). *Circulation.* 2003;107(24):3109–16.

123. Thune I, Furberg AS. Physical activity and cancer risk: dose-response and cancer, all sites and site-specific. *Med Sci Sports Exerc.* 2001;33(6 Suppl):S530–50; discussion S609–10.

124. Tobias DK, Zhang C, van Dam RM, Bowers K, Hu FB. Physical activity before and during pregnancy and risk of gestational diabetes mellitus: a meta-analysis. *Diabetes Care.* 2011;34(1):223–9.

125. Tuomilehto J, Lindstrom J, Eriksson JG, et al. Prevention of type 2 diabetes mellitus by changes in lifestyle among subjects with impaired glucose tolerance. *N Engl J Med.* 2001;344(18):1343–50.

126. U.S. Department of Health and Human Services, Centers for Disease Control and Prevention, National Center for Chronic Disease Prevention and Health Promotion, The President's Council on Physical Fitness and Sports. *Physical Activity and Health: A Report of the Surgeon General.* Atlanta (GA): President's Council on Physical Fitness and Sports; 1996. 278 p.

127. Wannamethee G, Shaper AG. Physical activity and stroke in British middle aged men. *BMJ.* 1992;304(6827):597–601.

128. Wannamethee SG, Shaper AG, Walker M. Changes in physical activity, mortality, and incidence of coronary heart disease in older men. *Lancet.* 1998;351(9116):1603–8.

129. Wei M, Gibbons LW, Kampert JB, Nichaman MZ, Blair SN. Low cardiorespiratory fitness and physical inactivity as predictors of mortality in men with type 2 diabetes. *Ann Intern Med.* 2000;132(8):605–11.

130. Weinstein AR, Sesso HD, Lee IM, et al. Relationship of physical activity vs body mass index with type 2 diabetes in women. *JAMA.* 2004;292(10):1188–94.

131. Weintraub WS, Daniels SR, Burke LE, et al. Value of primordial and primary prevention for cardiovascular disease: a policy

statement from the American Heart Association. *Circulation.* 2011;124(8):967–90.

132. Westerterp KR. Assessment of physical activity: a critical appraisal. *Eur J Appl Physiol.* 2009;105(6):823–8.

133. Whelton SP, Chin A, Xin X, He J. Effect of aerobic exercise on blood pressure: a meta-analysis of randomized, controlled trials. *Ann Intern Med.* 2002;136(7):493–503.

134. *WHO Global Recommendations on Physical Activity for Health* [Internet]. Geneva (Switzerland): World Health Organization; [cited 2011 Sep 2]. Available from: http://whqlibdoc.who.int/ publications/2010/9789241599979_eng.pdf

135. *WHO Mortality and burden of disease attributable to selected major risks* [Internet]. Geneva (Switzerland): World Health Organization; [cited 2011 Sep 2]. Available from: http://www .who.int/healthinfo/global_burden_disease/GlobalHealthRisks _report_full.pdf

136. Williams MA, Haskell WL, Ades PA, et al. Resistance exercise in individuals with and without cardiovascular disease: 2007 update: a scientific statement from the American Heart Association Council on Clinical Cardiology and Council on Nutrition, Physical Activity, and Metabolism. *Circulation.* 2007;116(5):572–84.

137. Williams PT. A cohort study of incident hypertension in relation to changes in vigorous physical activity in men and women. *J Hypertens.* 2008;26(6):1085–93.

138. Williams PT. Physical fitness and activity as separate heart disease risk factors: a meta-analysis. *Med Sci Sports Exerc.* 2001;33(5):754–61.

139. Wolin KY, Yan Y, Colditz GA, Lee IM. Physical activity and colon cancer prevention: a meta-analysis. *Br J Cancer.* 2009;100(4):611–6.

140. Woodcock J, Franco OH, Orsini N, Roberts I. Non-vigorous physical activity and all-cause mortality: systematic review and meta-analysis of cohort studies. *Int J Epidemiol.* 2011;40(1):121–38.

SELECTED REFERENCES FOR FURTHER READING

National diabetes fact sheet, 2011: National estimates and general information on diabetes and prediabetes in the United States [Internet]. Atlanta (GA): U.S. Department of Health and Human Services, Centers for Disease Control and Prevention; [cited 2011 Mar 10]. Available from: http://www.cdc.gov/diabetes/pubs/ factsheet11.htm

Pearson TA, Blair SN, SR Daniels, et al. AHA Guidelines for Primary Prevention of Cardiovascular Disease and Stroke: 2002 Update: Consensus Panel Guide to Comprehensive Risk Reduction for Adult Patients Without Coronary or Other Atherosclerotic Vascular Diseases. American Heart Association Science Advisory and Coordinating Committee. *Circulation.* 2002;106(3):388–91.

Report of the Institute of Medicine, the National Academy of Sciences. Adequacy of Evidence for Physical Activity Guidelines Development [Internet]. Washington (DC): National Academies Press; [cited 2011 Sep 2]. Available from: http://www.nap.edu/catalog/11819.html

United States, Public Health Service, Office of the Surgeon General, National Center for Chronic Disease Prevention and Health Promotion (U.S.), President's Council on Physical Fitness and Sports (U.S.). *Physical Activity and Health: A Report of the Surgeon General.* Atlanta, GA: U.S. Department of Health and Human Services, Centers for Disease Control and Prevention, National Center for Chronic Disease Prevention and Health Promotion, President's Council on Physical Fitness and Sports; 1996. 278 p. Available from: Supt. of Docs, Washington.

WHO Global Recommendations on Physical Activity for Health [Internet]. Geneva (Switzerland): World Health Organization; [cited 2011 Sep 2]. Available from: http://whqlibdoc.who.int/publications/ 2010/9789241599979_eng.pdf

INTERNET RESOURCES

- Exercise is Medicine: http://exerciseismedicine.org/index.htm
- National Center for Disease Prevention and Health Promotion, Nutrition and Physical Activity: http://www.cdc.gov/nccdphp/ dnpa/physical/index.htm
- National Coalition for Promoting Physical Activity: http://www .ncppa.org
- Public Health Agency of Canada, Physical Activity: http://www .phac-aspc.gc.ca/hp-ps/hl-mvs/pa-ap/03paap-eng.php
- United States Department of Health & Human Services: http://aspe .hhs.gov/health/reports/physicalactivity/
- US National Institutes of Health, ClincialTrials.gov, Action For Health in Diabetes: http://clinicaltrials.gov/ct2/show/record/ NCT00017953?term=Look+Ahead&rank=1
- World Health Organization: http://www.who.int/dietphysical activity/pa/en/index.html

Physical activity has been defined as bodily movement generated by skeletal muscles resulting in energy expenditure (14,15). The physical activity portion of energy expenditure can be further divided into spontaneous activities, including non-exercise activity thermogenesis (NEAT), such as fidgeting or work-related walking, and voluntary physical activity. Voluntary physical activity includes activities of daily living and those that require amounts of energy above that necessary to perform activities of daily living (54). This component of physical activity varies most among individuals (50).

The benefits of a physically active lifestyle are widely known (49,73). The American College of Sports Medicine's (ACSM) physical activity recommendations have evolved over time (3–5,23,49). Early recommendations focused on higher intensity physical activities to achieve significant or maximal improvements in physical fitness. In the mid-1990s, however, the emphasis shifted toward getting individuals to participate in moderate-intensity lifestyle physical activities to improve health. This change in emphasis was brought about by the realization that moderate-intensity lifestyle physical activities can contribute to health in a similar fashion to structured exercise programs (20). Since 2005, there has been an increase in research demonstrating the health hazards of sedentary behaviors (*e.g.*, sitting, watching a television, using a computer, playing video games). Individuals who spend a large percentage of their day sedentary have increases in metabolic risk factors including obesity, hypertension, dyslipidemia, impaired glucose tolerance, and C-reactive protein even after adjusting for the amount of moderate-to-vigorous physical activity they perform (26,41,47). A large prospective study showed that the combined time spent riding in automobiles and watching television was positively correlated to the risk of all-cause mortality (75). Although avoidance of sedentary behavior and engagement in moderate-intensity physical activity have significant health benefits, the most recent shift in the ACSM recommendations is the recognition that performing vigorous-intensity exercise likely yields greater benefits than moderate-intensity physical activity alone (22).

Given the positive health implications of physical activity, it is important to assess the frequency, intensity, time (duration), and type (*i.e.*, the *FITT* principle) of physical activities. Specific reasons to measure physical activity include the ability to investigate the direct relationship between physical activity and disease endpoints as well as the indirect relationship with disease through the effects of activity on diet or body weight (52). Additional reasons include being able to study physical activity patterns, determinants, and barriers in different groups and to evaluate physical activity interventions (2,76,77).

Various **subjective methods** and **objective methods** can be used to measure physical activity. When using subjective methods such as questionnaires or diaries, the physical activity assessment is based on the

KEY TERMS

Accelerometer: An instrument that assesses frequency, duration, and intensity of physical activity by measuring acceleration and deceleration of the body recorded as "counts." Values can be stored and then downloaded to a computer.

Heart rate monitor: An instrument that assesses heart rate (HR). HR is related to intensity of physical activity. Values can be stored and then downloaded to a computer.

Objective methods: Methods that are not influenced by perception; these methods include pedometers, accelerometers, and HR monitors.

Pedometer: An instrument that detects vertical accelerations of the body and records a "step" when vertical acceleration exceeds a threshold value.

Subjective methods: Methods that necessitate interpretation; these methods include self-reported measures from questionnaires and diaries.

TABLE 13-1. General Advantages and Disadvantages of Physical Activity Measures

Advantages	Disadvantages
Subjective: • Relatively inexpensive • Easy to administer • Data collected for many individuals • Can be ascertained with a few questions	**Subjective:** • Inaccurate recall • Fails to accurately capture all types of activity (*e.g.*, moderate, lifestyle, and occupational activity) • Not recommended for children younger than the age of 10 yr
Objective: • Not subject to recall error • Small and lightweight • Unobtrusive	**Objective:** • Specific types of activity not assessed (*e.g.*, water sports, arm exercise, inclined walking) • Extraneous variables may affect results • Usually more expensive than questionnaires

individual's perception of his or her level of activity. With objective methods, physical activity is assessed by an instrument, and the individual's interpretation and perception of physical activity are not taken into account.

Several of the advantages and disadvantages of using subjective and objective methods of assessment are listed in *Table 13-1*. The main advantage of using subjective measures, such as questionnaires or diaries, is the ability to administer the assessment relatively inexpensively to many individuals in a short amount of time. Disadvantages of subjective assessment include inaccurate recall that results in the overreporting or underreporting of physical activity and the inability to accurately capture all types of physical activity (*e.g.*, moderate, lifestyle, occupational). Unlike subjective assessment methods, recall error is not an issue for objective methods, such as **pedometers**, **accelerometers**, and **heart rate monitors**. These objective monitors, for the most part, are small, lightweight, and unobtrusive. The disadvantages of this type of assessment include the expense, the inability to assess specific types of activities (*e.g.*, swimming, weightlifting, and stationary cycling), and the potential effect of extraneous factors on the physical activity assessment results.

Regardless of the technique, because of day-to-day and seasonal variation, the method should reflect physical activity participation on the weekends and weekdays as well as each season of the year (45). It is also important to use a reliable and valid evaluation method. A reliable method is reproducible, giving the same results for a given amount of physical activity. A valid method is one that accurately measures what

it is intended to measure. Establishing validity of a physical activity measure is difficult because no true gold standard for quantifying physical activity exists (71). Methods of energy expenditure (*i.e.*, doubly labeled water, indirect and direct calorimetry) are often used to validate physical activity assessments. These measures are not gold standards for physical activity validation because physical activity encompasses movement, and energy expenditure takes into account movement and body mass (45). In addition, doubly labeled water and indirect calorimetry, although serving as good techniques for measurement of energy expenditure, provide no information on the types of activities performed or the context in which these activities are performed. Given these limitations, validity is indirectly established by comparing results with other physical activity measures as well as physiologic variables. To determine if a physical activity assessment tool is reliable, the reproducibility should be examined with a test–retest period of 2–4 wk. This period is sufficiently short that behaviors should not change, but it is long enough that the initial administration will not influence the second test (76). The following sections describe various valid and reliable subjective and objective methods of physical activity assessment as well as the various criteria to consider when deciding on the appropriate method to use.

SUBJECTIVE ASSESSMENT: SELF-REPORT MEASURES OF PHYSICAL ACTIVITY

Subjective physical activity measurements include questionnaires and diaries. The complexity of the questionnaire can vary from a single, physical activity–related question to a more thorough, detailed account regarding physical activity patterns (24,35,50,57,77). Even though a single-item questionnaire cannot provide a complete account of one's physical activity, it may be an adequate measure for classifying individuals into crude activity categories. For instance, a query about leisure-time physical activity on the U.S. Behavioral Risk Factor Surveillance System (BRFSS) (32) survey asks, "During the past 30 d, other than your regular job, did you participate in any physical activities or exercise such as running, calisthenics, golf, gardening, or walking for exercise?" A more comprehensive questionnaire takes into account the type of activity, how frequently it is performed over a certain time period, and the duration and intensity of the activity session (50). A physical activity diary can also range in complexity from one that has participants' record every activity every minute of the day to those that have participants' record activities in 4-h periods and can be as general as including only the intensity of the activity. One example is the ACTIVITYGRAM, a component of the FITNESSGRAM

TABLE 13-2. Advantages and Disadvantages of Specific Subjective Measures of Physical Activity

	Advantages	Disadvantages
Diary	• Suitable for large populations • Little expense • No observer or interviewer • Collected in many subjects at the same time • Specific activities and patterns can be recorded	• Large amount of data to process, increasing the time and expense • Participants' cooperation and motivation required • Longer collection period can result in less accurate data • Need to record throughout the year to get typical physical activity
Questionnaire	• Suitable for large populations • Specific activities can be recorded • Patterns of behavior not affected • Total energy expenditure may be estimated • Applicable to wide age range	• Inaccurate recall • May be burdensome • Must be age appropriate • Interviewer may be necessary for accuracy • Limited use with younger children (younger than the age of 10 yr)

assessment (81). Children are asked to record their activities in 30-min time blocks for this component. However, this may be further divided into 15-min intervals, depending on whether the activity was performed "all of the time" (given credit for entire 30 min) during the 30-min segment or "some of the time" (given credit for 15 min). Other examples of popular questionnaires and diaries are found in resources by Montoye et al. (45), Periera et al. (50), and Kriska and Caspersen (36). The following sections describe questionnaires and diaries as well as several advantages and disadvantages to using each (*Table 13-2*).

QUESTIONNAIRES

A physical activity questionnaire usually can be administered quickly and inexpensively, is reliable, and does not cause a person's normal daily activity habits to change (39). This type of instrument does not provide an absolute measurement of energy expenditure, but it allows energy expenditure to be estimated and for individuals to be ranked from least to most active (35). As soon as a person's relative activity level is known, it is possible to examine the associations between physical activity and various disease endpoints such as heart disease, diabetes, various types of cancer, and obesity (35).

Self-report measures, such as questionnaires, can be used by various age groups and may be modified based on the study purpose or population (35,59,82). When using a questionnaire to assess physical activity in young children, a proxy report (*e.g.*, time spent playing outside) can be used (58). Assessing physical activity level in women is an example of the importance of questionnaire modification based on the population. According to national data from 2000, women were almost 7% less active than men (6). This discrepancy may be partly attributable to the nature of the physical activity questions asked by national surveys rather than women's actual activity levels. Some women may spend a large part of their day involved in household, family, and transportation activities, which are not captured by national survey questions (1).

Limitations of questionnaires include recall bias, individuals' problems with accurately recalling information, and differing recollection based on factors such as the person's age and disease status. Sedentary and high-intensity activities are the most reliably recalled using self-reported methods (32,57,59). Difficulties remembering and accurately recording moderate physical activities, especially lifestyle activities, offer another challenge to using questionnaires to assess physical activity. Finally, individuals may feel compelled to give socially desirable answers to physical activity questions when responding directly to an interviewer. Overall, the evidence suggests that adults tend to overestimate their physical activity levels (59).

DIARIES

Collecting physical activity information with a diary allows for data collection from many participants at the same time and eliminates the expense associated with an interviewer or observer. With this method of assessment, specific activities are usually recorded on the diary; therefore, physical activity patterns can be determined. Given that participants are asked to record their activities throughout the day, it is important that they are cooperative and willing to perform the task accurately. Recording all activities can be quite tedious. Therefore, keeping a diary over long periods of time can result in inaccurate data collection. Three days of diary collection — 2 weekdays and 1 weekend day — are adequate to accurately assess physical activity patterns (11). The short, 3-d assessment time frame limits participant burden.

A limitation to using a diary is the time and expense it takes to process large amounts of data. In addition, the diary process should be completed at various times (seasons) throughout the year to help ensure that regular activity patterns are being ascertained. For example, in some areas of the country, physical activity levels are higher in the summer than in the winter (51). Another limitation of diaries is that subjects may alter their behavior in order to provide responses they deem to be more acceptable.

SUMMARIZING DATA

After the data have been collected with a diary or questionnaire, they can be summarized in several different ways. Physical activity can be expressed as time, kilocalories (kcal), and volume of activity calculated as the product of intensity and duration; such volume measures are often reported as metabolic equivalents (METs) of activity times duration in minutes (MET-min) or in hours (MET-h) (50). A MET is an estimate of intensity based on the ratio of working metabolic rate to resting metabolic rate. One MET is equivalent to an oxygen uptake of $3.5 \text{ mL} \cdot \text{kg}^{-1} \cdot \text{min}^{-1}$, which represents energy expended at rest for a reference human. For example, slow jogging at 4.6 mph (7.4 kph) has an average gross oxygen consumption of $28.2 \text{ mL} \cdot \text{kg}^{-1} \cdot \text{min}^{-1}$, or about 8 MET. *Figure 13-1* illustrates three potential ways to derive a physical activity summary score (50). The most basic way is to calculate total time spent in physical activity by multiplying the number of sessions per week of the activity by the time spent performing the activity each session. A second calculation weighs the time spent in the activity by an estimated metabolic cost of each activity (MET). An example of a calculation using METs (*Fig. 13-1*) follows. An individual reported jogging four times a week for 30 min a session. As shown at level 1 in the figure, this equates to 2 h a week of exercise. Multiplying the total time spent in jogging by its MET value of 8 results in an estimated energy expended from this activity of 16 MET-h $\cdot$ wk^{-1} (level 2; *Fig. 13-1*). Finally, if the individual's body mass is known, one can calculate the kilocalories per week expended during physical activity. The results from this calculation are provided at level 3 (*Fig. 13-1*). For an individual with a mass of 60 kg, this equates to 960 kcal $\cdot$ wk^{-1}.

Assumptions made when using these calculations include (a) MET values are representative of the way an activity is performed regardless of the skill level of the individual or pace of the activity, and (b) the metabolic cost of performing activities (in MET) is constant among individuals regardless of body weight (50). Note that the calculations in this example are based on the gross oxygen consumption of the individual during the activity, that is, including both the oxygen consumption needed for continuance of normal resting energy needs (1 MET) and the net additional oxygen consumption needed to perform the exercise (7 MET). If the information is to be used to determine potential weight loss from the exercise program, only the net value should be used (*i.e.*, 14 MET-h $\cdot$ wk^{-1}, or 840 kcal) because the resting energy expenditure would have occurred whether the individual exercised during those 2 h. The Compendium of Physical Activities compiled by Ainsworth et al. is a popular resource for obtaining MET values for a wide range of physical activities (2,16).

OBJECTIVE ASSESSMENT: DIRECT MEASUREMENT OF PHYSICAL ACTIVITY

Physical activity monitors, such as pedometers, accelerometers, and heart rate (HR) monitors, provide objective estimates of one's physical activity. Other objective measures of physical activity and energy expenditure — such as direct observation, doubly labeled water, and indirect calorimetry — are often used to estimate physical activity level; however, these costly methods may not always be practical with large groups of individuals. Direct observation is primarily used for physical activity assessment in

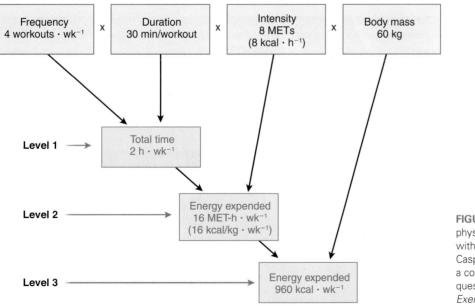

FIGURE 13-1. Ways to summarize physical activity data. Modified with permission from Kriska AM, Caspersen CJ. Introduction to a collection of physical activity questionnaires. *Med Sci Sports Exerc.* 1997;29(6, suppl):S5–9.

children over short periods. Examples of direct observation systems include the System for Observing Play and Leisure Activity in Youth (SOPLAY) and the Children's Activity Rating Scale (CARS) (44,53). Total energy expenditure measures, such as doubly labeled water, are limited because they do not allow for the determination of physical activity patterns (8). Different activity combinations or patterns (*e.g.*, a small amount of strenuous activity vs. a larger amount of moderate-intensity activity) can result in the same amount of energy expenditure (45). Many energy expenditure methods do not provide accurate estimates of absolute amount of physical activity (59).

Accelerometers and pedometers can accurately determine baseline and small changes in activity level (71). The cost of the instruments makes these measures potentially more expensive to administer than questionnaires. Unlike questionnaires, they are not subject to recall bias or inaccurate recall by participants. Physical activity monitors are also relatively easy to use, and participant language and reading ability are not issues. However, the monitors are designed to record ambulatory activity and cannot be worn while performing water activities. Therefore, they may not accurately detect movement from activities such as bicycling, weightlifting, or swimming (8). Wearable monitors appear to provide reasonable measures of ambulatory activity (45). Several methods of objective assessment of physical activity as well as the advantages and disadvantages of each are described subsequently and listed in *Table 13-3*.

PEDOMETERS

Pedometers detect vertical accelerations of the body and record a "step" when vertical acceleration exceeds a threshold value (80). These monitors are small and

relatively inexpensive but do not provide information as extensive as accelerometers. Some pedometers have proven to be quite accurate for recording the number of steps taken and distance walked at various walking paces (7,19,60). Pedometers are more reliable for faster walking and running paces compared with slower ones (6,80). Research has shown that a pedometer records a higher number of steps for walking compared with running for the same distance (7). This finding is not surprising given that the stride length is shorter when walking compared with running. The accuracy of the pedometer does not appear to differ based on the type of walking or running surface (7,80). Welk et al. (80) extended pedometer research to compare step counts with energy expenditure estimated from self-reported physical activities. They found that the relationship between pedometer step counts and energy expended in moderate-intensity activities was stronger than the relationship with energy expended in vigorous activities (80). Finally, some pedometers express energy expenditure in kilocalorie; however, these functions have not been as well validated as actual step counting. Hence, researchers recommend reporting pedometer data as "steps" because that is the most direct expression of what the pedometer measures (56,72).

For certain groups, special types of pedometers are needed. A problem with pedometers that use a horizontal spring-suspended lever arm to register steps is that they are much less sensitive if they are tilted away from the vertical plane. Thus, in adults who are obese, pedometers may undercount steps at slow walking speeds if the belt is tilted. However, a newer type of pedometer with a piezoelectric accelerometer mechanism (New Lifestyles NL-2000) overcomes this problem and is thus a good choice for monitoring ambulatory activity in obese individuals (18). Another problem with

TABLE 13-3. Advantages and Disadvantages of Specific Objective Measures of Physical Activity

	Advantages	Disadvantages
Pedometer	<ul><li>Instrument low-to-moderate expense</li><li>Small and lightweight</li><li>Unobtrusive</li><li>With proper instruction, is easy to use and provides immediate feedback</li></ul>	<ul><li>Detects only ambulatory activity</li><li>Cannot determine type, intensity, or pattern of activity</li><li>Cannot detect changes in terrain</li><li>Cannot be worn in the water</li><li>Can be worn on shoe or ankle during cycling</li></ul>
Accelerometer	<ul><li>Total energy expenditure may be estimated</li><li>Applicable to wide age range</li><li>Enjoyable with respect to amount of information provided</li></ul>	<ul><li>Detects only ambulatory activity</li><li>Cannot detect changes in terrain</li><li>Cannot be worn in the water or when cycling</li><li>Expense of instrument and hardware or software to process data</li><li>Cannot determine type of activity</li><li>Requires a computer to process and report data</li></ul>
Heart rate monitor	<ul><li>Physiologic marker</li><li>Can record and store heart rate data over an extended period of time</li><li>Can detect different intensities of activity</li></ul>	<ul><li>Influenced by factors not related to physical activity participation</li><li>Cannot determine type of activity</li><li>Hard to detect low intensity activities</li><li>Time and cost of processing data</li></ul>

waist-mounted pedometers is that they are not sensitive enough to detect steps taken in frail, older individuals who walk with a slow, shuffling gait. In this population, a comfortable, lightweight ankle-mounted device called the StepWatch 3 (Cyma Corporation, Seattle, WA) will record steps with a high level of accuracy, even at 1 mile $\cdot$ h^{-1} (31).

A new type of pedometer (Omron HJ-720 ITC) uses two piezoelectric accelerometers and can be worn in a pocket or attached to a belt. One advantage to this type of pedometer is that it can store 40 d of step data in 1-h increments, and the data can be downloaded to a computer. This pedometer has been validated against direct observation of step counts (28,83). The Omron HJ-720ITC pedometer greatly simplifies data management for clinical trials and it has the advantage of providing a completely objective measure of physical activity because a researcher need not rely on participants to record their steps each day. However, this Omron pedometer has a 4-s filter and does not count any steps that are taken in bouts of less than 4 s. Thus, it undercounts steps during intermittent activities (e.g., light housework) (62).

Limitations to using a pedometer for physical activity assessment include insensitivity to changes in walking speed and the inability of most pedometers to determine intensity or duration of the activity being performed (45). Even though the pedometer does not give a complete picture of physical activity patterns, step count results are highly related to physical activity assessments from various accelerometers, which provide a more thorough pattern of activity (8,40). Therefore, a pedometer is a practical and accurate means of assessing physical activity (9,67).

ACCELEROMETER-BASED ACTIVITY MONITORS

Accelerometer-based activity monitors can be worn on the trunk or limbs and measure movement based on acceleration and deceleration of the device. These measurements are proportional to muscular forces (45). Given this principle, most results from accelerometers are in proportion to energy expenditure and are used to ascertain the time, frequency, and duration of physical activity performed at various intensities (1,45). These types of activity patterns cannot be determined from doubly labeled water (8), although they can be determined by indirect calorimetry and measurement of HR.

Uniaxial monitors, such as the Caltrac (Muscle Dynamics, Torrance, CA) accelerometer and ActiGraph model 7164 (Actigraph, Pensacola, FL), measure movement in the vertical plane. Triaxial monitors, such as the Tritrac-R3D (Hemokinetics Inc., Madison, WI) and ActiGraph model GT3X+, measure movement in the vertical, horizontal, and mediolateral planes (21).

Advantages of the accelerometer-based device include its small size and ability to record data over long periods (e.g., several days or weeks) as well as the ability to download data and to segment physical activity periods (27). To reduce the expense of using this type of device, the same unit can be worn repeatedly by different participants. When using one monitor worn at different times for multiple participants, only small amounts of data can be collected at one time (71).

This type of objective assessment requires more time and resources than a pedometer because technical expertise, hardware, and software are needed to calibrate, input, download, and analyze data (70,71). Uniaxial accelerometers may not accurately detect movement from activities such as bicycling, weightlifting, or swimming (8). In addition, when worn on the hip, certain accelerometers may not accurately identify activity level on other areas of the body (78). Importantly, none are able to detect increased activity level resulting from upper body movement, carrying a load, or variations in the surface (e.g., climbing uphill vs. level ambulation) (27). Given the limitation of type of movement detected, Swartz et al. had participants wear monitors on the hip and wrist simultaneously and determined that the extra monitor slightly increased the accuracy of estimating the energy expenditure necessary to perform various physical activities (66). The small increases in accuracy reported with the additional monitor need to be weighed against the time, cost, and effectiveness of an additional monitor (66).

An additional limitation of this mode of measuring physical activity is the potential to misclassify one's activity levels. The accelerometer equations that estimate energy expenditure are typically derived from specific laboratory activities; therefore, they may not be applicable to free-living situations (19). For instance, accelerometer equations derived from treadmill walking and jogging have been shown to predict the energy cost of those activities quite accurately. However, when these same equations are applied to lifestyle activities such as gardening and housework, they tend to overestimate or underestimate the actual energy cost (8,78). The relationship between treadmill walking or running measured in a laboratory with an accelerometer and indirect calorimetry is stronger than that reported for moderate lifestyle activities (78).

Several investigators have developed accelerometer equations that are based on moderate-intensity lifestyle activities, including housework, yard work, and occupational tasks (27,66). These equations are generally more accurate for moderate-intensity lifestyle activities, but they tend to overpredict sedentary and light activities and to underpredict vigorous sports. For this reason, Crouter et al. (17) developed a new two-regression model that examines the variability in accelerometer counts and used this to determine whether an individual is performing (a) intermittent lifestyle activities or (b) dynamic, rhythmic locomotion such as walking or jogging. The model then uses either a walk/jog regression or an intermittent lifestyle regression to predict the energy cost from the mean accelerometer counts. The Crouter two-regression approach may provide a more accurate estimate of energy expenditure across a wide range of physical activities (17). However, this study has yet to be replicated at the time of this writing.

According to Welk et al., accelerometer-based devices give the most objective and detailed physical activity data for research purposes (78). Overall, they provide a useful measure of physical activity, but they are less accurate than other devices for determining total energy expenditure (27,78). In the future, it may be possible to improve estimations of physical activity by supplementing accelerometer data with questionnaire data. In addition, researchers are seeking to improve the accuracy of accelerometer-based devices by developing more sophisticated mathematic algorithms to convert acceleration data into energy expenditure (27,78). Pattern recognition shows tremendous promise for being able to identify the type and intensity of physical activities performed (55,63). This technique takes acceleration data stored at frequent intervals and uses the mathematical characteristics of the data to predict energy expenditure.

Accelerometer-based devices can also be used to assess the amount of time spent in sedentary behaviors. With the Actigraph GT1M, some researchers have defined inactivity as accelerometer count values less than 100 counts per minute because values lower than that indicates that a person is seated (42). The ActivPAL (PAL Technologies, Glasgow, UK) is a small device that can be affixed to the thigh and it contains an accelerometer that measures body posture to determine if a person is seated or upright. The accelerometer in this device can detect ambulation; hence, it is useful for those wishing to determine what percentage of the day is spent sitting, standing, and ambulating.

HEART RATE MONITORING

HR is linearly related to $\dot{V}O_2$ during aerobic activities; therefore, HR monitoring is another reasonable method of physical activity assessment (21). Other physiologic variables such as cardiac output, pulmonary ventilation, tidal volume, ventilatory rate, and arteriovenous oxygen difference also increase with increasing $\dot{V}O_2$ but are more difficult to measure. Thus, HR is one of the most practical physiologically based ways to estimate energy expenditure in the field (45). HR monitoring is "low cost, noninvasive, and able to give information of the pattern of physical activity" (65). As with accelerometers, HR recorders can store data, which allows for the estimation of frequency, duration, and intensity of physical activity for days and weeks. Strath et al. reported

a correlation of .87 when comparing the relationship between energy expenditure for lifestyle activities measured with indirect calorimetry and estimates from HR monitoring (65). This correlation is stronger than those reported between energy expenditure measured with indirect calorimetry and accelerometers for lifestyle activities (64).

Strath et al. (64) suggested that when subjects wear an Actigraph and an HR monitor simultaneously, energy expenditure estimation and classification of time spent in light, moderate, and hard activity were more accurate. Further research needs to be conducted, but it appears that HR monitors with additional types of activity assessment may be effective means of assessing physical activity (45,64).

A limitation to using HR monitors to assess physical activity is that factors such as ambient temperature, humidity, and high altitude will increase the HR response to exercise. In addition, emotional state, hydration status, type of contraction (static vs. dynamic), and the amount of muscle mass recruited will affect HR, independent of physical activity level (45). In addition, the HR response to a given physical activity challenge is highly individual, and to maximize accuracy, individualized HR-energy cost calibrations must be performed, which is time consuming. One practical approach would be to estimate the subject's $\dot{V}O_{2max}$ from the HR response to given submaximal loads, and use this value to allow translation of HR responses to energy expenditure. Finally, the specific type of activity cannot be determined by the HR monitor, and low intensity activities are hard to detect.

MONITORS THAT USE MULTIPLE INPUTS

Some physical activity monitors use a combination of accelerometer and physiological signals to predict energy expenditure. For instance, the SenseWear Pro 3 Armband (BodyMedia, Pittsburgh, PA) uses an accelerometer, plus sensors to detect heat flux across the skin and galvanic skin responses. The SenseWear Armband uses pattern recognition to detect the type of activities performed, which allows it to provide the user with more accurate energy expenditure data than accelerometer-based monitors. This device has been validated against indirect calorimetry during structured activity bouts (13) and against doubly labeled water in the free-living environment (30). The Actiheart (MetriSense, Cambridge, UK) is another device that uses a combination of accelerometer and physiological (HR) signals to estimate energy expenditure. Finally, the IDEEA monitor (Intelligent Device for Energy Expenditure and Physical Activity) (Minisun, Fresno, CA) takes acceleration signals from several accelerometers placed on different parts of the body and uses them to predict 40 different types of physical activities, postures, and gaits.

OTHER POTENTIAL METHODS

There are several other types of technologically advanced objective measures such as task-specific monitoring sensors and the global positioning system (GPS), which may be helpful for improving physical activity assessment in the future. Eventually, it may be possible to have sensors located on clothing and accessories that can monitor physiologic responses, such as HR and ventilation, and transmit the information to a computer (25). This information, along with that provided by a wearable digital camera that can provide pictures of the day's activities, could give an accurate, objective account of an individual's physical activities throughout the day (25). GPS is a satellite-based navigational system that uses signal information between satellites and receivers, worn by individuals, to ascertain the velocity and duration of displacement (25). Research studies to date support the ability of GPS to provide accurate assessments of speed, ranging from slow walking to fast running, as well as other biomechanical parameters (61,68). Currently, there are relatively inexpensive ($100) GPS units available that are lightweight, can be worn on the wrist, and provide speed, distance, and pace information while walking or running. However, GPS units cannot be used for stationary exercise and may be unable to be used indoors and in some outdoor settings. As these methods continue to become more feasible and their cost is reduced, they have the potential to expand our ability to accurately assess physical activity.

CHOOSING A METHOD

Various types of subjective and objective physical activity assessments have been described. There are several criteria to consider when choosing an assessment method. These criteria include the purpose of the assessment, cost, characteristics of the population being assessed, and the endpoints being evaluated. The method chosen should be valid and reproducible in a representative population (52). There are also additional considerations such as the assessment time frame and method of administration that should be taken into account when administering questionnaires.

PURPOSE

Regardless of one's health or fitness profession, at least one of the tools described in this chapter can help the professional achieve the purpose of assessing physical activity. For example, a health fitness specialist in a fitness center working with a new participant who would like to assess the client's past physical activity habits may want to use a past-year assessment tool such as the Modifiable Activity Questionnaire (50). This type of questionnaire allows the determination of the frequency and duration of an individual's specific activities performed over the past year to ascertain his or her usual physical activity habits. Knowing an individual's physical activity patterns is also helpful in developing an appropriate exercise program. If the purpose is monitoring a participant's physical activity level or change in physical activity level, one could use an objective measure or an activity log. If ambulatory activity is primarily being performed, then a participant could wear a pedometer and record the number of steps taken. For this method to be effective, the baseline number of steps the participant takes should be established. Then the monitor should be worn continuously or at various intervals over time to evaluate the maintenance or change in physical activity. If the activities primarily involve resistance training, it is important to use a log that includes the exercise performed, the amount of weight lifted, and the number of sets and repetitions performed. For monitoring general activity, logs can be completed by participants through the Internet at no cost. An example of this type of log can be found at http://www.presidentschallenge.org/tools-resources/forms.shtml. Versions of this log can either be printed out and completed or completed online. This type of log allows participants to record the type of physical activity as well as intensity and duration. Alternatively, there is an option for recording the number of pedometer steps taken each day.

COST

With all these measures, it is necessary to weigh the cost of assessment against the quality of data obtained. More expensive techniques usually provide more accurate data. Self-report methods to assess physical activity typically involve low-to-moderate costs, mostly for printing and data processing. Higher costs with diary administration relate to the large amounts of data to process. Interviewer-administered questionnaire expenses are predominantly attributable to personnel costs. The cost of using physical activity monitors depends on the expense associated with the instrument. Pedometers (~$10–$40, with some combination models costing as much as $70) are less expensive than accelerometers ($300–$450) and HR monitors ($200–$1,000). Accelerometers and HR monitors with data-storage capabilities also result in the additional cost of downloading, preparing, and analyzing the data.

CLINICAL POPULATIONS

As discussed previously, there are issues with accurately measuring moderate and lifestyle physical activities as well as physical activity in women. Therefore, it is crucial that methods used to assess physical activity levels accurately capture these types of activities. Similar issues exist when assessing physical activity in various ethnic or racial groups. It is important to determine the activities that contribute most to energy expenditure in the study population (34). For some minority groups, the activities include occupational activities, transportation, household chores, and caretaking, rather than sports and high-intensity leisure activities (34). Therefore, physical activity assessment tools should validly and reliably measure physical activity common to the population under study.

Age is also a consideration, especially in questionnaire administration. This method may not be appropriate for children younger than 10 yr old. For older individuals, it has been suggested that effective questionnaire administration should involve an interviewer. This mode of administration helps to clarify questions individuals may have. The type of domains assessed should be age appropriate (*i.e.*, in older adults, activities such as walking, light-to-moderate housework, and yard work may be the focus of the assessment), and recall time frames should be short (45). Older adults also tend to handle short, specific questions involving specific activities and periods (*e.g.*, minutes spent in an activity, times per week an activity is done) better than general, open-ended questions (45). If using an objective measure, pedometers may be as effective for assessing energy expenditure as accelerometers in older individuals if the activities predominantly involve walking rather than jogging, running, and upper-body motion. These instruments also appear to be appropriate in children (79).

ENDPOINTS

The endpoint being evaluated is also an important consideration when choosing a method to assess physical activity. For example, measuring lifetime patterns of physical activity may be important when examining the relationships between cancer and bone health (43,46,74). If the focus of the study is to establish a dose-response relationship with a health-related endpoint, a questionnaire, accelerometer, or HR monitor that allows for physical activity pattern determination is necessary. Finally, if the study goal is to determine the effectiveness of a physical activity intervention, comparing preintervention and postintervention data from questionnaires with shorter time frames (*e.g.*, past week or 3-d diary) or physical activity monitors should be appropriate. Exceptions to using a monitor include the evaluation of interventions that involve strength training or another type of nonambulatory activity not accurately assessed with a monitor.

CONSIDERATIONS FOR QUESTIONNAIRE AND DIARY USE

Time Frames

Time frames used when assessing physical activity vary from a diary that segments the day and has participants record their activities in 15-min intervals to questionnaires that ask about lifetime physical activity. The time frame assessed depends on the population and endpoint of interest to the researcher.

Shorter time frames are the easiest to recall; however, they may not give an accurate picture of typical physical activity patterns. There are certain endpoints that rely on recent physical activity to accurately predict risk because it may affect the outcome more than the history of physical activity. This finding is reflected in studies by Blair et al. and Paffenbarger et al. that demonstrated that changes in physical activity or fitness levels predict mortality risk (10,48). For example, a woman may be unfit at one point in time, but if her fitness level improves, her mortality risk is lower than someone who remained unfit. Relatively recent physical activity level, rather than physical activity history, was related to mortality. Questionnaires that cover shorter periods of time, however, may not provide an adequate representation of a person's normal activity level (*e.g.*, during bad weather, assessment of activities from the past week or past month may substantially underestimate one's activity level for the remainder of the year) (39). Physical activities performed over the past year may not be remembered as accurately, but they do provide a more complete physical activity profile. Lifetime physical activity may be important to assess for its relationship to certain types of cancer as well as bone health (43,46,74). Although this time frame might be the most difficult to recall accurately, several studies have reported reasonable reliability results for long-term physical activity recall (15,37,38). In addition, researchers have examined the validity of long-term recall (*i.e.*, 10–15 yr) and have found results comparable to that of questionnaires with shorter recall time frames (12,33,79).

Administration Techniques

Questionnaires are administered in various ways. Questionnaires that are interviewer-administered (either in person or over the telephone) take more time and are more costly than those that are self-administered. This method allows participants to clarify any issues and uncertainties about the questions, thereby reducing response errors.

Self-administered questionnaires are inexpensive and provide information comparable to that from interviewer-administered questionnaires (29). Using this method of administration, the questionnaire can either be given to participants or sent to them through the mail. These questionnaires can be easily administered to large groups of individuals in a short amount of time.

More recent advances in technology have made the Internet a viable means of questionnaire administration. With the popularity and widespread availability of computers and Internet access, this may be a cost-effective way to monitor activity levels. Potential uses include online questionnaire administration and continuous monitoring of physical activity (*e.g.*, online physical activity diaries). Further validation is needed for this potentially valuable method of recording and tracking physical activity behaviors.

SUMMARY

It is important to use a valid and reliable method of assessing physical activity that is appropriate for the population as well as the study endpoint. The advantages and disadvantages of each type of subjective and objective assessment have been introduced. Given these strengths and weaknesses, a combination of physical activity assessment methods may provide the most accurate estimate of physical activity. This combination approach to assessment has not been widely examined (46). However, based on the conclusion of various reports regarding the assessment of physical activity, using more than one method should increase the accuracy of the measurement (33,61,67,70,71). Treuth recently recommended that additional research should focus on applying different combinations of assessment techniques to larger samples as well as various age groups and special populations (69).

REFERENCES

1. Ainsworth BE. Issues in the assessment of physical activity in women. *Res Q Exerc Sport.* 2000;71(2 Suppl):S37–42.
2. Ainsworth BE, Haskell WL, Herrmann SD, et al. Compendium of physical activities: a second update of codes and MET values. *Med Sci Sports Exerc.* 2011;43(8):1575–81.
3. American College of Sports Medicine. The recommended quantity and quality of exercise for developing and maintaining fitness in healthy adults. *Med Sci Sports Exerc.* 1978;10(3):vii–x.
4. American College of Sports Medicine position stand. The recommended quantity and quality of exercise for developing and maintaining cardiorespiratory and muscular fitness in healthy adults. *Med Sci Sports Exerc.* 1990;22(2):265–74.
5. American College of Sports Medicine Position Stand. The recommended quantity and quality of exercise for developing and maintaining cardiorespiratory and muscular fitness, and flexibility in healthy adults. *Med Sci Sports Exerc.* 1998;30(6):975–91.
6. Barnes PM, Schoenborn CA, National Center for Health Statistics (U.S.), Centers for Disease Control and Prevention (U.S.). *Physical Activity among Adults, United States, 2000.* Hyattsville (MD): U.S. Dept. of Health and Human Services, Centers for Disease Control and Prevention, National Center for Health Statistics; 2003. 24 p.
7. Bassett DR Jr, Ainsworth BE, Leggett SR, et al. Accuracy of five electronic pedometers for measuring distance walked. *Med Sci Sports Exerc.* 1996;28(8):1071–7.
8. Bassett DR Jr, Ainsworth BE, Swartz AM, Strath SJ, O'Brien WL, King GA. Validity of four motion sensors in measuring moderate intensity physical activity. *Med Sci Sports Exerc.* 2000;32(9 Suppl):S471–80.
9. Bassett DR Jr, Strath SJ. Use of pedometers to assess physical activity. In: Welk G, editor. *Physical Activity Assessments for Health-Related Research.* Champaign: Human Kinetics; 2002. p. 213–25.
10. Blair SN, Kohl HW,3rd, Barlow CE, Paffenbarger RS Jr, Gibbons LW, Macera CA. Changes in physical fitness and all-cause mortality. A prospective study of healthy and unhealthy men. *JAMA.* 1995;273(14):1093–8.
11. Bouchard C, Tremblay A, Leblanc C, Lortie G, Savard R, Theriault G. A method to assess energy expenditure in children and adults. *Am J Clin Nutr.* 1983;37(3):461–7.
12. Bowles HR, FitzGerald SJ, Morrow JR Jr, Jackson AW, Blair SN. Construct validity of self-reported historical physical activity. *Am J Epidemiol.* 2004;160(3):279–86.
13. Calabro MA, Welk GJ, Eisenmann JC. Validation of the SenseWear Pro Armband algorithms in children. *Med Sci Sports Exerc.* 2009;41(9):1714–20.
14. Caspersen CJ, Powell KE, Christenson GM. Physical activity, exercise, and physical fitness: definitions and distinctions for health-related research. *Public Health Rep.* 1985;100(2):126–31.
15. Chasan-Taber L, Erickson JB, McBride JW, Nasca PC, Chasan-Taber S, Freedson PS. Reproducibility of a self-administered lifetime physical activity questionnaire among female college alumnae. *Am J Epidemiol.* 2002;155(3):282–9.
16. The Compendium of Physical Activities [Internet]. Washington (DC): President's Council on Physical Fitness and Sports; [cited 2011 June 6]. Available from: http://purl.access.gpo.gov/GPO/LPS53360
17. Crouter SE, Clowers KG, Bassett DR Jr. A novel method for using accelerometer data to predict energy expenditure. *J Appl Physiol.* 2006;100(4):1324–31.
18. Crouter SE, Schneider PL, Bassett DR Jr. Spring-levered versus piezo-electric pedometer accuracy in overweight and obese adults. *Med Sci Sports Exerc.* 2005;37(10):1673–9.
19. Crouter SE, Schneider PL, Karabulut M, Bassett DR Jr. Validity of 10 electronic pedometers for measuring steps, distance, and energy cost. *Med Sci Sports Exerc.* 2003;35(8):1455–60.
20. Dunn AL, Marcus BH, Kampert JB, Garcia ME, Kohl HW,3rd, Blair SN. Comparison of lifestyle and structured interventions to increase physical activity and cardiorespiratory fitness: a randomized trial. *JAMA.* 1999;281(4):327–34.
21. Freedson PS, Miller K. Objective monitoring of physical activity using motion sensors and heart rate. *Res Q Exerc Sport.* 2000;71 (2 Suppl):S21–9.
22. Garber CE, Blissmer B, Deschenes MR, et al. Quantity and quality of exercise for developing and maintaining cardiorespiratory, musculoskeletal, and neuromotor fitness in apparently healthy adults: guidance for prescribing exercise. *Med Sci Sports Exerc.* 2011; 43(7):1334–59.
23. Haskell WL, Lee IM, Pate RR, et al. Physical activity and public health: updated recommendation for adults from the American College of Sports Medicine and the American Heart Association. *Med Sci Sports Exerc.* 2007;39(8):1423–34.
24. Haskell WL, Taylor HL, Wood PD, Schrott H, Heiss G. Strenuous physical activity, treadmill exercise test performance and plasma high-density lipoprotein cholesterol.The Lipid Research Clinics Program Prevalence Study. *Circulation.* 1980;62(4 Pt 2):IV53–61.
25. Healey J. Future possibilities in electronic monitoring of physical activity. *Res Q Exerc Sport.* 2000;71(2 Suppl):S137–45.
26. Healy GN, Wijndaele K, Dunstan DW, et al. Objectively measured sedentary time, physical activity, and metabolic risk: the Australian Diabetes, Obesity and Lifestyle Study (AusDiab). *Diabetes Care.* 2008;31(2):369–71.
27. Hendelman D, Miller K, Baggett C, Debold E, Freedson P. Validity of accelerometry for the assessment of moderate intensity physical activity in the field. *Med Sci Sports Exerc.* 2000;32(9 Suppl):S442–9.
28. Holbrook EA, Barreira TV, Kang M. Validity and reliability of Omron pedometers for prescribed and self-paced walking. *Med Sci Sports Exerc.* 2009;41(3):670–4.
29. Jacobs DR Jr, Ainsworth BE, Hartman TJ, Leon AS. A simultaneous evaluation of 10 commonly used physical activity questionnaires. *Med Sci Sports Exerc.* 1993;25(1):81–91.
30. Johannsen DL, Calabro MA, Stewart J, Franke W, Rood JC, Welk GJ. Accuracy of armband monitors for measuring daily energy expenditure in healthy adults. *Med Sci Sports Exerc.* 2010; 42(11):2134–40.
31. Karabulut M, Crouter SE, Bassett DR Jr. Comparison of two waist-mounted and two ankle-mounted electronic pedometers. *Eur J Appl Physiol.* 2005;95(4):335–43.
32. Kimsey CD, Ham SA, Macera CA. Reliability of moderate and vigorous physical activity questions in the Behavioral Risk Factor

Surveillance System (BRFSS) [abstract]. *Med Sci Sports Exerc.* 2003;35(Suppl 5):S114.

33. Kohl HW,3rd, Kampert JB, Maasse LC. The accuracy of historical physical activity recall among middle-aged women and men [abstract]. *Med Sci Sports Exerc.* 1997;29(Suppl 5):S242.

34. Kriska A. Ethnic and cultural issues in assessing physical activity. *Res Q Exerc Sport.* 2000;71(2 Suppl):47–53.

35. Kriska AM, Bennett PH. An epidemiological perspective of the relationship between physical activity and NIDDM: from activity assessment to intervention. *Diabetes Metab Rev.* 1992;8(4):355–72.

36. Kriska AM, Caspersen CJ. Introduction to a collection of physical activity questionnaires. *Med Sci Sports Exerc.* 1997;29(6):S5–9.

37. Kriska AM, Knowler WC, LaPorte RE, et al. Development of questionnaire to examine relationship of physical activity and diabetes in Pima Indians. *Diabetes Care.* 1990;13(4):401–11.

38. Kriska AM, Sandler RB, Cauley JA, LaPorte RE, Hom DL, Pambianco G. The assessment of historical physical activity and its relation to adult bone parameters. *Am J Epidemiol.* 1988;127(5): 1053–63.

39. LaPorte RE, Montoye HJ, Caspersen CJ. Assessment of physical activity in epidemiologic research: problems and prospects. *Public Health Rep.* 1985;100(2):131–46.

40. Leenders NYJM, Sherman WM, Nagaraja HN. Comparisons of four methods of estimating physical activity in adult women. *Med Sci Sports Exerc.* 2000;32(7):1320–6.

41. Levine JA, Lanningham-Foster LM, McCrady SK, et al. Interindividual variation in posture allocation: possible role in human obesity. *Science.* 2005;307(5709):584–6.

42. Matthews CE, Chen KY, Freedson PS, et al. Amount of time spent in sedentary behaviors in the United States, 2003-2004. *Am J Epidemiol.* 2008;167(7):875–81.

43. Matthews CE, Shu XO, Jin F, et al. Lifetime physical activity and breast cancer risk in the Shanghai Breast Cancer Study. *Br J Cancer.* 2001;84(7):994–1001.

44. McKenzie TL, Marshall SJ, Sallis JF, Conway TL. Leisure-time physical activity in school environments: an observational study using SOPLAY. *Prev Med.* 2000;30(1):70–7.

45. Montoye HJ. *Measuring Physical Activity and Energy Expenditure.* Champaign (IL): Human Kinetics; 1996. 191 p.

46. Nieves JW, Grisso JA, Kelsey JL. A case-control study of hip fracture: evaluation of selected dietary variables and teenage physical activity. *Osteoporos Int.* 1992;2(3):122–7.

47. Owen N, Healy GN, Matthews CE, Dunstan DW. Too much sitting: the population health science of sedentary behavior. *Exerc Sport Sci Rev.* 2010;38(3):105–13.

48. Paffenbarger RS Jr, Hyde RT, Wing AL, Lee IM, Jung DL, Kampert JB. The association of changes in physical-activity level and other lifestyle characteristics with mortality among men. *N Engl J Med.* 1993;328(8):538–45.

49. Pate RR, Pratt M, Blair SN, et al. Physical activity and public health. A recommendation from the Centers for Disease Control and Prevention and the American College of Sports Medicine. *JAMA.* 1995;273(5):402–7.

50. Pereira MA, FitzerGerald SJ, Gregg EW, et al. A collection of Physical Activity Questionnaires for health-related research. *Med Sci Sports Exerc.* 1997;29(6 Suppl):S1–205.

51. Pivarnik JM, Reeves MJ, Rafferty AP. Seasonal variation in adult leisure-time physical activity. *Med Sci Sports Exerc.* 2003;35(6): 1004–8.

52. Pols MA, Peeters PH, Kemper HC, Grobbee DE. Methodological aspects of physical activity assessment in epidemiological studies. *Eur J Epidemiol.* 1998;14(1):63–70.

53. Puhl J, Greaves K, Hoyt M, Baranowski T. Children's Activity Rating Scale (CARS): description and calibration. *Res Q Exerc Sport.* 1990;61(1):26–36.

54. Ravussin E, Swinburn BA. Pathophysiology of obesity. *Lancet.* 1992;340(8816):404–8.

55. Rothney MP, Neumann M, Beziat A, Chen KY. An artificial neural network model of energy expenditure using nonintegrated acceleration signals. *J Appl Physiol.* 2007;103(4):1419–27.

56. Rowlands AV, Eston RG, Ingledew DK. Measurement of physical activity in children with particular reference to the use of heart rate and pedometry. *Sports Med.* 1997;24(4):258–72.

57. Sallis JF, Haskell WL, Wood PD, et al. Physical activity assessment methodology in the Five-City Project. *Am J Epidemiol.* 1985;121(1):91–106.

58. Sallis JF, Nader PR, Broyles SL, et al. Correlates of physical activity at home in Mexican-American and Anglo-American preschool children. *Health Psychol.* 1993;12(5):390–8.

59. Sallis JF, Saelens BE. Assessment of physical activity by self-report: status, limitations, and future directions. *Res Q Exerc Sport.* 2000;71(2 Suppl):1–14.

60. Schneider PL, Crouter SE, Lukajic O, Bassett DR Jr. Accuracy and reliability of 10 pedometers for measuring steps over a 400-m walk. *Med Sci Sports Exerc.* 2003;35(10):1779–84.

61. Schutz Y, Herren R. Assessment of speed of human locomotion using a differential satellite global positioning system. *Med Sci Sports Exerc.* 2000;32(3):642–6.

62. Silcott NA, Bassett DR Jr, Thompson DL, Fitzhugh EC, Steeves JA. Evaluation of the Omron HJ-720ITC pedometer under free-Living conditions. *Med Sci Sports Exerc.* 2011;43(9):1791–7.

63. Staudenmayer J, Pober D, Crouter S, Bassett D, Freedson P. An artificial neural network to estimate physical activity energy expenditure and identify physical activity type from an accelerometer. *J Appl Physiol.* 2009;107(4):1300–7.

64. Strath SJ, Bassett DR Jr, Thompson DL, Swartz AM. Validity of the simultaneous heart rate-motion sensor technique for measuring energy expenditure. *Med Sci Sports Exerc.* 2002;34(5):888–94.

65. Strath SJ, Swartz AM, Bassett DR Jr, O'Brien WL, King GA, Ainsworth BE. Evaluation of heart rate as a method for assessing moderate intensity physical activity. *Med Sci Sports Exerc.* 2000;32(9 Suppl):S465–70.

66. Swartz AM, Strath SJ, Bassett DR Jr, O'Brien WL, King GA, Ainsworth BE. Estimation of energy expenditure using CSA accelerometers at hip and wrist sites. *Med Sci Sports Exerc.* 2000;32 (9 Suppl):S450–6.

67. Taking steps toward increased physical activity using pedometers to measure and motivate [Internet]. Washington (DC): President's Council on Physical Fitness and Sports; [cited 2011 Jun 6]. Available from: http://purl.access.gpo.gov/GPO/LPS20620; http://purl.access.gpo.gov/GPO/LPS20620

68. Terrier P, Ladetto Q, Merminod B, Schutz Y. High-precision satellite positioning system as a new tool to study the biomechanics of human locomotion. *J Biomech.* 2000;33(12):1717–22.

69. Treuth MS. Applying multiple methods to improve the accuracy of activity assessments. In: Welk G, editor. *Physical Activity Assessments for Health-Related Research.* Champaign: Human Kinetics; 2002. p. 213–25.

70. Tudor-Locke C, Ainsworth BE, Thompson RW, Matthews CE. Comparison of pedometer and accelerometer measures of free-living physical activity. *Med Sci Sports Exerc.* 2002;34(12): 2045–51.

71. Tudor-Locke CE, Myers AM. Challenges and opportunities for measuring physical activity in sedentary adults. *Sports Med.* 2001;31(2):91–100.

72. Tudor-Locke CE, Myers AM. Methodological considerations for researchers and practitioners using pedometers to measure physical (ambulatory) activity. *Res Q Exerc Sport.* 2001;72(1):1–12.

73. U.S. Department of Health and Human Services, Centers for Disease Control and Prevention, National Center for Chronic Disease Prevention and Health Promotion, The President's Council on Physical Fitness and Sports. *Physical Activity and Health: A Report of the Surgeon General.* Atlanta, GA: President's Council on Physical Fitness and Sports; 1996. 278 p.

74. Vuillemin A, Guillemin F, Jouanny P, Denis G, Jeandel C. Differential influence of physical activity on lumbar spine and femoral neck bone mineral density in the elderly population. *J Gerontol A Biol Sci Med Sci.* 2001;56(6):B248–53.

75. Warren TY, Barry V, Hooker SP, Sui X, Church TS, Blair SN. Sedentary behaviors increase risk of cardiovascular disease mortality in men. *Med Sci Sports Exerc.* 2010;42(5):879–85.

76. Washburn RA, Heath GW, Jackson AW. Reliability and validity issues concerning large-scale surveillance of physical activity. *Res Q Exerc Sport.* 2000;71(2 Suppl):S104–13.

77. Weiss TW, Slater CH, Green LW, Kennedy VC, Albright DL, Wun CC. The validity of single-item, self-assessment questions as measures of adult physical activity. *J Clin Epidemiol.* 1990;43(11):1123–9.

78. Welk GJ, Blair SN, Wood K, Jones S, Thompson RW. A comparative evaluation of three accelerometry-based physical activity monitors. *Med Sci Sports Exerc.* 2000;32(9 Suppl):S489–97.

79. Welk GJ, Corbin CB, Dale D. Measurement issues in the assessment of physical activity in children. *Res Q Exerc Sport.* 2000;71 (2 Suppl):S59–73.

80. Welk GJ, Differding JA, Thompson RW, Blair SN, Dziura J, Hart P. The utility of the Digi-walker step counter to assess daily physical activity patterns. *Med Sci Sports Exerc.* 2000;32 (9 Suppl):S481–8.

81. Welk GJ, Morrow JR. Physical activity assessments. In: Meredith MD, Welk G, Cooper Institute for Aerobics Research, editors. *Fitnessgram Test Administration Manual.* 2nd ed. Champaign: Human Kinetics; 1999. p. 55–65.

82. Winters-Hart CS, Brach JS, Storti KL, Trauth JM, Kriska AM. Validity of a questionnaire to assess historical physical activity in older women. *Med Sci Sports Exerc.* 2004;36(12):2082–7.

83. Zhu W, Lee M. Invariance of wearing location of Omron-BI pedometers: a validation study. *J Phys Act Health.* 2010;7(6):706–17.

SELECTED REFERENCES FOR FURTHER READING

Lee I-M, Blair S, Manson J, Pafferbarger RS. Physical Activity and Health: Epidemiologic Methods and Studies. New York (NY): Oxford University Press; 2008.

Measurement of Physical Activity: The Cooper Institute Conference Series. Proceedings from the 9th Measurement and Evaluation Symposium. *Res Q Exerc Sport.* 2000;71(suppl 2).

Montoye HJ, Kemper HCG, Saris WHM, Washburn RA. *Measuring Physical Activity and Energy Expenditure.* Champaign (IL): Human Kinetics; 1996. 191 p.

National Center for Health Statistics. *Assessing Physical Fitness and Physical Activity in Population-Based Surveys.* Drury TF, editor. DHHS Pub. No. (PHS) 89-1253. Public Health Service. Washington (DC): U.S. Government Printing Office; 1989.

Pereira MA, FitzGerald SJ, Gregg EW, et al. A collection of physical activity questionnaires for health related research. *Med Sci Sports Exerc.* 1997;29(6):S1–205.

Welk GJ, editor. *Physical Activity Assessments for Health-Related Research.* Champaign (IL): Human Kinetics; 2002. 269 p.

INTERNET RESOURCES

- Centers for Disease Control and Prevention: Nutrition and Physical Activity: http://www.cdc.gov/nccdphp/dnpa/
- The Cooper Institute: http://www.cooperinst.org
- PACE Projects: http://www.paceproject.org
- Physical Activity Devices: http://wockets.wikispaces.com/Loggers
- The President's Challenge: http://www.presidentschallenge.org/activity_log/track_progress.aspx
- USC PRC Reports and Tools: http://prevention.sph.sc.edu/tools/index.htm

Nutritional Status and Chronic Diseases

Compelling evidence demonstrates that lifestyle changes such as dietary improvements, increased physical activity, and behavior modification can prevent or delay major chronic diseases, including cardiovascular disease (CVD), obesity, osteoporosis, and diabetes. Importantly, research confirms that the effects of dietary and other lifestyle changes (including exercise and weight loss) may be additive (16,25). At the same time that clinical and population studies have supported the importance of diet, the effects of nutrients and foods on genome stability, imprinting, expression, and viability have also correlated with dietary factors at the molecular level that lead to prevention of chronic diseases (186). Largely because of this emerging evidence, a paradigm shift in health care approaches has occurred toward early and aggressive prevention strategies. Accordingly, a greater proportion of the population will need behavioral strategies for lifestyle changes that positively affect chronic metabolic disease risk. Thus, the purpose of this chapter is to examine the relationship of diet and nutrition to chronic disease and to encourage health care professionals to promote healthier lifestyles.

Chronic metabolic diseases are often interrelated. For example, obesity is associated with the comorbidities of CVD, diabetes, and hypertension, all of which are characterized by increased morbidity and mortality risk from insulin resistance and its consequences (53). Increased levels of circulating free fatty acids associated with excess stored fat, particularly intra-abdominal, hepatic, pancreatic, and other depots, appear to contribute to systemic inflammation and heightened insulin resistance (6,56,107,155). A related condition known as metabolic syndrome encompasses most of these chronic conditions (3,55,72).

KEY TERMS

Antioxidants: Dietary components such as vitamins C and E, selenium, carotenoids, and other phytochemicals (chemicals from plants with antioxidant or hormone-like actions) that can protect DNA and cell membranes against oxidative damage from carcinogens.

Body mass index (BMI): A measure used to evaluate body mass; equal to body weight (in kilograms) divided by height^2 (in meters).

Cholesterol: A steroid alcohol present in human cells and blood that regulates membrane fluidity and functions as a precursor molecule in metabolism. As a constituent of low-density lipoprotein cholesterol (LDL-C), it contributes to plaque formation in arteries, and recommendations concerning maximal blood levels have been made as part of the National Cholesterol Education Program (NCEP) (133).

Diabetes: A state of elevated blood glucose levels (fasting ≥ 126 mg $\cdot$ dL^{-1}) associated with elevated glycated hemoglobin A1C (HbA1C), caused either by loss of insulin-producing cells in the pancreas (Type 1) or by peripheral insulin resistance (Type 2) (8).

Glycemic index (GI): The increase in blood sugar after ingestion of a food or food component compared with the increase after ingestion of glucose, which is assigned an index of 100, with foods being assigned higher and lower relative values. The glycemic response varies with the type of sugar, other food components, amount of carbohydrate, nature of the starch, and cooking or food processing.

Glycemic load: A value for each food that combines both the quality and quantity of carbohydrate to predict blood glucose responses to different types and amounts of food: (GI × the amount of carbohydrate) divided by 100.

High-density lipoprotein cholesterol (HDL-C): Compound that transports body cholesterol to other lipoproteins for disposal, contains a high proportion of phospholipids (30%) and protein (45%–50%), and generally decreases the risk of coronary artery disease (133).

Hypertension: Systolic blood pressure of 140 mm Hg or higher or a diastolic blood pressure of 90 mm Hg or greater (35 — update with JNC 8 in Spring 2012).

Impaired fasting glucose (IFG): A prediabetic condition in which the fasting blood sugar is elevated ($100–125$ mg $\cdot$ dL^{-1}) (8).

Impaired glucose tolerance (IGT): A prediabetic condition in which the blood sugar level is elevated ($140–199$ mg $\cdot$ dL^{-1}) after a 2-h glucose tolerance test (8).

Interesterified fats: The latest modified (stearic acid-rich) fats created by manufacturers to replace unhealthy trans fats in commercial food products. This newer fat may raise blood glucose and depress insulin action in humans similarly to trans fat (189).

Low-density lipoprotein cholesterol (LDL-C): Substance that is taken up by receptor and scavenger pathways in blood vessels, contains a high proportion of cholesterol (45%), and generally increases the risk of cardiovascular disease (CVD) (133).

Metabolic syndrome: A cluster of metabolic conditions, including obesity, IFG, elevated triglycerides, low levels of HDL-C, and hypertension, usually characterized by insulin resistance and a high risk of developing CVD or diabetes (72).

Monounsaturated fatty acids (MUFA): Fatty acids with one double bond within the carbon chain, prevalent in olive oil, canola oil, and high oleic acid oils. These fats are neutral or only slightly increase serum LDL-C levels.

Obesity: A marked excess of body fat, defined by the National Institutes of Health as a BMI of 30 kg $\cdot$ m^{-2} or more.

Omega-3 fatty acids: Fatty acids with the first double bond between carbon atoms located between the third and fourth carbons from the methyl end of the chain, including α-linolenic acid (ALA) and the three series such as eicosapentaenoic acid (EPA) and docosahexaenoic acid (DHA). These fats decrease the risk of CVD and are prevalent in fish and flaxseed, walnut, canola, and soybean oils.

Omega-6 fatty acids: Fatty acids with the first double bond between carbon atoms located between the sixth and seventh carbons from the methyl end of the chain, which are converted to hormone-like substances called eicosanoids. Sources of omega-6 fatty acids are corn, safflower, peanut, cottonseed, soybean, sesame, rapeseed, borage, and primrose oils.

Osteoporosis: A condition characterized by microarchitectural deterioration of bone tissue leading to decreased bone mass and increased bone fragility.

Overweight: A condition of excess body fat less marked than obesity, defined by the National Institutes of Health as a BMI of $25–29.9$ kg $\cdot$ m^{-2}.

Polyunsaturated fatty acids (PUFA): Fatty acids with two or more double bonds within the carbon chain. Foods with a high percentage of polyunsaturated fats include corn, safflower, peanut, cottonseed, soybean, fish, walnut, and flaxseed oils (86).

Prediabetes: The intermediate metabolic state between normal fasting blood glucose levels (<100 mg $\cdot$ dL^{-1}) and diagnosed diabetes (≥126 mg $\cdot$ dL^{-1}), which can include IGT, IFG, or a combination of both conditions. Individuals with prediabetes are considered to be at risk for developing Type 2 diabetes (134).

Saturated fatty acids (SFA): Fatty acids with single bonds between all carbons atoms, that is, the carbon atoms are attached to as many hydrogen atoms as possible (saturated). These fats increase serum LDL-C levels and are prevalent in animal fats, butter, meats, milk fat, cheeses, and tropical oils, such as palm, coconut, and palm kernel oil.

Trans fats: Fatty acids with a rearrangement of the bond between some of the carbon atoms to a form rarely found in natural foods. The change occurs because of processing such as hydrogenation (the addition of hydrogen to change texture and improve shelf life). Foods containing these fats include margarine, shortening, processed foods, and commercially baked or fried foods.

The National Cholesterol Education Program (NCEP) criteria (3,133) for the metabolic syndrome include any three of the following: large waist circumference (≥102 cm or 40 in. in men and ≥88 cm or 35 in. in women); high triglycerides (≥150 mg $\cdot$ dL^{-1}); low-serum, **high-density lipoprotein cholesterol (HDL-C)** levels (<40 mg $\cdot$ dL^{-1} for men and <50 mg $\cdot$ dL^{-1} for women); high blood pressure (BP; systolic ≥130 mm Hg or diastolic ≥85 mm Hg); and fasting plasma glucose concentration ≥100 mg $\cdot$ dL^{-1}. It is estimated that 34%

of American adults meet three or more of these criteria and have metabolic syndrome, thereby increasing their risk for CVD and Type 2 diabetes (55). Abdominal obesity has been the most common, followed by decreased HDL-C levels, hypertension, and elevated plasma triglycerides (52). As of 2011, an estimated 79 million Americans have **prediabetes** and another 25.8 million have diabetes (134). The risk for disease increases as the number of these characteristics accumulates, warranting the need for early intervention.

The prospective Insulin Resistance Atherosclerosis Study (145) found that the best predictor for developing the metabolic syndrome in adults without diabetes was waist circumference and that abdominal obesity may precede the development of other metabolic syndrome components. More recently, nonalcoholic fatty liver disease (NAFLD) has also emerged as a component of the metabolic syndrome, with elevated liver markers predicting its development (74). However, the existence of this syndrome remains controversial, with some arguing that it cannot be considered a "real" syndrome in a strict sense because, at present, no unifying mechanism explains it (187). Definition of metabolic syndrome varies as well, but a single set of cut points has now been agreed upon by the major national and international organizations for all components except waist circumference (3). However, adults may fare better in managing their disease risk when each metabolic component that is present is simply treated separately rather than focusing on treating the syndrome as a whole. In other research, the development of insulin resistance in young adulthood was strongly predicted from childhood adiposity and serum insulin levels and from being the offspring of a parent with Type 2 diabetes (147,185,186). This research underscores the need to address excess weight gain in children to manage metabolic risk factors.

Unfortunately, there is also no agreement about the optimal diet for preventing and treating chronic metabolic diseases, but recommendations from professional organizations and government institutes or agencies provide evidence-based guidelines, such as the guidelines for diabetes, obesity, and CVD given in *Table 14-1*. The American Dietetic Association (122) advocates the terminology *medical nutrition therapy* (MNT) for the nutritional diagnostic, therapeutic, and counseling services to accomplish the following:

- Effectively treat and manage disease conditions
- Reduce or eliminate the need for prescription drug use
- Help reduce complications in patients with disease
- Improve patients' overall health and quality of life

The MNT recommendations for obesity, diabetes, and CVD specify dietary proportions of macronutrients: carbohydrate, fat, and protein. The average diet in the United States (as of 2005–2006) for individuals older than 20 yr consisted of approximately 34% kcal from fat, 48% kcal from carbohydrates, 16% kcal from protein, and approximately 2% (females) to 4% (males) of kilocalories from alcohol (95). When a diet low in one macronutrient is promoted, other macronutrients are concomitantly increased at a given energy level; for example, a low-carbohydrate diet results in a higher fat and protein dietary intake (175). Therefore, frequent monitoring of fasting lipid panels may be indicated for persons at risk of chronic disease who choose a low-carbohydrate diet (12). Usually, slight-to-moderate changes in macronutrient proportions have little effect on short-term health parameters, such as serum lipids, but deleterious, long-term health effects may be possible. More research is needed.

The greatest similarities across national diet recommendations (see *Table 14-1*) for obesity, hypertension, CVD, and diabetes are the recommendations to maintain a healthy weight and to consume total dietary fat of approximately 30% kcal. The NCEP Therapeutic Lifestyle Changes (TLC) recommends a dietary fat intake of 25%–35% of daily kilocalories (133). The specified purpose of the TLC diet is for prevention and treatment of obesity, metabolic syndrome, and CVD. Although recommendations for specific diet components vary with disease risk, a healthy weight (or at least modest weight loss and prevention of further weight gain), is a primary step toward decreasing chronic disease risk. All calorie-restricted diets can be balanced to result in weight loss, regardless of their composition, but some diets meet nutrition needs with less health risk and should be the preferred choice for health professionals. A reasonable guide is the Institute of Medicine/National Academy of Sciences 2002 recommendation of acceptable macronutrient ranges of 20%–35% fat, 45%–65% carbohydrate, and 10%–35% protein (48).

CARDIOVASCULAR DISEASE AND DIET

Major CVDs leading to heart attacks and strokes are the leading cause of death and disability in the United States and worldwide (136). The World Health Organization currently attributes one-third of all global deaths to CVD. This ongoing and increasing health problem underscores the need to improve our communication of improved diet and lifestyle interventions. Disease progression occurs over a lifetime, and dietary changes must be maintained to be effective. Public health and clinical approaches alone have limitations. Therefore, the American Heart Association's (AHA) guide (151) for improving cardiovascular health at the community level advocates for concomitant and parallel public health and clinical approaches. They identify public health problems, including limited access to screening; limited long-term and effective strategies for diet and physical activity changes; poor identification of healthy food choices at grocery stores and restaurants; and lack of safe, attractive sites for physical activity in many communities. Clinical settings provide a complementary focus on individuals with high disease risk, but diet counseling and nutrition education are often inadequate and highly variable (151).

Diverse and interdisciplinary diet and lifestyle changes are required to address CVD risk. The AHA (14) recommends the following for the general population: consume an overall healthy diet; aim for a healthy body weight; aim for recommended levels of

TABLE 14-1. Medical Nutrition Therapy for Obesity/Metabolic Syndrome, Hypertension, Cardiovascular Disease, and Diabetes

Diagnostic Criteria and Risk Factors	Nutrition and Lifestyle Recommendations	Therapeutic Objectives	Practice Guidelines (References)
Obesity/metabolic syndrome Criteria for metabolic syndrome include any three of the following: Waist circumference: Men >102 cm (>40 in) Women >88 cm (>35 in) BP: ≥130/85 mm Hg Trig: ≥150 mg · dL^{-1} HDL-C: men <40 mg · dL^{-1}, women <50 mg · dL^{-1} FPG: ≥100 mg · dL^{-1} Other risk factors: BMI ≥30 kg · m^{-2}, sleep apnea, elevated CRP levels Hyperinsulinemia and insulin resistance may also be present	**Low calorie Step I diet and referral to dietitian** Lower risk individuals: 500–1,000 kcal · d^{-1} reduction, ≤30% fat, 8%–10% SFA, <300 mg cholesterol, 20–30 g fibers ~2.4 g Na, 1,000–1,500 mg Ca **Total Lifestyle Change (TLC) diet and referral to dietitian** (higher risk for heart disease or with diagnosed heart disease) Establish appropriate kilocalorie Rx with 50%–60% CHO, ~15% protein, 25%–35% total fat, <7% SFA, <200 mg cholesterol (**same as Step II diet**), PUFA (up to 10% of total kilocalories), MUFA (up to 20% of total kilocalories), 10–25 g viscous (soluble) fibers, 2 g plant stanols/sterols **Weight reduction, long-term control** 1–2 lb · wk^{-1} and gradually reach healthy BMI (<30 initially, then <25 kg · m^{-2}) **Increase physical activity** (~200 kcal · d^{-1}) **Smoking cessation**	1. Reasonable weight loss of 5%–10%, maintain healthy BMI, prevent weight gain 2. Primary: ↓ LDL-C to ↓ CAD risk Secondary: recognize and treat metabolic syndrome for further risk reduction Optimal BMI range: 18.5–24.9 kg · m^{-2} Target total cholesterol: <200 mg · m^{-2} Target TG: <150 mg · dL^{-1} Target LDL-C: <100 mg · dL^{-1} Target HDL-C: >40 mg · dL^{-1} (men) >50 mg · dL^{-1} (women) Target BP: <130/85 mm Hg Target FPG: <100 mg · dL^{-1}	NHLBI, NIH — *Clinical Guidelines on the Identification, Evaluation, and Treatment of Overweight and Obesity in Adults* (37) NCEP ATP III — Metabolic Syndrome Criteria and Therapeutic Lifestyle Changes (133) http://www.nhlbi.nih.gov/guidelines/obesity/ http://www.nhlbi.nih.gov/guidelines/cholesterol/ http://www.surgeongeneral.gov/topics/obesity
Hypertension BP classification: Normal: <120/80 mm Hg Pre-HTN: 120–139/80–89 mm Hg Stage 1 HTN: 140–159/ 90–99 mm Hg Stage 2 HTN: ≥160/100 mm Hg Risk of CVD, starting with 115/75 mm Hg, doubles with each increment of 20/10 mm Hg	**DASH diet and referral to dietitian** Establish appropriate kilocalorie Rx ≤2,400 mg Na, <30% total fat Limit alcohol: men ≤2, women ≤1 drink · d^{-1} Reduce dietary sodium and red meat intake Increase dietary calcium, magnesium, potassium, and fiber via fruits, vegetables, whole grains, reduced fat dairy, and lean protein Include fish, nuts, seeds, and dry beans weekly Choose plant fats and oils **Achieve and maintain healthy body weight** **Increase physical activity** **Smoking cessation**	1. Prevent progression to HTN in prehypertensive population 2. Decrease CVD complications and reduce cardiovascular and renal morbidity and mortality in hypertensive population Optimal BP: <120/80 mm Hg Goal of tx: BP <130/80 mm Hg (for patients with diabetes or chronic kidney disease) Goal of tx: BP <140/90 mm Hg (for patients with HTN)	NHLBI, NIH — Prevention, Detection, Evaluation, and Treatment of High Blood Pressure and DASH Eating Plan (214) http://www.nhlbi.nih.gov/guidelines/hypertension/jnc8/index http://www.nhlbi.nih.gov/health/public/heart/hbp/dash_brief.htm
Cardiovascular disease Abnormal blood lipid profile: Total cholesterol: ≥200 mg · dL^{-1} Triglyceride: ≥150 mg · dL^{-1} LDL-C: ≥100 mg · dL^{-1} HDL-C: men <40 mg · dL^{-1}, women <50 mg · dL^{-1} Other major CVD risk factors include the following: Obesity, inactive lifestyle, atherogenic diet Elevated BP, blood glucose, and homocysteine levels Hyperinsulinemia and insulin resistance may also be present	**AHA Dietary Guidelines and referral to dietitian** Establish appropriate kilocalorie Rx <6 g NaCl (<2,400 mg Na) <30% total fat, limit TFAs **(AHA population-wide recommendations for individuals at lower risk)** <10% SFA, <300 mg cholesterol **(AHA MNT for individuals at higher risk)** <7% SFA, <200 mg cholesterol Limit alcohol: men ≤2 drinks · d^{-1}, women ≤1 drink · d^{-1} Limit high-caloric/low-nutrient dense foods and beverages Increase intake of antioxidants, ω fatty acids, and fiber via variety of fruits, vegetables, whole grains, lower fat dairy, fish, legumes, nuts, plant fats, and oils **Achieve and maintain healthy body weight** **Increase physical activity: 30 min daily** of moderate-intensity exercise using large muscle groups (*i.e.*, walking or swimming) **Smoking cessation**	1. Reduce CVD risk, morbidity, and mortality by preventing or reducing the development of atherosclerotic disease and stroke 2. For overweight/obese patients, ↓ weight by 10% in first year of therapy Target total cholesterol: <160 mg · dL^{-1} (optimal) Total cholesterol: 160–199 mg · dL^{-1} (low-risk profile) Target LDL-C: <100 mg · dL^{-1} ≥2 CAD risk factors Target HDL-C: >40 (men), >50 (women) mg · dL^{-1} Goal BP: <140/90 or <130/85 mm Hg for patients with renal insufficiency, heart failure, or <130/80 mm Hg for patients with diabetes	AHA Dietary Guidelines, Revision 2002 (152) AHA Diet and Lifestyle Recommendations, 2006 (14) http://www.americanheart.org

(continued)

TABLE 14-1. Medical Nutrition Therapy for Obesity/Metabolic Syndrome, Hypertension, Cardiovascular Disease, and Diabetes *(Continued)*

Diagnostic Criteria and Risk Factors	Nutrition and Lifestyle Recommendations	Therapeutic Objectives	Practice Guidelines (References)
Diabetes Normoglycemia: FPG <100 mg · dL^{-1} 2-h PG <140 mg · dL^{-1} IFG (impaired fasting glucose): FPG 100–125 mg · dL^{-1} IGT (impaired glucose tolerance): 2-h PG 140–199 mg · dL^{-1} Diabetes: FPG ≥126 mg · dL^{-1} 2-h PG ≥200 mg · dL^{-1} Casual PG ≥200 mg · dL^{-1} (symptoms present)	**ADA Dietary Guidelines and referral to dietitian** Establish appropriate kilocalorie Rx, aiming for modest weight loss CHO should provide 50%–55% total kilocalorie, with intake of 14 g fibers per 1,000 kcal, 50% of grains as whole, and low glycemic index foods rich in fiber Monitoring carbohydrate intake is a key strategy in glycemic control Low-carbohydrate diets (total <130 g · d^{-1}) are not recommended 15%–20% protein; high-protein diets are not recommended as a method for weight loss at this time ~30% total fat, minimize TFAs <7% SFA, <200 mg cholesterol Limit alcohol: men ≤2, women <1 drink · d^{-1} Appropriate Rx may integrate any of the following established regimens: Low calorie Step I or Step II, TLC, DASH, AHA, or Mediterranean diets **Goals of MNT and self-management education:** • Attain and maintain recommended metabolic outcomes, including glucose, A1C, LDL-C, HDL-C, TG levels, BP, and body weight • Modify nutrient intake and lifestyle as appropriate for the prevention and treatment of obesity, dyslipidemia, HTN, CVD, depression, and nephropathy • Structured, intensive lifestyle programs involving participant education, individualized counseling, regular physical activity, and SMBG • Smoking cessation	1. Diabetes prevention: ↓ risk by encouraging physical activity and food choices that facilitate moderate weight loss (5%–7%) or at least prevent weight gain 2. Prevent and treat chronic complications and comorbidities of diabetes Target HbA1C: <7.0% Target FPG: 80–120 mg · dL^{-1} Target bedtime BG: 100–140 mg · dL^{-1} Target BP: <130/80 mm Hg Target blood lipids (mg · dL^{-1}): TG <150 LDL <100 HDL ≥40 (men), ≥50 (women) Target microalbumin: <30 µg · mg^{-1} creatinine	American Diabetes Association — "Nutrition Recommendations and Interventions for Diabetes" (12) Clinical Practice Guidelines http://www.diabetes.org American Dietetic Association — Nutrition Practice Guidelines at http://www.eatright.org

BP, blood pressure; Trig, triglyceride; HDL–C, high-density lipoprotein cholesterol; FPG, fasting plasma glucose; BMI, body mass index; CRP, C-reactive protein; SFA, saturated fatty acids; Na, sodium; Ca, calcium; Rx, prescription; CHO, carbohydrate; PUFA, polyunsaturated fatty acids; MUFA, monounsaturated fatty acids; LDL–C, low-density lipoprotein cholesterol; CAD, coronary artery disease; TG, triglyceride; NHLBI, National Heart, Lung and Blood Institute; NIH, National Institutes of Health; NCEP, National Cholesterol Education Program; ATP III, Adult Treatment Panel III; HTN, Hypertension; DASH, Dietary Approaches to Stop Hypertension; CVD, cardiovascular disease; tx, treatment; AHA, American Heart Association; NaCl, sodium chloride; TFA, trans fatty acid; MNT, medical nutrition therapy; PG, plasma glucose; SMBG, self-monitored blood glucose; HbA1C, hemoglobin A1C; BG, blood glucose.

low-density lipoprotein cholesterol (LDL-C), HDL-C, and triglycerides; aim for normal blood pressure; aim for a normal blood glucose level; be physically active; and avoid use of and exposure to tobacco products. To do so, they recommend that all individuals balance caloric intake and physical activity to achieve and maintain a healthy body weight; consume a diet rich in vegetables and fruits; choose whole-grain, high-fiber foods; consume fish, especially oily fish, at least twice a week; limit intake of saturated fatty acids (SFA) to 7% of energy, trans fat to 1% of energy, and cholesterol to 300 mg $\cdot$ d^{-1} by choosing lean meats and vegetable alternatives, fat-free (skim) or low-fat (1% fat) dairy products, and minimize intake of partially hydrogenated fats; minimize intake of beverages and foods with added sugars; choose and prepare foods with little or no salt; consume alcohol in moderation; and make healthy choices when eating outside the home.

CORONARY ARTERY DISEASE

Coronary artery disease (CAD), also known as coronary heart disease, includes the development of atherosclerosis with the potential negative outcome of clot formation, resulting in a myocardial infarction (MI) or heart attack (see *Chapter 6*). Risk factors for CAD include an abnormal lipid profile, obesity, inactive lifestyle, atherogenic diet, elevated blood glucose and homocysteine levels, and hyperinsulinemia and insulin resistance, to name a few (152). The INTERHEART study additionally listed smoking, hypertension, abdominal obesity, psychosocial factors, low consumption of fruits, vegetables and alcohol, and a lack of regular physical activity as risk factors for MI in men and women of all ages in 52 countries spanning all regions worldwide (217). The preferred lipid profile, recommended by the NCEP and others through 2011, includes a total cholesterol of 200 mg $\cdot$ dL^{-1} or less with a target of 160 mg $\cdot$ dL^{-1} with high CAD risk, triglycerides 150 mg $\cdot$ dL^{-1} or less, LDL-C 100 mg $\cdot$ dL^{-1} or less, and an HDL-C equal to or greater than 40 mg $\cdot$ dL^{-1} for women and 50 mg $\cdot$ dL^{-1} for men (14,133,152).

The primary dietary factors that prevent atherosclerotic lesions and abnormally elevated serum lipid levels include diets moderate or low in SFA and cholesterol, decreased trans fatty acid intake, increased omega-3 fatty acid intake, and greater monounsaturated fatty acids (MUFA) consumption (14,133,152). Vitamins decrease cardiovascular risk if patients consume an adequate food intake of antioxidants and dietary vitamins and minerals (*e.g.*, vitamin B$_{12}$, vitamin B$_6$, folate, magnesium). In addition, intake of fruits, vegetables, whole-grain breads, cereals, nuts, seeds, and other plant foods provides fiber, plant sterols and stanols, and phytochemicals (like flavonoids) that decrease cardiovascular risk are recommended. A variety of other foods and food components, such as alcohol and soy protein, have been investigated as a means to decrease risk (133). Dietary factors important for CVD risk also decrease clot formation, including regular consumption of fish sources containing high concentrations of omega-3 fatty acids and moderate alcohol intake.

Fats and Cholesterol

Saturated and Unsaturated

SFA, cholesterol, and high-fat diets are strongly associated with increased risk of CAD in susceptible persons (111,152). Changes in dietary cholesterol can dramatically alter serum LDL-C in a select segment of the population. Genetic explanations such as apoprotein E and E4 variants have been explored, but the results have been variable and remain unclear (133). Egg yolks are a rich source of cholesterol but are low in SFA. The role of eggs has been controversial, but current approaches emphasize limiting dietary intake to achieve 200–300 mg $\cdot$ d^{-1} of dietary cholesterol (no more than 100 mg per 1,000 kcal) (103,133). For reference, a large egg contains approximately 190 mg of cholesterol in the yolk.

Dietary SFA can be decreased by changing total fat intake to moderate- (<30% kcal) or low-fat (20% kcal) levels while altering the sources and types of fat to increase MUFA and polyunsaturated fatty acids (PUFA) intakes. SFA that need reduction include those with the greatest effect on increasing serum cholesterol and LDL-C: myristic and palmitic acids found in dairy products and meat (93) and trans fatty acids found in margarine, processed foods, and commercially baked or fried foods containing hydrogenated oils (92). The primary dietary MUFA is oleic (abundant in olive and canola oils and nuts), whereas linoleic (abundant in soybean and sunflower oils) is the comparable PUFA (14).

Exactly how dietary fat intake should be modified to lower cardiovascular risk remains controversial. For example, in the year 2006, the results were published from a large-scale, randomized controlled trial of 48,835 postmenopausal women aged 50–79 yr, of diverse backgrounds and ethnicities, who participated in the Women's Health Initiative Dietary Modification Trial (83). Intensive behavior modification in group and individual sessions was implemented to attempt to reduce total fat intake to 20% of calories and increase intakes of vegetables and fruits to five servings per day and grains to at least six daily servings in the intervention group (19,541 women). The comparison group (29,294 women) received diet-related education materials only. Over a mean of 8.1 yr, the dietary intervention did not significantly reduce the risk of CAD, stroke, or CVD and achieved only modest effects on CVD risk factors, although a trend toward greater reductions in CAD risk was observed in women with lower intakes of saturated fat or trans fat or higher intakes of vegetables and fruits. At the time participants were enrolled (1993–1998), though, far less was known about the health benefits of omega-3 and other fats, and intake of all types of fats declined as a result of the intervention, making definitive conclusions based on these findings problematic.

It is likely that dietary changes to lower LDL-C levels and cardiovascular risk involve more than a simple alteration in fat intake. By way of example, a randomized clinical trial (66) compared LDL-C changes from a low-fat diet (consistent with former AHA Step I guidelines that advocated avoiding SFA and cholesterol) to a low-fat diet incorporating considerably more vegetables, legumes, and whole grains, as per the AHA revised guidelines (14). After 4 wk in 120 individuals with hypercholesterolemia but otherwise healthy adults, aged 30–65 yr, the inclusion of more nutrient-dense, plant-based foods resulted in greater reductions in total cholesterol and LDL-C than a low-fat diet.

Along a similar vein, associations of dietary fat and specific types of fat with risk of CAD among 78,778 women in the Nurses' Health Study (144) initially free of CVD and diabetes in 1980 were studied, the finding being an inverse association between PUFA intake and CAD risk, particularly in overweight or younger women. In addition, a greater trans fat intake was associated with a higher risk, especially in younger women. A recent meta-analysis (130) of studies that investigated and quantified the effects of increased PUFA consumption, as a replacement for SFA, on CAD endpoints (MI and/or cardiac death) in eight randomized, controlled trials similarly concluded that rather than trying to lower PUFA consumption, a shift toward greater population PUFA consumption in place of SFA (particularly from animal sources) would significantly reduce rates of CAD by as much as 10% for each 5% energy of increased PUFA.

Omega-3 Fatty Acids

A type of PUFA, omega-3 fatty acids, is believed to exert a cardioprotective effect and reduce CAD risk by reducing elevated triglyceride levels, inhibiting platelet aggregation and formation of blood clots, lowering BP, preventing plaque formation, providing dysrhythmia protection, and promoting the health of the vascular endothelium in the coronary arteries (75). Omega-3s are found in plant foods (flaxseed, canola oil, soybean oil, walnuts, mustard seed oil, and some leafy vegetables) as α-linolenic acid (ALA) and in cold-water fish as the eicosanoids (eicosapentaenoic acid [EPA] and docosahexaenoic acid [DHA]). About 10% of the ALA that is consumed is converted in the body to EPA and DHA, depending on the presence of omega-6 fatty acids that compete for the same enzymes.

The evidence for benefits of omega-3 fatty acids from the diet and supplements has been mixed (104), but at least one meta-analysis supports a strong association between a lower CAD risk and higher intake

of fish (207). The investigators included 228,864 adult participants from 14 cohort and 5 case-control studies in which fish was consumed on a regular basis in the experimental group, whereas the comparison group consumed little or no fish. Overall, fish consumption was associated with a 20% reduction in the risk of fatal CAD and a 10% reduction in total CAD, both hypothesized to be related to omega-3 fatty acid intake. In addition, a systematic review of prospective cohort studies (119) found that high-risk populations had the most benefit from fish consumption, with 40–60 g of fish per day being associated with a 50% reduction in CAD death. Moreover, a secondary prevention trial, Diet and Reinfarction Trial (DART), found a 2-yr, 29% decrease in mortality for survivors of a first MI in individuals consuming fatty fish two times per week (31).

Supplemental omega-3 fatty acids apparently have similar benefits as fish consumption to reduce CVD mortality, stroke, and all-cause mortality (118,120,179). The largest supplement trial included 11,324 patients who were survivors of MI (118). The fish oil supplement group had a 20% reduction in total mortality, a 30% reduction in cardiovascular death, and a 45% decrease in sudden death 3.5 yr after supplementation began. Recent systematic reviews of prospective cohort studies, however, suggested that the benefits of fish oil are likely stronger in the secondary prevention of cardiovascular problems than primary (200), and that dietary supplementation with omega-3 fatty acids exerts similar benefits (120).

Current AHA guidelines recommend at least two servings of fish (preferably oily varieties, such as tuna, salmon, and mackerel) per week for adult, nonpregnant, or nursing patients without documented CAD (104). For patients with documented CAD, the recommendation is to consume a diet rich in ALA and 1 g of EPA and DHA per day, preferably from fish, but an omega-3 fatty acid supplement may be needed to meet this level. The use of supplements requires review by the patient's physician. Patients who use omega-3 fatty acids to lower triglyceride levels are recommended to take 2–4 g of EPA and DHA under their physician's care (104). The American Diabetes Association guidelines also recommend supplemental omega-3 fatty acids for patients with diabetes and severe hypertriglyceridemia, but recommend concomitant monitoring for potential increases in LDL-C (12).

Omega-6 Fatty Acids

Although a large body of literature has suggested that higher intakes of omega-6 (or n-6) PUFA may reduce CAD risk (77), some have recommended substantial reductions in its intake (178). Linoleic acid (LA), an 18-carbon fatty acid with two double bonds (18:2 omega-6), is the primary dietary omega-6 PUFA. LA cannot be synthesized in humans, although an intake of 0.5%–2.0% of energy is likely sufficient. After consumption, LA can be converted into the metabolically important omega-6 PUFA arachidonic acid (AA; 20:4 omega-6), the substrate for a wide array of reactive oxygenated metabolites (*e.g.*, eicosanoids and cytokines). LA accounts for 85%–90% of the dietary omega-6 PUFA and is found in vegetable oils (*e.g.*, corn, sunflower, safflower, soy). Based on an average intake of 2,000 kcal · d^{-1}, LA intake is 6.7% of energy. AA (0.15 g · d^{-1}) is consumed preformed in meat, eggs, and some fish, but most is derived from LA in the body.

Despite assertions that such PUFA are proinflammatory (178), in a recent study from Japan, AA supplementation (840 mg · d^{-1} for 4 wk) had no effect on any metabolic parameter or platelet function (105). Similarly, in observational studies including the Nurses' Health Study, higher omega-6 PUFA consumption was associated with unaltered or lower levels of inflammatory markers (144,158), even with LA intakes of up to 10%–12% of daily energy. A meta-analysis including six randomized, controlled trials indicated that replacing SFA with PUFA lowered the risk for CAD-related events by 24% (70). However, the AHA recently summarized a large body of evidence indicating that omega-6 fatty acids reduce inflammatory states and decrease the risk of coronary heart disease (77). In addition to lowering plasma LDL-C levels, omega-6 PUFA also may play a role in lowering blood pressure and diminishing adverse factors relating to insulin resistance. The AHA supports an omega-6 PUFA intake of at least 5%–10% of energy, implemented along with AHA lifestyle and dietary recommendations (14), stating that a reduction in omega-6 PUFA intakes from their current levels would be more likely to increase than to decrease risk for CAD. However, any recommendation to increase omega-6 PUFA intake should likely include a concomitant increase in omega-3 PUFA consumption (163).

Trans Fatty Acids and Interesterified Fats

Trans fatty acids behave similarly to saturated ones in many ways, such as increasing LDL-C level. However, they are even more destructive than saturated because they also lower HDL-C level (207) and are associated with an increased risk of CAD (144). The AHA recommends lowering intake of trans fatty acids to <1% of daily total calories, primarily by minimizing intake of partially hydrogenated fats used to prepare commercially fried and baked products (14). Efforts to reduce trans fatty acids typically rely on the substitution of partially hydrogenated fats with those made with liquid vegetable oils (with the exception of tropical fats); however, even if partially hydrogenated fats were removed from the food supply, it is estimated that trans fats still would represent close to 1% of total calories because some are produced from deodorization of vegetable oils, and meat and dairy products contain naturally occurring trans fatty acids (142). The introduction of mandatory trans fat labeling

that was implemented in the United States in 2006 has made it somewhat easier for consumers to choose products containing less of this fat.

A more recent concern is the substitution of interesterified fats for trans varieties of fat in commercial food products. This newer altered fat has preliminarily been shown to also negatively affect blood lipid levels and insulin action in humans more than saturated, but similar to trans, fat (189). Levels between 8% and 12% of daily total calories from interesterified fat that incorporated stearic acid (the typical diet provides about 2%–4% of energy from natural stearate fats) show the most deleterious effect (78). More research is clearly needed to assess their full health impact.

Carbohydrates and Fiber

Refined Carbohydrates and Whole Grains

Refined carbohydrates include those that have gone through enough manufacturing to remove many, if not all, of the original micronutrients and fiber and include white sugar, white flour, white rice, most pastas, and other plant-based carbohydrates. In 2009, AHA Dietary Guidelines (88) set recommended limits for the intake of added sugars, which are a significant source of empty calories and associated with greater overall calorie intake, higher body weights, and lower intakes of essential nutrients, particularly vitamins E, A, and C, and magnesium (121). Excess sugar consumption has also been linked to several metabolic abnormalities and adverse health conditions, including obesity, hyperlipidemias (*e.g.*, elevated triglyceride levels), CVD (3), and diabetes (84,88,205). These current guidelines recommend that no more than one-half of discretionary calories should come from added sugars, translating to a limit for most women of no more than 100 kcal · d^{-1} (about 6 tsp) and no more than 150 kcal (about 9 tsp) for men.

The same AHA guidelines (88) recommended a decrease in consumption of refined grains such as white bread and white rice to continue with previous advice to keep at least half of all grains whole. Evidence from observational studies has suggested that carbohydrate quality rather than absolute intake is associated with greater risk of chronic diseases. For example, a study involving a sample of 2,941 Framingham Offspring Participants examined cross-sectional associations between total carbohydrate and dietary glycemic index (GI) intakes and CVD risk factors (124). Dietary GI was positively associated with fasting triglycerides and insulin and inversely associated with HDL-C, suggesting that intake of a high GI diet unfavorably affects CVD risk factors and, therefore, substitution of high with low GI dietary carbohydrates may reduce the risk of CVD. Dietary patterns that are high in whole-grain products and fiber have been associated with increased diet quality and decreased risk of CVD (85). They also recommended that federal agencies develop a single definition for whole grains that is easily understood by consumers and can be adopted for use by the food industry.

Dietary Fiber

Although many studies have investigated the health benefits of fiber, a recent pooled analysis of 10 prospective cohort studies from the United States and Europe (154) examined the association between dietary fiber intake and the risk of CAD. Over 6–10 yr of follow-up, 5,249 incident total coronary cases and 2,011 coronary deaths occurred among 91,058 men and 245,186 women. After adjustment for demographics, **body mass index (BMI)**, and lifestyle factors, each 10-g $\cdot$ d^{-1} increment of energy-adjusted and measurement error-corrected total dietary fiber was associated with a 14% decrease in risk of all coronary events and a 27% decrease in risk of coronary death in both men and women. Thus, it appears that the consumption of dietary fiber from cereals and fruits is inversely associated with risk of CAD.

The AHA TLC diet recommends a total fiber intake of 20–30 g each day (133). Soluble fiber increases the excretion of cholesterol in the bile, and an intake of 10–25 g $\cdot$ d^{-1} is suggested. To increase intake of soluble fiber, include or increase servings of fruits (especially those with high pectin content, such as apples, strawberries, and citrus), vegetables, oats, oat bran, and beans. The remainder of daily fiber intake is insoluble fiber that is largely not digested, adds bulk to the stool, and contributes to correcting diarrhea and constipation. Wheat bran is a good source of insoluble fiber (133).

Other Plant Sources of Nutrients

Plant sources of nutrients and fiber combined in a dietary plan, the Portfolio, have produced significant reductions in LDL-C compared with the TLC diet and statin cholesterol-lowering drugs (87). The diet consists of 30 g of almonds; 2 g of plant sterols from enriched margarine; 35 g of soy protein; and 15 g of viscous fibers from sources such as oats, barley, eggplant, and okra. A study of 25 individuals with hyperlipidemia showed a 35% reduction of LDL-C after 2 wk of consuming the prepared diet compared to only a 12% reduction for individuals consuming the TLC diet (87). The benefit of these plant sources individually has been identified, and their inclusion is advocated in the TLC diet.

Plant Sterols and Stanols

Recommendations for dietary changes to decrease serum cholesterol include a greater intake of plant sterols. The plant kingdom contains several sterols that differ from cholesterol because of their ethyl or methyl groups or unsaturation in the side chain. The major plant sterols — sitosterol, stigmasterol, and campesterol — can be present in Western diets in amounts almost equal to dietary cholesterol. Sitosterol, the most prominent dietary sterol, with the saturated stanol derivative sitostanol, reduces the absorption of cholesterol and decreases blood cholesterol level. Several companies began marketing margarine, salad dressings, and other products containing either stanols or sterols made from soy and corn. An intake of 2–3 g $\cdot$ d^{-1}, or about two to three servings a day of products containing plant sterols and stanols, decreased both dietary and biliary cholesterol absorption. Serum cholesterol levels decreased by 10% and LDL-C decreased by 13% (34).

Other studies have suggested that elevated levels of plant sterols in the blood may actually cause CAD rather than preventing it. Researchers evaluated the association between plant sterols and CAD in a cohort of 1,242 subjects older than 65 yr participating in the Longitudinal Aging Study in Amsterdam (57). Concentrations of sitosterol, campesterol, brassicasterol, and stigmasterol plant sterols (and their ratios to cholesterol) were found to be slightly, but significantly, lower in patients with CAD. Moreover, high plasma concentrations of sitosterol were associated with a markedly reduced risk for CAD. Thus, these data suggest that plant sterols could have neutral or even protective effects on development of CAD, a finding that needs to be confirmed in intervention trials. Sitosterols and a sterol precursor, squalene, are present in both MUFA- and PUFA-containing vegetable oils and, thus, may be responsible for some of the variable cholesterol-lowering effects found in studies using these products. The levels of these sterols may also explain differences in study results with various sources and degrees of refinement of olive oil (111,148).

Recently, a meta-analysis including 14 randomized, controlled studies (n = 531 subjects) showed that there is no difference between plant sterols and plant stanols in their abilities to modify total cholesterol, LDL-C, HDL-C, or triglycerides (191). However, another meta-analysis of 114 studies confirmed that intakes of plant stanols in excess of 2 g $\cdot$ d^{-1} are associated with additional and dose-dependent reductions in LDL-C, possibly resulting in further reductions in the risk of CAD (131). In that analysis, the maximal LDL-C reductions for plant stanols (16.4%) and plant stanol ester (17.1%) were significantly greater than the maximal LDL-C reductions for plant sterols (8.3%) and plant sterol ester (8.4%).

Flavonoids

Flavonoids are another type of phytochemical (*Table 14-2*) or chemically varied compound present in fruits, vegetables, nuts, and seeds that have been inversely linked with CAD, cancer, and other health problems. In the Zutphen Elderly Study (80), the Seven Countries Study (89), and a cohort study in Finland (98), people with low intakes of flavonoids had a higher death rate from CAD than did those who consumed more flavonoids. The amounts of foods rich in flavonoids, such as intake of about 5–6 cups

TABLE 14-2. Examples of Phytochemical-Rich Foods

Phytochemical	Food Sources
Anthocyanidins	Berries, cherries, red grapes, red wine, tea
Ascorbic acid	Citrus, leafy green vegetables, broccoli, tomatoes, strawberries, melons
β-Carotene	Carrots, sweet potatoes, pumpkin, winter squash, cantaloupe, mango, papaya
Ellagic acid	Blueberries, strawberries
Flavonols (catechins, etc.)	Tea, cocoa, chocolate, apples, grapes
Flavanones	Citrus fruit
Flavones	Apple skins, berries, broccoli, celery, cranberries, grapes, lettuce, olives, onions, parsley
Isoflavones	Soy
Isothiocyanates, indole-3-carbinol	Cruciferous vegetables
Lutein, zeaxanthin	Green vegetables (kale, collards, spinach), corn, eggs, citrus
Lycopene	Tomatoes
Organosulfur compounds	Onions, garlic, leeks, chives
Proanthocyanidins	Cocoa, apples, strawberries, grapes, wine, peanuts, cinnamon
Quercetin	Red wine, tea

of tea per day, that have been effective in these studies are at levels greater than usual dietary intake.

The major flavonoid categories are flavones (apple skins, berries, broccoli, celery, cranberries, grapes, lettuce, olives, onions, parsley), catechins (red wine, tea), flavanones (citrus fruits, citrus peel), isoflavones (soy), and anthocyanidins (berries, cherries, red wine, red grapes, tea). Subdivisions of flavonoids include quercetin glucoside in onions and quercetin rutinoside in tea. Some flavonoids have toxic effects (gastrointestinal or allergic), especially if taken in large amounts (140). In addition, flavonoids have antioxidant properties. For example, the phenolic substances in red wine inhibit oxidation of human LDL-C. Flavonoids have also been shown to inhibit the aggregation and adhesion of platelets in the blood, which may be another way they lower the risk of CAD. Isoflavones in soy foods have been reported to lower plasma cholesterol level and to have effects similar to estrogen (140).

Although dietary flavonols and flavones, subgroups of flavonoids, have been suggested to decrease the risk of CAD, a recent prospective evaluation of their intake done using food frequency questionnaires from the Nurses' Health Study reported no association between flavonol or flavone intake and risk of nonfatal MI or fatal CAD (112). However, a weak reduction in risk for CAD death was found for a higher intake of kaempferol, an individual flavonol found primarily in broccoli and tea. Conversely, a recent prospective study examining 34,489 postmenopausal women in the Iowa Women's Health Study free of CVD also used food frequency questionnaires (128). Although the researchers found no association between flavonoid intake and stroke mortality, individual flavonoid-rich foods were associated with significant mortality

reduction from CAD and CVD including the following: added bran (lower risk of mortality from stroke and CVD); apples, pears, and red wine (CAD and CVD); grapefruit (CAD); strawberries (CVD); and chocolate (CVD). These results suggest that dietary intakes of specific flavanones, anthocyanidins, and certain foods rich in flavonoids may be associated with reduced risk of death as a result of CAD, CVD, and all causes.

Soy Protein

The U.S. Food and Drug Administration (FDA) approved the CVD health claim for soy protein, noting that when it is included in a low-fat and low-cholesterol diet, soy protein can lower total blood cholesterol and LDL-C levels (about 5% with 25 g · d^{-1}) without adversely affecting HDL-C levels (54). The FDA has stated that in order to claim the health effects of soy, a product must contain 6.25 g of soy protein or more, be low fat (less than 3 g), be low in SFA (less than 1 g), and low in cholesterol (less than 20 mg). Food sources of soy protein (serving size and grams of protein) include soybeans (1/2 cup = 30 g), soy flour (1/2 cup = 15 g), textured soy protein (1 cup dry = 12 g), soy milk (1/2 cup = 3 g), tofu (1/2 cup = 20 g), and tempeh (1/2 cup = 16 g), but soy sauce and soy oil do not contain protein (142).

Soy isoflavones, fiber, phytic acid, and saponins in combination with soy protein are probably involved in this lipid-lowering effect, although soy protein was identified as the active component rather than isoflavones, fiber, phytic acid, or saponins (54,152). However, recent meta-regression analyses showed a dose-response relation between soy protein and isoflavone supplementation and net changes in serum lipids (167). Soy protein supplementation reduces serum lipids among adults with or without hypercholesterolemia; therefore, replacing foods high in saturated fat, trans fat, and/or cholesterol with soy protein will likely have a beneficial effect on coronary risk factors. The AHA advocates a greater intake of soy products to enhance cardiovascular and overall health because of their high content of PUFA, fiber, vitamins, and minerals and low content of SFA (172).

Vitamins

Antioxidant Vitamins

Food sources of antioxidant vitamins, instead of supplements, are advised because of the positive potential health effects of other associated food components like flavones. Epidemiologic studies of vitamin supplementation with antioxidant vitamins, particularly vitamins C, E, and A, as well as β-carotene, have supported their possible role in reducing CVD risk, but randomized, controlled trials have challenged the benefits for vitamins A and E and β-carotene supplementation. Over a 5-yr period, the Heart Protection Study Collaborative Group (79) studied the effects of supplementation with vitamins E and C and β-carotene versus placebo on mortality and coronary events, finding no significant differences in any parameters for the 20,536 adults studied other than increased blood vitamin concentrations. The investigators reviewed the results for 6,000 patients with diabetes and 7,000 patients with no evidence of CAD and found no cardiovascular benefit from vitamin supplementation.

These results are in agreement with the Age-Related Eye Diseases (AREDs) study of the same vitamins in 4,500 older adults without any recent cardiovascular events (2). Similarly, the Primary Prevention Project (41) studied the effects of vitamin E and the α-tocopherol β-carotene (51) by investigating low-dose vitamin E and β-carotene supplementation and found no differences in CAD outcomes. Likewise, natural vitamin E, as opposed to synthetic products, produced no significant difference for CAD (216), and a recent meta-analysis also concluded that neither antioxidant nor B vitamin supplements have a protective effect against the progression of atherosclerosis or cardiovascular events (24). Thus, the preponderance of evidence from well-designed, large studies and meta-analyses of multiple studies has found no clear evidence of CAD benefits for antioxidant supplementation. Accordingly, the AHA does not recommend antioxidant supplements, but natural food sources of antioxidant nutrients principally from a variety of plant-derived foods such as fruits, vegetables, whole grains, and vegetable oils are recommended (14).

Vitamin D, Folate, and Vitamins B₆ and B₁₂

A growing body of epidemiological and clinical research has found an association between vitamin D deficiency and CVD, and the discovery of the vitamin D hormone functioning as an endocrine inhibitor of the renin-angiotensin system provides a possible explanation for this association (109). This vitamin is mainly synthesized in the skin by sunlight (UV light) irradiation; therefore, vitamin D status is influenced by geographic locations, seasonal changes, and skin pigmentations. A recent systematic review of 17 prospective studies and randomized trials (201) examined vitamin D supplementation, calcium supplementation, or both and subsequent cardiovascular events. These data suggested that vitamin D supplements at moderate-to-high doses may reduce CVD risk, whereas calcium supplements seem to have minimal effects. Another systematic review of 13 observational studies (14 cohorts) and 18 trials (160) found that lower 25-hydroxyvitamin D concentration was associated with incident CVD in 5 of 7 analyses that included 6 cohorts.

The role of various B vitamins in CAD has been investigated, primarily in association with their effects on levels of serum homocysteine, which have been considered to be a CAD risk factor, albeit not necessarily an independent one (198). Increased serum homocysteine is most often caused by a combination of a genetic variant of an enzyme in its metabolism or suboptimal nutritional status for folate and vitamins B_{12} and B_6. The conversion of the amino acid methionine to homocysteine is limited when adequate folic acid is available, and its conversion to less toxic compounds is promoted when vitamin B_6 is available. B_{12} is another cofactor in its metabolism, and it interacts with folic acid or substitutes for folic acid in some cases (115). A meta-analysis by Wald et al. (199) suggested that lowering homocysteine levels by 3 μmol $\cdot$ L^{-1} with increased folic acid intake would reduce the risk of ischemic heart disease by 16% and stroke by 24%. Similarly, the Nurses' Health Study showed that intake of folate and vitamin B_6 from the diet and supplements was associated with increased protection against CAD (168).

In contrast, a meta-analysis examining the effects of folate supplementation failed to show a reduced risk of CVD or all-cause mortality among participants with prior history of vascular disease who supplemented with enough folate to lower homocysteine (22). Moreover, the most recent related meta-analysis included eight homocysteine-lowering trials for preventing vascular disease, which comprised a total of 37,485 individuals and compared the effects of B vitamins on 5,074 CAD-related events; 1,483 stroke events; and 5,128 deaths (36). That analysis concluded that supplementation with B vitamins had no effect on the risks of cardiovascular events or total mortality rates, stating that available evidence does not support the routine use of B vitamins to prevent CVD.

Alcohol

The latest AHA dietary guidelines (14,102) continue to assert that moderate alcohol consumption (one drink per day for women and two drinks a day for men) reduces the overall risk of CAD, but the basis for the protective effect of alcohol remains unclear. Alcohol consumption beginning in middle age (ages 35–69 yr) may suffice for cardioprotection, while averting much of the risk of accidents and cancer associated with drinking alcohol (97,192). The phenolic compounds in red wine contribute to a greater coronary risk reduction than other alcohol sources, but other wines, beer, and spirits also reduce CAD risk. Alcohol has potentially negative consequences for individuals with diabetes, hypertension, cancer risk, and liver disease, however. Additional recommendations suggest that abstainers should not be encouraged to begin consuming alcohol for its purported health benefits and that those consuming alcohol should have their medications reviewed by their physicians for potential interactions (69,150).

Recommended Diets for Coronary Artery Disease

Patients who are at high risk of CAD or with diagnosed CAD can benefit from a nutrition plan that is consistent with the AHA Dietary Guidelines, including Step I and Step II diets (102,152) or the National Cholesterol Education Program; Adult Treatment Panel (NCEP ATP) III guidelines that use the TLC diet (133). The TLC diet replaced the Step II AHA diet and differs only in that the range of calories from fat is greater in the TLC diet to accommodate evidence that CAD risk can be reduced with a variety of dietary patterns (see *Table 14-1*). The Step II AHA/TLC diet has a lower SFA recommendation of 7% (vs. 10% for the Step I AHA diet) and a lower cholesterol recommendation of 200 mg $\cdot$ d^{-1} (down from 300 mg $\cdot$ d^{-1}). A meta-analysis of 37 studies (215) found that the stricter TLC diet reduced total serum cholesterol by 15% versus 10% and LDL-C by 16% versus 12% compared to the Step I, but that both diets reduced triglycerides by 8%. Whereas the Step I diet maintained HDL-C levels, the Step II and TLC diets led HDL-C to decrease by 7%. Thus, the AHA recommends the Step II/TLC diet for individuals who have CAD, who have a high risk of CAD, or who have not met the LDL-C goals with Step I (152).

Low-fat diets have an additional positive benefit when they contribute to weight loss, but any diet should be coupled with activity recommendations to maintain or improve the serum HDL-C level. Obesity decreases HDL-C levels as well so that the net effect of weight loss, when coupled with increased activity, is to improve cardiovascular health by decreasing LDL-C and increasing or maintaining HDL-C (133).

The Mediterranean diet may be useful for individuals who prefer a moderate fat intake with more added MUFA than the AHA or TLC diets (194); it also promotes positive cardiovascular benefits and approximates the Step I AHA diet with higher levels of MUFA, such as oleic acid, and polyunsaturated ALA. A traditional Mediterranean diet is composed of higher amounts of fruits, vegetables, bread and other cereals, potatoes, poultry, beans, nuts, fish, grains, dairy products, and moderate amounts of alcohol and olive oil. Given that it contains little red meat, this diet is naturally low in SFA and high in MUFA (mainly from olive oil), complex carbohydrates, fiber, β-carotene, vitamin C, and tocopherols.

A population-based study examined the effects of the Mediterranean diet on total mortality, cardiac mortality, and cancer mortality in 22,043 adults in Greece (195). The median follow-up was 44 mo, and adherence to the Mediterranean diet positively correlated with a reduction in total mortality, as well as death caused by CAD or cancer, even in individuals with diagnosed CAD at enrollment (194). Interestingly, the individual food groups contributing to the Mediterranean diet did not have a significant effect on total mortality unless they were integrated together into a diet.

A secondary prevention trial, the Lyon Diet Heart Study, with subjects who had a history of an initial MI, incorporated the Mediterranean diet with increased levels of ALA from fortified margarine, MUFA from olive oil, and omega-6 PUFA from rapeseed (canola) oil (43). The participants following the Mediterranean-style diet had 50%–70% lower risk of recurrent heart disease with risk reductions of the same size as those typically associated with statin drug therapy. This multifactorial dietary intervention study demonstrated a positive effect of decreasing the ratio of omega-6 to omega-3 fatty acids to 4:1 versus the typical Western diet ratio of 14–20:1. In accordance, updated dietary guidelines from January 2006 for secondary prevention of cardiovascular events in individuals with known CVD were issued (125). They reiterated that lowering SFA intake appears to reduce morbidity in such individuals and further advised the addition of Mediterranean dietary habits and increased omega-3 fats for individuals with a prior MI.

HYPERTENSION

Hypertension is the third leading cause of death in the world, with more than 1 billion individuals worldwide affected and approximately 65 million adults (~25% of individuals aged 18 yr and older) in the United States (35). High BP increases the risk of MI, heart failure, stroke, and kidney disease. Kottke et al. (101) identified high BP as a symptom of the "lifestyle syndrome," a cluster of conditions and diseases that result from consuming too many calories and too much SFA, sodium, and alcohol; not balancing caloric intake with physical activity; and using tobacco. Obesity is a major risk factor for hypertension that is addressed in the next section of this chapter.

Unfortunately, current knowledge about the prevention and treatment of hypertension with lifestyle changes and other effective early interventions has not been adequately translated to the public and to high-risk individuals. For example, Greenlund et al. (71) found that more than one-third of individuals with established stroke (secondary to elevated BP levels) did not receive advice from a health care professional on dietary or exercise changes that would benefit health and prevent stroke recurrence.

The latest report of the Joint National Committee on Prevention, Detection, Evaluation, and Treatment of High Blood Pressure (35) established the optimal BP as a systolic BP of 115 mm Hg and a diastolic of 75 mm Hg with the need to begin treatment when the patient has a systolic BP of 120–139 mm Hg or a diastolic BP of 80–89 mm Hg. This prehypertensive state initially requires health-promoting lifestyle modifications, rather than medications, to prevent CVD. This report also reiterates that in individuals older than age 50 yr, systolic BP readings greater than 140 mm Hg indicate a greater risk for CVD than elevations in diastolic BP. Moreover, starting with a BP of 115/75 mm Hg, CVD risk doubles for each increment of 20/10 mm Hg, and even individuals with normal BP levels at the age of 55 have a 90% lifetime risk of developing hypertension, which demonstrates that it is a widespread health problem.

For children, especially those with a higher risk of hypertension because of obesity, prevention is an ideal intervention. In the Bogalusa Heart Study (184–186), hypertension and obesity in parents and relatives increased the risk of the child's development of hypertension. Among elementary schoolchildren, elevated systolic and diastolic blood pressures were 4.5 and 2.4 times, respectively, more likely among obese than normal weight children. Figueroa-Colon et al. (61) found that 20%–30% of obese children aged 5–11 yr from a high-risk population had hypertension.

Benefits of Dietary Changes on Blood Pressure

Changes encompassing several dietary factors have lowered BP in hypertensive and normotensive individuals with systolic BP <160 mm Hg and diastolic BP of 80–95 mm Hg. Following the lifestyle modifications to manage hypertension (35) resulted in decreases in systolic BP of 5–20 mm Hg per 10 kg of weight loss, 8–14 mm Hg for adopting the DASH diet high in fruits and vegetables, 2–8 mm Hg for dietary sodium restriction, 4–9 mm Hg for 30 min · d^{-1} of physical activity, and 2–4 mm Hg for moderate alcohol consumption. In particular, the DASH diet significantly reduced systolic and diastolic BP by 5.5 and 3.0 mm Hg more than a control diet followed by participants who were normotensive (17). In participants with hypertension, following this diet without a specific salt restriction still reduced systolic and diastolic BP by 11.4 and 5.5 mm Hg, respectively, more than the control diet. The DASH diet was lower in fat and higher in vegetables, fruits, and low-fat dairy foods, and included whole grains, poultry, fish, and nuts. The diet was also rich in calcium, magnesium, and potassium. The control group had a diet composition typical of the average individual in the United States (low in fruits, vegetables, and dairy products, with an average fat content). The addition of a lower salt intake (1,500 mg · d^{-1}) resulted in a reduction in mean systolic BP of 7.1 mm Hg for participants without hypertension and 11.5 mm Hg in those with hypertension (17,173,214).

As further evidence of the importance of dietary interventions, the PREMIER Collaborative Research Group (16) compared the implementation of three interventions in a population of 810 adults at four clinical centers: (a) "established" (a behavioral intervention that implemented established recommendations), (b) established plus DASH diet, and (c) advice only. Both the established and the established/DASH diet interventions resulted in significant weight reduction, improved fitness, and lower sodium intake. Decreases in the prevalence of hypertension and increases in optimal BP were highly significant for the established/DASH intervention only.

Similarly, two independent systematic reviews of randomized, controlled trials (with 8 or more weeks followup and patients with a BP of at least 140/85 mm Hg) directly compared lifestyle, drug, and other interventions and concluded that in the short term, lifestyle treatment including a healthier diet may be effective at reducing BP for some individuals and may reduce, delay, or remove the need for long-term drug therapy in others (46,137). In fact, in the more recent of the two (46), robust effects were found for improved diet, aerobic exercise, alcohol and sodium restriction, and fish oil supplements, with mean reductions in systolic BP of 5.0, 4.6, 3.8, 3.6, and 2.3 mm Hg, respectively, and corresponding reductions in diastolic blood pressure, although supplements of potassium, magnesium, or calcium were unimportant.

However, Folsom et al. (64) recently studied whether a greater concordance with the DASH diet (using food frequency data) is associated with reduced incidence of self-reported hypertension and mortality from CVD in 20,993 women (initially aged 55–69 yr) followed from 1986 through 2002. In this case, a greater concordance with DASH guidelines was not independently associated with lesser hypertension or a reduced cardiovascular mortality, suggesting that a very high concordance, as achieved in the DASH trials, may be necessary to achieve measurable benefits from this diet. In most cases, the combination of lifestyle interventions results in additive effects and important implications for counseling patients.

Dietary Mineral Intake

Recommendations related to dietary minerals to positively influence hypertension include limiting daily sodium intake to <1,500 mg (<4 g salt) and increasing intake of food sources of calcium, magnesium, and potassium (35,133). The response to dietary sodium may vary with the degree of adiposity. For example, obese adolescents who changed from a high- to a low-salt diet had a significantly larger decrease in BP compared with an insignificant change among nonobese adolescents in one study (169).

The preponderance of a benefit from increasing minerals comes from potassium (206). Healthy food choices to provide the preferred mineral balance include an intake of five or more servings of fruits and vegetables, six or more servings of grains, and two to four servings of low-fat dairy products daily (35). The effect of dietary modifications varies among individuals because of genetic factors, age, medications, and other host factors. Two systematic reviews of the effects of reductions in dietary sodium or salt found minimal effects for normal and hypertensive patients, particularly of Caucasian ethnicity, but greater benefits for Asians and African Americans (90) including maintenance of a lower BP after antihypertensive drugs were discontinued (81). In addition, it appears that African Americans are particularly sensitive to the BP-lowering effects of reduced salt intake, increased potassium intake, and the DASH diet (15).

Dietary Supplements for Blood Pressure Management

Although most of the studies have focused to date on dietary interventions, increasing evidence indicates that vitamin D may influence the risk of hypertension, which is a major risk factor for CVD. A recent meta-analysis examined the association between blood 25-hydroxyvitamin D concentrations and hypertension (29). Of the 18 studies included, 4 were prospective studies and 14 were cross-sectional studies. The pooled odds ratio of hypertension was 0.73 for the highest versus the lowest category of blood 25-hydroxyvitamin D concentration. In a dose-response meta-analysis, the odds ratio for a 40 nmol $\cdot$ L^{-1} (16 ng $\cdot$ mL^{-1}) increment in blood 25-hydroxyvitamin D concentration was 0.84. These findings indicate that blood 25-hydroxyvitamin D concentration is inversely associated with hypertension.

Also of interest is the mineral magnesium. At onset of mild hypertension, correction of poor magnesium status can likely improve BP status. A comprehensive analytical review of 44 studies involving oral magnesium therapy for hypertension showed that supplements may enhance the BP lowering effect of antihypertensive medications in Stage 1 hypertensive subjects (170). Magnesium supplements above recommended dietary allowance (RDA) may be necessary to significantly lower high BP in the early stages unless individuals have been continuously treated with antihypertensive medications for at least 6 mo. Such medication use may lower by half the oral supplemental doses needed to significantly decrease high

blood pressure. Such therapies may have no effect in studies with normotensive subjects, and little has been studied to date about the effects in severe or complicated hypertension. By way of contrast, at least one study found no association among serum magnesium concentration and incident hypertension, CVD, and mortality in 3,531 middle-aged adult participants in the Framingham Heart Study offspring cohort (96).

OBESITY AND DIET

Obesity is a chronic, multifactorial problem largely caused by dietary and physical activity choices and influenced by a variety of other factors, some nonmodifiable (*e.g.*, genetics, sex, age, developmental stages) and others can be modified, such as medications, environmental contributions, and social considerations. The increased prevalence of obesity in the United States largely reflects a change in lifestyle patterns influenced by an overabundance of food choices, large portion sizes, and fast foods; industrialization, technology, and conveniences, which decrease opportunities and motivation for physical activity; and a decline in cigarette smoking (159,162,180). Approximately 14% of American adults are completely sedentary, and 38% spend insufficient time doing physical activity (162).

PREVALENCE, MORTALITY, AND MORBIDITY OF OBESITY

The prevalence of obesity and overweight in the United States has increased dramatically, with obesity (BMI $\geq$30 kg $\cdot$ m^{-2}) increasing from 13.4% in 1960 to 32.2% among adult men and 35.5% among adult women in 2008 (62). In addition, the incidence of severe obesity (BMI $\geq$35 kg $\cdot$ m^{-2} with comorbidities, or BMI $\geq$40 kg $\cdot$ m^{-2}) based on the 2003–2004 U.S. population data is 2.8% for men and 6.9% for women, concentrated more heavily in ethnic minority groups like African Americans and Latinos. Poor diet coupled with physical inactivity is the second leading cause of preventable death, underscoring the depth of this major public health challenge (4,129). Allison et al. (4) reported approximately 300,000 deaths from overweight and obesity in 1999. Mokdad et al. (129) then used the hazard ratios of that study along with the U.S. Centers for Disease Control and Prevention's (CDC) 1999 and 2000 National Heart and Nutrition Examination Survey (NHANES) data (135) to estimate that 400,000 U.S. deaths in the year 2000 were attributable to having a poor diet and being inactive, both lifestyles that contribute to excessive fat weight gain.

More recently, Danaei and colleagues (40) used data from 2005 from the National Center for Health Statistics to assert that tobacco smoking and high BP were responsible for the greatest number of deaths (an estimated 467,000 and 395,000 deaths, respectively, accounting for about one in five or six deaths in U.S. adults). Overweight obesity and physical inactivity were each responsible for nearly 1 in 10 deaths, and high dietary salt, low dietary omega-3 fats, and high dietary trans fats were the dietary risks with the highest mortality. Weight loss is also an effective treatment for hypertension, which is a significant CVD risk factor (82).

Available evidence does not support advising overweight or obese individuals who are otherwise healthy to lose weight as a means of prolonging life (76). However, obesity-associated diseases that increase morbidity include CAD, hypertension, stroke, sleep apnea, Type 2 diabetes, and certain types of cancer, such as endometrial, breast, prostate, and colon (162). The risks of obesity on health begin during pregnancy and extend throughout childhood into adulthood. Some of the obstetric and gynecologic risks include menstrual abnormalities, polycystic ovary syndrome, and shoulder dystopia in childbirth. Orthopedic problems are a common health consequence of obesity. For example, 30%–50% of children with slipped capital epiphyses and bilateral slipped capital epiphyses in one study were obese (49). Likewise, Blount disease (i.e., severe bowing of the legs) is greatly increased by childhood obesity. Adult musculoskeletal problems may include increased joint pain and back pain (28). Obesity also stimulates biliary excretion of cholesterol that increases the likelihood of gallstone formation, leading childhood and adult obesity to be associated with up to 33% of the cases of gallstones (1,21).

The impact of childhood obesity on the progression of the metabolic syndrome in adulthood is alarming. Pinhas-Hamiel et al. (157) estimated that about one-third of diabetes cases diagnosed in 10- to 19-yr-old children and young adults were associated with obesity. A review of dyslipidemias in adults aged 27–31 yr who were previously Bogalusa Heart Study participants reported that adult hyperinsulinemia was 12.6 times more likely in individuals who had been obese as children (65). In another study, adults who had been overweight adolescents had a 2.4 times increase in prevalence of total cholesterol values above 240 mg $\cdot$ dL^{-1}, a threefold increase in LDL-C values above 160 mg $\cdot$ dL^{-1}, and 8 times the incidence of low HDL-C levels (below 35 mg $\cdot$ dL^{-1}) (148). Modest weight loss of 5%–15% of body weight has beneficial effects on serum triglycerides, total cholesterol, BP, degenerative joint disease, gynecologic problems, insulin sensitivity, and glucose control and may lead to improvement or resolution of other comorbidities in both children and adults (44). In overweight adults with Type 2 diabetes, a meta-analysis examining the effectiveness of lifestyle and behavioral weight loss interventions revealed that multicomponent interventions, including very low or low-calorie diets,

may hold promise for achieving longer term weight loss and greater health benefits, particularly when combined with intense physical activity (141).

WEIGHT LOSS ISSUES AND DIETING

The 1998 Behavioral Risk Factor Surveillance Survey found that about one-third of U.S. adults were trying to lose weight and another third were trying to maintain weight at any one time (176). By 2002, that estimate had risen to 48% of women (but only 34% of men) being on a weight loss diet in the previous 12-mo period (204). Many types of weight loss and weight management programs are available, including balanced deficit diets, very low-calorie diets, gastric bypass surgery, and pharmacotherapy (37).

However, fewer than one-fourth of dieters chose to combine caloric restriction with levels of physical activity (300 or more minutes per week) recommended in the 2005 dietary guidelines by the U.S. Department of Health and Human Services and the U.S. Department of Agriculture (204). Furthermore, a systematic review assessed the effects of energy restriction (dieting) and exercise on fat-free mass (FFM) in overweight and obese middle-aged and older adults (202). On average, 81% of dieters (alone), but only 39% of dieting individuals who also exercised, lost 15% or more of their body weight as FFM. These findings suggest that exercise is an effective (and likely critical) tool to help men and postmenopausal women aged 50 yr and older preserve their FFM during moderate dieting-induced weight loss, which is important for combating sarcopenic obesity.

Although modest weight reductions have been observed in many weight loss studies, there is a lack of high-quality evidence to support the efficacy of weight loss programs, especially in older individuals (212). Even with programs that result in weight loss, the results are often short term, and regaining weight is a significant problem for most individuals who initially lose weight. The key to sustaining weight loss is to adopt permanent diet and physical activity changes. A more conservative means for achieving healthy body weight recommended by the American Dietetic Association's guidelines includes adoption of a healthful eating style with an energy intake that does not exceed expenditure (13). Individuals tracked by the National Weight Control Registry (211) (who have lost at least 10% of their initial body weight and kept it off for a minimum of 1 yr, although on average have lost 33 kg and kept the weight off for more than 5 yr) have certain behaviors in common. Most Registry members were found to rely heavily on high levels of daily physical activity (60 min $\cdot$ d^{-1} on average); eat low-calorie, low-fat foods; eat breakfast regularly; self-monitor body weight; and maintain a consistent eating pattern across weekdays and weekends.

OSTEOPOROSIS AND DIET

Osteoporosis contributed to more than 2 million fractures in the United States in 2005, and by 2025, annual fractures are projected to rise by almost 50%, most rapidly increasing for individuals 65–74 yr of age (increase >87%) and nearly 175% for Hispanic and other ethnic populations (30). American women aged 50 yr and older have an incidence of osteoporosis affecting 13%–18% of women with early decreases in porosity. Osteopenia is present in another 37%–50% of women with early decreases in porosity (114). Although the incidence is less in men, those older than 65 yr have approximately 30% of the hip fractures. Peak bone mass is usually achieved by age 30 yr for both men and women.

The risk factors for osteoporosis include genetics, diet, activity, lifestyle, hormone status, medication use, and some diseases (*Box 14-1*) (138). Genetic and environmental factors contribute to poor bone mass acquisition during adolescence and accelerated bone loss in perimenopausal women and men in the sixth decade and older. Contributing factors for reduced bone mass include hormone deficiencies, such as estrogen; inadequate calcium and vitamin D intake; tobacco and alcohol abuse; decreased physical activity; comorbidities like renal failure, hyperparathyroidism, and athletic amenorrhea; and medication effects, such as chronic steroid use. A follow-up of the Nurses' Health Study found that women with diets high in calcium and vitamin D tended to use more multivitamin, calcium, and estrogen supplements; women with the lowest intakes were more likely to smoke and consume alcohol (60).

Another compounding dietary factor may be excessive intake of phosphorus and possibly caffeine. Bone mineral density was measured at the spine and three hip sites in 1,413 women and 1,125 men in the Framingham Osteoporosis Study (196), and intake of colas and other soft drinks was determined using a food frequency questionnaire. Although total phosphorus intake was not significantly higher in daily cola consumers than nonconsumers, the calcium-to-phosphorus ratios were lower in female cola drinkers. However, the reported association between intake of colas, particularly caffeinated ones (but not other carbonated soft drinks), and low bone mass in women does not prove cause and effect. These findings may simply reflect the impact of a lower calcium intake (190). Two recent meta-analyses found no evidence that the dietary acid load from phosphate supplements or higher protein intake and diet acid load promotes skeletal bone mineral loss or osteoporosis (58,59). In fact, higher phosphate intakes (via supplements) were associated with decreased urine calcium and increased calcium retention (59). Thus, assertions that dairy products, meats, and grains are detrimental to bone health due to "acidic" phosphate content need reassessment.

CALCIUM BALANCE AND VITAMIN D

The FDA allowed a bone health claim for calcium-rich foods, and the National Institutes of Health Consensus Development Panel stated that a prolonged high calcium intake decreases osteoporosis (138). A high calcium intake does not protect a person against bone loss caused by hormonal changes, physical activity, or other causes, but may prevent osteoporosis caused by low calcium intake (190). Calcium supplementation in bone remodeling studies has shown an assimilation of additional calcium increases bone density by about 2%, but density does not continue to increase, and losses occur after supplementation ends (23,177).

BOX 14-1	Risk Factors for Osteoporosis (7,138)

Female sex	High caffeine intake
Petite body frame	High carbonated soda intake
White or Asian ancestry	Excessive alcohol use
Sedentary lifestyle or immobilization	Low body weight
Family history of osteoporosis	Anorexia nervosa
Nulliparity (female, never given birth)	Premenopausal amenorrhea (>1 yr)
Increasing age	Smoking
Lifelong low calcium intake	Postmenopausal status
Impaired calcium absorption	Long-term use of certain drugs
High protein intake	Renal disease
Vitamin A supplementation >3 mg · d^{-1}	Bariatric surgery

A systematic review of 15 randomized, controlled trials with 1,806 participants evaluated the use of calcium supplements versus usual dietary intake with placebo for at least 1 yr (177). The review confirmed that the percent change from baseline was 2.1% for total body bone density, with smaller increases for bone density for the lumbar spine (1.7%), hip (1.6%), and distal radius (1.9%). The data on vertebral and nonvertebral fractures were inconclusive. Peacock et al. (149) investigated the effects of supplementation with 750 mg · d^{-1} of calcium and 15 mg · d^{-1} oral 25-hydroxyvitamin D on hip bone density in men and women aged 60 yr or older over a 4-yr trial. The calcium group lost 1% in bone density, the placebo group lost 3%, and the vitamin D group lost 2.7%. Feskanich and colleagues (60) reported a lower risk of hip fracture with a higher calcium intake when there was a concurrent high intake of vitamin D. They confirmed the lack of a relationship between risk of fractures and calcium intake, but concluded that adequate vitamin D was associated with a lower occurrence of osteoporotic hip fractures. Likewise, a 2005 meta-analysis of randomized controlled trials conducted by Bischoff-Ferrari et al. (23) reached similar conclusions: in their analysis, oral vitamin D supplementation of 700–800 IU · d^{-1} appeared to lower the risk of hip and any nonvertebral fractures in ambulatory or institutionalized elderly persons, although 400 IU · d^{-1} appeared insufficient for fracture prevention. Decreased risk of fractures has been consistently shown for women who have higher milk or dairy food intake at age 30 yr or younger but not necessarily for women older than age 50 yr (203).

However, another meta-analysis, one focused on the need for additional calcium and designed to extend the findings of Bischoff-Ferrari et al., suggested that oral vitamin D appears to reduce the risk of hip fractures only when calcium supplementation is added (26). Others concur, and in most trials, the effects of vitamin D and calcium cannot be separated (39). Vitamin D (3) (>700 IU · d^{-1}) with calcium supplementation compared to placebo has a small beneficial effect on bone mineral density and reduces the risk of fractures and falls although benefit may be confined to specific subgroups. Vitamin D intake above current dietary reference intakes was not reported to be associated with an increased risk of adverse events.

Even after full skeletal growth is completed, the body loses calcium every day that must be replaced. The National Academy of Sciences recommends 1,000–1,200 mg · d^{-1} of calcium for adult men and women (47). Calcium supplements from unrefined oyster shell, bone meal, coral calcium, or dolomite without the United States Pharmacopeia (USP) symbol may contain higher levels of lead or other toxic metals and should be avoided, especially during pregnancy. Calcium from food and supplements is absorbed best when taken several times a day in amounts of 500 mg or less.

Calcium carbonate is absorbed best when taken with food; calcium citrate can be taken at any time (47).

Vitamin D, phosphorus, magnesium, zinc, boron, and fluoride are nutrients that are important for bone growth and maintenance, but they neither have to be consumed with calcium for absorption nor require supplementation unless the diet is inadequate in these nutrients. Vitamin D increases calcium absorption in the gastrointestinal tract, and an adequate vitamin D intake reduces nonvertebral fracture rates (165). Vitamin D intake (1 μg cholecalciferol = 40 IU vitamin D) recommendations were raised in 2010 by the FDA (Office of Dietary Supplements), are based on minimal sun exposure, and increase with age: 15 μg · d^{-1}, or 600 IU, for ages 1–70 yr, including pregnant and lactating women; and 20 μg · d^{-1}, or 800 IU, for anyone older than age 70 yr (171). These recommendations incorporate changes in absorption and use; a fourfold decrease in skin synthesis of vitamin D with aging; and decreased exposure to sunlight, particularly in the winter (47). Nutrient needs and osteoporosis may be affected by medications, such as corticosteroids (*e.g.*, prednisone), anticonvulsants, long-term heparin therapy, and excessive thyroxine therapy (7).

Dietary factors may alter calcium balance by decreasing calcium bioavailability or increasing urinary calcium excretion. Foods high in oxalates (*e.g.*, spinach, rhubarb, almonds) or in phytates (*e.g.*, legumes and wheat bran) contain calcium that is unavailable for absorption and may bind with calcium in the gut to reduce absorption. Dietary advice includes eating calcium-rich foods before or several hours after foods with phytates and oxalates or compensate for their reduced absorption with a higher calcium intake for the day. Protein, alcohol, and sodium may increase calcium excretion through the kidneys (47). Protein intakes of 2 g · kg^{-1} of body weight used by some athletes have the potential to decrease calcium balance. Alcohol also has a negative impact on osteoblast function, and higher sodium diets have also been shown to increase the loss of calcium in the urine (33).

OTHER FACTORS ASSOCIATED WITH OSTEOPOROSIS

Although some observational studies have found a relationship between increased hip fracture and excessive supplemental use of vitamin A (126,127), others have not. In the Nurses' Health Study (60), vitamin A intake of 1.5 mg · d^{-1} or more retinol (most common form of vitamin A) was associated with a relative risk of 1.64 for hip fracture, and 21% of subjects exceeded 3 mg · d^{-1}. On the other hand, the association between fasting serum retinyl esters and bone mineral density were examined in NHANES III (19), and although the prevalence of high fasting serum retinyl esters concentration and low bone mineral density were both substantial, no significant associations between them were evident in that study or others (190). More recently, serum retinyl esters were not found to be elevated in postmenopausal women despite intakes of total vitamin A that were nearly double the recommended amount (153). However, retinyl ester concentration (as a percentage of total vitamin A) has been marginally associated with osteoporosis and warrants further investigation.

Finally, eating disorders and the inability to maintain body mass promote osteoporosis. In addition to the impact of body mass, low-calorie diets and, particularly, low-carbohydrate diets that promote ketosis may have the potential to leach cationic minerals, such as calcium, from the bones (27). Patients who have recovered from anorexia nervosa require many years to improve their bone density, but may never completely recover (88). Along similar lines, female athletes with disordered eating and amenorrhea may develop low bone mineral density (the so-called female athlete triad) (67), although elite athletes with adequate calorie, vitamin, and mineral intake are two to three times less likely to experience thinning bones compared with similarly aged, nonathletic premenopausal women (193).

DIABETES AND DIET

Lifestyle interventions including dietary changes to prevent Type 2 diabetes are effective and are recommended for all patients with prediabetes or metabolic syndrome (134,197,210). Management of diabetes includes balancing diet, exercise, and medications to achieve treatment goals (11). A primary principle of diabetes management is the relationship of medication dosage, selection, and timing to dietary intake (especially carbohydrates) and physical activity (38). Patient preferences and lifestyle can be incorporated into a plan that typically focuses on consistency of dietary intake and exercise patterns balanced with medications.

PREVALENCE, CAUSES, AND SYMPTOMS OF DIABETES

Diabetes is a major cause of mortality and morbidity, with 231,404 deaths in 2007 attributable to diabetes in the United States alone, making it the seventh leading cause of death (134). However, studies have found that only 35%–40% of decedents with diabetes had it listed anywhere on the death certificate and about 10%–15% had it listed as the underlying cause of death (134). Overall, the risk for death among people with diabetes is about twice that of people of similar age but without diabetes. However, diabetes is frequently preventable with appropriate lifestyle improvements, as are many of its potential health complications (10,11,99,146,197).

Prevalence of Diabetes and Prediabetes

In 2011, the CDC estimated that 25.8 million Americans have diabetes, with 7 million of those individuals still undiagnosed (134). Another 79 million Americans aged 20 or older who are estimated to have prediabetes, characterized by impaired glucose tolerance (IGT) and/or impaired fasting glucose (IFG) levels, are at an elevated risk of developing Type 2 diabetes. Moreover, the worldwide incidence of diabetes between 2000 and 2030 is projected to more than double from 171 million to 366 million (209). Prediabetes has also become a concern in the pediatric population. Conditions of hyperinsulinemia and IFG have been directly related to overweight and obesity in children and adolescents (123).

Causes of Diabetes

Diabetes results from impairment of insulin secretion and defects in insulin action that likely occur simultaneously (8,134). Autoimmune processes with an absolute deficiency of insulin secretion characterize the less common Type 1 diabetes, but insulin resistance and an inadequate insulin secretion characterize the more prevalent Type 2 (90%–95% of cases). Type 2 diabetes has many different contributing causes, including obesity, especially abdominal distribution and intra-abdominal fat (which may increase insulin resistance), increasing age (*e.g.*, steep increase in incidence after age 45), and a sedentary lifestyle (210). Other risk factors for diabetes include previously identified IFG or IGT, history of gestational diabetes mellitus or delivery of a baby weighing more than 9 lb, hypertension ($\geq$140/90 mm Hg in adults), HDL-C of 35 mg $\cdot$ dL^{-1} or less or a triglyceride level of 250 mg $\cdot$ dL^{-1} or more, polycystic ovary syndrome, and a history of vascular disease (8,134).

Symptoms of Diabetes and Prediabetes

Acute symptoms of diabetes include hyperglycemia with polyuria, polydipsia, weight loss, sometimes polyphagia, and often blurred vision. Chronic hyperglycemia may lead to retarded growth and to increased incidence of infections. An asymptomatic period with IGT and/or IFG and potential organ changes without clinical symptoms may precede overt symptoms. The incidence of retinopathy, peripheral neuropathy, foot ulcers, lower limb amputation, autonomic neuropathy, gastroparesis, sexual dysfunction, peripheral vascular disease, MI, hyperlipidemia, periodontal disease, cerebrovascular disease, hypertension, hearing loss, pregnancy complications, and depression are well known to increase with a history of diabetes, particularly when blood glucose levels are not well controlled (9,32,52,68,116,132,166). Diabetic complications appear to be multifactorial in origin, but in particular, the biochemical process of advanced glycation (attachment of glucose to other molecules), which is accelerated in diabetes as a result of chronic hyperglycemia and increased oxidative stress, has been postulated to play a central role in these disorders through the formation of advanced glycated end products (68).

Symptoms associated with insulin resistance, which is frequently present in both Type 2 diabetes and prediabetes, include acanthosis nigricans (dark, thickened skin at the back of the neck or under the breasts), hypertension, dyslipidemia, and polycystic ovary syndrome. The visible presence of acanthosis nigricans correlated with higher insulin needs in a study of newly diagnosed Type 2 diabetes (113). The study found 36% of the 216 patients with newly diagnosed Type 2 diabetes and 54% of patients with a BMI of 30 kg $\cdot$ m^{-2} or higher manifested the skin changes.

LIFESTYLE MODIFICATION BENEFITS FOR DIABETES AND PREDIABETES

Several large, well-designed, randomized controlled studies have supported the value of lifestyle changes that include diet and physical activity to prevent diabetes in high-risk persons (99,146,197) (also see *Chapter 40*). Prescribed medications for the treatment of diabetes are intended to enhance the effect of lifestyle changes rather than to replace them (11). Screening for diabetes in high-risk groups is a cost-effective practice to allow for implementation of prevention strategies.

Diabetes Risk Reduction with Lifestyle Intervention

In the Finnish Diabetes Prevention Study, Tuomilehto et al. (197) found that intensive individualized diet and exercise instruction had a 58% relative reduction in the incidence of diabetes compared with brief diet and exercise counseling in 522 middle-aged men with IGT and obesity (mean BMI = 31 kg $\cdot$ m^{-2}). The average follow-up time was 3.2 yr. Halting the progression toward diabetes was strongly associated with accomplishment of one of the following goals: 5% weight reduction, fat intake <30% of calories, SFA intake <10% of calories, fiber intake of 15 g per 1,000 kcal or more, and physical activity in excess of than 150 min $\cdot$ wk^{-1}. Another study — the Da Qing, China study (146) of 520 normal-weight participants over 6 yr — found significant reductions in diabetes for a diet group (31%), exercise group (46%), and diet plus exercise (42%). Overall, the lifestyle intervention groups lost 3.4 kg more than the control subjects in the first year. Thus, this study underlines the value of lifestyle changes, especially exercise, for leaner subjects.

Similarly, the U.S. Diabetes Prevention Program, or DPP (99), supported the value of intensive diet and exercise interventions (58% relative reduction in progression to diabetes) compared with metformin (31% relative reduction in progression to diabetes) or

placebo medication interventions with standard diet and exercise. The 3,234 ethnically and racially diverse subjects at high risk for Type 2 diabetes development, with a mean age of 51 yr, were followed for weight and IGT for an average of 2.8 yr. The weight reduction goal of a loss of more than 7% of initial weight at 6 mo was met by 38% of the lifestyle change group, and the exercise goal of more than 150 min $\cdot$ wk^{-1} was maintained by 74% of the lifestyle change group. Over 3.2 yr of follow-up, results from 1,079 DPP "lifestyle arm" participants were analyzed, and it was determined that for every kilogram of weight loss, they experienced an average 16% reduction in risk after adjustment for changes in diet and activity (73). Both lower percentage of calorie intake from fat and increased physical activity predicted weight loss, but increased physical activity was critical for sustained weight loss. In addition, for the 495 participants not meeting the weight loss goal at end of the first year, achievement of physical activity goals still resulted in a 44% lower diabetes incidence.

Effect of Weight Loss on Diabetes Risk

The battle over whether weight loss or physical activity is more important in preventing diabetes continues. A recent study of 68,097 female nurses conducted by Rana et al. (164) attempted to determine the relative contribution of adiposity and physical inactivity to the development of Type 2 diabetes. In this prospective study, researchers estimated adiposity using BMI and waist circumference measurements, and physical activity was assessed through average hours of moderate or vigorous exercise and computation of a metabolic equivalent (MET) score. During 16 yr of follow-up (from 1986 to 2002), diabetes risk in these nurses increased progressively with increasing BMI and waist circumference and with decreasing physical activity levels. Compared with lean (BMI <25 kg $\cdot$ m^{-2}), physically active (exercise ≥21.8 MET $\cdot$ wk^{-1}) women, the relative risks of Type 2 diabetes were 16.8 times greater than for their obese (BMI ≥30 kg $\cdot$ m^{-2}) and inactive (exercise <2.1 MET h $\cdot$ wk^{-1}) counterparts; 10.7 for active, obese women; and 2.1 for lean, but inactive women. Both waist circumference and physical activity were independent predictors of Type 2 diabetes, but the association for waist circumference was substantially stronger, leading the investigators to conclude that the magnitude of risk for diabetes contributed by abdominal obesity may be much greater than for physical inactivity. However, a modest weight loss of 5%–7% of starting weight remains a recommended goal to decrease diabetes risk (12).

Physical Activity Lifestyle Recommendations

All forms of exercise training (aerobic, resistance, or both) appear to produce small benefits in overall blood glucose control for Type 2 individuals with diabetes similar to dietary, drug, and insulin treatments, although combined aerobic/resistance training is generally superior to aerobic or resistance training alone (181). In a joint position statement, the American Diabetes Association and the American College of Sports Medicine (38) recommend that most people with Type 2 diabetes should accumulate at least 150 min · wk^{-1} of aerobic exercise (*e.g.*, brisk walking, bicycling, jogging) at a moderate-to-vigorous intensity, spread over at least 3 d · wk^{-1} with no more than 2 consecutive days without exercise. They also recommend at least two weekly sessions of resistance exercise (exercise with free weights or weight machines), with each session consisting of at least one set of five or more different resistance exercises involving the large muscle groups. For most individuals with Type 2 diabetes, exercise reduces blood glucose levels and can be undertaken safely. Therefore, individuals who are willing to become educated and monitor themselves can increase their physical activity options, as well as make better dietary choices.

DIETARY CONCERNS SPECIFIC TO DIABETES

MNT has been shown to play a key role in preventing Type 2 diabetes, managing existing diabetes, and preventing or slowing the rate of development of diabetes complications (10,11). It is, therefore, important at all levels of diabetes prevention (see *Table 14-1*). Because overweight and obesity are closely associated with increasing diabetes risk, particular attention is paid to this area of MNT.

Carbohydrate, Fat, and Protein Intake

Specific nutrient intake, both macronutrients and micronutrients, has not been widely linked to the development of diabetes, but in a recent meta-analysis, higher consumption of sugar-sweetened beverages was associated with an increased risk for development of Type 2 diabetes and metabolic syndrome, possibly by providing excessive calories and large amounts of rapidly absorbable sugars (117). Even in specific high-risk populations, such as in Chinese adults, relatively frequent intake of soft drinks and juice has been associated with an increased risk for development of Type 2 diabetes (143).

Carbohydrate intake is the dietary component that is the most important determinant of acute blood glucose responses in individuals with diabetes (12). Surprisingly, studies have shown that simple and complex carbohydrates frequently yield similar glycemic responses, although considerable variability in the results exists (50). Thus, presently no evidence-based research conclusion supports improving blood sugar control with exclusive use of the GI, although choice of low-GI foods that are rich in fiber and other important nutrients and intake of a lower glycemic load (GL) are encouraged (12,20). Low-GI and/or low-GL diets are independently associated with a reduced risk of certain chronic diseases, likely through lower postprandial glycemia (20,124). In diabetes and heart disease, the protection is comparable with that seen for whole-grain and high-fiber intakes. A recent meta-analysis that included 974 subjects aged 42–87 yr reported that a low-GI diet, high in dairy and fruit but low in potatoes and cereals, is associated with improved insulin sensitivity and lipid metabolism and reduced chronic inflammation, which may lower risk of Type 2 diabetes and CVD development (50).

The American Diabetes Association "Nutrition Recommendations and Interventions for Diabetes Position Statement" (12) suggests that people with Type 2 diabetes can substitute MUFA in place of carbohydrates to reduce postprandial glycemia and triglyceridemia. A liberal intake of MUFA can promote weight gain, so this substitution should only be advised when carbohydrate calories are replaced by the same number of fat calories (175). A recent meta-analysis that included 19 studies and 306 patients with Type 2 diabetes examined different diets to determine the effect of replacing dietary fat with carbohydrate on glucose and lipid parameters (100). They found that replacing carbohydrate with fat calories (median carbohydrate/fat composition of diets was 58%/24% vs. 40%/40%) reduces insulin resistance, whereas the potential adverse effect on triglycerides from lower fat diets can be avoided by restricting energy intake enough to sustain weight loss. SFA intake should be limited to 7% of total daily energy intake in individuals with diabetes, and total fat intake should remain ~30% of total calories with minimal intake of trans fats. Cholesterol should be <200 mg · d^{-1}, particularly if LDL-C levels are above 100 mg · dL^{-1}. Intake of two or more servings of fish per week is recommended to provide heart-healthy PUFA omega-3s (12).

Protein intake is also a concern in the setting of diabetes because of the potential of exacerbating nephropathy. If renal function is normal, a protein intake of 15%–20% of total daily energy intake is acceptable, but at this time, high-protein diets are not recommended for individuals with diabetes (12). Microalbuminuria, or small amounts of albumin in the urine, is the first evidence of damage to the kidneys. Ethnicity appears to be an important factor in the incidence of kidney disease for people with Type 2 diabetes, given that it develops in 40%–50% of Native Americans, 20%–30% of African Americans and Latinos, and 10% of Caucasians with Type 2 diabetes. High-protein diets cause hyperfiltration in the kidneys and may potentially contribute to kidney failure for high-risk individuals. The American Diabetes Association (12) currently recommends protein intakes of 0.8–1.0 g · kg^{-1} of body mass per day for prevention of kidney disease and 0.8 g · kg^{-1} of good quality protein or about 10% of kilocalories for management of overt kidney disease.

Vitamin and Mineral Intake and Deficiency

Given the associations among Type 2 diabetes and CVD, hypertension, obesity, and even osteoporosis, the micronutrient advice given for these other disease states is particularly relevant to a diabetic population. Micronutrients decrease cardiovascular risk if individuals with diabetes consume an adequate food intake of antioxidants and dietary vitamins and minerals (*e.g.*, vitamin B_{12}, vitamin B_6, folate, magnesium), fiber, plant sterols and stanols, and phytochemicals (like flavonoids) that decrease cardiovascular risk, as recommended for the public at large (10,133,151). In addition, some unique micronutrient deficiencies are relevant to diabetes prevention and treatment.

Vitamin D and Vitamin Status

In individuals at high risk for developing Type 2 diabetes, a deficiency of vitamin D has been found to increase the risk of its onset in many observational studies (161). A recent systematic review of 13 observational studies (14 cohorts) and 18 trials conducted by Pittas et al. (160) reported a lower incident diabetes risk in the highest versus the lowest vitamin D status group in 3 of 6 analyses (from 4 different cohorts), although 8 trials found no effect of vitamin D supplementation on glycemia or incident diabetes. Type 2 diabetes has also been increasing in children and adolescents with combinations of risk factors, especially increasing rates of excessive weight and obesity. Low blood levels of 25-hydroxyvitamin D, common in the pediatric population at risk for diabetes (*e.g.*, older children, African Americans, children with increasing BMI), have been found to also be associated with worse insulin resistance in recent cross-sectional studies (94). Epidemiologic studies have also linked vitamin D deficiency to onset of Type 1 diabetes and an increased inflammatory state in such individuals (45).

Vitamin D has actions beyond playing a possible role in the onset of diabetes. The kidneys are involved in the biosynthesis of 1,25-dihydroxyvitamin D and the reuptake of filtered 25-hydroxyvitamin D from the proximal tubules; thus, vitamin D deficiency is highly prevalent in patients with kidney disease who suffer renal insufficiency (109,156). Moreover, low 25-hydroxyvitamin D levels have been associated with increased all-cause and cardiovascular mortality in individuals with chronic kidney disease, supportive of taking action to correct vitamin D deficiency in such patients, but far from conclusive about whether vitamin D supplementation improves their long-term survival (91,156).

Of note in patients with Type 2 diabetes, metformin use appears to reduce blood levels of folate and vitamin B_{12} and increase homocysteine levels, even in short-term trials (174,213). Therefore, regular measurement of blood levels, particularly of vitamin B_{12}, during long-term use of metformin is advised, along with possible supplementation with both folate and vitamin B_{12} to increase levels to normal (42).

Magnesium and Other Minerals

Another micronutrient of importance in the onset of Type 2 diabetes is magnesium. Seven cohort studies of magnesium intake, including four with intake from foods only and another three with magnesium from foods and supplements combined, were included in a recent meta-analysis with a total of 286,668 participants and 10,912 cases of diabetes (106). All but one study found an inverse relation between magnesium intake and relative risk of developing the disease, regardless of the magnesium source, suggesting that increased consumption of magnesium-rich foods like whole grains, beans, nuts, and green leafy vegetables may reduce the risk of Type 2 diabetes. Moreover, supplementing with oral magnesium for 4–16 wk (with, on average in nine studies, 360 mg $\cdot$ d^{-1}) may be effective in reducing fasting glucose levels and raising HDL-C in individuals with diagnosed Type 2 diabetes, although the long-term benefits and safety of magnesium treatment on glycemic control remain to be determined (182).

Although other minerals have been investigated for their antidiabetic qualities, including chromium, selenium, vanadium, zinc, and others, the evidence remains weak for supplementation with any specific minerals (besides magnesium) to prevent diabetes or significantly improve its management (5,208). On the contrary, a recent prospective study reported that increased dietary selenium intake was associated with an increased risk of Type 2 diabetes, not a lower one (188). Moreover, antagonistic interactions between molybdenum and copper have recently been identified as possibly playing a role in the progression of diabetes complications (63).

Use of Dietary Supplements

Use of multivitamin and mineral supplements has grown rapidly over the past several decades, and dietary supplements are now used by more than half of the adult population in the United States (139). Despite their widespread use, most studies do not provide strong evidence for beneficial health-related effects of supplements taken singly, in pairs, or in combinations of three or more (with the exception of vitamin D and calcium supplements in postmenopausal women), and the present evidence is insufficient to recommend either for or against the use in individuals with diabetes or in the public at large to prevent and manage chronic diseases (86,139). However, a recent study by Song et al. (183) that included a cohort of 232,007 older participants found that multivitamin/mineral supplement use was not associated with diabetes risk. The investigators reported a lower diabetes risk among frequent users of vitamin C or calcium supplements.

The use of dietary supplements by individuals with Type 2 diabetes was estimated at 8%–49% in a study that searched 12 databases for recent studies on supplement use (108). They identified the following dietary supplements as potentially beneficial for Type 2 diabetes treatment or prevention: vitamins C and E, α-lipoic acid, melatonin, red mold, emodin from aloe vera and Rheum officinale, astragalus, and cassia cinnamon. β-Carotene was shown to be ineffective in the prevention of Type 2 diabetes, and others have reported no effect of cinnamon supplementation on glucose or lipid parameters (18). The ingestion of vinegar may reduce postprandial glycemia in patients with Type 2 diabetes, but likely only when it is added to a high-GI meal (110). Given the high prevalence of use of supplements and the potential for select ones to be of benefit in the treatment or prevention of Type 2 diabetes (although more stringent research is needed to confirm this), health providers are advised to query patients about their self-prescribed use of such treatments and to investigate potential drug-nutritional supplement interactions.

SUMMARY

Dietary intervention is one tool in the arsenal of lifestyle changes that combine to effectively reduce the risk of chronic disease. Dietary treatment of the diet-related chronic diseases — CVD, obesity, osteoporosis, and diabetes — improves morbidity, mortality, and quality of life. Prevention efforts for at-risk youth also need to be increased if the potential benefits of healthy lifestyles are to be realized for the population as a whole.

REFERENCES

1. Acalovschi MV, Blendea D, Pascu M, Georoceanu A, Badea RI, Prelipceanu M. Risk of asymptomatic and symptomatic gallstones in moderately obese women: a longitudinal follow-up study. *Am J Gastroenterol*. 1997;92(1):127–31.

2. Age-Related Eye Disease Study Research Group. A randomized, placebo-controlled, clinical trial of high-dose supplementation with vitamins C and E and beta carotene for age-related cataract and vision loss: AREDS report no. 9. *Arch Ophthalmol*. 2001;119(10):1439–52.

3. Alberti KG, Eckel RH, Grundy SM, et al. Harmonizing the metabolic syndrome: a joint interim statement of the International Diabetes Federation Task Force on Epidemiology and Prevention; National Heart, Lung, and Blood Institute; American Heart Association; World Heart Federation; International Atherosclerosis Society; and International Association for the Study of Obesity. *Circulation*. 2009;120(16):1640–5.

4. Allison DB, Fontaine KR, Manson JE, Stevens J, VanItallie TB. Annual deaths attributable to obesity in the United States. *JAMA*. 1999;282(16):1530–8.

5. Althuis MD, Jordan NE, Ludington EA, Wittes JT. Glucose and insulin responses to dietary chromium supplements: a meta-analysis. *Am J Clin Nutr*. 2002;76(1):148–55.

6. Alvehus M, Buren J, Sjostrom M, Goedecke J, Olsson T. The human visceral fat depot has a unique inflammatory profile. *Obesity (Silver Spring)*. 2010;18(5):879–83.

7. American College of Obstetricians and Gynecologists, Women's Health Care Physicians. ACOG practice bulletin. Clinical management guidelines for obstetrician-gynecologists. Number 50, January 2003. *Obstet Gynecol*. 2004;103(1):203–16.

8. American Diabetes Association. Diagnosis and classification of diabetes mellitus. *Diabetes Care*. 2011;34 Suppl 1:S62–9.

9. American Diabetes Association. Implications of the diabetes control and complications trial. *Diabetes Care*. 2003;26 Suppl 1:S25–7.

10. American Diabetes Association. Nutrition Recommendations and Interventions for Diabetes: a position statement of the American Diabetes Association. *Diabetes Care*. 2007;30 Suppl 1:S48–65.

11. American Diabetes Association. Standards of medical care in diabetes—2011. *Diabetes Care*. 2011;34 Suppl 1:S11–61.

12. American Diabetes Association, Bantle JP, Wylie-Rosett J, et al. Nutrition recommendations and interventions for diabetes: a position statement of the American Diabetes Association. *Diabetes Care*. 2008;31 Suppl 1:S61–78.

13. American Dietetic Association. Position of the American Dietetic Association: integration of medical nutrition therapy and pharmacotherapy. *J Am Diet Assoc*. 2003;103(10):1363–70.

14. American Heart Association Nutrition Committee, Lichtenstein AH, Appel LJ, et al. Diet and lifestyle recommendations revision 2006: a scientific statement from the American Heart Association Nutrition Committee. *Circulation*. 2006;114(1):82–96.

15. Appel LJ, Brands MW, Daniels SR, et al. Dietary approaches to prevent and treat hypertension: a scientific statement from the American Heart Association. *Hypertension*. 2006;47(2):296–308.

16. Appel LJ, Champagne CM, Harsha DW, et al. Effects of comprehensive lifestyle modification on blood pressure control: main results of the PREMIER clinical trial. *JAMA*. 2003;289(16):2083–93.

17. Appel LJ, Moore TJ, Obarzanek E, et al. A clinical trial of the effects of dietary patterns on blood pressure. DASH Collaborative Research Group. *N Engl J Med*. 1997;336(16):1117–24.

18. Baker WL, Gutierrez-Williams G, White CM, Kluger J, Coleman CI. Effect of cinnamon on glucose control and lipid parameters. *Diabetes Care*. 2008;31(1):41–3.

19. Ballew C, Galuska D, Gillespie C. High serum retinyl esters are not associated with reduced bone mineral density in the Third National Health and Nutrition Examination Survey, 1988–1994. *J Bone Miner Res*. 2001;16(12):2306–12.

20. Barclay AW, Petocz P, McMillan-Price J, et al. Glycemic index, glycemic load, and chronic disease risk—a meta-analysis of observational studies. *Am J Clin Nutr*. 2008;87(3):627–37.

21. Barlow SE, Dietz WH. Obesity evaluation and treatment: Expert Committee recommendations. The Maternal and Child Health Bureau, Health Resources and Services Administration and the Department of Health and Human Services. *Pediatrics*. 1998;102(3):E29.

22. Bazzano LA, Reynolds K, Holder KN, He J. Effect of folic acid supplementation on risk of cardiovascular diseases: a meta-analysis of randomized controlled trials. *JAMA*. 2006;296(22):2720–6.

23. Bischoff-Ferrari HA, Willett WC, Wong JB, Giovannucci E, Dietrich T, Dawson-Hughes B. Fracture prevention with vitamin D supplementation: a meta-analysis of randomized controlled trials. *JAMA*. 2005;293(18):2257–64.

24. Bleys J, Miller ER,3rd, Pastor-Barriuso R, Appel LJ, Guallar E. Vitamin-mineral supplementation and the progression of atherosclerosis: a meta-analysis of randomized controlled trials. *Am J Clin Nutr*. 2006;84(4):880,887; quiz 954–5.

25. Blumenthal JA, Babyak MA, Hinderliter A, et al. Effects of the DASH diet alone and in combination with exercise and weight loss on blood pressure and cardiovascular biomarkers in men and women with high blood pressure: the ENCORE study. *Arch Intern Med*. 2010;170(2):126–35.

26. Boonen S, Lips P, Bouillon R, Bischoff-Ferrari HA, Vanderschueren D, Haentjens P. Need for additional calcium to reduce the risk of

hip fracture with vitamin d supplementation: evidence from a comparative metaanalysis of randomized controlled trials. *J Clin Endocrinol Metab*. 2007;92(4):1415–23.

27. Bray GA. Low-carbohydrate diets and realities of weight loss. *JAMA*. 2003;289(14):1853–5.

28. Brown WJ, Dobson AJ, Mishra G. What is a healthy weight for middle aged women? *Int J Obes Relat Metab Disord*. 1998;22(6):520–8.

29. Burgaz A, Orsini N, Larsson SC, Wolk A. Blood 25-hydroxyvitamin D concentration and hypertension: a meta-analysis. *J Hypertens*. 2011;29(4):636–45.

30. Burge R, Dawson-Hughes B, Solomon DH, Wong JB, King A, Tosteson A. Incidence and economic burden of osteoporosis-related fractures in the United States, 2005–2025. *J Bone Miner Res*. 2007;22(3):465–75.

31. Burr ML, Fehily AM, Gilbert JF, et al. Effects of changes in fat, fish, and fibre intakes on death and myocardial reinfarction: diet and reinfarction trial (DART). *Lancet*. 1989;2(8666):757–61.

32. Buse JB, Ginsberg HN, Bakris GL, et al. Primary prevention of cardiovascular diseases in people with diabetes mellitus: a scientific statement from the American Heart Association and the American Diabetes Association. *Circulation*. 2007;115(1):114–26.

33. Carbone LD, Barrow KD, Bush AJ, et al. Effects of a low sodium diet on bone metabolism. *J Bone Miner Metab*. 2005;23(6):506–13.

34. Cater NB. Plant stanol ester: review of cholesterol-lowering efficacy and implications for coronary heart disease risk reduction. *Prev Cardiol*. 2000;3(3):121–30.

35. Chobanian AV, Bakris GL, Black HR, et al. The Seventh Report of the Joint National Committee on Prevention, Detection, Evaluation, and Treatment of High Blood Pressure: the JNC 7 report. *JAMA*. 2003;289(19):2560–72.

36. Clarke R, Halsey J, Bennett D, Lewington S. Homocysteine and vascular disease: review of published results of the homocysteine-lowering trials. *J Inherit Metab Dis*. 2011;34(1):83–91.

37. *Clinical Guidelines on the Identification, Evaluation, and Treatment of Overweight and Obesity in Adults* [Internet]. Bethesda (MD): National Institutes of Health; National Heart, Lung, and Blood Institute; 1998 [cited 2011 Jan 19]. 228 p. Available from: http://www.nhlbi.nih.gov/guidelines/obesity/ob_home.htm

38. Colberg SR, Sigal RJ, Fernhall B, et al. Exercise and type 2 diabetes: the American College of Sports Medicine and the American Diabetes Association: joint position statement. *Diabetes Care*. 2010;33(12):e147–67.

39. Cranney A, Horsley T, O'Donnell S, et al. Effectiveness and safety of vitamin D in relation to bone health. *Evid Rep Technol Assess (Full Rep)*. 2007;(158):1–235.

40. Danaei G, Ding EL, Mozaffarian D, et al. The preventable causes of death in the United States: comparative risk assessment of dietary, lifestyle, and metabolic risk factors. *PLoS Med*. 2009;6(4):e1000058.

41. de Gaetano G, Collaborative Group of the Primary Prevention Project. Low-dose aspirin and vitamin E in people at cardiovascular risk: a randomised trial in general practice. Collaborative Group of the Primary Prevention Project. *Lancet*. 2001;357(9250):89–95.

42. de Jager J, Kooy A, Lehert P, et al. Long term treatment with metformin in patients with type 2 diabetes and risk of vitamin B-12 deficiency: randomised placebo controlled trial. *BMJ*. 2010;340:c2181.

43. de Lorgeril M, Salen P, Martin JL, Monjaud I, Delaye J, Mamelle N. Mediterranean diet, traditional risk factors, and the rate of cardiovascular complications after myocardial infarction: final report of the Lyon Diet Heart Study. *Circulation*. 1999;99(6):779–85.

44. Deitel M. How much weight loss is sufficient to overcome major co-morbidities? *Obes Surg*. 2001;11(6):659.

45. Devaraj S, Yun JM, Duncan-Staley CR, Jialal I. Low vitamin D levels correlate with the proinflammatory state in type 1 diabetic subjects with and without microvascular complications. *Am J Clin Pathol*. 2011;135(3):429–33.

46. Dickinson HO, Mason JM, Nicolson DJ, et al. Lifestyle interventions to reduce raised blood pressure: a systematic review of randomized controlled trials. *J Hypertens*. 2006;24(2):215–33.

47. *Dietary Reference Intakes for Calcium, Phosphorus, Magnesium, Vitamin D, and Fluoride* [Internet]. Washington (DC): National Academy Press; 1997 [cited 2011]. 448 p. Available from: http://www.nap.edu/catalog.php?record_id=5776

48. *Dietary Reference Intakes for Energy, Carbohydrate, Fiber, Fat, Fatty Acids, Cholesterol, Protein, and Amino acids* [Internet]. Washington (DC): National Academies Press; 2005 [cited 2011]. 1357 p. Available from: http://www.nap.edu/catalog.php?record_id=10490

49. Dietz WH. Health consequences of obesity in youth: childhood predictors of adult disease. *Pediatrics*. 1998;101(3 Pt 2):518–25.

50. Du H, van der ADL, van Bakel MM, et al. Glycemic index and glycemic load in relation to food and nutrient intake and metabolic risk factors in a Dutch population. *Am J Clin Nutr*. 2008;87(3):655–61.

51. The effect of vitamin E and beta carotene on the incidence of lung cancer and other cancers in male smokers. The Alpha-Tocopherol, Beta Carotene Cancer Prevention Study Group. *N Engl J Med*. 1994;330(15):1029–35.

52. Egede LE. Diabetes, major depression, and functional disability among U.S. adults. *Diabetes Care*. 2004;27(2):421–8.

53. Einhorn D, Reaven GM, Cobin RH, et al. American College of Endocrinology position statement on the insulin resistance syndrome. *Endocr Pract*. 2003;9(3):237–52.

54. Erdman JW Jr. AHA Science Advisory: soy protein and cardiovascular disease: a statement for healthcare professionals from the Nutrition Committee of the AHA. *Circulation*. 2000;102(20):2555–9.

55. Ervin RB. Prevalence of metabolic syndrome among adults 20 years of age and over, by sex, age, race and ethnicity, and body mass index: United States, 2003–2006. *Natl Health Stat Report*. 2009;(13):1–7.

56. Fabbrini E, Magkos F, Mohammed BS, et al. Intrahepatic fat, not visceral fat, is linked with metabolic complications of obesity. *Proc Natl Acad Sci U S A*. 2009;106(36):15430–5.

57. Fassbender K, Lutjohann D, Dik MG, et al. Moderately elevated plant sterol levels are associated with reduced cardiovascular risk—the LASA study. *Atherosclerosis*. 2008;196(1):283–8.

58. Fenton TR, Eliasziw M, Lyon AW, Tough SC, Hanley DA. Meta-analysis of the quantity of calcium excretion associated with the net acid excretion of the modern diet under the acid-ash diet hypothesis. *Am J Clin Nutr*. 2008;88(4):1159–66.

59. Fenton TR, Lyon AW, Eliasziw M, Tough SC, Hanley DA. Meta-analysis of the effect of the acid-ash hypothesis of osteoporosis on calcium balance. *J Bone Miner Res*. 2009;24(11):1835–40.

60. Feskanich D, Willett WC, Colditz GA. Calcium, vitamin D, milk consumption, and hip fractures: a prospective study among post-menopausal women. *Am J Clin Nutr*. 2003;77(2):504–11.

61. Figueroa-Colon R, Franklin FA, Lee JY, Aldridge R, Alexander L. Prevalence of obesity with increased blood pressure in elementary school-aged children. *South Med J*. 1997;90(8):806–13.

62. Flegal KM, Carroll MD, Ogden CL, Curtin LR. Prevalence and trends in obesity among US adults, 1999–2008. *JAMA*. 2010;303(3):235–41.

63. Flores CR, Puga MP, Wrobel K, Garay Sevilla ME, Wrobel K. Trace elements status in diabetes mellitus type 2: possible role of the interaction between molybdenum and copper in the progress of typical complications. *Diabetes Res Clin Pract*. 2011;91(3):333–41.

64. Folsom AR, Parker ED, Harnack LJ. Degree of concordance with DASH diet guidelines and incidence of hypertension and fatal cardiovascular disease. *Am J Hypertens*. 2007;20(3):225–32.

65. Freedman DS, Dietz WH, Srinivasan SR, Berenson GS. The relation of overweight to cardiovascular risk factors among children and adolescents: the Bogalusa Heart Study. *Pediatrics*. 1999;103(6 Pt 1):1175–82.

66. Gardner CD, Coulston A, Chatterjee L, Rigby A, Spiller G, Farquhar JW. The effect of a plant-based diet on plasma lipids in hypercholesterolemic adults: a randomized trial. *Ann Intern Med.* 2005;142(9):725–33.

67. Gibson JH, Mitchell A, Harries MG, Reeve J. Nutritional and exercise-related determinants of bone density in elite female runners. *Osteoporos Int.* 2004;15(8):611–8.

68. Goh SY, Cooper ME. Clinical review: the role of advanced glycation end products in progression and complications of diabetes. *J Clin Endocrinol Metab.* 2008;93(4):1143–52.

69. Goldberg IJ, Mosca L, Piano MR, et al. AHA Science Advisory: wine and your heart: a science advisory for healthcare professionals from the Nutrition Committee, Council on Epidemiology and Prevention, and Council on Cardiovascular Nursing of the American Heart Association. *Circulation.* 2001;103(3):472–5.

70. Gordon DJ. Lowering cholesterol and total mortality. In: Rifkin BM, editor. *Lowering Cholesterol in High-Risk Individuals and Populations.* New York: Marcel Dekker, Inc; 1995. p. 33–48.

71. Greenlund KJ, Giles WH, Keenan NL, Croft JB, Mensah GA. Physician advice, patient actions, and health-related quality of life in secondary prevention of stroke through diet and exercise. *Stroke.* 2002;33(2):565–70.

72. Grundy SM, Cleeman JI, Daniels SR, et al. Diagnosis and management of the metabolic syndrome: an American Heart Association/National Heart, Lung, and Blood Institute Scientific Statement. *Circulation.* 2005;112(17):2735–52.

73. Hamman RF, Wing RR, Edelstein SL, et al. Effect of weight loss with lifestyle intervention on risk of diabetes. *Diabetes Care.* 2006;29(9):2102–7.

74. Hanley AJ, Williams K, Festa A, Wagenknecht LE, D'Agostino RB Jr, Haffner SM. Liver markers and development of the metabolic syndrome: the insulin resistance atherosclerosis study. *Diabetes.* 2005;54(11):3140–7.

75. Harper CR, Jacobson TA. The fats of life: the role of omega-3 fatty acids in the prevention of coronary heart disease. *Arch Intern Med.* 2001;161(18):2185–92.

76. Harrington M, Gibson S, Cottrell RC. A review and meta-analysis of the effect of weight loss on all-cause mortality risk. *Nutr Res Rev.* 2009;22(1):93–108.

77. Harris WS, Mozaffarian D, Rimm E, et al. Omega-6 fatty acids and risk for cardiovascular disease: a science advisory from the American Heart Association Nutrition Subcommittee of the Council on Nutrition, Physical Activity, and Metabolism; Council on Cardiovascular Nursing; and Council on Epidemiology and Prevention. *Circulation.* 2009;119(6):902–7.

78. Hayes KC, Pronczuk A. Replacing trans fat: the argument for palm oil with a cautionary note on interesterification. *J Am Coll Nutr.* 2010;29(3 Suppl):253S–84S.

79. Heart Protection Study Collaborative Group. MRC/BHF Heart Protection Study of antioxidant vitamin supplementation in 20,536 high-risk individuals: a randomised placebo-controlled trial. *Lancet.* 2002;360(9326):23–33.

80. Hertog MG, Feskens EJ, Hollman PC, Katan MB, Kromhout D. Dietary antioxidant flavonoids and risk of coronary heart disease: the Zutphen Elderly Study. *Lancet.* 1993;342(8878):1007–11.

81. Hooper L, Bartlett C, Davey SG, Ebrahim S. Advice to reduce dietary salt for prevention of cardiovascular disease. *Cochrane Database Syst Rev.* 2004;(1):CD003656.

82. Horvath K, Jeitler K, Siering U, et al. Long-term effects of weight-reducing interventions in hypertensive patients: systematic review and meta-analysis. *Arch Intern Med.* 2008;168(6):571–80.

83. Howard BV, Van Horn L, Hsia J, et al. Low-fat dietary pattern and risk of cardiovascular disease: the Women's Health Initiative Randomized Controlled Dietary Modification Trial. *JAMA.* 2006;295(6):655–66.

84. Hu FB, Malik VS. Sugar-sweetened beverages and risk of obesity and type 2 diabetes: epidemiologic evidence. *Physiol Behav.* 2010;100(1):47–54.

85. Hu FB, Willett WC. Optimal diets for prevention of coronary heart disease. *JAMA.* 2002;288(20):2569–78.

86. Huang HY, Caballero B, Chang S, et al. Multivitamin/mineral supplements and prevention of chronic disease. *Evid Rep Technol Assess (Full Rep).* 2006;(139):1–117.

87. Jenkins DJ, Kendall CW, Marchie A, et al. The effect of combining plant sterols, soy protein, viscous fibers, and almonds in treating hypercholesterolemia. *Metabolism.* 2003;52(11):1478–83.

88. Johnson RK, Appel LJ, Brands M, et al. Dietary sugars intake and cardiovascular health: a scientific statement from the American Heart Association. *Circulation.* 2009;120(11):1011–20.

89. Joshipura KJ, Hu FB, Manson JE, et al. The effect of fruit and vegetable intake on risk for coronary heart disease. *Ann Intern Med.* 2001;134(12):1106–14.

90. Jurgens G, Graudal NA. Effects of low sodium diet versus high sodium diet on blood pressure, renin, aldosterone, catecholamines, cholesterols, and triglyceride. *Cochrane Database Syst Rev.* 2004;(1):CD004022.

91. Kandula P, Dobre M, Schold JD, Schreiber MJ Jr, Mehrotra R, Navaneethan SD. Vitamin D supplementation in chronic kidney disease: a systematic review and meta-analysis of observational studies and randomized controlled trials. *Clin J Am Soc Nephrol.* 2011;6(1):50–62.

92. Katan MB. Trans fatty acids and plasma lipoproteins. *Nutr Rev.* 2000;58(6):188–91.

93. Katan MB, Zock PL, Mensink RP. Dietary oils, serum lipoproteins, and coronary heart disease. *Am J Clin Nutr.* 1995;61 (6 Suppl):1368S–73S.

94. Kelly A, Brooks LJ, Dougherty S, Carlow DC, Zemel BS. A cross-sectional study of vitamin D and insulin resistance in children. *Arch Dis Child.* 2011;96(5):447–52.

95. *Key Statistics from NHANES 2005–2006* [Internet]. Atlanta (GA): Centers for Disease Control and Prevention, U.S. Department of Health and Human Services; [cited 2011 Mar 10]. 7 p. Available from: http://www.ars.usda.gov/SP2UserFiles/Place/12355000/pdf/0506/Table_2_NIF_05.pdf

96. Khan AM, Sullivan L, McCabe E, Levy D, Vasan RS, Wang TJ. Lack of association between serum magnesium and the risks of hypertension and cardiovascular disease. *Am Heart J.* 2010;160(4):715–20.

97. Klatsky AL, Armstrong MA, Friedman GD. Red wine, white wine, liquor, beer, and risk for coronary artery disease hospitalization. *Am J Cardiol.* 1997;80(4):416–20.

98. Knekt P, Jarvinen R, Reunanen A, Maatela J. Flavonoid intake and coronary mortality in Finland: a cohort study. *BMJ.* 1996; 312(7029):478–81.

99. Knowler WC, Barrett-Connor E, Fowler SE, et al. Reduction in the incidence of type 2 diabetes with lifestyle intervention or metformin. *N Engl J Med.* 2002;346(6):393–403.

100. Kodama S, Saito K, Tanaka S, et al. Influence of fat and carbohydrate proportions on the metabolic profile in patients with type 2 diabetes: a meta-analysis. *Diabetes Care.* 2009;32(5):959–65.

101. Kottke TE, Stroebel RJ, Hoffman RS. JNC 7—it's more than high blood pressure. *JAMA.* 2003;289(19):2573–5.

102. Krauss RM, Eckel RH, Howard B, et al. AHA Dietary Guidelines: revision 2000: a statement for healthcare professionals from the Nutrition Committee of the American Heart Association. *Circulation.* 2000;102(18):2284–99.

103. Kris-Etherton P, Daniels SR, Eckel RH, et al. Summary of the scientific conference on dietary fatty acids and cardiovascular health: conference summary from the nutrition committee of the American Heart Association. *Circulation.* 2001;103(7):1034–9.

104. Kris-Etherton PM, Harris WS, Appel LJ, American Heart Association. Nutrition Committee. Fish consumption, fish oil, omega-3 fatty acids, and cardiovascular disease. *Circulation.* 2002;106(21):2747–57.

105. Kusumoto A, Ishikura Y, Kawashima H, Kiso Y, Takai S, Miyazaki M. Effects of arachidonate-enriched triacylglycerol supplementation on serum fatty acids and platelet aggregation in healthy male subjects with a fish diet. *Br J Nutr.* 2007;98(3):626–35.

106. Larsson SC, Wolk A. Magnesium intake and risk of type 2 diabetes: a meta-analysis. *J Intern Med.* 2007;262(2):208–14.

107. Le KA, Ventura EE, Fisher JQ, et al. Ethnic differences in pancreatic fat accumulation and its relationship with other fat depots and inflammatory markers. *Diabetes Care.* 2011;34(2):485–90.

108. Lee T, Dugoua JJ. Nutritional supplements and their effect on glucose control. *Curr Diab Rep.* 2011;11(2):142–8.

109. Li YC. Molecular mechanism of vitamin D in the cardiovascular system. *J Investig Med.* 2011;59(6):868–71.

110. Liatis S, Grammatikou S, Poulia KA, et al. Vinegar reduces postprandial hyperglycaemia in patients with type II diabetes when added to a high, but not to a low, glycaemic index meal. *Eur J Clin Nutr.* 2010;64(7):727–32.

111. Lichtenstein AH, Deckelbaum RJ. AHA Science Advisory. Stanol/sterol ester-containing foods and blood cholesterol levels. A statement for healthcare professionals from the Nutrition Committee of the Council on Nutrition, Physical Activity, and Metabolism of the American Heart Association. *Circulation.* 2001;103(8):1177–9.

112. Lin J, Rexrode KM, Hu F, et al. Dietary intakes of flavonols and flavones and coronary heart disease in US women. *Am J Epidemiol.* 2007;165(11):1305–13.

113. Litonjua P, Pinero-Pilona A, Aviles-Santa L, Raskin P. Prevalence of acanthosis nigricans in newly-diagnosed type 2 diabetes. *Endocr Pract.* 2004;10(2):101–6.

114. Looker AC, Wahner HW, Dunn WL, et al. Updated data on proximal femur bone mineral levels of US adults. *Osteoporos Int.* 1998;8(5):468–89.

115. Lowering blood homocysteine with folic acid based supplements: meta-analysis of randomised trials. Homocysteine Lowering Trialists' Collaboration. *BMJ.* 1998;316(7135):894–8.

116. Malik S, Wong ND, Franklin S, Pio J, Fairchild C, Chen R. Cardiovascular disease in U.S. patients with metabolic syndrome, diabetes, and elevated C-reactive protein. *Diabetes Care.* 2005;28(3):690–3.

117. Malik VS, Popkin BM, Bray GA, Despres JP, Willett WC, Hu FB. Sugar-sweetened beverages and risk of metabolic syndrome and type 2 diabetes: a meta-analysis. *Diabetes Care.* 2010;33(11):2477–83.

118. Marchioli R, Barzi F, Bomba E, et al. Early protection against sudden death by n-3 polyunsaturated fatty acids after myocardial infarction: time-course analysis of the results of the Gruppo Italiano per lo Studio della Sopravvivenza nell'Infarto Miocardico (GISSI)-Prevenzione. *Circulation.* 2002;105(16):1897–903.

119. Marckmann P, Gronbaek M. Fish consumption and coronary heart disease mortality. A systematic review of prospective cohort studies. *Eur J Clin Nutr.* 1999;53(8):585–90.

120. Marik PE, Varon J. Omega-3 dietary supplements and the risk of cardiovascular events: a systematic review. *Clin Cardiol.* 2009;32(7):365–72.

121. Marriott BP, Olsho L, Hadden L, Connor P. Intake of added sugars and selected nutrients in the United States, National Health and Nutrition Examination Survey (NHANES) 2003–2006. *Crit Rev Food Sci Nutr.* 2010;50(3):228–58.

122. McCabe-Sellers BJ, Skipper A, American Dietetic Association. Position of the American Dietetic Association: integration of medical nutrition therapy and pharmacotherapy. *J Am Diet Assoc.* 2010;110(6):950–6.

123. McCance DR, Pettitt DJ, Hanson RL, Jacobsson LT, Bennett PH, Knowler WC. Glucose, insulin concentrations and obesity in childhood and adolescence as predictors of NIDDM. *Diabetologia.* 1994;37(6):617–23.

124. McKeown NM, Meigs JB, Liu S, et al. Dietary carbohydrates and cardiovascular disease risk factors in the Framingham offspring cohort. *J Am Coll Nutr.* 2009;28(2):150–8.

125. Mead A, Atkinson G, Albin D, et al. Dietetic guidelines on food and nutrition in the secondary prevention of cardiovascular disease—evidence from systematic reviews of randomized controlled trials (second update, January 2006). *J Hum Nutr Diet.* 2006;19(6):401–19.

126. Melhus H, Michaelsson K, Kindmark A, et al. Excessive dietary intake of vitamin A is associated with reduced bone mineral density and increased risk for hip fracture. *Ann Intern Med.* 1998;129(10):770–8.

127. Michaelsson K, Lithell H, Vessby B, Melhus H. Serum retinol levels and the risk of fracture. *N Engl J Med.* 2003;348(4):287–94.

128. Mink PJ, Scrafford CG, Barraj LM, et al. Flavonoid intake and cardiovascular disease mortality: a prospective study in postmenopausal women. *Am J Clin Nutr.* 2007;85(3):895–909.

129. Mokdad AH, Marks JS, Stroup DF, Gerberding JL. Actual causes of death in the United States, 2000. *JAMA.* 2004;291(10):1238–45.

130. Mozaffarian D, Micha R, Wallace S. Effects on coronary heart disease of increasing polyunsaturated fat in place of saturated fat: a systematic review and meta-analysis of randomized controlled trials. *PLoS Med.* 2010;7(3):e1000252.

131. Musa-Veloso K, Poon TH, Elliot JA, Chung C. A comparison of the LDL-cholesterol lowering efficacy of plant stanols and plant sterols over a continuous dose range: results of a meta-analysis of randomized, placebo-controlled trials. *Prostaglandins Leukot Essent Fatty Acids.* 2011;85(1):9–28.

132. Nathan DM, Cleary PA, Backlund JY, et al. Intensive diabetes treatment and cardiovascular disease in patients with type 1 diabetes. *N Engl J Med.* 2005;353(25):2643–53.

133. National Cholesterol Education Program (NCEP) Expert Panel on Detection, Evaluation, and Treatment of High Blood Cholesterol in Adults (Adult Treatment Panel III). Third Report of the National Cholesterol Education Program (NCEP) Expert Panel on Detection, Evaluation, and Treatment of High Blood Cholesterol in Adults (Adult Treatment Panel III) final report. *Circulation.* 2002;106(25):3143–421.

134. *National Diabetes Fact Sheet, 2011: National Estimates and General Information on Diabetes and Prediabetes in the United States* [Internet]. Atlanta (GA): U.S. Department of Health and Human Services, Centers for Disease Control and Prevention; 2011 [cited 2011 Mar 10]. 12 p. Available from: http://www.cdc.gov/diabetes/pubs/factsheet11.htm

135. National Health Interview Survey Web site [Internet]. Atlanta (GA): Centers for Disease Control and Prevention, National Center for Health Statistics; [cited 2007 Aug 15]. Available from: http://www.cdc.gov/nchs/nhis.htm

136. *NCHS Health E-Stats: Mortality from Major Cardiovascular Diseases: United States, 2007* [Internet]. Atlanta (GA): Centers for Disease Control and Prevention, National Center for Health Statistics; 2010 [cited 2011 Mar 10]. 3 p. Available from: http://www.cdc.gov/nchs/data/hestat/cardio2007/cardio2007.htm

137. Nicolson DJ, Dickinson HO, Campbell F, Mason JM. Lifestyle interventions or drugs for patients with essential hypertension: a systematic review. *J Hypertens.* 2004;22(11):2043–8.

138. NIH Consensus Development Panel on Osteoporosis Prevention, Diagnosis, and Therapy. Osteoporosis prevention, diagnosis, and therapy. *JAMA.* 2001;285(6):785–95.

139. NIH state-of-the-science conference statement on multivitamin/mineral supplements and chronic disease prevention. *NIH Consens State Sci Statements.* 2006;23(2):1–30.

140. Nijveldt RJ, van Nood E, van Hoorn DE, Boelens PG, van Norren K, van Leeuwen PA. Flavonoids: a review of probable mechanisms of action and potential applications. *Am J Clin Nutr.* 2001;74(4):418–25.

141. Norris SL, Zhang X, Avenell A, et al. Long-term effectiveness of lifestyle and behavioral weight loss interventions in adults with type 2 diabetes: a meta-analysis. *Am J Med.* 2004;117(10):762–74.

142. Nutrient Data Laboratory Web site [Internet]. Washington (DC): U.S. Department of Agriculture, Agricultural Research Service; [cited 2007 Aug 15]. Available from: http://www.nal.usda.gov/fnic/foodcomp/search/

143. Odegaard AO, Koh WP, Arakawa K, Yu MC, Pereira MA. Soft drink and juice consumption and risk of physician-diagnosed incident type 2 diabetes: the Singapore Chinese Health Study. *Am J Epidemiol.* 2010;171(6):701–8.

144. Oh K, Hu FB, Manson JE, Stampfer MJ, Willett WC. Dietary fat intake and risk of coronary heart disease in women: 20 years of follow-up of the nurses' health study. *Am J Epidemiol.* 2005;161(7):672–9.

145. Palaniappan L, Carnethon MR, Wang Y, et al. Predictors of the incident metabolic syndrome in adults: the Insulin Resistance Atherosclerosis Study. *Diabetes Care.* 2004;27(3):788–93.

146. Pan XR, Li GW, Hu YH, et al. Effects of diet and exercise in preventing NIDDM in people with impaired glucose tolerance. The Da Qing IGT and Diabetes Study. *Diabetes Care.* 1997;20(4):537–44.

147. Pankow JS, Jacobs DR Jr, Steinberger J, Moran A, Sinaiko AR. Insulin resistance and cardiovascular disease risk factors in children of parents with the insulin resistance (metabolic) syndrome. *Diabetes Care.* 2004;27(3):775–80.

148. Patel S. Sitosterolaemia. Dietary cholesterol absorption. *Lancet.* 2001;358 Suppl:S63.

149. Peacock M, Liu G, Carey M, et al. Effect of calcium or 25OH vitamin D3 dietary supplementation on bone loss at the hip in men and women over the age of 60. *J Clin Endocrinol Metab.* 2000;85(9):3011–9.

150. Pearson TA. Alcohol and heart disease. *Circulation.* 1996;94(11):3023–5.

151. Pearson TA, Bazzarre TL, Daniels SR, et al. American Heart Association guide for improving cardiovascular health at the community level: a statement for public health practitioners, healthcare providers, and health policy makers from the American Heart Association Expert Panel on Population and Prevention Science. *Circulation.* 2003;107(4):645–51.

152. Pearson TA, Blair SN, Daniels SR, et al. AHA guidelines for primary prevention of cardiovascular disease and stroke: 2002 update: consensus panel guide to comprehensive risk reduction for adult patients without coronary or other atherosclerotic vascular diseases. American Heart Association Science Advisory and Coordinating Committee. *Circulation.* 2002;106(3):388–91.

153. Penniston KL, Weng N, Binkley N, Tanumihardjo SA. Serum retinyl esters are not elevated in postmenopausal women with and without osteoporosis whose preformed vitamin A intakes are high. *Am J Clin Nutr.* 2006;84(6):1350–6.

154. Pereira MA, O'Reilly E, Augustsson K, et al. Dietary fiber and risk of coronary heart disease: a pooled analysis of cohort studies. *Arch Intern Med.* 2004;164(4):370–6.

155. Petersen KF, Dufour S, Savage DB, et al. The role of skeletal muscle insulin resistance in the pathogenesis of the metabolic syndrome. *Proc Natl Acad Sci U S A.* 2007;104(31):12587–94.

156. Pilz S, Tomaschitz A, Friedl C, et al. Vitamin D status and mortality in chronic kidney disease. *Nephrol Dial Transplant.* 2011;26(11):3603–9.

157. Pinhas-Hamiel O, Dolan LM, Daniels SR, Standiford D, Khoury PR, Zeitler P. Increased incidence of non-insulin-dependent diabetes mellitus among adolescents. *J Pediatr.* 1996;128(5 Pt 1):608–15.

158. Pischon T, Hankinson SE, Hotamisligil GS, Rifai N, Willett WC, Rimm EB. Habitual dietary intake of n-3 and n-6 fatty acids in relation to inflammatory markers among US men and women. *Circulation.* 2003;108(2):155–60.

159. Pi-Sunyer FX. The fattening of America. *JAMA.* 1994;272(3):238–9.

160. Pittas AG, Chung M, Trikalinos T, et al. Systematic review: vitamin D and cardiometabolic outcomes. *Ann Intern Med.* 2010;152(5):307–14.

161. Pittas AG, Lau J, Hu FB, Dawson-Hughes B. The role of vitamin D and calcium in type 2 diabetes. A systematic review and meta-analysis. *J Clin Endocrinol Metab.* 2007;92(6):2017–29.

162. Plodkowski RA, St Jeor ST. Medical nutrition therapy for the treatment of obesity. *Endocrinol Metab Clin North Am.* 2003;32(4):935–65.

163. Ramsden CE, Hibbeln JR, Majchrzak SF, Davis JM. n-6 fatty acid-specific and mixed polyunsaturate dietary interventions have different effects on CHD risk: a meta-analysis of randomised controlled trials. *Br J Nutr.* 2010;104(11):1586–600.

164. Rana JS, Li TY, Manson JE, Hu FB. Adiposity compared with physical inactivity and risk of type 2 diabetes in women. *Diabetes Care.* 2007;30(1):53–8.

165. Reid IR. The roles of calcium and vitamin D in the prevention of osteoporosis. *Endocrinol Metab Clin North Am.* 1998;27(2):389–98.

166. Renard CB, Kramer F, Johansson F, et al. Diabetes and diabetes-associated lipid abnormalities have distinct effects on initiation and progression of atherosclerotic lesions. *J Clin Invest.* 2004;114(5):659–68.

167. Reynolds K, Chin A, Lees KA, Nguyen A, Bujnowski D, He J. A meta-analysis of the effect of soy protein supplementation on serum lipids. *Am J Cardiol.* 2006;98(5):633–40.

168. Rimm EB, Willett WC, Hu FB, et al. Folate and vitamin B6 from diet and supplements in relation to risk of coronary heart disease among women. *JAMA.* 1998;279(5):359–64.

169. Rocchini AP, Key J, Bondie D, et al. The effect of weight loss on the sensitivity of blood pressure to sodium in obese adolescents. *N Engl J Med.* 1989;321(9):580–5.

170. Rosanoff A. Magnesium supplements may enhance the effect of antihypertensive medications in stage 1 hypertensive subjects. *Magnes Res.* 2010;23(1):27–40.

171. Ross AC, Institute of Medicine (U.S.), Committee to Review Dietary Reference Intakes for Vitamin D and Calcium. *Dietary Reference Intakes for Calcium and Vitamin D.* Washington, DC: National Academies Press; 2011 [cited 2011 Mar 18]. 1132 p. http://www.nap.edu/catalog.php?record_id=13050#toc

172. Sacks FM, Lichtenstein A, Van Horn L, et al. Soy protein, isoflavones, and cardiovascular health: an American Heart Association Science Advisory for professionals from the Nutrition Committee. *Circulation.* 2006;113(7):1034–44.

173. Sacks FM, Svetkey LP, Vollmer WM, et al. Effects on blood pressure of reduced dietary sodium and the Dietary Approaches to Stop Hypertension (DASH) diet. DASH-Sodium Collaborative Research Group. *N Engl J Med.* 2001;344(1):3–10.

174. Sahin M, Tutuncu NB, Ertugrul D, Tanaci N, Guvener ND. Effects of metformin or rosiglitazone on serum concentrations of homocysteine, folate, and vitamin B12 in patients with type 2 diabetes mellitus. *J Diabetes Complications.* 2007;21(2):118–23.

175. Scott B, Perumean-Chaney S, St. Jeor S. Relationship of body mass index to energy density and diet composition in a free-living population. *Topics in Clinical Nutrition.* 2002;17(4):38–46.

176. Serdula MK, Mokdad AH, Williamson DF, Galuska DA, Mendlein JM, Heath GW. Prevalence of attempting weight loss and strategies for controlling weight. *JAMA.* 1999;282(14):1353–8.

177. Shea B, Wells G, Cranney A, et al. Calcium supplementation on bone loss in postmenopausal women. *Cochrane Database Syst Rev.* 2004;(1):CD004526.

178. Simopoulos AP. The importance of the omega-6/omega-3 fatty acid ratio in cardiovascular disease and other chronic diseases. *Exp Biol Med (Maywood).* 2008;233(6):674–88.

179. Singh RB, Niaz MA, Sharma JP, Kumar R, Rastogi V, Moshiri M. Randomized, double-blind, placebo-controlled trial of fish oil and mustard oil in patients with suspected acute myocardial infarction: the Indian experiment of infarct survival—4. *Cardiovasc Drugs Ther.* 1997;11(3):485–91.

180. Smiciklas-Wright H, Mitchell DC, Mickle SJ, Goldman JD, Cook A. Foods commonly eaten in the United States, 1989–1991 and 1994–1996: are portion sizes changing? *J Am Diet Assoc.* 2003;103(1):41–7.

181. Snowling NJ, Hopkins WG. Effects of different modes of exercise training on glucose control and risk factors for complications in type 2 diabetic patients: a meta-analysis. *Diabetes Care*. 2006;29(11):2518–27.

182. Song Y, He K, Levitan EB, Manson JE, Liu S. Effects of oral magnesium supplementation on glycaemic control in Type 2 diabetes: a meta-analysis of randomized double-blind controlled trials. *Diabet Med*. 2006;23(10):1050–6.

183. Song Y, Xu Q, Park Y, Hollenbeck A, Schatzkin A, Chen H. Multivitamins, individual vitamin and mineral supplements, and risk of diabetes among older U.S. adults. *Diabetes Care*. 2011;34(1):108–14.

184. Srinivasan SR, Bao W, Wattigney WA, Berenson GS. Adolescent overweight is associated with adult overweight and related multiple cardiovascular risk factors: the Bogalusa Heart Study. *Metabolism*. 1996;45(2):235–40.

185. Srinivasan SR, Frontini MG, Berenson GS, Bogalusa Heart Study. Longitudinal changes in risk variables of insulin resistance syndrome from childhood to young adulthood in offspring of parents with type 2 diabetes: the Bogalusa Heart Study. *Metabolism*. 2003;52(4):443,50; discussion 451–3.

186. Srinivasan SR, Myers L, Berenson GS. Predictability of childhood adiposity and insulin for developing insulin resistance syndrome (syndrome X) in young adulthood: the Bogalusa Heart Study. *Diabetes*. 2002;51(1):204–9.

187. Stolar M. Metabolic syndrome: controversial but useful. *Cleve Clin J Med*. 2007;74(3):199,202,205–8.

188. Stranges S, Sieri S, Vinceti M, et al. A prospective study of dietary selenium intake and risk of type 2 diabetes. *BMC Public Health*. 2010;10:564.

189. Sundram K, Karupaiah T, Hayes KC. Stearic acid-rich interesterified fat and trans-rich fat raise the LDL/HDL ratio and plasma glucose relative to palm olein in humans. *Nutr Metab (Lond)*. 2007;4:3.

190. Suzuki Y, Whiting SJ, Davison KS, Chilibeck PD. Total calcium intake is associated with cortical bone mineral density in a cohort of postmenopausal women not taking estrogen. *J Nutr Health Aging*. 2003;7(5):296–9.

191. Talati R, Sobieraj DM, Makanji SS, Phung OJ, Coleman CI. The comparative efficacy of plant sterols and stanols on serum lipids: a systematic review and meta-analysis. *J Am Diet Assoc*. 2010;110(5):719–26.

192. Thun MJ, Peto R, Lopez AD, et al. Alcohol consumption and mortality among middle-aged and elderly U.S. adults. *N Engl J Med*. 1997;337(24):1705–14.

193. Torstveit MK, Sundgot-Borgen J. Low bone mineral density is two to three times more prevalent in non-athletic premenopausal women than in elite athletes: a comprehensive controlled study. *Br J Sports Med*. 2005;39(5):282,287; discussion 282–7.

194. Trichopoulou A, Bamia C, Trichopoulos D. Mediterranean diet and survival among patients with coronary heart disease in Greece. *Arch Intern Med*. 2005;165(8):929–35.

195. Trichopoulou A, Costacou T, Bamia C, Trichopoulos D. Adherence to a Mediterranean diet and survival in a Greek population. *N Engl J Med*. 2003;348(26):2599–608.

196. Tucker KL, Morita K, Qiao N, Hannan MT, Cupples LA, Kiel DP. Colas, but not other carbonated beverages, are associated with low bone mineral density in older women: the Framingham Osteoporosis Study. *Am J Clin Nutr*. 2006;84(4):936–42.

197. Tuomilehto J, Lindstrom J, Eriksson JG, et al. Prevention of type 2 diabetes mellitus by changes in lifestyle among subjects with impaired glucose tolerance. *N Engl J Med*. 2001;344(18):1343–50.

198. Ueland PM, Refsum H, Beresford SA, Vollset SE. The controversy over homocysteine and cardiovascular risk. *Am J Clin Nutr*. 2000;72(2):324–32.

199. Wald DS, Law M, Morris JK. Homocysteine and cardiovascular disease: evidence on causality from a meta-analysis. *BMJ*. 2002;325(7374):1202.

200. Wang C, Harris WS, Chung M, et al. n-3 Fatty acids from fish or fish-oil supplements, but not alpha-linolenic acid, benefit cardiovascular disease outcomes in primary- and secondary-prevention studies: a systematic review. *Am J Clin Nutr*. 2006;84(1):5–17.

201. Wang L, Manson JE, Song Y, Sesso HD. Systematic review: vitamin D and calcium supplementation in prevention of cardiovascular events. *Ann Intern Med*. 2010;152(5):315–23.

202. Weinheimer EM, Sands LP, Campbell WW. A systematic review of the separate and combined effects of energy restriction and exercise on fat-free mass in middle-aged and older adults: implications for sarcopenic obesity. *Nutr Rev*. 2010;68(7):375–88.

203. Weinsier RL, Krumdieck CL. Dairy foods and bone health: examination of the evidence. *Am J Clin Nutr*. 2000;72(3):681–9.

204. Weiss EC, Galuska DA, Khan LK, Serdula MK. Weight-control practices among U.S. adults, 2001–2002. *Am J Prev Med*. 2006;31(1):18–24.

205. Welsh JA, Sharma A, Abramson JL, Vaccarino V, Gillespie C, Vos MB. Caloric sweetener consumption and dyslipidemia among US adults. *JAMA*. 2010;303(15):1490–7.

206. Whelton PK, He J, Cutler JA, et al. Effects of oral potassium on blood pressure. Meta-analysis of randomized controlled clinical trials. *JAMA*. 1997;277(20):1624–32.

207. Whelton SP, He J, Whelton PK, Muntner P. Meta-analysis of observational studies on fish intake and coronary heart disease. *Am J Cardiol*. 2004;93(9):1119–23.

208. Wiernsperger N, Rapin J. Trace elements in glucometabolic disorders: an update. *Diabetol Metab Syndr*. 2010;2:70.

209. Wild S, Roglic G, Green A, Sicree R, King H. Global prevalence of diabetes: estimates for the year 2000 and projections for 2030. *Diabetes Care*. 2004;27(5):1047–53.

210. Williamson DF, Vinicor F, Bowman BA, Centers For Disease Control And Prevention Primary Prevention Working Group. Primary prevention of type 2 diabetes mellitus by lifestyle intervention: implications for health policy. *Ann Intern Med*. 2004;140(11):951–7.

211. Wing RR, Phelan S. Long-term weight loss maintenance. *Am J Clin Nutr*. 2005;82(1 Suppl):222S–5S.

212. Witham MD, Avenell A. Interventions to achieve long-term weight loss in obese older people: a systematic review and meta-analysis. *Age Ageing*. 2010;39(2):176–84.

213. Wulffele MG, Kooy A, Lehert P, et al. Effects of short-term treatment with metformin on serum concentrations of homocysteine, folate and vitamin B12 in type 2 diabetes mellitus: a randomized, placebo-controlled trial. *J Intern Med*. 2003;254(5):455–63.

214. *Your Guide to Lowering Your Blood Pressure with DASH Eating Plan* [Internet]. Washington (DC): U.S. Department of Health and Human Services; 2006 [cited 2011]. 64 p. Available from: http://www.nhlbi.nih.gov/health/public/heart/hbp/dash/new_dash.pdf

215. Yu-Poth S, Zhao G, Etherton T, Naglak M, Jonnalagadda S, Kris-Etherton PM. Effects of the National Cholesterol Education Program's Step I and Step II dietary intervention programs on cardiovascular disease risk factors: a meta-analysis. *Am J Clin Nutr*. 1999;69(4):632–46.

216. Yusuf S, Dagenais G, Pogue J, Bosch J, Sleight P. Vitamin E supplementation and cardiovascular events in high-risk patients. The Heart Outcomes Prevention Evaluation Study Investigators. *N Engl J Med*. 2000;342(3):154–60.

217. Yusuf S, Hawken S, Ounpuu S, et al. Effect of potentially modifiable risk factors associated with myocardial infarction in 52 countries (the INTERHEART study): case-control study. *Lancet*. 2004;364(9438):937–52.

SELECTED REFERENCES FOR FURTHER READING

American Diabetes Association, Bantle JP, Wylie-Rosett J, et al. Nutrition recommendations and interventions for diabetes: a position statement of the American Diabetes Association. *Diabetes Care*. 2008;31(Suppl 1):S61–78.

Appel LJ, Brands MW, Daniels SR, et al. Dietary approaches to prevent and treat hypertension: a scientific statement from the American Heart Association. *Hypertension.* 2006;47(2):296–308.

Colberg SR, Sigal RJ, Fernhall B, et al. Exercise and type 2 diabetes: the American College of Sports Medicine and the American Diabetes Association: joint position statement. *Diabetes Care.* 2010;33(12):e147–67.

National Cholesterol Education Program (NCEP) Expert Panel on Detection, Evaluation, and Treatment of High Blood Cholesterol in Adults (Adult Treatment Panel III). Third Report of the National Cholesterol Education Program (NCEP) Expert Panel on Detection, Evaluation, and Treatment of High Blood Cholesterol in Adults (Adult Treatment Panel III) final report. *Circulation.* 2002;106(25):3143–421.

NIH Consensus Development Panel on Osteoporosis Prevention, Diagnosis and Therapy. Osteoporosis prevention, diagnosis, and therapy. *JAMA.* 2001;285(19):785–95.

U.S. Department of Health and Human Services. *Your Guide to Lowering Your Blood Pressure with DASH.* Bethesda, MD: National Heart, Lung, and Blood Institute Information Center; 2006. 56 p.

INTERNET RESOURCES

- American Diabetes Association: http://www.diabetes.org
- American Dietetic Association: http://www.eatright.org
- American Heart Association: http://www.heart.org
- American Stroke Association: http://www.strokeassociation.org
- Centers for Disease Control and Prevention. Division of Nutrition, Physical Activity and Obesity: http://www.cdc.gov/nccdphp/dnpao/index.html
- Centers for Disease Control and Prevention. Preventing Chronic Diseases: Investing Wisely in Health: Preventing Obesity and Chronic Diseases through Good Nutrition and Physical Activity: http://www.cdc.gov/nccdphp/publications/factsheets/Prevention/pdf/obesity.pdf
- National Cholesterol Education Program. Third Report of the Expert Panel on Detection, Evaluation, and Treatment of High Blood Cholesterol in Adults (Adult Treatment Panel III): http://www.nhlbi.nih.gov/guidelines/cholesterol
- National Heart Lung and Blood Institute. Clinical Guidelines on the Identification, Evaluation, and Treatment of Overweight and Obesity in Adults: http://www.nhlbi.nih.gov/guidelines/obesity
- National Heart Lung and Blood Institute. The Eighth Report of the Joint National Committee on Prevention, Detection, Evaluation, and Treatment of High Blood Pressure (JNC 8): http://www.nhlbi.nih.gov/guidelines/hypertension/jnc8/index.htm
- National Osteoporosis Foundation: http://www.nof.org
- U.S. Department of Agriculture, Agricultural Research Service. Nutrient Data Laboratory. Washington, DC: http://www.nal.usda.gov/fnic/foodcomp/search/
- U.S. Department of Health and Human Services. Your Guide to Lowering Your Blood Pressure with DASH Eating Plan. Washington, DC: http://www.nhlbi.nih.gov/health/public/heart/hbp/dash/new_dash.pdf

15

Assessment of Nutritional Status

Accurate **dietary assessment** is a challenge because of the day-to-day variation in the type and amount of foods and beverages people consume, the difficulty in describing and recalling these items, and the difficulty in estimating portion size. Furthermore, the lack of a single "best" method or gold standard to measure diet, the cost and amount of time to collect and process the data, and the need to translate the data to meaningful feedback using nutrient and food databases are hurdles that must be overcome (21). Despite these challenges, dietary assessment can provide worthwhile information if the assessment is conducted with the appropriate tool and both the interviewer and client understand the level of detail required to accurately assess intake.

Fitness professionals may provide dietary guidance to clients who are generally healthy. Many of these clients are interested in improving their diets to lose weight, improve sports performance, or prevent the development of chronic diseases. There are, however, circumstances under which the fitness professional should refer clients to a registered or licensed dietitian. Clients who have special dietary needs, such as people with diabetes, renal problems, eating disorders, or other similar serious medical conditions, should be referred to a registered or licensed dietitian. To locate dietitians to whom clients can be referred, check with local hospitals to find out if they provide outpatient services. Also, go to the American Dietetic Association's Web site at www.eatright.org. Look for the "Find a Registered Dietician" section and enter the client's city and state or zip code.

The objectives of this chapter are to (a) explain the steps and purpose of dietary assessment; (b) identify the strengths and weaknesses of the various dietary assessment tools, including when each should be used; and (c) discuss the analysis and evaluation of dietary intake and how to provide beneficial feedback to clients. Practical tips are provided to illustrate main concepts; (d) discuss the concept of referring patients to an appropriate professional when necessary for nutritional counseling.

THE STEPS OF DIETARY ASSESSMENT

Conducting a dietary assessment to estimate intake involves (a) identifying the purpose of the dietary assessment, (b) selecting the appropriate diet assessment tool,

KEY TERMS

Diet history: A type of dietary assessment that uses a combination of several diet assessment methods to provide a detailed assessment of health habits and usual eating patterns.

Diet record: A diary type of dietary assessment that provides details about all foods and beverages consumed over a defined time.

Dietary assessment: The use of any of the various methods to describe or quantify intake of foods and beverages in humans.

Dietary reference intakes: Science-based recommendations for intake of nutrients that consider risk of dietary deficiencies, protection against chronic diseases, and adverse dietary health risks. Three types of dietary reference intakes are published by the

U.S. government: recommended dietary allowance, adequate intake, and tolerable upper intake level.

Food frequency questionnaire: A type of dietary assessment that is designed to measure general dietary patterns over a defined period of time. Food frequency questionnaires have two parts, which are a defined food list of interest and a frequency response section for reporting how often each food of interest is eaten.

Observation: A type of dietary assessment in which a trained observer records all foods, beverages, and amounts consumed by an individual or group during mealtime.

24-hour recall: A type of dietary assessment method that relies on a person's recall and reporting of food and beverage intake in a defined (usually prior) day.

(c) obtaining the dietary intake data from the individual, (d) analyzing the dietary intake data, (e) evaluating the diet, and (f) providing useful feedback. Each of these steps is described in detail in this chapter.

IDENTIFYING THE PURPOSE OF DIETARY ASSESSMENT

A **dietary assessment** is performed to evaluate the quality and quantity of foods and beverages consumed by individuals. A dietary assessment is one of several indicators of nutritional status, which also include anthropometrics, biochemical data, clinical data, and social history information that may impact the ability to purchase and prepare healthy foods (5). Dietary assessment may be conducted to evaluate an individual's intake in a counseling setting or for research purposes. Many of the diet assessment tools may be used for both purposes; however, this chapter focuses on individual dietary assessment.

The benefits to assessing an individual's diet include the ability to identify food consumption patterns, inadequate or excessive intakes of certain foods or food groups, and issues related to portion size. An individual may seek a diet assessment for several reasons: to assist with a weight-loss program; to learn how to lower fat intake, decrease calories, or increase fruit and vegetable consumption; to improve overall diet; or to optimize dietary intake for athletic performance. In addition, when the diet assessment is used as a part of counseling, the individual may become more aware of his or her intake habits, and this information can be a useful teaching tool.

SELECTING THE APPROPRIATE DIETARY ASSESSMENT TOOL

Dietary assessment methods include diet records, 24-hour recall, food frequency questionnaires (FFQs), diet history, and observation. Each of these methods have strengths and weaknesses, so selection of the appropriate dietary assessment tool depends on whether the information collected will be for an individual or group and the reason for the assessment. Understanding the strengths and weaknesses of the tools used in each step of the dietary assessment process helps ensure that the most appropriate method is used. Certain types of dietary assessment tools may not be appropriate for use with children, persons with memory problems, persons with low literacy levels, or individuals with visual or hearing impairment. This section begins with the methods most likely to be used for assessing individual dietary intake in a fitness setting and concludes with the tools used less commonly. A brief description of each tool, how it should be administered, and its strengths and weaknesses are discussed. The sections that follow provide specific information on analyzing the dietary intake data, evaluating the diet, and providing useful feedback to the client.

Diet Records

Diet records are based on the report of actual intake over a specific number of days, typically 3–4 d and not more than 7 d. When selecting days, it is ideal to include at least one weekend day. The individual records all foods and beverages consumed for a predetermined number of days, with specific details and portion sizes (21). The data are then coded and averaged over the number of days collected. The respondent may also be encouraged to write down information about where, when, and with whom the foods were eaten. This method may be used with nonliterate populations by using tape recorders to record intake.

It is critical to remember that one day of intake does not provide an accurate assessment of usual dietary intake. The number of days of intake necessary to assess an individual's intake varies by the nutrient. Collecting more than 1 d of intake allows estimations of the within-person error, which can assist in determining the number of days to estimate true intake (22). The number of days necessary to estimate usual intake of energy and the macronutrients ranges from 3 to 10 d (3); to estimate many of the micronutrients requires even more days.

The strengths of the diet record are that it provides quantitatively accurate information for the time that the diet record is kept, and that by recording foods when they are consumed, the participant does not rely on memory to recall the information (21). Eating behaviors and patterns can also be addressed with this assessment tool. The limitations of this tool include a high respondent burden because of the need to keep the record with them at all times and record everything that is eaten, usually immediately after consumption. Additionally, the process of recording the items consumed can alter eating behaviors; respondents must be motivated and literate; and coding of the data is time-consuming (3). Collecting too few days of intake will not provide an accurate assessment of an individual's usual intake, and caution should be used when providing feedback to acknowledge the shortcomings of this assessment method.

24-Hour Recall

The 24-hour recall is a popular method to assess current dietary intake. In a structured interview, the respondent is asked to recall all foods and beverages consumed in the past 24 h, including the amount consumed and details on the method of preparation. A single 24-hour recall provides an estimate of actual intake for a specific day but is not appropriate for estimating usual intake because of the daily variation in diet. To estimate usual intake, several 24-hour recalls would need to be collected, with the actual number depending on the nutrient of interest. However, in a research setting, a single 24-hour recall collected from groups of individuals can be used to adequately assess average intake of the groups.

The 24-hour recall is the dietary assessment method used by the U.S. Department of Agriculture (USDA) to assess the nutrient intakes of Americans in the current national nutrition survey known as *What We Eat in America* (18). To obtain the necessary level of detail on each recall, the USDA has developed a five-step multiple-pass method to administer the tool (7). The five steps include a quick list, a forgotten foods list, time and occasion, detail cycle, and the final review probe. The accuracy of the five-step method has been tested in women who are normal, overweight, and obese and was found to assess mean intake within 10% of actual intake that was measured by direct observation (7).

When used for counseling, the 24-hour recall is useful as a method to discuss general eating patterns, keeping in mind that a single day is not representative of overall diet. The 24-hour recall can be completed relatively quickly — in about 20 min. For some populations, this method may not be ideal because of poor memory or difficulty with estimating amounts. This method does not alter usual diet, although individuals may underreport or overreport foods that are more "socially desirable" to appear healthier.

Food Frequency Questionnaire

The FFQ is a checklist from which foods, beverages, and supplements frequently consumed are selected to assess usual intake of particular foods or food groups over a specific time (5,22). In research, this method is useful for assessing the relationship between diet and disease because it can be used to rank individuals by high and low intake. The FFQ may either be interviewer administered or self-administered, will not alter usual diet, and depending on the size of the questionnaire and takes between 20 and 30 min to complete.

The FFQ is composed of a food list, options for reporting the frequency of intake, and options for portion size. The food list used must be representative of the population being studied to ensure that the foods or food groups that are popular sources of nutrient intake are represented. This food list may be subdivided by food groups and typically contain 100–125 foods. The options used for collecting data about frequency of consumption include daily, weekly, monthly, and yearly; and the options depend on the purpose for assessing the diet.

An FFQ may or may not contain portion-size options. A nonquantitative FFQ only requires the individual to provide information about the frequency of consumption. For example, the individual would specify only if he or she ate or drank that item over a specified period (day, week, or month). A semiquantitative FFQ inquires about the frequency of consumption of a prespecified amount of food or beverage (21). Prespecified amounts, such as a slice of bread or glass of milk, are easier to report than items not typically consumed or easily quantifiable, such as chicken (21). A quantitative FFQ asks the individual

to complete information on a portion size, but the portion-size options can range from small, medium, or large, to open-ended questions (22).

The FFQ relies on memory and may be challenging for participants to estimate the foods and beverages consumed over a prespecified length of time. The FFQ may require less administrative time than other methods because answers to the FFQ can be entered on scan sheets and the data entered directly into a database.

Diet History

The diet history is a combination of several diet assessment tools used together to collect data regarding an individual's food habits, eating patterns, dietary restrictions, and other factors influencing nutrient intake (5). The diet history was originally used in human growth and development studies to assess an individual's usual meal patterns, food preparation practices, and intake over a certain time, such as a month or year (4). The diet history may include a 24-hour recall, a food frequency check list, and a 3–7 d food diary. Nutrition knowledge and training are generally necessary to probe for personal dietary habits and patterns. Some data, such as portion sizes, are subject to interpretation. Also, after data are collected, they must be coded and analyzed — processes that are labor intensive, difficult, and expensive.

Observation

Likely, the best method to determine an individual's actual intake is to directly observe a client during several days and record all foods and beverages consumed; however, this is not a realistic option in a free-living population. Using this method, a trained observer records all foods, beverages, and amounts consumed by an individual or group during mealtime. To accurately determine the amount consumed, the observer must know the exact amount the individual or group is served, which is why this method works well in controlled situations, such as metabolic units, institutionalized populations, and schools. The interviewer does not interact with the individuals consuming the food. This method is more often used to assess intake of a group because it is typically conducted during one period. The benefit of the observation method is the accuracy of the dietary intake data collected for the time assessed. The main limitations of this method are that it is very labor intensive and is not appropriate for assessing usual intake.

Summary of Dietary Assessment Tools

As illustrated by the descriptions, benefits, and limitations of each diet assessment tool, the choices for assessing diet are varied. Each dietary assessment tool has strengths and weaknesses. The 24-hour recall or diet record may be most useful because of the ease of administration and the amount of data that can be collected quickly. Thus, the remaining sections in this chapter focus specifically on these two methods. It is important for fitness professionals to realize that the processes associated with assessing dietary intake are quite complicated and require a good bit of training and practice. This chapter provides an overview of the process, but readers are encouraged to work with dietitians or other nutrition specialists to hone their skills in this area. It should also be noted that fitness professionals should consult state laws regarding providing nutritional counseling to clients.

OBTAINING THE DIETARY INTAKE

This section focuses on the steps that can be incorporated into dietary assessment to optimize the data quality obtained from 24-hour recalls and diet records. These steps include providing detailed, verbal and written, easy-to-understand instructions to the client about recording intake and estimating portion size; probing either during the interview or after the completed recall has been received to elicit the necessary detail about intake and portion size; and scanning the completed assessment for missing values and outliers.

Completing the 24-Hour Recall and Diet Record

Usually, the 24-hour recall is completed by the interviewer and does not require instructions for the client. The client is asked to recall all foods and beverages consumed in the past 24 h and to estimate the portion size of each item. The interviewer is responsible for recording the intake and probing for as much detail as possible. *Table 15-1* contains a list of probing questions that will help with this task. It is important to ask open-ended questions, as well as portray a nonjudgmental expression when inquiring about an individual's intake (21).

When a client is asked to keep a diet record for a predetermined number of days, detailed instructions are very useful because clients are typically sent home with a blank diary to complete. *Box 15-1* provides instructions for recording food intake. The instructions should include general information about how to complete the record as well as the contact information of an individual able to assist with the process, if necessary. In addition, instructions for keeping the diet record should be reviewed with the client to reinforce the importance of the exercise, answer questions, explain the level of detail needed for accurate assessment, and remind the client not to omit foods or beverages or change intake.

Recording Portion Size

The importance of estimating portion size should be emphasized to the client. The expanding portion sizes of foods and beverages coupled with the decrease in

physical activity (and, thus, energy expenditure) are likely contributors to the current epidemic of overweight and obesity in the United States (23). Recent analyses from past national nutrition surveys indicate an increase in the portion size of several foods eaten inside and outside the home (17,20). Because weight reduction is a common reason for seeking dietary advice, inaccurate assessment of portion size may hide opportunities for improvement or modification of diet.

The estimation of portion size is one of the most challenging components of dietary assessment. Portion size can be determined by weighing food portions; visually estimating weights of foods; and making visual estimates of size through the use of household measures, food models, or photographs (24). The interviewer may suggest that the client use common household items, such as scales, measuring cups, or a ruler, to assist with estimating portion size. Additionally, the client may be asked to bring in recipes and food labels. Given that portion size is difficult to estimate and mistakes are often encountered during this step, a list of probes to assist with estimating portion size has been provided in *Table 15-2*. Specific attention should be given to the common mistake of confusing fluid and weight ounces when describing portion size.

ANALYZING THE DIETARY INTAKE

After dietary intake has been recorded and reviewed, the contents of the diet need to be analyzed. The goal of this step is to translate the food and beverage consumption data to nutrient intake or food group information, using nutrient composition or food group databases, respectively. Several resources are available to analyze dietary data, such as computerized database software, nutrient composition tables, and food manufacturer data.

Nutrient Composition Databases

Quantitative dietary assessment through repeated contact with subjects by telephone or in-person interviews is expensive. The use of computerized databases for online dietary assessment not only reduces costs but also has several other advantages. Web-based programs can be accessed from any geographic location with little effort, simplifying the acquisition of repeated diet measures by eliminating the logistics involved in arranging appointments and personal interviews (1). Online nutrient databases provide easy access to food pictures, which may reduce the reading level needed to complete an FFQ or estimate portion sizes in a 24-hour food recall (2). In addition, online nutrition assessments can be tailored to individual populations. The Pacific Tracker, for example, contains local foods found in the diets of Pacific Island populations (15). Several online diet analysis programs are available at low cost or no charge from

TABLE 15-1. Probes for Identifying Details of Foods

Type of Information	Did You Specify?
Grains and Cereals	
Bread or tortilla	Brand, type (*e.g.*, diet, regular, wheat, whole wheat, rye, flour vs. corn)
Bakery items	Brand, type (bran, blueberry), how prepared (cake, raised), toppings
Cereal	Brand, type, anything added during preparation or consumption (sugar, fat)
Pasta, rice, and other grains	Brand; fat or salt added
Vegetables and Fruits	
Vegetables and fruit	Fresh, frozen, canned, dried; brand name; cooked or raw; juice: added sugar; salads: what was in salad; added fats, oils, or other toppings (*e.g.*, croutons, sauces, bacon)
Dairy	
Milk	Brand, percent fat, anything added
Cheese	Brand, type (cheddar, American, cottage), version (lite, low fat, low sodium)
Yogurt	Brand, version, frozen or regular
Nondairy	Brand, powder or liquid
Other (ice cream, cream)	Brand, version, type, flavor
Meat, Poultry, and Fish	
Fresh cuts	Type of cut (*e.g.*, T-bone, sirloin, thigh, breast, salmon, haddock) Fat trimmed or skin removed, before or after cooking Is reported weight for cooked or raw, with or without bone? Percent lean (hamburger) How prepared (baked, grilled, fried, barbecue) Fat, sauces and seasonings used during cooking
Cold cuts	Brand, version (*e.g.*, lite hot dog, bun length, foot long), type (*e.g.*, beef, turkey)
Canned tuna and salmon	Type (solid white, chunk light), packed in oil or water, reduced salt
Oils, Spreads, and Dressings	
Margarine	Brand, type (stick, tub, liquid), version (whipped, diet, lite)
Oils	Brand, type (corn, canola, olive)
Mayonnaise/salad dressings	Brand, type or flavor, version (low fat, nonfat, cholesterol free)
Other	
Mixed dishes	Is recipe included, brand, principal components
Pizza	Brand, thin or thick crust, toppings, diameter (*e.g.*, 16 in, 20 in), how many pieces eaten
Soup	Brand or homemade, type or flavor, creamed, water or milk added
Other	Brand; include recipe, if possible; principal components; gravies and sauces
Beverages	Brand, sweetened or unsweetened, alcohol, diet or low calorie, decaffeinated
Eggs	Whole, egg substitute, brand, how prepared
Crackers, snacks, chips	Brand, type, how prepared (*e.g.*, microwave popcorn), size, handfuls, bowls (vitamins B_1 and B_2 food models, cups or ounces if they read it off the bag)
Pies, cakes	Brand, type, one or two crusts or layers, type of frosting

the Internet. MyPlate.gov, the USDA nutrition guide replacing MyPyramid, contains a free dietary analysis tool that assesses daily food consumption, physical activity, and energy status interactively.

Additionally, in April 2003, the USDA made publicly available a user-friendly interface for downloading and using the Survey Nutrient Database, which is the most authoritative nutrient database available. The 2010 updated database includes more than 7,538 foods. The nutrient database displays individual food reports of all the foods in the database as well as nutrient lists for selected foods and nutrients.

Government Guidelines

The Dietary Guidelines for Americans have been the cornerstone of federal nutrition policy and nutrition education since 1980 (20). The guidelines reflect a

BOX 15-1 Instructions for Recording Intake

GENERAL INSTRUCTIONS FOR KEEPING A DIET RECORD

Write legibly.

Record for the specific number of days.

Record each meal, snack, and beverage *immediately* after you eat it. See the following instructions.

Record each food on a separate line.

Leave one or two blank lines after each meal or snack.

If additional space is required for the same day, continue on an extra page.

INSTRUCTIONS FOR RECORDING FOODS

Write down every bit of food and beverage that goes into your mouth — even snacks — for the entire day! Fully describe everything you eat and drink *in detail*

(*e.g.*, chicken thigh, skin not eaten; decaffeinated coffee; low-calorie French dressing; low-fat mayonnaise; whole milk).

Specify preparation methods (*e.g.*, whether meat is breaded and fried, broiled, or baked; vegetables cooked with fat).

List each separate ingredient for mixed dishes (sandwiches, casseroles, salads) on a separate line.

Record exact amounts of food and beverages. If possible, weigh and measure your foods. Example: ½ cup cereal and ½ cup 2% milk. Attach food labels or recipes, if possible.

Include anything that you add to your food at the table (*e.g.*, baked potato with 1 tbsp butter; coffee with 1 tsp sugar).

Try not to modify your eating habits.

---

consensus of the most current science and medical knowledge available. To account for ongoing research efforts in nutrition and health, the guidelines are updated every 5 yr. The government convenes a panel of nutrition, medical, and epidemiologic experts to review the existing guidelines in light of new scientific data. The panel's recommendations are reviewed by government agencies and then provided to the public for comment. In addition, testing is done to determine consumer understanding of the guidelines before they are made final. The latest revision of Dietary Guidelines was made public in 2010.

The intent of the Dietary Guidelines is to summarize and synthesize knowledge about individual nutrients and food components into an interrelated set of recommendations for healthy eating that can be adopted by the public (8). The recommendations are based on the preponderance of scientific evidence for lowering risk of chronic disease and promoting health. It is important to remember that these are integrated messages that should be implemented as a whole. Taken together, they encourage most Americans to eat fewer calories, be more active, and make wiser food choices (see Chapters 4 and 14 in this *Resource Manual* for more details on nutritional recommendations).

Food Guide Pyramid and MyPlate

The Food Guide Pyramid was developed in 1992 as a graphic way to translate the Dietary Guidelines into practical recommendations for foods consumers need to eat daily to get the nutrients they require for good health. In 2005, the USDA replaced the Food Guide Pyramid with a new MyPyramid icon consistent with the recommendations of the 2005 Dietary Guidelines for Americans. The new icon incorporated a person climbing steps to stress physical activity, the narrowing of each food group from bottom to top to suggest moderation, and food bands of differing widths to indicate how much food a person should consume from each food group (16).

In 2011, the USDA replaced MyPyramid with a new generation food icon called MyPlate (6). The plate icon is designed to be an uncomplicated visual cue to help consumers build a healthy plate consistent with the 2010 Dietary Guidelines for Americans. One-half of the plate consists of fruits and vegetables; the other half is divided into grains and protein. The plate is accompanied by a

TABLE 15-2. Portion Size Probes

Portion Sizes

How Many?	Discrete Numbers
Food model	Usual kitchen measures (*e.g.*, cup, tablespoon, teaspoon, ounces) Ounces — fluid or weighed Reasonable Portion of model
Thickness of food or amount of ice in drink	Meat Cakes, brownies Unsliced bread Cubes or crushed A lot of ice, a little ice If the subject knows *exactly* how much he or she drank (*e.g.*, one 12-oz can), you do not need to know if ice was used

smaller circle representing dairy intake, such as a glass of low-fat/nonfat milk or a yogurt cup.

The Web site MyPlate.gov contains much of the same information that was previously available on MyPyramid. Although the icon is different, information about what and how much to eat has not changed. Tools based on MyPyramid, such as MyPyramidTracker, are imbedded in the MyPlate site and continue to be readily available. Over time, these tools will be updated to incorporate the MyPlate icon.

Dietary Reference Intakes

Evaluating clients' diets by analyzing the foods consumed is an adequate and efficient way to determine their dietary needs. However, some clients may want information regarding specific nutrients. For example, a man with a family history of early heart attacks who is trying to lower his blood cholesterol level may want to evaluate his saturated fat intake. A postmenopausal woman may want to know how much calcium she is getting to determine if she should take a calcium supplement. MyPlate includes nutrient analysis software that allows users to compare specific nutrients, such as saturated fat or calcium, to the recommended intake based on their personal profile. The software is consumer friendly and easy to use.

In an effort to make public health recommendations based on the latest research on nutrient needs, the federal government periodically commissions leading scientists in various areas of nutrient research to review the literature and establish estimates of nutrient intakes that can be used to assess and plan diets for generally healthy people. These are called the dietary reference intakes (DRIs) (9–14). For macronutrients such as carbohydrate, fat, and protein, Acceptable Macronutrient Distribution Ranges (AMDRs) have recently been established (14).

The DRIs include three classifications that are of interest to fitness professionals. First, the recommended dietary allowances (RDAs) and adequate intakes (AIs) can both be used as goals for clients. The RDAs are set to meet the nutrient needs of almost all individuals in a particular group (age, sex, pregnant, etc.). Second, when scientists establish an AI instead of an RDA for a nutrient, it is because they believe that the AI is adequate to meet the needs of all individuals in a group, but there are not sufficient data to establish an RDA for that particular nutrient. For some nutrients, there are enough data that support the setting of a tolerable upper intake level (UL). This level is the maximum daily intake that is likely to pose no risk or adverse effects. In most cases, the UL includes total daily intake from food, water, and supplements. Not all nutrients (*e.g.*, thiamin, vitamin B_{12}, vitamin K) have a UL established for them, but that does not mean that it is safe to take them in amounts above the RDA or AI.

EVALUATING DIETARY INTAKE

After the results of a qualitative or quantitative analysis have been determined, the next step is to compare the results with dietary recommendations. Food and nutrient needs differ based on sex, age, physical activity level, life stage, and health status. Since the 1940s, the federal government has established guidelines for food and nutrient intake. Initially, the guidelines were designed to reduce the prevalence of nutrient deficiencies. As such, the dietary recommendations were used to establish policies for many federal aid programs, such as the National School Lunch and the Women, Infants, and Children (WIC) programs. Dietary recommendations are still used for this purpose, but as the prevalence of chronic diseases, such as coronary heart disease, stroke, cancer, diabetes, and obesity, has grown in the past 50 yr, the guidelines shifted to a dual focus of preventing deficiencies and promoting health.

In addition to providing the basis for many federal nutrition programs, current public health dietary recommendations are used as a basis for nutrition label information, military rations, the development of some food and nutritional products, and evaluation of the adequacy of intake for individuals and groups. The remainder of this section focuses on food and nutrient guidelines that fitness professionals would most likely use for evaluating dietary intake of individuals. Practical recommendations for using these guidelines are also provided. Diet can be evaluated at either the food or nutrient level by using MyPlate. For the former, one would use the food search tool. For the latter, one would use the nutrient analysis tool. Regardless of which information is desired, the steps are the same.

1. Convert foods and amounts eaten into food group servings or nutrients.
2. Determine the recommended intake of food groups or nutrients.
3. Compare the amount eaten with recommendations to determine dietary inadequacies.

Although these steps appear to be simple, the diet assessment process is not simplistic and can be fraught with missing information, errors, and miscalculations, as described in earlier sections of this chapter. These errors can be compounded when dietary assessment is done by people with little or no training or experience. If fitness professionals feel uncomfortable with any part of this process, they should consult with, or refer their clients to, a registered dietitian. In addition, in many states, only registered dieticians or licensed nutritionists are legally able to analyze diets and counsel clients regarding their diet. It is recommended that the exercise professional investigate the law in the state in which they are practicing to determine their scope of practice with respect to nutrition counseling.

Converting Foods and Amounts Eaten

Calculate nutrient intake by hand or by using computer software. The former requires one to list each food and the amount eaten. Then use a reference guide, such as *Bowes and Church* (19), to look up the amount of different nutrients in each food. Using computer software can be faster and more accurate than the hand-tabulation method. After entering the foods and amount eaten into the dietary analysis software, it calculates the quantity consumed for dozens of nutrients for each food. The software then sums the quantity of each nutrient for all foods to generate a total daily intake for each nutrient. Many programs calculate an average nutrient intake amount for multiple days of food data as well.

Determine the Recommended Intake

In step one, determine nutrient intake either by hand calculation or by computer. Likewise, in step two, look up a client's intake need for most nutrients in consideration. Review the tables, and take note that nutrient needs sometimes differ from one age category to another or between sexes. Computerized dietary analysis software contains DRI information for each nutrient.

Compare the Amount Eaten with Recommendations

Determining nutrient adequacy simply means comparing actual intake with nutrient recommendations for a person based on his or her age and sex. Most nutrient analysis software programs have a database of the DRIs against which nutrient intake is compared. These applications often provide a tabular and graphic presentation of the adequacy of a client's intake compared with the nutrient needs of someone of the same sex and age. These are often given as percentages of recommended intake. For example, *Figure 15-1* shows a graph that many applications may use.

This example shows that the client did not meet her nutrient needs at exactly 100% for a single nutrient. Does this mean she is nutritionally at risk? How should this be interpreted? There are several things to consider:

1. Dietary assessment information: The report generated from either a 24-hour recall or diet record is an estimate of nutrient intake and is only as good as the completeness of the data provided, the accuracy of the data entry, and the quality of the analysis software used to analyze the intake.
2. Number of days recorded: One day's food record can have a high degree of variability compared with

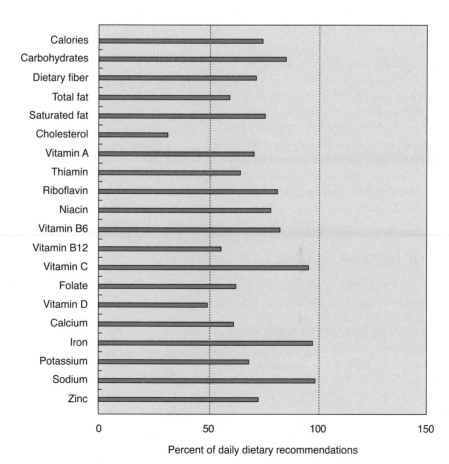

FIGURE 15-1. Sample nutrient analysis report.

another day's. What a client eats today may be very different from what he or she eats tomorrow or the next day, and what is eaten in a single day is not likely to affect one's health positively or negatively. Smoothing out the highs and lows in the daily variability of nutrient intake by averaging the nutrient values across several days will be helpful.

3. Typical of usual intake: If the day (or days) the client recorded were not very typical of his or her usual eating pattern, then the analysis may be skewed. For example, a client usually has a bowl of cereal and skim milk every morning, but on two of the days he recorded, he only ate a granola bar as he commuted to the courthouse for jury duty.

4. Accurate portion descriptions: Often people guess at the size of their portions or misinterpret information provided on their measuring tools.

5. Data entry errors: Making a mistake in entering the many foods in a client's dietary intake record is common. For example, misplacement of a decimal point can make 0.75 cup of Brussels sprouts 7.5 cups of sprouts! When the results seem skewed, review the data entered to make sure the correct food option and portion amount were entered.

If reviewing these issues does not at least somewhat account for any nutrient values below or above the recommended levels, it is rarely cause for alarm. Deficiency is not a concern until an individual is chronically lower than 66% of recommended intake. Excessive intake can occur when a client chronically consumes levels higher than the UL from both diet and supplements.

In summary, this section has provided a step-by-step process for evaluating dietary intake. The fitness professional can use a food-focused evaluation process or a nutrient-focused evaluation process, both using the DRIs available through MyPlate. The professional translates the dietary evaluation into practical recommendations for changing food intake and works with clients to help them set attainable personal goals for dietary improvement.

PROVIDING USEFUL DIETARY FEEDBACK

After the clients' diet is analyzed and evaluated, the next step is to educate them about the aspects of their diet that need to be changed to improve dietary intake. There are two components of giving feedback. The first is the content or the information given. The second component is the process or the way in which the information is provided.

Feedback Content

The task is to inform clients of the gaps that occur in their diets based on what they reported eating and what is recommended for them. These gaps can be characterized as underconsumption or overconsumption of foods or nutrients. Feedback can be given to close such gaps using specific foods and MyPlate's food groups. *Box 15-2* provides a list of practical recommendations for improving intake of foods in different food groups.

If the client's diet has been evaluated using nutrient analysis, it is necessary to convert nutrient needs to food-based recommendations. For example, if it has been determined that a client is eating too much saturated fat, recommend that the client reduce the intake of whole-milk dairy products, including cheese; choose smaller portions of red meat; choose red meats less often; choose fish, skinless poultry, and complementary bean and grain dishes more often; and limit butter and foods with hydrogenated fats. If a client needs to increase her fiber intake, the fitness professional could advise that she eat more whole-grain products, fruits, vegetables, legumes, and nuts.

The Process of Giving Feedback

Identifying the gaps in what a client eats and what is recommended is the first step in providing dietary guidance. Working with the client to determine a plan for closing the gaps is the next step. This step requires an understanding about the behavior change process, and although this is covered elsewhere in this book, listed in the following sections are several change strategies that fitness professionals can use to help clients succeed at improving their eating habits. It is important to note that the process is done collaboratively between professionals and clients. Simply telling clients what they need to change without providing assistance on how to do it is not an effective way of giving feedback.

Educate on Dietary Gaps

This step provides the process in which the client is informed of his or her dietary needs. It is important to share all needs while being mindful not to overwhelm the client. Many clients are tempted to totally overhaul their eating habits based on the information provided. Point out early on in the feedback process that it is best that they choose one or two areas that they want to work on at first. After they have had success making those changes, they can refocus their efforts to address other areas.

Assess Readiness to Change

Clients may be more ready to change some aspects of their diet than others. For example, a client may be more willing to incorporate more whole grains than increase dairy foods. It is important that the fitness professional determine which of the dietary improvement areas the client is most ready to change. This strategy has been discussed as it relates to physical activity readiness in

| BOX 15-2 | **Dietary Feedback Tips** |

BREAD, CEREAL, PASTA, AND RICE

Most Americans meet the recommended dietary intake of 6 oz of grains per day. Because people often misjudge serving sizes, overconsumption of grains is common. A 1-oz serving of grain is considered to be 1 slice of bread, 1 cup of ready-to-eat cereal, or ½ cup cooked rice or pasta. At least one-half of all grains eaten should be whole grains.

Decrease Servings

- Monitor portion sizes. Large portions contribute to weight gain. Visualize your plate divided into four equal parts. Pasta servings should equal one-fourth of the plate, with the remaining sections devoted to protein sources and vegetables. Measure cereal, rice, and pasta to become familiar with actual serving sizes.

Increase Whole Grains

- Start the day with a whole-grain breakfast cereal. Look for one that has at least 5 g of fiber per serving.
- Use 100% whole wheat bread.
- Make oatmeal a regular part of your diet.
- Switch to whole-grain pastas, such as whole-grain spaghetti and whole-grain macaroni.
- Try new whole grains such as bulgur (wheat berries), barley, amaranth, spelt, and quinoa in place of rice or pasta or as side dishes and salads.

VEGETABLES

Few people eat enough vegetables, and the vegetables they do eat are often limited to a few kinds, such as potatoes, corn, and iceberg lettuce.

Increase Servings

- Double and triple up on servings at meals.
- Order a side of vegetables when eating out.
- Enjoy large salads as a meal instead of a sandwich or burger. They can often count as two to four servings, depending on the size.
- Try vegetable juices as a refreshing alternative to soda.
- Eat vegetables and low-fat dips as healthy snack.
- Add extra veggies to soups, stews, and casseroles.

Other Suggestions

- Choose a variety of vegetables. Challenge your taste buds with sweet potatoes, rutabagas, Hubbard squash, kale, and other nutrient-packed veggies.

- Choose colorful vegetables such as carrots, spinach, and tomatoes. Often, the more color, the more nutrients.
- Use canned or frozen vegetables to speed up the preparation process. Look for choices with no added sodium.

FRUITS

As with vegetables, fruits are underconsumed by most adults. They are packed with many nutrients.

Increase Servings

- Start your day with a glass of orange or grapefruit juice.
- Snack on fresh or dried fruits instead of chips or candy bars.
- Serve fruit as dessert and help yourself to seconds.

Other Suggestions

- Like vegetables, choose a rainbow of colors.
- Pack frozen fruit in your lunch bag, and it will be thawed by the time the noon hour rolls around.

MEAT, POULTRY, FISH, EGGS, DRIED BEANS, AND MEAT ALTERNATIVES

Most people eat adequate amounts of meat and poultry, and some people eat these foods in excess.

Limit Meat Group Foods That Are High in Total and Saturated Fat

- Choose lean cuts of red meat. Cuts with the words "loin" or "round" in the name are usually good choices. Wild game (i.e., venison, bison) is leaner than beef.
- Choose ground beef that is at least 95% lean. Note that "% lean" for ground beef refers to the weight of the product including water. A "90% lean" ground beef has 10% of the weight as fat, but 47% of the calories as fat.
- Trim visible fat from meat and poultry before cooking.
- Substitute two egg whites for one whole egg.
- Choose reduced-fat processed meats, cold cuts, and sausages. Check the Nutrition Facts label.

Choose Lean Meats and Meat Alternatives

- Fish and shellfish are healthy food options. However, the presence of mercury in seafood can be a health issue, particularly for children and women of childbearing age. Avoid swordfish, shark, tilefish, and king mackerel. Choose fish and shellfish low in mercury, such as shrimp, canned tuna, tilapia, and salmon.

| **BOX 15-2** | **Dietary Feedback Tips (*Continued*)** |

Opt for fish that is baked, broiled, or grilled, rather than fried.

- Give meat alternatives a try. Sausages, burgers, and chicken tenders are all available in veggie versions, and many grocery stores carry them. Look in the freezer section. Remember, do not expect them to taste just like meat, but enjoy them for their own delicious flavor.
- Eat several meatless meals each week. Look in cookbooks or online for vegetarian recipes.
- Get a leg up with legumes. Try different types of dried beans, peas, and lentils as meat substitutes in soups, salads, or casseroles.

MILK, YOGURT, AND CHEESE

Dairy foods are often overlooked by many adults who think only children need milk. Even people who are lactose intolerant can (and should) enjoy dairy foods by using specially prepared dairy products.

Choose Low-fat and Nonfat Dairy Foods

- Use skim or 1% milk or yogurt.
- Use reduced fat cheese or smaller serving of regular cheese.
- Go easy on regular ice cream. Try low-fat or fat-free versions. Sorbet and sherbet are other low-fat choices.

Increase Dairy Foods

- Make hot cereals and condensed soups with skim milk instead of water.
- Enjoy fruit and low-fat yogurt smoothies for a quick, delicious meal or snack.
- Drink low-fat milk with meals instead of soda.

FATS, OILS, AND SWEETS

Foods in this category are high in calories, and many do not provide much in the way of nutrients; that is, they provide essentially empty calories. So, these foods should be used sparingly.

Limit Empty Calories

- Choose fruits and vegetables as snacks instead of candy.
- Cut amount of fat or oil called for in a recipe by one-fourth or one-third.
- Replace regular soda or sweetened soft drinks with diet versions or fruit juices or low-fat milk.

Other Ideas

- When choosing a fat for cooking, select vegetable oils, such as canola or olive oil, instead of using lard, butter, or shortening.
- Retrain your sweet tooth by gradually removing high-sugar foods from your diet.

Chapter 44 of this *Resource Manual* and can easily be adapted to assessing readiness to change diet.

Set Goals

People who are successful at changing habits challenge themselves by setting goals. However, it is not enough to simply state: "I want to eat better." Effective goals are those that are realistic (are within a client's reach), specific (defined in behavioral terms), and measurable (will be able to know whether or not it was attained). Ask clients to state some short-term (1-d to 1-mo) and long-term (more than 1-mo) goals for the dietary improvement areas they are ready to change. Here is an example of a good goal: "On the fifth of the next 7 d, I will eat at least five servings of fruits and vegetables." It is *realistic* because the client was already eating three servings on most, but not all days. In addition, the client recognizes that it is not likely that he is going to be able to get five servings every day, so he set the goal at 5 d. The goal is *specific* because it states what aspect of the diet (fruits and vegetables) he is going to change and to what extent. Finally, it is *measurable* because he defined

a time frame (*i.e.*, the next 7 d) and quantified the specific parameters of the goal.

Define an Action Plan

A goal is hollow unless it has an action plan to back it up. An action plan identifies the specific strategies the client is going to use to attain his or her goal. Using the example goal given previously, the client identified the following action plan:

> Go to the store on my way home to buy orange juice, fresh strawberries, carrots, premixed salad, and frozen vegetables. Have orange juice for breakfast every morning. Take strawberries and carrots to work for snacks. Eat a big salad at lunch or dinner every weekday. Double up on servings of vegetables at dinner.

Identify a Self-monitoring Strategy

Daily logging helps clients identify whether they are on track toward their goals. Not only does self-monitoring help clients keep a record of what they are doing to attain their goals, but it can also prompt them to make better choices. Unlike keeping diet records for a dietary analysis, when clients are focusing on a specific goal, such as eating five or more servings of fruits and vegetables per day, they only need to focus on recording that specific behavior, simplifying the recording process a great deal.

Arrange Follow-up

Before the feedback session with a client has ended, a follow-up appointment should be set. The follow-up can be done face to face, by telephone, or by electronic means, such as fax or e-mail. The important thing is that clients know the availability of the fitness professional to discuss the success or difficulties they had with attaining their goals. This session is a good time to praise clients for their attainment of goals, problem solve difficulties, and set new goals. Many clients find the accountability of a follow-up contact to be very motivating. As stated earlier, this presentation is a rather simplistic overview of the process for helping clients take the information provided about their dietary needs and applying it to their particular lifestyle. The behavior change principles described in Chapters 45–47 of this *Resource Manual* give a much more thorough review of the change process.

SUMMARY

This chapter is intended to serve as a resource for fitness professionals interested in assessing diet by providing the descriptions of the diet assessment tools and their benefits and limitations. The steps to dietary assessment include identifying the purpose of diet assessment, selecting the appropriate diet assessment tool, obtaining the dietary intake from the individual, analyzing the data, evaluating the diet, and providing useful feedback. Assessing diet is a complex task and requires follow through with each step to assist clients with reaching their goals.

REFERENCES

1. Arab L, Wesseling-Perry K, Jardack P, Henry J, Winter A. Eight self-administered 24-hour dietary recalls using the Internet are feasible in African Americans and Whites: the energetics study. *J Am Diet Assoc.* 2010;110(6):857–64.
2. Beasley JM, Davis A, Riley WT. Evaluation of a web-based, pictorial diet history questionnaire. *Public Health Nutr.* 2009;12(5):651–9.
3. Buzzard M. 24-hour dietary recall and food record methods. In: Willett W, editor. *Nutritional Epidemiology.* 2nd ed. New York: Oxford University Press; 1998. p. 50–73.
4. Byers T, Marshall J, Anthony E, Fiedler R, Zielezny M. The reliability of dietary history from the distant past. *Am J Epidemiol.* 1987;125(6):999–1011.
5. Charney P, Malone A, American Dietetic Association. *ADA Pocket Guide to Nutrition Assessment.* 2nd ed. Chicago (IL): American Dietetic Association; 2009. 214 p.
6. ChooseMyPlate.gov [Internet]. Alexandria (VA): U.S. Department of Agriculture; [cited 2011 Sep 1]. Available from: http://www.choosemyplate.gov/

7. Conway JM, Ingwersen LA, Vinyard BT, Moshfegh AJ. Effectiveness of the US Department of Agriculture 5-step multiple-pass method in assessing food intake in obese and nonobese women. *Am J Clin Nutr.* 2003;77(5):1171–8.
8. Dietary Guidelines for Americans [Internet]. Washington (DC): U.S. Department of Health and Human Services and U.S. Department of Agriculture; [cited 2011 Mar 31]. Available from: http://www.cnpp.usda.gov/DGAs2010-PolicyDocument.htm
9. Dietary reference intakes: for calcium, phosphorus, magnesium, vitamin D, and fluoride [Internet]. Washington (DC): National Academy Press; [cited 2012 Apr 11]. Available from: http://www.nap.edu/catalog.php?record_id=5776
10. Dietary reference intakes for energy, carbohydrate, fiber, fat, fatty acids, cholesterol, protein, and amino acids [Internet]. Washington (DC): National Academies Press; [cited 2011]. Available from: http://www.nap.edu/catalog.php?record_id=10490
11. Dietary reference intakes for thiamin, riboflavin, niacin, vitamin B6, folate, vitamin B12, pantothenic acid, biotin, and choline [Internet]. Washington (DC): National Academy Press; [cited 2012 Apr 11]. Available from: http://www.nap.edu/catalog.php?record_id=6015
12. Dietary reference intakes for vitamin A, vitamin K, arsenic, boron, chromium, copper, iodine, iron, manganese, molybdenum, nickel, silicon, vanadium, and zinc: a report of the Panel on Micronutrients, Subcommittees on Upper Reference Levels of Nutrients and of Interpretation and Uses of Dietary Reference Intakes, and the Standing Committee on the Scientific Evaluation of Dietary Reference Intakes, Food and Nutrition Board, Institute of Medicine [Internet]. Washington (DC): National Academy Press; [cited 2012 Apr 11]. Available from: http://www.nap.edu/catalog.php?record_id=10026
13. Dietary reference intakes for vitamin C, vitamin E, selenium, and carotenoids: a report of the Panel on Dietary Antioxidants and Related Compounds, Subcommittees on Upper Reference Levels of Nutrients and of Interpretation and Use of Dietary Reference Intakes, and the Standing Committee on the Scientific Evaluation of Dietary Reference Intakes, Food and Nutrition Board, Institute of Medicine [Internet]. Washington (DC): National Academy Press; [cited 2012 Apr 11]. Available from: http://www.nap.edu/catalog.php?record_id=9810
14. Dietary reference intakes for water, potassium, sodium, chloride, and sulfate [Internet]. Washington (DC): National Academies Press; [cited 2012 Apr 11]. Available from: http://www.nap.edu/catalog.php?record_id=10925
15. Murphy S, Blitz C, Novotny R. Pacific Tracker (PacTrac): an interactive dietary assessment program at the CRCH website. *Hawaii Med J.* 2006;65(6):175–8.
16. MyPyramid USDA's New Food Guidance System [Internet]. Beltsville (MD): U.S. Department of Agriculture and Center for Nutrition Policy & Promotion [cited 2011 Sep 7]. Available from: healthymeals.nal.usda.gov/hsmrs/Louisiana/10080.ppt
17. Nielsen SJ, Popkin BM. Patterns and trends in food portion sizes, 1977–1998. *JAMA.* 2003;289(4):450–3.
18. Nutrient Intakes from Foods: Mean Amounts Consumed per Individual, by Gender and Age, What We Eat in America, NHANES2007–2008 [Internet]. Washington (DC): U.S. Department of Agriculture, Agriculture Research Service; [cited 2011 Mar 16]. Available from: http://www.ars.usda.gov/SP2UserFiles/Place/12355000/pdf/0708/Table_1_NIN_GEN_07.pdf
19. Pennington JAT, Douglass JS. *Bowes & Church's Food Values of Portions Commonly Used.* 18th ed. Baltimore (MD): Lippincott Williams & Wilkins; 2004. 452 p.
20. Smiciklas-Wright H, Mitchell DC, Mickle SJ, Goldman JD, Cook A. Foods commonly eaten in the United States, 1989–1991 and 1994–1996: are portion sizes changing? *J Am Diet Assoc.* 2003;103(1):41–7.
21. Thompson FE, Byers T. Dietary assessment resource manual. *J Nutr.* 1994;124(11 Suppl):2245S–317S.

22. Willett WC. Nature of variation in the diet. In: Willett WC, editor. *Nutritional Epidemiology*. 2nd ed. New York: Oxford University Press; 1998. p. 33–49.

23. Young LR, Nestle M. The contribution of expanding portion sizes to the US obesity epidemic. *Am J Public Health*. 2002;92(2):246–9.

24. Young LR, Nestle MS. Portion sizes in dietary assessment: issues and policy implications. *Nutr Rev*. 1995;53(6):149–58.

SELECTED REFERENCES FOR FURTHER READING

Charney P, Malone A. *ADA Pocket Guide to Nutrition Assessment*. 2nd ed. Chicago (IL): American Dietetic Association; 2009. 214 p.

Pennington JA, Douglass JS. *Bowes & Church's Food Values of Portions Commonly Used*. 18th ed. Baltimore (MD): Lippincott Williams & Wilkins; 2004.

INTERNET RESOURCES

- American Dietetic Association: http://www.eatright.org
- Dietary Reference Intakes (DRI) and Recommended Dietary Allowances (RDA): http://www.nal.usda.gov/fnic/etext/000108.html
- MyPlate: http://www.myplate.gov
- Nutrition and Your Health: Dietary Guidelines for Americans 2010 http://www.healthierus.gov/dietaryguidelines

Psychosocial Status and Chronic Disease

Chronic diseases such as cardiovascular disease (CVD), cancer, chronic obstructive pulmonary disease (COPD), and diabetes account for more than 70% of all deaths in the United States (108). Consequently, the alleviation of chronic disease and risk associated with these diseases is a priority of the Year 2020 Health Objectives for the nation (108). Chronic diseases typically progress through a series of stages characterized by increased morbidity and disability. Whereas the term *disease* is commonly used to describe pathologic or physiologic changes in the body, *illness* refers to the individual's ensuing adaptation to the disease.

Physical limitations and emotional issues surrounding chronic illness can have a devastating effect on the patient's quality of life. These diseases cause major limitations in about 1 of every 10 Americans or 25 million individuals (108). The influence of emotional distress on chronic illness is often not as recognized compared with other risk factors (100) despite a rapidly growing body of evidence showing a reciprocal relationship between psychosocial factors and chronic disease progression, in which emotional distress can be both a cause and consequence of chronic illness.

This chapter is directed to clinical exercise professionals to provide an overview into the psychology and mental health aspects of disease prevention. This chapter is intended to serve as a quick reference guide for those who need relevant information for professional and public education. This chapter does not provide a comprehensive review of the psychosocial literature associated with chronic disease. Instead, it focuses on the major chronic illnesses that account for much of the morbidity and mortality in the U.S. adult population, including CVD, stroke, heart failure, diabetes, COPD, and asthma.

This chapter reviews epidemiologic and clinical research investigating the relationship between emotional distress and chronic disease. The evidence linking psychosocial factors to the onset and progression of chronic disease is examined. In addition to the three psychosocial domains identified in the Surgeon General's Report on Mental Health (148) — life stress, depression, and anxiety — consideration is given to the role of low social support and other psychological states and traits (*e.g.*, hostility).

This chapter also describes the impact of psychosocial and behavioral interventions on emotional distress.

KEY TERMS

Anxiety: A perception of fear or apprehension that is accompanied by a state of heightened physiologic arousal that may include a surge in heart rate, sweating, and tensing of muscles.

Depression: The presence of a depressed mood or a markedly decreased interest in all activities, persisting for at least 2 wk and accompanied by at least four of the following additional symptoms: changes in appetite, sleep disturbance, fatigue, psychomotor retardation or agitation, feelings of guilt or worthlessness, difficulty concentrating, and suicidal thoughts.

Hostility: An attitude of cynicism and mistrust that may provoke feelings of anger, irritation, and impatience.

Life stress: A combination of negative physiologic, cognitive, emotional, and behavioral responses that occur in response to an individual's unique perception of life events.

Psychological states: Transient changes in mood that may reflect a person's circumstance at a particular point in time.

Psychological traits: Persistent and stable enduring attributes or predispositions of an individual (*e.g.*, type A pattern, which may be characterized by an over commitment to work or completing tasks, competitiveness, an exaggerated need to achieve, free-floating hostility, and a propensity to become easily angered or annoyed).

Social support: An affiliation with social networks that provide emotional support and assistance with aspects of daily living.

Particular attention is given to the role of cognitive behavioral therapy (CBT) because of its general application to numerous chronic conditions. CBT is a counseling method that is used by trained mental health specialists to change ineffective or unrealistic thought patterns and subsequently modify behavior. Consideration is also given to motivational interviewing, which has demonstrated success in the treatment of substance abuse (122) and which has been shown to improve a wide range of problem behaviors in medical settings (21,22,38,60, 76,98,123,130,150,151). Motivational interviewing is a patient-centered, directive method of communication that can be used by a wide variety of trained health care providers to enhance an individual's intrinsic motivation to change unhealthful behavior by exploring and resolving ambivalence (102). Finally, this chapter briefly reviews the direct role exercise may have in the reduction of emotional distress.

CHRONIC DISEASE AND ILLNESS

CARDIOVASCULAR DISEASE

Approximately 16.3 million Americans have coronary heart disease (CHD); 7.0 million have cerebrovascular disease, and 5.8 million have heart failure (126). CVD is the most prevalent chronic illness in the United States (147). Research investigating the relationship of psychosocial factors and CVD provides a wealth of information about the assessment and treatment of this chronic condition. Thus, a large portion of this chapter focuses on the CVD literature.

Evidence indicates there is a relationship between chronic life stress at work and the development of CVD. Stressful life events include the breakup of intimate personal relationships, death of a family member or friend, economic hardship, role conflict, work overload, racism and discrimination, poor physical health, accidental injuries, and intentional assaults of physical safety (62,83,87). Stressful life events may also reflect past events. Severe trauma in childhood including sexual and physical abuse may persist as stressors into adulthood or may make individuals more vulnerable to ongoing stress (19). Each individual exhibits a unique response to stressful life events that includes some combination of physiologic, cognitive, emotional, and behavioral characteristics that may be harmful to susceptible individuals.

In a meta-analysis of five different populations numbering more than 12,000 individuals and covering an 18- to 30-yr period, work stress was associated with higher levels of cholesterol, systolic blood pressure (BP), and smoking behavior (118). Monotonous work, high-paced work, and job burnout have been correlated with an increased incidence of CHD (3). High-demand jobs with low decision latitude have been associated with a fourfold increased risk of cardiovascular-related death (72). Work stress associated with high demand and low reward has also resulted in an increase in cardiac events (17,137) and the progression of carotid atherosclerosis (97). Researchers have identified that in a working population compared with a nonworking population, there is a 33% increase in relative risk of disease onset on Mondays (158). In a study involving a sample of 170,000 men and women, death from CVD was 20% above the daily average on Mondays for those younger than the age of 50 yr (41). In the 20-yr follow-up of the Framingham Heart Study, the incidence of angina was two times greater among those who exhibited higher levels of worry, dissatisfaction with work, feeling undue time pressure, and competitive drive (39). Together, these studies indicate that there is strong association between this form of chronic stress and the development of CVD. Almost four decades ago, Holmes and Rahe (120) developed the Recent Life Change Questionnaire to assess the severity of typical stressful life events. Whereas the death of a spouse, divorce, and loss of a job were considered high stress, vacations and holidays were given a lower weighting. A retrospective recall found that elevated scores on the survey were associated with higher rates of myocardial infarction (MI) or sudden cardiac death at 6-mo follow-up (158).

Acute stress has been implicated in the triggering of cardiovascular events. Epidemiologic evidence has revealed that life-threatening situations such as earthquakes (73,91,141,144) and war (7,101) are associated with increased rates of MI and cardiac mortality. This observation does not appear to be limited to life-threatening situations. An increase in the rate of hospital admissions for MI and sudden cardiac death has been reported after important national soccer games (26,159). In an examination of the acute effect of anger as a trigger of MI, retrospective interviews of 1,623 patients who have experienced MI identified a greater than twofold relative risk of MI after an episode of anger (103). Cross-sectional studies have yielded evidence that acute negative emotional states such as anger, anxiety, and frustration (55) are associated with myocardial ischemia. In an observational clinical cohort study of acute coronary syndrome (ACS), the risk of anger onset compared with no anger was 2.06 (139). Anger was more common in patients who are younger and socioeconomically deprived who primarily presented with an ST-elevation MI. Platelet reactivity with mental stress has been positively correlated with hostile personality traits contributing to the association with anger (139). Moreover, emotional stress may induce transient ischemia and disturb autonomic function leading to arrhythmias.

Depression takes a monumental toll on human suffering, lost productivity, and death. Data from surveys undertaken by the U.S. Centers for Disease Control and Prevention indicate that 6.8% of adults in the United States had depression in the 2 wk prior to being surveyed (28). The prevalence of depression among patients with CVD is three times higher than the general population, and assessments among MI patients suggest that as many as 15%–20% of hospitalized patients meet criteria for major depression (93). When unrecognized, depression can result in excessive health care use.

Depression affects more than 120 million people worldwide (92). Major depression is the most well-known mood disorder, but there are others, including bipolar disorder (one or more episodes of mania) and dysthymia (a chronic but less severe form of major depression) (148). Episodes of major depression are characterized by the presence of a depressed mood or a markedly decreased interest in all activities, persisting for at least 2 wk and accompanied by at least four of the following additional symptoms: changes in appetite, sleep disturbance, fatigue, psychomotor retardation or agitation, feelings of guilt or worthlessness, problems concentrating, and suicidal thoughts. It is estimated that depression will rank as the leading cause of disease burden by 2030 (92).

The causes of depression are not fully known. Depression may be triggered by stressful life events, enduring stressful social conditions (*e.g.*, poverty, discrimination), neurochemical imbalance in the brain, maladaptive cognitions, or a combination of these factors and is twice as common in women as men. It is also correlated with other mental disorders associated with adverse cardiovascular outcomes such as anxiety (93).

Depression tends to be underdiagnosed and under-treated in patients with CVD. Fewer than 25% of patients with major depression are recognized as being depressed by their cardiologists or general internists, and only about 50% of patients diagnosed as depressed receive treatment (99). The reasons for this finding are not clear, although it has been suggested that physicians may have difficulty differentiating between the symptoms of depression and those related to the disease (29). Depression in patients with CHD is associated with a worse prognosis, and studies suggest there is a doubling in risk of CVD events in the 1–2 yr following an MI (93). Epidemiologic evidence demonstrates a significant prospective relationship between the occurrence of depression, or depressive symptoms, and the incidence of future cardiac events among both healthy (2,6) and CVD populations (5,45,47). Patients with CVD and depression compared to nondepressed patients have higher levels of biomarkers known to predict CVD events and promote atherosclerosis. Patients who are depressed show reduced heart rate variability, hypothalamic-pituitary-adrenal axis dysfunction, increased plasma platelet factor 4 and B thromboglobulin, impaired vascular function, and increased levels of C-reactive protein, interleukin-6 (IL-6) levels, intracellular adhesion molecule-1, and fibrinogen levels (93).

Anxiety disorders are the most prevalent mental disorders in adults (122), affecting twice as many women as men. These disorders include panic disorder, phobias, obsessive-compulsive disorder, posttraumatic stress disorder, and generalized anxiety disorder. It is estimated that 18.1% of the U.S. adult population have anxiety disorders (28). Underlying this heterogeneous group of disorders is a state of heightened arousal or fear in relation to stressful events or feelings. The biological manifestations of anxiety, which are grounded in the "fight-or-flight" response, are unmistakable: they include surge in heart rate, sweating, and tensing of muscles. The Harvard Mastery of Stress Study, one of the longest prospective studies ever conducted in this field, revealed that severe anxiety and conflict with hostility were significant predictors of CVD and risk of overall future illness (131).

Social support has been widely recognized as an independent predictor of health and well-being in both general and clinical populations (69,146), especially among patients with cardiac disease. Social isolation indicating few close relationships or social ties is associated with an increase in all cause and CVD mortality (9,64) and predicts 1-yr mortality after MI as strongly as other risk factors (104). Low social support has also been prospectively associated with poor clinical prognosis among patients with heart failure (106) and stable CVD (20,63,116,157).

There are two broad categories of social support. Structural support refers to social networks and includes such indices as marital status, number of friends, and participation in church or civic organizations. Functional support refers to the perception of support and includes such elements as instrumental support (*e.g.*, having someone who can assist in activities of daily living) and emotional support (*e.g.*, having someone to talk to and whom you believe loves or cares for you) (148).

Studies on animals (70) and humans (4,11,33,67,82, 116,128) have identified that psychological stress has an adverse impact on the cardiovascular system. The mechanism by which stress may influence the development of atherosclerosis involves a complex interaction of sympathetic arousal, hypothalamic stimulation, and adrenergic and neurohormonal responses that lead to increased BP, increased circulating catecholamine levels, and increased platelet activity (30,107,153). The resulting increased shearing forces of blood on the arterial wall lead to endothelial injury and arterial wall damage. Thus, chronic exposure to psychological stress promotes the development of atherosclerosis that may result in vasospasm (160), myocardial ischemia (15), coronary artery occlusion, MI, and increased incidence of ventricular arrhythmia, a known risk factor for sudden coronary death (31). These pathophysiologic mechanisms have been schematized by Rozanski et al. (129) in *Figure 16-1*.

Although conclusions regarding the mechanisms by which more chronic psychosocial factors contribute to cardiac events are not definitive, considerable evidence points to several mechanisms likely to be involved in the

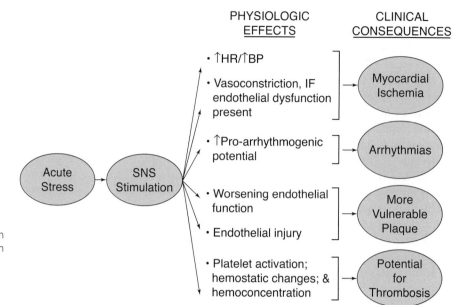

FIGURE 16-1. Pathophysiologic effects of acute psychosocial stress. Sympathetic nervous system (SNS) stimulation emanating from acute stress leads to a variety of effects, ranging from heart rate (HR) and blood pressure (BP) stimulation to direct effects on coronary vascular endothelium. Clinical consequences of these effects include myocardial ischemia, cardiac arrhythmias, and fostering of more vulnerable coronary plaques and hemostatic changes. These changes form a substrate for development of acute myocardial infarction and sudden cardiac death. (Adapted with permission from Rozanski A, Blumenthal JA, Kaplan J. Impact of psychological factors on the pathogenesis of cardiovascular disease and implications for therapy. *Circulation.* 1999;99:2192–217.)

impact of depression on the prognosis of patients with established CVD. For example, it has been shown that patients with depression exhibit increased sympathetic nervous system outflow and decreased parasympathetic function (153). This combination can lead to ventricular arrhythmias, platelet activation and aggregation, and increased myocardial oxygen consumption. These kinds of reactions could contribute to the pathophysiologic processes involved in the development of both CVD and MI. Increased activation of the pituitary adrenal axis in patients with depression has also been shown to produce high levels of cortisol (79), which can potentiate and prolong the effects of catecholamines (152).

Depression has been shown to be a predictor of poor adherence to a wide variety of medical treatments (25,36,103). A meta-analysis by Di Matteo et al. revealed that patients with chronic disease and depression were three times more likely to be nonadherent with medical treatment than patients without depression (35). Moreover, tobacco use and lack of exercise and attention to dietary factors may also contribute to the development and progression of CAD in patients with depression (93). Consequently, depression may indirectly promote the progression of chronic illness by preventing adherence to other treatment regimens, such as healthy eating, physical activity and exercise, taking medications appropriately, abstaining from smoking, managing stress, and moderating alcohol consumption.

Psychosocial and Behavioral Interventions

Psychosocial and behavioral intervention trials in patients with CVD have reported mixed success. In a study of 107 patients with heart disease with exercise-induced ischemia, a CBT-based approach to stress management

was associated with improved psychosocial measures, a reduction in mental stress-induced ischemia (14), and fewer clinical events after a 5-yr follow-up when compared with exercise therapy alone or usual care (12). In a review of other studies involving similar populations, CBT interventions have been reported to improve quality of life and reduce mortality in patients with heart disease (96). However, in the Enhancing Recovery in Coronary Heart Disease (ENRICHD) Trial, a multicenter trial involving 2,481 patients who have experienced MI with depression or low social support, CBT reduced depression levels but failed to yield a significant reduction in all-cause mortality and cardiac morbidity (8). Other trials (46,68) have also reported negative findings, and the failure of these brief interventions to alter psychosocial risk factors such as anxiety and depression may have been responsible for the lack of effect on "hard" clinical endpoints, such as mortality and morbidity. A post hoc analysis of the ENRICHD Trial revealed that patients who were treated with selective serotonin reuptake inhibitors (SSRIs) irrespective of assignment to CBT or usual care had a 42% reduction in deaths or recurrent MI compared to patients not receiving antidepressants (93).

The role of exercise as a stand-alone intervention in the prevention and management of CVD is well documented (24,145). However, it should be recognized that there is uncertainty about the extent to which clinical outcomes may have been directly or indirectly affected by improved psychosocial status as a result of exercise. Regardless, it is safe to conclude that exercise therapy added to a multi-intervention approach that includes behavioral cardiac risk modification, education, and counseling may enhance the improvements in CVD outcomes reported in exercise-only interventions (24). This finding is exemplified by the Lifestyle Heart Trial, which demonstrated that an intervention composed of exercise therapy, group support meetings, education and skills training in a low-fat diet, and daily stress management (*i.e.*, yoga-derived stretching, breathing, meditation, imagery, and relaxation techniques) could assist a highly motivated group of patients with CVD to make comprehensive changes in lifestyle. Arteriographic data identified an average arterial stenosis regression from 40.0% to 37.8% in the intervention group compared with a progression from 42.7% to 46.1% in a usual care group at a 1-yr follow-up (114). A 5-yr follow-up showed continued progression in the control group and regression in the intensive lifestyle intervention group (115). Motivating patients with CVD to adopt and maintain comprehensive changes in lifestyle is a challenge that faces health care professionals, and motivational interviewing is an innovative approach that has demonstrated efficacy in brief consultations. Scales et al. (136) found that compared with traditional cardiac rehabilitation, adding motivational interviewing coupled with brief skills-building sessions significantly lowers stress and enhances multiple health-related behaviors for patients with CVD.

STROKE

Stroke and heart failure are especially important cardiovascular conditions that deserve attention because of the psychological sequelae associated with these chronic conditions and the need for more effective interventions. Stroke is the third leading cause of death in the United States behind CVD and all cancers and the leading cause of long-term disability (126). Each year, 795,000 people experience a new or recurrent stroke. The direct and indirect cost of stroke in 2007 was $40.9 billion (126).

The most common psychological reaction in individuals suffering a stroke is depression. The incidence of depression ranges from 25% to 79%, with most studies showing a rate of approximately 30% (75). The large variation in incidence is due to the timing of assessment relative to stroke onset and the instruments used to assess depression. A debate also exists whether depression following a stroke is organic or a result of the psychosocial adjustment required by the disease (75). Several factors may contribute to depression following a stroke, including institutionalization, prestroke alcohol use, impairment of activities of daily living, and perception of social support. Poststroke depression has been found to be higher among older adults with similar chronic conditions causing similar physical disabilities (75). Finally, assessing depression following a stroke is complicated by the fact that patients may exhibit lethargy, memory impairment, and difficulties because of dysphagia and/or other cognitive losses. Thus, family members and caregivers may need to help in the assessment process. Instruments such as the Center for Epidemiological Studies Depression Scale (CES-D) (119), used in epidemiologic studies of stroke;

the Post-Stroke Depression Rating Scale (50); and the Structured Assessment of Depression in Brain Damaged Individuals (54) may help to define the nature and severity of poststroke depression.

Assessment and treatment is critical in this population as patients with poststroke depression use more health care resources. In a study of 2,405 veterans with poststroke depression, compared with 2,257 with other mental conditions, patients with poststroke depression had more inpatient hospitalization days and outpatient visits in the first 3 yr following a stroke, even after adjustment for mental health clinic visits (52).

Psychological and Behavioral Interventions

Few intervention studies have shown success in decreasing depression in patients following a stroke. Psychological interventions have involved the use of health care disciplines, such as social workers and nurses, to provide counseling and support for patients following a stroke; CBT by therapists; and pharmacologic agents, such as the use of nortriptyline and SSRIs (75,95,121). In a Cochrane review of interventions to treat depression after stroke involving nine trials and 780 subjects, Hackett and colleagues found no strong evidence of benefit of either pharmacotherapy or psychotherapy to enable complete remission of depression following stroke (57). However, patients did show improvement in scores on depression rating scales. In a merged analysis of three studies, Kimura et al. using the Hamilton interview found that patients treated with nortriptyline compared with those in placebo groups showed significant reductions in depression scores as well as improvements in anxiety (74). More recently, Williams showed in a randomized controlled trial that a case management approach that included SSRIs not only decreased depression but also the likelihood of remission when compared to usual care as well (156).

Because CBT by trained therapists has been shown to be an effective treatment in the general population and the elderly, it certainly deserves greater attention in patients with depression following a stroke. To date, only a handful of studies with a small number of mildly to moderately patients with depression have been undertaken to determine the effects of CBT (8). Few studies have shown success, although investigators agree that further study is needed because of the success of using problem solving, a component of CBT to improve family function after a stroke. Problem solving has also been shown to reduce depression in institutionalized older adults.

HEART FAILURE

Heart failure is a condition affecting more than 5.8 million patients in the United States alone, and the prevalence of heart failure is expected to increase substantially as the population ages (126). By 2030, it is estimated that

40.5% of the U.S. population will have some form of CVD, with heart failure increasing by 25% (59). Like other chronic conditions such as stroke, heart failure is associated with disability and decline causing significant psychological distress (48).

Depression, anxiety, and social isolation are common in patients with heart failure. In a meta-analysis of 36 studies, Rutledge et al. (132) found that depression was present in 21.5% of patients with heart failure, varying by the use of questionnaires versus diagnostic interviews (33.6% and 19.3%, respectively). Their results also indicate that depression is associated with a higher death rate (relative risk [RR] = 2.1; 95% confidence interval [CI], 1.7–2.6) and a trend toward increased health care use, hospitalization rates, and emergency room visits. Depression has been documented in both acute heart failure (66,144) and in those with chronic heart failure (149,155).

Although much less well studied, anxiety is also common in patients with heart failure. Anxiety is typically defined as a negative affective state with a component of fear because of an inability to predict, control, or obtain desired results in upcoming situations (67). Using the State-Trait Anxiety Scale to measure anxiety in 291 patients with heart disease hospitalized as a result of cardiac events, Jiang et al. found that 29% had a state-A score ≥40, and 28% had a trait-A score ≥40. These scores (≥40) have previously shown a threefold increased risk of cardiac events in patients who have experience MI. However, although relatively prevalent in this population with heart failure and closely associated with depression, Jiang et al. did not find anxiety was highly correlated with mortality (66).

Konstam and colleagues (80) assessed both self-reported depression and anxiety in the Studies of Left Ventricular Dysfunction (SOLVD) trial as part of several psychological factors that might predict readmission and death. In this trial, neither depression nor anxiety was associated with worse outcomes (80). More recently, 153 patients in the Sudden Cardiac Death in Heart Failure Trial (SCD-HeFT) participated in the Psychosocial Factors in Outcome Study (PFOS), which investigated the prevalence of depression and anxiety and the relationship of psychological factors to mortality in outpatients with heart failure. Although anxiety scores (≥40) measured by the State-Trait Anxiety Scale were high (45%), anxiety did not predict mortality (48). Thus, although these studies show a high prevalence of anxiety, it does not appear to reflect a worse heart failure outcome for patients with this condition.

A few studies have also shown a relationship between social support and heart failure and its relationship to mortality. For example, it has been shown that individuals who live alone with heart failure have a greater likelihood of developing depression within 1 yr (58). After controlling for depression and heart failure severity, social isolation was also noted to increase mortality in outpatients with heart failure (106). Finally, after controlling for demographics, medical characteristics, and depression, emotional support — defined as the number of people available to talk over problems — was also an independent predictor of mortality in patients hospitalized with heart failure (84).

Psychosocial and Behavioral Interventions

Depression and anxiety in heart failure both appear to be associated with sympathetic activation and catecholamine release as well as abnormal platelet reactivity (65,132). Depression is associated with elevations of proinflammatory cytokines, including IL-6, tumor necrosis factor-α (TNF-α), and IL-1B. Exercise programs following heart failure appear to reduce IL-6 and TNF-α levels in heart failure. Whether exercise and pharmacologic treatments for depression reduce symptoms and inflammation, showing a favorable outcome on morbidity and mortality in heart failure has not been well studied. Findings from Heart Failure–A Controlled Trial to Investigate the Outcomes of Exercise Training (HF ACTION) did not support a reduction in overall mortality from exercise in patients with heart failure (112).

Although many more studies are needed with larger sample sizes to look at the effects of intervening in patients with heart failure with depression, anxiety, and social isolation to determine the effects on clinical outcomes, relief of symptoms may support patients with heart failure now. Thus, the use of CBT and exercise training may be appropriate interventions. SSRIs may also be used to treat depression and anxiety in this population (75,95).

DIABETES

Diabetes is a chronic disease caused by insulin deficiency, resistance to insulin action, or both. The prevalence of diabetes in the United States in 2010 was 25.8 million, which includes 18.8 million diagnosed new cases and 7.0 million undiagnosed cases. Diabetes is the leading cause of new cases of blindness and kidney failure, and 60%–70% of individuals with diabetes have mild-to-severe forms of nervous system damage (34). Stress, depression, and anxiety are more prevalent among patients with diabetes than the general population (117,125,140).

Evidence suggests that stress may precipitate the onset of diabetes or compromise glucose control after the disease is established (140). Glucose toxicity resulting from chronic, intermittent, stress-induced elevations in blood glucose further compromises the ability of the pancreas to secrete insulin (88), leading to the progression of the disease. However, evidence characterizing the effects of stress in Type 1 diabetes is inconsistent. Human studies have shown that stress can stimulate hyperglycemia or hypoglycemia or have no effect at all on glycemic status in established diabetes. More consistent evidence supports the role of stress in Type 2 diabetes. Animal and human studies suggest that individuals with Type 2 diabetes have altered adrenergic sensitivity in the pancreas, which could make them particularly sensitive to stressful life events. However, although substantial data link stress to the expression or control of Type 2 diabetes (53), further evidence is needed. Moreover, few studies have followed patients long enough to determine the long-term consequences of stress in patients with diabetes.

Psychosocial and Behavioral Interventions

The few studies involving psychosocial and behavioral interventions in patients with diabetes have involved CBT, coping skills, empowerment, and diabetes management training. These approaches have been found to decrease diabetes-related anxiety and avoidance behaviors; enhance quality of life, coping ability, and emotional well-being; and, most importantly, improve self-care and glycemic control (53).

The Diabetes Prevention Program (DPP) Research Group (77) demonstrated the strong effect that physical activity and weight loss can exert in preventing the onset of diabetes in high-risk adults. Compared with usual care, there was a 58% reduction in the onset of diabetes over a period of approximately 3 yr among individuals who were supported in their efforts to follow a healthful lifestyle. Although the intervention did not directly target stress management, these individuals received regular weekly support from a case manager and additional meetings with an exercise specialist, dietitian, and behavioral counselor. An intervention involving medication alone reduced the incidence of new cases by 31% (77). In another randomized controlled trial, the Finnish Diabetes Prevention Study (DPS), investigators used behavior modification techniques similar to the DPP that focused on intensively changing lifestyle. At the end of 4.5 yr of follow-up, the DPS found that participants in the lifestyle intervention group who succeeded in increasing their physical activity were least likely to develop diabetes after controlling for changes in diet (90). Both the DPP and the DPS support the impact of lifestyle changes on preventing Type 2 diabetes. Whether these types of interventions and other psychological/behavioral interventions can affect the status or complications in people with already established Type 2 diabetes is largely unknown.

CHRONIC OBSTRUCTIVE PULMONARY DISEASE

COPD is characterized by the presence of airflow obstruction resulting from chronic bronchitis and emphysema, two diseases that often coexist (147). COPD is the fourth leading cause of death in the United States and worldwide, currently affecting 13.1 million adults in the United States older than the age of 18 yr (143). Moreover, morbidity and mortality have not significantly declined in the past 20 yr, and because of an aging population with debilitating illness, COPD is expected to increase and become the third leading cause of death by 2020 (109). COPD rank as the fourth leading cause of death in the United States (78).

Common psychological reactions among patients with COPD include anger, frustration, guilt, dependency, and embarrassment (56,134). However, the most frequently observed psychological symptoms among patients with COPD are depression and anxiety. A meta-analysis of 13 studies involving 900 subjects demonstrated a prevalence rate of depression of 40% (Johannes). One of the best studies of depression in COPD was a cross-sectional trial of 1,224 Veterans Administration patients with COPD. Investigators used the Structured Clinical ID (SCID) interview and found that 39% were diagnosed with depression (111).

One of the main problems of measuring depression in patients with COPD is the overlap of symptoms of depression and COPD. Increased fatigue, sleep, and appetite problems and difficulties concentrating are associated with both depression and COPD, making the diagnosis difficult. Using instruments to address the overlap between depression and COPD may help to address this problem.

Depression can be aggravated in patients with COPD because of worsening dyspnea and fatigue and perceived poor health, which in turn may decrease functional capacity and exercise tolerance. Therefore, it is important for clinicians to monitor quality of life over time to intervene appropriately. Depression has also been associated with a poorer survival and longer hospitalization stays. In a study of 376 consecutive patients with COPD who were hospitalized and followed for 1 yr, Ng and colleagues (110) found that the prevalence of depression on admission to hospital was 44.4%. Multivariate analysis revealed that depression was significantly associated with mortality (hazard rates, 1.93; CI, 1.04–3.58), a longer index stay (mean, 1.1 more days; $P = .02$) and total stay (mean, 3.0 more days; $P = .047$), and worse physical and social functioning assessed by the St. George Respiratory Questionnaire (110).

Anxiety is another common psychological consequence of COPD. The prevalence of generalized anxiety in patients with COPD ranges from 10% to 33% and the prevalence of panic attacks ranges from 8% to 67% (61). Dyspnea in conjunction with fear of suffocation and death is a source of significant anxiety in this population (134). Dyspnea increases during acute exacerbations of COPD with intractable dyspnea being associated with anxiety. Moreover, feelings of anger and frustration are potent triggers of anxiety that may heighten dyspnea (61).

Psychosocial and Behavioral Interventions

The use of antidepressants and CBT in patients with COPD is rare and heterogeneous in results, making it difficult to draw conclusions on the effectiveness of these therapies (49). Trials have been burdened by small sample size, lack of sound diagnostic tools to identify depression, patient nonadherence, and for CBT confounding results due to the overlap of both depression and anxiety with less optimal treatment of depression (49). However, pulmonary rehabilitation programs have been shown to reduce both depression and anxiety and improve quality of life, even if patients did not show significant improvements in exercise performance (110). No study to date has shown that psychotherapeutic interventions in depressed patients with COPD have been able to reduce mortality and hospitalizations.

Treatment studies involving patients with COPD have also shown that psychosocial intervention combined with exercise therapy improves mood, anxiety, and neurocognitive functioning (81). Psychological interventions on their own have been noted to reduce breathlessness and general disability and improve quality of life (124,127). In comparison, exercise-based interventions have tended to show additional benefits (40), with relief of dyspnea and improved functioning and control of the disease (10). However, these studies have been limited by small sample sizes, and as such, large-scale clinical trials are required before definitive conclusions can be drawn.

A Cochrane review indicated that patients who participated in pulmonary rehabilitation showed clinically significant improvements in patient-reported symptoms of dyspnea and fatigue as well as disease-specific and general quality of life. However, to date, it is unclear how pulmonary rehabilitation improves health-related quality of life (105). One of the largest studies of patients with COPD undertaking pulmonary rehabilitation was performed with 590 patients who participated in 24 wk of rehabilitation at the University of California, San Diego (154). These investigators found the 6-minute walk test, quality of life as measured by the Medical Outcomes Study SF-36, and the perception of dyspnea with activities of daily living all improved after 12 wk of rehabilitation and were maintained at 24 wk. The authors recommend that patients participate in supervised pulmonary rehabilitation for at least 24 wk to gain and maintain optimal benefits (154).

ASTHMA

Asthma is a lung disease with recurrent exacerbations of airflow constriction, mucous secretion, and chronic inflammation of the airways, resulting in reduced airflow that causes symptoms of wheezing, coughing, chest tightness, and difficulty breathing. In 2009, the prevalence of asthma was 8.2% of the U.S. population or 24.6 million people. Prevalence among children younger than 18 yr of age was 9.6% and among adults was 7.7% (27).

Research has demonstrated an association between emotional stress and various indices of impaired airway function, including increased breathlessness (dyspnea) and bronchoconstriction in patients with asthma (1). As with patients with COPD, anxiety is common in patients with asthma, with panic disorder being particularly prevalent (89). The prevalence of anxiety from the use of different surveys is 16%–52% (142). Anxiety appears to be related to excessive use of bronchodilators, greater prescriptions for corticosteroid medication, more frequent hospital readmissions, and more lengthy hospitalizations, independent of pulmonary impairment (71). It has been well documented that individuals who have asthma also have a reduced quality of life, and quality of life tends to be lower in those with severe asthma (113). Ford et al., for example, showed that patients with asthma had a reduced quality of life compared with individuals who had never experienced asthma, and they experienced an average of 10 d of impaired physical or mental health; almost double that of those who had never had asthma (44).

Numerous studies report that the prevalence of depression in those with asthma ranges from 14% to 41% (85). The large variation in prevalence relates to three issues: symptoms of asthma linked to depression may be misinterpreted; use of corticosteroids, which has been hypothesized as a link between asthma and depression; and a positive feedback loop in which depression leads to nonadherence with asthma treatment, which then exacerbates asthma that leads to increased depression, resulting in worsened outcomes (89). In addition, there has been a dearth of quality studies reviewing depression in those with asthma. Most studies are cross sectional or retrospective in design, making it difficult to interpret the results.

Psychosocial and Behavioral Interventions

A limited number of psychological intervention studies have been done with patients with asthma. Therapies such as training in CBT, stress management, yoga, biofeedback, and symptom perception have been shown to reduce measures of asthma morbidity and improve patient quality of life (90). In addition, because of its complex medication regimen, adherence has been one of the main foci of behavioral interventions (36,89). The primary intervention used is asthma education and management, which has been shown to improve measures such as frequency of asthma attacks and symptoms, medication adherence, and self-management skills (89). Although it is still unclear if exercise interventions for individuals with asthma improve pulmonary function and bronchial responsiveness, there is very good evidence that exercise training improves quality of life (135).

EXERCISE THERAPY TO REDUCE EMOTIONAL DISTRESS

The association between regular exercise and mood has been recognized since the late 1970s; however, the role of exercise as a clinical treatment for psychiatric disorders has only been explored recently (18). One of the original long-term prospective studies, the Alameda County Study (23), found that compared with individuals who were active at baseline, inactive participants were at a greater risk for high depression scores 9 yr later. In addition, participants who increased their exercise levels across the first 9 yr of the study were at no greater risk for depression after 18 yr than those who exercised throughout the study. However, those who became inactive after the first 9 yr were more likely to become depressed after 18 yr relative to active participants. A meta-analysis of clinical trials (86) found that compared with no treatment, exercise reduced depression and was equally as effective as cognitive therapy. Also, evidence from cross-sectional and prospective studies suggests a dose-response effect of physical activity on depressive and anxiety disorders, although this relationship has not yet been found in clinical trials (37). Exercise has been shown to improve stress management ability, general feelings of well-being, self-esteem (43), and muscular tension (32). Clinically, exercise training potentially offers a vehicle for nonspecific psychological therapy. It also offers a specific psychological treatment that may be particularly effective for patients for whom more conventional psychological interventions are less acceptable (133).

A variety of mechanisms has been suggested for the therapeutic effects of exercise, including alterations in the central monoamine systems, improved regulation of the hypothalamic-pituitary-adrenal axis, and increased β-endorphin levels. However, to date, there are no known studies that have directly assessed the mechanisms behind the exercise–mood relationship (18). Exercise training has also been shown to attenuate the cardiovascular response to emotional stressors (13,16,51,138). This response includes a decreased β-adrenergic myocardial response to physical or behavioral challenges and an acute prophylactic effect in reducing BP response to psychological stressors (16,94). In addition, there may be indirect effects of exercise on emotional distress. For example, the addition of diagnostic exercise testing can reassure anxious patients of safety and improve self-confidence (42). In summary, although good evidence suggests that increased physical activity and exercise training improve psychological distress, more high-quality studies are needed to identify if there is a dose-response relationship and to identify the mechanisms by which exercise exerts its antidepressant and anxiolytic affects.

SUMMARY

Psychosocial factors such as depression, anxiety, and low perceived social support are common among patients living with chronic illness and appear to be both a cause and a consequence of several chronic medical conditions. However, future prospective studies that include valid measures to assess psychosocial factors and clinical outcomes associated with chronic illness are needed to further our understanding in this field of research.

Most people with psychosocial risk factors do not present themselves to mental health services for treatment. Therefore, systems need to be established to help non–mental health professionals, such as exercise specialists, find ways to screen for emotional distress and recognize potential symptoms. Consideration should also be given to developing improved liaison relationships with psychological or behavioral specialists to facilitate more specialized interventions when appropriate. Individual or group CBT-based interventions have shown to be particularly effective in this regard. In addition, non–mental health specialists need to be encouraged and supported to develop skills that will enable them to better promote healthful behavior and emotional functioning in the overall treatment of individuals with chronic illness. For example, motivational interviewing, noted in *Chapter 45*, is one of several useful approaches that can be used by exercise professionals to meet this challenge.

REFERENCES

1. Affleck G, Apter A, Tennen H, et al. Mood states associated with transitory changes in asthma symptoms and peak expiratory flow. *Psychosom Med.* 2000;62(1):61–8.
2. Anda R, Williamson D, Jones D, et al. Depressed affect, hopelessness, and the risk of ischemic heart disease in a cohort of U.S. adults. *Epidemiology.* 1993;4(4):285–94.
3. Appels A, Schouten E. Burnout as a risk factor for coronary heart disease. *Behav Med.* 1991;17(2):53–9.
4. Bacon SL, Watkins LL, Babyak M, et al. Effects of daily stress on autonomic cardiac control in patients with coronary artery disease. *Am J Cardiol.* 2004;93(10):1292–4.
5. Barefoot JC, Helms MJ, Mark DB, et al. Depression and long-term mortality risk in patients with coronary artery disease. *Am J Cardiol.* 1996;78(6):613–7.
6. Barefoot JC, Schroll M. Symptoms of depression, acute myocardial infarction, and total mortality in a community sample. *Circulation.* 1996;93(11):1976–80.
7. Bergovec M, Mihatov S, Prpic H, Rogan S, Batarelo V, Sjerobabski V. Acute myocardial infarction among civilians in Zagreb city area. *Lancet.* 1992;339(8788):303.
8. Berkman LF, Blumenthal J, Burg M, et al. Effects of treating depression and low perceived social support on clinical events after myocardial infarction: the Enhancing Recovery in Coronary Heart Disease Patients (ENRICHD) Randomized Trial. *JAMA.* 2003;289(23):3106–16.
9. Berkman LF, Glass T, Brissette I, Seeman TE. From social integration to health: Durkheim in the new millennium. *Soc Sci Med.* 2000;51(6):843–57.
10. Berry MJ, Walschlager SA. Exercise training and chronic obstructive pulmonary disease: past and future research directions. *J Cardiopulm Rehabil.* 1998;18(3):181–91.

11. Blazer DG. Social support and mortality in an elderly community population. *Am J Epidemiol.* 1982;115(5):684–94.

12. Blumenthal JA, Babyak M, Wei J, et al. Usefulness of psychosocial treatment of mental stress-induced myocardial ischemia in men. *Am J Cardiol.* 2002;89(2):164–8.

13. Blumenthal JA, Fredrikson M, Kuhn CM, Ulmer RL, Walsh-Riddle M, Appelbaum M. Aerobic exercise reduces levels of cardiovascular and sympathoadrenal responses to mental stress in subjects without prior evidence of myocardial ischemia. *Am J Cardiol.* 1990;65(1):93–8.

14. Blumenthal JA, Jiang W, Babyak MA, et al. Stress management and exercise training in cardiac patients with myocardial ischemia. Effects on prognosis and evaluation of mechanisms. *Arch Intern Med.* 1997;157(19):2213–23.

15. Blumenthal JA, Jiang W, Waugh RA, et al. Mental stress-induced ischemia in the laboratory and ambulatory ischemia during daily life. Association and hemodynamic features. *Circulation.* 1995;92(8):2102–8.

16. Boone JB Jr, Probst MM, Rogers MW, Berger R. Postexercise hypotension reduces cardiovascular responses to stress. *J Hypertens.* 1993;11(4):449–53.

17. Bosma H, Peter R, Siegrist J, Marmot M. Two alternative job stress models and the risk of coronary heart disease. *Am J Public Health.* 1998;88(1):68–74.

18. Brosse AL, Sheets ES, Lett HS, Blumenthal JA. Exercise and the treatment of clinical depression in adults: recent findings and future directions. *Sports Med.* 2002;32(12):741–60.

19. Browne A, Finkelhor D. Impact of child sexual abuse: a review of the research. *Psychol Bull.* 1986;99(1):66–77.

20. Brummett BH, Barefoot JC, Siegler IC, et al. Characteristics of socially isolated patients with coronary artery disease who are at elevated risk for mortality. *Psychosom Med.* 2001;63(2):267–72.

21. Burke BL, Arkowitz H, Dunn C. The effectiveness of motivational interviewing and its adaptations: what we know so far. In: Miller WR, Rollnick S, editors. *Motivational Interviewing: Preparing People for Change.* 2nd ed. New York: Guilford Press; 2002. p. 217–250.

22. Burke BL, Arkowitz H, Menchola M. The efficacy of motivational interviewing: a meta-analysis of controlled clinical trials. *J Consult Clin Psychol.* 2003;71(5):843–61.

23. Camacho TC, Roberts RE, Lazarus NB, Kaplan GA, Cohen RD. Physical activity and depression: evidence from the Alameda County Study. *Am J Epidemiol.* 1991;134(2):220–31.

24. *Cardiac Rehabilitation Clinical Practice Guideline: AHCPR Pub. No. 96-0673* [Internet]. Rockville, MD: Agency for Health Care Policy and Research, National Heart, Lung and Blood Institute; 1995 [cited 2012 Apr 11]. Available from: http://www.ncbi.nlm.nih.gov/books/NBK12243/

25. Carney RM, Freedland KE, Eisen SA, Rich MW, Jaffe AS. Major depression and medication adherence in elderly patients with coronary artery disease. *Health Psychol.* 1995;14(1):88–90.

26. Carroll D, Ebrahim S, Tilling K, Macleod J, Smith GD. Admissions for myocardial infarction and World Cup football: database survey. *BMJ.* 2002;325(7378):1439–42.

27. Centers for Disease Control and Prevention. CDC Health Disparities and Inequalities Report—United States, 2011: current asthma prevalence—United States, 2006–2008. *MMWR.* 2011;60(Suppl):1–113.

28. Centers for Disease Control and Prevention. Mental illness surveillance among adults in the United States. *MMWR.* 2011;60 (Suppl):1–29.

29. Clarke DM. Psychological factors in illness and recovery. *N Z Med J.* 1998;111(1076):410–2.

30. Coumel P, Leenhardt A. Mental activity, adrenergic modulation, and cardiac arrhythmias in patients with heart disease. *Circulation.* 1991;83(4 Suppl):II58–70.

31. Davis AM, Natelson BH. Brain-heart interactions. The neurocardiology of arrhythmia and sudden cardiac death. *Tex Heart Inst J.* 1993;20(3):158–69.

32. De Vries HA, Adams GM. Electromyographic comparison of single doses of exercise and meprobamate as to effects on muscular relaxation. *Am J Phys Med.* 1972;51(3):130–41.

33. Deanfield JE, Shea M, Kensett M, et al. Silent myocardial ischaemia due to mental stress. *Lancet.* 1984;2(8410):1001–5.

34. *Diabetes Statistics* [Internet]. Alexandria, VA: American Diabetes Association; [cited 2011 Sep 22]. Available from: http://www.diabetes.org/diabetes-basics/diabetes-statistics/

35. DiMatteo MR, Lepper HS, Croghan TW. Depression is a risk factor for noncompliance with medical treatment: meta-analysis of the effects of anxiety and depression on patient adherence. *Arch Intern Med.* 2000;160(14):2101–7.

36. Dunbar J. Predictors of patient adherence: patient characteristics. In: Shumaker SA, Schron EB, Ockene JK, editors. *The Handbook of Health Behavior Change.* New York: Springer Pub. Co; 1990. p. 348–360.

37. Dunn AL, Trivedi MH, O'Neal HA. Physical activity dose-response effects on outcomes of depression and anxiety. *Med Sci Sports Exerc.* 2001;33(6 Suppl):S587–97; discussion 609–10.

38. Dunn C, Deroo L, Rivara FP. The use of brief interventions adapted from motivational interviewing across behavioral domains: a systematic review. *Addiction.* 2001;96(12):1725–42.

39. Eaker ED, Abbott RD, Kannel WB. Frequency of uncomplicated angina pectoris in type A compared with type B persons (the Framingham Study). *Am J Cardiol.* 1989;63(15):1042–5.

40. Emery CF, Schein RL, Hauck ER, MacIntyre NR. Psychological and cognitive outcomes of a randomized trial of exercise among patients with chronic obstructive pulmonary disease. *Health Psychol.* 1998;17(3):232–40.

41. Evans C, Chalmers J, Capewell S, et al. "I don't like Mondays"-day of the week of coronary heart disease deaths in Scotland: study of routinely collected data. *BMJ.* 2000;320(7229):218–9.

42. Ewart CK, Taylor CB, Reese LB, DeBusk RF. Effects of early postmyocardial infarction exercise testing on self-perception and subsequent physical activity. *Am J Cardiol.* 1983;51(7):1076–80.

43. Fillingim RB, Blumenthal JA. The use of aerobic exercise as a method of stress management. In: Lehrer PM, Woolfolk RL, editors. *Principles and Practice of Stress Management.* 2nd ed. New York: Guilford Press; 1993. p. 443–462.

44. Ford ES, Mannino DM, Homa DM, et al. Self-reported asthma and health-related quality of life: findings from the behavioral risk factor surveillance system. *Chest.* 2003;123(1):119–27.

45. Frasure-Smith N, Lesperance F, Juneau M, Talajic M, Bourassa MG. Gender, depression, and one-year prognosis after myocardial infarction. *Psychosom Med.* 1999;61(1):26–37.

46. Frasure-Smith N, Lesperance F, Prince RH, et al. Randomised trial of home-based psychosocial nursing intervention for patients recovering from myocardial infarction. *Lancet.* 1997;350 (9076):473–9.

47. Frasure-Smith N, Lesperance F, Talajic M. Depression and 18-month prognosis after myocardial infarction. *Circulation.* 1995;91(4):999–1005.

48. Friedmann E, Thomas SA, Liu F, et al. Relationship of depression, anxiety, and social isolation to chronic heart failure outpatient mortality. *Am Heart J.* 2006;152(5):940.e1–8.

49. Fritzsche A, Clamor A, von Leupoldt A. Effects of medical and psychological treatment of depression in patients with COPD—a review. *Respir Med.* 2011;105(10):1422–33.

50. Gainotti G, Azzoni A, Razzano C, Lanzillotta M, Marra C, Gasparini F. The Post-Stroke Depression Rating Scale: a test specifically devised to investigate affective disorders of stroke patients. *J Clin Exp Neuropsychol.* 1997;19(3):340–56.

51. Georgiades A, Sherwood A, Gullette EC, et al. Effects of exercise and weight loss on mental stress-induced cardiovascular responses in individuals with high blood pressure. *Hypertension.* 2000;36(2):171–6.

52. Ghose SS, Williams LS, Swindle RW. Depression and other mental health diagnoses after stroke increase inpatient and outpatient medical utilization three years poststroke. *Med Care.* 2005;43(12): 1259–64.

53. Gonder-Frederick LA, Cox DJ, Ritterband LM. Diabetes and behavioral medicine: the second decade. *J Consult Clin Psychol.* 2002;70(3):611–25.

54. Gordon WA, Hibbard MR. Poststroke depression: an examination of the literature. *Arch Phys Med Rehabil.* 1997;78(6):658–63.

55. Gullette EC, Blumenthal JA, Babyak M, et al. Effects of mental stress on myocardial ischemia during daily life. *JAMA.* 1997;277(19):1521–6.

56. Guyatt GH, Townsend M, Berman LB, Pugsley SO. Quality of life in patients with chronic airflow limitation. *Br J Dis Chest.* 1987;81(1):45–54.

57. Hackett ML, Anderson CS, House AO. Interventions for treating depression after stroke. *Cochrane Database Syst Rev.* 2004;(3): CD003437.

58. Havranek EP, Spertus JA, Masoudi FA, Jones PG, Rumsfeld JS. Predictors of the onset of depressive symptoms in patients with heart failure. *J Am Coll Cardiol.* 2004;44(12):2333–8.

59. Heidenreich PA, Trogdon JG, Khavjou OA, et al. Forecasting the future of cardiovascular disease in the United States: a policy statement from the American Heart Association. *Circulation.* 2011; 123(8):933–44.

60. Hettema J, Steele J, Miller WR. Motivational interviewing. *Annu Rev Clin Psychol.* 2005;1:91–111.

61. Hill K, Geist R, Goldstein RS, Lacasse Y. Anxiety and depression in end-stage COPD. *Eur Respir J.* 2008;31(3):667–77.

62. Holmes TH, Rahe RH. The Social Readjustment Rating Scale. *J Psychosom Res.* 1967;11(2):213–8.

63. Horsten M, Mittleman MA, Wamala SP, Schenck-Gustafsson K, Orth-Gomer K. Depressive symptoms and lack of social integration in relation to prognosis of CHD in middle-aged women. The Stockholm Female Coronary Risk Study. *Eur Heart J.* 2000;21(13):1072–80.

64. House JS. Social isolation kills, but how and why? *Psychosom Med.* 2001;63(2):273–4.

65. James PN, Anderson JB, Prior JG, White JP, Henry JA, Cochrane GM. Patterns of drug taking in patients with chronic airflow obstruction. *Postgrad Med J.* 1985;61(711):7–10.

66. Jiang W, Alexander J, Christopher E, et al. Relationship of depression to increased risk of mortality and rehospitalization in patients with congestive heart failure. *Arch Intern Med.* 2001;161(15):1849–56.

67. Jiang W, Babyak M, Krantz DS, et al. Mental stress—induced myocardial ischemia and cardiac events. *JAMA.* 1996;275(21):1651–6.

68. Jones DA, West RR. Psychological rehabilitation after myocardial infarction: multicentre randomised controlled trial. *BMJ.* 1996;313(7071):1517–21.

69. Kaplan GA, Salonen JT, Cohen RD, Brand RJ, Syme SL, Puska P. Social connections and mortality from all causes and from cardiovascular disease: prospective evidence from eastern Finland. *Am J Epidemiol.* 1988;128(2):370–80.

70. Kaplan JR, Manuck SB, Clarkson TB, Lusso FM, Taub DM. Social status, environment, and atherosclerosis in cynomolgus monkeys. *Arteriosclerosis.* 1982;2(5):359–68.

71. Kaptein AA. Psychological correlates of length of hospitalization and rehospitalization in patients with acute, severe asthma. *Soc Sci Med.* 1982;16(6):725–9.

72. Karasek R, Baker D, Marxer F, Ahlbom A, Theorell T. Job decision latitude, job demands, and cardiovascular disease: a prospective study of Swedish men. *Am J Public Health.* 1981;71(7):694–705.

73. Katsouyanni K, Kogevinas M, Trichopoulos D. Earthquake-related stress and cardiac mortality. *Int J Epidemiol.* 1986;15(3):326–30.

74. Kimura M, Tateno A, Robinson RG. Treatment of poststroke generalized anxiety disorder comorbid with poststroke depression: merged analysis of nortriptyline trials. *Am J Geriatr Psychiatry.* 2003;11(3):320–7.

75. Kneebone II, Dunmore E. Psychological management of post-stroke depression. *Br J Clin Psychol.* 2000;39(Pt 1):53–65.

76. Knight KM, McGowan L, Dickens C, Bundy C. A systematic review of motivational interviewing in physical health care settings. *Br J Health Psychol.* 2006;11(Pt 2):319–32.

77. Knowler WC, Barrett-Connor E, Fowler SE, et al. Reduction in the incidence of type 2 diabetes with lifestyle intervention or metformin. *N Engl J Med.* 2002;346(6):393–403.

78. Kochanek KD, Smith BL. Deaths: preliminary data for 2002. *Natl Vital Stat Rep.* 2004;52(13):1–47.

79. Koetnansky R. Catecholamines-corticosteroid interactions. In: Usdin E, Kvetnanský R, Kopin IJ, editors. *Catecholamines and Stress: Recent Advances: Proceedings of the Second International Symposium on Catecholamines and Stress, Held in Smolenice Castle, Czechoslovakia, September 12–16, 1979.* New York: Elsevier/North-Holland; 1980. p. 7.

80. Konstam V, Salem D, Pouleur H, et al. Baseline quality of life as a predictor of mortality and hospitalization in 5,025 patients with congestive heart failure. SOLVD Investigations. Studies of Left Ventricular Dysfunction Investigators. *Am J Cardiol.* 1996;78(8):890–5.

81. Kozora E, Tran ZV, Make B. Neurobehavioral improvement after brief rehabilitation in patients with chronic obstructive pulmonary disease. *J Cardiopulm Rehabil.* 2002;22(6):426–30.

82. Krantz DS, Helmers KF, Bairey CN, Nebel LE, Hedges SM, Rozanski A. Cardiovascular reactivity and mental stress-induced myocardial ischemia in patients with coronary artery disease. *Psychosom Med.* 1991;53(1):1–12.

83. Krieger N, Rowley DL, Herman AA, Avery B, Phillips MT. Racism, sexism, and social class: implications for studies of health, disease, and well-being. *Am J Prev Med.* 1993;9(6 Suppl):82–122.

84. Krumholz HM, Butler J, Miller J, et al. Prognostic importance of emotional support for elderly patients hospitalized with heart failure. *Circulation.* 1998;97(10):958–64.

85. Lavoie KL, Bacon SL, Barone S, Cartier A, Ditto B, Labrecque M. What is worse for asthma control and quality of life: depressive disorders, anxiety disorders, or both? *Chest.* 2006;130(4):1039–47.

86. Lawlor DA, Hopker SW. The effectiveness of exercise as an intervention in the management of depression: systematic review and meta-regression analysis of randomised controlled trials. *BMJ.* 2001;322(7289):763–7.

87. Lazarus RS, Folkman S. *Stress, Appraisal, and Coping.* New York (NY): Springer Pub. Co; 1984. 445 p.

88. Leahy JL. Natural history of beta-cell dysfunction in NIDDM. *Diabetes Care.* 1990;13(9):992–1010.

89. Lehrer P, Feldman J, Giardino N, Song HS, Schmaling K. Psychological aspects of asthma. *J Consult Clin Psychol.* 2002; 70(3):691–711.

90. Lehrer P, Smetankin A, Potapova T. Respiratory sinus arrhythmia biofeedback therapy for asthma: a report of 20 unmedicated pediatric cases using the Smetankin method. *Appl Psychophysiol Biofeedback.* 2000;25(3):193–200.

91. Leor J, Kloner RA. The Northridge earthquake as a trigger for acute myocardial infarction. *Am J Cardiol.* 1996;77(14):1230–2.

92. Lepine JP, Briley M. The increasing burden of depression. *Neuropsychiatr Dis Treat.* 2011;7(Suppl 1):3–7.

93. Lichtman JH, Bigger JT Jr, Blumenthal JA, et al. Depression and coronary heart disease: recommendations for screening, referral, and treatment: a science advisory from the American Heart Association Prevention Committee of the Council on Cardiovascular Nursing, Council on Clinical Cardiology, Council on Epidemiology and Prevention, and Interdisciplinary Council on Quality of Care and Outcomes Research: endorsed by the American Psychiatric Association. *Circulation.* 2008;118(17):1768–75.

94. Light KC, Obrist PA, James SA, Strogatz DS. Cardiovascular responses to stress: II. Relationships to aerobic exercise patterns. *Psychophysiology.* 1987;24(1):79–86.

95. Lincoln NB, Flannaghan T. Cognitive behavioral psychotherapy for depression following stroke: a randomized controlled trial. *Stroke*. 2003;34(1):111–5.

96. Linden W. Psychological treatments in cardiac rehabilitation: review of rationales and outcomes. *J Psychosom Res*. 2000;48(4–5):443–54.

97. Lynch J, Krause N, Kaplan GA, Salonen R, Salonen JT. Workplace demands, economic reward, and progression of carotid atherosclerosis. *Circulation*. 1997;96(1):302–7.

98. Martins RK, McNeil DW. Review of motivational interviewing in promoting health behaviors. *Clin Psychol Rev*. 2009;29(4):283–93.

99. Mayou R, Foster A, Williamson B. Medical care after myocardial infarction. *J Psychosom Res*. 1979;23(1):23–6.

100. McKenna MT, Taylor WR, Marks JS, Koplan JP. Current issues and challenges in chronic disease control. In: Brownson RC, Remington PL, Davis JR, editors. *Chronic Disease Epidemiology and Control*. 2nd ed. Washington: American Public Health Association; 1998. p. 1–26.

101. Meisel SR, Kutz I, Dayan KI, et al. Effect of Iraqi missile war on incidence of acute myocardial infarction and sudden death in Israeli civilians. *Lancet*. 1991;338(8768):660–1.

102. Miller WR, Rollnick S. *Motivational Interviewing: Preparing People for Change*. 2nd ed. New York (NY): Guilford Press; 2002. 428 p.

103. Mittleman MA, Maclure M, Sherwood JB, et al. Triggering of acute myocardial infarction onset by episodes of anger. Determinants of Myocardial Infarction Onset Study Investigators. *Circulation*. 1995;92(7):1720–5.

104. Mookadam F, Arthur HM. Social support and its relationship to morbidity and mortality after acute myocardial infarction: systematic overview. *Arch Intern Med*. 2004;164(14):1514–8.

105. Moullec G, Laurin C, Lavoie KL, Ninot G. Effects of pulmonary rehabilitation on quality of life in chronic obstructive pulmonary disease patients. *Curr Opin Pulm Med*. 2011;17(2):62–71.

106. Murberg TA, Bru E. Social relationships and mortality in patients with congestive heart failure. *J Psychosom Res*. 2001;51(3):521–7.

107. Naesh O, Haedersdal C, Hindberg I, Trap-Jensen J. Platelet activation in mental stress. *Clin Physiol*. 1993;13(3):299–307.

108. *National Center for Chronic Disease Prevention and Health Promotion 2009. The Power of Prevention: Chronic Disease . . . The Challenge of the 21st Century* [Internet]. Atlanta, GA: Centers for Disease Control and Prevention; 2009 [cited 2011 Oct 4]. 18 p. Available from: http://www.cdc.gov/

109. National Center for National Health Statistics. United States, 2002. *Natl Vital Stat Rep*. 2005;53(17):9.

110. Ng TP, Niti M, Tan WC, Cao Z, Ong KC, Eng P. Depressive symptoms and chronic obstructive pulmonary disease: effect on mortality, hospital readmission, symptom burden, functional status, and quality of life. *Arch Intern Med*. 2007;167(1):60–7.

111. Norwood R. Prevalence and impact of depression in chronic obstructive pulmonary disease patients. *Curr Opin Pulm Med*. 2006;12(2):113–7.

112. O'Connor CM, Whellan DJ, Lee KL, et al. Efficacy and safety of exercise training in patients with chronic heart failure: HF-ACTION randomized controlled trial. *JAMA*. 2009;301(14):1439–50.

113. Opolski M, Wilson I. Asthma and depression: a pragmatic review of the literature and recommendations for future research. *Clin Pract Epidemiol Ment Health*. 2005;1:18.

114. Ornish D, Brown SE, Scherwitz LW, et al. Can lifestyle changes reverse coronary heart disease? The Lifestyle Heart Trial. *Lancet*. 1990;336(8708):129–33.

115. Ornish D, Scherwitz LW, Billings JH, et al. Intensive lifestyle changes for reversal of coronary heart disease. *JAMA*. 1998;280(23):2001–7.

116. Orth-Gomer K, Unden AL, Edwards ME. Social isolation and mortality in ischemic heart disease. A 10-year follow-up study of 150 middle-aged men. *Acta Med Scand*. 1988;224(3):205–15.

117. Peyrot M, Rubin RR. Levels and risks of depression and anxiety symptomatology among diabetic adults. *Diabetes Care*. 1997;20(4):585–90.

118. Pieper C, LaCroix AZ, Karasek RA. The relation of psychosocial dimensions of work with coronary heart disease risk factors: a meta-analysis of five United States data bases. *Am J Epidemiol*. 1989;129(3):483–94.

119. Radloff LS. The CES-D Scale: a self-report depressive scale for research in the general population. *J Appl Psychol Meas*. 1977;1:385–401.

120. Rahe RH, Romo M, Bennett L, Siltanen P. Recent life changes, myocardial infarction, and abrupt coronary death. Studies in Helsinki. *Arch Intern Med*. 1974;133(2):221–8.

121. Ramasubbu R. Relationship between depression and cerebrovascular disease: conceptual issues. *J Affect Disord*. 2000;57(1–3):1–11.

122. Regier DA, Farmer ME, Rae DS, et al. Comorbidity of mental disorders with alcohol and other drug abuse. Results from the Epidemiologic Catchment Area (ECA) Study. *JAMA*. 1990;264(19):2511–8.

123. Resnicow K, Davis R, Rollnick S. Motivational interviewing for pediatric obesity: Conceptual issues and evidence review. *J Am Diet Assoc*. 2006;106(12):2024–33.

124. Rietveld S, Everaerd W, Creer TL. Stress-induced asthma: a review of research and potential mechanisms. *Clin Exp Allergy*. 2000;30(8):1058–66.

125. Robinson N, Fuller JH. Role of life events and difficulties in the onset of diabetes mellitus. *J Psychosom Res*. 1985;29(6):583–91.

126. Roger VL, Go AS, Lloyd-Jones DM, et al. Heart disease and stroke statistics—2012 update: a report from the American Heart Association. *Circulation*. 2012;125(1):e2–220.

127. Rose C, Wallace L, Dickson R, et al. The most effective psychologically-based treatments to reduce anxiety and panic in patients with chronic obstructive pulmonary disease (COPD): a systematic review. *Patient Educ Couns*. 2002;47(4):311–8.

128. Rozanski A, Bairey CN, Krantz DS, et al. Mental stress and the induction of silent myocardial ischemia in patients with coronary artery disease. *N Engl J Med*. 1988;318(16):1005–12.

129. Rozanski A, Blumenthal JA, Kaplan J. Impact of psychological factors on the pathogenesis of cardiovascular disease and implications for therapy. *Circulation*. 1999;99(16):2192–217.

130. Rubak S, Sandbaek A, Lauritzen T, Christensen B. Motivational interviewing: a systematic review and meta-analysis. *Br J Gen Pract*. 2005;55(513):305–12.

131. Russek LG, King SH, Russek SJ, Russek HI. The Harvard Mastery of Stress Study 35-year follow-up: prognostic significance of patterns of psychophysiological arousal and adaptation. *Psychosom Med*. 1990;52(3):271–85.

132. Rutledge T, Reis VA, Linke SE, Greenberg BH, Mills PJ. Depression in heart failure a meta-analytic review of prevalence, intervention effects, and associations with clinical outcomes. *J Am Coll Cardiol*. 2006;48(8):1527–37.

133. Salmon P. Effects of physical exercise on anxiety, depression, and sensitivity to stress: a unifying theory. *Clin Psychol Rev*. 2001;21(1):33–61.

134. Sandhu HS. Psychosocial issues in chronic obstructive pulmonary disease. *Clin Chest Med*. 1986;7(4):629–42.

135. Satta A. Exercise training in asthma. *J Sports Med Phys Fitness*. 2000;40(4):277–83.

136. Scales R, Lueker RD, Atterbom HA. Motivational interviewing and skills-based counseling to change multiple lifestyle behaviors [abstract]. *Ann Behav Med*. 1998;22D:68.

137. Siegrist J, Peter R, Junge A, Cremer P, Seidel D. Low status control, high effort at work and ischemic heart disease: prospective evidence from blue-collar men. *Soc Sci Med*. 1990;31(10):1127–34.

138. Sothmann MS, Hart BA, Horn TS. Plasma catecholamine response to acute psychological stress in humans: relation to aerobic fitness and exercise training. *Med Sci Sports Exerc*. 1991;23(7):860–7.

139. Strike PC, Perkins-Porras L, Whitehead DL, McEwan J, Steptoe A. Triggering of acute coronary syndromes by physical exertion and anger: clinical and sociodemographic characteristics. *Heart.* 2006;92(8):1035–40.

140. Surwit RS, Schneider MS, Feinglos MN. Stress and diabetes mellitus. *Diabetes Care.* 1992;15(10):1413–22.

141. Suzuki S, Sakamoto S, Miki T, Matsuo T. Hanshin-Awaji earthquake and acute myocardial infarction. *Lancet.* 1995;345(8955):981.

142. Thomas M, Bruton A, Moffat M, Cleland J. Asthma and psychological dysfunction. *Prim Care Respir J.* 2011;20(3):250–6.

143. *Trends in COPD (Chronic Bronchitis and Emphysema): Morbidity and Mortality* [Internet]. Washington, DC: American Lung Association, Epidemiology and Statistics Unit Research and Program Services Division; 2011 [cited 2012 Apr 11]. 28 p. Available from: http://www.lungusa.org/finding-cures/our-research/trend-reports/copd-trend-report.pdf

144. Trichopoulos D, Katsouyanni K, Zavitsanos X, Tzonou A, Dalla-Vorgia P. Psychological stress and fatal heart attack: the Athens (1981) earthquake natural experiment. *Lancet.* 1983;1(8322):441–4.

145. U.S. Department of Health and Human Services, Centers for Disease Control and Prevention, National Center for Chronic Disease Prevention and Health Promotion, The President's Council on Physical Fitness and Sports. *Physical Activity and Health: A Report of the Surgeon General.* Atlanta, GA: President's Council on Physical Fitness and Sports; 1996. 278 p.

146. Uchino BN, Cacioppo JT, Kiecolt-Glaser JK. The relationship between social support and physiological processes: a review with emphasis on underlying mechanisms and implications for health. *Psychol Bull.* 1996;119(3):488–531.

147. United States, Office of Public Health and Science, United States, Office of Disease Prevention and Health Promotion. *Healthy People 2010 Objectives: Draft for Public Comment.* Washington, DC: U.S. Department of Health and Human Services, Office of Public Health and Science: For sale by the U.S. G.P.O., Supt. of Docs; 1998.

148. United States, Public Health Service, Office of the Surgeon General, Center for Mental Health Services (U.S.), National Institute of Mental Health (U.S.). *Mental Health: A Report of the Surgeon General.* Rockville, MD: U.S. Department of Health and Human Services, U.S. Public Health Service; For sale by the Supt. of Docs; 1999. 487 p.

149. Vaccarino V, Kasl SV, Abramson J, Krumholz HM. Depressive symptoms and risk of functional decline and death in patients with heart failure. *J Am Coll Cardiol.* 2001;38(1):199–205.

150. Van Dorsten B. The use of motivational interviewing in weight loss. *Curr Diab Rep.* 2007;7(5):386–90.

151. VanWormer JJ, Boucher JL. Motivational interviewing and diet modification: a review of the evidence. *Diabetes Educ.* 2004;30(3):404,406, 408–10, 414–6 passim.

152. Veith RC, Lewis N, Linares OA, et al. Sympathetic nervous system activity in major depression. Basal and desipramine-induced alterations in plasma norepinephrine kinetics. *Arch Gen Psychiatry.* 1994;51(5):411–22.

153. Verrier RL, Dickerson LW. Autonomic nervous system and coronary blood flow changes related to emotional activation and sleep. *Circulation.* 1991;83(4 Suppl):II81–9.

154. Verrill D, Barton C, Beasley W, Lippard WM. The effects of short-term and long-term pulmonary rehabilitation on functional capacity, perceived dyspnea, and quality of life. *Chest.* 2005;128(2):673–83.

155. Westlake C, Dracup K, Fonarow G, Hamilton M. Depression in patients with heart failure. *J Card Fail.* 2005;11(1):30–5.

156. Williams LS, Kroenke K, Bakas T, et al. Care management of post-stroke depression: a randomized, controlled trial. *Stroke.* 2007;38(3):998–1003.

157. Williams RB, Barefoot JC, Califf RM, et al. Prognostic importance of social and economic resources among medically treated patients with angiographically documented coronary artery disease. *JAMA.* 1992;267(4):520–4.

158. Willich SN, Lowel H, Lewis M, Hormann A, Arntz HR, Keil U. Weekly variation of acute myocardial infarction. Increased Monday risk in the working population. *Circulation.* 1994;90(1):87–93.

159. Witte DR, Bots ML, Hoes AW, Grobbee DE. Cardiovascular mortality in Dutch men during 1996 European football championship: longitudinal population study. *BMJ.* 2000;321(7276):1552–4.

160. Yeung AC, Vekshtein VI, Krantz DS, et al. The effect of atherosclerosis on the vasomotor response of coronary arteries to mental stress. *N Engl J Med.* 1991;325(22):1551–6.

SELECTED REFERENCES FOR FURTHER READING

Kneebone I, Dunmore E. Psychological management of post-stroke depression. *Br J Clin Psychol.* 2000;39:53–65.

Opolski M, Wilson M. Asthma and depression: a pragmatic review of the literature and recommendations for future research. *Clin Pract Epidemiol Ment Health.* 2005;1:1–7.

Rutledge T, Reis VA, Linke SE, et al. Depression in heart failure: a meta-analytic review of prevalence, intervention effects, and associations with clinical outcomes. *J Am Coll Cardiol.* 2006;48:1527–37.

Smith TW, Kendall P, Keefe F, editors. Behavioral medicine and clinical health psychology. *J Consult Clin Psychol* [special issue]. 2002;70:459–856.

INTERNET RESOURCES

- Cognitive Behavior Therapy: http://www.cognitive-behavior-therapy.org
- Mental Health: A Report of the Surgeon General: http://www.surgeongeneral.gov/library/mentalhealth/home.html
- Motivational Interviewing: http://www.motivationalinterviewing.org

Assessment of Psychosocial Status

This chapter focuses on assessment and treatment of common psychosocial and psychological correlates of cardiovascular disease (CVD), stroke, chronic obstructive pulmonary disease (COPD), and metabolic disease (obesity and diabetes), with an emphasis on **stress**, **anxiety**, and **depression** (SAD).

The development of behaviorally based management and prevention strategies for chronic disease is becoming an urgent priority, not only for health care providers, but as a matter of social and economic policy as well. The costs associated with health care are already staggering and will continue to increase in the coming years, fueled

KEY TERMS

Anxiety: Distressful emotional state marked by excessive anticipatory worry and tension.

Cognitive behavior therapy (CBT): A widely practiced, empirically validated method for treating common psychological disorders, including anxiety and depression. CBT focuses on helping patients become aware of how thoughts influence feelings and behavior and how dysfunctional thoughts become linked to anxiety and depression. *Cognitive restructuring* is the general term used to describe CBT techniques designed to lessen the grip of maladaptive thought patterns on emotional states. CBT is strongly influenced both by behavior therapy and social cognitive theory.

Depression: A pervasive, enduring mood characterized by a low self-esteem, low energy, physical lethargy, and emotional distress. Isolated episodes of a depressed mood are common; when frequent or prolonged, they may signify major depressive disorder, a *DSM-IV-TR* subcategory of the mood disorders.

Diagnostic and Statistical Manual of Mental Disorders, Fourth Edition (DSM-IV): The current standard for psychiatric diagnosis, published by the American Psychiatric Association (APA) in 1994 and used by virtually all mental health professionals. A text revision (*DSM-IV-TR*) published in 2000 updated background information but did not alter diagnostic criteria (12,13).

Mindfulness: Mindfulness, a term originally derived from Buddhist philosophy, is defined as nonjudgmental awareness of the present-moment experience (154). Behavioral medicine interventions have been

developed based on principles of mindfulness meditation, and a growing body of research has demonstrated their beneficial effects on a variety of physical and psychological conditions.

Mood disorder: A diagnostic term in the *DSM-IV-TR* denoting a group of psychological disorders marked by disruption of normal mood (prevailing emotional tone) and affect (fluctuating emotional state). The most common mood disorders are major depressive disorder, bipolar disorder, dysthymic disorder, and cyclothymic disorder.

Perceived self-efficacy (PSE): The self-assessment of one's capabilities to perform or regulate behavior, based in Bandura's social cognitive theory. Perceived self-efficacy is the most influential psychological variable on a range of health and wellness behaviors.

Psychological disorder: A general term in the *DSM-IV-TR* used to denote a state of maladjustment marked by (a) subjective distress and/or (b) functional impairment in activities of daily life. One or both of these criteria must be met, in addition to the criteria for specific disorders, in order for a person to be diagnosed with a psychological or mental disorder.

Social cognitive/social learning theory: Fundamental theories of behavior by Bandura that emphasize the role of social mediating factors on psychological development and learning.

Stress: The subjective experience of feeling overloaded or overwhelmed that results when personal resources (psychological or otherwise) are insufficient to meet existing challenges of daily life.

by our historic allegiance to end-state or tertiary models of medical care, an aging population, and spiraling costs of surgical, pharmacologic, and increasingly sophisticated technologic interventions (49). There is also an urgent need for prevention and long-term management strategies, especially for those diseases that are strongly correlated with lifestyle behavior patterns and that are the focus of this chapter: CVD, stroke, COPD, obesity, and diabetes. Extensive research conducted in behavioral medicine and health psychology has documented the influence of psychological and social factors on illness, health, and well-being. The underlying model driving much of this research emphasizes the contributions of biological, psychological, and social influences on health and illness and is referred to as the biopsychosocial model (102).

All health care professionals need to be familiar with ways in which biological, social, and psychological factors interact, producing illness, the cultural context of disease. The purpose of this chapter is to provide exercise professionals with an overview of clinical assessment and intervention strategies for three common forms of emotional distress, originally highlighted in the 1999 U.S. Surgeon General's Report on Mental Health, and which continue to be of widespread concern in contemporary society: stress, anxiety, and depression, designated by the acronym "SAD." Significant distress may warrant a formal psychological clinical assessment, and it is useful to know some basic diagnostic nomenclature related to common psychological disorders, especially those involving anxiety and depression. It is also important to have a working knowledge of empirically validated interventions that have been developed to treat both clinically significant and subclinical manifestations of emotional distress.

This knowledge can be helpful in three ways. First, exercise professionals need to have a basic understanding of how SAD affect physical capabilities related to exercise testing and programming, both at a general level and in the context of specific disease. Knowing how to make appropriate adjustments or accommodations in designing exercise programs and determining how best to teach and motivate clients who are anxious, depressed, or highly stressed is important. Individualizing exercise protocols is significant. Second, and perhaps more significant, exercise professionals need to be familiar with research documenting the positive effects of physical activity (*Table 17-1*) on SAD and be able to apply this knowledge effectively with individual clients of increasingly diverse medical, social, and cultural backgrounds. In the case of patients diagnosed with anxiety or mood disorders, the latter being an umbrella term that encompasses depression, the exercise professional may be able to forge a collaboration with mental health professionals responsible for primary treatment of the disorder, in much the same way that productive working alliances

TABLE 17-1. Benefits of Physical Activity

Self-administration
Social acceptability
Decreased physical health risks
Ancillary strength and conditioning benefits
Convenience
Low cost
Minimal side effects

Adapted from Buckworth J, Dishman RK. *Exercise Psychology*. Champaign (IL): Human Kinetics; 2002. p. 13.

are often formed with physicians treating patients for heart disease, hypertension, or diabetes. This process can aid in tailoring general exercise guidelines (122) to the needs of specific individuals.

Physical activity is important as a form of complementary health for both medically and psychologically based conditions. With regard to the latter, both cost and social stigma inhibit many people from seeking treatment. For such individuals, being physically active can do much to reduce emotional distress in a cost-effective manner.

Finally, knowledge about psychological conditions and how emotional distress is affected by common diseases is essential information. This knowledge may help the exercise professional determine when consultation with mental health professionals may be warranted for clients whose medical management and exercise programming appear to be compromised. Working in a broad biopsychosocial framework is believed to counteract the common tendency to become overly focused on the physical aspects of medical conditions.

This chapter begins by addressing common assessment procedures to clarify emotional distress patterns and determine whether formal clinical diagnoses are warranted. The next section focuses on a discussion of contemporary intervention models used to treat both clinical and subclinical manifestations of emotional distress. The final section of this chapter considers the implications of emotional distress in the context of four specific medical conditions: CVD, stroke, COPD, and the most common metabolic disorders: diabetes, obesity, and the metabolic syndrome (MS).

SURGEON GENERAL'S MENTAL HEALTH REPORT: LIFE STRESS, ANXIETY, DEPRESSION

The 1999 Surgeon General's report provided a detailed overview of mental health issues in the United States just before the millennium (282). Based on a public health perspective, this report emphasized the need not only for epidemiologic monitoring and access to clinical mental health services but health promotion and disease prevention initiatives as well. The report cited statistics underscoring the debilitating nature of mental disorders, which, at the time, ranked second only to CVD in terms of years lost to premature death and disability. The corresponding economic costs associated with mental illnesses are substantial and have been documented elsewhere (186). The report defined mental health as ". . . the successful performance of mental function resulting in productive activities, fulfilling relationships with other people, and the ability to adapt to change and to cope with adversity" (282). The report also described a continuum linking mental health and mental illness, using language compatible with the *Diagnostic and Statistical Manual of Mental Disorders, Fourth Edition, Text Revision (DSM-IV-TR)* diagnostic system for diagnosing mental disorders, in addition to subclinical manifestations of distress not meeting formal diagnostic criteria. Finally, this report advocated a unified view of mind and body compatible with the biopsychosocial perspective described earlier (102) as a way of broadening the perspective on health and medical care and reducing the social stigma attached to mental distress. This finding is the most significant aspect of the report because it clearly supports the use of empirically validated psychosocial interventions in the context of treating known medical conditions. Both before and following publication of the Surgeon General's report, this integrative mind/body perspective has gradually been supplanting the historic, dichotomous view of mind and body as separate entities (151).

The Surgeon General's report was followed 2 yr later by a report focusing on mental health needs in the context of cultural diversity (283). There are widely acknowledged disparities in health care services, delivery, and utilization. This report, although not as widely publicized as its predecessor, warrants careful attention in terms of the health and medical needs of clients from diversified cultural and racial backgrounds. Both reports have played an important role in stimulating thinking and research about how best to meet the psychological health needs of an increasingly diversified population.

THE BACKGROUND OF HEALTH PSYCHOLOGY AND BEHAVIORAL MEDICINE

Extensive research and clinical work in health psychology and behavioral medicine echo the sentiments of the Surgeon General's report. Three key principles in particular reflect an emerging consensus concerning the nature and maintenance of mental health: first, that mind and body interact reciprocally; second, that participatory health care is superseding medical disease management; and third, that the immune system serves as a critical point of integration between mind and body. The first principle concerns the reciprocal interaction between mental and physical health, a cornerstone not only of

contemporary mental health practices (245), but also of research on the interconnections between personality (115) and exercise (203) and health. Of interest in this regard is a comment in the introduction to *DSM-IV* that the term *mental disorder* suggests an unfortunate distinction "that is a reductionistic anachronism of mind/body dualism" (12). It is also worth noting that the American College of Sports Medicine (ACSM) subsequently released a consensus statement aimed at physicians that advocated an integrative perspective on the care of athletes (143). This statement noted that physical injuries often have significant psychological sequelae and emphasized that psychological factors are related to injury vulnerability and rehabilitation outcomes.

Infectious diseases no longer pose the greatest threats to health, as they did in the late 19th and much of the 20th century (104,116). Today, lifestyle factors result in chronic cardiovascular and metabolic diseases, which, along with cancer, are among the leading causes of mortality. As a result, lifestyle modifications and management of psychosocial factors are achieving parity with medical management of most chronic illnesses and offer enormous physical, psychological, and economic benefits to help prevent these conditions from developing in the first place. However, convincing people to take an active stance regarding health maintenance and disease management/prevention has proven to be a significant challenge. One reason is that the concept of health itself has traditionally been defined as the absence of disease, a rather impoverished concept that does not offer any positive attributes to be cultivated in a proactive manner. Fortunately, contemporary formulations of health have expanded this early definition to include social and psychological factors that can be cultivated and contribute to an overall sense of well-being (185). A second factor acting against the proactive adoption of health behaviors concerns behavioral passivity, reflected, for example, in chronically low rates of regular physical activity (58) and, more generally, poor compliance with health care recommendations aimed at improving overall health (92,195).

There is substantial evidence that health promotion and a capacity for self-regulation are interrelated, much of it based on the research of psychologist Albert Bandura, a prominent figure in the area of social learning theory (32) and social cognitive theory (31). According to Bandura, self-regulation is a key factor not only in managing existing medical conditions but in disease prevention as well. Models of self-regulation entail three components: (a) monitoring health behavior, (b) goal setting, and (c) proactive enlistment of social and other resources to foster goal attainment (28). A discussion of the role of self-regulation and a related psychological characteristic, self-efficacy, will be presented later in this chapter. It is important to remember that intervention strategies based on social cognitive principles can be very effective in helping overcome behavioral passivity. Social cognitive theory underlies virtually all current intervention models in health psychology and behavioral medicine.

The third principle in contemporary health research concerns the critical role of research on ways the immune system influences mind/body interactions (76). Psychoneuroimmunology, the study of brain, immune system, and behavior interactions (183,296), emerged in research by Ader and Cohen (4) and documents ways in which the immune and nervous systems interact to affect emotions, behavior, and cognitive (thought) processes. Stress affects the immune system via the hypothalamic-pituitary-adrenal (HPA) axis (199,243) and accounts for the well-known observation that periods of high stress heighten susceptibility to illness. Social factors play a key role in mediating the effects of stress, either positively or negatively, as documented in extensive research by Cohen, Kiecolt-Glazer, and others (76,160). Other research in this area has documented the impact of immune system activity on mood states via production of cytokines as part of a restorative system that promotes an adaptive sort of depression associated with heart disease and athletic overtraining (182). Collectively, research in the area of psychoneuroimmunology has established a solid foundation for clinical health care practice that incorporates a range of psychosocial interventions, in addition to primary medical care.

The 1999 Surgeon General's report on mental health articulated a clear need for clinical services and resources to address a major health issue with psychological, social, and economic implications. Much still needs to be done to meet these needs. As noted in the *Healthy People 2010, Midcourse Review* (284), in the area of mental health and mental disorders, only 1 of 14 goals had been met or exceeded. In addition to traditional clinical services, more and better quality research (203) is needed to further document the impact of physical activity as an effective intervention for both clinically significant and subclinical conditions and ease the burden of delivering mental health services. Greater attention to disparities affecting access to health, wellness, and medical care is urgently needed, as is updated research pertaining to correlates of physical activity (277) to assist in the delivery of individually oriented, widely disseminated mental health resources. In the remainder of this chapter, the focus is on three key aspects of distress identified in the Surgeon General's report as affecting a significant percentage of the population, in terms of either diagnosable psychological disorders or subclinical patterns of distress: SAD.

ASSESSMENT OF SOCIAL INFLUENCES ON EMOTIONAL DISTRESS

People experience significant fluctuations in both negative and positive emotions as a function of interpersonal influences. Extensive research has revealed that social influences can markedly affect psychological stress in either positive or negative ways. For example, researchers have demonstrated that the immune system interacts with the central nervous system (CNS), which is the conduit through which social and other environmental stimuli are processed (4,160,243). Social support can help strengthen immune system responses, reduce stress reactivity, and help mitigate the impact of CVD, AIDS, COPD, cancer, and other challenging illnesses (4,76,160,243,279). Social support has been identified as a key variable affecting the onset, course, and outcome of heart disease (255), and it has been found to affect the immune system and metabolic conditions as well (280). Social relationships influence local immune inflammatory responses related to disease progression and aging (159). Virtually, all conceptual models of healthy psychological adjustment (*e.g.*, social cognitive theory) (27) and emotional adaptation (169), as well as systems of psychotherapy, incorporate social/interpersonal influences as an essential component.

The implications of the social/interpersonal influences for all health care providers are clear. First, it is important to be aware of, and sensitive to, the social context of health care services delivery. Interpersonal aspects of interactions between patients and professionals have a significant impact on the initiation, cultivation, and maintenance of health care practice. Second, social influences outside the immediate context of health care systems exert a powerful influence on health and psychological well-being. Finally, even though psychological, like medical, diagnoses are applied to the individual they should be viewed in a broader context that includes interpersonal and social influences. In fact, as noted later in the discussion of clinical diagnosis, the *DSM-IV* diagnostic system includes a provision for rating the severity of psychosocial stressors that may affect the onset, course, and outcome of various disorders.

The field of psychological assessment has a long history that can be traced at least back to research on individual differences in mental abilities by Sir Francis Galton in England in the mid-19th century. Subsequently, Freudian psychodynamic psychology stimulated interest in hypothetical unconscious forces believed to influence much of conscious behavior. This interest led to the development of projective tests that were believed capable of clarifying nonconscious drives and motives and found favor in early clinical assessments. Research on personality traits (relatively enduring predispositions) emerged in the mid-20th century, stimulated by the work of Allport (9), who analyzed and grouped thousands of terms in the English language into core dimensions or factors to describe individual differences. At present, the predominant model of personality structure with broadest clinical application is the five-factor model of McCrae et al., which is rooted in Allport's earlier work

TABLE 17-2. Five Factor Model of Personality

Factor 1:	Neuroticism	Worry, anxiety prone
Factor 2:	Extraversion	Socially outgoing, gregarious
Factor 3:	Openness	Nondefensive, inquisitive
Factor 4:	Agreeableness	Socially oriented
Factor 5:	Conscientiousness	Dependable, reliable

Reprinted with permission from Costa PT, McCrae RR. Personality assessment in psychosomatic medicine. *Adv Psychosom Med.* 1987;17:71–82.

(81,189). The five-factor model (outlined in *Table 17-2*), using the statistical technique of factor analysis, has identified dimensions that appear to reflect common, fundamental characteristics that are relatively enduring in nature. This model has been used extensively in personality research in various contexts, including health and physical activity (233).

In behavioral medicine, interest in personality traits and medical conditions was initially high (116) and continues to attract interest (176). Perhaps best known in this regard is research on the type A personality pattern originally identified by Friedman and Rosenman (117) as predictive of heart disease. The original conception of the type A individual hypothesized that disease risk was due to a combination of impatience, low frustration tolerance, a fast-paced lifestyle, and poorly modulated anger. Anger and hostility have also been identified as key disease risk factors (34), a finding that has since been found to be of moderate predictive use in clinical applications. Subsequent research suggests that the relationship between personality and disease is highly complex, with multiple causal pathways at work in the development of medical problems (115). On the positive side, research by Antonovsky and others has focused on identifying personality traits associated with health, rather than illness. The salutogenic model of health developed by Antonovsky (18) focuses on a trait termed *sense of coherence* (17) to explain the capacity of some individuals to remain physically and psychologically healthy despite exposure to chronically stressful circumstances.

Collectively, much of the research on personality and psychological trait factors, especially in the early years, focused on internal processes hypothesized to influence overt behavior. This research evolved independently of behavioral psychology, which emphasized the influence of external forces on behavior. This artificial dichotomy has gradually been bridged in contemporary psychology, beginning with Mischel's person by situation interactionist model of personality (200,201). Assessments conducted by clinical and health psychologists use a wide range of both trait and state measures, although the latter tend to predominate in health care settings where the emphasis is on relatively rapid assessment and circumscribed treatment of what is often transient psychological distress. Most clinics have neither time nor resources to conduct extensive assessments required to diagnose disorders rooted in personality patterns, nor are they equipped to offer the sort of long-term treatment that these conditions tend to necessitate.

SAD are examples of state-like conditions that are the focus of considerable contemporary clinical interest. Recent epidemiologic data suggest that mood and anxiety disorders are highly prevalent, along with substance-use disorders (157), cutting across cultural and racial boundaries (246). It is important to have a practical understanding of each condition, as well as knowledge about how depression and anxiety are related to other mental and medical disorders.

PSYCHOSOCIAL MODELS OF HEALTH BEHAVIOR

The gradual merging of research on personality traits and emotional states that emphasized the influence of social and other environmental influences eventually led to the formulation of behaviorally based models that combined the influence of both groups of factors. As previously noted, a key figure in this evolution was Albert Bandura, whose (29) formulation of social learning theory (32) and social cognitive theory (31) both emphasize the reciprocal interaction among cognitive processes, social influences, and behavioral inclinations. Bandura's research focused on how many behavioral responses are learned simply via observation and served as a critical bridge between early behavioral and current cognitive formulations of behavior acquisition and modifications that emphasize the influence of social mediators. He is best known for the concept of perceived self-efficacy (PSE), which refers to one's perception of having the necessary capabilities to learn and navigate the many challenges of daily life (30). Social cognitive theory is perhaps the most influential contemporary model of health behavior, and self-efficacy is the most widely researched and extensively validated variable in clinical health research.

There are other influential models of socially based health behavior as well, including the theory of reasoned action (105) and a closely related variant, the theory of planned behavior (6). The theory of reasoned action posited that the *intention* to perform a behavior is of primary importance in determining health behavior. The theory of planned behavior adds the dimension of "perceived control" as an additional influential factor. Subsequent research using both models has found them to be of varying utility in predicting patterns of health behavior adoption (45).

In addition, the transtheoretical model (TTM) is a highly influential model of health behavior (224). TTM is an overarching, integrative model of health behavior interventions that incorporates many different intervention techniques and conceptual approaches into a longitudinal approach that takes into account stages of readiness for change with respect to physical activity and other health behaviors. There are five stages: (a) precontemplation, (b) contemplation, (c) preparation, (d) action, and (e) maintenance. A key feature of this model is that it proposes a progressive shift from verbal strategies (*i.e.*, education, motivational) to behaviorally based therapies (such as selective reinforcement), controlling environmental stimuli with each succeeding stage, although both types of strategies may be concurrently implemented (95). State-wise progression is mediated by a cognitively based process termed decisional balance, which evaluates positive and negative aspects of the associated changes. Progression from one stage to another is typically not linear but rather marked by a series of advances and declines (225). Originally developed as model to guide therapy for eliminating negative health behaviors such as smoking, drug use, and risky sexual practices (226), the TTM has more recently been applied to cultivating positive behaviors as well, including exercise, where it appears to be moderately effective (263).

IMPLICATIONS FOR CLINICAL ASSESSMENT

Emotional distress can vary considerably in intensity and persistence. Emotional ups and downs are normal; what sets them apart from psychological disorders is the level of associated subjective distress. Intensity, duration, and functional impairment should all be assessed to determine the significance of negative emotional states. The health advantages of balanced, positive emotions are well documented and appear to comprise a biologically based dimension of psychological "resilience" that favorably impacts not only physiological and immune functions but patterns of social engagement as well (270).

Measures of psychological and emotional states can be rated on dimensional scales that assess intensity and pervasiveness. A variety of scales have been developed, primarily for use in clinical research, to assess depression, anxiety, stress, anger, and many other emotional characteristics linked to emotional distress. However, such scales do not provide a sufficient basis for clinical diagnosis, which involves a formal evaluative process conducted by a mental health professional. From a medical perspective, the purpose of diagnosis is to identify the underlying cause(s) of symptoms and specify treatment. Diagnosing psychological disorders serves a similar purpose, although it is seldom possible to isolate a specific cause because psychological disorders involve multiple contributory factors consistent with the biopsychosocial model. As a result, interventions frequently

entail multiple components as well. For example, the diagnosis of depression, a mood disorder, might involve a coordinated treatment plan involving psychotherapy, antidepressant medication, and exercise.

Whereas clinical research scales used to assess emotional states tend to be dimensional in nature, the *DSM-IV* is categorically based. It was developed by the American Psychiatric Association and is compatible with the International Classification of Diseases (ICD) system, published by the World Health Organization. The *DSM-IV* is strongly oriented toward an epidemiologic/disease model, employing standardized, symptom-based diagnostic criteria for each psychological disorder. The *DSM-IV* is multiaxial, comprising five independent dimensions or axes (*Table 17-3*). Axes I and II focus on psychological diagnoses, and Axis III identifies any health-related problems or conditions. Axis IV addresses psychosocial and environmental factors contributing to diagnosis. Axis V assesses functional capabilities and resultant *prognosis* (*i.e.*, anticipated outcome), based on an evaluation of psychosocial stressors evident at the time of diagnosis. A rating scale, the Global Assessment of Functioning (GAF), is used for this purpose.

The *DSM-IV* is currently the most widely used clinical standard for diagnosing mental disorders, although

TABLE 17-3. *DSM-IV* Axes

Axis I	• Contains the majority of mental disorders, having a clear-cut onset and course (*e.g.*, mood, substance abuse, anxiety disorders) • Multiple diagnoses are common, with high comorbidity of mood and anxiety disorders (158)
Axis II	• Pervasive, long-standing conditions (*e.g.*, personality disorders) • Personality disorders include acute maladaptive reactions and stable patterns of maladjustment that solidify with age (73) • Frequently co-occur with Axis I disorders (131)
Axis III	• Medical conditions contributing to onset, course, or outcome of a mental disorder • Based on International Classification of Disease (ICD) system
Axis IV	• Psychosocial and environmental factors contributing to diagnosis • Includes problems with social support, educational, occupation, or economic factors
Axis V	• Clinician's rating of overall adjustment • Used to help plan treatment and assess prognosis • Uses Global Assessment of Functioning (GAF) scale, a 100-point measure ranging from seriously impaired functioning (*e.g.*, persistent risk of harming self or others; unable to care for self) to highly adaptive behavior

DSM-IV, *Diagnostic and Statistical Manual of Mental Disorders, Fourth Edition.*

Adapted from American Psychiatric Association. *Diagnostic and Statistical Manual of Mental Disorders.* 4th ed. Text Revision. Washington (DC): American Psychiatric Association; 2000.

it is not without critics (43,106). The diagnosis of mental disorders requires evidence of an established percentage of symptoms relative to the total, which constitutes a diagnostic threshold, below which the term *subclinical* is often used. In addition, to qualify as a mental disorder, symptoms must be present for time periods that vary with specific disorders. Clarifying periods help differentiate, for example, transient periods of depressed mood or anxiety that everyone experiences from more enduring periods of emotional distress that do not spontaneously resolve. Currently, a revision of the *DSM-IV* is underway, with a planned release date of 2013. The new version will incorporate evolving scientific understanding of psychological disorders and improve the utility of the diagnostic system. Proposed changes include the addition of new diagnoses, alteration of existing diagnostic criteria, changes to the current multiaxial structure, and incorporation of dimensional assessment to complement categorical information. Information about proposed changes can be accessed at http://www.dsm5.org (82).

DSM-IV–based diagnoses typically draw on multiple sources of information and may include data from clinical interviews, questionnaires to assess state and/or personality factors, case history material, collateral reports, and other sources. The use of multiple sources of information aids the process of cross-validating clinical impressions by avoiding excessive reliance on any single type of data. Thus, although questionnaires used to assess depression or anxiety may provide useful information, they are not sufficient to diagnose psychological disorders in either category.

Exercise professionals are likely to work with individuals experiencing emotional distress, both at the level of subclinical intensity and with psychological disorders based on *DSM-IV* criteria. An understanding of common forms of distress and related psychological disorders, especially anxiety and depression, and the ways each of these affect behavior, cognitive processes, and emotional states is increasingly important owing to the widespread prevalence of these conditions. For years, anxiety and depression-related disorders, along with substance-use disorders, have been, and continue to be, the most prominent areas of clinical practice and research (37).

DEPRESSION

The key feature of depression is a negative emotional state marked by feelings of sadness and unhappiness, often accompanied by self-criticism and low self-esteem. Depressive spectrum disorders, collectively referred to as mood disorders in *DSM-IV*, are among the most common mental disorders, affecting approximately 10% of the population (157). Depressive spectrum disorders, along with bipolar disorder, a condition marked by mood swings ranging from depression to mania, extract

a significant toll on work productivity (156) and social engagement (145). Depression is also linked to several chronic illnesses, including heart disease (14,216), and tends to have adverse effects on spouses and others who potentially could serve as sources of social support (70,262). People who are depressed typically experience a loss of physical and mental energy needed to handle everyday situations and often present as lethargic or tired. A related term, *melancholia*, describes a pattern of such chronic and pervasive sadness that it appears to be almost "characterological" in nature. The concept of depression is intimately related to loss, bringing to mind states of grief or bereavement that would occur naturally in the context of, for example, the death of a loved one or the reaction to a catastrophic natural disaster, such as Hurricane Katrina. But such events are seldom at the root of sustained clinical depression, for which concepts such as loss or the perception of declining capabilities has more to do with negative self-appraisals, a pessimistic view of the world, and feelings of helplessness and hopelessness about the future. People who are depressed find that it blunts other emotional reactions, including bereavement (125). Psychiatrist Aaron Beck termed this the *cognitive triad of depression*, a central concept in cognitive therapy for depression and other emotional disorders first formulated in the 1960s. This theory has undergone progressive evolution (41,42,72) to the point to which it is the most widely used, empirically validated clinical practice model. Persistence and severity of symptoms form the basis for diagnosing an actual disorder as opposed to a subclinical state. In addition to heightened risk of suicide, depression is accompanied by significant health risks for heart disease (14,64) and other chronic health impairments.

Other early and influential models of depression by Seligman and Lewinsohn emphasized, respectively, the importance of powerlessness, termed *learned helplessness*, and withdrawal from sources of behavioral reinforcement as important psychological contributors to depression (175,251,278). These models all converge in their emphasis on the importance of social factors with respect to onset, course, and amelioration of depressive symptoms. A review of the literature on social functioning in depression (145) described it as a prominent feature of depression and noted that neither pharmacologic nor psychological interventions effective in relieving cognitive and physical impairments necessarily restore social functioning to predepression levels.

Biological theories of depression have emphasized the role of neurotransmitter deficiencies, in particular biogenic amines, as a key contributory factor. Norepinephrine and serotonin are brain neurotransmitters that are the principal target of pharmacologic interventions to increase their activity level. Initially employing tricyclic antidepressants and later monoamine oxidase inhibitors (MAOIs), contemporary pharmacologic interventions for depression now favor selective serotonin reuptake inhibitors (SSRIs) for routine cases (125). There is also evidence associating depression with dysregulation of the HPA axis, a key mediator of stress reactivity (199).

An important relative of depression in medical and athletic settings involves intense fatigue and mental exhaustion. Appels (20) devised a measure of vital exhaustion (the Maastricht Questionnaire) that was found to predict myocardial infarction (MI) in patients with heart disease (163). Similarly, athletic overtraining involves symptoms of depression, especially chronic fatigue, along with performance decrements and other impairments collectively labeled the *overtraining syndrome* (23,174), which involves dysregulation of the HPA stress reactivity system (191). An intriguing explanation for this syndrome has been offered by Nesse, who views depression as an adaptive response to overexertion that promotes energy conservation and restoration (205). Interesting support for this hypothesis comes from studies suggesting that production of cytokines in immunologic responses to inflammation signal a need for reallocating energy and reducing behavioral activation to fight infection, resulting in what is termed *sickness behavior* (86). Cytokine levels are elevated in clinical depression, and their production may be precipitated by stress (231), lending credibility to this energy conservation hypothesis concerning depression-like behavior. The distinction between classic clinical depression and symptoms associated with CVD is currently the focus of significant research and analysis (87).

Depression is a mood disorder, of which the chief characteristic is relatively persistent alteration in mood or emotional tone. *Table 17-4* depicts the three broad classes of mood disorders. To screen for depression, a two-item questionnaire has recently been proposed, inquiring whether within the preceding month patients have experienced either (a) "little interest or pleasure in doing things" or (b) "feeling down, depressed, or hopeless" (60). However, it should be noted that an actual diagnosis of depression can only be made by a health care professional, using the criteria set forth in the *DSM-IV*.

ANXIETY

The term *anxiety* is related to fear, in that both conditions generally involve heightened activation of the sympathetic nervous system (SNS). They differ in that anxiety is future oriented, whereas fear is a reaction to

TABLE 17-4. Classes of Mood Disorders	
Class	**Diagnoses Included**
Depressive (or unipolar) disorders	**Major depressive disorder** • Most common mood disorder; at least one major episode • Two or more weeks of either diminished pleasure/interest in normal activities or depressed mood, and four of the following: weight change (<5% per month), altered sleep patterns, increased/decreased motor activity, fatigue, feeling worthless/guilty, poor concentration, persistent thoughts of death or suicide
	Dysthymic disorder • Chronically depressed for at least 2 yr, and two of the following: altered appetite, minimal/excessive sleep, constant fatigue, poor self-esteem, hopelessness
	Depressive disorder not otherwise specified (NOS) • Atypical manifestations of depression • Often linked to other mental disorders
Bipolar disorders	**Bipolar I** • Episodes of mania (heightened energy and expansive mood) that alternate with depressive episodes • Previously known as manic-depressive illness
	Bipolar II • Periods of depression alternate with hypomanic episodes (less extreme elevations of mood and energy)
	Cyclothymic disorder • Chronic (at least 2 yr) fluctuations in mood, alternating between hypomanic and depressive symptoms
	Bipolar disorder NOS • Atypical alternating mood patterns
Mood disorders that are due to a medical condition or substance abuse	• Mood disorders associated with **medical condition** (*e.g.*, degenerative neurologic disorders, stroke, cancers)
	• Mood disorders associated with **substance use** (resulting from states of intoxication, withdrawal, or medication side effects)
	• Symptoms can be depressive or manic-like.

Adapted from American Psychiatric Association. *Diagnostic and Statistical Manual of Mental Disorders*. 4th ed. Text Revision. Washington (DC): American Psychiatric Association; 2000.

TABLE 17-5. Subtypes of *DSM-IV* Anxiety Disorders

Panic disorder with or without agoraphobia	*Panic attacks:* • Brief, unexpected, intense episodes of SNS activation peaking within a 10-min period • Anxious apprehension about attacks or their reoccurrence
	Agoraphobia: • Situational avoidance (being in a crowd, being outdoors, etc.) perceived as risky and difficult to escape from • May be diagnostically linked to panic disorder but can be diagnosed independently
Phobias	• Extreme anticipatory fear of specific objects or situations evoking anxiety symptoms comparable to panic attacks • Typically accompanied by recognition that fear is excessive or unwarranted • May become conditioned to virtually any object or situation
Obsessive-compulsive disorder	• Recurrent, uncontrolled obsessions (thoughts, impulses, images) and/or compulsions (repetitive behaviors) • Obsessions/compulsions generally acknowledged as unnecessary
Posttraumatic stress disorder	• Reexperiencing prior traumatic, catastrophic stressors 1 mo or more after the event (termed *acute stress disorder* if reaction occurs within 1 mo) • Avoidance of circumstances or cues related to trauma • Persisting, heightened SNS activation is common
Generalized anxiety disorder	• Broadly based apprehension, unattached to specific object or situation • Heightened vigilance with moderately elevated SNS activation and chronic anticipatory worry

DSM-IV, *Diagnostic and Statistical Manual of Mental Disorders, Fourth Edition*; SNS, sympathetic nervous system.

Adapted from American Psychiatric Association. *Diagnostic and Statistical Manual of Mental Disorders.* 4th ed. Text Revision. Washington (DC): American Psychiatric Association; 2000.

present threat or danger. Anxious people worry extensively about real or imagined future events over which they believe they have little control. Chronic anxiety is characterized by persisting apprehension that may or may not be attached to a specific source of concern. A focused object of concern is termed a *phobia*; anxiety that is not attached to a specific object or situation is described as *free floating* or *generalized anxiety*.

Anxiety is extremely common and is often referred to as the "common cold of psychopathology." Clinically, anxiety has high rates of comorbidity with other mental disorders, especially mood disorders. A large sample (46,114) survey conducted by the National Institute on Alcohol Abuse and Alcoholism (NIAAA) reported a 12-mo prevalence of any form of anxiety disorder to be 11.1% (131). Efforts to control anxiety consume billions of dollars and double the cost for medical patients afflicted with anxiety (36). Anxiety symptoms are common secondary reactions to many medical disorders and appear to be predictive of coronary heart disease (CHD) risk independent of clinical depression (35), and even in healthy individuals, they are associated with inflammation and coagulation markers (221).

One reason for anxiety's prominence as a clinical disorder is that it is related to activation of the SNS. Normal SNS activation is adaptive and even protective, as when a reflexive fight-or-flight reaction is triggered in a risky or dangerous situation. Elevated heart rate, peripheral vasodilation, altered breathing, and diaphoresis are correlates of SNS activation (287). Activation of the SNS is normally balanced with that of the parasympathetic nervous system (PNS), which exerts a counterbalancing effect of

energy restoration and recovery. A cardinal feature of most anxiety is unwarranted SNS activation in response to anticipated risk or danger, implying that it is (a) cognitively mediated and (b) future oriented. Either chronic or episodic SNS activation under circumstances that pose no immediate danger can be highly debilitating and lead to additional anxiety, typically in the form of worry (52), as well as being associated with heightened hypertension risk related to both CHD and metabolic disorders (132).

The following are the primary subtypes of anxiety disorders in the *DSM-IV*: panic disorder with/without agoraphobia, phobias (agoraphobia, specific phobia, social phobia), obsessive-compulsive disorder, posttraumatic stress disorder, and generalized anxiety disorder (*Table 17-5*). As with mood disorders, there are additional subtypes related to medical conditions and substance-use disorders, and with atypical symptoms (*i.e.*, not otherwise specified [NOS]).

As with mood disorders, anxiety disorders can be a result of certain medical conditions or psychoactive substances, including some medications. Panic attacks may be mistakenly perceived as heart attacks, owing to the prominence of tachycardia in conjunction with sudden SNS hyperactivation. For example, one study (295) found that roughly one-third of emergency room visits for chest pain were linked to either panic disorder or depression. It is also the case that both anxiety and depression, either subclinical variants or diagnosable disorders, can occur as secondary reactions to the stress associated with many medical disorders. As a result, it is important for exercise professionals to be sensitive to possible interactions between medical and psychological factors that contribute to the individual's overall level of adaptation. In addition, knowledge about side effects of pharmacotherapy for anxiety disorders is warranted (207), which is commonly employed either singly or in combination with psychotherapy (cognitive behavior therapy [CBT]). A brief screening measure for anxiety (60) poses three questions concerning symptoms within the preceding month: "being bothered by 'nerves,' or feeling anxious or on edge," "worrying about a lot of different things," and "having an anxiety attack (suddenly feeling fear or panic)."

STRESS

The term *stress* is interpreted in many different ways but is rooted in engineering terminology, where it refers to deformation of an object (such as a steel beam) in response to an imposed load. In health and medicine, the concept of stress is related to Bernard and Cannon's concept of internal responses that maintain physiologic balance despite environmental changes, which Cannon termed *homeostasis* and popularized in an early book (62). Lazarus et al. (173) define stress as the result of a cognitive appraisal process comparing situational demands with available coping resources; high stress occurs when perceived demands exceed resources. According to Lazarus (169,171), stress is highly integrated with emotion, defined as "an organized, psychophysiologic reaction to ongoing relationships with the environment" (172). This conception is useful because everyday experience is marked by a range of emotional reactions to situations that pose challenges and evoke coping responses. Increasingly, research in this area is incorporating positive (*e.g.*, hope, love) as well as negative (*e.g.*, fear, anger, anxiety) emotions into the overall model (170).

Early interest in stress was stimulated by Selye, who formulated the general adaptation syndrome (GAS) based on early animal studies suggesting that a variety of physical stressors elicited a common, characteristic physiologic response pattern. There are three phases in the GAS: alarm, reaction, and exhaustion. The alarm phase entails physiologic arousal that increases metabolism and heightens vigilance and is preparatory in nature. This phase is followed by sustained activation that underlies coping responses, followed by a phase of exhaustion and recovery. Chronic stress overloads the GAS, which functions best when only episodically activated. Selye distinguished between stress and eustress, the latter a positive response, as a way of emphasizing the possible adaptive, as well as maladaptive, aspects. Selye's research highlighted the importance of the HPA axis, which triggers secretion of cortisol from the adrenal cortex in response to prolonged stress. Research clearly demonstrates the key role of the HPA axis integrating the nervous, endocrine, and immune systems (199).

The HPA neuroendocrine axis and SNS make up two somewhat independent systems activated in response to stressful and/or anxiety-provoking circumstances. Functionally, it can be difficult to differentiate stress and anxiety because both involve states of heightened physiologic arousal. One difference is cognitive: Anxiety is a response to anticipated risk or threat, whereas stress involves a state of physiologic adaptation to immediate concerns. Second, whereas anxiety is perceptible and unpleasant, signaled by SNS activation, stress reactions may involve less obvious patterns of arousal that evolve into chronically elevated activation in response to cortisol secretion. Third, stress has positive aspects in relation to, for example, exercise and performance contexts. Psychological and physiologic correlates of stress occur in a time-limited context that challenges coping resources and evokes adaptive emotional responses (170). Recently, the concepts of allostasis (stability in the context of change) and allostatic load (cumulative, pathologic stress adaptation) have been used to characterize neurologically based hormonal and cognitive changes reflecting adaptation to chronically variable environmental circumstances (190). Trait-based behavioral variations may predispose individuals to different stress-based diseases as a result of cumulative allostatic load (164).

Stress is associated with a range of health risk factors. Research in this area began with Holmes and Rahe's use of the Social Readjustment Rating Scale (SRRS) to predict illness onset (146), although this produced only modest correlations because of individual differences in response to specific stressful events. In order to address this issue, measures of perceived stress such as the widely used Perceived Stress Scale (PSS) (77) were developed, which accounted for individual variations in the perception of stressful events. Stress is a commonly reported stimulus to overeating and has been shown to increase intake in less healthy food selections (133,297). In addition, stress influences blood lipid levels via increased concentration of cortisol, catecholamines, and fatty acids (56). And as previously noted, various types of stressors can weaken immune system responses to viruses and other opportunistic pathogens (74,75,249). Psychosocial stressors have also been found to impede recovery from intensive training in athletes (219).

Stress and coping are inextricably linked, and many different strategies and programs have been developed outside the context of formal psychotherapy to help people manage stress. Lazarus characterizes coping simply as how people manage stressful life events (171). In earlier writings (169,173), he used the terms *emotion focused* and *problem focused* to describe common ways of coping, the former involving cognitive interpretive strategies to reduce the emotional impact of stress, the latter taking direct action to deal with a stressor. Both are typically used at various times in the course of managing stressful events. Exercise (94) and meditation (154) are but two of many techniques found useful in helping to manage stress. Despite its pervasive nature, stress does not have a corresponding discrete *DSM-IV* diagnosis. However, **posttraumatic stress disorder** and **acute stress disorder** are considered Axis I disorders involving reactions to specific catastrophic events well in excess of the severity needed to activate the HPA axis. In these disorders, symptoms may persist and often emerge well after the stressful event, whereas chronic stress reflects the cumulative impact of multiple day-to-day events that, either singly or collectively, overtax coping resources. One relevant *DSM-IV* diagnosis is psychological factors affecting physical condition, an Axis I disorder including what were previously referred to as psychosomatic disorders, reflecting the interplay between psychological and physical symptoms, and frequently attributed to stress (272). However, such interactions are based largely on correlational epidemiologic studies and await verification via more rigorous research methodology (158).

INTERVENTION MODELS AND STRATEGIES

The term *psychosocial intervention* is very broad and encompasses ways of helping people deal with emotional distress that include, but are not limited to, psychotherapy. Although pharmacotherapy is an obvious and well-proven means of providing relief for depression, anxiety, and other emotional disorders, there is increasing evidence that interpersonally based therapeutic interventions not only have strong empirical support (67), but also exert their effects at a neurobiological level (256).

Health care professionals are increasingly likely to encounter patients battling anxiety, depression, stress, and other challenging conditions in the context of treating primary diseases (166). Psychological problems cut across socioeconomic, cultural, and all other levels of society (139) and are of sufficient prevalence that there are not nearly enough psychotherapists to address these needs (224). Formal training in psychotherapy normally involves either medical or postgraduate education, the latter leading to either a master's or doctorate degree. The practice of psychotherapy is regulated in most cases by state boards that grant licenses or certificates to practice. There are, however, many ways in which health care professionals without such formal training can at least be sensitive to the psychosocial needs of their clients, know how to make appropriate referrals when warranted, and frequently intervene in effective ways to reduce clients' distress.

Psychotherapy incorporates aspects of interpersonal relationships common to other professional relationships, including those with health care providers. Several key factors have emerged that help account for its impact, including the therapeutic relationship,

expectancy placebo factors, characteristics of the patient and extra therapeutic elements, and specific techniques (25). Self-disclosure is an important aspect of patient characteristics. Pennebaker, among others, has extensively documented the positive effects of both written and verbal narratives of stressful events on health and well-being, including immune system activity (217).

Although there are many forms of psychotherapy, virtually all employ (a) an emotionally charged relationship with a therapist, (b) a healing environment, (c) a conceptual rationale, and (d) procedures or techniques to provide relief (112). This section focuses on CBT, the most widely practiced form of psychotherapy, with well-validated applications for treating stress (192), depression (41), and anxiety (36). Useful reference texts include a recent description of CBT techniques for wide ranging clinical issues (209) and a compilation of diagnostically oriented conceptualizations and therapy narratives (38).

Psychosocial interventions, including CBT, have solid empirical support (67) and broad application in health, medical, and psychiatric settings. Psychological interventions are also efficient and cost-effective means of treating emotional disorders (204), primarily in terms of reducing inpatient hospitalization time and work-related impairments for even serious psychological conditions (120). Psychosocial treatment for depression is a viable alternative to pharmacotherapy in primary care practice (247), a finding that has held up following additional clinical trials (264). In the area of behavioral medicine, Friedman et al. enumerated six routes through which psychosocial interventions could help contain costs, including (a) fostering active patient involvement in health and medical care; (b) reducing the negative and additive impact of stress on disease; (c) modifying overt behavior associated with destructive lifestyle patterns necessitating expensive end-stage medical care; (d) providing social support to buffer the impact of critical medical procedures, including cardiac surgery and cesarean sections; (e) identifying and treating psychological disorders underlying medical symptoms; and (f) reducing primary care usage by patients whose primary needs are emotional in nature, but expressed physically (somatization) (119).

COGNITIVE BEHAVIOR THERAPY

Cognitive behavior therapy (CBT) is a problem-oriented, time-limited intervention model that views psychological distress as the result of negative thoughts based on either conscious or nonconscious unrealistic underlying assumptions about the world (cognitive schemas), such as "People should always treat me well" or "I should be perfect" (97,192) (*Table 17-6*). Clinically, its historical roots are in behaviorism, which emphasizes modifying overt behaviors rather than thought patterns (113). CBT also incorporates social behavioral models, especially

TABLE 17-6. Key Components of Cognitive Behavior Therapy

- Form supportive, working relationship with patients.
- Treat patients as active collaborators in learning new skills.
- Promote self-efficacy by helping patients develop capabilities and self-confidence.
- Be aware of how thoughts, behavior, and emotions interact to affect motivation, learning, and retention.
- Listen to how patients talk about themselves for indications of positive or negative cognitions associated with distress (anxiety, depression, stress).
- Foster skills that have present-moment relevance.
- Provide encouragement and support in situations that evoke unwarranted anxiety and avoidant tendencies.
- Encourage patients to develop self-assessment and self-reinforcement capabilities as a means of promoting developmental autonomy.
- Use a "building block" approach to skill development: Break challenging tasks down into readily mastered components that build confidence and promote self-efficacy.
- Help patients enlist social support in learning and maintaining new skills.

social learning and social cognitive theory (31,32), in terms of its emphasis on mediating factors such as self-efficacy to foster change in the face of depression, anxiety, or stress. CBT has widespread endorsement in behavioral medicine settings (101), perhaps because of its practical nature and amenability to empirical validation.

CBT combines cognitive restructuring with modifying underlying assumptions about the world reflected in conscious thought patterns and behaviorally based exposure. CBT encourages direct experience with the source of one's fear, using exposure techniques to treat psychological problems (55). These components are often accompanied by training in relaxation techniques, such as progressive muscle relaxation (PMR) and diaphragmatic breathing. Proponents of CBT have emphasized its specificity in treating anxiety, depression, and other disorders, akin to the medical model of diagnosis and treatment (37), but there is active debate whether such efficacy is due to specific or common factors characteristic of virtually all forms of psychotherapy (210,291). In fact, Barlow and others note that the concept of discrete *DSM-IV* diagnostic categories tends to accentuate differences that are difficult to empirically justify and, consequently, that developing specific treatment protocols for each disorder appears unwarranted (39). For example, the consistently high reported concordance between depression (mood) and anxiety disorders is consistent with this view (157). Barlow et al. have recently proposed a unified treatment model of CBT (39) with three factors: (a) modify antecedent cognitive appraisals that contribute to anticipatory emotional distress; (b) encourage acceptance, rather than avoidance or suppression, of unpleasant emotional states; and (c) encourage behavioral activation in domains not limited by the disordered emotion. Practically, this entails helping people become aware of and limit negative anticipatory appraisals in circumstances otherwise likely to elicit stressful, depressive, or anxious reactions; encourage openness to emotional experiences, whether positive or negative; and facilitate active engagement in daily life. Of particular relevance for patients with the chronic illnesses described in this chapter, CBT has been validated for use with older patients, who are most vulnerable to these conditions (268).

Consistent with this unified treatment model, CBT is currently evolving in the direction of acceptance and mindfulness-based models of psychotherapy advocated by Hayes and others (137,138,248). These developments reflect the interesting confluence of diverse influences, including cognitive theories of language and Buddhist meditation practices, united in the belief that detaching from and being less reactive to (hence accepting of) and aware (mindful) of thoughts and other elements of experience is therapeutically beneficial. Applications of this model in behavioral medicine, sports performance, and addiction treatment are now appearing in the literature (8,123,147,241). Of particular relevance are results of a recent study (96) reporting short-term autonomic and cardiovascular benefits from one component of a stress reduction protocol based on this model.

One particularly noteworthy psychosocial intervention based on the principles of mindfulness and acceptance is a group-based intervention known as Mindfulness-Based Stress Reduction, or MBSR (154,242). MBSR, originally developed for use among chronic pain patients, is a time-limited behavioral medicine intervention that makes use of meditation-based practices designed to increase focused awareness in the present moment. Mindfulness interventions have been making rapid headway in the practice of clinical psychology in recent years, where they have been effectively applied in work with depression, anxiety, and stress (242). Gardner and Moore (124) have developed an intervention program for athletically based coaching as well, and it is evident that this intervention model will achieve increasing prominence in the future. Mindfulness-based clinical interventions are especially notable in that they include both cognitive and somatic elements of potentially great significance for physical activity and exercise. Among these are the body scan (a narrative that directs attention inwardly to somatic cues), hatha yoga (gentle stretching, with mindful attention), and sitting meditation. Mindfulness shows great potential for work in health, wellness, exercise adherence (281), and athletic contexts. Interventions that focus on specific forms of psychological distress have been developed in recent years, including those that are the focus of attention here: anxiety (213), depression

TABLE 17-7. Acceptance and Mindfulness-Based Interventions

- Clinician and client both practice mindful (present moment) awareness

- Emphasize present-moment, nonjudgmental awareness of challenging circumstances

- Encourage moment-by-moment awareness of thoughts, emotions, and physical sensations

- Teach clients to observe thoughts and emotions without getting "caught up" in them or being judgmental

- Employ "beginner's mind" attitude to work with challenging situations by seeing things with a fresh perspective, as if for the first time

- Cultivate the ability to respond skillfully to challenges, rather than reacting as if on "auto pilot"

- Limit excess physiological activation through formal and informal mindfulness practices

- Encourage greater acceptance of current difficulties as a prelude to meaningful change

(248), and stress (154). A broad range of clinical practitioners are beginning to employ mindfulness and acceptance-based practices, key elements of which are summarized in *Table 17-7*.

CBT interventions continue to be successfully used in medical and health applications, including reducing depression among individuals with HIV diagnosis (16,144), preventing defibrillator shock (68), responding discriminatively to sudden chest pain (235), encouraging older adults to exercise (141), and reducing stress-related injury and illness among athletes (218). In general, CBT has attained parity with pharmacotherapy for treating depression and anxiety, and involving patients in the decision process is one way to enhance active engagement in treatment. CBT is a practical, problem-oriented form of psychotherapy. The basic principles can be readily applied in health and wellness, as well as in clinical settings.

EXERCISE AND PSYCHOSOCIAL FACTORS

Exercise professionals are in an especially advantageous position to help clients deal with symptoms of anxiety, depression, and stress because exercise and physical activity have well-documented positive effects on these conditions. Physical activity has well-documented, positive effects on brain functions underlying emotional health throughout the lifespan regarding neurotransmitters, nerve cell generation, and brain blood flow (91). However, the effects of SAD on exercise motivation need to be taken into account to increase the likelihood of exercise initiation and maintenance. There are numerous cognitive and behavioral determinants of physical activity (59,254), and it is important to have a working

knowledge of how these can affect day-to-day behavior. Stress-prone individuals are vulnerable to fatigue and unfavorable appraisals of their capacity to cope with the inevitable challenges in becoming and staying physically active. Anxiety triggers apprehension and worry about future outcomes, even in the context of potentially enjoyable activities, whereas depression saps both psychological and physical energy, triggering pessimistic cognitive appraisals and crippling self-doubts. All three undermine self-efficacy in different ways.

However, there is growing evidence that physical activity can help reduce distress associated with symptoms of stress (236), anxiety (178), and depression (211), and exercise guidelines for work with clinical populations have been published (198). Early research showed that exercise alleviated negative emotional states, but only with nonclinical samples (*i.e.*, physically fit individuals and athletes who completed state-based measures of emotionality prior to and following bouts of high-intensity exercise). Comparatively few studies were conducted with clinical populations. Furthermore, the absence of conceptual models linking emotions to physical activity and lack of integration with extant psychiatric diagnostic nomenclature limited clinical applications of the early research literature. Finally, SAD are associated with advanced age, which imposes its own constraints on physical activity.

Despite these caveats, there is increasing evidence from recent longitudinal epidemiologic and clinical studies attesting to the positive effects of physical activity based on clinical samples to reinforce the conclusions of earlier studies (40,136). Evidence in support of the beneficial effects of clinical interventions as an adjunct to standard medical or psychiatric care continues to steadily accumulate (273). In addition, contemporary conceptually driven models integrating physical activity, neurobiological structures, cognitive functions, and emotional reactivity have stimulated research on the impact of even low-intensity or dose activity on emotional states (100). The emergence of the interdisciplinary field of "exercise" psychology, with a corresponding emphasis on health optimization in clinical settings that has occurred in recent years, has developmental roots in exercise physiology, behavioral medicine, and health psychology. However, the impact of physical activity across the full spectrum of both anxiety and mood clinical disorders has not been systematically evaluated, being limited largely to panic disorder (208) and moderate-intensity depression (211). One study evaluating the relationship between regular physical activity and mental health found that exercise is positively associated with decreased major depression and anxiety disorders (128).

Exercise professionals need to integrate knowledge of exercise prescription techniques with sensitivity to psychosocial factors when designing programs for patients who present with symptoms of stress, anxiety, and/or depression. The importance of gauging the impact of exercise — itself a stressor — on overall cumulative stress level (*i.e.*, allostatic load) cannot be overstated. The common channel factor here is the HPA axis, which, as noted earlier, is designed to modulate the impact of short-term rather than chronic stress. Although it has been hypothesized that exercise-based stress may reduce the impact of stress in other modalities (the cross-stressor adaptation hypothesis), supportive evidence is equivocal (94,261), although research is ongoing (260). Although this hypothesis has some validity with respect to people who are physically fit, adjusting exercise prescriptions in response to varying self-reported stress is recommended (1), especially to avoid overtaxing unfit patients or those with chronic medical conditions whose immune system may be compromised either by the disease or as a result of treatment side effects.

It may seem paradoxical that physical activity appears to reduce symptoms of both anxiety and depression, the latter involving heightened SNS arousal, the former a reduction in overall activation. Psychological benefits accrue from both aerobic and nonaerobic forms of exercise, eliminating physiologic conditioning *per se* as the principal explanatory factor (222). In part, this finding can be explained by nonspecific aspects of any psychological intervention described earlier (25), including expectancy factors and a positive therapeutic relationship. Physical activity may be beneficial in other ways as a temporary distraction (26,229) and as a way to enhance self-efficacy (30), the perception of fitness (222), and perhaps even alterations in trait factors as well (88), independent of measurable changes in fitness. Physiologically, regular physical activity helps modulate SNS and HPA activation, a contributing factor to both anxiety and depression spectrum disorders. Furthermore, as noted earlier, the high comorbidity of depression and anxiety disorders suggests at least a partial underlying etiologic commonality. It has been suggested that a unifying factor concerning the benefits of physical activity may in fact lead to an overarching increase in stress resilience, mediated by both cognitive and physiologic mechanisms (240). Finally, neurocognitive changes associated with exercise suggest a generalized positive impact on CNS functioning that may indeed have implications for emotional, cognitive, and behavioral well-being (269).

A particular challenge facing exercise professionals is how to help emotionally distressed patients work with the low level of physical conditioning common in anxiety and depression (187,228). Exacerbating this problem is the inevitable experience of most individuals initiating exercise programs; that the experience is not particularly pleasant and that perceptible benefits take time to accrue. Self-consciousness and skill

TABLE 17-8. Guidelines for the Treatment of Emotional Distress

- Know symptoms of common psychological disorders and medications used to treat them.
- Listen attentively to patients without minimizing their concerns; know how and where to refer patients for professional help if needed.
- Conduct thorough assessment of physical capabilities and motivational factors. Anxiety is linked to worry and fear, depression to self-criticism, both of which can decrease motivation.
- Encourage enjoyable, nonthreatening, easily accessible exercise; link it to being active outside scheduled sessions.
- Eliminate obstacles, establish reasonable goals, and help patients integrate physical activity into daily life.
- Incorporate patients in planning and assessing of exercise programs to enhance active collaboration and counteract passivity associated with anxious worry and depressive pessimism.
- Adopt a nonjudgmental, problem-solving stance when difficulties with compliance arise. Emphasize immediate benefits rather than long-term outcomes; minimize significance of lapses.
- Watch for resistance to change that can sabotage progress; address it directly and collaboratively. Reinforce positive behaviors unrelated to depression or anxiety to sidestep negative effects on motivation.

Adapted from O'Neal HA, Dunn AL, Martinsen EW. Depression and exercise. *Int J Sport Psychol.* 2000;31:110–35.

deficits are also potential issues to be faced. Anxious individuals — those with panic disorder in particular — may be conditioned to experience physiologic arousal as both unpleasant and, because of prior elicitation during panic attacks, embarrassing or even dangerous. Anticipating the worst, they may worry about the possibility of injury or other negative outcomes. And those who experience chronic SNS activation may find even modest exercise-induced stimulation excessive rather than invigorating. Depressed individuals pose unique challenges as well (250), in terms of low motivation, chronic inactivity, and a pessimistic view of the world. In working with depressed or anxious patients, the recommendations listed in *Table 17-8*, although developed primarily for depressed individuals (211), are useful in either case. Especially important in this work is anticipating and making allowances for cognitively based motivational barriers to progress when initiating exercise programs (24). For example, one recent study showed that a values-based wellness intervention elicited improvements in fitness and reductions in perceived barriers to exercising (57).

Finally, emerging clinical practice and research on mindfulness emphasizes the value of keeping one's attention focused in the present moment. Being mindful can help anxious or depressed patients avoid being distracted by past or future concerns and help cultivate an appreciation for present-moment experience. Currently, applications of mindfulness in exercise tend to emphasize non-Western practices such as sitting meditation, yoga, and tai chi (168), but in fact, a much broader framework exists in Western psychology underlying its incorporation into many other aspects of daily life (241).

CLINICAL APPLICATIONS

CARDIOVASCULAR DISEASE

Psychosocial interventions for patients with CVD have involved both preventive and postmyocardial infarct applications. CVD and related vascular diseases are adversely associated with psychological functioning, cognitive impairments, and even risk of dementia (129). Beginning with early efforts to identify psychological precursors of cardiac events (34,117,118), accumulating data have shown that psychosocial factors, stress, and emotional reactivity in particular are significant predictors of CVD risk. Moreover, emotional distress has been associated with heightened risk of sudden cardiac death (22,155,267). A related factor, heightened cardiovascular reactivity, may be a risk factor as well, although supportive evidence has been considered equivocal (165). Recently, however, convincing evidence links depression and dysfunctional autonomic nervous system activity with both mortality and morbidity associated with CVD (64). In addition, attitudinal factors including optimism/pessimism and hostility have historically been correlated with physiological CVD risk, although not yet causally linked (275). These relationships may be mediated in part by immune system dysregulation, marked by cytokine production, which has deleterious cardiac effects and produces depression symptoms (215).

More recent research continues to validate this relationship, particularly with respect to anxiety and depression. Rozanski et al. (237) cited evidence linking CVD risk to the following five domains: (a) depression, (b) anxiety, (c) personality traits, (d) social isolation, and (e) chronic stress. All of these factors appear to contribute to endothelial damage as a function of stress and, among some individuals, SNS hyperactivation. An analysis of data from the Normative Aging Study, a longitudinal study of aging in men, revealed a dose-response relationship between negative emotionality and CVD incidence (276). A more recent study derived from this database revealed that anxiety and a factor characterized as "general emotional distress" was a significant predictor of CVD risk. Similar results were also recently reported from a moderately sized sample of men and women in the Pittsburgh Healthy Heart Project, where it was reported that somatic symptoms of depression in particular compared with measures of anxiety and hostility are linked to early-stage CVD (271). Research has documented a diverse biological substrate contributing to *both* cardiovascular and mood regulation that includes the HPA axis, proinflammatory cytokines, neurotransmitter systems, and other components (134).

Overall, studies of patients with CVD support the value of psychosocial, lifestyle, and related complementary interventions. An early meta-analysis based on 23 randomized control studies (177) concluded that adding a psychosocial intervention component to standard cardiac care not only reduced psychological distress, but mortality and morbidity as well. Several specific outcome studies are especially notable. The Stanford Coronary Risk Intervention Project (SCRIP) employed a multicomponent treatment package to reduce multiple CVD risk factors via lifestyle modification involving diet, exercise, and medication. Over a 4-yr period, there was a significant decline in coronary artery stenosis, documented by angiography.

Ornish and colleagues (212) reported that radical lifestyle alterations over a 5-yr period in patients with known CVD showed an angiographically documented slight reduction in coronary artery stenosis compared with a significant increase in patients receiving usual medical care. Intervention components consisted of a low-fat vegetarian diet, aerobic exercise, smoking cessation, and stress-reduction training in the context of a supportive social milieu. Coronary perfusion abnormalities also decreased as a result of the intervention (130). The Ornish program has subsequently been employed in multiple clinical settings, and a recent composite analysis based on data from eight independent medical centers reported positive changes in both physiologic (lipids, body fat, blood pressure) and psychosocial (quality of life, stress, depression, hostility) measures (7).

Multicomponent interventions such as these are clearly effective in reducing CVD risk but make it difficult to specify the nature of the treatment effects. Nonetheless, they underscore the importance of lifestyle factors in risk management, an obvious point of emphasis in any exercise program for medical patients. It is also important to emphasize that CVD is frequently accompanied by emotional reactivity (stress, anxiety, depression) reflecting either the primary (stress-based) impact of the disease itself or a secondary reaction, and that this emotional reactivity should be addressed either in terms of the general guidelines previously enumerated or via referral to an appropriate mental health specialist. Although exercise may be an effective antidote for depression, dealing with cognitively based motivational factors requires interpersonal skill, sensitivity, and patience. Exercise professionals working with CVD (and other controlled chronic illnesses) would do well to augment their training in developing aerobic, strength, and flexibility programs with relaxation and other stress management skills. Of clinical significance is evidence that depressive symptoms may reflect "vital exhaustion," an inflammation-based precursor of MI in some patients (20,21). Similar issues arise with patients with post-MI or ischemic CVD, exacerbated by the psychological trauma of an acute, life-threatening event. Depression in particular as well as anxiety and other manifestations of emotional stress are both common and persistent in the aftermath of MI, and depression is predictive of subsequent 18-mo cardiac mortality (114). Depressed patients are also less likely to follow through on recommendations to reduce risk of subsequent MIs (299).

However, despite widespread prevalence, there is presently no consensus concerning the relationship between CVD-based depression syndrome and standard psychiatric diagnosis with respect to underlying cause(s) or optimal treatment (149). Nonetheless, the frequency with which this condition is encountered makes clinical management a high priority (223). The American Association of Cardiovascular and Pulmonary Rehabilitation (AACVPR) issued a position statement advocating early screening and treatment of post-MI depression (142) in the context of cardiac rehabilitation. Both antidepressants (SSRIs) and CBT, either singly or in combination, were identified as effective treatment options. Naturally, prevention of CVD is highly desirable, and a recent review of the literature on risk reduction strategies highlighted the importance of behavioral strategies, including goal setting and feedback, that could readily be implemented by health and fitness specialists (78).

The effects of psychosocial interventions have been studied following both MI and ischemia (46,48). Ischemic heart disease is of particular interest because of its close association with stress and further complications, including MI. In a landmark study, the effects of aerobic exercise and a stress management program (SMP) on postischemic patients were compared with usual medical care over a 5-yr period in older male and female patients with CVD (46). The SMP was based on cognitive/social learning principles (similar to CBT) and also included training in PMR and electromyography (EMG) biofeedback. Participants in the SMP experienced fewer subsequent cardiac events and also incurred lower medical costs. This study was subsequently replicated using a stronger research design (48), at which time both SMP and exercise were found to reduce depression, distress, and cardiovascular abnormalities in comparison with usual medical care. Components of the SMP that could be adapted for use with exercise patients include (a) education concerning stress and cardiac function, (b) training in learning to recognize the impact of negative thoughts and acquire relaxation skills, and (c) establishing a supportive social network.

Similar results for patients with post-MI were reported by the same research group in a large-scale, multicenter, randomized control trial to evaluate the impact of exercise and CBT on post-MI depression, mortality, and subsequent adverse events in older men and women. The Enhancing Recovery in Coronary Heart Disease (ENRICHD) study found that aerobic exercise in particular was helpful in reducing mortality and subsequent infarction in patients with post-MI with either depression or low social support (47). In contrast, neither medication nor CBT for depression affected mortality more than usual care, but patients who were unresponsive to either intervention had elevated risk of late mortality (63). In a separate analysis, CBT was found to have a modest positive impact on quality of life (196).

Neither CBT nor other psychosocial interventions are really intended to directly affect biological markers of health or disease, and it is no surprise when such negative findings are reported, as was recently the case (71). Rather, such practices are more likely to affect psychological mediators, such as self-efficacy and self-regulatory skills, which in turn affect motivation and treatment adherence (258). The impact of such interventions can be further amplified if implemented not only by patients, but by family members as well, who are also otherwise vulnerable to emotional distress and ineffective coping strategies (262).

STROKE

CVD including stroke, ranks second worldwide in all-cause mortality (53). Stroke has devastating consequences, and prevention is not only desirable but also feasible in the majority of cases. Pharmacologic treatments for precursors of stroke including hypertension, clot formation, and elevated lipids are routinely recommended (53), but diet, exercise, stress management, and other lifestyle modifications contribute significant protective effects as well. Management of emotional problems is also important because prospective studies have linked anxiety, depression, and anger to the development of hypertension, a precursor of stroke (153,238).

In addition to physical and cognitive impairments, stroke impairs psychological functioning. Depression is a common sequel, and it appears appropriate to consider psychosocial interventions in the aftermath (206). Poststroke depression is related to both cerebral localization and secondary emotional reactions. In addition, management must take into account the degree of cognitive and motor impairment present; obviously, presence of aphasia and other communicative impediments would interfere with psychotherapy. However, for patients without disabling language impairments, cognitively oriented interventions are recommended (162). A recent review and formulation of a biosocial approach to poststroke depression (188) recommended increasing emphasis on cognitive and behavioral management strategies in addition to pharmacotherapy. The behaviorally oriented model of depression proposed by Lewinsohn et al. (175) is potentially applicable because of its emphasis on formulating pleasant experiences and positively reinforcing social interactions. An added advantage of such an approach is that it can incorporate caregivers and others in the patient's network as therapeutic resources. Reducing risk of subsequent stroke is another important intervention target, as suggested by results of a health promotion program for African American stroke survivors, in which a 12-wk intervention showed significant, positive changes in lipid levels, fitness, strength, and social isolation (234). Clearly, however, prevention of stroke is preferable to postincident intervention, and exercise specialists are a key resource in encouraging those at risk to develop healthy lifestyle patterns to reduce contributory risk factors.

CHRONIC OBSTRUCTIVE PULMONARY DISEASE

COPD, defined as "nonreversible pulmonary function impairment," is the fourth leading cause of death in the United States (69). Like CVD and stroke, it takes a substantial personal, social, and economic toll, owing to the debilitating symptoms, functional impairment, and need for long-term care. The clinical course of COPD is a spiraling cycle that begins with dyspnea and progresses through reduced physical activity, deconditioning, and ultimately to a state of disability (19). Guidelines for clinical care (227) have traditionally emphasized smoking cessation, pharmacologic management, and pulmonary rehabilitation. Training to minimize dyspnea and promote physical activity is an important treatment component and appears to be effective if consistently used (239). However, the cost of such interventions can be substantial to begin with and escalate over time (220) and may not address psychological factors (depression and anxiety) that can limit treatment adherence and exacerbate symptomatology.

Psychosocial interventions designed to foster active self-management and to limit the adverse impact of depression and anxiety are a relatively recent addition to clinical practice that appear to be effective if consistently used (239). Incorporating psychosocial interventions into routine COPD rehabilitation is of relatively recent origin, despite the fact that both depression and anxiety are common comorbid factors that markedly attenuate quality of life (83) and may interfere not only with rehabilitation, but also with effective self-regulation of lifestyle behaviors. For example, smoking is strongly linked to COPD; the 2002 National Health Interview Survey reported that 36.2% of adults with COPD were smokers. In addition, it is astonishing that only half reported trying to stop smoking, and of these, only 14.6% succeeded in eliminating this life-threatening habit (244). Significantly, this same survey reported that fewer than 25% of current smokers or recent quitters reported receiving cessation advice from health care professionals, but even advice and social support may not be enough to help patients change their behavior (293). Ironically, smoking is negatively associated with long-term treatment participation, according to interviews conducted with long-term (11-yr) survivors involved in the Lung Health Study (259).

Shortness of breath (dyspnea), a key symptom of COPD, creates acute distress symptoms of anxiety with both sensory and cognitive components (65). Not surprisingly, anxiety disorder in patients with COPD reportedly occurs at two to three times the rate of the general population and significantly more frequently than in most other medical conditions (54). This finding may in part account for high rates of emergency room visits and use of other forms of health care resources, which to some extent can be contained by applying a model of chronic illness management used successfully with other diseases that encourages informed decision making, self-management, and use of authoritative information (3).

Both CBT and SSRI antidepressants have been effectively used to treat psychosocial distress in COPD, although medications sometimes used to treat depression and anxiety, including tricyclic antidepressants and benzodiazepines, are not recommended (60). CBT helps reduce the impact of negative, sometimes catastrophic, thinking by teaching patients to monitor (*i.e.*, notice) rather than become preoccupied with mental rumination. It is also paired with some form of relaxation training to help counteract accompanying SNS activation. These techniques are helpful with older adults (269) and especially applicable with patients with COPD. In one study, a 2-h, group-based CBT session teaching cognitive and relaxation strategies with follow-up home practice for 6 wk reduced anxiety and depression symptoms significantly more than an education-only control condition (167). A promising intervention currently under way uses a group-based CBT intervention to foster increased compliance with physical activity recommendations in patients with COPD, using a model successful with other chronic medical conditions (111). At this time, however, there is limited research on the efficacy of behavioral medicine interventions for COPD (33), despite their widespread and effective application with other clinical populations. Effective management of negative affect associated with COPD is especially important, in light of evidence that depression in particular appears to be an independent risk factor for mortality in this population (89).

METABOLIC DISEASE

Diabetes

Physical activity and metabolism are interdependent, and physical inactivity is associated with physiologic changes that alter energy balance, increase insulin resistance, promote muscle atrophy, and consequently further reduce exercise capacity (44). In diabetes, metabolic processes are disrupted either because of inadequate pancreatic insulin secretion (Type 1) or resistance to cellular insulin absorption (Type 2); gestational diabetes is another form associated with pregnancy. The long-term consequences of uncontrolled diabetes are profound, resulting in chronic disability and global systemic failure. Among its effects are vision loss (as a result of retinopathy), kidney failure, peripheral neuropathy, and CNS dysfunction affecting multiple organs and functions (10). Type 1 diabetes can be managed with supplementary insulin, but the process of monitoring and stabilizing insulin levels requires constant attention and care. Type 2 diabetes is strongly influenced by diet and physical activity and thus potentially can be controlled by lifestyle adjustments. Both Type 2 diabetes and obesity are reaching epidemic proportions in Westernized countries, affecting not only adults but increasingly children as well, diminishing health-related quality of life in the process (257). Along with increased prevalence overall, ethnic disparities are increasing as well, based on data comparing Caucasian, African American, and Hispanic Americans (298).

The problem of insulin resistance is of relatively recent origin and has profound implications for health on a global scale (292) because it is linked to a lethal syndrome of risk factors, including obesity, elevated low-density lipoprotein (LDL) cholesterol, low high-density lipoprotein (HDL) cholesterol, hyperglycemia, hypertension associated with Type 2 diabetes, and CVD (193).

The American Diabetes Association (ADA) recognizes physical activity as a potential therapeutic agent for both Type 1 and Type 2 diabetes, provided it is preceded by a thorough medical assessment to evaluate cardiovascular, retinal, and CNS status. Prescriptive guidelines have been recently updated by the ACSM and ADA (79). Recent ADA guidelines continue to emphasize the importance of physical activity in diabetes management plans, along with (minimal) screening for psychosocial factors related to negative emotional states, attitudinal factors, cognitive functioning, and overall quality of life (11).

The potential of physical activity for insulin regulation warrants consideration of psychosocial factors related to motivation, self-efficacy, and self-regulation. Both cognitive and behavioral strategies appear to be helpful in this regard for Type 2 diabetes (161). Depression is a key factor, affecting more than 25% of patients with Types 1 and 2 diabetes and having a negative impact on insulin, medication, and dietary management (180), all of which in turn affect physical activity level, and the relationship is reciprocal. The presence of depression in diabetes is associated with functional disability — the capacity or lack thereof to carry out daily activities (99). The prevalence of depression in patients with diabetes is at least twice that of the nondiabetic population, and it has been found to have adverse effects on glycemic control,

complications, and negative outcomes (232). A recent review of psychological complications linked to diabetes (5) concluded that although several moderator variables (including age, sex, and social support) influence the nature and severity of such impairments, educating patients and physicians about their manifestations and effects is critically important. Treatment options include CBT, family/social, and problem-oriented interventions. Several studies employing CBT-based interventions support this recommendation.

The effects of a group-based diabetic education program plus CBT (compared with education alone) on major depression in patients with Type 2 diabetes was evaluated in one study (181). More than three-fourths of those in the CBT group showed a significant decline on depression scores, versus approximately one-fourth of those in the education-only condition. Significantly, glycemic levels (glycosylated hemoglobin, HbA1C) improved as well, suggesting improved self-management.

More recently, short-term, group-based CBT was effective in improving self-efficacy and mood in adult patients with Type 1 diabetes with poor glycemic control, nearly half of whom likely experienced clinically significant depression (286). However, the treatment effect of CBT did not differ from that of an education-based control group, nor was there a significant improvement in glycemic control. Self-care behavior was the target of a short-term, CBT-based intervention in adult patients with diabetes, who attended six sessions focusing on obstacles to self-care, cognitive factors, and ways to promote self-regulation. At the program's conclusion, participants showed an improvement in goal setting, and those who engaged in self-monitoring (using activity records) achieved the greatest behavioral changes. In general, lifestyle programs focusing on psychosocial factors, diet, weight management, and physical activity are effective in managing diabetes (particularly Type 2) and, as an added bonus, reducing CVD risk (148). Regardless of the intervention modality employed (pharmacotherapy, psychotherapy, combined), adequate glycemic control is vital (285).

Obesity

Like diabetes, obesity is a health problem of epidemic proportions. It is associated with risk of metabolic and other disorders, and rates of both obesity and diabetes are increasing in virtually all segments of the population (202), although there are some indications that prevalence rates are beginning to stabilize (294). Currently, more than half of the U.S. population is classified as overweight (body mass index [BMI] = 25.0–29.9 kg · m^{-2}) or obese (BMI $\geq$ 30 kg · m^{-2}). To counteract excess weight, the ACSM advocates combining increased energy expenditure with reduced intake to effect controlled, gradual loss (98), and there is ample evidence that physical activity lowers insulin resistance, a stimulus to weight gain (90,126). Empirically validated procedures to control obesity include bariatric surgery, pharmacotherapy, and behavioral strategies (80), nonsurgical methods potentially being of comparable efficacy (50). However, losing weight and, more importantly, keeping it off is not easy, despite potential benefits that include improved quality of life (214). For this reason, behavioral and cognitive behavioral interventions have been developed to enhance motivation and persistence, along with many other motivational strategies (274). Early behavioral models focused on environmental cues, such as stimuli to eating, and advocated controlling exposure, whereas subsequent interventions adopted a broader focus, incorporating emotional and cognitive factors (84,109). These elements are integrated into CBT via strategies that include (a) self-monitoring of dysfunctional thoughts, (b) controlling access to eating cues (stimulus control), (c) cognitive restructuring related to maladaptive beliefs about weight and how to control it, (d) effective stress management, and (e) social support (110,289).

Structured interventions based on CBT have tended to emphasize in particular the common problem of regaining weight previously lost. Long-term weight maintenance may entail a combination of ongoing weight monitoring, cognitive strategies to help avoid negative thinking that can cause relapses, and behavioral programming to control energy expenditure and intake (80). They may also help manage depression, which has been found to have a reciprocal relationship with obesity (179). Despite such efforts, long-term compliance tends to be low (194), but it can be improved when CBT is embedded in an interdisciplinary treatment framework, including nutritional counseling and exercise, as reported in one study that involved an initial 6-wk hospitalization stay (127). Following up behavioral intervention with a program of monitored physical activity has also been shown to be effective in long-term weight loss (288), further underscoring the importance of physical activity in managing obesity, especially at relatively high volumes (152). However, physical activity alone does not appear to ensure weight loss maintenance, as reported by a recent study comparing the effects of a CBT-based intervention with a behaviorally oriented program emphasizing physical activity, which found that the cognitively based intervention results in significantly greater weight loss and maintenance (266). The social cognitive concept of "self-regulatory efficacy" (perceived capacity to manage the challenges of weight management) appears to be especially important in this regard (15).

Collectively, these studies suggest that cognitive-based strategies are helpful in controlling obesity, especially in the context of an integrative management program that includes, but is not limited to, physical activity. Both psychological (253) and activity-based

(252) interventions are empirically validated weight management strategies, the effects of which appear to be most likely sustained when they are combined. A recent review of both short- and long-term results of behavioral/cognitive behavioral interventions advocated an approach that is (a) goal oriented; (b) process oriented; and (c) strives for small, incremental changes (290). The emphasis on "process" factors is especially relevant for clinical exercise specialists working with obese patients. It advocates helping patients specify what it is they want to modify and how to bring this about based on an analysis of behavior chains that can lead to episodes of overeating or other behaviors incompatible with goals (e.g., lose weight, alter body composition). Consistent with previous recommendations, the basic intervention model teaches self-monitoring, stimulus control, and cognitive restructuring in the context of programs designed to provide structure and social support. Early interventions, aimed at children and adolescence, are of particular importance as a means of reducing adult-onset obesity risk through long-term, concerted interventions targeting both psychosocial and behavioral correlates of the problem (265).

Metabolic Syndrome

Much of what has been said about diabetes and obesity can be applied to the MS, a related and potentially lethal mix of central obesity plus two of several additional conditions (elevated triglycerides, low HDL-C, high blood pressure, and elevated fasting glucose level), according to the International Diabetes Federation (IDF) consensus statement (150). A similar definition, focusing on cholesterol management, was previously formulated by the National Cholesterol Education Program Adult Treatment Panel III (103) and is widely cited. An epidemiologic study (2) reported that IDF-based prevalence rates may be even higher than the figure of nearly 25% reported using adult treatment panel (ATP) III criteria (107). It is especially alarming not only that the MS is increasing rapidly in adults, but that childhood obesity, now at an epidemic level, is an early risk factor (51). Prevalence rates are also high in African American women (73), and MS appears to be a risk factor for cognitive decline in later adulthood (135). Onset of symptoms in childhood is especially significant, in light of emerging evidence that set points for related circadian rhythms, and stress reactivity patterns may be established during these early years (61).

Psychosocial interventions for MS have focused on behavioral, cognitive, and emotional aspects. It has recently been hypothesized that SNS overactivation may be a significant contributor (184), and consequently, management techniques to reduce SNS activation are likely to prove helpful. According to these authors, both diet and physical activity can have this effect, but in addition, CBT-based interventions should be considered as well. Significantly, depression has recently been shown to be an MS risk factor (140), independent of variations in clinical definitions (230).

Because of the multifaceted nature of MS, it is important to integrate intervention strategies (66). As with the other metabolic disorders discussed in this section, weight management is of critical importance and can best be achieved via CBT-based strategies for increasing energy output via physical activity and reducing weight via controlling eating patterns. Concurrent management of emotional disorders, especially depression, via CBT and/or pharmacotherapy should be considered a primary factor for immediate attention, as should treatment of hypertension, which places patients at risk for further cardiovascular complications, including stroke and diabetes (121).

The MS calls for radical lifestyle changes that can be a daunting challenge for health care professionals and patients alike. Weight management and increasing physical activity are of fundamental importance, but it is important to have an overall plan that addresses the many complications that accompany this disorder. An extremely useful overview of lifestyle interventions has recently been proposed (108) that is relevant not only for MS specifically but also for the spectrum of metabolic conditions discussed in this chapter. The key components of this intervention model are as follows:

1. Preliminary assessment of obesity level, eating and exercise patterns, emotional status, and degree of motivation.
2. Lifestyle interventions, incorporating (a) setting reasonable goals for weight loss, (b) raising self-awareness as a means of enhancing self-regulation, (c) developing a problem-solving attitude toward common compliance problems, (d) stress management skills, (e) cognitive restructuring, (f) relapse prevention strategies, (g) social support, (h) behavioral contracting to increase health-oriented behaviors, and (i) pharmacotherapy as needed.

SUMMARY

Psychosocial interventions can have a significant impact on increasing healthy behaviors and eliminating those that are harmful. All of the diseases discussed in this chapter — CVD, stroke, COPD, diabetes, obesity, and the MS — are largely preventable via healthy lifestyle patterns (85). Unfortunately, we are currently facing the prospect of increases in most of these conditions because of an aging population, lack of prevention-oriented initiatives at a sociocultural level, and an overall largely sedentary population (93). Moreover, there has been insufficient progress on amelioration of psychological conditions, including the SAD trio (stress, anxiety, depression) discussed here, despite the

attention called to these conditions by the U.S. Surgeon General years ago in the context of an integrated view of mental and physical health. In addition, the recent *Healthy People 2010, Midcourse Review* (282) revealed that of 14 objectives related to promoting mental health and treating mental illness, only 3 had moved toward or met the targeted goal.

There are, however, some promising developments, including the implementation of the Mental Health Parity and Addiction Equity Act (MHPAEA) of 2008 (197), which requires that group health insurance plans have financial requirements and treatment limitations that are no more restrictive for psychological treatment than those for medical care. There is also a clear trend toward greater integration of psychosocial interventions with traditional medical treatment of chronic disease, consistent with Engel's biopsychosocial model (102). Clinical exercise professionals can play an important role in this more integrative management of chronic illnesses by developing a sensitivity to psychologically based impediments to physical activity, knowing when to refer patients for mental health services, and incorporating basic elements of the cognitive behavioral and mindfulness- and acceptance-based perspectives described here into their day-to-day work as a way of encouraging self-efficacy and self-regulatory capacities.

REFERENCES

1. Adams KJ, Salmon P. Acute adjustments for stress. *Strength Cond J.* 2002;24(1):63–4.
2. Adams RJ, Appleton S, Wilson DH, et al. Population comparison of two clinical approaches to the metabolic syndrome: implications of the new International Diabetes Federation consensus definition. *Diabetes Care.* 2005;28(11):2777–9.
3. Adams SG, Smith PK, Allan PF, Anzueto A, Pugh JA, Cornell JE. Systematic review of the chronic care model in chronic obstructive pulmonary disease prevention and management. *Arch Intern Med.* 2007;167(6):551–61.
4. Ader R, Cohen N. Behaviorally conditioned immunosuppression. *Psychosom Med.* 1975;37(4):333–40.
5. Adili F, Larijani B, Haghighatpanah M. Diabetic patients: psychological aspects. *Ann N Y Acad Sci.* 2006;1084:329–49.
6. Ajzen I. *Attitudes, Personality, and Behavior.* U.S. ed. Chicago (IL): Dorsey Press; 1988. 175 p.
7. Aldana SG, Greenlaw R, Thomas D, et al. The influence of an intense cardiovascular disease risk factor modification program. *Preventive Cardiology.* 2004;7(1):19–25.
8. Allen NB, Chambers R, Knight W, Melbourne Academic Mindfulness Interest Group. Mindfulness-based psychotherapies: a review of conceptual foundations, empirical evidence and practical considerations. *Aust N Z J Psychiatry.* 2006;40(4):285–94.
9. Allport GW. *Personality: A Psychological Interpretation.* New York (NY): H. Holt and Company; 1937. 588 p.
10. American Diabetes Association. Diagnosis and classification of diabetes mellitus. *Diabetes Care.* 2007;30 Suppl 1:S42–7.
11. American Diabetes Association. Standards of medical care in diabetes—2011. *Diabetes Care.* 2011;34 Suppl 1:S11–61.
12. American Psychiatric Association, American Psychiatric Association, Task Force on DSM-IV. *Diagnostic and Statistical Manual of Mental Disorders: DSM-IV.* 4th ed. Washington (DC): American Psychiatric Association; 1994. 886 p.

13. American Psychiatric Association, American Psychiatric Association, Task Force on DSM-IV. *Diagnostic and Statistical Manual of Mental Disorders: DSM-IV-TR*. 4th ed. Washington (DC): American Psychiatric Association; 2000. 943 p.

14. Anda R, Williamson D, Jones D, et al. Depressed affect, hopelessness, and the risk of ischemic heart disease in a cohort of U.S. adults. *Epidemiology*. 1993;4(4):285–94.

15. Annesi JJ, Whitaker AC. Psychological factors discriminating between successful and unsuccessful weight loss in a behavioral exercise and nutrition education treatment. *Int J Behav Med*. 2010;17(3):168–75.

16. Antoni MH, Baggett L, Ironson G, et al. Cognitive-behavioral stress management intervention buffers distress responses and immunologic changes following notification of HIV-1 seropositivity. *J Consult Clin Psychol*. 1991;59(6):906–15.

17. Antonovsky A. The structure and properties of the sense of coherence scale. *Soc Sci Med*. 1993;36(6):725–33.

18. Antonovsky A. *Unraveling the Mystery of Health: How People Manage Stress and Stay Well*. 1st ed. San Francisco (CA): Jossey-Bass; 1987. 218 p.

19. Anzueto A. Clinical course of chronic obstructive pulmonary disease: review of therapeutic interventions. *Am J Med*. 2006;119 (10 Suppl):46–53.

20. Appels A. Psychological prodromata of myocardial infarction and sudden death. *Psychother Psychosom*. 1980;34(2–3):187–95.

21. Appels A, Bar FW, Bar J, Bruggeman C, de Baets M. Inflammation, depressive symptomtology, and coronary artery disease. *Psychosom Med*. 2000;62(5):601–5.

22. Appels CW, Bolk JH. Sudden death after emotional stress: a case history and literature review. *Eur J Intern Med*. 2009;20(4):359–61.

23. Armstrong LE, VanHeest JL. The unknown mechanism of the overtraining syndrome: clues from depression and psychoneuroimmunology. *Sports Med*. 2002;32(3):185–209.

24. Artal M. Exercise against depression. *Phys Sportsmed*. 1998;26(10):55–60.

25. Asay TP, Lambert MJ. The empirical case for the common factors in therapy: quantitative findings. In: Hubble MA, Duncan BL, Miller SD, editors. *The Heart & Soul of Change: What Works in Therapy*. Washington: American Psychological Association; 1999. p. 23–55.

26. Bahrke MS, Morgan WP. Anxiety reduction following exercise and meditation. *Cognitive Ther Res*. 1978;2(4):323–33.

27. Bandura A. Health promotion by social cognitive means. *Health Educ Behav*. 2004;31(2):143–64.

28. Bandura A. The primacy of self-regulation in health promotion. *Appl Psychol*. 2005;54(2):245–54.

29. Bandura A. *Principles of Behavior Modification*. New York (NY): Holt, Rinehart and Winston; 1969. 677 p.

30. Bandura A. *Self-Efficacy: The Exercise of Control*. New York (NY): W.H. Freeman; 1997. 604 p.

31. Bandura A. *Social Foundations of Thought and Action: A Social Cognitive Theory*. Englewood Cliffs (NJ): Prentice-Hall; 1986. 617 p.

32. Bandura A. *Social Learning Theory*. Englewood Cliffs (NJ): Prentice Hall; 1977. 247 p.

33. Baraniak A, Sheffield D. The efficacy of psychologically based interventions to improve anxiety, depression and quality of life in COPD: a systematic review and meta-analysis. *Patient Educ Couns*. 2011;83(1):29–36.

34. Barefoot JC, Dahlstrom WG, Williams RB Jr. Hostility, CHD incidence, and total mortality: a 25-year follow-up study of 255 physicians. *Psychosom Med*. 1983;45(1):59–63.

35. Barger SD, Sydeman SJ. Does generalized anxiety disorder predict coronary heart disease risk factors independently of major depressive disorder? *J Affect Disord*. 2005;88(1):87–91.

36. Barlow DH. *Anxiety and Its Disorders: The Nature and Treatment of Anxiety and Panic*. 2nd ed. New York (NY): Guilford Press; 2002. 704 p.

37. Barlow DH. *Clinical Handbook of Psychological Disorders: A Step-by-Step Treatment Manual*. 3rd ed. New York (NY): Guilford Press; 2001. 659 p.

38. Barlow DH. *Clinical Handbook of Psychological Disorders: A Step-by-Step Treatment Manual*. 4th ed. New York (NY): Guilford Press; 2008. 722 p.

39. Barlow DH, Allen LB, Choate ML. Toward a unified treatment for emotional disorders. *Behav Ther*. 2004;35(2):205–30.

40. Bartholomew JB, Morrison D, Ciccolo JT. Effects of acute exercise on mood and well-being in patients with major depressive disorder. *Med Sci Sports Exerc*. 2005;37(12):2032–7.

41. Beck AT. *Cognitive Therapy of Depression*. New York (NY): Guilford Press; 1979. 425 p.

42. Beck AT. *Depression: Clinical, Experimental, and Theoretical Aspects*. New York (NY): Hoeber Medical Division, Harper & Row; 1967. 370 p.

43. Beutler LE, Malik ML. The emergence of dissatisfaction with the DSM. In: Beutler LE, Malik ML, editors. *Rethinking the DSM: A Psychological Perspective*. Washington: American Psychological Association; 2002. p. 3–16.

44. Biolo G, Ciocchi B, Stulle M, et al. Metabolic consequences of physical inactivity. *J Ren Nutr*. 2005;15(1):49–53.

45. Blue CL. The predictive capacity of the theory of reasoned action and the theory of planned behavior in exercise research: an integrated literature review. *Res Nurs Health*. 1995;18(2):105–21.

46. Blumenthal JA, Babyak M, Wei J, et al. Usefulness of psychosocial treatment of mental stress-induced myocardial ischemia in men. *Am J Cardiol*. 2002;89(2):164–8.

47. Blumenthal JA, Babyak MA, Carney RM, et al. Exercise, depression, and mortality after myocardial infarction in the ENRICHD trial. *Med Sci Sports Exerc*. 2004;36(5):746–55.

48. Blumenthal JA, Sherwood A, Babyak MA, et al. Effects of exercise and stress management training on markers of cardiovascular risk in patients with ischemic heart disease: a randomized controlled trial. *JAMA*. 2005;293(13):1626–34.

49. Bodenheimer T. High and rising health care costs. Part 2: technologic innovation. *Ann Intern Med*. 2005;142(11):932–7.

50. Bond DS, Phelan S, Leahey TM, Hill JO, Wing RR. Weight-loss maintenance in successful weight losers: surgical vs non-surgical methods. *Int J Obes (Lond)*. 2009;33(1):173–80.

51. Boney CM, Verma A, Tucker R, Vohr BR. Metabolic syndrome in childhood: association with birth weight, maternal obesity, and gestational diabetes mellitus. *Pediatrics*. 2005;115(3):e290–6.

52. Borkovec TD, Inz J. The nature of worry in generalized anxiety disorder: a predominance of thought activity. *Behav Res Ther*. 1990;28(2):153–8.

53. Brass LM. Strategies for primary and secondary stroke prevention. *Clin Cardiol*. 2006;29(10 Suppl):II21–7.

54. Brenes GA. Anxiety and chronic obstructive pulmonary disease: prevalence, impact, and treatment. *Psychosom Med*. 2003;65(6):963–70.

55. Brewin CR. Theoretical foundations of cognitive-behavior therapy for anxiety and depression. *Annu Rev Psychol*. 1996;47:33–57.

56. Brindley DN, McCann BS, Niaura R, Stoney CM, Suarez EC. Stress and lipoprotein metabolism: modulators and mechanisms. *Metabolism*. 1993;42(9 Suppl 1):3–15.

57. Brinthaupt TM, Kang M, Anshel MH. A delivery model for overcoming psycho-behavioral barriers to exercise. *Psychol Sport Exerc*. 2010;11(4):259–66.

58. Brownson RC, Boehmer TK, Luke DA. Declining rates of physical activity in the United States: what are the contributors? *Annu Rev Public Health*. 2005;26:421–43.

59. Buckworth J, Dishman RK. *Exercise Psychology*. Champaign (IL): Human Kinetics; 2002. 330 p.

60. Burgess A, Kunik ME, Stanley MA. Chronic obstructive pulmonary disease: assessing and treating psychological issues in patients with COPD. *Geriatrics*. 2005;60(12):18–21.

61. Cagampang FR, Poore KR, Hanson MA. Developmental origins of the metabolic syndrome: body clocks and stress responses. *Brain Behav Immun.* 2011;25(2):214–20.

62. Cannon WB. *The Wisdom of the Body.* New York (NY): W.W. Norton & Company; 1939. 315 p.

63. Carney RM, Blumenthal JA, Freedland KE, et al. Depression and late mortality after myocardial infarction in the Enhancing Recovery in Coronary Heart Disease (ENRICHD) study. *Psychosom Med.* 2004;66(4):466–74.

64. Carney RM, Freedland KE, Veith RC. Depression, the autonomic nervous system, and coronary heart disease. *Psychosom Med.* 2005;67 Suppl 1:S29–33.

65. Carrieri-Kohlman V, Donesky-Cuenco D, Park SK, Mackin L, Nguyen HQ, Paul SM. Additional evidence for the affective dimension of dyspnea in patients with COPD. *Res Nurs Health.* 2010;33(1):4–19.

66. Cassells HB, Haffner SM. The metabolic syndrome: risk factors and management. *J Cardiovasc Nurs.* 2006;21(4):306–13.

67. Chambliss DL, Baker MJ, Baucom DH, et al. Update on empirically validated therapies, II. *Clin Psychol.* 1998;51(1):3–16.

68. Chevalier P, Cottraux J, Mollard E, et al. Prevention of implantable defibrillator shocks by cognitive behavioral therapy: a pilot trial. *Am Heart J.* 2006;151(1):191.

69. *Chronic Obstructive Pulmonary Disease Surveillance—United States, 1971–2000* [Internet]. Atlanta, GA: Centers for Disease Control and Prevention, U.S. Department of Health and Human Services; 2002 [cited 2007 May 25]. Available from: http://www.cdc.gov/mmwr/preview/mmwrhtml/ss5106a1.htm

70. Chung ML, Moser DK, Lennie TA, Rayens MK. The effects of depressive symptoms and anxiety on quality of life in patients with heart failure and their spouses: testing dyadic dynamics using Actor-Partner Interdependence Model. *J Psychosom Res.* 2009;67(1):29–35.

71. Claesson M, Birgander LS, Jansson JH, et al. Cognitive-behavioural stress management does not improve biological cardiovascular risk indicators in women with ischaemic heart disease: a randomized-controlled trial. *J Intern Med.* 2006;260(4):320–31.

72. Clark DA, Beck AT, Alford BA. *Scientific Foundations of Cognitive Theory and Therapy of Depression.* New York (NY): John Wiley; 1999. 494 p.

73. Clark LA. Assessment and diagnosis of personality disorder: perennial issues and an emerging reconceptualization. *Annu Rev Psychol.* 2007;58:227–57.

74. Cohen S. Keynote Presentation at the Eight International Congress of Behavioral Medicine: the Pittsburgh common cold studies: psychosocial predictors of susceptibility to respiratory infectious illness. *Int J Behav Med.* 2005;12(3):123–31.

75. Cohen S, Frank E, Doyle WJ, Skoner DP, Rabin BS, Gwaltney JM Jr. Types of stressors that increase susceptibility to the common cold in healthy adults. *Health Psychol.* 1998;17(3):214–23.

76. Cohen S, Herbert TB. Health psychology: psychological factors and physical disease from the perspective of human psychoneuroimmunology. *Annu Rev Psychol.* 1996;47:113–42.

77. Cohen S, Kamarck T, Mermelstein R. A global measure of perceived stress. *J Health Soc Behav.* 1983;24(4):385–96.

78. Cohen SM, Kataoka-Yahiro M. Themes in the literature related to cardiovascular disease risk reduction. *J Cardiovasc Nurs.* 2009;24(4):268–76.

79. Colberg SR, Sigal RJ, Fernhall B, et al. Exercise and type 2 diabetes: the American College of Sports Medicine and the American Diabetes Association: joint position statement. *Diabetes Care.* 2010;33(12):e147–67.

80. Cooper Z, Fairburn CG. A new cognitive behavioural approach to the treatment of obesity. *Behav Res Ther.* 2001;39(5):499–511.

81. Costa PT Jr, McCrae RR. Personality assessment in psychosomatic medicine. Value of a trait taxonomy. *Adv Psychosom Med.* 1987;17:71–82.

82. *Cross-Cutting Dimensional Assessment in DSM-5. American Psychiatric Association DSM-5 Development* [Internet]. Arlington, VA: American Psychiatric Association [cited 2011 Apr 25]. Available from: http://www.dsm5.org

83. Cully JA, Graham DP, Stanley MA, et al. Quality of life in patients with chronic obstructive pulmonary disease and comorbid anxiety or depression. *Psychosomatics.* 2006;47(4):312–9.

84. Dalle Grave R, Calugi S, Centis E, El Ghoch M, Marchesini G. Cognitive-behavioral strategies to increase the adherence to exercise in the management of obesity. *J Obes.* 2011;2011:1–11.

85. Danaei G, Ding EL, Mozaffarian D, et al. The preventable causes of death in the United States: comparative risk assessment of dietary, lifestyle, and metabolic risk factors. *PLoS Med.* 2009;6(4):e1000058.

86. Dantzer R, Kelley KW. Twenty years of research on cytokine-induced sickness behavior. *Brain Behav Immun.* 2007;21(2):153–60.

87. Davidson KW, Rieckmann N, Rapp MA. Definitions and distinctions among depressive syndromes and symptoms: implications for a better understanding of the depression-cardiovascular disease association. *Psychosom Med.* 2005;67 Suppl 1:S6–9.

88. De Moor MH, Beem AL, Stubbe JH, Boomsma DI, De Geus EJ. Regular exercise, anxiety, depression and personality: a population-based study. *Prev Med.* 2006;42(4):273–9.

89. de Voogd JN, Wempe JB, Postema K, et al. More evidence that depressive symptoms predict mortality in COPD patients: is type D personality an alternative explanation? *Ann Behav Med.* 2009;38(2):86–93.

90. DeFronzo RA, Sherwin RS, Kraemer N. Effect of physical training on insulin action in obesity. *Diabetes.* 1987;36(12):1379–85.

91. Deslandes A, Moraes H, Ferreira C, et al. Exercise and mental health: many reasons to move. *Neuropsychobiology.* 2009;59(4):191–8.

92. DiMatteo MR. Variations in patients' adherence to medical recommendations: a quantitative review of 50 years of research. *Med Care.* 2004;42(3):200–9.

93. Dishman RK, Buckworth J. Increasing physical activity: a quantitative synthesis. *Med Sci Sports Exerc.* 1996;28(6):706–19.

94. Dishman RK, Jackson EM. Exercise, fitness, and stress. *Int J Sport Psychol.* 2000;31(2):175–203.

95. Dishman RK, Vandenberg RJ, Motl RW, Nigg CR. Using constructs of the transtheoretical model to predict classes of change in regular physical activity: a multi-ethnic longitudinal cohort study. *Ann Behav Med.* 2010;40(2):150–63.

96. Ditto B, Eclache M, Goldman N. Short-term autonomic and cardiovascular effects of mindfulness body scan meditation. *Ann Behav Med.* 2006;32(3):227–34.

97. Dobson DJG, Dobson KS. *Evidence-Based Practice of Cognitive-Behavioral Therapy.* New York (NY): Guilford Press; 2009. 322 p.

98. Donnelly JE, Blair SN, Jakicic JM, et al. American College of Sports Medicine Position Stand. Appropriate physical activity intervention strategies for weight loss and prevention of weight regain for adults. *Med Sci Sports Exerc.* 2009;41(2):459–71.

99. Egede LE. Diabetes, major depression, and functional disability among U.S. adults. *Diabetes Care.* 2004;27(2):421–8.

100. Ekkekakis P, Acevedo EO. Affect responses to acute exercise: toward a psychobiological dose-response model. In: Acevedo EO, Ekkekakis P, editors. *Psychobiology of Physical Activity.* Champaign: Human Kinetics; 2006. p. 91–109.

101. Emmelkamp PM, van Oppen P. Cognitive interventions in behavioral medicine. *Psychother Psychosom.* 1993;59(3–4):116–30.

102. Engel GL. The need for a new medical model: a challenge for biomedicine. *Science.* 1977;196(4286):129–36.

103. Expert Panel on Detection, Evaluation, and Treatment of High Blood Cholesterol in Adults. Executive Summary of the Third Report of the National Cholesterol Education Program (NCEP) Expert Panel on Detection, Evaluation, and Treatment of High Blood Cholesterol in Adults (Adult Treatment Panel III). *JAMA.* 2001;285(19):2486–97.

104. Fedder DO, Desai H, Maciunskaite M. Putting a public health face on clinical practice: potential for using an infectious disease management model for chronic disease prevention. *Dis Manage Health Outcomes.* 2006;14(6):329–33.

105. Fishbein M. A theory of reasoned action: some applications and implications. *Nebr Symp Motiv.* 1980;27:65–116.

106. Follette WC. Introduction to the special section on the development of theoretically coherent alternatives to the DSM system. *J Consult Clin Psychol.* 1996;64(6):1117–9.

107. Ford ES, Giles WH, Dietz WH. Prevalence of the metabolic syndrome among US adults: findings from the third National Health and Nutrition Examination Survey. *JAMA.* 2002;287(3):356–9.

108. Foreyt JP. Need for lifestyle intervention: how to begin. *Am J Cardiol.* 2005;96(4A):11E–4E.

109. Foreyt JP, Goodrick GK. Evidence for success of behavior modification in weight loss and control. *Ann Intern Med.* 1993;119 (7 Pt 2):698–701.

110. Foreyt JP, Poston WS,2nd. What is the role of cognitive-behavior therapy in patient management? *Obes Res.* 1998;6 Suppl 1:18–22S.

111. Foy CG, Wickley KL, Adair N, et al. The Reconditioning Exercise and Chronic Obstructive Pulmonary Disease Trial II (REACT II): rationale and study design for a clinical trial of physical activity among individuals with chronic obstructive pulmonary disease. *Contemp Clin Trials.* 2006;27(2):135–46.

112. Frank JD, Frank J. *Persuasion and Healing: A Comparative Study of Psychotherapy.* 3rd ed. Baltimore (MD): Johns Hopkins University Press; 1991. 343 p.

113. Franks CM. *Behavior Therapy: Appraisal and Status.* New York (NY): McGraw-Hill; 1969. 730 p.

114. Frasure-Smith N, Lesperance F, Talajic M. Depression and 18-month prognosis after myocardial infarction. *Circulation.* 1995; 91(4):999–1005.

115. Friedman HS. The multiple linkages of personality and disease. *Brain Behav Immun.* 2008;22(5):668–75.

116. Friedman HS. Personality and disease: overview, review, and preview. In: Friedman HS, editor. *Personality and Disease.* New York: Wiley; 1990. p. 3–13.

117. Friedman M, Rosenman RH. Association of specific overt behavior pattern with blood and cardiovascular findings; blood cholesterol level, blood clotting time, incidence of arcus senilis, and clinical coronary artery disease. *J Am Med Assoc.* 1959;169(12):1286–96.

118. Friedman M, Rosenman RH. *Type A Behavior and Your Heart.* 1st ed. New York (NY): Knopf; 1974. 319 p.

119. Friedman R, Sobel D, Myers P, Caudill M, Benson H. Behavioral medicine, clinical health psychology, and cost offset. *Health Psychol.* 1995;14(6):509–18.

120. Gabbard GO, Lazar SG, Hornberger J, Spiegel D. The economic impact of psychotherapy: a review. *Am J Psychiatry.* 1997;154(2):147–55.

121. Ganne S, Arora S, Karam J, McFarlane SI. Therapeutic interventions for hypertension in metabolic syndrome: a comprehensive approach. *Expert Rev Cardiovasc Ther.* 2007;5(2):201–11.

122. Garber CE, Blissmer B, Deschenes MR, et al. Quantity and quality of exercise for developing and maintaining cardiorespiratory, musculoskeletal, and neuromotor fitness in apparently healthy adults: guidance for prescribing exercise. *Med Sci Sports Exerc.* 2011;43(7):1334–59.

123. Gardner FL, Moore ZE. A mindfulness-acceptance-commitment-based approach to athletic performance enhancement: theoretical considerations. *Behavior Therapy.* 2004;35(4):707–23.

124. Gardner FL, Moore ZE. *The Psychology of Enhancing Human Performance: The Mindfulness-Acceptance-Commitment (MAC) Approach.* New York (NY): Springer; 2007. 289 p.

125. Gelenberg AJ, Hopkins HS. Assessing and treating depression in primary care medicine. *Am J Med.* 2007;120(2):105–8.

126. Gill JM, Malkova D. Physical activity, fitness and cardiovascular disease risk in adults: interactions with insulin resistance and obesity. *Clin Sci (Lond).* 2006;110(4):409–25.

127. Golay A, Buclin S, Ybarra J, et al. New interdisciplinary cognitive-behavioural-nutritional approach to obesity treatment: a 5-year follow-up study. *Eat Weight Disord.* 2004;9(1):29–34.

128. Goodwin RD. Association between physical activity and mental disorders among adults in the United States. *Prev Med.* 2003; 36(6):698–703.

129. Gorelick PB, Scuteri A, Black SE, et al. Vascular contributions to cognitive impairment and dementia: a statement for healthcare professionals from the American Heart Association/American Stroke Association. *Stroke.* 2011;2011:1–11.

130. Gould KL, Ornish D, Scherwitz L, et al. Changes in myocardial perfusion abnormalities by positron emission tomography after long-term, intense risk factor modification. *JAMA.* 1995;274(11): 894–901.

131. Grant BF, Hasin DS, Stinson FS, et al. Co-occurrence of 12-month mood and anxiety disorders and personality disorders in the US: results from the national epidemiologic survey on alcohol and related conditions. *J Psychiatr Res.* 2005;39(1):1–9.

132. Grassi G. Sympathetic overdrive and cardiovascular risk in the metabolic syndrome. *Hypertens Res.* 2006;29(11):839–47.

133. Greeno CG, Wing RR. Stress-induced eating. *Psychol Bull.* 1994; 115(3):444–64.

134. Grippo AJ, Johnson AK. Stress, depression and cardiovascular dysregulation: a review of neurobiological mechanisms and the integration of research from preclinical disease models. *Stress.* 2009; 12(1):1–21.

135. Hao Z, Wu B, Wang D, Liu M. Association between metabolic syndrome and cognitive decline: a systematic review of prospective population-based studies. *Acta Neuropsychiatrica.* 2011;23(2):69–74.

136. Harris AHS, Cronkite R, Moos R. Physical activity, exercise coping, and depression in a 10-year cohort study of depressed patients. *J Affect Disord.* 2006;93(1–3):79–85.

137. Hayes SC. Acceptance and commitment therapy, relational frame theory, and the third wave of behavioral and cognitive therapies. *Behav Ther.* 2004;35(4):639–65.

138. Hayes SC, Follette VM, Linehan M. *Mindfulness and Acceptance: Expanding the Cognitive-Behavioral Tradition.* New York (NY): Guilford Press; 2004. 319 p.

139. Hays PA. *Addressing Cultural Complexities in Practice: A Framework for Clinicians and Counselors.* 1st ed. Washington (DC): American Psychological Association; 2001. 239 p.

140. Heiskanen TH, Niskanen LK, Hintikka JJ, et al. Metabolic syndrome and depression: a cross-sectional analysis. *J Clin Psychiatry.* 2006;67(9):1422–7.

141. Herning MM, Cook JH, Schneider JK. Cognitive behavioral therapy to promote exercise behavior in older adults: implications for physical therapists. *J Geriatr Phys Ther.* 2005;28(2):34–8.

142. Herridge ML, Stimler CE, Southard DR, King ML, AACVPR Task Force. Depression screening in cardiac rehabilitation: AACVPR Task Force Report. *J Cardiopulm Rehabil.* 2005;25(1):11–3.

143. Herring SA, Boyajian-O'Neill LA, Coppel DB, et al. Psychological issues related to injury in athletes and the team physician: a consensus statement. *Med Sci Sports Exerc.* 2006;38(11):2030–4.

144. Himelhoch S, Medoff DR, Oyeniyi G. Efficacy of group psychotherapy to reduce depressive symptoms among HIV-infected individuals: a systematic review and meta-analysis. *AIDS Patient Care STDS.* 2007;21(10):732–9.

145. Hirschfeld RM, Montgomery SA, Keller MB, et al. Social functioning in depression: a review. *J Clin Psychiatry.* 2000;61(4):268–75.

146. Holmes TH, Rahe RH. The social readjustment rating scale. *J Psychosom Res.* 1967;11(2):213–8.

147. Hoppes K. The application of mindfulness-based cognitive interventions in the treatment of co-occurring addictive and mood disorders. *CNS Spectr.* 2006;11(11):829–51.

148. Horton ES. Effects of lifestyle changes to reduce risks of diabetes and associated cardiovascular risks: results from large scale efficacy trials. *Obesity (Silver Spring).* 2009;17 Suppl 3:S43–8.

149. Huffman JC, Smith FA, Quinn DK, Fricchione GL. Post-MI psychiatric syndromes: six unanswered questions. *Harv Rev Psychiatry*. 2006;14(6):305–18.

150. *The IDF Consensus Worldwide Definition of the Metabolic Syndrome* [Internet]. Brussels (Belgium): International Diabetes Federation; 2006 [cited 2008 Apr 3]. 24 p. Available from: http://www.idf .org/webdata/docs/MetS_def_update2006.pdf

151. Institute of Medicine (U.S.), Committee on Health and Behavior: Research, Practice, and Policy. *Health and Behavior: The Interplay of Biological, Behavioral, and Societal Influences*. Washington (DC): National Academy Press; 2001. 377 p.

152. Jakicic JM, Otto AD. Treatment and prevention of obesity: what is the role of exercise? *Nutr Rev*. 2006;64(2 Pt 2):S57–61.

153. Jonas BS, Franks P, Ingram DD. Are symptoms of anxiety and depression risk factors for hypertension? Longitudinal evidence from the National Health and Nutrition Examination Survey I Epidemiologic Follow-up Study. *Arch Fam Med*. 1997;6(1):43–9.

154. Kabat-Zinn J. *Full Catastrophe Living: Using the Wisdom of Your Body and Mind to Face Stress, Pain, and Illness*. New York (NY): Delacorte Press; 1990. 453 p.

155. Kawachi I, Sparrow D, Vokonas PS, Weiss ST. Symptoms of anxiety and risk of coronary heart disease. The Normative Aging Study. *Circulation*. 1994;90(5):2225–9.

156. Kessler RC, Akiskal HS, Ames M, et al. Prevalence and effects of mood disorders on work performance in a nationally representative sample of U.S. workers. *Am J Psychiatry*. 2006;163(9):1561–8.

157. Kessler RC, Chiu WT, Demler O, Merikangas KR, Walters EE. Prevalence, severity, and comorbidity of 12-month DSM-IV disorders in the National Comorbidity Survey Replication. *Arch Gen Psychiatry*. 2005;62(6):617–27.

158. Ketterer MW, Mahr G, Goldberg AD. Psychological factors affecting a medical condition: ischemic coronary heart disease. *J Psychosom Res*. 2000;48(4–5):357–67.

159. Kiecolt-Glaser JK, Gouin JP, Hantsoo L. Close relationships, inflammation, and health. *Neurosci Biobehav Rev*. 2010;35(1):33–8.

160. Kiecolt-Glaser JK, Newton TL. Marriage and health: his and hers. *Psychol Bull*. 2001;127(4):472–503.

161. Kirk AF, Mutrie N, Macintyre PD, Fisher MB. Promoting and maintaining physical activity in people with type 2 diabetes. *Am J Prev Med*. 2004;27(4):289–96.

162. Kneebone II, Dunmore E. Psychological management of post-stroke depression. *Br J Clin Psychol*. 2000;39(Pt 1):53–65.

163. Kop WJ, Appels AP, Mendes de Leon CF, de Swart HB, Bar FW. Vital exhaustion predicts new cardiac events after successful coronary angioplasty. *Psychosom Med*. 1994;56(4):281–7.

164. Korte SM, Koolhaas JM, Wingfield JC, McEwen BS. The Darwinian concept of stress: benefits of allostasis and costs of allostatic load and the trade-offs in health and disease. *Neurosci Biobehav Rev*. 2005;29(1):3–38.

165. Krantz DS, Manuck SB. Acute psychophysiologic reactivity and risk of cardiovascular disease: a review and methodologic critique. *Psychol Bull*. 1984;96(3):435–64.

166. Krishnan KR. Treatment of depression in the medically ill. *J Clin Psychopharmacol*. 2005;25(4 Suppl 1):S14–8.

167. Kunik ME, Braun U, Stanley MA, et al. One session cognitive behavioural therapy for elderly patients with chronic obstructive pulmonary disease. *Psychol Med*. 2001;31(4):717–23.

168. La Forge R. Aligning mind and body: exploring the disciplines of mindful exercise. *ACSM's Health Fit J*. 2005;9(5):7–14.

169. Lazarus RS. *Emotion and Adaptation*. New York (NY): Oxford University Press; 1991. 557 p.

170. Lazarus RS. How emotions influence performance in competitive sports. *Sport Psychol*. 2000;14(3):229–52.

171. Lazarus RS. *Stress and Emotion: A New Synthesis*. New York (NY): Springer; 1999. 342 p.

172. Lazarus RS. Toward better research on stress and coping. *Am Psychol*. 2000;55(6):665–73.

173. Lazarus RS, Folkman S. *Stress, Appraisal, and Coping*. New York (NY): Springer; 1984. 445 p.

174. Lehmann M, Foster C, Keul J. Overtraining in endurance athletes: a brief review. *Med Sci Sports Exerc*. 1993;25(7):854–62.

175. Lewinsohn PM, Weinstein MS, Shaw DA. Depression: a clinical-research approach. In: Rubin RD, Franks CM, Association for Advancement of Behavior Therapy, editors. *Advances in Behavior Therapy, 1968; Symposium Held in San Francisco, August 1968*. New York: Academic Press; 1969. p. 231–240.

176. Lewis M, Sutton A. Understanding exercise behavior: examining the interaction of exercise motivation and personality in predicting exercise frequency. *J Sport Behav*. 2011;34(1):82–97.

177. Linden W, Stossel C, Maurice J. Psychosocial interventions for patients with coronary artery disease: a meta-analysis. *Arch Intern Med*. 1996;156(7):745–52.

178. Long BC, van Stavel R. Effects of exercise training on anxiety: a meta-analysis. *J Appl Sport Psychol*. 1995;7(2):167–89.

179. Luppino FS, de Wit LM, Bouvy PF, et al. Overweight, obesity, and depression: a systematic review and meta-analysis of longitudinal studies. *Arch Gen Psychiatry*. 2010;67(3):220–9.

180. Lustman PJ, Clouse RE. Depression in diabetic patients: the relationship between mood and glycemic control. *J Diabetes Complications*. 2005;19(2):113–22.

181. Lustman PJ, Griffith LS, Freedland KE, Kissel SS, Clouse RE. Cognitive behavior therapy for depression in type 2 diabetes mellitus. A randomized, controlled trial. *Ann Intern Med*. 1998;129(8): 613–21.

182. Maier SF, Watkins LR. Cytokines for psychologists: implications of bidirectional immune-to-brain communication for understanding behavior, mood, and cognition. *Psychol Rev*. 1998;105(1):83–107.

183. Maier SF, Watkins LR, Fleshner M. Psychoneuroimmunology. The interfaces between behavior, brain, and immunity. *Am Psychol*. 1994;49(12):1004–17.

184. Mancia G, Bousquet P, Elghozi JL, et al. The sympathetic nervous system and the metabolic syndrome. *J Hypertens*. 2007;25(5):909–20.

185. Manderscheid RW, Ryff CD, Freeman EJ, McKnight-Eily LR, Dhingra S, Strine TW. Evolving definitions of mental illness and wellness. *Prev Chronic Dis*. 2010;7(1):1–6.

186. Marcotte DE, Wilcox-Gok V. Estimating earnings losses due to mental illness: a quantile regression approach. *J Ment Health Policy Econ*. 2003;6(3):123–34.

187. Martinsen EW. Exercise and depression. *Int J Sport Exerc Psychol*. 2005;3(4):469–83.

188. Mast BT, Vedrody S. Poststroke depression: a biopsychosocial approach. *Curr Psychiatry Rep*. 2006;8(1):25–33.

189. McCrae RR, Allik I. *The Five-Factor Model of Personality Across Cultures*. New York (NY): Kluwer Academic; 2002. 333 p.

190. McEwen BS. Protective and damaging effects of stress mediators: central role of the brain. *Dialogues Clin Neurosci*. 2006;8(4):367–81.

191. Meeusen R. Physical activity and neurotransmitter release. In: Acevedo EO, Ekkekakis P, editors. *Psychobiology of Physical Activity*. Champaign: Human Kinetics; 2006. p. 129–143.

192. Meichenbaum D. *Cognitive-Behavior Modification: An Integrative Approach*. New York (NY): Plenum Press; 1977.

193. Meigs JB. Epidemiology of the insulin resistance syndrome. *Curr Diab Rep*. 2003;3(1):73–9.

194. Melchionda N, Besteghi L, Di Domizio S, et al. Cognitive behavioural therapy for obesity: one-year follow-up in a clinical setting. *Eat Weight Disord*. 2003;8(3):188–93.

195. Melzer K, Kayser B, Pichard C. Physical activity: the health benefits outweigh the risks. *Curr Opin Clin Nutr Metab Care*. 2004; 7(6):641–7.

196. Mendes de Leon CF, Czajkowski SM, Freedland KE, et al. The effect of a psychosocial intervention and quality of life after acute myocardial infarction: the Enhancing Recovery in Coronary Heart Disease (ENRICHD) clinical trial. *J Cardiopulm Rehabil*. 2006;26(1):9,13; quiz 14–5.

197. *The Mental Health Parity and Addiction Equity Act of 2008. Employee Benefits Security Administration* [Internet]. Washington, DC: U.S. Department of Labor; 2010 [cited 2011 Apr 14]. Available from: http://www.dol.gov/ebsa/newsroom/fsmhpaea.html

198. Meyer T, Broocks A. Therapeutic impact of exercise on psychiatric diseases: guidelines for exercise testing and prescription. *Sports Med.* 2000;30(4):269–79.

199. Miller GE, Chen E, Zhou ES. If it goes up, must it come down? Chronic stress and the hypothalamic-pituitary-adrenocortical axis in humans. *Psychol Bull.* 2007;133(1):25–45.

200. Mischel W. *Personality and Assessment.* New York (NY): Wiley; 1968. 365 p.

201. Mischel W, Shoda Y. A cognitive-affective system theory of personality: reconceptualizing situations, dispositions, dynamics, and invariance in personality structure. *Psychol Rev.* 1995;102(2):246–68.

202. Mokdad AH, Ford ES, Bowman BA, et al. Prevalence of obesity, diabetes, and obesity-related health risk factors, 2001. *JAMA.* 2003;289(1):76–9.

203. Morgan WP. Methodological considerations. In: Morgan WP, editor. *Physical Activity and Mental Health.* Washington: Taylor & Francis; 1997. p. 3–32.

204. MumFord E, Schlesinger HJ, Glass GV, Patrick C, Cuerdon T. A new look at evidence about reduced cost of medical utilization following mental health treatment. 1984. *J Psychother Pract Res.* 1997;7(1):68,86; discussion 65–7.

205. Nesse RM. Is depression an adaptation? *Arch Gen Psychiatry.* 2000;57(1):14–20.

206. Nicholl CR, Lincoln NB, Muncaster K, Thomas S. Cognitions and post-stroke depression. *Br J Clin Psychol.* 2002;41(Pt 3):221–31.

207. Nutt DJ, Ballenger JC, Sheehan D, Wittchen HU. Generalized anxiety disorder: comorbidity, comparative biology and treatment. *Int J Neuropsychopharmacol.* 2002;5(4):315–25.

208. O'Connor PJ, Raglin JS, Martinsen EW. Physical activity, anxiety and anxiety disorders. *Int J Sport Psychol.* 2000;31(2):136–55.

209. O'Donohue W, Fisher JE. *Cognitive Behavior Therapy: Applying Empirically Supported Techniques in Your Practice.* Hoboken (NJ): John Wiley & Sons; 2008. 642 p.

210. Ogden J. Some problems with social cognition models: a pragmatic and conceptual analysis. *Health Psychol.* 2003;22(4):424–8.

211. O'Neal HA, Dunn AL, Martinsen EW. Depression and exercise. *Int J Sport Psychol.* 2000;31(2):110–35.

212. Ornish D, Scherwitz LW, Billings JH, et al. Intensive lifestyle changes for reversal of coronary heart disease. *JAMA.* 1998;280(23):2001–7.

213. Orsillo SM, Roemer L. *Acceptance and Mindfulness-Based Approaches to Anxiety: Conceptualization and Treatment.* New York (NY): Springer; 2005. 375 p.

214. Pan HJ, Cole BM, Geliebter A. The benefits of body weight loss on health-related quality of life. *J Chin Med Assoc.* 2011;74(4):169–75.

215. Pasic J, Levy WC, Sullivan MD. Cytokines in depression and heart failure. *Psychosom Med.* 2003;65(2):181–93.

216. Patten SB, Williams JV, Lavorato DH, Modgill G, Jette N, Eliasziw M. Major depression as a risk factor for chronic disease incidence: longitudinal analyses in a general population cohort. *Gen Hosp Psychiatry.* 2008;30(5):407–13.

217. Pennebaker JW. *Emotion, Disclosure & Health.* Washington (DC): American Psychological Association; 1995. 337 p.

218. Perna FM, Antoni MH, Baum A, Gordon P, Schneiderman N. Cognitive behavioral stress management effects on injury and illness among competitive athletes: a randomized clinical trial. *Ann Behav Med.* 2003;25(1):66–73.

219. Perna FM, McDowell SL. Role of psychological stress in cortisol recovery from exhaustive exercise among elite athletes. *Int J Behav Med.* 1995;2(1):13–26.

220. Pierson DJ. Clinical practice guidelines for chronic obstructive pulmonary disease: a review and comparison of current resources. *Respir Care.* 2006;51(3):277–88.

221. Pitsavos C, Panagiotakos DB, Papageorgiou C, Tsetsekou E, Soldatos C, Stefanadis C. Anxiety in relation to inflammation and coagulation markers, among healthy adults: the ATTICA study. *Atherosclerosis.* 2006;185(2):320–6.

222. Plante TG. Could the perception of fitness account for many of the mental and physical health benefits of exercise? *Adv Mind Body.* 1999;15(4):291–5.

223. *Post-myocardial Infarction Depression* [Internet]. Rockville (MD): Agency for Healthcare Research and Quality; 2005 [cited 2011 Jul 29]. 310 p. Available from: http://purl.access.gpo.gov/GPO/PS61014

224. Prochaska JO. How do people change, and how can we change to help many more people? In: Hubble MA, Duncan BL, Miller SD, editors. *The Heart & Soul of Change: What Works in Therapy.* Washington: American Psychological Association; 1999. p. 227–55.

225. Prochaska JO, Di Clemente CC. Transtheoretical therapy: toward a more integrative model of change. *Psychotherapy.* 1982;19(3): 276–88.

226. Prochaska JO, Johnson S, Lee P. The transtheoretical model of behavior change. In: Shumaker SA, editor. *The Handbook of Health Behavior Change.* 2nd ed. New York: Springer Pub. Co; 1998. p. 59–84.

227. Pulmonary rehabilitation: joint ACCP/AACVPR evidence-based guidelines. ACCP/AACVPR Pulmonary Rehabilitation Guidelines Panel. American College of Chest Physicians. American Association of Cardiovascular and Pulmonary Rehabilitation. *Chest.* 1997;112(5):1363–96.

228. Raglin JS. Anxiolytic effects of physical activity. In: Morgan WP, editor. *Physical Activity and Mental Health.* Washington: Taylor & Francis; 1997. p. 107–126.

229. Raglin JS, Morgan WP. Influence of vigorous exercise on mood state. *Behav Ther.* 1985;8(9):179–83.

230. Raikkonen K, Matthews KA, Kuller LH. Depressive symptoms and stressful life events predict metabolic syndrome among middle-aged women: a comparison of World Health Organization, Adult Treatment Panel III, and International Diabetes Foundation definitions. *Diabetes Care.* 2007;30(4):872–7.

231. Raison CL, Capuron L, Miller AH. Cytokines sing the blues: inflammation and the pathogenesis of depression. *Trends Immunol.* 2006;27(1):24–31.

232. Reddy P, Ford D, Dunbar JA. Improving the quality of diabetes care in general practice. *Aust J Rural Health.* 2010;18(5):187–93.

233. Rhodes RE, Smith NE. Personality correlates of physical activity: a review and meta-analysis. *Br J Sports Med.* 2006;40(12):958–65.

234. Rimmer JH, Braunschweig C, Silverman K, Riley B, Creviston T, Nicola T. Effects of a short-term health promotion intervention for a predominantly African-American group of stroke survivors. *Am J Prev Med.* 2000;18(4):332–8.

235. Robertson N. Unexplained chest pain: a review of psychological conceptualizations and treatment efficacy. *Psychol Health Med.* 2006;11(2):255–63.

236. Rostad FG, Long BC. Exercise as a coping strategy for stress: a review. *Int J Sport Psychol.* 1996;27(2):197–222.

237. Rozanski A, Blumenthal JA, Kaplan J. Impact of psychological factors on the pathogenesis of cardiovascular disease and implications for therapy. *Circulation.* 1999;99(16):2192–217.

238. Rutledge T, Hogan BE. A quantitative review of prospective evidence linking psychological factors with hypertension development. *Psychosom Med.* 2002;64(5):758–66.

239. Salman GF, Mosier MC, Beasley BW, Calkins DR. Rehabilitation for patients with chronic obstructive pulmonary disease: meta-analysis of randomized controlled trials. *J Gen Intern Med.* 2003; 18(3):213–21.

240. Salmon P. Effects of physical exercise on anxiety, depression, and sensitivity to stress: a unifying theory. *Clin Psychol Rev.* 2001;21(1): 33–61.

241. Salmon P, Sephton S, Weissbecker I, Hoover K, Ulmer C, Studts JL. Mindfulness meditation in clinical practice. *Cogn Behav Pract.* 2004;11(4):434–46.

242. Salmon PG, Sephton SS, Dreeben SJ. Mindfulness-based stress reduction. In: Herbert JD, editor. *Acceptance and Mindfulness in Cognitive Behavior Therapy: Understanding and Applying the New Therapies.* Hoboken: Wiley; 2010. p. 132–163.

243. Sapolsky RM. *Why Zebras Don't Get Ulcers.* 3rd ed. New York (NY): Times Books; 2004. 539 p.

244. Schiller JS, Ni H. Cigarette smoking and smoking cessation among persons with chronic obstructive pulmonary disease. *Am J Health Promot.* 2006;20(5):319–23.

245. Schneiderman N, Siegel SD. Mental and physical health influence each other. In: Lilienfeld SO, O'Donohue WT, editors. *The Great Ideas of Clinical Science: 17 Principles that Every Mental Health Professional should Understand.* New York: Routledge; 2007. p. 329–346.

246. Schraufnagel TJ, Wagner AW, Miranda J, Roy-Byrne PP. Treating minority patients with depression and anxiety: what does the evidence tell us? *Gen Hosp Psychiatry.* 2006;28(1):27–36.

247. Schulberg HC, Katon W, Simon GE, Rush AJ. Treating major depression in primary care practice: an update of the agency for health care policy and research practice guidelines. *Arch Gen Psychiatry.* 1998;55(12):1121–7.

248. Segal ZV, Williams JMG, Teasdale JD. *Mindfulness-Based Cognitive Therapy for Depression: A New Approach to Preventing Relapse.* New York (NY): Guilford Press; 2002. 351 p.

249. Segerstrom SC, Miller GE. Psychological stress and the human immune system: a meta-analytic study of 30 years of inquiry. *Psychol Bull.* 2004;130(4):601–30.

250. Seime RJ, Vickers KS. The challenges of treating depression with exercise: from evidence to practice. *Clin Psychol: Sci Pr.* 2006;13(2):194–7.

251. Seligman MEP. *Helplessness: On Depression, Development, and Death.* New York (NY): W.H. Freeman; 1992. 250 p.

252. Shaw K, Gennat H, O'Rourke P, Del Mar C. Exercise for overweight or obesity. *Cochrane Database Syst Rev.* 2006;(4):CD003817.

253. Shaw K, O'Rourke P, Del Mar C, Kenardy J. Psychological interventions for overweight or obesity. *Cochrane Database Syst Rev.* 2005;(2):CD003818.

254. Sherwood NE, Jeffery RW. The behavioral determinants of exercise: implications for physical activity interventions. *Annu Rev Nutr.* 2000;20:21–44.

255. Shumaker SA, Czajkowski SM. *Social Support and Cardiovascular Disease.* New York (NY): Plenum Press; 1994. 360 p.

256. Siegel DJ. An interpersonal neurobiology approach to psychotherapy. *Psychiat Ann.* 2006;36(4):248–56.

257. Sikdar KC, Wang PP, MacDonald D, Gadag VG. Diabetes and its impact on health-related quality of life: a life table analysis. *Qual Life Res.* 2010;19(6):781–7.

258. Sniehotta FF, Scholz U, Schwarzer R, Fuhrmann B, Kiwus U, Voller H. Long-term effects of two psychological interventions on physical exercise and self-regulation following coronary rehabilitation. *Int J Behav Med.* 2005;12(4):244–55.

259. Snow WM, Connett JE, Sharma S, Murray RP. Predictors of attendance and dropout at the Lung Health Study 11-year follow-up. *Contemp Clin Trials.* 2007;28(1):25–32.

260. Sothmann MS. The cross-stressor adaptation hypothesis and exercise training. In: Acevedo EO, Ekkekakis P, editors. *Psychobiology of Physical Activity.* Champaign: Human Kinetics; 2006. p. 149–160.

261. Sothmann MS, Buckworth J, Claytor RP, Cox RH, White-Welkley JE, Dishman RK. Exercise training and the cross-stressor adaptation hypothesis. *Exerc Sport Sci Rev.* 1996;24:267–87.

262. Spangenberg JJ, Theron JC. Stress and coping strategies in spouses of depressed patients. *J Psychol.* 1999;133(3):253–62.

263. Spencer L, Adams TB, Malone S, Roy L, Yost E. Applying the transtheoretical model to exercise: a systematic and comprehensive review of the literature. *Health Promot Pract.* 2006;7(4):428–43.

264. Spielmans GI, Berman MI, Usitalo AN. Psychotherapy versus second-generation antidepressants in the treatment of depression: a meta-analysis. *J Nerv Ment Dis.* 2011;199(3):142–9.

265. Spruijt-Metz D. Etiology, treatment and prevention of obesity in childhood and adolescence: a decade in review. *J Res Adolesc.* 2011;21(1):129–52.

266. Stahre L, Tarnell B, Hakanson CE, Hallstrom T. A randomized controlled trial of two weight-reducing short-term group treatment programs for obesity with an 18-month follow-up. *Int J Behav Med.* 2007;14(1):48–55.

267. Stalnikowicz R, Tsafrir A. Acute psychosocial stress and cardiovascular events. *Am J Emerg Med.* 2002;20(5):488–91.

268. Stanley MA, Beck JG, Novy DM, et al. Cognitive-behavioral treatment of late-life generalized anxiety disorder. *J Consult Clin Psychol.* 2003;71(2):309–19.

269. Stein DJ, Collins M, Daniels W, Noakes TD, Zigmond M. Mind and muscle: the cognitive-affective neuroscience of exercise. *CNS Spectr.* 2007;12(1):19–22.

270. Steptoe A, Dockray S, Wardle J. Positive affect and psychobiological processes relevant to health. *J Pers.* 2009;77(6):1747–76.

271. Stewart JC, Janicki DL, Muldoon MF, Sutton-Tyrrell K, Kamarck TW. Negative emotions and 3-year progression of subclinical atherosclerosis. *Arch Gen Psychiatry.* 2007;64(2):225–33.

272. Stoudemire A, Hales RE. Psychological and behavioral factors affecting medical conditions and DSM-IV. An overview. *Psychosomatics.* 1991;32(1):5–13.

273. Strohle A. Physical activity, exercise, depression and anxiety disorders. *J Neural Transm.* 2009;116(6):777–84.

274. Svensson M, Lagerros YT. Motivational technologies to promote weight loss—from internet to gadgets. *Patient Educ Couns.* 2010;79(3):356–60.

275. Tindle H, Davis E, Kuller L. Attitudes and cardiovascular disease. *Maturitas.* 2010;67(2):108–13.

276. Todaro JF, Shen BJ, Niaura R, Spiro A,3rd, Ward KD. Effect of negative emotions on frequency of coronary heart disease (The Normative Aging Study). *Am J Cardiol.* 2003;92(8):901–6.

277. Trost SG, Owen N, Bauman AE, Sallis JF, Brown W. Correlates of adults' participation in physical activity: review and update. *Med Sci Sports Exerc.* 2002;34(12):1996–2001.

278. Turner RW, Ward MF, Turner DJ. Behavioral treatment for depression: an evaluation of therapeutic components. *J Clin Psychol.* 1979;35(1):166–75.

279. Uchino BN. Social support and health: a review of physiological processes potentially underlying links to disease outcomes. *J Behav Med.* 2006;29(4):377–87.

280. Uchino BN, Cacioppo JT, Kiecolt-Glaser JK. The relationship between social support and physiological processes: a review with emphasis on underlying mechanisms and implications for health. *Psychol Bull.* 1996;119(3):488–531.

281. Ulmer CS, Stetson BA, Salmon PG. Mindfulness and acceptance are associated with exercise maintenance in YMCA exercisers. *Behav Res Ther.* 2010;48(8):805–9.

282. United States, Public Health Service, Office of the Surgeon General, Center for Mental Health Services (U.S.), National Institute of Mental Health (U.S.). *Mental Health: A Report of the Surgeon General.* Rockville, MD: U.S. Department of Health and Human Services, U.S. Public Health Service; 1999. 487 p.

283. United States, Public Health Service, Office of the Surgeon General, Center for Mental Health Services (U.S.), United States, Substance Abuse and Mental Health Services Administration. *Mental Health: Culture, Race, and Ethnicity: A Supplement to Mental Health: A Report of the Surgeon General.* Rockville, MD: U.S. Department of Health and Human Services, U.S. Public Health Service; 2001. 204 p.

284. U.S. Department of Health and Human Services. *Healthy People 2010, Midcourse Review.* Washington, DC: U.S. Department of Health and Human Services; 2006. 976 p.

285. van der Feltz-Cornelis CM, Nuyen J, Stoop C, et al. Effect of interventions for major depressive disorder and significant depressive symptoms in patients with diabetes mellitus: A systematic

review and meta-analysis. *Gen Hosp Psychiatry*. 2010;32(4): 380–95.

286. van der Ven NC, Hogenelst MH, Tromp-Wever AM, et al. Short-term effects of cognitive behavioural group training (CBGT) in adult Type 1 diabetes patients in prolonged poor glycaemic control. A randomized controlled trial. *Diabet Med*. 2005;22(11):1619–23.

287. Vander AJ, Sherman JH, Luciano DS. *Human Physiology: The Mechanism of Body Function*. 8th ed. Boston (MA): WCB McGraw-Hill; 2001. 818 p.

288. Villanova N, Pasqui F, Burzacchini S, et al. A physical activity program to reinforce weight maintenance following a behavior program in overweight/obese subjects. *Int J Obes (Lond)*. 2006;30(4):697–703.

289. Wadden TA, Butryn ML. Behavioral treatment of obesity. *Endocrinol Metab Clin North Am*. 2003;32(4):981,1003, x.

290. Wadden TA, Crerand CE, Brock J. Behavioral treatment of obesity. *Psychiatr Clin North Am*. 2005;28(1):151,70, ix.

291. Wampold BE. *The Great Psychotherapy Debate: Models, Methods, and Findings*. Mahwah (NJ): Lawrence Erlbaum Associates; 2001. 263 p.

292. Wilcox G. Insulin and insulin resistance. *Clin Biochem Rev*. 2005;26(2):19–39.

293. Wilson JS, Fitzsimons D, Bradbury I, Stuart Elborn J. Does additional support by nurses enhance the effect of a brief smoking cessation intervention in people with moderate to severe chronic obstructive pulmonary disease? A randomised controlled trial. *Int J Nurs Stud*. 2008;45(4):508–17.

294. Yanovski SZ, Yanovski JA. Obesity prevalence in the United States—up, down, or sideways? *N Engl J Med*. 2011;364(11):987–9.

295. Yingling KW, Wulsin LR, Arnold LM, Rouan GW. Estimated prevalences of panic disorder and depression among consecutive patients seen in an emergency department with acute chest pain. *J Gen Intern Med*. 1993;8(5):231–5.

296. Zachariae R. Psychoneuroimmunology: a bio-psycho-social approach to health and disease. *Scand J Psychol*. 2009;50(6): 645–51.

297. Zellner DA, Loaiza S, Gonzalez Z, et al. Food selection changes under stress. *Physiol Behav*. 2006;87(4):789–93.

298. Zhang Q, Wang Y, Huang ES. Changes in racial/ethnic disparities in the prevalence of Type 2 diabetes by obesity level among US adults. *Ethn Health*. 2009;14(5):439–57.

299. Ziegelstein RC, Fauerbach JA, Stevens SS, Romanelli J, Richter DP, Bush DE. Patients with depression are less likely to follow recommendations to reduce cardiac risk during recovery from a myocardial infarction. *Arch Intern Med*. 2000;160(12): 1818–23.

SELECTED REFERENCES FOR FURTHER READING

Lox CL, Ginis KAM, Petruzello SJ. *The Psychology of Exercise: Integrating Theory and Practice*. 3rd ed. Scottsdale (AZ): Holcomb Hathaway, Publishers; 2010. 464 p.

Sarafino EP, Smith TW. *Health Psychology: Biopsychosocial Interactions*. 7th ed. New York (NY): John Wiley & Son; 2011.

INTERNET RESOURCES

- American Psychological Association (APA): http://www.apa.org
- National Alliance on Mental Illness (NAMI): http://www.nami.org
- National Institute of Mental Health (NIMH): http://www.nimh.gov
- National Library of Medicine (NLM): http://www.nlm.nih.gov/medlineplus/mentalhealth.html

Body Composition Status and Assessment

Body composition describes the relative proportions of fat, bone, and muscle mass in the human body. Measurement of body composition is a standard component of testing and evaluation for exercise professionals (51). Valuable information regarding percent body fat, fat distribution, body segment girth, and lean tissue mass may be gained through body composition assessment. Such information may be pertinent to athletic performance and for reducing risk factors associated with musculoskeletal injury and disease. This chapter discusses body composition assessment and compares commonly used measurement techniques.

RATIONALE FOR BODY COMPOSITION ASSESSMENT

The assessment of body composition has many benefits in children, adolescent, adult, and elderly populations.

Body fat percentage estimation provides vital information concerning health and fitness. An excess amount of body fat, or obesity, is linked to several diseases including Type 2 diabetes mellitus, hypertension, hyperlipidemia, cardiovascular disease (CVD), and certain types of cancer (19), thereby leading to increased morbidity and mortality. The mortality rate increases by 50%–100% when the body mass index (BMI) is equal to or greater than 30 kg · m^{-2}. Central or visceral obesity serves as platform for a cascade of events that can result in a variety of health problems. In addition to the greater risk of serious illness, obesity poses other mechanical limitations that limit performance of activities of daily living. Obesity has been linked to disc degeneration and low back pain (70), increased risk of bone and joint injury and osteoarthritis (15,125), and reduced cognitive performance (43). Because of the current epidemic

KEY TERMS

Anthropometry: Measurements of the human body including height, weight, circumferences, girths and skinfolds.

Bland-Altman analysis: A statistical procedure used to compare a test criterion with a standard criterion indicating the level of agreement between the two methods.

Body fat percentage: Fat mass expressed as a percentage of total body mass. Percent body fat can only be estimated because no direct measurement methods are available for living organisms.

Body mass index (BMI): BMI is used to assess an individual's mass (kilogram) relative to height (meters squared) (BMI = mass [kg]/height [m^2]) and is a measure of stockiness not body fat. (Also known as the Quetelet index.)

Component-based methods: A system of detailed taxonomies that separates the body into different components (*e.g.*, fat tissue, lean tissue, bone density, body water).

Obesity: A major public health concern affecting more than 90 million Americans in which an excess of nonessential body fat is observed.

Overweight: A weight in excess of a recommended range or standard.

Property-based methods: Measurement of specific properties such as body volume, decay properties of specific isotopes, or electrical resistance.

Standard error of estimate (SEE): A statistic used to express the amount of variability (error) from predictions. The prediction error of a test score can be expressed as the SEE. Similar to the standard deviation, the SEE is generally expressed as a ± around the mean score. Using the bell-shaped curve for normal distribution, ±1 SEE unit refers to 68% of the population — that is, 68% of the population will be within the score ± the SEE. For example, a predicted percent body fat of 20 ± 3.5% means that 68% of the population studied will have a percent body fat between 16.5% and 23.5%.

of obesity in the United States, detection of obesity is of primary importance for health and exercise science professionals.

Body composition assessment is useful for those individuals with a low, as well as high, body fat percentage. During times of malnutrition (*e.g.*, eating disorders) and in some weight-controlled sports, body fat levels and water content can fall to dangerously low levels. Sports such as gymnastics, wrestling, and bodybuilding require athletes to compete at either low weight or with minimal body fat. For wrestling, the American College of Sports Medicine (ACSM) has documented via a position stand the "weight cutting" procedures commonly used by wrestlers and the low percent body fat recorded in some wrestlers in season (89). Procedures such as excessive exercise; fasting; food restriction; and various dehydration techniques, such as rubber suits, steam rooms, and pharmaceutical use, elicit rapid weight loss, much of which comes in the form of water weight, which poses inherent health risks. Regular body composition assessment can be used as a monitoring tool to benefit these individuals. With some methodologies, not only can percent body fat be estimated, but total body water (TBW) can be estimated as well. In fact, the National Collegiate Athletic Association (NCAA) has recommended assessing body composition preseason in wrestling to establish a minimum body weight for each wrestler (fat-free mass [FFM] + 5% body fat) (9).

Measurement of muscle mass and bone mineral density (BMD) have several important ramifications. In the clinical setting, assessment of muscle mass and BMD can be used to assess the effects of aging and disease. *Sarcopenia* is the degenerative loss of skeletal muscle mass and strength as a result of aging and reduced physical activity. A progressive reduction in BMD — that is, osteopenia and osteoporosis — may occur with aging and physical inactivity. Sarcopenia reduces the ability to perform activities of daily living; alters metabolism, muscle, and bone function; and increases the risk of musculoskeletal injury (21,66). Thus, body composition assessment in the clinical setting can be used to monitor the progression of disease or muscle/bone enhancement as a result of therapeutic or pharmaceutical intervention. Body composition assessment is particularly important in populations with pulmonary disease because prolonged use of steroid therapies adversely affects BMD, often resulting in increased risk of falls, broken bones, or compression fractures of the spine. In apparently healthy or athletic populations, body composition assessment can be used to quantify changes in muscle mass and BMD as a result of physical training (12). These measurements may be used for individualization of exercise prescriptions and for training program evaluation.

LEVELS OF BODY COMPOSITION

Body composition may be described at five levels: atomic, molecular, cellular, tissue, and whole body (75,92). Basic elements are found at the atomic level. Of all the elements found in nature, about 50 are found in the human body. Of these, oxygen, carbon, hydrogen, and nitrogen account for >95% of body mass, and other key elements such as sodium, potassium, phosphorous, calcium, chloride, magnesium, and sulfur raise the total to nearly 99.5% of body mass (75). At the molecular level, the major components are water, lipids, protein, minerals, and carbohydrates. At the cellular level, the critical components are the cell mass (*e.g.*, muscle, nerve, connective tissue, adipocytes), extracellular fluid, and extracellular solids. At the tissue level, body composition analyses focus on skeletal muscle, bone, blood, visceral organs, and adipose tissue. Adipose tissue includes adipocytes with collagenous fibers, fibroblasts, capillaries, and extracellular fluid. Lastly, the whole-body level entails body mass, size, stature, volume, density, and proportions. Most body composition assessments discussed in this chapter involve measurements at the whole-body level.

BODY COMPOSITION MODELS

Body composition methods can be categorized as being direct, indirect, or doubly indirect (124). A direct method (chemical analysis of the whole body or cadaver) is not suitable in the living human body. Thus, indirect or doubly indirect methods are preferred. Indirect methods (*e.g.*, hydrostatic weighing [HW]) were derived from the direct method, and doubly indirect methods (*e.g.*, skinfolds) were generally derived from an indirect method. Therefore, doubly indirect methods are generally prone to greater measurement error in comparison to the direct method. *Table 18-1* categorizes many popular body composition assessment methods into indirect or doubly indirect.

Indirect methods are based on either property or component (49) approaches. Property-based methods involve the measurement of specific properties, such as body volume, decay properties of specific isotopes, or electrical resistance (*e.g.*, estimation of TBW from tritium dilution). The development of in vivo neutron activation analysis, for example, has made possible nondestructive chemical analysis by measuring the radiation given off during the decay of excited atoms (25). Component-based methods depend on well-established models, usually ratios of measurable quantities to components that are assumed to be constant, both within and between individuals. The measured quantity is first assessed using a property-based method, and the component is estimated by application of the model. Thus, FFM can be estimated from TBW by use of tritium dilution, and subsequently, fat mass can be calculated.

TABLE 18-1. Categorization of Common Body Composition Assessment Techniques

Assessment Technique	Method	Component Model
Skinfolds	Doubly indirect	Largely 2C (some multiple C equations)
Bioelectrical impedance	Doubly indirect	3C
Near-infrared interactance	Doubly indirect	2C
Hydrodensitometry	Indirect	2C
CT and MRI scans	Indirect	Multiple C
Plethysmography: air displacement	Indirect	2C
Dual-energy X-ray absorptiometry (DEXA)	Indirect	3C

Method: direct, indirect, or doubly indirect (see text for complete explanation). Component model: 2C (two compartment), 3C (three compartment), multiple C (more than 2C) (see text for complete explanation).

Two types of mathematical approaches are used to estimate body composition with property- and component-based methods. The model approach, which depends on the ratio between a particular constituent and the component of interest, was illustrated earlier. In the second approach, regression analysis is used with experimental data to derive an equation that relates a measured property or component to an unknown (estimated) component. Equations for estimating percent body fat from skinfold thickness or bioelectrical impedance are developed in this manner — for example, doubly indirect. Direct methods represent the most fundamental approach to assessment, property-based methods are one step removed, and component-based methods are two steps removed. Assessment methods are structured so that measurement errors are propagated from level to level.

Different models have been proposed for characterizing human body composition by compartments with the sum totaling the individual's body mass. The two-compartment (2C) model partitions body mass into fat mass and FFM (13,110) and has the widest application to body composition analysis. This model is limited by the assumptions that water and mineral contents of the body remain constant throughout life and between all individuals, and that the density of FFM is constant among all individuals. The assumption related to FFM composition is known to be violated by age, sex, pregnancy, weight loss, some states of disease, and racial/ethnic differences (69).

Multicompartment models have been developed because of violation of the inherent assumptions of the 2C model. These models divide the body into more than two compartments and require fewer assumptions about the composition of the FFM. Thus, multicompartment models may provide more accurate results. However, their application requires additional measurements (*e.g.*, TBW, bone mineral content); therefore, the theoretic reduction in total error may be offset by an increased technical error in measuring multiple components. Multicompartment models include the three-compartment (3C), four-compartment (4C), and five-compartment (5C) models. Regression equations are developed with three, four, or five components to increase the accuracy of body fat estimation. The 3C model includes fat mass, but also partitions FFM into TBW and dry FFM. Thus, the addition of TBW (*i.e.*, by isotope dilution) is added to the 2C model. The 4C model partitions body mass into fat mass, TBW, BMD, and the residual dry FFM. Thus, the addition of BMD (via dual-energy X-ray absorptiometry [DEXA]) is added to the 3C model. In addition, 4C models (7,48) often serve as the criterion model for body composition measurement in validation studies. The measurement of soft tissue mineral content (via in vivo neutron analysis or by using a prediction equation based on neutron analysis) has been added to 4C models to generate a criterion 5C model (80,108,123). Soft tissue minerals constitute a mass of ~400 g in adults and have a relatively high density; thus, it can improve a model by its addition (123). The choice of an appropriate model depends on the component of FFM that is expected to vary the most from population norms. When equipment is limited and 3C, 4C, and 5C models are not feasible, population-specific equations (using a 2C model) that are adjusted for differences in FFM can be used to improve accuracy (see *GETP9 Table 4-4*). Population-specific equations appropriate for children and older adults, various racial or ethnic groups, athletic groups, and some clinical populations should result in more accurate estimates than generalized equations (51,72).

METHODOLOGIES IN BODY COMPOSITION ASSESSMENT

There are no direct in vivo methods available to measure different body composition compartments. Rather, most body composition measurements involve indirect assessment or estimation. Comparative studies between different methods are numerous because each method has advantages and disadvantages. Critical to these comparisons is the establishment of a criterion or standard method. Evaluation of each technique for accuracy, validity, and reliability is critical for assessment. The decision on which method to use depends on several factors, including the needs of the individual, purpose of the evaluation, cost of the measurements or equipment needed, availability of each assessment tool, training of the technician, and the weighed advantages/disadvantages of each. In this chapter, each body composition assessment tool listed next is discussed. These basic and advanced measures include the following:

- Height
- Body mass
- BMI
- Waist and hip circumferences
- Hydrodensitometry (underwater weighing)
- Skinfold assessments
- Bioelectrical impedance
- Near-infrared interactance (NIR)
- Air displacement plethysmography (ADP)
- Computed tomography (CT) scans and positron emission tomography (PET)
- Magnetic resonance imaging (MRI) and spectroscopy
- Ultrasound
- Isotopic dilution
- DEXA
- Three-dimensional body scanning

HEIGHT, BODY MASS, AND BODY MASS INDEX

Anthropometry is the measurement of the human body using simple physical techniques. Height should be assessed with a stadiometer (a vertical ruler mounted on a wall with a wide horizontal headboard). Although many commercial scales have an attached vertical ruler, these devices are less reliable and not recommended. Standards for height measurements include the following: (a) subject removes shoes, (b) subject stands straight up with heels together, (c) subject takes a deep breath and holds it, and (d) subject stands with head level, looking straight ahead. The height of the subject is then recorded in inches or centimeters. Failure to follow these standards reduces reliability and accuracy. Height can vary slightly throughout the day with variations in fluid content of the spine's intervertebral discs and is affected by activity level (weight-bearing, upright exercise increases spinal disc compression, which can slightly reduce height). Height is typically greatest in the morning (when intervertebral disc fluid content is highest), so selecting a standard time and monitoring preactivity level increases reliability when multiple measures are taken from the same individual over time.

Body mass is best measured on a calibrated scale with a beam and moveable weights. If other types of commercial scales are used, it is recommended they be calibrated using standardized weights or compared with the measured value from the beam-type scale. Clothing is the major measurement issue for body mass assessment. The type and amount of clothing must be standardized (*Box 18-1*). Ideally, measurements should be completed with minimal clothing. However, this recommendation may not be feasible in some instances, so a facility should adopt the most reasonable clothing policy for their population. Individuals should remove their shoes and any excess layers of clothing (*e.g.*, coats), empty their pockets, and remove jewelry and cell phones. A reasonable standard in many fitness environments is shorts and a T-shirt. Body mass can change at various times of day because of meal/beverage consumption, urination, defecation, and potential dehydration/water loss. Thus, a standard time (*e.g.*, early in the morning) relative to exercise and nutritional intake will increase the consistency of measurements. Body weight is recorded in the English unit of pounds, and body mass is recorded in the metric unit of kilograms. The term *body weight* is often used interchangeably with body mass, but they represent different properties of matter. Body mass is the quantity of matter the human body possesses, whereas body weight is the force of gravity acting on that mass, that is, body weight is equivalent to mass $\times$ acceleration due to gravity. (The English unit for mass is the seldom used term "slugs." The metric unit for weight is the same as for force, newtons).

Body mass index (BMI) is used to assess an individual's mass relative to height (BMI = body mass/height

BOX 18-1	Standards for Basic Body Composition Measurements	
MEASUREMENT	**INSTRUMENT**	**STANDARDIZATION**
Waist circumference	Tension-controlled tape	See *GETP9 Box 4-1*
Weight	Balance beam scale	Nude or hospital gown or Facility-developed standard
Height	Stadiometer	No shoes, heels together, after a deep inhalation, head level

squared; kg · m^{-2}). BMI has been used to determine risk of developing Type 2 diabetes, hypertension, and CVD according to standards developed by the Expert Panel on the Identification, Evaluation, and Treatment of Overweight and Obesity in Adults (85). BMI has also been shown to consistently relate to insulin resistance, dyslipidemia, and hypertension in children (36). According to current BMI standards (kg · m^{-2}), (a) individuals with a BMI <18.5 are classified as underweight; (b) a BMI of 18.5–24.9 is normal; (c) a BMI of 25.0–29.9 indicates overweight; and (d) a BMI of 30.0 or more is obese, with 30.0–34.9 being grade I obesity, 35.0–39.9 being grade II obesity, and 40.0 or more being grade III (morbid) obesity. Thus, a BMI range of 30.0–39.9 indicates a moderate risk for disease development, whereas a BMI ≥40 indicates a high risk of developing metabolic disease. Criticisms of the use of BMI are that it is a relatively poor predictor of **body fat percentage** and it may result in inaccurate classifications (normal, overweight, obese) for some individuals, particularly those who are muscular. The standard error of estimate (SEE) for predicting percent body fat from BMI is ±5%, thereby demonstrating the criticism of BMI to be valid. The error is particularly high when BMI equations are used to predict percent body fat in athletic populations (e.g., body builders) (119). The primary advantages of BMI are that it is a relatively easy measure to obtain and it is useful for categorizing the extent of overweight and obesity in large populations.

The accuracy of BMI is highly questionable in athletes and individuals who exercise regularly as has been shown in adolescent (96) and adult athletes (63). In a study examining body composition in National Football League (NFL) players, every player (including kickers and punters) was classified as overweight or obese using BMI, despite having body fat percentages of 6.3%–18.5% (with offensive linemen at 25.1%) (63). Thus, BMI is not a particularly useful body composition analysis tool in resistance-trained populations. Misclassification of body weight is not prevalent in nonathletic adult populations who are weight stable or who have gained weight in their adult years. Thus, BMI should provide a reasonably accurate classification in these individuals.

CIRCUMFERENCES

Circumferences, or girths, are used to estimate body composition and provide specific reference to the distribution of fat in the body. The pattern of body fat distribution is an important predictor of the health risks associated with obesity. Increased fat distribution on the trunk (android obesity) is positively correlated with an increased risk of hypertension, metabolic syndrome, Type 2 diabetes, dyslipidemia, coronary artery disease, and premature death when compared with individuals whose fat is distributed in the hip and thigh region (gynoid obesity) (34).

Using circumference measures as a means for estimating body composition has the advantage of being easy to learn, quick to complete, and inexpensive. Various translational equations are available for men and women to convert girth measurements to body fat estimations across a range of ages (116,117). Accuracy of circumference measures vary but can range within 2.5%–4.0% of the body composition derived from hydrostatic densitometry if precise circumference measures are obtained and the subject's characteristics match those of the original validation population. An improvement in measurement accuracy can occur when duplicate measurements are obtained at each site using a cloth tape measure with a spring-loaded handle (e.g., Gulick tape measure). In addition, measurements should be obtained in a rotational order instead of consecutively.

Waist circumference can be used as an indicator of disease risk, as abdominal obesity has been identified as a predictor of disease. Although all fitness assessments should include a minimum of waist circumference or BMI, it is preferable that both be performed when evaluating for risk classification. The classification of disease risk based on both BMI and waist circumference is shown in *Table 4-1* of the *GETP9*. In addition, risk classification is now available for adults based on waist circumference measures (see *Table 4-3* of GETP9).

WAIST-TO-HIP RATIO

The waist-to-hip ratio (WHR) is a ratio measurement of the circumference of the waist to that of the hip and is an indicator of body fat distribution. A high WHR ratio may indicate visceral obesity. Visceral obesity increases the risk of hypertension, Type 2 diabetes, hyperlipidemia, metabolic syndrome, and CVD. Standardization of circumference measurement technique for the WHR is critical for accuracy and reliability. The waist circumference is measured around the smallest area of the waist, typically approximately 1 in (2.54 cm) above the umbilicus or navel. The hip circumference is taken around the largest area of the buttocks. Multiple measurements are taken until each is within 5 mm (~0.25 in) of each other. Young adults are at a very high risk for disease when WHR values are greater than 0.95 for men and 0.86 for women. These values rise to 1.03 and 0.90, respectively, for ages 60–69 yr (50).

HYDRODENSITOMETRY (UNDERWATER OR HYDROSTATIC WEIGHING)

Underwater or HW (also known as hydrodensitometry) has been considered the criterion method for body composition analysis even though it is an indirect method. HW is based on Archimedes' principle for determining body density (BD). Archimedes' principle states that a body immersed in water is subjected to a buoyant force that results in a loss of weight equal to the weight of the displaced water. Subtracting the body weight measured in the water during submersion from the body weight measured on land provides the weight of the displaced water. Body fat contributes to buoyancy because the assumed density of fat ($0.9007 \text{ g} \cdot \text{cm}^{-3}$) is less than water ($1 \text{ g} \cdot \text{cm}^{-3}$), whereas FFM (assumed to average $1.100 \text{ g} \cdot \text{cm}^{-3}$) exceeds the density of water. Density is inversely related to body fat. Thus, HW is based on the equation: body density = mass $\cdot$ volume^{-1}. A volumetric analysis of the body is possible with HW because body volume can be determined via hydrodensitometry or ADP. BD is then converted to percent body fat using a 2C (fat and FFM) model equation, such as the Siri (110) or Brozek (13) BD equations. Other popular methods of body composition analysis (*e.g.*, skinfolds, bioelectrical impedance) are validated against HW.

Several variables must be known to use HW. These include the following:

1. Residual volume — the amount of air remaining in the lungs following full exhalation. Residual volume can be measured or predicted using a combination of age, sex, and height. If a client does not fully exhale during underwater weighing, the additional air left in the lungs increases buoyancy, which will erroneously increase the estimated body fat.
2. Density of the water — this varies inversely with water temperature; thus, water temperature must be measured and the density adjusted accordingly.
3. The amount of trapped gas in the gastrointestinal system — typically an estimated constant of 100 mL is used, introducing a source of error.
4. Dry body weight — the client should be naked for greatest accuracy but is typically measured with minimal, skintight clothing.
5. Body (wet) weight fully submerged in water — the client must wear exactly the same clothing as for the dry measurement.

BD may then be calculated and converted to percent body fat using a 2C model prediction equation.

When performing HW, the subjects should wear a tight-fitting bathing suit that traps little air, remove all jewelry, and have urinated/defecated before assessment. In addition, the subject should be 2–12 h postabsorptive and avoid foods that may have increased gas in the gastrointestinal tract. Menstruation may pose a problem for women because of associated water gain; thus, women should try to avoid being tested within 7 d of menstruation. The equipment used for HW may vary. The tank can be made of stainless steel, fiberglass, ceramic tile, Plexiglas, or other material and should be at least 4 ft × 5 ft (42). A chair suspended from a scale or force transducer is needed to allow subjects to be weighed while completely submerged underwater. The subject is weighed on land to determine dry weight

and the associated mass. The temperature of the water should be between 33° and 36° C, and the density can be determined based on temperature. Subjects enter the tank; remove potential trapped air from the skin, hair, suit, etc.; and attain a seated position. Once seated and chair height adjusted, the subject fully exhales as much air as possible and leans forward to become fully submerged. The subject should be weighed 5–10 times while submerged underwater for 5–10 s per trial. Movement in the chair should be minimized to reduce scale fluctuations. The highest of the weights or the average of the three highest weights is used for analysis. The weight of the chair in addition to any weight belts used to ensure complete submersion when determining underwater weight are subtracted from the subject's weight. Residual lung volume can be measured directly (which increases accuracy) in some systems or estimated based on height and age:

- Men: RV (L) = [0.019 × ht (cm)] + [0.0155 × age (yrs)] − 2.24   (11)
- Women: RV (L) = [0.032 × ht (cm)] + [0.009 × age (yrs)] − 3.90   (87)

BD may then be calculated using the following equation:

- BD = Mass in air / [([Mass in air − Mass in water] / Water density)
  − (RV + 100 mL)]
  Masses are recorded in grams
  RV is recorded in milliliter

Body fat can then be calculated using either the Siri (110) or Brozek (13) equations:

- Siri: % Fat = $\dfrac{457}{\text{BD}}$ − 414.2
- Brozek: % Fat = $\dfrac{457}{\text{BD}}$ − 450

The test–retest reliability of HW is high (R = 0.95) (72). High correlation coefficients and similar percent body fat estimates have been shown between HW and a 4C model in athletes (119). Although the density of lean tissue is assumed to be $1.100 \text{ g} \cdot \text{cm}^{-3}$ for all subjects in the Siri and Brozek equations, this value differs in African Americans ($>1.10 \text{ g} \cdot \text{cm}^{-3}$) and in children and the elderly ($<1.10 \text{ g} \cdot \text{cm}^{-3}$), which is a major source of error if population-specific equations are not used with these groups (76). In addition, the density of FFM varies between individuals, resulting in a body fat SEE of about $\pm 2.7\%$, even when the technique is performed flawlessly (72). Major practical limitations to HW include space and plumbing requirements, the cost and specialized use of the equipment needed, the time involved in each measurement, the need for an accurate residual volume measurement, and the inherent fear and discomfort many individuals have being fully submerged in water.

The last issue may prevent the client from fully exhaling, invalidating the test. Because of these limitations, HW is not used in many fitness or medical centers.

SKINFOLD MEASUREMENT

One of the more popular and practical methods used to estimate percent fat is the skinfold thickness measurement. Skinfold measurement predicts percent body fat reasonably well if performed properly by a trained technician using a high-quality skinfold caliper (*i.e.*, a Lange or Harpenden caliper that provides a constant pressure of ~10 g · mm^{-2} across its range of movement). However, skinfold analysis provides only an estimate of BD and percent body fat, typically based on correlation with the 2C model. Skinfold analysis is based on the principle that the amount of subcutaneous fat (fat immediately below the skin) is directly proportional to the total amount of body fat. The proportion of subcutaneous to total fat varies with sex, age, race or ethnicity, and other factors. Numerous regression equations using a combination of multiple skinfold sites have been developed to predict BD and fat. These multiple regression equations are either general or population specific for sex, age, race or ethnicity, and activity or sport status.

The number of sites needs to be predetermined based on the regression equation or methods used (*i.e.*, three-, four-, or seven-site skinfold). A fold of skin is firmly grasped between the thumb and index finger of the left hand (about 8 cm apart on a line perpendicular to the long axis of the site) and lifted away from the body while the subject is relaxed. Palpation of the fold ensures that subcutaneous tissue (skin, fat) is measured and not skeletal muscle. For individuals who are obese, a large grasping area (*i.e.*, >8 cm) may be needed. While the caliper dial is facing up, the jaws of the caliper are opened and placed over the skinfold 1 cm below the fingers of the tester directly at the designated anatomical site. The grip of the caliper is released, and the skinfold measurement is subsequently taken within 2–3 s while the tester's other hand maintains the grasp of the skinfold. All measurements are taken on the right side of the body in duplicate or triplicate for consistency between measurements to the nearest 0.5 mm. If there is more than a 2-mm difference between readings, then a fourth measurement may be needed. It is important to rotate through the measurement sites as opposed to taking two or three measurements sequentially from the same site (see *Fig. 18-1* for a description of selected skinfold sites). Each site is averaged, and then the sites are summed to estimate percent body fat via a regression equation or prediction table. *Box 18-2* lists generalized equations that allow calculation of body composition from skinfolds, whereas population-specific equations are provided in *Table 4-4* of *GETP9*. The specific skinfold equation used must match the anatomic measurement description specific to the equation, as there are reported differences in skinfold anatomic site descriptions and

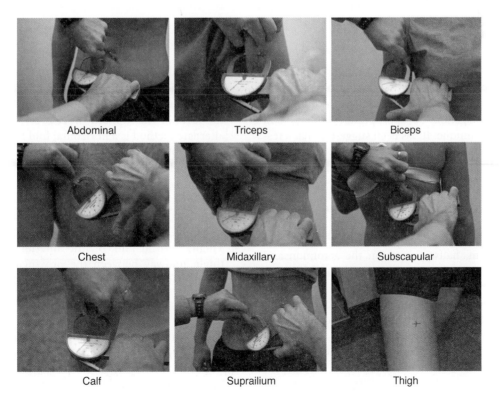

FIGURE 18-1. Skinfold measures.

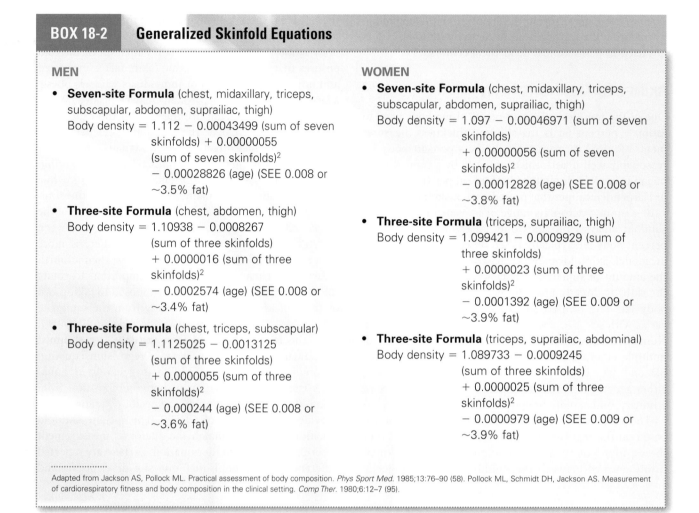

BOX 18-2 | Generalized Skinfold Equations

MEN

- **Seven-site Formula** (chest, midaxillary, triceps, subscapular, abdomen, suprailiac, thigh)
  Body density = 1.112 − 0.00043499 (sum of seven skinfolds) + 0.00000055 (sum of seven skinfolds)² − 0.00028826 (age) (SEE 0.008 or ~3.5% fat)

- **Three-site Formula** (chest, abdomen, thigh)
  Body density = 1.10938 − 0.0008267 (sum of three skinfolds) + 0.0000016 (sum of three skinfolds)² − 0.0002574 (age) (SEE 0.008 or ~3.4% fat)

- **Three-site Formula** (chest, triceps, subscapular)
  Body density = 1.1125025 − 0.0013125 (sum of three skinfolds) + 0.0000055 (sum of three skinfolds)² − 0.000244 (age) (SEE 0.008 or ~3.6% fat)

WOMEN

- **Seven-site Formula** (chest, midaxillary, triceps, subscapular, abdomen, suprailiac, thigh)
  Body density = 1.097 − 0.00046971 (sum of seven skinfolds) + 0.00000056 (sum of seven skinfolds)² − 0.00012828 (age) (SEE 0.008 or ~3.8% fat)

- **Three-site Formula** (triceps, suprailiac, thigh)
  Body density = 1.099421 − 0.0009929 (sum of three skinfolds) + 0.0000023 (sum of three skinfolds)² − 0.0001392 (age) (SEE 0.009 or ~3.9% fat)

- **Three-site Formula** (triceps, suprailiac, abdominal)
  Body density = 1.089733 − 0.0009245 (sum of three skinfolds) + 0.0000025 (sum of three skinfolds)² − 0.0000979 (age) (SEE 0.009 or ~3.9% fat)

Adapted from Jackson AS, Pollock ML. Practical assessment of body composition. *Phys Sport Med*. 1985;13:76–90 (58). Pollock ML, Schmidt DH, Jackson AS. Measurement of cardiorespiratory fitness and body composition in the clinical setting. *Comp Ther*. 1980;6:12–7 (95).

---

measurement techniques. Therefore, major limitations to the skinfold procedure are the amount of technician training in equation selection, accuracy of skinfold site measurement, selection of appropriate calipers, and measurement technique. It has been suggested that a tester measure approximately 50–100 individuals to attain a high level of competency (42). Common sites assessed are as follows:

- Abdominal: Vertical fold; 2 cm to the right of the umbilicus
- Triceps: Vertical fold; on the posterior midline of the upper arm, halfway between the acromion and olecranon processes, with the arm hanging freely to the side of the body
- Biceps: Vertical fold; on the anterior aspect of the arm over the belly of the biceps muscle, 1 cm above the level used to mark the triceps site
- Chest/pectoral: Diagonal fold; one-half the distance between the anterior axillary line and the nipple (men) or one-third the distance between the anterior axillary line and the nipple (women)

- Medial calf: Vertical fold; at the maximum circumference of the calf on the midline of its medial border
- Midaxillary: Vertical fold; on the midaxillary line at the level of the xiphoid process of the sternum (an alternate method is a horizontal fold taken at the level of the xiphoid/sternal border in the midaxillary line)
- Subscapular: Diagonal fold (at a 45-degree angle), 1–2 cm below the inferior angle of the scapula
- Suprailiac: Diagonal fold; in line with the natural angle of the iliac crest taken in the anterior axillary line immediately superior to the iliac crest
- Thigh: Vertical fold; on the anterior midline of the thigh, midway between the proximal border of the patella and the inguinal crease (hip)

Reliability and accuracy of skinfold measurement are specific to the skinfold regression equation used. Variability in percent body fat prediction from skinfold analysis is approximately ±3.5% (SEE), assuming that appropriate techniques and equations have been used (72). In those with abdominal subcutaneous fat that is not easily grasped because of marked abdominal obesity, skinfold assessment may not be accurate, and other body composition assessment techniques may be required. Skinfold analysis has been shown to overestimate BD in individuals who are overweight and obese compared to ADP (104), thus resulting in an underestimation of percent body fat.

BIOELECTRICAL IMPEDANCE

Bioelectrical impedance analysis (BIA) is a noninvasive and easy-to-administer body composition assessment tool. A variety of different BIA analyzers are commercially available that range in utility and price. The premise underlying this procedure is that fat-free tissue in the body is proportional to the electrical conductivity of the body (6). A small electrical current is sent through the body (from ankle to wrist with some units, or from hand to hand or foot to foot), and the impedance to that current is measured. The theory underlying BIA is that lean tissue (mostly water and electrolytes) is a good electrical conductor (low impedance), whereas fat is a poor electrical conductor and acts as impedance to electrical current. BIA estimates TBW and uses equations for percent body fat (using a 3C model) based on assumptions about hydration levels and the exact water content of various tissues (50). A single-frequency (50 kHz), low-level current (500 mA) is used to measure whole-body impedance using electrodes placed on two distant peripheral sites. Unlike lower frequency current (<50 kHz), which flows through the extracellular fluid, higher frequencies penetrate the cell membranes and flow through both the intracellular and extracellular fluid. Thus, total body impedance at the constant frequency of 50 kHz primarily reflects the volumes of water (intracellular and extracellular fluid) and muscle compartments constituting the FFM. Most studies examining BIA have used the equation: $V = pL^2 \cdot R^1$, where V is the volume of the conductor (i.e., TBW), p is the specific resistance of the tissue, L is the length of the conductor, and R is the observed resistance (42).

Potential limitations to single-frequency BIA analyzers are that they cannot distinguish between intracellular and extracellular water components (69) and they assume the body to be a single cylinder with constant resistivity (106). Other BIA analyzers have been developed to address these limitations. Multifrequency BIA analyzers (also known as bioimpedance spectroscopy) allow for partitioning intracellular and extracellular components (6,69,74) as a range from low to high frequencies are used. Common analyzers studied typically use ~50 frequencies ranging from 5 to 1,000 kHz, whereas newer models use up to ~256 frequencies ranging from 4 to 1,000 kHz. They may be less affected by hydration status and may provide a better estimate of FFM. Multiple-frequency BIA may enhance the clinical application of BIA to assess changes and shifts between intracellular and extracellular fluid compartments associated with certain diseases as well as accurate measurements of hydration status. Both have been shown to provide accurate assessment of TBW compared to deuterium dilution (82). Multisegmental BIA analyzers are also available that assume the body is made up of five groups (arms, trunk, and legs) of heterogeneous cylinders rather than a single cylinder (69). They typically use eight electrodes with detection on both sides of the body. The multisegmental BIA analyzers may have greater impact when examining overweight and obese populations who possess large variations in regional body fat. Multisegmental BIA analyzers also have the capacity to conduct multifrequency impulses, thereby expanding their operational range. However, recent evidence shows that, in comparison to DEXA, multisegmental BIA overestimated percent body fat in individuals who are obese by ~3.4% but was valid when examining individuals who are normal and overweight (106) and was valid in assessing body composition changes in patients undergoing hemodialysis (38).

The methods used in single-frequency BIA testing are relatively simple. The subject lies supine on a nonconductive surface with arm and legs at the side, not in contact with the rest of the body. The right hand and foot are prepared with an alcohol pad and allowed to dry. Source electrodes are placed on the distal metacarpal of the right index finger and the distal metatarsal of the right big toe, and the reference (detecting) electrodes are placed on the right wrist (bisecting the ulnar and radial styloid processes) and the right ankle (midpoint on the line bisecting the medial and lateral malleoli). The voltage drop between reference electrodes is the impedance. Newer BIA equipment is simpler to use and requires the subject to either stand on an electronic digital platform scale with built-in stainless steel footpad electrodes or hold the BIA analyzer in both hands. Accuracy among different BIA models varies greatly.

Most BIA machines use different equations that account for the differences in water content and BD between different sexes, ages, and races or ethnicities as well as by physical activity status. The BIA technology has been shown to be reliable for single measurements and measurements taken up to 5 d (42). It is important when performing a BIA assessment that the subject has not eaten or consumed a beverage within 4 h of the test, has not exercised within 12 h of the test, has not consumed alcohol or diuretics before testing, has completely voided the bladder within 30 min of the test, and has had minimal consumption of diuretic agents, such as chocolate or caffeine. In addition, glycogen stores can affect impedance and can be a factor during times of weight loss. If possible, BIA measurements should not be taken before menstruation to avoid the possible effects of water retention in women. BIA manufacturers also recommend avoiding this method of body composition assessment with pregnant women and those with implanted electrical devices, such as a pacemaker. The reported SEE for BIA is between ±1.8% and 6.3%, which is greater than that reported for skinfold analysis (42,81,83). Although high correlations between BIA and other criterion methods have been established, percent body fat from BIA appears to be consistently overestimated for lean individuals and underestimated for persons who are obese. In athletes, BIA has been shown to significantly underestimate percent body fat when compared with HW (20) but compared favorably to ADP for body fat percentage measurement in adolescent volleyball players (96). Compared with DEXA, BIA has been shown to underestimate percent body fat and overestimate lean tissue mass (10). However, BIA has been shown to detect similar changes in percent body fat during weight loss comparable with the magnitude of change determined via DEXA (37). BIA has compared favorably to a 3C reference method in estimating percent body fat in college men and women (81,83). Subject factors, technical skill, the prediction equation used, and the instruments used all affect the accuracy of BIA. To reduce measurement error, analyzers should be calibrated before measurement, and the same instrument, or at least brand when applicable, should be used when following changes in body composition for a given individual. Hydration, temperature, and exercise status must be controlled to stabilize resistance measurements. Technician error is minor if standard procedures for subject and electrode positioning are followed. Finally, error can be reduced by selecting appropriate prediction equations according to age, sex, ethnicity, and level of physical activity and by using an equation developed on a BIA unit similar to the one being used for testing.

NEAR-INFRARED INTERACTANCE

NIR is based on principles of light absorption and reflection using near-infrared spectroscopy to provide information about the chemical composition of the body. A light wand device is positioned perpendicularly on a body part (typically on the anterior midline of the biceps brachii, midway between the antecubital fossa and the acromion process), and infrared light is emitted at specific wavelengths (either two or six wavelengths, depending on the device). The absorption of the infrared beam is measured via a silicon-based detector and is then expressed as optical densities. Prediction equations estimate percent body fat via optical density, sex, height, and body weight. Some research indicates that NIR is valid and reliable for body composition assessment in female athletes (35). However, the SEE associated with NIR has been shown to be higher than other assessment tools (i.e., skinfolds and BIA) (11,35). NIR has been shown to overestimate percent body fat in women who are obese (90) and in young wrestlers (56). Even when NIR equations are adjusted for constant error values, the error rate in youth

wrestlers is still approximately 2%–3% (55), suggesting unacceptable prediction errors for these populations. Two studies examining the six-wavelength model (using a 3C model criterion standard) showed that NIR underestimated percent fat by nearly 2% in college men with a large (>4%) SEE but provided valid percent fat measure in college women (81,83). In addition, NIR has been shown to be least effective for monitoring body composition changes following resistance and aerobic training (12). Some commercial versions of NIR are portable and require minimal technician training, making them attractive to the health and fitness industry. However, a major limitation is the relatively small sampling area on the body for NIR absorption. The SEE reported for NIR varies more than ±5.0 percent body fat (27). Thus, the high SEE reported in most NIR studies questions the use of this body composition assessment technique in healthy, athletic, or clinical populations.

AIR DISPLACEMENT PLETHYSMOGRAPHY

Body volume can be measured by air displacement rather than water displacement. ADP is an alternative body composition assessment technique to HW for individuals who may experience difficulty with HW. This technique offers several advantages over other reference methods. ADP is usually a quick and comfortable assessment, is noninvasive, and accommodates children, adults, obese, elderly, and disabled individuals (31). However, a major disadvantage for ADP is initial cost of purchasing the ADP unit.

ADP is performed with the BOD POD system (Life Measurement Instruments, Concord, CA) which uses a dual-chamber (e.g., 450 L for the subject test chamber, 300 L for the reference chamber) plethysmograph that measures body volume via changes in air pressure, that is, using Boyle's law ($P_1 \cdot P_2^{-1} = V_2 \cdot V_1^{-1}$), within a closed 2C chamber. A plethysmograph is an instrument for measuring volume or changes in volume. The ADP system also includes an electronic weighing scale, computer, and software. The volume of air displaced is equal to body volume and is calculated indirectly by subtracting the volume of air remaining in the chamber when the subject is inside from the volume of air in the chamber when it is empty. A diaphragm (which separates the two internal chambers) oscillates back and forth to create volume changes that produce pressure changes in the two chambers. Thoracic gas volume is measured during normal breathing via the "panting" method, in which the subject breathes normally into a tube connected within the chamber, followed by three small puffs after the airway tube becomes momentarily occluded at the midpoint of exhalation. Thoracic gas volume could also be predicted or retrieved from a previous test. Corrected body volume (raw body volume − thoracic gas volume) is then calculated (42). Sources of error include (a) interlaboratory variation, (b) variations in testing conditions, (c) performing testing while not in a fasting state, (d) air that is not accounted for in the lungs or that is trapped within clothing and bodily hair, and (e) body moisture and/or increased body temperature (31,32). The Pea Pod (Life Measurement Instruments, Concord, CA) can be used to measure body composition in infants weighing up to 17.6 lb. The Pea Pod has been shown to provide accurate and reliable body composition data in infants (26).

The subject needs to wear a bathing suit (or minimal clothing, such as Lycra biking shorts) and a swim cap and then sits quietly during testing while a minimum of two measurements (within 150 mL of each other) are taken. It is essential that the subject minimizes the volume of isothermal air via tight clothing and swim caps. Loose clothing (T-shirts, shorts, hospital scrubs) overestimates BD and underestimates percent body fat by 4%–11% compared to subject testing in spandex (105). Percent body fat may be underestimated by ~3%–5% if a swimming cap is not worn and the subject has hair covering a large portion of the face (52,91). The type of cap plays a role in accuracy of the measurement as recent evidence has shown that silicone swim caps compress the scalp better than Lycra caps, yielding a 1.2% difference in percent body fat (91). Percent body fat can be overestimated by 2.0%–3.7% when lung volume is intentionally altered during measurement (114).

After BD has been determined, percent body fat can be calculated. Most prediction equations used to convert BD to percent body fat using ADP are similar to HW, although BD measured via ADP does result in consistently higher values compared with HW (42). ADP is effective for measuring changes over time provided standardized techniques are used. Reliability of ADP in adults is good (within-subject coefficients of variation [CVs] = 1.7%–4.3%) (4,18,31). In addition, ADP has been shown to be valid in comparison to HW and DEXA. In comparison to HW, ADP ranges −4.0% to 1.9% with SEEs of 1.8%–2.3% in adults and −2.9% to 2.6% with SEEs of 3.3% in children (31). In comparison to DEXA, ADP ranges −3.0% to 2.2% with SEEs of 2.4%–3.7% in adults and −3.9% to −0.1% with SEEs of 3.4%–4.1% in children (3,31). In comparison to 3C models, ADP produces similar percent body fat measurements in college men and women, SEE of 1.9%–2.4% (81,83). In comparison to 4C models, ADP underestimates percent body fat by nearly 2% in women (33). ADP has been shown to be valid in comparison to HW in subjects classified as overweight (BMI = 27.1 kg · m^{-2}), obese (BMI = 34.0 kg · m^{-2}), and morbidly obese (BMI = 47.2 kg · m^{-2}) (40). Compared with HW and DEXA, ADP produces similar measurements (percent body fat = 0.5%, SEE = 2.9%) in collegiate female athletes (4) and collegiate wrestlers (20), overestimates percent body fat in collegiate female athletes (120), and underestimates percent body fat by about 2% in collegiate football players (18). Last, ADP is an effective body composition assessment technique for

monitoring changes during weight loss. In comparison with DEXA, ADP assessment of percent body fat during weight loss programs of 8 wk to 16 mo produces similar absolute changes, although ADP underestimated percent body fat by 2%–4% (78,128); overestimates percent body fat by about 5% (37); and produces similar percent fat changes (102) in the preexperimental and postexperimental periods.

COMPUTED TOMOGRAPHY SCANS, POSITRON EMISSION TOMOGRAPHY, AND MAGNETIC RESONANCE IMAGING AND SPECTROSCOPY

Cross-sectional imaging of the whole body for body composition analysis has been used since 1979 via CT (47,109). All major organs and tissues can be accurately viewed with CT, MRI, and related technologies. These imaging techniques produce scans that noninvasively quantify the volume of certain body tissues, such as regional fat distribution. A total body composition analysis is possible with sequential "slicing" through the body and assumptions for tissue densities used in calculation. Tissue area within the scan is calculated by segmentation techniques. Fat and lean tissue can be quantified by selecting regions of interest. Area can be determined by multiplying the number of pixels by their known area. Both MRI and CT scans have been validated compared with cadavers for determining interstitial and subcutaneous adipose tissue (79). MRI and CT scans provide relevant clinical information on skeletal muscle and bone density, and subcutaneous and visceral fat.

For CT scans, the system is composed of a cylindrical housing that contains a rotating X-ray unit. The X-ray passes through the subject and creates cross-sectional slices approximately 10-mm thick. The image represents a two-dimensional map of pixels corresponding to a three-dimensional section of volume elements (voxels). Each pixel has a numeric value called the *attenuation coefficient* that helps differentiate tissues based on the density and electrons per unit mass (42), and an image is created via a process known as *windowing*. The pixel is displayed according to the mean attenuation of the tissue(s) on a scale from most to least attenuating using *Hounsfield units* (HU), named after Geoffrey Hounsfield who first introduced CT in 1971 (47). For example, HUs for water, air, adipose tissue, and all other lean tissues and organs are 0, −1,000, −190 to −30, and −29 to 151, respectively (16). Tissue area and volume are then calculated. CT scans are very accurate and reliable with low coefficients of variation reported for subcutaneous and visceral adipose tissue determination (16). However, CT scanning exposes individuals to moderate-to-large amounts of radiation (2.7–10.0 mSv for a whole-body scan) that can limit its use in children and special adult populations, and it is limited for assessment of fat in nonadipose tissues (*e.g.*, heart, liver, skeletal muscle) (109). CT scans are costly, and many individuals have limited access to CT units.

PET is a nuclear imaging technique often combined with CT scanning to determine brown fat content in human tissues and organs (47). PET provides greater precision at the organ and tissue levels than other scanning methods. A metabolic tracer, usually fluorodeoxyglucose (^{18}F-FDG), is injected into the circulation, incorporates into various organs and tissues, and the subject is then scanned. ^{18}F-FDG is a glucose analog that is taken up by glucose-requiring cells in a manner similar to glucose. As the tracer decays, it emits a positron (electron antagonist) that moves within the organ or tissue, interacts with electrons, and produces γ-photons, which are detected during scanning and converted to an image. Because brown adipose tissue plays an important role in thermogenesis and is metabolically active (uses glucose), the use of PET-CT has been instrumental in the study of metabolism (98).

Body composition assessment with MRI has been in use since 1984 (47,109). For MRI scans, the image is based on proton density and relaxation times generating contrasts between adipose and lean tissues. Relaxation times represent the rate by which absorbed energy is released. The image is created by interaction of hydrogen atoms via the magnet creating a magnetic field. With the hydrogen protons aligned within the field, a pulsed radio frequency is applied causing the hydrogen protons to absorb energy, and an image is generated. The image is made up of T1 (time required for protons to return to original position, longitudinal relaxation) and T2 (images generated that provide information on tissue differences, transverse relaxation) information. MRI scans are accurate and have been shown to yield small CVs (109). However, they are costly and can be problematic for large individuals who may feel claustrophobic in a closed system. In addition, MRI has not been useful for determining lipid or water content in skeletal muscle. However, chemical shift imaging techniques such as *magnetic resonance spectroscopy* (^{1}H-MRS) can provide assessment of tissue lipid content. ^{1}H-MRS can separate, characterize, and record chemical signals within each voxel (109). Metabolites are identified by their frequency and expressed as the frequency shift relative to water (109). The chemical shift is expressed in parts per million (ppm), which for fat is around 1.25 ppm, whereas water = 4.26 ppm (109). After data correction, ^{1}H-MRS can be used as an accurate tool to assess lipid content at the tissue and organ levels.

ULTRASOUND

The use of ultrasound for body composition assessment has been in existence for many years. Ultrasound provides sonic energy at frequencies well above the audible range in humans (20 Hz–20 kHz) (42). The sonic energy (pulse or vibration) is propagated through the tissues at a specific velocity. For example, skeletal muscle has a density of 1.07 g · cm^{-3} and a velocity of 1,570 m · s^{-1}, whereas fat has a density of 0.90 g · cm^{-3} and a velocity of 1,440 m · s^{-1} (42). The pattern produced depends on its wavelength (frequency) and the density of the tissues. Part of the energy is reflected while the rest is refracted where the tissue density dictates the magnitude of reflection. Pulsed ultrasound imaging technology measures the reflection. In A-mode ultrasound, a pulse is sent from the probe through the subject and back (similar to an echo), and the depth (time of echo) is visually shown on an oscilloscope. B-mode ultrasound collects similar information but adds the positioning of the echo in a two-dimensional plane as well as the memory to recall previous echoes. The probe (transducer) is coupled to an echo camera that converts the impulses into a recognizable image. B-mode ultrasonography is the most practical for body composition assessment.

The reliability and validity of B-mode ultrasound body fat measurements have been established. Reliability coefficients >0.90 for various regions measured have been reported (8,42). Research has validated ultrasound compared with other techniques (46,60) and has shown ultrasound to produce similar percent fat estimates as DEXA in athletes (93) and adolescents who are obese (94). Compared to skinfolds, ultrasound has shown high correlation coefficients (46,60) and may be more accurate for measuring actual subcutaneous fat thickness (126). In fact, B-mode ultrasound has been shown to be superior to skinfolds for measuring subcutaneous fat in adults and children who are obese (64,103) and reliable and valid for measuring visceral fat (1,112). Total percent body fat can be predicted via regression equations (using various sites of subcutaneous fat measurements) that estimate BD similar to skinfold analysis (28,93). Critical to reliable ultrasonic measurement is standardization of technique. The technician needs to be able to standardize the exact site locations of measurement and apply uniform and constant pressure on the probe throughout because an imbalance can alter adipose tissue distribution significantly (42).

ISOTOPIC DILUTION

Isotopic dilution enables measurement of TBW and estimation of FFM and percent body fat. Isotopic dilution also serves as a criterion model for TBW estimation via BIA and bioimpedance spectroscopy. Determination of TBW (in addition to FFM and fat mass assessments) has important clinical and performance relevance. For example, TBW assessment has been measured as a correlation tool to help monitor upper-body power changes in judo athletes who frequently lose weight prior to competition (107). TBW is calculated from the compartment volume, which is the ratio of the dose of a tracer to its concentration in the bodily compartment after equilibration is achieved within the body (42). Common tracers used in isotopic dilution are D_2O, ^{18}O, and tritiated water (^3H_2O). Sodium bromide has also been used as a tracer to detect extracellular water content; intracellular water content can subsequently be determined by subtracting the extracellular component from TBW. Following a baseline fluid sample (blood, urine, saliva), a tracer dose of labeled water is given. A second fluid sample (administered about 2–4 h after equilibration) is collected and then analyzed via mass spectroscopy or gas chromatography (42). TBW may be calculated by dilution space (L)/1.041 (118). Because the mean hydration fraction of FFM is about 73.2%, FFM = TBW (kg)/0.732 (118), and fat mass may be calculated by subtracting FFM from total body mass.

Test–retest reliability of isotopic dilution is very good. However, isotopic dilution does have a few limitations. Technical errors can occur with the methodology. Hydrogen tracers (2%–4%) may exchange with nonaqueous hydrogen, thereby altering fat mass by up to 1.4 kg and percent body fat by approximately 2% (42). Correction factors (0.5%–4.0%) may be needed to account for errors in the calculation of isotopic dilution space. In addition, isotopic dilution is costly, which may further limit its use.

DUAL-ENERGY X-RAY ABSORPTIOMETRY

DEXA is based on a 3C model of total body mineral stores, FFM, and fat mass. The principle of absorptiometry is based on exponential attenuation of X-rays at two energies as they pass through the body. Modern DEXA technology has developed from single-photon absorptiometry used in the 1960s and subsequent dual-photon absorptiometry (DPA) (47). DEXA machines are commonly used in hospitals and research facilities and have replaced DPA (which uses a radionuclide, such as gadolinium, to generate γ-rays) in many settings since 1989 (47,59). In comparison, DEXA offers better precision, improved spatial resolution, reduced radiation exposure, and decreased scan times compared to DPA (77). X-rays are generated at two energies (either alternating voltages or constant potentials) via a low-current X-ray tube located underneath the DEXA machine. A detector positioned overhead on the scanning arm and interface with a computer is also needed for scanning an image. Following system calibration and removal of metallic objects from the subject, the subject is instructed to lie motionless on a scanning bed and is secured with Velcro straps on the lower leg and feet. The individual is then scanned rectilinearly from head to toe for 5–25 min, depending on the type of scan. Newer DEXA units have greatly reduced total scan time, making the technique more practical and easy to administer. The X-rays are delivered at two photon energies (between 38 and 140 keV, depending on the manufacturer), and the differential attenuation is used to estimate bone mineral content and soft tissue composition (a 2C model). Soft tissue measurements can only be made in regions where no bone is present. The ratio of soft tissue attenuation of the low- and high-energy beams is measured as follows: soft tissue attenuation (low and high energy) = proportion of fat (fat attenuation) + proportion of lean tissue (attenuation of lean tissue) (59). Thus, a 3C model is seen as soft tissue mass is divided into FFM and fat mass. Lohman (72) reported a precision for the DEXA technique of about 1% with a SEE of about 1.8% body fat. A DEXA scan generates pertinent information regarding the masses (g) of fat, lean tissue, and bone mineral content and density for the total body and for specific regions (e.g., the head, trunk, limbs) (Fig. 18-2).

DEXA has many advantages for measurement of body composition. DEXA is easy to administer, and subjects have a higher comfort level compared with other techniques, such as HW. DEXA software provides a great deal of information for the user. Regional body composition measurements are particularly attractive for clinical and research utilities. For example, BMD assessments of the lumbar spine, proximal femur, and forearm are useful in the diagnosis of osteoporosis (2). DEXA has been shown to be a very reliable analytic tool for body composition measurements in clinical populations, including those with gastrointestinal, renal, endocrinologic, pulmonary, hepatic, bone, neuromuscular, and metabolic/nutritional disorders (2). Regional measurement of FFM is attractive for examining the effects of various exercise programs, such as resistance training on muscular hypertrophy (121). DEXA uses low-level radiation and is safe, fast, and accurate. A whole-body measurement is <5–7 μSv, which is close to background radiation levels (6–20 μSv) (29,59) and far less than CT scans (2.7–10.0 mSv) (67,109), chest X-ray (12–50 μSv), and lumbar spine X-ray (700–820 μSv) (2,28).

There are some limitations associated with DEXA measurements. An individual's size is of some concern. A very tall person or individual of large weight (e.g., >300 lb) may extend beyond the measurable range on the scanner table or have to maintain a "cramped" position, which can distort regional measurements. Often, individuals who are morbidly obese may not be able to be scanned due to these limitations. The DEXA instruments (General Electric Lunar, Hologic, and Norland) are large and expensive, although the machines are becoming more accessible in number. Because of the expense of the DEXA equipment, these machines are typically found in a clinical or research setting. Because of its emission of low-level radiation, several states require a physician's prescription in order to perform DEXA scans. This requirement could limit the use of DEXA primarily to the research setting. DEXA assumes the same amount of fat lies over bone as over neighboring bone-free tissue, which could potentially reduce accuracy in the limb and trunk regions (39). An increase in tissue anterior-posterior thickness in individuals who are obese could also reduce accuracy via attenuation of the dual-energy rays (39). Variations in percent body fat determined via DEXA (compared to a 4C model) have been shown to correlate to anterior-posterior chest depth in individuals who are obese (65). DEXA unit algorithms appear more accurate (as the assumption of density is not violated) when the subject's anterior-posterior thickness ≤20 cm; thus, error rate increases as anterior-posterior thickness increases (109). DEXA assumes a constant hydration state (73.2%) and electrolyte content in lean tissue; thus, a change in hydration status could have a small effect of soft tissue attenuation and percent body fat determination (39,59,109). Lastly, user error can occur when delineating regional measurements, thereby demonstrating the importance of a single technician for sequential testing.

There is some concern over the lack of standardization between DEXA equipment manufacturers. Differences exist in hardware, calibration methodology, and software that elicit different body composition results between instruments (2,39,62,115). The imaging geometry — the older style pencil versus the fan beam — may be a source of variation. A pencil beam is coupled to a single detector and scans the whole body in a raster, whereas a fan beam is coupled to a multidetector (because Z/X-rays overlap) linear array that distributes the X-rays across a wider area for a whole-body scan (2). Fan beam systems also have a higher X-ray flux and better image quality (2). Different manufacturers have different arrangements for X-ray distribution, number, and alignment of detectors (72). Genton et al. (39) reported that fat mass varied between DEXA devices of different manufacturers and with different software used by the same manufacturer by 0.4–4.4 kg (0.5%–6.9%). In addition, body fat

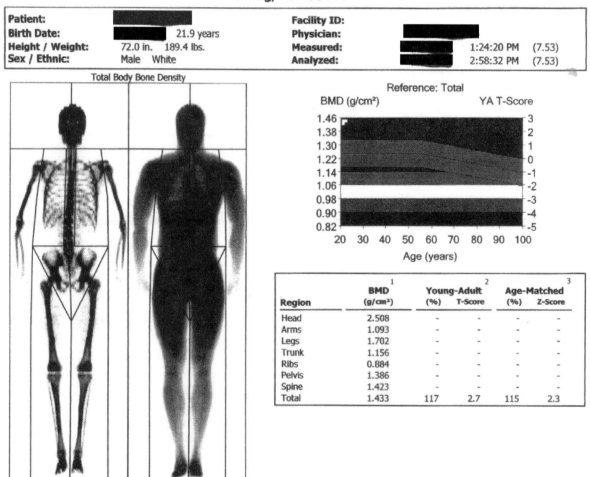

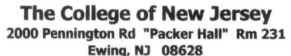

FIGURE 18-2. Sample DEXA scan report.

ANCILLARY RESULTS [Total Body]

Region	BMD (g/cm²)[1]	Young-Adult[2] (%)	Young-Adult[2] T-Score	Age-Matched[3] (%)	Age-Matched[3] Z-Score	BMC (g)	Area (cm²)
Head	2.508	-	-	-	-	595	237
Arms	1.093	-	-	-	-	544	497
Legs	1.702	-	-	-	-	1,515	890
Trunk	1.156	-	-	-	-	1,357	1,174
Ribs	0.884	-	-	-	-	491	555
Pelvis	1.386	-	-	-	-	539	389
Spine	1.423	-	-	-	-	328	230
Total	1.433	117	2.7	115	2.3	4,011	2,799

BODY COMPOSITION

Region	Tissue (%Fat)	Region (%Fat)	Tissue (g)	Fat (g)	Lean (g)	BMC (g)	Total Mass (kg)
Left Arm	9.1	8.6	5,162	467	4,695	266	-
Left Leg	19.2	18.2	14,288	2,737	11,551	735	-
Left Trunk	18.5	17.8	19,948	3,685	16,263	699	-
Left Total	17.0	16.2	42,201	7,164	35,037	2,013	-
Right Arm	9.1	8.6	5,415	490	4,925	278	-
Right Leg	19.2	18.2	14,929	2,861	12,068	780	-
Right Trunk	18.5	17.8	18,381	3,394	14,987	658	-
Right Total	17.0	16.2	41,054	6,973	34,081	1,998	-
Arms	9.1	8.6	10,577	958	9,619	544	-
Legs	19.2	18.2	29,216	5,598	23,619	1,515	-
Trunk	18.5	17.8	38,330	7,079	31,251	1,357	-
Total	17.0	16.2	83,255	14,137	69,118	4,011	87.3

FIGURE 18-2. *Continued.*

measurements have been shown to vary by about 1.7% when repeated measurements are taken on different DEXA machines from the same manufacturer (113). CVs between DEXA devices have been reported to be <5.2% (22,44), although the CV may be <1% when the same device is used (86). Thus, for high reliability of measurements, it is strongly recommended that DEXA scans be performed on the same instrument for repeated intra-subject measurements.

DEXA has been shown to correlate highly with HW and other multicompartment models (4C) in athletes and in young, middle-aged, or elderly men and women. However, Bland-Altman analyses have shown that DEXA typically registered higher body fat percentages (1%–2%) for total body measurements (61,86,119) and may longitudinally overestimate fat mass loss and underestimate fat mass gains during precompetition training in elite judo athletes (101). This procedure is commonly used to assess how well an experimental result compares with a result obtained from a more sophisticated or criterion method. DEXA has been shown to overestimate percent body fat in young (±4.5%) and elderly (±2.2%) women,

but to underestimate percent body fat in young (±0.9%) and elderly men (±1.7%) (17). DEXA correlates strongly, but also underestimates, total fat mass by approximately 0.7 kg (100). In men and women who are obese, DEXA correlates highly and produces similar mean percent body fat data to a 4C model; however, individual differences of −3% to 4% were shown between measurements taken via DEXA and calculated from a 4C model (65). In one investigation, when lard was added to either the trunk or thigh regions, DEXA was able to quantify the additional mass as 96% fat (61) but was only able to identify approximately 62% of lard in the trunk as fat and >80% in the legs in another study (100). Regional body composition assessment has produced varying results, although DEXA is valid for measuring abdominal adiposity (41). In some studies, DEXA has been shown to underestimate central body fat (41,42) and to overestimate fat mass in the thigh and calf areas compared with CT scans (100). It is important to note that DEXA alone cannot distinguish intra-abdominal from subcutaneous fat (59). DEXA has been shown to be a reliable tool for monitoring body composition changes over time (128) but may be limited when

BOX 18-3	Summary of Body Composition Techniques

SKINFOLD ANALYSIS

- Highly regarded technique yet prone to many sources of error
- Technician training and anatomic site selection important
- Equation(s) selected should be specific to population tested
- Many skinfold formulas exist from 1 to 10 sites
- Standard error of estimate (SEE) is approximately ±3.5% (differs with each equation)

BIOELECTRICAL IMPEDANCE

- Less technician training required compared with skinfold measurement
- Numerous pretest control conditions need to be followed by the client (anything that affects hydration status)
- SEE is approximately ±3.5%–5.0% (differs with each equation)

HYDRODENSITOMETRY

- Procedure is time consuming
- Equipment is fairly expensive and requires adequate space, plumbing, and high maintenance
- Often considered the criterion-referenced standard
- Some clients may not be able to perform the procedure (complete water submersion at full exhalation)
- Requires measurement of residual lung volume (additional equipment needed)
- SEE is approximately ±2.5% when performed correctly

NEAR-INFRARED INTERACTANCE

- Limited research on this procedure compared with other techniques

- Very little technician training needed
- SEE is approximately ±5% (differs with each equation)

CLINICAL ASSESSMENT PROCEDURES: COMPUTED TOMOGRAPHY SCANS AND MAGNETIC RESONANCE IMAGING SCANS

- Procedures are time consuming
- Equipment is very expensive and is accessible only in clinical facilities
  - CT scans expose subjects to moderate-to-high levels of radiation
- Have numerous clinical applications
  - Advances in technology have made it possible to assess organ- and tissue-level fat content
- SEE is not yet fully developed (more research data are needed)

PLETHYSMOGRAPHY: AIR DISPLACEMENT

- Equipment is expensive and is generally accessible only in research facilities
- No physical performance requirements for client (advantage compared with hydrodensitometry)
- Require special clothing (tight-fitting Lycra-type material)
- SEE is approximately ±2.2%–3.7% (more research data are needed)

DUAL-ENERGY X-RAY ABORPTIOMETRY

- Equipment is expensive and is generally accessible only in clinical or research facilities
- Has more clinical utility than just percent body fat (also bone density)
- Can provide regional measurements on the body
- SEE is approximately ±1.8% (more research data are needed)

---

monitoring athletes with low percent body fat (101) and has been shown to be more sensitive for assessing small changes in body composition in postmenopausal women than HW and other multicompartment methods (57). *Box 18-3* summarizes the pros and cons of body composition techniques. These limitations in part prevent DEXA assessment from being considered the "gold standard" for body composition assessment.

THREE-DIMENSIONAL BODY SCANNING

Various imaging techniques have been developed to assess body shapes and dimensions via scanners that are based on laser scanning, structured light, or stereo vision

systems (129). Three-dimensional photonic scanning (3DPS; Hamamatsu Photonics, Japan) uses high-speed digital cameras and triangular algorithms to detect the positions of laser light points projected onto the surface of an object and reflected to the cameras (122). Software connects the points to generate a three-dimensional image that is used to determine values for body circumferences, lengths, widths, volume, and thickness (122). More than 2 million data points are generated in a 10-s scan. Size of a segment scanned is calculated from all detected data points at that level, and distance between two points is determined from all data points on a line between the points. Stereo vision systems (3DSV) use two slightly separated cameras at different views to generate disparity (relative displacement of objects from the two images), which is used to calculate depth (129), and a projector to form a stereo head. Multiple stereo heads are used during a total body scan, and body volumes and circumferences can be mathematically determined.

For total body scanning, subjects stand motionless in the center of the scanner with arms and legs abducted so they are not touching the trunk/legs while wearing tight clothing with head caps (similar to ADP). Multiple scans are taken, and body volume and density are calculated for subsequent determination of percent body fat. Studies have shown 3DPS and 3DSV systems to provide reliable body composition measures (88,129). Compared to HW, 3DPS produced statistically similar percent body fat measures but slightly greater body volume (122). 3DPS also produced larger body circumference measurements compared to those data obtained from use of a tape measure (122). Compared to ADP, 3DSV produced similar body volume and percent body fat values, although (in comparison to tape measures) hip circumference and waist depth values were significantly higher (129). Nevertheless, most studies generally agree that three-dimensional imaging systems do provide valid and reliable body fat percent measurements.

BODY COMPOSITION ASSESSMENT IN CHILDREN AND ADOLESCENTS

Approximately 17% (12.5 million) of children and adolescents aged 2–19 yr in the United States are considered obese (84), with the numbers rising annually. The prevalence of metabolic syndrome in children is approximately 4%, with estimates reaching as high as 50% in obese youth populations (45). With the rise in childhood obesity in the United States, body composition measurement in children and adolescents has become a very important assessment tool. However, these populations can be difficult to assess because of the effects of growth/maturation on FFM, fat mass, and hydration state.

Several studies have examined skinfolds, BMI, the waist-to-height ratio (WHtR), ADP, BIA, HW, ultrasound, and DEXA assessments in children and adolescents. BMI has been shown to be weakly associated with percent body fat in several studies examining children; however, accuracy improves as it is used in children with higher body fat (36). BMI has not been shown to be a good measure of body fat in adolescent athletes (96). The WHtR has been used in some studies in a similar manner to BMI and has shown to be strongly correlated to metabolic disease (36). In comparison to 4C models, DEXA and ADP have correlated very highly (30,111), but DEXA has been shown to underestimate percent body fat in lean subjects and overestimate percent body fat (while underestimating lean tissue mass) in children and adolescent who are obese (30,111,127). Overall, percent body fat obtained

with DEXA has been approximately 1.0%–1.7% higher than in 4C models (30,111). DEXA and ultrasound have shown similar percent body fat measurements in adolescents who are obese (94). Skinfolds are commonly used and have been shown to correlate highly with DEXA (14). However, selection of the appropriate equation is critical, as more than 15 researchers have developed specific equations for children and adolescents, but few have correlated well to DEXA (99). Several studies have shown ADP and skinfolds to provide accurate assessments of body composition in children compared with DEXA (23,24), with absolute percent body fat values higher in DEXA (71). However, BIA has been shown to underestimate percent body fat considerably (23) (sometimes by as much as 12.8%) to overestimate FFM (54) and to overestimate changes in percent body fat over time (24). In children and adolescents who are obese, ADP has been shown to correlate highly with DEXA, with absolute percent body fat values being higher in DEXA by about 3%–5% (68,97). HW has been shown to produce similar percent body fat values compared with DEXA (71) but to underestimate percent body fat (30) in children. HW has been considered unsuitable in children because of the difficulty in following the procedures of being submerged underwater and exhaling completely (23,30,111).

BODY FAT PREDICTION EQUATION SELECTION

Since the early 1950s, more than 100 regression equations have been developed to predict BD and percent body fat. Prediction equations may be either general or population specific. Population-specific equations may underestimate or overestimate body composition if they are applied to individuals from other populations. In contrast, generalized equations can replace several equations as they can be applied to diverse populations. Generalized equations are developed from heterogeneous samples and account for differences in age, sex, ethnicity, and other characteristics by including these variables as predictors in the equation.

To develop prediction equations, it is necessary to select a large representative sample of a specific population. The predictor variables (*e.g.*, height and weight, sex, age, race or ethnicity, skinfolds, or bioelectrical impedance) and the criterion estimates of body composition are measured in the same subjects, and the equation is developed using appropriate statistical methods. The usefulness of the equation depends on the strength of association between the variables and the accuracy with which the dependent variable is estimated. Useful equations give estimates of percent fat or FFM that are reasonably well correlated ($r > 0.80$) with the criterion measure. Moreover, the means and standard deviations of the estimated and criterion scores should be nearly equal, and the SEE for predicting the criterion from the estimated values is between ±2.5% and 3.5% for percent body fat (5). To select the most appropriate equation, the following questions should be considered (5):

1. To whom is the specific percent body fat equation applicable? Age, ethnicity, sex, physical activity level, and estimated amount of body fat all influence which equation should be used.
2. Was an appropriate compartment model used to develop the equation? Errors from the compartment model contribute to the equation's total error. For example, multicompartment models require fewer assumptions and give more accurate reference measurements than methods based on the 2C model. Equations derived from 3C, 4C, and 5C models should be used in populations for whom the assumptions underlying the 2C model are not valid.
3. Was a representative sample of the population studied? Large, randomly selected samples are needed to ensure that the data are representative of the population. If random sampling is not possible and convenience samples are used, the prediction equation may be acceptable as long as a sufficient number of subjects are studied. Large sample sizes yield stable and valid equations.
4. How were the predictor variables measured? When any equation is applied, it is important that the predictor variables be measured in the same way as the original investigators to minimize prediction errors.
5. Was the equation cross-validated in another sample of the population? Investigator/laboratory differences can reduce equation accuracy. Thus, the equation should be cross-validated in other samples of the same population.
6. Does the equation give accurate estimates of percent body fat? In validation studies, when estimating body fat, the multiple correlations between variables should be $R^2 > 0.80$, and SEEs should range from 2.5% to 3.5%.

INTERPRETATION OF BODY FAT PERCENTAGE ESTIMATES

Interpretation of body fat percentage estimates is complicated by three factors: (a) there are no universal standards for percent body fat that have been established and accepted; (b) all methods of measurement are indirect, so error needs to be considered; and (c) there is no universally accepted criterion measurement method.

BODY FAT PERCENTAGE STANDARDS

Although national standards have been developed and accepted for BMI and waist circumference (*GETP9 Table 4-1*; *Fig. 18-3*), none exist for estimates of body fat

Women

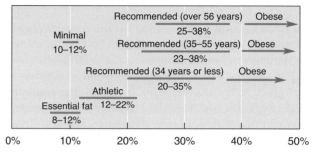

Men

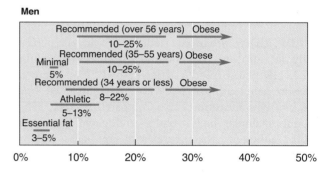

FIGURE 18-3. Percent body fat standards for men and women.

percentage. Thus, practitioners must choose from many classifications proposed by textbook authors, researchers, and programs (53,73). Standards may be based on health or physical performance, but only sex is considered a differentiating factor in percent body fat classifications. However, it is well known that body fat increases with age from the late teens/early 20s up to the sixth decade of life. The magnitude of increase in body fat with age is associated with lifestyle factors that affect energy intake and expenditure and is not likely to represent a normal response to biologic aging.

Since 1981, releases of the *ACSM Guidelines for Exercise Testing and Prescription* have included the normative-based standards developed by the Cooper Institute in Dallas, Texas. These norms were revised in 1994 and were developed using skinfold measurements to estimate body fat percentage in a population of predominately white and college-educated men and women (*GETP9 Tables 4-5* and *4-6*). These norms provide percentiles that differ by sex and age (ranging from 20 to 79 yr). The average (50th percentile) for young (20–29 yr) men and women is 16.6% and 21.0%, respectively. The average increases to 24.1% and 30.4% for elderly (70–79 yr) men and women, respectively (73).

MEASUREMENT ERROR CONSIDERATIONS

Body fat percentage data should be presented and interpreted with the SEE term for the methods used (*e.g.*, 22% ± 3.5%). Minimally, ±1 SEE unit should be used; however, if the 95% confidence interval (CI) limits are desired, then ±2 SEE units are required. A major concern in interpreting body fat percentage values is the relatively large SEE of the measurements (*e.g.*, ±3.5% for skinfold equations). A 45-yr-old woman who had a percent body fat of 28.5% based on skinfold measurements (35th percentile) could be as low as 21.5% (70th percentile) or as high as 35.5% (10th percentile) when considering the 95% CI (±2 SEE). Because of the lack of accepted national standards and the large SEE, interpretation of percent body fat estimates needs to be done with caution and shared with clients only after careful explanation of the meaning of the values. The most appropriate use of these estimates may be for serial measurements over time to evaluate responses to diet or physical activity where the same measurement procedure (*i.e.*, instrument and technician) is used.

SUMMARY

Excess body fat is detrimental to overall health and physical performance. Measurement and quantification of body fat is of great importance for allied health professionals, fitness practitioners, and athletic personnel. In most nonathletic adults, a reasonable assessment of excess weight (fat) status can be determined from simple measurements of height, weight, and waist circumference. These measurements are easy to obtain, do not require extensive training to perform, and do not require expensive equipment. Advanced body composition estimates can be made when specific information is needed, equipment is available, and trained technicians perform the assessments. It is important for users of these advanced body fat estimation methods to understand the error associated with these measurements, to use the SEE in reporting body composition results, and to strictly adhere to the procedures outlined in this chapter when assessing body composition.

REFERENCES

1. Abe T, Kawakami Y, Sugita M, Yoshikawa K, Fukunaga T. Use of B-mode ultrasound for visceral fat mass evaluation: comparisons with magnetic resonance imaging. *Appl Human Sci.* 1995;14(3):133–9.
2. Albanese CV, Diessel E, Genant HK. Clinical applications of body composition measurements using DXA. *J Clin Densitom.* 2003;6(2):75–85.
3. Ball SD, Altena TS. Comparison of the Bod Pod and dual energy x-ray absorptiometry in men. *Physiol Meas.* 2004;25(3):671–8.
4. Ballard TP, Fafara L, Vukovich MD. Comparison of Bod Pod and DXA in female collegiate athletes. *Med Sci Sports Exerc.* 2004;36(4):731–5.
5. *Basic Data on Anthropometric Measurements and Angular Measurements of the Hip and Knee Joints for Selected Age Groups 1–74 Years of Age, United States, 1971–1975* [Internet]. Hyattsville, MD: U.S. Department of Health and Human Services, Public Health Service, Office of the Assistant Secretary of Health, National Center for Health Statistics; For sale by the Supt. of Docs, U.S. Govt. Print. Off; 1981 [cited 2011 Jan 13]. 76 p. Available from: http://www.cdc.gov/nchs/data/series/sr_11/sr11_219.pdf

6. Baumgartner RN. Electrical impedance and total body electrical conductivity. In: Roche AF, Heymsfield S, Lohman TG, editors. *Human Body Composition.* Champaign: Human Kinetics; 1996. p. 79–107.
7. Baumgartner RN, Heymsfield SB, Lichtman S, Wang J, Pierson RN,Jr. Body composition in elderly people: effect of criterion estimates on predictive equations. *Am J Clin Nutr.* 1991;53(6):1345–53.
8. Bellisari A, Roche AF, Siervogel RM. Reliability of B-mode ultrasonic measurements of subcutaneous adipose tissue and intra-abdominal depth: comparisons with skinfold thicknesses. *Int J Obes Relat Metab Disord.* 1993;17(8):475–80.
9. Benson M. Committee refines wrestling safety rules. *NCAA News.* 1998;35(16):114.
10. Bolanowski M, Nilsson BE. Assessment of human body composition using dual-energy x-ray absorptiometry and bioelectrical impedance analysis. *Med Sci Monit.* 2001;7(5):1029–33.
11. Boren HG, Kory RC, Syner JC. The veterans administration-army cooperative study of pulmonary function. II. The lung volume and its subdivisions in normal men. *Am J Med.* 1966;41(1):96–114.
12. Broeder CE, Burrhus KA, Svanevik LS, Volpe J, Wilmore JH. Assessing body composition before and after resistance or endurance training. *Med Sci Sports Exerc.* 1997;29(5):705–12.
13. Brozek J, Grande F, Anderson JT, Keys A. Densitometric analysis of body composition: revision of some quantitative assumptions. *Ann N Y Acad Sci.* 1963;110:113–40.
14. Buison AM, Ittenbach RF, Stallings VA, Zemel BS. Methodological agreement between two-compartment body-composition methods in children. *Am J Hum Biol.* 2006;18(4):470–80.
15. Chan G, Chen CT. Musculoskeletal effects of obesity. *Curr Opin Pediatr.* 2009;21(1):65–70.
16. Chowdhury B, Sjostrom L, Alpsten M, Kostanty J, Kvist H, Lofgren R. A multicompartment body composition technique based on computerized tomography. *Int J Obes Relat Metab Disord.* 1994;18(4):219–34.
17. Clasey JL, Kanaley JA, Wideman L, et al. Validity of methods of body composition assessment in young and older men and women. *J Appl Physiol.* 1999;86(5):1728–38.
18. Collins MA, Millard-Stafford ML, Sparling PB, et al. Evaluation of the BOD POD for assessing body fat in collegiate football players. *Med Sci Sports Exerc.* 1999;31(9):1350–6.
19. Despres JP, Lemieux I. Abdominal obesity and metabolic syndrome. *Nature.* 2006;444(7121):881–7.
20. Dixon CB, Deitrick RW, Pierce JR, Cutrufello PT, Drapeau LL. Evaluation of the BOD POD and leg-to-leg bioelectrical impedance analysis for estimating percent body fat in National Collegiate Athletic Association Division III collegiate wrestlers. *J Strength Cond Res.* 2005;19(1):85–91.
21. Dutta C. Significance of sarcopenia in the elderly. *J Nutr.* 1997;127(5 Suppl):992S–3S.
22. Economos CD, Nelson ME, Fiatarone MA, et al. A multi-center comparison of dual energy X-ray absorptiometers: in vivo and in vitro soft tissue measurement. *Eur J Clin Nutr.* 1997;51(5):312–7.
23. Eisenmann JC, Heelan KA, Welk GJ. Assessing body composition among 3- to 8-year-old children: anthropometry, BIA, and DXA. *Obes Res.* 2004;12(10):1633–40.
24. Elberg J, McDuffie JR, Sebring NG, et al. Comparison of methods to assess change in children's body composition. *Am J Clin Nutr.* 2004;80(1):64–9.
25. Ellis KJ. Whole-body counting and neutron activation analysis. In: Roche AF, Heymsfield S, Lohman TG, editors. *Human Body Composition.* Champaign: Human Kinetics; 1996. p. 45–61.
26. Ellis KJ, Yao M, Shypailo RJ, Urlando A, Wong WW, Heird WC. Body-composition assessment in infancy: air-displacement plethysmography compared with a reference 4-compartment model. *Am J Clin Nutr.* 2007;85(1):90–5.
27. Erickson JM, Stout JR, Eveertouch TK, Housh TJ, Johnson GO, Worrell N. Validity of self-assessment techniques for estimating

percent body fat in men and women. *J Strength Cond Res.* 1998;12(4):243–7.

28. Fanelli MT, Kuczmarski RJ. Ultrasound as an approach to assessing body composition. *Am J Clin Nutr.* 1984;39(5):703–9.

29. Fewtrell MS, British Paediatric & Adolescent Bone Group. Bone densitometry in children assessed by dual x ray absorptiometry: uses and pitfalls. *Arch Dis Child.* 2003;88(9):795–8.

30. Fields DA, Goran MI. Body composition techniques and the four-compartment model in children. *J Appl Physiol.* 2000;89(2): 613–20.

31. Fields DA, Goran MI, McCrory MA. Body-composition assessment via air-displacement plethysmography in adults and children: a review. *Am J Clin Nutr.* 2002;75(3):453–67.

32. Fields DA, Higgins PB, Hunter GR. Assessment of body composition by air-displacement plethysmography: influence of body temperature and moisture. *Dyn Med.* 2004;3(1):3.

33. Fields DA, Wilson GD, Gladden LB, Hunter GR, Pascoe DD, Goran MI. Comparison of the BOD POD with the four-compartment model in adult females. *Med Sci Sports Exerc.* 2001;33(9): 1605–10.

34. Folsom AR, Kaye SA, Sellers TA, et al. Body fat distribution and 5-year risk of death in older women. *JAMA.* 1993;269(4):483–7.

35. Fornetti WC, Pivarnik JM, Foley JM, Fiechtner JJ. Reliability and validity of body composition measures in female athletes. *J Appl Physiol.* 1999;87(3):1114–22.

36. Freedman DS, Sherry B. The validity of BMI as an indicator of body fatness and risk among children. *Pediatrics.* 2009;124 Suppl 1:S23–34.

37. Frisard MI, Greenway FL, Delany JP. Comparison of methods to assess body composition changes during a period of weight loss. *Obes Res.* 2005;13(5):845–54.

38. Furstenberg A, Davenport A. Comparison of multifrequency bioelectrical impedance analysis and dual-energy X-ray absorptiometry assessments in outpatient hemodialysis patients. *Am J Kidney Dis.* 2011;57(1):123–9.

39. Genton L, Hans D, Kyle UG, Pichard C. Dual-energy X-ray absorptiometry and body composition: differences between devices and comparison with reference methods. *Nutrition.* 2002;18(1): 66–70.

40. Ginde SR, Geliebter A, Rubiano F, et al. Air displacement plethysmography: validation in overweight and obese subjects. *Obes Res.* 2005;13(7):1232–7.

41. Glickman SG, Marn CS, Supiano MA, Dengel DR. Validity and reliability of dual-energy X-ray absorptiometry for the assessment of abdominal adiposity. *J Appl Physiol.* 2004;97(2):509–14.

42. Graves JE, Kanaley JA, Garzarella L, Pollock ML. Anthropometry and body composition assessment. In: Maud PJ, Foster C, editors. *Physiological Assessment of Human Fitness.* 2nd ed. Champaign: Human Kinetics; 2006. p. 185–225.

43. Gunstad J, Paul RH, Cohen RA, Tate DF, Spitznagel MB, Gordon E. Elevated body mass index is associated with executive dysfunction in otherwise healthy adults. *Compr Psychiatry.* 2007;48(1):57–61.

44. Guo Y, Franks PW, Brookshire T, Antonio Tataranni P. The intra- and inter-instrument reliability of DXA based on ex vivo soft tissue measurements. *Obes Res.* 2004;12(12):1925–9.

45. Harrell JS, Jessup A, Greene N. Changing our future: obesity and the metabolic syndrome in children and adolescents. *J Cardiovasc Nurs.* 2006;21(4):322–30.

46. Haymes EM, Lundegren HM, Loomis JL, Buskirk ER. Validity of the ultrasonic technique as a method of measuring subcutaneous adipose tissue. *Ann Hum Biol.* 1976;3(3):245–51.

47. Heymsfield SB. Development of imaging methods to assess adiposity and metabolism. *Int J Obes (Lond).* 2008;32 Suppl 7:S76–82.

48. Heymsfield SB, Lichtman S, Baumgartner RN, et al. Body composition of humans: comparison of two improved four-compartment models that differ in expense, technical complexity, and radiation exposure. *Am J Clin Nutr.* 1990;52(1):52–8.

49. Heymsfield SB, Wang ZM, Withers RT. Multicomponent molecular level models of body composition. In: Roche AF, Heymsfield S, Lohman TG, editors. *Human Body Composition.* Champaign: Human Kinetics; 1996. p. 129–147.

50. Heyward VH, Stolarczyk LM. *Applied Body Composition Assessment.* Champaign (IL): Human Kinetics; 1996. 221 p.

51. Heyward VH, Wagner DR. *Applied Body Composition Assessment.* 2nd ed. Leeds (United Kingdom): Human Kinetics; 2004. 268 p.

52. Higgins PB, Fields DA, Hunter GR, Gower BA. Effect of scalp and facial hair on air displacement plethysmography estimates of percentage of body fat. *Obes Res.* 2001;9(5):326–30.

53. Hoffman J. *Norms for Fitness, Performance, and Health.* Champaign (IL): Human Kinetics; 2006. 221 p.

54. Hosking J, Metcalf BS, Jeffery AN, Voss LD, Wilkin TJ. Validation of foot-to-foot bioelectrical impedance analysis with dual-energy X-ray absorptiometry in the assessment of body composition in young children: the EarlyBird cohort. *Br J Nutr.* 2006;96(6): 1163–8.

55. Housh TJ, Johnson GO, Housh DJ, et al. Accuracy of near-infrared interactance instruments and population-specific equations for estimating body composition in young wrestlers. *J Strength Cond Res.* 2004;18(3):556–60.

56. Housh TJ, Stout JR, Johnson GO, Housh DJ, Eckerson JM. Validity of near-infrared interactance instruments for estimating percent body fat in youth wrestlers. *Pediatr Exerc Sci.* 1996;8(1):69–76.

57. Houtkooper LB, Going SB, Sproul J, Blew RM, Lohman TG. Comparison of methods for assessing body-composition changes over 1 y in postmenopausal women. *Am J Clin Nutr.* 2000; 72(2):401–6.

58. Jackson AS, Pollock ML. Practical assessment of body composition. *Phys Sportsmed.* 1985;13(5):76,80;82–90.

59. Jebb SA. Measurement of soft tissue composition by dual energy X-ray absorptiometry. *Br J Nutr.* 1997;77(2):151–63.

60. Jones PR, Davies PS, Norgan NG. Ultrasonic measurements of subcutaneous adipose tissue thickness in man. *Am J Phys Anthropol.* 1986;71(3):359–63.

61. Kohrt WM. Preliminary evidence that DEXA provides an accurate assessment of body composition. *J Appl Physiol.* 1998;84(1): 372–7.

62. Koo WWK, Hammami M, Shypailo RJ, Ellis KJ. Bone and body composition measurements of small subjects: discrepancies from software for fan-beam dual energy X-ray absorptiometry. *J Am Coll Nutr.* 2004;23(6):647–50.

63. Kraemer WJ, Torine JC, Silvestre R, et al. Body size and composition of National Football League players. *J Strength Cond Res.* 2005;19(3):485–9.

64. Kuczmarski RJ, Fanelli MT, Koch GG. Ultrasonic assessment of body composition in obese adults: overcoming the limitations of the skinfold caliper. *Am J Clin Nutr.* 1987;45(4):717–24.

65. LaForgia J, Dollman J, Dale MJ, Withers RT, Hill AM. Validation of DXA body composition estimates in obese men and women. *Obesity (Silver Spring).* 2009;17(4):821–6.

66. Lane JM, Serota AC, Raphael B. Osteoporosis: differences and similarities in male and female patients. *Orthop Clin North Am.* 2006;37(4):601–9.

67. Laskey MA. Dual-energy X-ray absorptiometry and body composition. *Nutrition.* 1996;12(1):45–51.

68. Lazzer S, Bedogni G, Agosti F, De Col A, Mornati D, Sartorio A. Comparison of dual-energy X-ray absorptiometry, air displacement plethysmography and bioelectrical impedance analysis for the assessment of body composition in severely obese Caucasian children and adolescents. *Br J Nutr.* 2008;100(4):918–24.

69. Lee SY, Gallagher D. Assessment methods in human body composition. *Curr Opin Clin Nutr Metab Care.* 2008;11(5):566–72.

70. Liuke M, Solovieva S, Lamminen A, et al. Disc degeneration of the lumbar spine in relation to overweight. *Int J Obes (Lond).* 2005;29(8):903–8.

71. Lockner DW, Heyward VH, Baumgartner RN, Jenkins KA. Comparison of air-displacement plethysmography, hydrodensitometry, and dual X-ray absorptiometry for assessing body composition of children 10 to 18 years of age. *Ann N Y Acad Sci.* 2000;904:72–8.

72. Lohman TG. *Advances in Body Composition Assessment.* Champaign (IL): Human Kinetics Publishers; 1992. 150 p.

73. Lohman TG, Houtkooper LB, Going SB. Body composition assessment: body fat standards and methods in the field of exercise and sports medicine. *ACSM Health Fitness J.* 1997;1:30–5.

74. Lukaski HC, Siders WA. Validity and accuracy of regional bioelectrical impedance devices to determine whole-body fatness. *Nutrition.* 2003;19(10):851–7.

75. Malina RM. Body composition in athletes: assessment and estimated fatness. *Clin Sports Med.* 2007;26(1):37–68.

76. Malina RM. Regional body composition: age, sex, and ethnic variation. In: Roche AF, Heymsfield S, Lohman TG, editors. *Human Body Composition.* Champaign: Human Kinetics; 1996. p. 217–255.

77. Mazess RB, Barden HS. Measurement of bone by dual-photon absorptiometry (DPA) and dual-energy X-ray absorptiometry (DEXA). *Ann Chir Gynaecol.* 1988;77(5–6):197–203.

78. Minderico CS, Silva AM, Teixeira PJ, Sardinha LB, Hull HR, Fields DA. Validity of air-displacement plethysmography in the assessment of body composition changes in a 16-month weight loss program. *Nutr Metab (Lond).* 2006;3:32.

79. Mitsiopoulos N, Baumgartner RN, Heymsfield SB, Lyons W, Gallagher D, Ross R. Cadaver validation of skeletal muscle measurement by magnetic resonance imaging and computerized tomography. *J Appl Physiol.* 1998;85(1):115–22.

80. Moon JR, Eckerson JM, Tobkin SE, et al. Estimating body fat in NCAA Division I female athletes: a five-compartment model validation of laboratory methods. *Eur J Appl Physiol.* 2009;105(1):119–30.

81. Moon JR, Hull HR, Tobkin SE, et al. Percent body fat estimations in college women using field and laboratory methods: a three-compartment model approach. *J Int Soc Sports Nutr.* 2007;4:16.

82. Moon JR, Tobkin SE, Roberts MD, et al. Total body water estimations in healthy men and women using bioimpedance spectroscopy: a deuterium oxide comparison. *Nutr Metab (Lond).* 2008;5:7.

83. Moon JR, Tobkin SE, Smith AE, et al. Percent body fat estimations in college men using field and laboratory methods: a three-compartment model approach. *Dyn Med.* 2008;7:7.

84. National Health and Nutrition Examination Survey Web site [Internet]. Atlanta (GA): Centers for Disease Control and Prevention; [cited 2011 Jan 19]. Available from: http://www.cdc.gov/nchs/nhanes.htm

85. National Heart, Lung, and Blood Institute, National Institute of Diabetes and Digestive and Kidney Diseases (U.S.). *Clinical Guidelines on the Identification, Evaluation, and Treatment of Overweight and Obesity in Adults: The Evidence Report.* Bethesda, MD: National Institutes of Health, National Heart, Lung, and Blood Institute; 1998. 228 p.

86. Norcross J, Van Loan MD. Validation of fan beam dual energy x ray absorptiometry for body composition assessment in adults aged 18–45 years. *Br J Sports Med.* 2004;38(4):472–6.

87. O'Brien RJ, Drizd TA. Roentgenographic determination of total lung capacity: normal values from a National Population Survey. *Am Rev Respir Dis.* 1983;128(5):949–52.

88. Olivares J, Wang J, Yu W, et al. Comparisons of body volumes and dimensions using three-dimensional photonic scanning in adult Hispanic-Americans and Caucasian-Americans. *J Diabetes Sci Technol.* 2007;1(6):921–8.

89. Oppliger RA, Case HS, Horswill CA, Landry GL, Shelter AC. American College of Sports Medicine position stand. Weight loss in wrestlers. *Med Sci Sports Exerc.* 1996;28(6):ix–xii.

90. Panotopoulos G, Ruiz JC, Guy-Grand B, Basdevant A. Dual x-ray absorptiometry, bioelectrical impedance, and near infrared interactance in obese women. *Med Sci Sports Exerc.* 2001;33(4):665–70.

91. Peeters MW, Claessens AL. Effect of different swim caps on the assessment of body volume and percentage body fat by air displacement plethysmography. *J Sports Sci.* 2011;29(2):191–6.

92. Pietrobelli A, Wang Z, Heymsfield SB. Techniques used in measuring human body composition. *Curr Opin Clin Nutr Metab Care.* 1998;1(5):439–48.

93. Pineau JC, Filliard JR, Bocquet M. Ultrasound techniques applied to body fat measurement in male and female athletes. *J Athl Train.* 2009;44(2):142–7.

94. Pineau JC, Lalys L, Bocquet M, et al. Ultrasound measurement of total body fat in obese adolescents. *Ann Nutr Metab.* 2010;56(1):36–44.

95. Pollock ML, Schmidt DH, Jackson AS. Measurement of cardiorespiratory fitness and body composition in the clinical setting. *Comp Ther.* 1980;6:12–7.

96. Portal S, Rabinowitz J, Adler-Portal D, et al. Body fat measurements in elite adolescent volleyball players: correlation between skinfold thickness, bioelectrical impedance analysis, air-displacement plethysmography, and body mass index percentiles. *J Pediatr Endocrinol Metab.* 2010;23(4):395–400.

97. Radley D, Gately PJ, Cooke CB, Carroll S, Oldroyd B, Truscott JG. Percentage fat in overweight and obese children: comparison of DXA and air displacement plethysmography. *Obes Res.* 2005;13(1):75–85.

98. Richard D, Picard F. Brown fat biology and thermogenesis. *Front Biosci.* 2011;16:1233–60.

99. Rodriguez G, Moreno LA, Blay MG, et al. Body fat measurement in adolescents: comparison of skinfold thickness equations with dual-energy X-ray absorptiometry. *Eur J Clin Nutr.* 2005;59(10):1158–66.

100. Salamone LM, Fuerst T, Visser M, et al. Measurement of fat mass using DEXA: a validation study in elderly adults. *J Appl Physiol.* 2000;89(1):345–52.

101. Santos DA, Silva AM, Matias CN, Fields DA, Heymsfield SB, Sardinha LB. Accuracy of DXA in estimating body composition changes in elite athletes using a four compartment model as the reference method. *Nutr Metab (Lond).* 2010;7:22.

102. Sasai H, Nakata Y, Nemoto M, et al. Air displacement plethysmography for estimating body composition changes with weight loss in middle-aged Japanese men. *Obes Facts.* 2010;3(6):357–62.

103. Semiz S, Ozgoren E, Sabir N. Comparison of ultrasonographic and anthropometric methods to assess body fat in childhood obesity. *Int J Obes (Lond).* 2007;31(1):53–8.

104. Shafer KJ, Siders WA, Johnson LK, Lukaski HC. Body density estimates from upper-body skinfold thicknesses compared to air-displacement plethysmography. *Clin Nutr.* 2010;29(2):249–54.

105. Shafer KJ, Siders WA, Johnson LK, Lukaski HC. Interaction of clothing and body mass index affects validity of air-displacement plethysmography in adults. *Nutrition.* 2008;24(2):148–54.

106. Shafer KJ, Siders WA, Johnson LK, Lukaski HC. Validity of segmental multiple-frequency bioelectrical impedance analysis to estimate body composition of adults across a range of body mass indexes. *Nutrition.* 2009;25(1):25–32.

107. Silva AM, Fields DA, Heymsfield SB, Sardinha LB. Body composition and power changes in elite judo athletes. *Int J Sports Med.* 2010;31(10):737–41.

108. Silva AM, Minderico CS, Teixeira PJ, Pietrobelli A, Sardinha LB. Body fat measurement in adolescent athletes: multicompartment molecular model comparison. *Eur J Clin Nutr.* 2006;60(8):955–64.

109. Silver HJ, Welch EB, Avison MJ, Niswender KD. Imaging body composition in obesity and weight loss: challenges and opportunities. *Diabetes Metab Syndr Obes.* 2010;3:337–47.

110. Siri WE. The gross composition of the body. *Adv Biol Med Phys.* 1956;4:239–80.

111. Sopher AB, Thornton JC, Wang J, Pierson RN,Jr, Heymsfield SB, Horlick M. Measurement of percentage of body fat in 411 children and adolescents: a comparison of dual-energy X-ray absorptiometry with a four-compartment model. *Pediatrics.* 2004;113(5):1285–90.

112. Stolk RP, Wink O, Zelissen PM, Meijer R, van Gils AP, Grobbee DE. Validity and reproducibility of ultrasonography for the measurement of intra-abdominal adipose tissue. *Int J Obes Relat Metab Disord.* 2001;25(9):1346–51.

113. Tataranni PA, Pettitt DJ, Ravussin E. Dual energy X-ray absorptiometry: inter-machine variability. *Int J Obes Relat Metab Disord.* 1996;20(11):1048–50.

114. Tegenkamp MH, Clark RR, Schoeller DA, Landry GL. Effects of covert subject actions on percent body fat by air-displacement plethysmography. *J Strength Cond Res.* 2011;25(7):2010–7.

115. Tothill P, Avenell A, Reid DM. Precision and accuracy of measurements of whole-body bone mineral: comparisons between Hologic, Lunar and Norland dual-energy X-ray absorptiometers. *Br J Radiol.* 1994;67(804):1210–7.

116. Tran ZV, Weltman A. Generalized equation for predicting body density of women from girth measurements. *Med Sci Sports Exerc.* 1989;21(1):101–4.

117. Tran ZV, Weltman A. Predicting body composition of men from girth measurements. *Hum Biol.* 1988;60(1):167–75.

118. Tylavsky FA, Lohman TG, Dockrell M, et al. Comparison of the effectiveness of 2 dual-energy X-ray absorptiometers with that of total body water and computed tomography in assessing changes in body composition during weight change. *Am J Clin Nutr.* 2003;77(2):356–63.

119. van Marken Lichtenbelt WD, Hartgens F, Vollaard NB, Ebbing S, Kuipers H. Body composition changes in bodybuilders: a method comparison. *Med Sci Sports Exerc.* 2004;36(3):490–7.

120. Vescovi JD, Hildebrandt L, Miller W, Hammer R, Spiller A. Evaluation of the BOD POD for estimating percent fat in female college athletes. *J Strength Cond Res.* 2002;16(4):599–605.

121. Volek JS, Ratamess NA, Rubin MR, et al. The effects of creatine supplementation on muscular performance and body composition responses to short-term resistance training overreaching. *Eur J Appl Physiol.* 2004;91(5–6):628–37.

122. Wang J, Gallagher D, Thornton JC, Yu W, Horlick M, Pi-Sunyer FX. Validation of a 3-dimensional photonic scanner for the measurement of body volumes, dimensions, and percentage body fat. *Am J Clin Nutr.* 2006;83(4):809–16.

123. Wang Z, Pi-Sunyer FX, Kotler DP, et al. Multicomponent methods: evaluation of new and traditional soft tissue mineral models by in vivo neutron activation analysis. *Am J Clin Nutr.* 2002;76(5):968–74.

124. Wang ZM, Heshka S, Pierson RN,Jr, Heymsfield SB. Systematic organization of body-composition methodology: an overview with emphasis on component-based methods. *Am J Clin Nutr.* 1995;61(3):457–65.

125. Wearing SC, Hennig EM, Byrne NM, Steele JR, Hills AP. Musculoskeletal disorders associated with obesity: a biomechanical perspective. *Obes Rev.* 2006;7(3):239–50.

126. Weits T, van der Beek EJ, Wedel M. Comparison of ultrasound and skinfold caliper measurement of subcutaneous fat tissue. *Int J Obes.* 1986;10(3):161–8.

127. Wells JC, Haroun D, Williams JE, et al. Evaluation of DXA against the four-component model of body composition in obese children and adolescents aged 5–21 years. *Int J Obes (Lond).* 2010;34(4):649–55.

128. Weyers AM, Mazzetti SA, Love DM, Gomez AL, Kraemer WJ, Volek JS. Comparison of methods for assessing body composition changes during weight loss. *Med Sci Sports Exerc.* 2002;34(3):497–502.

129. Xu B, Yu W, Yao M, Pepper MR, Freeland-Graves JH. Three-dimensional surface imaging system for assessing human obesity. *Opt Eng.* 2009;48(10):nihpa156427.

SELECTED REFERENCES FOR FURTHER READING

American College of Sports Medicine. *ACSM's Guidelines for Exercise Testing and Prescription.* 8th ed. Philadelphia (PA): Lippincott Williams & Wilkins; 2008. 400 p.

American College of Sports Medicine. *ACSM's Health-Related Physical Fitness Assessment Manual.* 3rd ed. Philadelphia (PA): Lippincott Williams & Wilkins; 2009. 224 p.

Heymsfield SB, Lohman T, Wang Z, Going SB. *Human Body Composition.* 2nd ed. Champaign (IL): Human Kinetics; 2005. 536 p.

Heyward VH, Wagner DR. *Applied Body Composition Assessment.* 2nd ed. Champaign (IL): Human Kinetics; 2004. 280 p.

Hoffman J. *Norms for Fitness, Performance, and Health.* Champaign (IL): Human Kinetics; 2006. 232 p.

Lohman TG, Roche AF, Martorell R, editors. *Anthropometric Standardization Reference Manual.* Champaign (IL): Human Kinetics; 1988. 184 p.

Maud PJ, Foster C. *Physiological Assessment of Human Fitness.* 2nd ed. Champaign (IL): Human Kinetics; 2006. 328 p.

National Heart, Lung, and Blood Institute. *Clinical Guidelines on the Identification, Evaluation, and Treatment of Overweight and Obesity in Adults: The Evidence Report.* Bethesda, MD: National Institutes of Health, National Heart, Lung, and Blood Institute, U.S. Department of Health and Human Services, Public Health Service; 1998. 262 p.

INTERNET RESOURCES

- Body Composition Tests: http://www.americanheart.org/presenter.jhtml?identifier=4489
- Body Fat Lab: http://www.shapeup.org/bodylab/default.php
- Centers for Disease Control and Prevention. Childhood Obesity: http://www.cdc.gov/obesity/childhood/index.html
- National Center for Health Statistics. National Health and Nutrition Examination Survey: http://http://www.cdc.gov/nchs/nhanes.htm
- National Heart Lung and Blood Institute. Clinical Guidelines on the Identification, Evaluation, and Treatment of Overweight and Obesity in Adults: http://www.nhlbi.nih.gov/guidelines/obesity/ob_home.htm
- National Institutes of Health. Calculate Your Body Mass Index: http://www.nhlbi.nih.gov/guidelines/obesity/bmi_tbl.htm

19

Exercise Program Safety and Emergency Procedures

The risk of sudden cardiac death or other injury during activity is always a concern in both the clinical and health/fitness settings. Although injuries are far more prevalent during exercise, exercise-related deaths can occur. Exercise-related deaths in persons younger than 40 yr are most often related to hereditary or congenital abnormalities (33). In contrast, coronary artery disease (CAD) is the most common exertion-related cardiovascular event in older individuals. Although studies have demonstrated that the risk of sudden cardiac death is transiently elevated during moderate-to-vigorous exercise compared with low-intensity activity or no exertion, habitual activity has been shown to reduce this transient risk (1,36). In addition, studies of both men and women have shown that, regardless of cardiovascular risk factors or the presence of cardiovascular disease, functional capacity is inversely related to both CAD and all-cause mortality rates (19,20). Studies investigating the incidence of exercise-related deaths suggest that, with the exception of individuals with diagnosed or occult heart disease, the benefits of vigorous-intensity exercise outweigh the risks (33). Moderate-intensity exercise is generally appropriate for individuals with heart disease, and recent studies with patients with heart disease have safely and effectively employed vigorous-intensity exercise, even among elderly patients with heart failure (37).

Although the benefits of habitual exercise have been shown to outweigh the risks, exercise professionals in clinical and fitness facilities have an obligation to their clients to provide the safest possible training and testing environments while minimizing the legal and personal liability associated with adverse outcomes. The best approach to management of emergencies is prevention through the following:

- Screening for cardiovascular risk factors, signs and symptoms, and fall risk before exercise and exercise testing
- Selection of appropriate exercise testing protocols
- Participant education to minimize the risk of sudden cardiac death and injury
- Appropriate participant supervision and monitoring
- Exercise equipment that is safely designed and positioned in a well-lit and ventilated area
- Development of a data-based exercise prescription for clients

KEY TERMS

Asystole: A form of cardiac arrest in which the heart has no mechanical activity, usually due to ventricular fibrillation.

Automated external defibrillator (AED): A portable device that identifies heart rhythms amenable to shock, directs the response, and delivers the appropriate shock.

Biphasic defibrillators: These use a biphasic waveform in which current flows in two directions rather than one (as in a conventional monophasic defibrillator).

Implantable cardioverter defibrillator (ICD): A small cardiac defibrillator implanted beneath the skin capable of delivering a shock to the heart if a malignant arrhythmia develops. Most can also provide backup pacing (pacemaker) if heart rate becomes too slow.

Occult: A medical condition that is hidden or difficult to detect.

Pulseless electrical activity: Organized electrical activity without a palpable pulse.

Sudden cardiac arrest (SCA): A cardiac emergency in which an individual develops an abnormal heart rhythm, preventing the effective pumping of blood.

Ventricular fibrillation (VF): An abnormal, unsynchronized fast heart rate originating in the ventricles that causes the heart to quiver rather than pump blood, resulting in zero cardiac output and sudden cardiac death.

Ventricular tachycardia (VT): An abnormally fast heart rate originating from the ventricles that typically compromises cardiac output; VT may deteriorate into a more chaotic rhythm called ventricular fibrillation.

However, given that exercise-related emergencies and injuries are not always preventable, all facilities should have policies and procedures to manage medical emergencies. The purpose of this chapter is to provide recommendations and resources that address the management of both life-threatening (major) and non–life-threatening (minor) medical emergencies.

SAFETY AND EMERGENCY PROGRAMMING

All facilities should have written emergency plans for medical complications. *Box 19-1* contains a list of questions to facilitate the preparation of an emergency plan. The plan should list specific responsibilities of each staff member, emergency equipment, and a predetermined contact for emergency response. Emergency plans including numbers for emergency medical services, police, building security, and the fire department should be posted next to all telephones. If paramedics or code teams are used for emergency response, it is imperative that they know the location and hours of the facility. First-aid kits, first-responder blood-borne pathogen kits, medical gloves, a blood pressure kit with stethoscope, an automated external defibrillator (AED) or manual defibrillator, oxygen, crash cart with medications and supplies, cardiopulmonary resuscitation (CPR) masks, and resuscitation bags as recommended based on the level of the facility as outlined in the American College of Sports Medicine (ACSM)/American Heart Association (AHA) Joint Position Statement (*Table 19-1*) must be readily available and transportable (5).

Facilities that perform maximal exercise tests or offer medically supervised cardiac or pulmonary rehabilitation programs should have all emergency equipment and drugs outlined for Level 5 facilities. Defibrillators, AEDs, crash carts (supplies and medication), oxygen tanks, and first-aid kits should be checked daily. Their storage areas must be clearly labeled with appropriate signage. A specific person should be assigned the task of daily equipment maintenance and documentation of all equipment checks.

In most facilities, the medical director or a risk management or safety committee is formed to oversee the development and revision of policies and procedures for medical emergencies. Regular periodic review of the emergency plan is recommended to ensure that all appropriate steps are outlined. The plan should be practiced with both announced and unannounced drills on a quarterly basis or more often, depending on staff turnover. All new employees and contractors should receive specific training regarding emergency procedures with documentation of training. Strategies for coping with potential and common injuries in the exercise, rehabilitation, and exercise testing settings should also be rehearsed. During the rehearsal or practice sessions, the supervisor presents a mock emergency, giving the staff information about the victim as the emergency unfolds; drills are practiced until the staff can effectively manage the emergency in a timely manner. All mock codes and other emergencies should be documented on a written report that includes a brief description of the drill, list of staff participating in the drill, documentation of each employee's competence, and any further training requirements. Each drill should be evaluated and recommendations for change documented and implemented.

Emergency plans should delineate procedures for both minor and major medical incidents. Minor medical events are not life or limb threatening and can be initially managed within the facility, but they may be referred to a medical resource. Major medical emergencies that occur in the nonmedical setting require an initial response by the staff followed by immediate transport to a medical facility. In the clinical setting outside the hospital, the physician or other medical staff should determine whether to transport the patient to a hospital. In the health/fitness setting without a physician, if there is any doubt about the status of the individual, he or she should be transported to a hospital. Emergency plans vary according to the type and size of facility, staff, location (hospital, physician's office, or fitness center), and local emergency response system. At least one staff member trained in the emergency plan and certified in CPR/AED and first aid should be on duty at all times in the health/fitness facility. This individual must be capable of assuming responsibility for management of all aspects of minor and major medical emergencies within the facility. Both the AHA and American Red Cross (ARC) offer CPR for the layman and health care provider. Because a medical emergency may arise at any time and any location, all employees including secretarial, janitorial, and child care staff should be certified in CPR/AED operation through an accredited training organization. Facilities with aquatic areas should require water safety or lifeguard certification for all exercise instructors and staff working in the area so that someone who is trained to perform a water rescue and is CPR/AED certified is available at all times the pool is open. Records of current certification and credentials for employees and consultants or contract staff should be kept with the emergency plan and/or personnel files.

CLINICAL EXERCISE TESTING LABORATORIES

The guidelines for emergency planning outlined earlier are also applicable to the clinical exercise testing laboratory. In the clinical setting (exercise testing or exercise rehabilitation), at least one staff member should be certified in advanced cardiac life support (ACLS) and licensed to administer medications (32). ACLS training is available through the AHA. However, in addition to standard 12-lead monitoring with or without gas exchange measurements, laboratories that use other cardiac imaging

BOX 19-1   Strategies for Developing an Emergency Care Plan

- Who is the staff member in charge of the facility's emergency plan and programming and is there physician oversight (medical director)?
- Is an outline of the entire emergency care plan displayed and accessible at a central staff location?
- Are different emergency procedures developed and posted for various areas within the facility (testing areas, pool, weight room, outdoor areas, and gymnasium)?
- What care will be provided?
- Who will render care?
- Are all staff and supervisors certified in first aid, CPR, AED, and/or ACLS as appropriate?
- Is there a plan for public access defibrillation (PAD)?
- Is staff training documented in personnel files or the emergency procedure plan?
- Have all staff received training for OSHA's blood-borne pathogen guidelines and procedures?
- Are the responsibilities of individual staff members identified (*e.g.*, team leader, captain, medical liaison)?
- Is there a manager/team leader available during all hours of operation to oversee a medical emergency?
- Who will activate EMS? Are telephone numbers for emergency procedures clearly posted?
- Are all staff members familiar with the information to be provided to EMS over the telephone, and is this information posted next to the phone?
    Type of emergency (injury, illness)
    Current status of involved or injured individuals
    Type of assistance being given
    Exact location of the facility and the afflicted individual within the facility
    Specific point of entry into the facility
    Telephone number being used
- Who will supervise the other activity areas if supervisors must leave to assist at an accident scene?
- Who will help with crowd control?
- Who has access to keys for locked areas or doors?
- Who will direct ambulance, EMS, or the code team to the emergency scene?
- Have the facility administrators invited representatives from EMS to become familiar with the floor plan and activities of the facility?
- Are emergency response training sessions conducted regularly (at least once every 3 mo) and documented?
- Does emergency training consists of both announced and unannounced mock drills?
- Are emergency drills and training documented and evaluated with recommendations for necessary changes?

- Is EMS involved in the training and conduction of drills?
- Do all staff members know the location and have easy access to first-aid kits, latex or similar gloves, AED, splints, stretchers, fire extinguishers, and other emergency equipment?
- Are emergency equipment and supplies clearly labeled and routinely checked, and do they receive routine maintenance?
- Is the facility conducting and documenting cardiovascular risk screening of all new members, guests, and patients?
- Are persons at high risk directed to seek facilities providing appropriate levels of care and staff supervision?
- Are appropriate documents (health appraisal, physician permission to participate, assumption of risk or waiver, informed consent, emergency information, and advanced directives) completed and accessible to staff in the event of an emergency?
- Have staff members been appropriately informed of orthopedic or other health problems, including cognitive problems such as dementia or Alzheimer disease, that might affect participation?
- Are emergency notification cards on file for each participant that include telephone numbers of family members, physician names, telephone numbers with special instructions, and alternative telephone numbers if primary contacts are unavailable? Patients/members should be encouraged to update this information on a regular basis.
- Are properly documented injury and accident reports including statements by the injured and witnesses and their contact information completed and stored in an appropriate secure location for review and follow-up by administration?
- Is there a plan for collecting facts and data after the accident including interviewing witnesses, retention of any broken equipment parts, and taking photographs if appropriate (*e.g.*, if exercise equipment malfunction were a potential concern)?
- Was the accident/injury report submitted to the facility's insurance administrator and legal counsel in a timely manner (within 24 h of the accident) and marked as "privileged and confidential" when appropriate?
- Are employees given appropriate protocols for handling inquiries made by media and other representatives regarding the incident?

Adapted from Peterson JA, Tharrett SJ, American College of Sports Medicine. *ACSM's Health/Fitness Facility Standards and Guidelines.* 4th ed. Champaign (IL): Human Kinetics; 2011. 211 p.

TABLE 19-1. Emergency Plans and Equipment for Health/Fitness Facilities

	Level 1	Level 2	Level 3	Level 4	Level 5
Type of facility	Unsupervised exercise room (*e.g.*, hotel, commercial building)	Single exercise leader	Fitness center for general membership	Fitness center offering special programs for clinical populations	Medically supervised clinical exercise program (*e.g.*, cardiac rehabilitation)
Personnel	None	Exercise leader; recommended: medical liaison	General manager; H/F instructor; exercise leader; recommended: medical liaison	General manager; exercise specialist; H/F instructor; medical liaison	General manager; exercise specialist; H/F instructor; exercise leader; medical liaison
Emergency plan	Present	Present	Present	Present	Present
Emergency equipment	Telephone in room	Telephone; signs	Telephone; signs	Telephone; signs	Telephone; signs
	Signs; encouraged: PAD plan with AED as part of the composite PAD plan in the host facility (hotel, commercial building)	Encouraged: BP kit, stethoscope, PAD plan with AED	Encouraged: BP kit, stethoscope, PAD plan with AED (the latter is strongly encouraged in facilities with membership >2,500 and those in which EMS response time is expected to be <5 min from recognition of arrest)	BP kit stethoscope; strongly encouraged: PAD plan with AED	BP kit, stethoscope, oxygen, crash cart defibrillator

H/F, health and fitness; PAD, public access to defibrillation; BP, blood pressure.

Reprinted with permission from American College of Sports Medicine, American Heart Association. American College of Sports Medicine and American Heart Association joint position statement: automated external defibrillators in health/fitness facilities. *Med Sci Sports Exerc.* 2002;34(3):561–4.

modalities — such as echocardiography and nuclear and pharmacologic studies — should have additional policies and procedures to manage emergencies unique to these modalities. In addition to policies and procedures specific to indications/contraindications for exercise testing, exercise protocol selection, and test termination, protocols for the administration of contrast agents and medications such as dobutamine, atropine, dipyridamole, and adenosine should be outlined with procedures for managing adverse reactions to any of these agents. Exercise testing should be supervised by an appropriately trained physician with ACLS certification. The AHA has established minimal competencies for physicians who supervise and interpret exercise tests (27). Some laboratories require the physician to be present during testing; however, exercise testing may be safely performed by properly trained nurses, exercise physiologists, physician assistants, and nurse practitioners with sufficient

knowledge of exercise physiology (12) under the supervision of a physician who is in the immediate vicinity to respond to emergencies.

LIFE-THREATENING EMERGENCIES

CLINICAL EXERCISE REHABILITATION PROGRAMS

In the clinical setting such as exercise testing laboratories and cardiac rehabilitation programs, standing orders to manage a variety of potentially life-threatening emergencies such as hypotension, hypoglycemia, bronchospasm, arrhythmia, angina, transient ischemic attack, and cardiac arrest should be included in the policies and procedures manual. An example of an emergency standing order is shown in *Figure 19-1*. In addition to

Ventricular Ectopy Symptomatic?	
Yes	**No**
1. Stop activity.	1. Stop exercise if new ventricular ectopy.
2. Sit patient down.	2. Notify physician if new ventricular ectopy.
3. Check vitals (heart rate, blood pressure, and oximetry), rhythm, and responsiveness and document.	3. Check vitals and document.
4. Notify physician and get 12-lead EKG tracing for physician.	4. Document rhythm.
5. Transfer to emergency room if unresolved.	5. Observe.
6. Initiate ACLS tachycardia or pulseless arrest protocol if patient is symptomatic or becomes unconscious.	

FIGURE 19-1. Standing orders for the management of ventricular ectopy. *EKG*, electrocardiogram.

the equipment and drugs required for ACLS protocols, other drugs and equipment may be required depending on the setting, types of activities, types of patients, and the facilities' emergency procedures. Equipment such as defibrillators, oxygen tanks, suction, and glucometers should be checked and documented daily. Expiration dates on ACLS drugs and non-ACLS medications used during stress testing should be checked regularly by staff or pharmacy and discarded and replaced when expired. *Table 19-2* outlines common life-threatening emergencies, associated signs and symptoms, and the appropriate acute response.

In clinical settings located outside the hospital, the emergency medical system (EMS) may be summoned rather than the code team. Emergency procedure plans will differ between programs depending on staffing, physician availability, hours of operation, access to emergency equipment, and location. For this reason, each area/program within the same facility should have its own emergency plan (*i.e.,* hospital-based vs. free-standing cardiac rehabilitation program vs. exercise testing laboratory). Many disciplines are involved in the execution of an emergency plan in the clinical setting; each staff member has a specific role to perform. It is unfortunate, however, that often the response to life-threatening emergencies is disorganized and chaotic. For an optimal emergency response and outcome, it is imperative that all team members participate in practicing emergency procedures together. The practice sessions should include the most skilled individuals such as the team leader as well as less skilled team members. Emergency drills should focus on the team aspects of resuscitative efforts (13).

In cardiac and pulmonary rehabilitation programs, a physician should be available for medical consultation, (2) and a physician-directed emergency response team must be immediately available to respond to emergencies during patient care hours. All nursing staff and licensed physical therapists trained in ACLS may perform defibrillation per ACLS protocol and licensing practice acts as allowable by jurisdictional law. The clinical staff including physicians, nurses, exercise physiologists, and physical therapists should be trained in ACLS. There should be at least one (preferably two) licensed and trained ACLS personnel and a physician immediately available when high-risk patients are exercising or participating in graded exercise tests. Patient information including advanced directives should be readily accessible during an emergency.

After an emergency (major or minor), an accident/incident report should be completed and filed with the appropriate department for review and evaluation. *Box 19-2* provides a list of items that should be addressed in this report for both clinical and nonclinical settings. The American Association of Cardiovascular and Pulmonary Rehabilitation has published guidelines for cardiac (2) and pulmonary (3) rehabilitation programs that provide sample emergency reports for documentation of mock codes, equipment checks, emergencies, and in-service training. In addition to incident reports, the team leader should gather team members to critique the code and debrief team members. The debriefing session provides an opportunity for education, allows the team members to express their feelings (anxiety, fear, grief, etc.), and facilitates improved future resuscitative attempts (13).

COMMUNITY SETTINGS

Nonclinical settings such as recreational and fitness facilities without access to a CPR code team or physician also need a set of emergency procedures to manage life-threatening and non–life-threatening events until an emergency team arrives. Emergency numbers should be posted in areas designated for fitness evaluations as well as exercise training. The 911 operator should be provided with a brief description of the problem as an advanced life support unit is dispatched in the event of a cardiac event or respiratory arrest. In non–life-threatening situations such as seizures or bodily injury, a basic life support unit is often dispatched. The life-threatening emergencies, associated signs and symptoms, and the appropriate acute responses in *Table 19-2* apply to the health/fitness as well as clinical setting; however, depending on the availability of emergency equipment, staff training, and licensure, all of the responses to a specific emergency may not be possible or legally appropriate. *Box 19-3* lists emergency equipment that should be available in the health/fitness setting.

In addition to waivers of liability and/or assumption of risk documents, facilities should have a signed medical release that provides authorization to release the victim's medical history and emergency contacts in the event that the emergency renders the victim unresponsive. Medical histories and other health care information should be kept in a locked file that is accessible to appropriate staff in the event of an emergency. When possible, a senior staff member should assume control of the emergency response, complete an accident/incident report after the emergency, and file the report with the facility's director. Depending on the type of incident, the facility's insurance carrier may also need to be alerted.

The director or senior staff member should follow-up with the victim or family regarding the victim's medical status as permitted by law and as the victim and family are willing to disclose information. Any information provided should be documented in the victim's personal file. The Health Insurance Portability and Accountability Act (HIPAA) does not allow private health information to be released to anyone except the medical director unless the

TABLE 19-2. Acute Responses for Cardiopulmonary and Metabolic Conditions/Emergencies

Condition	Definition/Signs and Symptoms	Acute Care
Dizziness/fainting Syncope	Disoriented; confused; skin color — pale; rapid, irregular pulse; weak Temporary loss of consciousness	Determine responsiveness, place supine with legs elevated, administer oral fluids if conscious, begin emergency breathing or compressions as needed, and check blood sugar if patient does not respond immediately. Activate EMS.
Hypoglycemia	Low blood sugar. Profuse sweating, tachycardia, hunger, blurred or double vision, tremors, headache, confusion, seizure, unconsciousness, sudden moodiness	Check blood sugar, administer 5–20 g (6) of CHO (4 oz or ½ cup regular soda or orange juice or three glucose tablets) if conscious. Repeat in 15 min if continued hypoglycemia. Consume meal or snack to prevent recurrence. If unconscious, use glucagon emergency kit if trained, if not, activate EMS.
Hyperglycemia	Abnormally high blood sugar. Nausea, polyuria, blurred vision, lethargy, sweet fruity breath, vomiting, hyperventilation	Postpone exercise if an individual is not feeling well or tests positive for urinary ketones (4). Stop activity if symptoms persist, turn head to side if vomiting, check blood sugar, and administer large amounts of noncaloric or low-calorie fluids orally if conscious. Continue to monitor blood glucose. Trained professionals may give insulin to lower blood sugar; activate EMS.
Angina	Pain/pressure in the chest, neck, jaw, arm and/or back; sweating; denial of medical problem; nausea; shortness of breath	Stop activity; place in seated or supine position (whichever is most comfortable); check pulse, blood pressure, and rhythm if possible; give nitroglycerin and oxygen per ACLS protocol if known history of CAD. Activate EMS or physician evaluation (unless patient is diagnosed with chronic stable angina, which is relieved with rest and/or medication). Get 12-lead EKG.
Sudden cardiac arrest	An abnormal heart rhythm usually caused by lack of oxygen to the heart; victim may be unresponsive without breathing or pulse.	Activate EMS, CAB (chest compressions, airway, rescue breathing); when AED/manual defibrillator is available, defibrillate shockable rhythms; continue CPR as indicated.
Dyspnea	Labored breathing. Hyperventilation, dizziness, wheezing, coughing, loss of coordination	Stop activity. Maintain open airway, assist with administration of bronchodilator if prescribed (18). Try pursed-lip breathing; move into a more relaxed position; if no relief, activate EMS and transport.
Tachypnea	Abnormally rapid respiration rate. Hyperventilation	Stop activity. Maintain open airway; treat cause if known; if signs/symptoms persist, activate EMS.
Stroke or TIA	Lack of oxygen to the brain. May cause symptoms such as drowsiness, confusion, severe headache with no known cause, nausea, or loss of vision and voluntary movement, muscle weakness, slurred speech, loss of coordination, or facial droop	Activate EMS; note time symptoms started. Start CPR if needed; check glucose if possible. Monitor vitals and signs/symptoms; give oxygen if hypoxic.
Hypertension	High blood pressure — if resting SBP >200 or DBP >110. SBP >250 or DBP >115 without symptoms of stroke or TIA during exercise test or SBP >200 and/or DBP >105 during exercise bout	Do not exercise. Alert provider or take to ER. Stop activity; monitor vitals and signs/symptoms. If BP does not drop quickly, alert physician or take to ER.
Hypotension	Low BP that causes symptoms such as syncope, dizziness, and fatigue.	Stop activity. Place in a supine position, elevate legs, assess vital signs, and give oral fluids if conscious. Activate EMS if symptoms do not resolve and BP does not improve. Treat the cause.
Tachycardia	Resting HR ≥100 bpm or abnormally high HR given the condition (anxiety, exercise, etc.). Other signs and symptoms such as dyspnea or angina may be present.	Stop activity. Assess vital signs, secure airway, give oxygen, and identify the rhythm. Activate EMS or obtain physician evaluation, follow ACLS guidelines for tachycardia, and treat contributing factors.
Bradycardia	Resting HR <60 bpm with symptoms; it is not unusual for patients on β-blockers or athletic individuals to have slow resting HRs without symptoms.	Stop activity. Maintain airway, check vital signs, give oxygen, and identify rhythm. Check for signs of poor perfusion; activate EMS.

(continued)

TABLE 19-2. Acute Responses for Cardiopulmonary and Metabolic Conditions/Emergencies (*Continued*)

Condition	Definition/Signs and Symptoms	Acute Care
Exertional rhabdomyolysis	Muscle pain, swelling and weakness, dark urine	Activate EMS and transport to hospital immediately, cool, and administer oral fluids if conscious.
Hyperthermia	Heat injury	
Heat cramps	Painful, involuntary, isolated muscle spasms most commonly affecting calves, arms, abdominal, and back muscles	Stop activity. Administer chilled oral electrolyte-carbohydrate fluids; application of ice and massage followed by gentle stretching; monitor vitals and hydration status.
Heat exhaustion	Heavy sweating, pale, muscle spasms, headache, nausea, loss of consciousness, dizziness, tachycardia, hypotension, headache, fatigue	Stop activity and move to cool area; remove clothes; cool with cool spray; encourage cool electrolyte-carbohydrate drinks but avoid chilling the victim. Monitor core temperature, refer for physician evaluation, or activate EMS if no rapid improvement.
Heat stroke	Hot, dry skin but can be sweating; dyspnea; tachycardia; confusion; dizziness; syncope; seizure; often unconscious with core body temperature >40° C (104° F)	Activate EMS and immediately move to cool area, remove clothing, dowse with cool water (ice water bath to chin preferred), or wrap in cool wet sheets. Administer fluids if conscious; monitor core temperature and vitals.
Hypothermia	Body temperature falls below 35° C or 95° F, shivering, loss of coordination, muscle stiffness, and lethargy, decrease in mental function, disorientation	Activate EMS and move to a warm place. Remove any wet clothing and replace with dry, warm clothing and cover with blankets or warm water to rewarm gradually. Monitor vital signs; give hot liquids.

CHO, carbohydrate; CAD, coronary artery disease; EKG, electrocardiogram; TIA, transient ischemic attack; SBP, systolic blood pressure; DBP, diastolic blood pressure; ER, emergency room; BP, blood pressure; HR, heart rate; bpm, beats per minute.

Adapted from Markenson D, Ferguson JD, Chameides L, et al. Part 17: first aid: 2010 American Heart Association and American Red Cross Guidelines for First Aid. Circulation. 2010;122(18 Suppl 3):S934–46.

victim has signed the appropriate authorization allowing a medical director designate to release the information. As in the clinical setting, an accident/incident report (see *Box 19-2*) should be completed by a senior staff member. *ACSM's Health/Fitness Facility Standards and Guidelines* (24) contains examples of emergency procedures and incident reports specific to the fitness setting that can be used as a template. Emergency drills and daily equipment checks of AEDs and first-aid kits should also be documented.

BOX 19-2 **Information Pertinent to an Incident Report**

- Date, time of the incident
- Location of incident
- Person/patient involved in the incident and contact information
- Witnesses to the incident and contact information
- Details of the incident
- Staff and their actions taken in response to the incident
- Signature of staff person completing the report
- Outcomes of the incident including follow-up communication with the victim or victim's family
- Clinical settings should attach EKG's, code form, and other medical information to the incident report

EKG, electrocardiogram.

Adapted from Peterson JA, Tharrett SJ, American College of Sports Medicine. *ACSM's Health/Fitness Facility Standards and Guidelines.* 4th ed. Champaign (IL): Human Kinetics; 2011. 211 p. and American Association of Cardiovascular and Pulmonary Rehabilitation. *Guidelines for Cardiac Rehabilitation and Secondary Prevention Programs.* 4th ed. Champaign (IL): Human Kinetics; 2004. 280 p.

BOX 19-3 **Emergency Equipment and Supplies for a Health/Fitness Facility**

- Automated external defibrillator (AED) with adult and pediatric attenuator pads (as appropriate)
- Cardiopulmonary resuscitation (CPR) barrier masks
- Blood pressure kit with aneroid sphygmomanometer and stethoscope
- First-aid kit
- First-responder blood-borne pathogen kits (often part of first-aid kit)
- 10% bleach — 10 parts water to 1 part bleach to clean up blood or body fluids (may be part of blood-borne pathogen kit)
- Flashlight with extra batteries
- Biohazard waste bags
- Accident report form

SUDDEN CARDIAC ARREST

Sudden cardiac arrest (SCA) is caused by factors such as heart disease, rhythm disturbances, and congenital abnormalities. More than 300,000 Americans have an out-of-hospital arrest each year, with an estimated national survival rate of 7.9% (28). During SCAs caused by abnormal heart rhythms such as pulseless ventricular tachycardia (VT) and ventricular fibrillation (VF), blood is not effectively pumped when the heart beats in an uncoordinated fashion causing both the pulse and breathing to stop. Death can occur within minutes after the first symptoms appear, especially if intervention does not occur. If the heart is electrically shocked using an AED soon after the onset of cardiac arrest, normal rhythm may be restored (16). For every minute that defibrillation is delayed, there is a 7%–10% reduction in the chance of survival in cases of witnessed VF if no CPR is provided (16). If CPR is provided until defibrillation can be performed, survival rates can double or triple (17). In cases where SCA is not caused by pulseless VT/VF such as asystole, victims do not benefit from AEDs. Note that all victims of SCA have the best chance of survival when the following actions are performed immediately: activation of the EMS system, CPR with emphasis on chest compressions, and rapid use of an AED when appropriate. When these steps are performed appropriately, witnessed out-of-hospital survival rates for SCA due to VF can approach 50% (26), indicating the need for community access to AEDs and layman training. Worth noting, in 2010 the AHA changed the CPR sequence to chest compressions, airway, breathing (CAB) from the traditional airway, breathing, and compressions (ABCs) protocol for adults, children, and infants (7). *Figure 19-2* (34) emphasizes the importance of chest compressions recommending that all rescuers, even untrained, provide chest compressions for victims of cardiac arrest. After CPR is started, rapid defibrillation using an AED is the next critical step in responding to SCA.

AUTOMATED EXTERNAL DEFIBRILLATORS

An AED is a portable device that identifies heart rhythms amenable to defibrillation, uses audiovisual prompts to direct the correct response, and delivers the appropriate shock. Even children can be trained to operate AEDs safely and effectively (14). Courses that incorporate AED training into traditional CPR training are available to the public through the ARC and AHA. The Cardiac Arrest Survival Act (2000) extends Good Samaritan protection to AED users. Furthermore, all 50 states have enacted defibrillator laws or adopted regulations to encourage the use and maintenance of AEDs (30). Trial court verdicts on AEDs suggest that organizations/facilities adopting AED programs have a lower risk of liability than those who do not. The ACSM and AHA's joint position statement on AEDs in health/fitness facilities (5) makes recommendations for the use and purchase of AEDs in both the clinical and fitness settings. The position statement recommends that AEDs be placed in health/fitness facilities with more than 2,500 members, facilities that offer programs for clinical or elderly populations, and those with an anticipated response time (from cardiac arrest to delivery of the first shock) greater than 5 min. In addition, unsupervised facilities are encouraged to purchase AEDs as part of their emergency plans. AEDs should be placed in well-marked, easily accessible locations near telephones. It should take no more than 1.5 min for a responder to retrieve the AED and reach the victim (24). Optimal response time should determine the number of AEDs placed in a facility. Facilities where children are present (including child care and exercise activities) should be aware of new AHA guidelines regarding AEDs. For children aged 1–8 yr, the AHA recommends the use of pediatric attenuator electrode pads when using an AED; however, if pads are not available, the AED may still be used (17). A manual defibrillator is preferred for infants <1 yr, but if unavailable, an AED with pediatric attenuator pads may be used. In the absence of AEDs with attenuator pads, AEDs have been used without adverse outcomes in infants. It is important to note that in the pediatric and infant populations, respiratory arrest is the most common cause of cardiac arrest, not life-threatening arrhythmias as is the case with adults. As more data become available, recommendations for the use of AEDs will be updated, necessitating periodic revision of policies and procedures for emergencies. Appendix B of the ACSM's *GETP9* (23) outlines general guidelines and special considerations regarding AEDs and CPR.

In addition to the use of AEDs in the lay community and outpatient and chronic care units, many medical

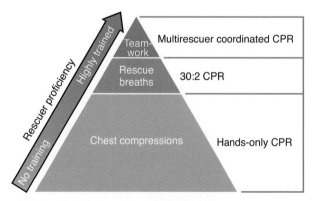

FIGURE 19-2. Building blocks of CPR. Reprinted with permission from Travers AH, Rea TD, Bobrow BJ, et al. Part 4: CPR overview: 2010 American Heart Association Guidelines for Cardiopulmonary Resuscitation and Emergency Cardiovascular Care. *Circulation.* 2010;122(18 Suppl 3):S676–84.

facilities have replaced conventional manual defibrillators with AEDs or devices, which have both manual defibrillation and AED modes. Studies comparing the use of AEDs to manual defibrillators in hospitals report mixed results with respect to survival rates to discharge (17). Factors such as delayed time to defibrillation in unmonitored hospital beds and diagnostic facilities versus monitored hospital beds and the use of monophasic defibrillators versus biphasic AEDs may have contributed to the differences in results. Biphasic AEDs/defibrillators that use two phases of reversed current allow the use of lower energy shocks and have higher or equivalent efficacy for terminating VF than conventional monophasic defibrillators. Furthermore, replacement of defibrillators with AEDs in areas where staff members have little training in rhythm recognition and/or defibrillator use is infrequent may facilitate early defibrillation.

All medical devices including AEDs and manual defibrillators are subject to malfunction. Many defibrillators perform automated checks for readiness; however, it is important to use user checklists to reduce equipment malfunction as well as operator errors. Most reported malfunctions are attributed to failure to maintain the AED or power supply (17). In addition to daily equipment checks, it is important for facilities to respond to advisory alerts. A study (29) that investigated the number of AED recalls over a 10-yr period reported that 21.2% of AEDs distributed during the study period were recalled. U.S. Food and Drug Administration (FDA) advisories are issued when a device has the potential to malfunction even when risk of failure is less than 1%. Although a recall does not necessarily indicate device failure, the need for diligent maintenance and equipment checks cannot be underestimated. Data suggest that although the number of AED advisories and AEDs affected by advisories has increased, the total number of device malfunctions is small compared with the number of lives saved (29). However, although medical devices are registered with the manufacturer when implanted in patients, no process exists for AEDs, making it difficult to track devices and end users. Because of the rapid growth in AED use, this presents a challenge for both the FDA and manufacturers to develop a reliable reporting system to ensure timely and accurate communication to potential users regarding advisory defects. For this reason, it is important for facilities to be vigilant about responding to advisory alerts and performing daily equipment checks.

IMPLANTABLE CARDIOVERTER DEFIBRILLATORS AND SUDDEN CARDIAC ARREST

Just as an AED recognizes shockable rhythms and delivers a life-saving shock, implantable cardioverter defibrillators (ICDs) can do the same when surgically implanted. The ICD is placed underneath the patient's skin, and lead wires from the device are attached directly to the heart, usually through the subclavian vein. ICDs are used to treat life-threatening arrhythmias in patients with heart failure and other cardiac disease. In addition to the delivery of cardioversion/defibrillation shocks, the ICD can be programmed to provide overdrive pacing to convert sustained VT or provide backup pacing for bradycardia. According to the AHA, nearly 5.8 million Americans are living with heart failure and 10 of every 1,000 persons older than the age of 65 yr will develop heart failure (28). To reduce the risk of sudden cardiac death, many patients with heart failure are implanted with ICDs. Given that Medicare and insurance companies reimburse for limited ($\leq$12 wk) supervised training in a cardiac rehabilitation program, even the health/fitness professional may train patients with ICDs or supervise workout areas where members with ICDs are exercising. For this reason, it is not only important for exercise professionals in the clinical setting but also for those working with special populations in the nonclinical setting to have a basic understanding of ICDs when conducting risk factor screening, corresponding with clinical health care professionals regarding exercise prescriptions, and responding to emergencies.

The exercise specialist should have knowledge of each patient's ICD program settings. For pacemakers, the upper rate limit for patients with complete heart block and the type of programmability or rate-responsive pacing should be used when developing the exercise prescription. Maximal exercise heart rate should be set at least 10–15 beats per minute below the ICD discharge heart rate (2) to reduce the risk of inappropriate shocks. Inappropriate shocks can be painful, anxiety provoking, and induce life-threatening arrhythmias. Several recent studies (11,35) report that atrial fibrillation/flutter, supraventricular tachycardia, as well as abnormal sensing can trigger inappropriate shocks. A magnet can be used to terminate inappropriate shocks; however, only a physician/provider with electrophysiology training should decide if the use of a magnet is appropriate. Any ICD malfunction or shock should be immediately reported to the patient's electrophysiologist so it can be interrogated to determine if the settings need to be adjusted or if there are problems with lead displacement (any position change in the pacemaker or leads).

One valid concern when working with individuals with ICDs is the possibility of ICD discharge when the exercise professional is touching the patient. Generally, contact during ICD discharge has been considered safe and the feeling reported as a slight tingling sensation (31). There are, however, documented reports of rescuer shock while performing chest compressions during cardiac arrest. The most serious injury involved nerve damage in the hand/wrist area when the defibrillator discharged as the patient's rhythm changed from pulseless electrical activity (PEA) to VF. For this reason, when performing CPR on individuals with ICDs, the use of a magnet to inactivate the device may reduce the risk of rescuer injury. In the event that an ICD fails, an AED or manual defibrillator should be used to convert pulseless VT/VF. Care should be taken to avoid placement of paddles over the ICD. Paddles/pads should be positioned 10 cm from the pulse generator and implanted electrodes (10).

OTHER MEDICAL CONCERNS

FIRST-AID KITS

First-aid kits are vital to an appropriate emergency response. The Occupational Safety and Health Administration (OSHA) provides general standards for work site first-aid kits and employee training based on the degree of hazard, location, facility size, amount of staff training, and availability of professional medical service including EMS response time (8) and recommends the minimum requirements set forth by the American National Standards Institute (ANSI) (15). These supplies are required items to treat major wounds, cuts and abrasions, minor burns, and eye injuries. There are three ANSI classifications for first-aid kits, depending on whether the kit is used indoors or outdoors and if it needs to be portable. The contents of first-aid kits in health care versus fitness facilities may be quite different, as many of the items in a standard first-aid kit may be readily available in the medical setting. In the health/fitness setting, first-aid kits are a necessity. The number of kits and amount of supplies should depend on the number of members; types of activities performed, which determine types of potential injuries; the layout of the facility; response time; level of staff training; and whether activities are indoors and/or outdoors (8). *Box 19-4* lists a sample of kit contents adequate to respond to a variety of injuries and emergencies.

All first-aid kits should also be stocked with CPR barrier masks. The ARC Web site (http://www.redcross.org) is a good resource for additional recommendations and for first-aid kits tailored for different settings (home vs. work site). The ARC offers various levels of training for first aid, CPR, and blood-borne pathogens. Although it is not necessary to keep an aneroid sphygmomanometer and blood pressure cuff in the first-aid kit, it should be readily accessible to monitor vitals.

BLOOD-BORNE PATHOGENS

Universal blood-borne pathogen precautions were developed by the U.S. Centers for Disease Control and Prevention (CDC) as an aggressive set of guidelines to protect employees from blood-borne pathogens, such as HIV and hepatitis B virus. Recommendations include the use of gloves, masks, gowns, and other barriers whenever it is possible for an individual to come in contact with blood and other body fluids. OSHA issued a regulation in 1991 requiring the adoption of universal precautions for occupational exposure to blood-borne pathogens (22). The standard also mandates annual training and documentation of training for all employees who could potentially be exposed to blood-borne pathogens.

Staff members should always use latex or other similar type gloves and appropriate barriers when treating skin wounds and handling items such as mouthpieces, resuscitation bags, and equipment that may have been exposed to blood-borne pathogens or other body fluids. Biohazard kits should be available to all employees who may be exposed to

---

BOX 19-4	**Sample Contents of a First-Aid Kit for a Fitness Facility**

- Sterile first-aid dressings in sealed envelope (2″ × 2″ for small wounds; 4″ × 4″ and 8″ × 10″ for larger wounds and for compress to stop bleeding)
- Tongue blades
- Bandage scissors
- Tweezers
- Eyewash solution
- Safety pins
- Ace bandage
- Band-Aids
- Roller bandage 1″ × 5 yd (for finger)
- Roller bandage 2″ × 5 yd to hold dressings in place
- Adhesive tape
- Triangular bandages for a sling or as a covering over a larger dressing

- Splints 0.25″ thick, 0.50″ wide, 12″–15″ long for splinting broken arms and legs
- 70% isopropyl alcohol and tincture green soap in a covered container for cleaning or sealed towelette
- Ice packs (chemical ice bags) to reduce swelling
- Insect bite kit (facilities with outdoor activities)
- Several pairs of disposable gloves
- Waterless hand wash
- First-aid instruction booklet
- Space blanket (facilities with outdoor activities)
- Resuscitation equipment (resuscitation bag or pocket mask)
- Directions for requesting emergency assistance posted on or next to first-aid kit

blood, cerebrospinal fluid, pleural fluid, saliva, or any body fluid with visible blood. These kits should contain disposable paper towels, a spray bottle with 10% bleach solution, hydrogen peroxide, assorted sizes of gloves, disposable gauze and towels, red biohazard bags, gowns, masks, and face shields (21). Hands should always be washed according to guidelines established by the CDC's Healthcare Infection Control Practices Advisory Committee (9) immediately after providing any type of care.

MUSCULOSKELETAL INJURIES

Most musculoskeletal injuries seen in the exercise setting are non–life-threatening, although they require a prompt emergency response to optimize outcomes and minimize liability. Injuries may be the result of a single traumatic event or chronic, repetitive, submaximal forces that lead to inflammation and pain. Strains, sprains, and fractures are often caused by an acute event, whereas injuries such as tendonitis, shin splints, plantar fasciitis, and stress fractures are examples of chronic "overuse" injuries. A description of the characteristics and appropriate first-aid procedures for common exercise-related musculoskeletal injuries are outlined in *Table 19-3*. The RICE protocol (25) outlined in *Table 19-4* involves the use of rest, ice, compression, and elevation and is the appropriate treatment for most acute musculoskeletal injuries.

When used properly, the RICE treatment regimen reduces the total amount of tissue damage, decreases swelling and pain, and aids in controlling the inflammatory

TABLE 19-3. Acute Responses for Common Musculoskeletal Injuries/Emergencies

Injury	Description	Signs/Symptoms	Acute Care
Blisters/corns	Closed skin wounds	Pain, swelling, infection	Clean with antiseptic soap. Apply sterile dressing, antibiotic ointment.
Lacerations/abrasions	Open skin wounds	Pain, redness, bleeding, swelling, mild fever	Follow universal precautions to prevent the transfer of blood-borne pathogens. Apply direct pressure to stop bleeding. Irrigate with large volumes of water to remove debris. Clean with soap or sterile saline; apply antibiotic ointment and sterile dressing for abrasions and superficial injuries. Refer to physician for stitches/tetanus. Wash your hands immediately after providing care.
Strain[a]	A stretch or tear in a muscle, tendon, and/or fascia		
Grade I	Affects only a few fibers	Mild discomfort, pain, tightness, possible localized spasms	RICE (see *Table 19-4* for definitions and protocol)
Grade II	More extensive damage to more fibers	Loss of function, swelling, bruising, and localized tenderness	RICE; refer for physician evaluation
Grade III	Severe tear or complete rupture	Palpable defect, complete loss of function, severe pain, swelling, and bruising	Immobilization, RICE, prompt physician evaluation as surgery may be required.
Sprain[a]	A stretch or tear to the ligaments and stabilizing connective tissues of a joint		
Grade I	Slight tear or stretch without joint instability	Minimal pain, swelling, little or no loss of function, slight or no bruising	RICE
Grade II	Partial tear	Bruising, moderate pain, swelling, difficulty with weight bearing, and some loss of function	RICE, physician evaluation
Grade III	Complete tear	Severe pain, swelling, bruising, unable to bear weight on the joint	Immobilization, RICE, prompt physician evaluation
Stress fracture	Microscopic damage to the bone due to repetitive stress	Insidious onset of pain that persists when attempting activity, point-specific tenderness	Physician evaluation, rest, non–weight-bearing activities
Simple acute fracture	Sudden break of a bone	Swelling, bruising, disability, pain	Immobilize joint with padded splint in position found if warranted, physician evaluation, X-rays

[a]Signs and symptoms for each grade include those for the grade below the one listed (*i.e.*, grade II includes those of grades I and II; grade III includes signs and symptoms listed under grades I, II, and III).

TABLE 19-4. RICE Protocol for Acute Injuries

Treatment	Purpose	Application
Rest	Pain control, prevention of reinjury	Complete rest, immobilization, or reduction in training intensity, duration, frequency, or use of non–weight-bearing activities, depending on severity of injury
Ice	Reduction of pain, swelling, inflammation, spasms, and bleeding	Immediately post injury, 10–20 min, two to three times per day; use plastic bag, ice and water mixture; place a thin towel between skin and ice bag
Compression	Reduction of swelling	Elastic wrap/compression sleeve
Elevation	Reduction of swelling	Elevate extremity above heart level

Adapted from Markenson D, Ferguson JD, Chameides L, et al. Part 17: first aid: 2010 American Heart Association and American Red Cross Guidelines for First Aid. *Circulation.* 2010;122(18 Suppl 3):S934–46; and Prentice WE, Arnheim DD. *Arnheim's Principles of Athletic Training: A Competency-Based Approach.* 14th ed. New York (NY): McGraw-Hill Higher Education; 2011. 940 p.

response, which results in quicker rehabilitation and recovery. Improper care or delay in treatment may cause additional pain, swelling, and damage of healthy tissues resulting in secondary hypoxic injury (cell death because of lack of oxygen) even after bleeding is controlled. The initial RICE treatment protocol should be continued for 24–72 h after injury. The use of an ice water mixture is preferable to ice only or refreezable gel packs for 10–20 min (18).

PREVENTING EXERCISE-RELATED EMERGENCIES

One of the major priorities in both the clinical and non-clinical settings is the prevention of emergencies and injuries through the development of policies and procedures that address risk factor screening, data-based exercise prescription, patient orientation and education, and training and competencies for both staff and consultants/contractors relative to patient risk status. The program director and/or office of human resources should verify that staff credentials include certifications and licensure appropriate for the patient population at that facility. Appropriate levels of supervision and staffing relative to the number of members/patients and facility layout and size, as well as equipment maintenance and selection, should also be addressed. The facility floor plan should provide for adequate space and appropriate traffic flow to prevent exercise-related injuries and facilitate a prompt emergency response. For a detailed discussion of these topics, the reader is referred to *ACSM's Health/Fitness Facility Standards and Guidelines* (24). Finally, documentation and referral to an appropriate medical professional is crucial when the exercise professional recognizes early signs and symptoms of potential medical problems or the patient/client reports them. Because it is impossible to prevent all exercise-related emergencies and injuries, the policies and procedures addressed in this chapter should be used as a template for the development of an emergency plan specific to each facility and area within the facility to effectively manage various medical emergencies.

SUMMARY

First and foremost, every clinical, fitness, and recreational facility should have a thorough set of policies and procedures in place and readily accessible to staff in the event of an emergency. They should follow national standards and guidelines, satisfy accrediting organizations, and provide a safe and effective exercise environment for all participants. Policies and procedures should be reviewed and revised on a regular basis. Employee training and rehearsal of procedures for managing both major and minor medical events should be conducted at orientation for employees and contractors and on a regular schedule thereafter to maintain optimal skill levels. In addition, all aspects of the emergency plan should be followed and documented to ensure participant safety, meet best practice guidelines, and limit both professional and personal liability.

REFERENCES

1. Albert CM, Mittlem an MA, Chae CU, Lee IM, Hennekens CH, Manson JE. Triggering of sudden death from cardiac causes by vigorous exertion. *N Engl J Med.* 2000;343(19):1355–61.
2. American Association of Cardiovascular and Pulmonary Rehabilitation. *Guidelines for Cardiac Rehabilitation and Secondary Prevention Programs.* 4th ed. Champaign (IL): Human Kinetics; 2004. 280 p.
3. American Association of Cardiovascular and Pulmonary Rehabilitation. *Guidelines for Pulmonary Rehabilitation Programs.* 3rd ed. Champaign (IL): Human Kinetics; 2004. 188 p.
4. American College of Sports Medicine, American Diabetes Association. Exercise and type 2 diabetes: American College of Sports Medicine and the American Diabetes Association: joint position statement. *Med Sci Sports Exerc.* 2010;42(12):2282–303.
5. American College of Sports Medicine, American Heart Association. American College of Sports Medicine and American Heart Association joint position statement: automated external defibrillators in health/fitness facilities. *Med Sci Sports Exerc.* 2002;34(3):561–4.
6. American Diabetes Association. Standards of medical care in diabetes—2010. *Diabetes Care.* 2010;33 Suppl 1:S11–61.
7. Berg RA, Hemphill R, Abella BS, et al. Part 5: adult basic life support: 2010 American Heart Association Guidelines for Cardiopulmonary Resuscitation and Emergency Cardiovascular Care. *Circulation.* 2010;122(18 Suppl 3):S685–705.
8. *Best Practices Guide: Fundamentals of a Workplace First-Aid Program* [Internet]. Washington, DC: U.S. Department of Labor, Occupational Safety and Health Administration; 2006 [cited 2011 Jan 31]. 28 p. Available from: http://purl.access.gpo.gov/GPO/LPS73422

9. Boyce JM, Pittet D, Healthcare Infection Control Practices Advisory Committee, HICPAC/SHEA/APIC/IDSA Hand Hygiene Task Force. Guideline for hand hygiene in health-care settings. Recommendations of the Healthcare Infection Control Practices Advisory Committee and the HICPAC/SHEA/APIC/IDSA Hand Hygiene Task Force. Society for Healthcare Epidemiology of America/Association for Professionals in Infection Control/Infectious Diseases Society of America. *MMWR Recomm Rep.* 2002;51(RR-16):1,45, quiz CE1–4.

10. Bukhari A, Garg S, Mehta Y. Anaesthetic management of patients with implantable cardioverter defibrillator. *Ann Card Anaesth.* 2005;8(1):61–3.

11. Daubert JP, Zareba W, Cannom DS, et al. Inappropriate implantable cardioverter-defibrillator shocks in MADIT II: frequency, mechanisms, predictors, and survival impact. *J Am Coll Cardiol.* 2008;51(14):1357–65.

12. Fletcher GF, Balady GJ, Amsterdam EA, et al. Exercise standards for testing and training: a statement for healthcare professionals from the American Heart Association. *Circulation.* 2001;104(14):1694–740.

13. Guidelines 2000 for Cardiopulmonary Resuscitation and Emergency Cardiovascular Care. Part 6: advanced cardiovascular life support: section 7: algorithm approach to ACLS emergencies. The American Heart Association in collaboration with the International Liaison Committee on Resuscitation. *Circulation.* 2000;102(8 Suppl):I136–65.

14. Gundry JW, Comess KA, DeRook FA, Jorgenson D, Bardy GH. Comparison of naive sixth-grade children with trained professionals in the use of an automated external defibrillator. *Circulation.* 1999;100(16):1703–7.

15. International Safety Equipment Association, American National Standards Institute. *American National Standard—Minimum Requirements for Workplace First Aid Kits.* Arlington (VA): International Safety Equipment Association; 2003. 16 p.

16. Larsen MP, Eisenberg MS, Cummins RO, Hallstrom AP. Predicting survival from out-of-hospital cardiac arrest: a graphic model. *Ann Emerg Med.* 1993;22(11):1652–8.

17. Link MS, Atkins DL, Passman RS, et al. Part 6: electrical therapies: automated external defibrillators, defibrillation, cardioversion, and pacing: 2010 American Heart Association Guidelines for Cardiopulmonary Resuscitation and Emergency Cardiovascular Care. *Circulation.* 2010;122(18 Suppl 3):S706–19.

18. Markenson D, Ferguson JD, Chameides L, et al. Part 17: first aid: 2010 American Heart Association and American Red Cross Guidelines for First Aid. *Circulation.* 2010;122(18 Suppl 3):S934–46.

19. Mora S, Redberg RF, Cui Y, et al. Ability of exercise testing to predict cardiovascular and all-cause death in asymptomatic women: a 20-year follow-up of the lipid research clinics prevalence study. *JAMA.* 2003;290(12):1600–7.

20. Myers J, Prakash M, Froelicher V, Do D, Partington S, Atwood JE. Exercise capacity and mortality among men referred for exercise testing. *N Engl J Med.* 2002;346(11):793–801.

21. National Safety Council. *Bloodborne Pathogens.* Boston (MA): Jones and Bartlett Publishers; 1993. 71 p.

22. *The OSHA Bloodborne Pathogens Standard* [Internet]. Washington, DC: U.S. Department of Labor, Occupational Safety and Health Administration. Available from: http://www.osha.gov/

23. Pescatello LS, Arena R, Riebe D, American College of Sports Medicine. *ACSM's Guidelines for Exercise Testing and Prescription.* 9th ed. Philadelphia (PA): Lippincott Williams & Wilkins; 2012. 380 p.

24. Peterson JA, Tharrett SJ, American College of Sports Medicine. *ACSM's Health/Fitness Facility Standards and Guidelines.* 4th ed. Champaign (IL): Human Kinetics; 2011. 211 p.

25. Prentice WE, Arnheim DD. *Arnheim's Principles of Athletic Training: A Competency-Based Approach.* 14th ed. New York (NY): McGraw-Hill Higher Education; 2011. 940 p.

26. Rea TD, Helbock M, Perry S, et al. Increasing use of cardiopulmonary resuscitation during out-of-hospital ventricular fibrillation arrest: survival implications of guideline changes. *Circulation.* 2006;114(25):2760–5.

27. Rodgers GP, Ayanian JZ, Balady G, et al. American College of Cardiology/American Heart Association Clinical Competence Statement on Stress Testing. A Report of the American College of Cardiology/American Heart Association/American College of Physicians-American Society of Internal Medicine Task Force on Clinical Competence. *Circulation.* 2000;102(14):1726–38.

28. Roger VL, Go AS, Lloyd-Jones DM, et al. Heart disease and stroke statistics—2012 update: a report from the American Heart Association. *Circulation.* 2012;125(1):e2–220.

29. Shah JS, Maisel WH. Recalls and safety alerts affecting automated external defibrillators. *JAMA.* 2006;296(6):655–60.

30. *State Laws on Cardiac Arrest and Defibrillators* [Internet]. Denver, CO: National Conference of State Legislators; 2009 [cited 2011 Mar 4]. Available from: http://www.ncsl.org/default.aspx?tabid=14506

31. Stockwell B, Bellis G, Morton G, et al. Electrical injury during "hands on" defibrillation—a potential risk of internal cardioverter defibrillators? *Resuscitation.* 2009;80(7):832–4.

32. Thomas RJ, King M, Lui K, et al. AACVPR/ACC/AHA 2007 performance measures on cardiac rehabilitation for referral to and delivery of cardiac rehabilitation/secondary prevention services. *Circulation.* 2007;116(14):1611–42.

33. Thompson PD, Franklin BA, Balady GJ, et al. Exercise and acute cardiovascular events placing the risks into perspective: a scientific statement from the American Heart Association Council on Nutrition, Physical Activity, and Metabolism and the Council on Clinical Cardiology. *Circulation.* 2007;115(17):2358–68.

34. Travers AH, Rea TD, Bobrow BJ, et al. Part 4: CPR overview: 2010 American Heart Association Guidelines for Cardiopulmonary Resuscitation and Emergency Cardiovascular Care. *Circulation.* 2010;122(18 Suppl 3):S676–84.

35. van Rees JB, Borleffs CJ, de Bie MK, et al. Inappropriate implantable cardioverter-defibrillator shocks: incidence, predictors, and impact on mortality. *J Am Coll Cardiol.* 2011;57(5):556–62.

36. Whang W, Manson JE, Hu FB, et al. Physical exertion, exercise, and sudden cardiac death in women. *JAMA.* 2006;295(12):1399–403.

37. Wisloff U, Stoylen A, Loennechen JP, et al. Superior cardiovascular effect of aerobic interval training versus moderate continuous training in heart failure patients: a randomized study. *Circulation.* 2007;115(24):3086–94.

SELECTED REFERENCES FOR FURTHER READING

American Heart Association. *ACC/AHA 2002 Guideline Update for Exercise Testing. A report of the American College of Cardiology/American Heart Association Task Force on Practice Guidelines (Committee on Exercise Testing)* [Internet]. Dallas, TX: American College of Cardiology, American Heart Association; 2002 [cited 2011 Apr 27]. Available from: http://www.americanheart.org/downloadable/heart/1032279013658exercise.pdf

INTERNET RESOURCES

- American Association of Cardiovascular and Pulmonary Rehabilitation: http://www.aacvpr.org
- American Heart Association: http://www.americanheart.org
- American Red Cross: http://www.redcross.org/services/hss/courses/workplace.html
- Occupational Safety and Health Administration: http://www.osha.gov/

ACKNOWLEDGMENT

Jennifer Eakins for her expertise and assistance with new AHA CPR guidelines.

Exercise Testing

MADELINE PATERNOSTRO BAYLES, PhD, FACSM, ACSM-CES, ACSM-PD, *Section Editor*

Exercise is considered a safe activity for most individuals. However, risks such as sudden cardiac death (SCD) and myocardial infarction are increased when initiating an exercise program or performing an exercise test (36). The benefits and risks associated with physical activity and exercise testing are discussed in *Chapter 1* of ACSM's *Guidelines for Exercise Testing and Prescription, 9th edition (GETP9)*. The preparticipation health screen assists in identifying the risk of an untoward event associated with starting an exercise program or performing an exercise test by identifying known diseases and risk factors for coronary artery disease. Furthermore, identification of additional factors that require special consideration when developing an appropriate exercise prescription and exercise program can optimize adherence, minimize risk, and maximize benefits. The purposes of the preparticipation health screen include the following:

- Identification of individuals with medical contraindications that require exclusion from exercise programs until those conditions have been abated or controlled
- Recognition of persons with clinically significant diseases or conditions who should participate in a medically supervised exercise program
- Detection of individuals who should undergo a medical evaluation and/or exercise testing before initiating an exercise program or increasing the frequency, intensity, or duration of their current program (28)

This chapter will focus on preparticipation health screening for (a) individuals beginning an exercise program, (b) athletes participating in sports, and (c) individuals prior to completing an exercise test. In addition to preparticipation health screening, aspects of the preexercise evaluation will be discussed.

PREPARTICIPATION HEALTH SCREENING BEFORE BEGINNING AN EXERCISE PROGRAM

Minimal recommendations for initiating a low intensity or moderate intensity exercise program include a preparticipation health screening and American College of Sports Medicine (ACSM) risk classification. Individuals classified with low risk can safely begin an exercise program at intensities up to vigorous, whereas those classified with moderate risk can safely begin at intensities up to moderate, without consultation of a physician. Individuals currently having signs or symptoms or previously diagnosed cardiovascular, pulmonary, or metabolic disease (high risk classification) should consult their physician prior to initiating an exercise program (*Chapter 2, GETP9*). Preparticipation health screenings are either self-administered or performed by an appropriately trained health care professional. A self-administered questionnaire such as the American Heart Association (AHA)/ACSM Health/Fitness Facility Preparticipation Screening Questionnaire (2) or Physical Activity Readiness Questionnaire (PAR-Q) (9) are considered the minimally accepted screening tools that apprise an individual to follow up with a qualified professional prior to initiating an exercise program. The AHA/ACSM Health/Fitness Facility Preparticipation Screening Questionnaire and PAR-Q

KEY TERMS

Aneroid: Without fluid; denoting a form of barometer without mercury, in which the varying air pressure is indicated by a pointer governed by the movement of the elastic wall of an evacuated chamber. Also used to denote a mercury-free pressure gauge used with some sphygmomanometers.

Coarctation: Pertaining to a constriction, stricture, or stenosis.

Peripheral: Situated nearer the periphery of an organ or part of the body in relation to a specific reference point; opposite of *central*.

Sudden Cardiac Death (SCD): natural death due to cardiac causes, heralded by abrupt loss of consciousness within 1 h of the onset of symptoms; preexisting heart disease may have been known to be present, but the time and mode of death are unexpected (23).

screening tools are provided in *Chapter 2* of *GETP9* and explained in more detail in *Chapter 11* of this resource Manual. ACSM risk classification identifies risk based on the presence or absence of CVD risk factors, signs or symptoms, and/or known cardiovascular, pulmonary, or metabolic disease (*Chapter 2, GETP9*).

PREPARTICIPATION SCREENING FOR COMPETITIVE ATHLETES

Sudden death in young competitive athletes has sparked interest in prevention of these untimely deaths. The AHA released recommended guidelines for preparticipation screenings for cardiovascular abnormalities in competitive athletes in 2007 (19). Currently, high schools and colleges do not have mandated standards for screening athletes. Generally, athletes are cleared to participate in sports by a physician or other trained health care provider. However, past medical history and physical examination alone are not sufficiently sensitive in detecting cardiovascular abnormalities that are linked to sudden death in youth athletes. The AHA recommends a 12-element Preparticipation Cardiovascular Screening of Competitive Athletes, which is presented in *Table 20-1*. Should an athlete have any one or more of the 12 items, a referral for a cardiovascular evaluation is recommended (19). Electrocardiogram (ECG) screening is not a component of the 12-item AHA screening recommendations. ECG screening may increase detection of athletes with potentially lethal cardiovascular disorders. However, widespread implementation in the United States is limited by current resources (31).

PREEXERCISE EVALUATION PRIOR TO BEGINNING AN EXERCISE PROGRAM

The preexercise evaluation generally includes a past medical history, physical examination, an exercise test, and/or laboratory test (5). The preexercise evaluation guides the health fitness professional in making decisions regarding the individual's optimal care (28).

IMPORTANCE OF PREEXERCISE EVALUATION

The focus of the preexercise evaluation is on detection of risk factors that can be directly modified (26). According to the American Thoracic Society and American College of Chest Physicians (5), a comprehensive preexercise evaluation allows the clinician to do the following:

- Determine reasons for clinical exercise testing
- Form a clinical diagnosis
- Determine medications that may alter heart rate and blood pressure (BP) responses to exercise
- Identify risk factors for cardiovascular, pulmonary, musculoskeletal, and metabolic disorders

TABLE 20-1. The 12-Element American Heart Association Recommendations for Preparticipation Cardiovascular Screening of Competitive Athletes

Medical history[a]

Personal history

1. Exertional chest pain/discomfort
2. Unexplained syncope/near-syncope[b]
3. Excessive exertional and unexplained dyspnea/fatigue, associated with exercise
4. Prior recognition of a heart murmur
5. Elevated systemic blood pressure

Family history

6. Premature death (sudden and unexpected, or otherwise) before age 50 years as a result of heart disease in ≥1 relative
7. Disability from heart disease in a close relative <50 years of age
8. Specific knowledge of certain cardiac conditions in family members: hypertrophic or dilated cardiomyopathy, long-QT syndrome or other ion channelopathies, Marfan syndrome, or clinically important arrhythmias

Physical examination

9. Heart murmur[c]
10. Femoral pulses to exclude aortic coarctation
11. Physical stigmata of Marfan syndrome
12. Brachial artery blood pressure (sitting positions)[d]

[a]Parental verification is recommended for high school and middle school athletes.

[b]Judged not to be neurocardiogenic (vasovagal); of particular concern when related to exertion.

[c]Auscultation should be performed in both supine and standing positions (or with Valsalva maneuver), specifically to identify murmurs of dynamic left ventricular outflow tract obstruction.

[d]Preferably taken in both arms.

Reprinted with permission from Maron BJ, Thompson PD, Ackerman MJ, et al. Recommendations and considerations related to preparticipation screening for cardiovascular abnormalities in competitive athletes: 2007 update: a scientific statement from the American Heart Association Council on Nutrition, Physical Activity, and Metabolism: endorsed by the American College of Cardiology Foundation. *Circulation*. 2007;115(12):1643–55.

Accurate, yet simple methods of risk assessment are important for individual care (8). Evidence suggests that an aggressive risk factor management program clearly improves survival rates, reduces recurrent events and the need for interventional procedures, and improves the quality of life for individuals with atherosclerosis. However, reports indicate a large proportion of individuals for whom therapies are indicated are *not* receiving those therapies in actual clinical practice (35,37). Therefore, a link is missing between the knowledge of risk factor management and the actual practice of risk factor management. The AHA and American College of Cardiology continue to urge all health care settings to have a specific plan to identify persons with known risk factors, provide health care providers with useful reminder clues based on the guidelines, and continuously assess the outcomes achieved in providing all appropriate therapies to all of the individuals who can benefit from them (35). Furthermore, the health fitness professional should focus on identifying individuals at an earlier stage of the disease process and encourage participation in a comprehensive cardiovascular risk reduction program so that individuals may realize the benefits that primary prevention can provide (26). Many times, the health fitness professional is the first to identify individuals in need of risk factor reduction.

The health fitness professional should create an environment supportive of risk factor change, including long-term reinforcement of adherence to lifestyle and drug interventions. Because risk factors have heredity and environmental factors, not only should risk factor reduction be implemented for the individual but also a family-centered approach to primary prevention is recommended. The family-centered approach would include avoidance of tobacco (including secondhand smoke), healthy dietary patterns, weight control, and regular, appropriate exercise (26).

PAST MEDICAL HISTORY

The past medical history of the individual initiates the preexercise evaluation process (5,26) and may include the following information:

- Demographic information (individual's name, address, admission date, date of birth, etc.)
- Medical diagnosis, past and present conditions, or diseases
- Recent or past surgeries
- Current medications (antiplatelet agents/anticoagulants, angiotensin-converting enzyme [ACE] inhibitors, β-blockers, etc.) (10)
- Medical test results (laboratory such as HbA1C, radiologic test, etc.)
- Functional status/activity level
- Social history (cultural/religious beliefs that could affect care, available social support)
- Employment status (full time or part time, retired or student, workplace demands)
- General health status (rating of the individual's health during the past year)
- Social/health habits (past and current alcohol, tobacco, and exercise habits) (5,10,16)
- Family health history (heart disease, diabetes, arthritis, osteoporosis, and other conditions)
- Individual goals (16)

Components of the medical history are further explained in *Box 3.1* of *GETP9*. All information obtained in the past medical history is used to provide quality care in determination of functional goals/outcomes for the individual.

PHYSICAL EXAMINATION

After obtaining past medical history, each individual is risk classified to determine necessary components of the physical examination (5,26). Components of the preexercise test physical examination are located in *Box 3.2* of *GETP9*.

Heart Rate Examination

Exercise professionals can obtain an index of resting heart rate by measuring peripheral pulses. The two most commonly used anatomical sites for palpation are the carotid and radial arteries. The radial pulse (wrist pulse) is felt by palpating the radial artery and is pictured in *Figure 20-1*. The radial artery is a smaller, terminal branch of the brachial artery located on the lateral side (thumb side) of the wrist (22).

The carotid pulse (neck pulse) is felt by palpating the common carotid artery on the side of the neck and is illustrated in *Figure 20-2*. The common carotid artery lies in the groove between the trachea and the infrahyoid muscles and is easily palpated just deep to the anterior border of the sternocleidomastoid muscle (22).

Other anatomic landmarks for palpation of heart rate include the brachial, femoral, popliteal, tibialis posterior, and dorsalis pedis artery, which are illustrated in *Figure 20-3*. The procedure for taking a pulse for determination of heart rate is as follows:

1. Locate an anatomic palpation site.
2. Place the index and third finger over the palpation site (avoid using the thumb).
3. Gently press down with the two fingers over the palpation site.
4. Count the number of pulsations for a specific period (*e.g.*, 10, 15, 20, or 30 seconds).
5. Begin counting the first pulsation as 0 when timing is initiated simultaneously or, if a lag time occurs after the start time and the first pulsation, begin with the number 1 for determining number of pulsations.
6. Multiply the number of pulsations in a given period by the appropriate factor to yields beats per minute (*e.g.*, pulsations times four when a 15-s count was used).

Accuracy of heart rate increases with longer palpation times. For instance, taking heart rate for 30 s yields a heart rate accurate to ±2 bpm, whereas taking it for 10 s

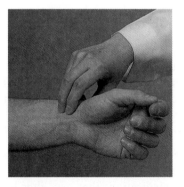

FIGURE 20-1. Palpation site for radial pulse. (Reprinted with permission from Bickley LS, Szilagyi P. *Bates' Guide to Physical Examination and History Taking.* 8th ed. Philadelphia [PA]: Lippincott Williams & Wilkins; 2003.)

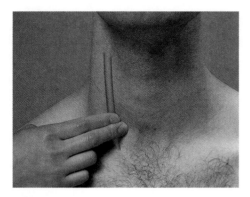

FIGURE 20-2. Palpation site for carotid pulse. (Reprinted with permission from Bickley LS, Szilagyi P. *Bates' Guide to Physical Examination and History Taking.* 8th ed. Philadelphia [PA]: Lippincott Williams & Wilkins; 2003.)

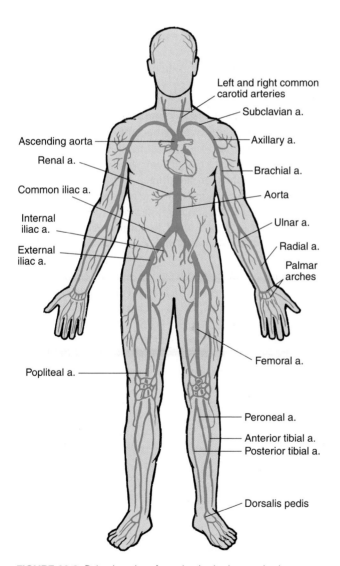

Left and right common carotid arteries

Subclavian a.

Ascending aorta

Renal a.

Axillary a.

Common iliac a.

Brachial a.

Internal iliac a.

Aorta

External iliac a.

Ulnar a.

Radial a.

Palmar arches

Popliteal a.

Femoral a.

Peroneal a.

Anterior tibial a.
Posterior tibial a.

Dorsalis pedis

FIGURE 20-3. Palpation sites for pulse in the human body. (Adapted with permission from *Stedman's Medical Dictionary.* 27th ed. Baltimore [MD]: Lippincott Williams & Wilkins; 2000.)

is only accurate to ±6 bpm. During exercise, it may be more practical to use brief counting periods because of the high heart rate. Moreover, heart rate will decrease rapidly once exercise has stopped. Thus, if the immediate post-exercise heart rate is used as an indicator of exercise intensity, a brief counting period is needed.

During an exercise test, palpation of a peripheral pulse may be difficult because of the individual's movement. Other options for monitoring an exercise heart rate are ECG monitoring, electronic heart rate monitors, and stethoscope auscultation at the point of maximal intensity.

Blood Pressure Examination

The accuracy of BP measurements is critical in the clinical setting (20). The gold standard for determining arterial BP is direct intra-arterial measurement with a catheter. However, this method is inappropriate for most settings due to its high risk of hemorrhage. The indirect method is the most commonly used method of measurement (27). The standard instruments for indirect BP measurement include auscultatory (manual) and oscillometric (automated) devices. Auscultatory devices include aneroid, mercury, and hybrid sphygmomanometers. Anaeroid devices measure pressure by a mechanical system of metal bellows that expand as the cuff pressure increases and a series of levers that register the pressure on a circular scale. These devices have decreased accuracy over time (especially after being dropped) and require calibrating at regular intervals. Mercury sphygmomanometers have a simplistic design leading to negligible differences in accuracy for different brands. However, mercury devices are being phased out because of environmental concerns. Hybrid sphygmomanometers combine features of both electronic and auscultatory devices. The mercury column is replaced by an electronic pressure gauge similar to what is used in automatic devices (29).

The use of automatic devices has increased in home and clinical settings. The variability and reliability of automated BP readings is often questioned. The AHA recommends automatic, cuff-style, upper arm monitors instead of wrist and/or finger monitors because of its decreased reliability (4). Further recommendations include choosing a validated monitor, ensuring that the monitor is validated for special needs (*e.g.,* pregnancy, elderly) and that the cuff fits appropriately. Skirton et al. (34) recommend the use of auscultatory devices over automatic devices in specific circumstances, such as management of hypertension, following trauma or where there is a potential for the individual's condition to deteriorate because of reduced reliability measures.

BP measurements are obtained when an artery is occluded by an inflatable cuff, and BP is determined either oscillometrically or by auscultation of Korotkoff sounds (6). The most common method used for BP determination is auscultation of the brachial artery (33), as shown in *Figure 20-4*. Other auscultation sites include the ankle or thigh, which may be necessary for individuals with peripheral arterial disease in determining ankle brachial index or in individuals that are morbidly obese (13). Proper procedures for a resting BP assessment are presented in *Box 3-4 of GETP9*. Improper assessment procedures lead to inaccurate measurements, which may lead to an underestimation or overestimation of the individual's true BP. Common BP procedure mistakes include using an inappropriately sized cuff, failing to allow adequate rest before the measurement, deflating the cuff too fast, not measuring in both arms, and failing to palpate maximal systolic pressure before auscultation (21). When choosing a BP cuff, the cuff and bladder must fit appropriately. A bladder that is too small will lead to an overestimation of BP, whereas a bladder that is too large will lead to an underestimation of BP. Recommended bladder dimensions are presented in *Table 20-2* (6). Considerable BP variability can occur with ventiation, emotion, exercise, meals, tobacco, alcohol, temperature, bladder distension, and pain. Furthermore, BP can be influenced by age, race, and circadian rhythm variation. Ideally, the individual should be relaxed in a quiet room at a comfortable temperature with a short rest period before BP measurement (6). The examination should include an appropriate measurement of BP, with verification in the contralateral arm (33). BP measurements should be modified in persons with mastectomy (13), lymphedema (13,18), or arteriovenous fistulas (11,13) so that measurements are taken on the unaffected arm (18). BP measurements may be taken in the lower extremity (*e.g.*, thigh or calf muscle) if an individual is suspected of having coarctation of the aorta or other type of obstructive aortic disease (13). Although measurements of BP can be taken in the lower extremity and forearm, the AHA contends that the accuracy of this procedure has not been verified (27).

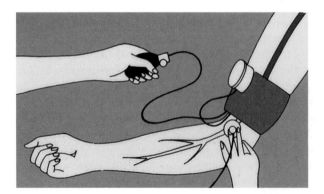

FIGURE 20-4. Blood pressure assessment in upper arm. (Adapted with permission from Weber J, Kelley J. *Health Assessment in Nursing*. 2nd ed. Philadelphia [PA]: Lippincott Williams & Wilkins; 2003.)

TABLE 20-2. Acceptable Bladder Dimensions (in cm) for Arms of Different Sizes[a]

Cuff	Bladder Width (cm)	Bladder Length (cm)	Arm Circumference Range at Midpoint (cm)
Newborn	3	6	≤6
Infant	5	15	6–15[b]
Child	8	21	6–15[b]
Small adult	10	24	22–26
Adult	13	30	27–34
Large adult	16	38	35–44
Adult thigh	20	42	45–52

[a]There is some overlapping of the recommended range for arm circumferences to limit the number of cuffs; it is recommended that the larger cuff be used when available.

[b]To approximate the bladder width: arm circumference ratio of 0.40 more closely in infants and children, additional cuffs are available.

The posture of the subject during BP measurement should be noted, that is supine, sitting, or standing. Sitting is most commonly used, except when examining orthostatic tolerance. When the arm is supported at heart level, the BP should be similar in all three positions (provided a brief period has passed following a change in position to allow for baroreceptor reflex control of BP). To assess the possibility of orthostatic intolerance, BP is measured supine and then standing. A normal response is for the BP to not change (or rise slightly because of the muscular effort of standing). A drop in BP in the standing position (sometimes accompanied by dizziness) indicates orthostatic intolerance (postural hypotension), and may be caused by antihypertensive drugs and certain medical conditions (*e.g.*, diabetic autonomic neuropathy) (6).

Supporting the arm during BP assessment is necessary to prevent possible increases (up to 10%) in diastolic blood pressure (DBP) associated with an isometric muscle action of the unsupported arm. Furthermore, placing the arm in a dependent position below the level of the heart leads to an overestimation of systolic blood pressure (SBP) and DBP, whereas raising the arm leads to an underestimation of SBP and DBP, both caused by gravitationally derived hydrostatic pressure differences between the heart and the arm. Many BP devices are inaccurate if the wrist is not held at the heart level during measurement (6).

During BP assessment, the BP cuff is inflated above the individual's SBP, which leads to complete artery occlusion and an elimination of audible sounds. Once the cuff pressure decreases to the individual's SBP, turbulent, intermittent blood flow in the artery causes audible sounds (Korotkoff sounds). The SBP is determined when the first of two or more Korotkoff sounds are heard (phase 1). Turbulent blood flow continues until the cuff pressure reaches the individual's DBP; at that time, smooth (laminar) blood flow occurs, and the Korotkoff sounds disappear. The DBP is determined just before the disappearance of Korotkoff sounds (phase 5) (33). A description of auscultatory sounds are presented in *Table 20-3* (3,7). During exercise, some individuals produce Korotkoff sounds at cuff pressures well below DBP. In such cases, the examiner should listen for a transition to muffled sounds (phase 4) and note that value as DBP.

In addition to listening to Korotkoff sounds, palpation is useful in individuals in whom auscultatory endpoints are difficult to judge (*e.g.*, during exercise, pregnant, etc.). With this technique, the brachial artery is palpated during BP assessment. The cuff is inflated to approximately 30 mm Hg above the point at which the pulse disappears. The cuff is then slowly deflated and the observer determines the SBP at which the pulse reappears. Palpation is important because phase 1 sounds sometimes disappear as pressure is reduced and then reappear at a lower level, leading to SBP being underestimated unless already determined by palpation (7).

Ambulatory BP monitoring is useful for evaluation of "white-coat" hypertension. Ambulatory BP is taken every 15–30 min during the day to determine BP in a 24-h period. Generally, ambulatory BP values will be lower than clinic readings (33). Evidence also supports the use of automated BP devices with individuals resting alone in a quiet examining room, which almost eliminates the white coat response (25).

According to the Seventh Report of the Joint National Committee on Prevention, Detection, Evaluation, and Treatment of High Blood Pressure (JNC7) (33), all individuals with documented hypertension should have a physical examination that includes the following:

- Examination of optic fundi
- Calculation of body mass index
- Auscultation for carotid, abdominal, and femoral bruits
- Palpation of the thyroid gland
- Examination of the heart and lungs
- Examination of the abdomen for enlarged kidneys, masses, and abnormal aortic pulsation
- Palpation of the lower extremities for edema and pulses
- A neurologic assessment

Laboratory Tests

Additional laboratory tests may be necessary based on information obtained from the past medical history. Cholesterol testing is outlined by the National Cholesterol Education Program (NCEP) and classifications are presented in *Table 3.2* of the *GETP9*. Further blood profile analysis may provide useful information regarding the individual's overall health status. *Table 3.3* of the *GETP9* provides normal ranges for selected blood chemistries.

RISK CLASSIFICATION

The exercise test is considered a diagnostic tool rather than a therapy tool and thus does not have a direct effect on individual outcomes. The risk of exercise testing in appropriately selected candidates is extremely low. The main argument for not performing an exercise test in many clinical situations is that the test would not be cost-effective in that given situation (1).

Risk classification is important for identifying individuals for whom physician supervision is recommended during maximal and submaximal exercise. A detailed risk classification process is located in *Chapter 2* and *Chapter 3* of *GETP9*. Individuals unable to exercise because of physical limitations, such as arthritis, severe peripheral vascular disease, severe chronic obstructive pulmonary disease, or general debility, should undergo pharmacologic stress testing in combination with an imaging modality (1).

Pulmonary risk factors that may require consultation with medical personnel before exercise testing include asthma, exercise-induced asthma/bronchospasm, extreme dyspnea at rest or during exercise, bronchitis, or emphysema. Individuals with pulmonary risk factors should have spirometry (see *Table 3.4* of *GETP9*) and maximal voluntary ventilation (MVV) measured. Furthermore, if hypoxemia is suspected, preexercise arterial blood gases should be obtained (5).

Metabolic risk factors that may require consultation with medical personnel before exercise testing include

TABLE 20-3. Korotkoff Sounds (3,7)	
Phase 1 (SBP)	First, initial sound of faint, repetitive, and clear tapping sounds. The phase 1 sounds approximate the SBP — the maximum pressure that occurs near the end of systole of the left ventricle.
Phase 2	A soft tapping or murmur sound that has a swishing quality. Phase 2 sounds begin 10–15 mm Hg after the onset of sound or below the phase 1 sound.
Phase 3	Return of loud, tapping sounds, which are crisper and louder than phase 1 or 2 sounds.
Phase 4 (true DBP)	Sounds become muffled and are less distinct and less audible. Sounds may be described as soft or blowing.
Phase 5 (clinical DBP)	Complete disappearance of sound that usually occurs 8–10 mm Hg from phase 4.

SBP, systolic blood pressure; DBP, diastolic blood pressure.

metabolic syndrome, obesity, thyroid disease, kidney disease, diabetes, glucose intolerance, and/or hypoglycemia. Before exercise testing, laboratory tests should be obtained to ensure that the individual's blood chemistry profiles are within normal limits.

Musculoskeletal risk factors that may require consultation with medical personnel before exercise testing include acute/chronic back pain, osteoarthritis, rheumatoid arthritis, osteoporosis, and/or joint inflammation/pain. Modifications to the exercise test may be necessary to avoid exacerbating musculoskeletal problems.

CLIENT PREPARATION

BEFORE TESTING

Each individual should be carefully prepared before all exercise testing. Ideally, a detailed set of instructions should be provided to the individual when the testing appointment is made. Verbal and written instructions are recommended to reduce test anxiety and to standardize the response to testing. Instructions before testing should include avoiding eating and smoking for a minimum of 3 h before testing and 8 h before nuclear imaging study. Individuals should wear comfortable footwear and loose-fitting clothing. Each individual should be instructed on whether medications should be tapered, discontinued, or continued for the test based on physician orders. Individuals should avoid unusual physical efforts for at least 12 h before testing (12,30).

A past medical history and physical examination that focuses on risk factors should be conducted before the exercise test to determine any risk factors, signs and symptoms of cardiovascular, pulmonary, metabolic, musculoskeletal, and neurological conditions (30). Furthermore, contraindications to testing should be determined before exercise testing (12). Contraindications to exercise testing are located in *GETP9, Chapter 3 (Box 3.5)*. In addition, determining the individual's current physical activity level can aid in the selection of an appropriate testing protocol. Informed consent (see *GETP9, Chapter 3 Figure 3.1*) should be signed and included in the exercise test record. The informed consent must accurately describe all procedures and potential risks/benefits associated with these procedures. Specific instructions should be given on how to perform the exercise test, purpose of the test, and a brief demonstration of the test procedure (*e.g.*, walking on treadmill, riding bicycle). Furthermore, any questions that the individual has should be addressed (12,30).

Individuals undergoing an exercise stress test with ECG should follow skin preparation guidelines to ensure adequate monitoring during the test. Improper skin preparation can lead to ECG artifact. Electrode resistance should be reduced to ≤5000 Ω by removing the superficial layer of skin. The area where electrodes

will be applied should be shaved and cleaned with an alcohol-saturated gauze pad to remove oil from the skin. Once the skin has dried, the electrode-placement areas should be rubbed with fine sandpaper or a commercially prepared abrasive to remove the superficial layer of skin (12,30).

After obtaining a supine ECG, a standing ECG and BP are recorded to determine vasoregulatory abnormalities and positional changes. Once a standing ECG and BP are obtained, the individual should be instructed, using verbal and written explanations, on all scales that will be used. The subjective rating of intensity of exertion is obtained with the Borg scale of perceived exertion (see *Chapter 4* of *GETP9, Table 4.7*) (12). Depending on the individual's past medical history and current signs/symptoms, other scales such as dyspnea, pain, claudication, and angina (see *Chapter 5* of *GETP9, Figure 5.4*) may be necessary.

PROTOCOL SELECTION

Protocol selection is an important consideration that should be based on the individual's past medical history, preparticipation screening, and physical examination. The health care provider must determine which device (treadmill, cycle ergometer, etc.) is most appropriate and then determine an appropriate protocol (1). Protocols for clinical exercise testing include a low-load initial warm-up, a progressive uninterrupted exercise with increasing loads and adequate time interval in each stage, and a recovery period (12). The exercise protocols can be submaximal or symptom-limited. Submaximal protocols have a predetermined endpoint, often defined as a peak heart rate of 120 bpm or 70% of the predicted maximum heart rate or a peak metabolic equivalent (MET) level of 5 (1,14). Symptom-limited tests continue until the individual presents with signs or symptoms that require termination of exercise testing (1,15). The treadmill, cycle ergometer, and arm ergometer are used for dynamic exercise testing. Treadmills are the most common modality for exercise testing in the United States. One major limitation of using a cycle ergometer for exercise testing is that quadriceps muscle fatigue often occurs before the subject reaches maximum oxygen uptake (1).

The most commonly used protocols following an acute myocardial infarction include the modified Bruce, the modified Naughton, and the standard Bruce (1,14). Much of the published data regarding stress testing, however, are based on the Bruce protocol. Protocols with the largest increments in work rate, like the Bruce protocol, demonstrate decreased ratios of oxygen uptake to work rate (12,24). An optimum protocol selection will include testing that lasts 6–12 min and can be adjusted to the subject's capabilities (12).

Ramping treadmill or cycle ergometer protocols offer the advantage of steady gradual increases in work rate and enhanced estimation of functional capacity (1,24). These protocols start at relatively low treadmill speeds, and the speed is gradually increased until the individual is at a comfortable walking pace. The incline or grade is progressively increased at fixed intervals (*e.g.*, 60 s), starting at 0% grade. The increase in grade is determined based on the person's estimated functional capacity so that the test will be completed in 6–12 min. Steady states are not reached in ramp protocols. Underestimation or overestimation of functional capacity will result if the test is prematurely terminated or if the test becomes too long (12). Ramp protocols have not been widely studied in patients early after myocardial infarction. Exercise capacity should be reported in estimated METs of exercise. Furthermore, the specific protocol and the minutes of exercise duration should be recorded (1).

The 6-min walk test is a functional test that can be used to evaluate exercise capacity in individuals with cardiopulmonary dysfunction and other clinical diagnoses such as obesity (17,32). This protocol uses a submaximal level of stress, and ECG monitoring is normally not used, thus limiting its diagnostic value (12). Protocols for arm ergometry testing require that the subject is seated upright with the fulcrum of the handle adjusted at shoulder height. The arm should be slightly bent at the elbow during the farthest extension movements. Cycling speed of 60–75 rpm must be maintained, with a work rate increase of 10 W per 2-min stage (12,30).

Cycle Ergometer

Cycle ergometers must have handlebars and an adjustable seat. The main advantage of cycle ergometer testing is that upper-body motion is reduced, making it easier to obtain BP measurements and to record the ECG. A disadvantage of cycle ergometer testing is the discomfort and fatigue of the quadriceps muscle. Because of leg fatigue, subjects unaccustomed to cycling exercise may stop the exercise test before reaching a true $\dot{V}O_{2max}$ (12). Cycle ergometry is an alternative for individuals with orthopedic, peripheral vascular, or neurologic limitations that restrict weight-bearing exercise. Work intensity is adjusted by changes in resistance and/or cycling pedal rate. Work rate is typically calculated in watts or kilopond-meters per minute (kpm $\cdot$ min^{-1}).

Stationary bicycles used for exercise testing are either mechanically braked or electronically braked. Mechanically braked ergometers require that a specified cycling rate be maintained to keep a constant work rate (*e.g.*, Monark). Electronically braked ergometers automatically adjust internal resistance to maintain specified work rates according to the cycling rate. Either type of stationary bicycle is used for exercise testing as long as the ergometer has the capability to adjust the work rate in specific increments either automatically or manually (30).

Treadmill

Treadmills used for exercise testing should have front and/or side rails. Subjects should be encouraged to minimize handrail holding during testing, using only their fingers to maintain balance once they are accustomed to walking on the treadmill (12). A treadmill should be electrically driven and accommodate up to at least 157.5 kg (350 lb) (30). The treadmill should be able to change speed and grades (12). Treadmill speed should range between 26.8 m $\cdot$ min^{-1} (1 mph) and at least 214.4 m $\cdot$ min^{-1} (8 mph). The elevation or grade should be electronically controlled and be able to move from no elevation to 20% elevation. All facilities should make sure that treadmills meet electrical safety standards according to the model of treadmill used. The treadmill platform should be a minimum of 127 cm (50 in) in length and 40.64 cm (16 in) in width. Models with side platforms are recommended to allow the individual to adapt to the moving belt before stepping onto the belt. All treadmills must have a visible emergency stop button that is accessible to staff and to the client. Many models also have a clip-on emergency stop apparatus so that if the client moves too far away, the magnet will pull away from the treadmill and stop the treadmill (*e.g.*, if the client is falling) (30).

Arm Ergometer

Arm exercise testing is an alternative mode for testing of individuals with lower-extremity impairments. Arm ergometers are either mechanically braked or electronically braked similar to the cycle ergometers (30). Protocols may begin in the range of 20–25 W and increase by 10–20 W per stage, which typically lasts for 2 min (12). BP should be evaluated regularly. At lower resistance levels, this may be done by removing one hand for BP evaluation while continuing to crank with the other hand. However, at higher resistances, this becomes difficult, and often an intermittent protocol is implemented, with approximately 1 min of rest between stages to take BP.

CALIBRATION OF TESTING EQUIPMENT

Each facility should record dates that equipment calibrations are performed as part of the facility's quality assurance procedures. At a minimum, equipment should be calibrated on a monthly basis and more frequently if many tests are performed. The product's operation manual, provided by the manufacturer, will provide specific directions on calibration and preventive maintenance. The user must assure that all measurements are accurate and maintain a calibration logbook so that long-term trends can be monitored (5). General calibration procedures are provided in the next section of this chapter for the treadmill, bicycle ergometery, arm ergometer, and indirect calorimetry systems.

Treadmill

Both speed and grade/incline must be calibrated on the treadmill. To calibrate speed, the treadmill belt length is measured. Normally, the manufacturer will supply the belt length, but if this information is not available, the belt can be measured with a measuring tape. To calibrate speed, a reference mark is made on the belt, the treadmill is turned on at a specified speed (*e.g.*, 2 miles $\cdot$ h^{-1} or 53.6 m $\cdot$ min^{-1}), and treadmill belt revolutions are counted for 1 min. The following equation is used to calculate the actual treadmill speed in English units (as most exercise protocols in the United States are performed in English units):

$$\frac{\text{Belt length (inches)} \times \text{number of revolutions per minute}}{1,056}$$

The constant of 1,056 represents the conversion of inches per minute to miles per hour.

The actual treadmill speed is compared with the speed indicator on the treadmill. If these values are different, the treadmill will need to be calibrated according to the manufacturer recommendations. These calibration procedures should be repeated for several different speeds that are commonly used in exercise testing protocols. Initially, the speed calibration should be performed without a subject on the treadmill. After the initial calibration, a moderately heavy subject (75–100 kg) should walk on the treadmill and the speed re-measured to ensure it is maintained (30).

To calibrate treadmill grade/incline, first set the treadmill elevation to 0%, and place a carpenter's level on the treadmill. If the treadmill is not level, adjust its support legs until it is. Next, mark two widely separated points along the length of the treadmill. Elevate the treadmill to 20% grade, and measure the height of each point above the floor, and measure the distance along the floor between the two points. The grade is determined as:

$$\frac{(\text{Height 1} - \text{Height 2})}{(\text{Distance along floor})}$$

If the actual result is not 20%, the elevation meter should be adjusted. Note that treadmill grade is the tangent of the angle the treadmill makes with the floor (height/floor length), not the sine of the angle (height divided by treadmill belt length). A check of 5%, 10%, and 15% grade is recommended (30). Most of today's equipment contains an electronic calibration procedure. Often speed or grade adjustments require engineering assistance.

Ergometers

Ergometers are either mechanically braked or electronically braked. Each type of ergometer requires different calibration techniques. The workload on mechanically braked ergometers depends on resistance and cycling rate in revolutions per minute^{-1}. Therefore, the belt tension must be adjusted appropriately, and the flywheel should be cleaned to ensure smooth operation. Electronically braked ergometers normally require special instruments to calibrate, thus calibration procedures are normally provided by the manufacturer.

During calibration of the mechanically braked ergometer, the belt is removed from the flywheel. The pendulum weight is set at 0, and a known weight (*e.g.*, 3 kg, 5 kg) is attached to the belt. A reading of the weight on the ergometer should correspond to the known weight added to the belt. If the scale shows an incorrect reading, the adjusting screw on the ergometer should be turned until the scale reads the appropriate value (3).

If an ergometer has a lateral friction device, the ergometer is placed on two chairs so that the brake scale plate is vertical. The brake regulator is released, and a known metric weight is hung on the brake arm using a wire S-hook. The fastening screw of the shock absorber is loosened, and the scale should correspond to the exact amount of the weight attached to the brake arm. The pointer should always be read from directly above. If the scale is inaccurate, the regulating nut should be turned. When the pointer indicates the same figure as the weight attached, the ergometer is correctly calibrated (30).

Electrocardiograph

Electrocardiograph machines should be calibrated before exercise testing. Each machine will have a 1-mV button to press. Once the button is pressed, the stylus should deflect 10 mm on the ECG paper. If the stylus does not deflect 10 mm, follow the calibration procedures supplied by the manufacturer to correct discrepancies.

Gas Exchange Analysis

The analysis of respiratory gases was once limited to specialized laboratories, but is now increasingly available in both clinical and health fitness settings. Today, there are several manufacturers of integrated gas analysis systems (also known as metabolic carts) that allow cardiorespiratory exercise testing to be administered by persons of various academic backgrounds. Although these systems can produce valid and reliable data, this is dependent on proper maintenance, calibration, and testing procedures. Staff members need to participate in equipment training sessions provided by the manufacturer (30). Calibration involves the measurement of ventilatory flow, the analysis of oxygen and carbon dioxide, and the timing (*i.e.*, phase delay) of the two.

Staff should know the typical physiological response of the individuals being tested, to include normal resting values of ventilation, oxygen consumption and respiratory exchange ratio, and expected increases in these values during exercise. This knowledge can be useful to check the system during a test. If non-physiological data are observed at rest or during exercise, sources of error can be considered (*e.g.*, air leak around the mask) and corrected, or a test can be restarted or rescheduled if necessary.

Sphygmomanometer

The aneroid sphygmomanometer can be calibrated using the standard mercury sphygmomanometer. The needle on the aneroid sphygmomanometer should read zero when no air pressure is inside the cuff. *Figure 20-5* is a drawing of the calibration setup. Steps for calibration include the following (3):

1. Wrap the aneroid sphygmomanometer cuff around a large can or bottle (similar in circumference to the upper arm). Be sure that the aneroid gauge is readable.
2. Connect the tube from the aneroid sphygmomanometer cuff that would go from the hand bulb to one end of the Y connector. *Note:* Some stethoscopes may have a Y connector on them that could be used for this purpose.
3. Connect the other end of the Y connector to the tube that would go from the hand bulb to the mercury sphygmomanometer.
4. Connect the third end of the Y connector to a hand bulb (an extra piece of tubing may be necessary to do this).
5. Pump the hand bulb so that a reading is obtained on the aneroid gauge (*e.g.*, 60 mm Hg).
6. Observe and record the level of the mercury in the mercury sphygmomanometer.
7. Deflate the bladder and repeat the same procedure several more times choosing different pressures throughout the expected measurement range.

A mathematical correction formula can be determined based on the differences between the aneroid and mercury sphygmomanometers. For instance, if the aneroid sphygmomanometer always reads 4 mm Hg low, then add 4 mm Hg to every pressure recorded with that aneroid sphygmomanometer, However, if the readings are variable and >4 mm Hg in disagreement, the aneroid sphygmomanometer should be repaired prior to using (3).

Automatic BP monitors need to be tested, validated and approved by the Association for the Advancement of Medical Instrumentation, the British Hypertension Society and the International Protocol for the Validation of Automated BP Measuring Device (4). All automated devices should follow manufacturer's recommendation for calibration protocols.

SUMMARY

Preparticipation health screenings help identify risk factors for individuals beginning an exercise program, competing in athletics, or completing an exercise test. Risk factor identification is based on the individual's past medical history and physical examination. The pre-exercise evaluation assists the health care professional in determining which protocol and modality to use for the individual's exercise test. Furthermore, the health care professional should understand proper calibration and use of all equipment commonly used for exercise testing.

REFERENCES

1. *ACC/AHA 2002 Guideline Update For Exercise Testing: A Report of the American College of Cardiology/American Heart Association Task Force on Practice Guidelines* (Committee on Exercise Testing) [Internet]. Washington (DC): American College of Cardiology; [cited 2011 Feb 28]. Available from: http://www.americanheart.org/downloadable/heart/1032279013658exercise.pdf
2. American College of Sports Medicine Position Stand and American Heart Association. Recommendations for cardiovascular screening, staffing, and emergency policies at health/fitness facilities. *Med Sci Sports Exerc.* 1998;30(6):1009–18.
3. American College of Sports Medicine. *ACSM's Health-Related Physical Fitness Assessment Manual.* 3rd ed. Baltimore (MD): Lippincott Williams & Wilkins; 2010. 224 p.
4. American Heart Association Web site [Internet]. Dallas (TX): American Heart Association; [cited 2011 Mar 15]. Available from: http://www.heart.org/HEARTORG/
5. American Thoracic Society, American College of Chest Physicians. ATS/ACCP Statement on cardiopulmonary exercise testing. *Am J Respir Crit Care Med.* 2003;167(2):211–77.
6. Beevers G, Lip GY, O'Brien E. ABC of hypertension. Blood pressure measurement. Part I-sphygmomanometry: factors common to all techniques. *BMJ.* 2001;322(7292):981–5.
7. Beevers G, Lip GY, O'Brien E. ABC of hypertension: Blood pressure measurement. Part II-conventional sphygmomanometry: technique of auscultatory blood pressure measurement. *BMJ.* 2001;322(7293):1043–7.
8. Braunwald E, Antman EM, Beasley JW, et al. American College of Cardiology/American Heart Association Task Force on Practice Guidelines (Committee on the Management of Patients With Unstable Angina). ACC/AHA guideline update for the management of patients with unstable angina and non-ST-segment elevation myocardial infarction—2002: Summary article: A report of the American College of Cardiology/American Heart Association Task Force on Practice Guidelines (Committee on the Management of Patients With Unstable Angina). *Circulation.* 2002;106(14):1893–900.

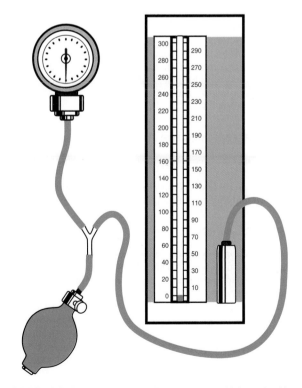

FIGURE 20-5. Blood pressure calibration setup. (Adapted with permission from *ACSM's Health Related Physical Fitness Assessment Manual.* 2nd ed.)

9. Canadian Society for Exercise Physiology Web site [Internet]. Gloucester (Ontario): Canadian Society for Exercise Physiology; [cited 2007 May 21]. Available from: http://www.csep.ca/english/view.asp?x=1

10. *Clinical Guidelines on the Identification, Evaluation, and Treatment of Overweight and Obesity in Adults* [Internet]. Bethesda (MD): National Institutes of Health; National Heart, Lung, and Blood Institute; [cited 2011 Jan 19]. Available from: http://www.nhlbi.nih.gov/guidelines/obesity/ob_home.htm

11. EMSWORLD [Internet]. Calverton (MD): Cygnus Interactive: a Division of Cygnus Business Media; [cited 2011 Apr 12]. Available from: http://www.emsresponder.com/publication/article.jsp?pubId=1&id=1799

12. Fletcher GF, Balady GJ, Amsterdam EA, et al. Exercise standards for testing and training: a statement for health care professionals from the American Heart Association. *Circulation.* 2001;104(14):1694–740.

13. Gardner AW. Exercise training for patients with peripheral artery disease. Activite physique pour des patients souffrant d arteriopathie. *Physician & Sportsmedicine.* 2001;29(8):25,28;31–32;35.

14. Hamm LF, Crow RS, Stull GA, Hannan P. Safety and characteristics of exercise testing early after acute myocardial infarction. *Am J Cardiol.* 1989;63(17):1193–7.

15. Jain A, Myers GH, Sapin PM, O'Rourke RA. Comparison of symptom-limited and low level exercise tolerance tests early after myocardial infarction. *J Am Coll Cardiol.* 1993;22(7):1816–20.

16. Kettenbach G. *Writing SOAP Notes: With Patient/Client Management Formats.* 3rd ed. Philadelphia (PA): F.A. Davis Company; 2004. 215 p.

17. Larsson UE, Reynisdottir S. The six-minute walk test in outpatients with obesity: reproducibility and known group validity. *Physiother Res Int.* 2008;13(2):84–93.

18. *Lymphedema: What Every Woman With Breast Cancer Should Know* [Internet]. Oklahoma City (OK): American Cancer Society; [cited 2007 Apr 2]. Available from: http://www.cancer.org/docroot/CRI/content/CRI_2_6X_Lymphedema_5.asp?sitearea=

19. Maron BJ, Thompson PD, Ackerman MJ, et al. Recommendations and considerations related to preparticipation screening for cardiovascular abnormalities in competitive athletes: 2007 update: a scientific statement from the American Heart Association Council on Nutrition, Physical Activity, and Metabolism: endorsed by the American College of Cardiology Foundation. *Circulation.* 2007; 115(12):1643–455.

20. McAlister FA, Straus SE. Evidence based treatment of hypertension. Measurement of blood pressure: an evidence based review. *BMJ.* 2001;322(7291):908–11.

21. McKay DW, Campbell NR, Parab LS, Chockalingam A, Fodor JG. Clinical assessment of blood pressure. *J Hum Hypertens.* 1990;4(6):639–45.

22. Moore KL, Agur AMRD, Dalley AF. *Essential Clinical Anatomy.* 4th ed. Philadelphia (PA): Lippincott Williams & Wilkins; 2010.

23. Myerburg RJ, Catellanos A. Cardiac arrest and current cardiac death. In: Braunwald E, editor. *Heart Disease: A Textbook of Cardiovascular Medicine.* 5th ed. Philadelphia: Saunders; 1997. p. 742–779.

24. Myers J, Buchanan N, Walsh D, et al. Comparison of the ramp versus standard exercise protocols. *J Am Coll Cardiol.* 1991;17(6):1334–42.

25. Myers MG, Valdivieso M, Kiss A. Use of automated office blood pressure measurement to reduce the white coat response. *J Hypertens.* 2009;27(2):280–6.

26. Pearson TA, Blair SN, Daniels SR, et al. AHA Guidelines for Primary Prevention of Cardiovascular Disease and Stroke: 2002 Update: Consensus Panel Guide to Comprehensive Risk Reduction for Adult Patients Without Coronary or Other Atherosclerotic Vascular Diseases. American Heart Association Science Advisory and Coordinating Committee. *Circulation.* 2002;106(3):388–91.

27. Perloff D, Grim C, Flack J, et al. Human blood pressure determination by sphygmomanometry. *Circulation.* 1993;88(5 Pt 1):2460–70.

28. Pescatello LS, Arena R, Riebe D, American College of Sports Medicine. *ACSM's Guidelines for Exercise Testing and Prescription.* 9th ed. Philadelphia (PA): Lippincott Williams & Wilkins; 2012. 380 p.

29. Pickering TG, Hall JE, Appel LJ, et al. Recommendations for blood pressure measurement in humans and experimental animals: Part 1: Blood pressure measurement in humans: a statement for professionals from the Subcommittee of Professional and Public Education of the American Heart Association Council on High Blood Pressure Research. *Circulation.* 2005;111(5):697–716.

30. Pina IL, Balady GJ, Hanson P, Labovitz AJ, Madonna DW, Myers J. Guidelines for clinical exercise testing laboratories. A statement for health care professionals from the Committee on Exercise and Cardiac Rehabilitation, American Heart Association. *Circulation.* 1995;91(3):912–21.

31. Rao AL, Standaert CJ, Drezner JA, Herring SA. Expert opinion and controversies in musculoskeletal and sports medicine: preventing sudden cardiac death in young athletes. *Arch Phys Med Rehabil.* 2010;91(6):958–62.

32. Rasekaba T, Lee AL, Naughton MT, Williams TJ, Holland AE. The six-minute walk test: a useful metric for the cardiopulmonary patient. *Intern Med J.* 2009;39(8):495–501.

33. *The Seventh Report of the Joint National Committee on Prevention, Detection, Evaluation, and Treatment of High Blood Pressure* [Internet]. Bethesda (MD): National Institutes of Health; National Heart, Lung, and Blood Institute; [cited 2011 Jan 19]. Available from: http://www.nhlbi.nih.gov/guidelines/hypertension/

34. Skirton H, Chamberlain W, Lawson C, Ryan H, Young E. A systematic review of variability and reliability of manual and automated blood pressure readings. *J Clin Nurs.* 2011;20(5–6):602–14.

35. Smith SC Jr, Blair SN, Bonow RO, et al. AHA/ACC Scientific Statement: AHA/ACC guidelines for preventing heart attack and death in patients with atherosclerotic cardiovascular disease: 2001 update: A statement for healthcare professionals from the American Heart Association and the American College of Cardiology. *Circulation.* 2001;104(13):1577–9.

36. Thompson PD. Cardiovascular risks of exercise: Avoiding sudden death and myocardial infarction. Risques cardiovasculaires dus a l'activite physique: Comment eviter la mort subite et l'infarctus du myocarde? *Physician & Sportsmedicine.* 2001;29(4):33,34; 37–38;41–42;44;47.

37. Vulic D, Lee BT, Dede J, Lopez VA, Wong ND. Extent of control of cardiovascular risk factors and adherence to recommended therapies in US multiethnic adults with coronary heart disease: from a 2005–2006 national survey. *Am J Cardiovasc Drugs.* 2010;10(2):109–14.

SELECTED REFERENCES FOR FURTHER READING

Chung EK, Tighe D. *A Pocket Guide to Stress Testing.* Oxford (England): Blackwell Science; 1997.

Ellestad MH. *Stress Testing: Principles and Practice.* 5th ed. New York (NY): Oxford University Press, Inc; 2003.

INTERNET RESOURCES

• American Heart Association. AHA/ACSM Scientific Statement: Recommendations for Cardiovascular Screening, Staffing, and Emergency Policies at Health/Fitness Facilities: http://circ.ahajournals.org/content/97/22/2283

• American Heart Association. ACC/AHA 2002 Guideline Update for Exercise Testing: Summary Article : A Report of the American College of Cardiology/American Heart Association Task Force on Practice Guidelines: http://circ.ahajournals.org/content/106/14/1883.full.pdf+html?sid=a619b0e3-f38f-49cd-9312-ed87e52e2e55

• American Thoracic Society. ATS/ACCP Statement on Cardiopulmonary Exercise Testing: http://www.thoracic.org/statements/resources/pfet/cardioexercise.pdf

Cardiorespiratory and Health-Related Physical Fitness Assessments

CARDIORESPIRATORY AND HEALTH-RELATED PHYSICAL FITNESS ASSESSMENT

The potential to assess levels of physical fitness begins with understanding what comprises physical fitness. The U.S. Surgeon General's report, Physical Activity and Health, defines physical fitness as "a set of attributes that people have or achieve that relates to the ability to perform physical activity" (22). There are numerous components of physical fitness, including cardiorespiratory capacity and endurance; muscular strength and endurance; flexibility, agility, balance, reaction time, and body composition; among others. Some experts have focused on five components as being health-related: cardiorespiratory fitness (CRF), muscular strength, muscular endurance, flexibility, and body composition (1). However, other aspects may be important as well, such as balance in the prevention of falls.

The traditional health-related components of physical fitness have a strong relationship with good health, are characterized by an ability to perform daily activities with vigor, and demonstrate the traits and capacities associated with a reduction in risk for developing diseases associated with physical inactivity (22). Individually and collectively, the health-related components of physical fitness relate closely with disease prevention and health promotion, and can each be modified with regular physical activity and exercise to positively affect disease risk (22).

The health benefits associated with regular physical activity and exercise (*Box 21-1*) are apparent. However, emphasis has been placed on the measurement of health-related physical fitness rather than on skill-related physical fitness (agility, balance, coordination, speed, power, reaction time) (6). As the definition offered by the U.S. Centers for Disease Control and Prevention states, "the five health-related components of physical fitness are more important to public health than are the components

KEY TERMS

Blood pressure: The force of blood against the walls of the arteries and veins created by the heart as it pumps blood to the body.

Body composition: The relative proportion of fat to fat-free tissue in the body.

Cardiac output (CO): The product of heart rate multiplied by stroke volume; the volume of blood pumped by the heart per min.

Cardiorespiratory capacity: The greatest ability of the body to perform large muscle, dynamic exercise as supported by aerobic metabolism and the heart's delivery of blood flow.

Cardiorespiratory endurance: The ability to perform large muscle, dynamic, moderate-to-high intensity exercise for prolonged periods.

Flexibility: The maximum range of motion of a joint.

Heart rate (HR): The number of times the heart contracts per unit time, usually expressed in beats per minute.

Maximal oxygen consumption ($\dot{V}O_{2max}$): The maximal rate of oxygen that can be used for production of adenosine triphosphate (ATP) during exercise.

Muscular endurance: The ability of a muscle group to perform repeated contractions over a period of time sufficient to cause muscular fatigue or to maintain a specific percentage of maximum voluntary contraction for a prolonged period of time.

Muscular strength: The maximal force (expressed in newtons or pounds) that can be generated by a specific muscle or muscle group.

Risk classification: Modeling that attempts to classify individuals (based on health conditions) into low, moderate, and high risk for untoward events during exercise.

Stroke volume (SV): The volume of blood ejected per heartbeat.

BOX 21-1	**Benefits of Regular Physical Activity and/or Exercise**[a]

IMPROVEMENT IN CARDIORESPIRATORY FUNCTION

- Increased maximal oxygen uptake because of both central and peripheral adaptations
- Lower minute ventilation at a given submaximal intensity
- Lower myocardial oxygen cost for a given absolute submaximal intensity
- Lower heart rate and blood pressure at a given submaximal intensity
- Increased capillary density in skeletal muscle
- Increased exercise threshold for the accumulation of lactate in the blood
- Increased exercise threshold for the onset of disease signs or symptoms (*e.g.*, angina pectoris, ischemic ST-segment depression, claudication)

REDUCTION IN CORONARY ARTERY DISEASE RISK FACTORS

- Reduced resting systolic/diastolic pressures
- Increased serum high-density lipoprotein cholesterol and decreased serum triglycerides
- Reduced total body fat, reduced intra-abdominal fat
- Reduced insulin needs, improved glucose tolerance

DECREASED MORTALITY AND MORBIDITY

- Primary prevention (*i.e.*, interventions to prevent an acute cardiac event)

- Lower death rates from coronary artery disease
- Lower incidence rates for combined cardiovascular diseases, coronary artery disease, cancer of the colon, and Type 2 diabetes
- Secondary prevention (*i.e.*, interventions after a cardiac event [to prevent another])
- Cardiovascular and all-cause mortality are reduced in post-myocardial infarction patients who participate in cardiac rehabilitation exercise training, especially as a component of multifactorial risk factor reduction
- Randomized controlled trials of cardiac rehabilitation exercise training involving postmyocardial infarction patients do not support a reduction in the rate of nonfatal reinfarction

OTHER POSTULATED BENEFITS

- Decreased anxiety and depression
- Enhanced feelings of well-being
- Enhanced performance of work, recreational, and sport activities

....

[a]Adapted from United States Department of Health and Human Services: Physical Activity and Health: A Report of the Surgeon General Atlanta (GA): US Department of Health and Human Services, Centers for Disease Control and Prevention, National Center for Chronic Disease Prevention and Health Promotion, 1996; and Garber CE, Blissmer B, Deschenes MR, et al. Quantity and quality of exercise for developing and maintaining cardiorespiratory, musculoskeletal, and neuromotor fitness in apparently healthy adults: Guidance for prescribing exercise. *Med Sci Sports Exerc.* 2011;43:1334–59.

---

related to athletic ability" (22). Thus, physical fitness assessment and programming on both the primary and secondary intervention levels provide a foundation to improve health, and should, therefore, focus on the components of health-related physical fitness.

The purpose of this chapter is to provide a detailed description of how to assess each component of health-related physical fitness in presumably healthy adults. *Figure 21-1* provides a summary of tests that may be used

to measure each individual component of health-related physical fitness.

REASONS FOR THE ASSESSMENT OF HEALTH-RELATED FITNESS

To determine the effectiveness of a preventive or rehabilitative fitness program, it is essential that a baseline evaluation is completed and that periodic follow-up

Cardiorespiratory Fitness:
- Field Tests: *i.e.*, Step Tests, 1.5 Mile Walk/Run, 1 Mile Walk Test
- Submaximal Tests: *i.e.*, YMCA Submaximal Cycle Test & Astrand-Rhyming Cycle Test
- Maximal Tests: Graded Exercise Test

Body Composition:
- Height/Weight & Body Mass Index
- Circumferences & Waist-to-Hip Ratio
- Skinfolds
- Bioelectrical Impedance
- Underwater Weighing
Flexibility:
- Sit and Reach Test
- Modified Sit and Reach Test

Muscular Strength:
- Hand Grip Test
- 1-RM (repetition maximum)
Muscular Endurance:
- Sit-ups
- Curl-ups
- Pushups
- YMCA Bench Press Test

FIGURE 21-1. Summary of Tests for Measuring Each Component of Health-Related Physical Fitness (Source: American College of Sports Medicine. *Health-Related Physical Fitness Assessment Manual.* 3rd ed. Philadelphia [PA]: Lippincott Williams & Wilkins; 2010.)

measurements of the health-related components of physical fitness are made. Additional reasons for measurement of health-related fitness include the following (1):

- To educate participants about their current level of health-related physical fitness
- To provide data that are helpful in developing an exercise prescription that addresses all of the components of fitness
- To evaluate an exercise program's effectiveness
- To motivate participants by establishing reasonable and attainable fitness goals
- To classify the participant's cardiovascular risk

BASIC PRINCIPLES AND GUIDELINES SURROUNDING HEALTH-RELATED FITNESS TESTING

The ideal approach to identifying an individual's physical fitness is to assess each component of health-related physical fitness separately, then compare the individual's assessment data with normative data for each component. The information obtained from fitness testing, in combination with the individual's health and medical information, can then be used by the health and fitness professional to identify and assist in achieving specific fitness goals. Although several tests are available for each fitness component, consideration of a multitude of issues needs to occur prior to determining the appropriate task. These include the following:

- Ease of test administration (How easy is it for the client to perform the test? Can the test administrator and the client interact during the test?)
- Ease of normative data comparison (How applicable and well-developed are the normative standards for any given mode of testing?)
- Economic issues such as the cost of the test, equipment, and personnel
- Validity and reliability of test results
- Client needs, preferences, current fitness level, and risk classification

The ideal health-related physical fitness test is reliable, valid, objective, relatively inexpensive, and easy to administer. It should provide information on an individual's current state of fitness and should be able to reflect any change related to participation in physical activity or exercise. Additionally, the information obtained from the fitness test should be comparable to a previously completed fitness evaluation or available normative data.

PREACTIVITY SCREENING

Preactivity screening gathers pertinent demographic, medical, and personal information that is then used to reduce the occurrence of unwanted and potentially dangerous events during a fitness assessment or exercise session.

The primary reasons for conducting preactivity screening include the following (1):

- Identification of medical contraindications (reasons not to test) to performing specific health-related fitness assessments
- Identification of those clients who should receive a medical evaluation before participating in specific health-related fitness assessments
- Identification of those clients who should be medically supervised during health-related fitness assessments
- Identification of any other health/medical concern or condition that may alter testing format (e.g., diabetes mellitus, orthopedic injuries, readiness for exercise)

PRETEST INSTRUCTIONS

Pretest instructions are to be provided and adhered to before arrival at the testing facility. Care should be taken to ensure client safety and comfort before administering a fitness test. At a minimum, it is recommended that individuals complete a questionnaire, such as the Physical Activity Readiness Questionnaire (PAR-Q) (see *GETP9*, *Chapter 2*, and *Chapter 20* of this *Resource Manual*). A listing of preliminary instructions can be found in *GETP9 Chapter 3* under Participant Instructions. These instructions, however, should be modified to meet needs and circumstances of the testing situation. Guidelines for preactivity screening are listed in *Box 21-2*.

TEST ENVIRONMENT

To minimize test anxiety, it is recommended that the test environment be controlled, including room temperature and ventilation. The test procedures should be well explained, and the test environment should be quiet and private. The room should be equipped with a comfortable seat and/or examination table to be used for resting blood pressure (BP), heart rate (HR), and/or electrocardiographic (ECG) recordings. The professional conducting the test should be relaxed and confident. Testing procedures should not be rushed, and all procedures must be clearly explained before initiating the process. The participant should confirm understanding of the testing procedures, and informed consent should be obtained before continuing with the procedures. General pretest instructions are provided in *Box 21-3*. *Box 21-4* provides recommendations for maintaining a conducive testing environment, and *Box 21-5* lists pretest organization and order of testing procedures.

BOX 21-2 Guidelines for Preactivity Screening

- Consult a physician before participating in health-related physical fitness assessment or any exercise program:
  - If you have cardiovascular, pulmonary, or metabolic disease
  - If you have signs or symptoms of disease
  - If you have two or more risk factors for cardiovascular disease and plan to perform vigorous physical activity
  - If you are in doubt about your health status
- Conduct a medical history/health habits questionnaire including but not limited to:
  - Family history
  - History of various diseases and illnesses, including cardiovascular disease
- Surgical history
- Past and present health behaviors/habits (such as a history of cigarette smoking and physical inactivity)
- Current use of various drugs and/or medications
- Specific history of any signs or symptoms suggesting cardiovascular disease or any other chronic disease
- Physical Activity Readiness Questionnaire (PAR-Q; a minimal standard for entry into a moderate-intensity exercise program; see the ACSM/AHA form in *GETP9 Figure 2.1*)
- Medical/health examination

Reprinted with permission from American College of Sports Medicine. *Health-Related Physical Fitness Assessment Manual.* 3rd ed. Philadelphia (PA): Lippincott Williams & Wilkins; 2010.

BOX 21-3 General Pretest Instructions to the Participant

1. Wear loose-fitting, comfortable clothes that will easily allow for participation in an exercise test.
2. Avoid food, alcohol, and caffeine for at least 3 h before the fitness assessment.
3. Drink plenty of fluids in the 24 h preceding the assessment.
4. Avoid strenuous exercise on the day of the test.
5. Sleep for at least 6 to 8 h the night before the test.
6. All pretest instructions should be provided to the participant ahead of time and adhered to by the participant before his or her arrival at the testing facility.

Reprinted with permission from American College of Sports Medicine. *Health-Related Physical Fitness Assessment Manual.* 3rd ed. Philadelphia (PA): Lippincott Williams & Wilkins; 2010.

BOX 21-4 Recommendations for Maintaining an Environment Conducive to Effective, Low-Anxiety, Health-Related Fitness Testing

1. Maintain room temperature of 68°F–72°F (20°C–22°C) and humidity of <60%.
2. Room should be private, quiet, and well ventilated.
3. Test subject should be made comfortable during resting measures and all nonstrenuous assessment procedures.
4. Test administrator should be relaxed and confident.

Reprinted with permission from from American College of Sports Medicine. *Health-Related Physical Fitness Assessment Manual.* 3rd ed. Philadelphia (PA): Lippincott Williams & Wilkins; 2010.

BOX 21-5 The Pretest Organization and Order of Testing Procedures

- Assure all forms, score sheets, tables, graphs, and other testing documents are organized and available for the test's administration.
- Calibrate all equipment a minimum of once each month to ensure accuracy (*e.g.*, metronome, cycle ergometer, treadmill, sphygmomanometer, skinfold calipers).
- The test session should be reasonably paced and not rushed for time.
- The participant should receive a clear explanation of all procedures associated with the assessment process (and informed consent obtained).
- Resting measures (including heart rate, blood pressure, body composition assessment) should be performed first, followed by cardiorespiratory fitness assessment, then tests of muscular fitness and flexibility.
- Organize equipment so that tests can follow in sequence without stressing the same muscle group repeatedly.

Reprinted with permission from American College of Sports Medicine. *Health-Related Physical Fitness Assessment Manual.* 3rd ed. Philadelphia (PA): Lippincott Williams & Wilkins; 2010.

TEST ORDER

To prepare for testing, the following should be completed before the participant arrives at the test site (*GETP9, Chapter 4*):

- Assure that all forms, score sheets, tables, graphs, and other testing documents are organized and available for the test's administration.
- Equipment should have been calibrated within the past month to ensure accuracy (*e.g.*, metronome, cycle ergometer, treadmill, sphygmomanometer, skinfold calipers).
- Testing equipment should be organized in a sequence that prevents stressing the same muscle group repeatedly.
- Have appropriate informed consent form available.
- Ensure that the appropriate room temperature (68° to 72° F [20° to 22° C]) and humidity (<60%) are maintained.

During the administration of multiple tests, the sequence can be very important. Testing order should include resting measurements of HR, BP, height, weight, and body composition, followed by tests of CRF, muscular fitness, and flexibility. When multiple fitness components are assessed in a single session, the order of the testing is extremely important. For example, testing CRF after assessing muscular fitness (which elevates HR) can produce inaccurate results. Likewise, perspiration may make skinfold assessment more difficult.

To preserve the validity and reliability of fitness assessment results, professionals are encouraged to pay close attention to the details throughout the entire assessment to minimize variance in test results. These recommendations, and those identified previously in this chapter, can save the test administrator time and allow for a more relaxed environment for the test participant.

RISK CLASSIFICATION

The American College of Sports Medicine (ACSM) has a specific set of guidelines for preactivity screening termed *risk classification* (see *Chapters 2* and *3* in *GETP9*). There are three risk categories (low, moderate, and high risk). Risk classification is used to help determine an appropriate course of action for an individual by identifying the need for a medical examination and the level of physician supervision before proceeding with a health-related physical fitness test.

Risk classification and medical clearance prior to exercise testing should also coincide with the gathering of information to identify signs and symptoms or known history of cardiovascular, pulmonary, and/or metabolic disease in the test participants. ACSM, in collaboration with other national organizations, provides test administrators with guidelines for recognizing and understanding the impact on exercise testing of these signs and symptoms (3). *Chapter 2* of *GETP9* provides guidelines for risk classification (see especially *Tables 2.2* and *2.3* and *Figure 2.4*) and assists in identifying individuals who may be candidates for physician supervision during an exercise test.

RESTING MEASURES: MEASUREMENT OF RESTING HEART RATE, BLOOD PRESSURE, AND BODY COMPOSITION

RESTING HEART RATE, STROKE VOLUME, AND CARDIAC OUTPUT

HR is the number of times the heart contracts per unit time, usually expressed in beats per minute. Stroke volume (SV) is the volume of blood ejected from the heart per beat. Cardiac output (CO) is the product of HR multiplied by SV, or the volume of blood pumped by the heart per minute. Chronic exercise training improves CRF in part by increasing maximal SV and, thus, maximal CO. These changes also result in a lower resting and exercise HR, which can be used as an indicator of improved CRF.

HR can be measured using manual palpation, via an HR monitor (14), by auscultation with a stethoscope, or use of an ECG. For greater accuracy, it is recommended that resting HR be measured by palpation at the radial artery for a full 60-s period prior to health-related fitness testing. More detailed information regarding HR measurement can be found in *Chapter 20* of this *Resource Manual*.

RESTING BLOOD PRESSURE

BP is defined as the force of blood, in millimeters of mercury (mm Hg), against the walls of the arteries and veins created by the heart as it pumps blood through the body. BP is created and altered by changes in the diameter of the more elastic blood vessels as they constrict and relax in response to various stimuli (such as blood volume, stress, and blood flow changes related to the support of bodily functions like digestion and exercise). Atherosclerosis, caused by plaque buildup, can also cause changes in BP by narrowing the diameter of the blood vessels and making them less pliant. The process for accurately measuring resting BP can be found in *Chapter 20* of this *Resource Manual* and in *Chapter 3* of ACSM's *Health-Related Physical Fitness Assessment Manual, Third Edition*.

BP assessment during exercise is more challenging than at rest. Although the technique used for measuring BP during exercise is the same as that used for resting measurement, significant practice is required to master this skill.

Exercise BP is an important physiological indicator of an individual's work intensity during exercise and may reflect inappropriate responses requiring test termination. Systolic BP serves as an indicator of left ventricular function during exercise and should rise with exercise intensity. Diastolic

BP, however, typically remains constant during dynamic exercise, although it may increase or decrease slightly.

DETERMINATION OF BODY COMPOSITION

Body composition is the relative proportion of fat to fat-free tissue in the body. It is an important measure because excess body fat, particularly when located centrally around the abdomen, is associated with increased disease risk (8,20). Estimation of body composition can be accomplished using both laboratory and field techniques that vary in terms of complexity, cost, and accuracy. Detailed descriptions of these techniques are available in *Chapter 18* of this Resource Manual.

CARDIORESPIRATORY FITNESS

CRF is determined by one's ability to aerobically perform dynamic exercise utilizing large muscle groups. The maximum ability to do such exercise is defined as cardiorespiratory capacity, which is associated with maximal oxygen consumption ($\dot{V}O_{2max}$), whereas the ability to maintain a submaximal intensity for prolonged periods is defined as cardiorespiratory endurance. The ability to perform such exercise depends on the functional ability of the pulmonary, cardiovascular, and skeletal muscle systems. The term cardiorespiratory "fitness" is commonly used synonymously with cardiorespiratory "capacity," with cardiovascular endurance being considered another aspect of fitness, just as muscular fitness is often divided into the components of muscular strength and muscular endurance.

CRF is well established as a health-related index of fitness, as (a) a low level of CRF is associated with a markedly increased cardiovascular and all-cause mortality, (b) increasing CRF results in a reduction in all-cause mortality, and (c) high levels of CRF are related to increased levels of habitual physical activity, which in turn is correlated with significant health benefits (4,5,22). The assessment of CRF is fundamentally important as part of a primary or secondary prevention program.

REASONS FOR MEASURING CARDIORESPIRATORY FITNESS

Identification of CRF can assist the professional by providing valuable information that can be used to determine the intensity, duration, and mode of exercise recommended as part of an exercise program. Additionally, the measurement of CRF following the initiation of an exercise training program can serve as motivation to the client as reason for continuing with a regular exercise program and may encourage the addition of other modes of exercise to improve overall fitness. Lastly, the assessment of CRF can assist in identifying, diagnosing, and prognosing health/medical situations.

HOW CARDIORESPIRATORY FITNESS IS MEASURED AND EXPRESSED: MAXIMAL OXYGEN CONSUMPTION

$\dot{V}O_{2max}$ is widely considered the best measure of CRF. $\dot{V}O_{2max}$ is the product of maximal CO ($L \cdot min^{-1}$) and maximal arteriovenous oxygen difference ($mL \cdot O_2$ per L blood). Variations resulting from sex, age, and fitness level are noted in $\dot{V}O_{2max}$ and result primarily from differences in maximal CO. Thus, the functional capacity of the heart is the primary determinant of $\dot{V}O_{2max}$.

$\dot{V}O_{2max}$ is measured using open-circuit spirometry, which requires the subject to breathe through a low-resistance mouthpiece with his or her nose occluded (or to breathe through a facemask that covers mouth and nose) while pulmonary ventilation and expired fractions of oxygen (O_2) and carbon dioxide (CO_2) are measured. Today, the measurement of $\dot{V}O_{2max}$ is less labor intensive in that data printouts and detailed graphics are provided on a breath-by-breath basis (11). However, this test remains highly specialized, and the administration of the test and interpretation of results should be reserved for trained professionals with a thorough understanding of exercise science. Additionally, because of the costs associated with the equipment, space, and personnel needed to complete this testing, $\dot{V}O_{2max}$ testing is generally reserved for research or clinical laboratory settings.

$\dot{V}O_{2max}$ can be estimated using various submaximal and maximal exercise tests. Although not as accurate as directly measuring $\dot{V}O_{2max}$, these tests provide validated estimates by examining (a) the physiologic response to submaximal exercise (*e.g.*, HR at a specified power output) as compared with correlations with directly measured $\dot{V}O_{2max}$, or (b) test performance measures (*e.g.*, distance completed within a specified amount of time) as compared with correlations with directly measured $\dot{V}O_{2max}$.

Because of the numerous options for assessing CRF, the choice of which test to use is important. Some factors to consider when choosing test type are the following (1):

- Length of the test
- Willingness of the participant
- Cost of the test to administer
- What personnel are needed (*i.e.*, qualifications)
- What equipment and facilities are needed for the test
- Whether physician supervision is needed
- Whether there are any safety concerns
- Needs to be met to preserve accuracy of the data being collected

CONTRAINDICATIONS TO EXERCISE TESTING

Before initiating an exercise test, the risk for performing the test must be weighed against the potential benefits. *Box 3.5* in *GETP9* lists both relative and absolute contraindications to exercise testing. Performing the preexercise test evaluation and the careful review of prior medical history, as described in the *GETP9* and in related chapters of this manual, assists in identifying potential contraindications to exercise testing and increases the safety of the exercise test.

Individuals identified as having absolute contraindications should not be tested until such conditions are stabilized or adequately treated. Those with relative contraindications may be tested only after careful evaluation to determine if the benefits obtained from test completion outweigh the risk involved. However, certain clinical situations may preclude the use of contraindications to determine testing risk — such as soon after acute myocardial infarction, revascularization procedure, or bypass surgery — or to determine the need for, or benefit of, drug therapy.

MAXIMAL VERSUS SUBMAXIMAL EXERCISE TESTING

The use of maximal or submaximal exercise testing depends on the information desired, the personnel available to perform the test, and the equipment available for testing purposes. Maximal exercise testing offers increased sensitivity in the diagnosis of coronary artery disease in asymptomatic individuals and provides a better estimate of $\dot{V}O_{2max}$ (see *Chapter 5* of *GETP9*). The disadvantage, however, of using maximal exercise testing to determine $\dot{V}O_{2max}$ is that clients are required to exercise to the point of volitional fatigue, thus potentially requiring medical supervision (see *Chapter 2* of *GETP9*) and the availability of emergency equipment. Only subjects classified in the low risk category may be maximally tested without physician supervision.

Submaximal exercise can provide reasonable estimates of $\dot{V}O_{2max}$ by considering test duration at a given workload on an ergometer and using the established prediction equations found in *Chapter 4* of ACSM's *GETP9*. Additionally, submaximal exercise testing estimates $\dot{V}O_{2max}$ through the determination of the HR response to one or more submaximal work rates. Lastly, the use of submaximal BP, workload, rating of perceived exertion (RPE), and other subjective indices (pain/discomfort) can provide valuable information regarding the client's functional response to exercise.

The following are assumed to have been met when estimating $\dot{V}O_{2max}$ from the submaximal HR response (*GTEP9, Chapter 4*):

- A steady-state HR (HR_{ss}) is achieved and is consistent for each work rate
- HR and work rate exists as a linear relationship
- The $\dot{V}O_{2max}$ is indicated by the maximal workload
- There is a uniform maximal HR for a given age
- Mechanical efficiency is the same for everyone
- The subject is not on medications that alter HR

To the extent that these assumptions are not true for a given subject, the estimation of $\dot{V}O_{2max}$ from submaximal data will be inaccurate.

Submaximal exercise tests are typically performed on low- to moderate-risk individuals, based on ACSM guidelines for risk classification. General Procedures for Submaximal Testing of Cardiorespiratory Fitness, which provides professionals with a quick-reference guide to test administration, can be found in *Box 4.4* of *GETP9*.

PRETEST INSTRUCTIONS FOR CARDIORESPIRATORY FITNESS ASSESSMENT

To standardize the testing conditions, increase the predictive accuracy for identifying CRF, and ensure the safety of the client, the following general instructions should be provided (*GETP9, Chapter 3*):

- Abstain from eating at least 4 h before testing (although clients who experience hypoglycemia may be advised to have a light, healthy snack of protein and carbohydrate combination 2–3 h before the test, and all clients should be encouraged to eat something light and well balanced in the 12 h preceding the 4-h pretest fast).
- Abstain from strenuous exercise for at least 24 h before the test.
- Abstain from consuming caffeine-containing products for a minimum of 12–24 h before the test.
- Abstain from using products containing nicotine for at least 3 h and from consuming alcohol for at least 24 h before the test.
- Consult the test administrator and/or physician for advice on the use of medications before testing (medications affecting resting or exercise HR, such as β-blockers, may affect test accuracy).

TEST MODE FOR MEASURING CARDIORESPIRATORY FITNESS: PROCEDURES AND PROTOCOLS FOR STEP TESTS, FIELD TESTS, SUBMAXIMAL EXERCISE TESTS, AND MAXIMAL EXERCISE TESTS

Step Tests

Step tests have been used for fitness testing for more than 50 yr. Step tests are practical for exercise testing in that they can be used in a field or laboratory setting, can be submaximal or maximal in nature, require little or no testing equipment, are easily transportable, require little practice, and are usually of short duration. Unlike traditional fitness testing, evaluation of CRF from step tests is usually done via the evaluation of recovery HR. The Queens College (or McArdle) Step Test is described in detail in *Box 21-6*. Other common step protocols are also available (*i.e.*, Forestry Test and Harvard Step Test) and differ from the Queens College step test in either step

---

BOX 21-6 **Queens College Step Test**

The Queens College Step Test is also known as the McArdle Step Test.

1. The step test requires that the individual step up and down on a standardized step height of 16.25 in (41.25 cm) for 3 min. (Many gymnasium bleachers have a riser height of 16.25 in.)
2. The men step at a rate (cadence) of 24 per min, whereas the women step at a rate of 22 per min. This cadence should be closely monitored and set with the use of an electronic metronome. A 24 per min cadence means that the complete cycle of step up with one leg, step up with the other, step down with the first leg, and finally step down with the last leg is performed 24 times in a minute (up one leg, up the other leg, down the first leg, down the other leg). Commonly, we set the metronome at a cadence of four times the step rate, in this case 96 beats per min for men, to coordinate each leg's movement with a beat of the metronome. The women's step rate would be 88 beats per min. Although it may be possible to test more than one patient at a time, depending on equipment, it would be difficult to test men and women together.
3. After the 3 min are up, the patient stops and palpates the pulse or has the pulse taken (at the radial

site, preferably) while standing within the first 5 s. A 15-s pulse count is then taken. Multiply this pulse count by 4 to determine heart rate (HR) in beats per minute (bpm). The recovery HR should occur between 5 and 20 s of immediate recovery from the end of the step test.

The subject's $\dot{V}O_{2max}$ in mL · kg^{-1} · min^{-1} is determined from the recovery HR by the following formulas:

For men:

$$\dot{V}O_{2max} \text{ (mL · kg}^{-1} \cdot \text{min}^{-1}) = 111.33 - (0.42 \cdot HR)$$

For women:

$$\dot{V}O_{2max} \text{ (mL · kg}^{-1} \cdot \text{min}^{-1}) = 65.81 - (0.1847 \cdot HR)$$

HR = recovery HR (bpm)

For example:

If a man finished the test with a recovery HR of 144 bpm (36 beats in 15 seconds), then:

$$\dot{V}O_{2max} \text{ (mL · kg}^{-1} \cdot \text{min}^{-1}) = 111.33 - (0.42 \cdot 144)$$
$$= 50.85 \text{ mL · kg}^{-1} \cdot \text{min}^{-1}$$

Reprinted with permission from American College of Sports Medicine. *Health-Related Physical Fitness Assessment Manual.* 3rd ed. Philadelphia (PA): Lippincott Williams & Wilkins; 2010.

---

height and/or test time (1). Also, the Canadian Home Fitness test has demonstrated that testing for CRF can be performed on a large scale and at a low cost (21).

Field Tests for the Prediction of Cardiorespiratory Fitness

Field tests may be used to measure CRF in large groups of apparently healthy subjects. Field tests offer many benefits over other forms of laboratory testing in that they are easy to administer, are inexpensive, and can be performed wherever a measured distance is available.

Several disadvantages are associated with using field tests for the prediction of CRF, including the inability to control the setting and the potential for the tests to become maximal or near maximal tests. In addition, field tests are unmonitored and can be highly affected by an individual's motivation or pacing ability. Thus, for these reasons, the vigorous field tests (such as running tests) are not recommended for individuals at moderate to high risk of cardiovascular or musculoskeletal complications.

Field tests can utilize various modes of exercise, including walking, running, a walk-run, cycling, and swimming. The most common field tests used for the prediction of CRF, however, are those requiring a timed completion of

a set distance (*i.e.*, 1.5-mile run) or a maximal distance measurement (*i.e.*, 12-min run). *Box 21-7* provides procedures for the 1.5-mile run and the 12-min walk/run test, and *Box 21-8* gives the Rockport 1-mile walk test procedures.

SUBMAXIMAL EXERCISE TESTS FOR THE PREDICTION OF CARDIORESPIRATORY FITNESS

Submaximal exercise testing can be a valid and reliable method for predicting CRF when done in a laboratory setting. These exercise tests usually involve use of a step test, treadmill, or cycle ergometer. The cycle ergometer is the most preferred mode for laboratory testing because of its ability to reproduce work output. For more information about work output and choice of testing mode, consult *ACSM's Health-Related Physical Fitness Assessment Manual, Third Edition* (1). *Box 4.4* of *GETP9* provides general procedures for submaximal exercise testing using a cycle ergometer.

To achieve valid results during submaximal exercise testing, it is essential that an accurate measurement of HR is achieved. Typically, HR is obtained by palpation; however, the accuracy of this method varies with the experience and technique of the fitness professional.

BOX 21-7   1.5-Mile Run and 12-Minute Walk/Run Test Procedures

1.5-MILE RUN TEST

This test is contraindicated for unconditioned beginners, individuals with symptoms of heart disease, and those with known heart disease or risk factors for heart disease. Your patient should be able to jog for 15 min continuously to complete this test and obtain a reasonable prediction of their aerobic capacity.

1. Ensure that the area for performing the test measures out to be 1.5 miles in distance. A standard quarter-mile track would be ideal (6 laps = 1.5 miles).
2. Inform the patient of the purposes of the test and the need to pace over the 1.5-mile distance. Effective pacing and the subject's motivation are key variables in the outcome of the test.
3. Have the patient start the test; start a stopwatch to coincide with the start. Give your patient feedback on time to help them with pacing.
4. Record the total time to complete the test and use the formula below to predict cardiorespiratory fitness in $mL \cdot kg^{-1} \cdot min^{-1}$

For men and women:

$$\dot{V}O_{2max} \ (mL \cdot kg^{-1} \cdot min^{-1}) = 3.5 + 483/Time$$

Time = time to complete 1.5 miles in nearest hundredth of a minute

For example:

If time to complete 1.5 miles was 11:12 (11 min and 12 s), then the time used in the formula would be 11.2 (12/60 = 0.2).

$$\dot{V}O_{2max} \ (mL \cdot kg^{-1} \cdot min^{-1}) = 3.5 + 483/11.2$$
$$= 46.6 \ mL \cdot kg^{-1} \cdot min^{-1}$$

12-MINUTE WALK/RUN TEST PROCEDURES

A popular variation of the 1.5-mile run test is the 12-min walk/run test popularized by Dr. Ken Cooper of the Aerobics Institute in Dallas, Texas. This test requires the patient to cover the maximum distance in 12 min by either walking, running, or using a combination of walking and running. The distance covered in 12 min needs to be measured and expressed in meters.

The prediction of aerobic capacity from the 12-min walk/run test is:

$$\dot{V}O_{2max} \ (mL \cdot kg^{-1} \cdot min^{-1})$$
$$= (distance \ in \ meters - 504.9)/44.73$$

Reprinted with permission from American College of Sports Medicine. *Health-Related Physical Fitness Assessment Manual.* 3rd ed. Philadelphia (PA): Lippincott Williams & Wilkins; 2010.

BOX 21-8   Rockport 1-Mile Walk Test Procedure

This test may be useful for those who are unable to run because of a low fitness level and/or injury. The patient should be able to walk briskly (get their exercise heart rate [HR] above 120 bpm) for 1 mile to complete this test.

1. The 1-mile walk test requires that the subject walk 1 mile as fast as possible around a measured course. The patient must not break into a run! Walking can be defined as having contact with the ground at all times (running involves an airborne phase). The time to walk this 1 mile is measured and recorded.
2. Immediately at the end of the 1-mile walk, the patient counts the recovery HR or pulse for 15 sec and multiplies by 4 to determine a 1-min recovery HR (bpm). In another version of the test, HR is measured in the final minute of the 1-mile walk (during the last quarter mile).

The formula for $\dot{V}O_{2max}$, $mL \cdot kg^{-1} \cdot min^{-1}$ is sex specific (*i.e.*, the constant of 6.315 is added to the formula for men only).

$$\dot{V}O_{2max} \ (mL \cdot kg^{-1} \cdot min^{-1}) = 132.853 - (0.1692 \cdot WT) -$$
$$(0.3877 \cdot AGE) + (6.315, \ for \ men) -$$

$$(3.2649 \cdot TIME) - (0.1565 \cdot HR)$$

WT = weight in kilograms

AGE = in years

TIME = time for 1 mile in nearest hundredth of a minute (*e.g.*, 15:42 = 15.7)

HR = recovery HR in bpm

This formula was derived on apparently healthy individuals ranging in age from 30 to 69 yr of age.

For example:

32-yr-old male; 68 kg (150 lbs)

1 mile = 10:35 (10.58); HR = 136

$$\dot{V}O_{2max} \ (mL \cdot kg^{-1} \cdot min^{-1}) = 132.853 - (0.1692 \cdot 68) -$$
$$(0.3877 \cdot 32) + (6.315) - (3.2649 \cdot 10.58) -$$
$$(0.1565 \cdot 136) = 59.4 \ mL \cdot kg^{-1} \cdot min^{-1}$$

Reprinted with permission from American College of Sports Medicine. *Health-Related Physical Fitness Assessment Manual.* 3rd ed. Philadelphia (PA): Lippincott Williams & Wilkins; 2010.

Alterations to palpation that may increase accuracy of HR measurement include the use of an ECG, HR monitor, or a stethoscope.

Additionally, submaximal HR response can be altered by several environmental (*i.e.*, heat and humidity), dietary (*i.e.*, caffeine, time since last meal), and behavioral (*i.e.*, anxiety, smoking, previous activity) factors (see pretest instructions earlier in this chapter) that must be controlled for, as previously discussed.

Assumptions of Submaximal Prediction of Cardiorespiratory Fitness

The following list of assumptions is specific to submaximal testing (1).

- A linear (straight line) relationship exists between $\dot{V}O_2$ and HR within the range of 110–150 bpm. It is at this point that SV has reached a plateau (approximately 40%–50% of max), and the HR and oxygen consumption track linearly.
- Maximum HR (HR_{max}), which must be predicted for submaximal ergometer testing, can be estimated or predicted as a function of age (*e.g.*, $HR_{max} = 220 - $ age). Unfortunately, a large variation exists in the age-prediction of HR_{max}, and this assumption may provide for the greatest source of error in the submaximal prediction of CRF.
- HR_{ss} can be achieved in 3–4 min at a constant, submaximal work output. HR_{ss} is ensured by consecutive HR measurements being within five beats of each other. Thus, the achievement of HR_{ss} during the protocol is essential for valid results.
- A cadence of 50 revolutions per minute (rpm) is typically considered comfortable and mechanically efficient in most individuals. It is assumed that each subject expends the same amount of energy and has the same absolute oxygen requirements at the same work output on the cycle. Maintaining a constant pedal rate on a mechanically braked ergometer is essential to ensure a constant power output.
- The HR at two separate work outputs can be plotted as the $HR-\dot{V}O_2$ relationship and extrapolated to the estimated HR_{max}. The YMCA submaximal cycle ergometer protocol and the Bruce submaximal treadmill protocol are both multistage tests that utilize a minimum of two stages to predict CRF. The Åstrand protocol prediction is based on the HR_{ss} at a single work stage.

Sources of Error in Submaximal Prediction

A submaximal exercise test requires predetermined test endpoints for satisfactory completion of the test. General indications for stopping an exercise test in low-risk adults can be found in *Box 4.5* of *GETP9*. In addition to terminating the test because of completion of the protocol, the health/fitness professional should consider test termination if the client's HR exceeds 70% of HR reserve or 85% of his or her age-predicted HR_{max} because this exposes the subject to near maximal exertion and increases the risk of cardiovascular or orthopedic complications.

Submaximal Protocols for Predicting Cardiorespiratory Fitness

As discussed previously in this chapter, various modes of exercise can be used in the completion of submaximal exercise tests. Most common modes of exercise for laboratory-based exercise testing include the motor-driven treadmill and the mechanically braked cycle ergometer. Although both provide adequate mechanisms for completion of submaximal testing, each has inherent advantages and disadvantages that must be considered. Common protocols utilized in predicting CRF using submaximal exercise testing can be found in *Boxes 21-9* through *21-12*, *Table 21-1*, and *Figure 21-2*.

MAXIMAL EXERCISE TESTING

Maximal exercise testing is the most challenging of all physical fitness assessment tests for both the client and the test technician. Also called a graded exercise test (GXT) or stress test, these tests use incremental changes in workload until peak exertion/exhaustion is achieved. Although many exercise professionals may not be involved in maximal exercise testing, they should be aware of the purposes, procedures, protocols, and contraindications to this type of exercise test. More information on maximal exercise testing can be found in *Chapters 23* and *24* of this *Resource Manual*.

Purposes of Maximal Exercise Testing

The maximal GXT has four primary purposes:

1. Screening for the presence of disease
2. Diagnosis of a disease when symptoms are present
3. Prognosis of the patient relative to coronary artery disease and/or other disease history
4. Guiding the management of an individual, including for use in prescribing exercise

Procedures for Maximal Exercise Testing

Decisions concerning the use of a maximal GXT include the identification of who should have the test, whether a physical examination should be performed before the test, whether a physician should be present for the test, and what personnel will be needed to conduct the test.

Who Should Have a Maximal Graded Exercise Test?

ACSM's *GETP9* addresses the appropriate candidates for a maximal GXT by applying the concept of risk

BOX 21-9 Submaximal Cycle Ergometer Test Procedures: Multistage Protocol

In summary, the client performs a multistage protocol based on the response to the first stage. The total test may last from 6 to 12 min

1. Explain the test to your client. Be sure you have adequately screened your client via a Health History Questionnaire and/or a PAR-Q and performed ACSM risk classification. *Note:* Physician supervision is not necessary with submaximal testing in low- and moderate-risk adults. More information on this can be found in ACSM's GETP9.

2. In addition, you should have already ensured that your client has followed some basic pretest instructions for this submaximal test: wearing comfortable clothing; having plenty of fluids beforehand; avoiding alcohol, tobacco, and caffeine within 3 h of the test; avoiding strenuous exercise on the day of the test; and having adequate sleep the night before the test.

3. Explain informed consent. The safety of this test is reported as >300,000 tests performed without a major complication. It is very important that the client understands that he or she is free to stop the test at any time, but he or she is also responsible for informing you of any and all symptoms that might develop.

4. You should also discuss with your client the concept of your general preparedness to handle any emergencies. The details of general preparedness include the testing environment and emergency plan/procedures. Also, an explanation of the rating of perceived exertion (RPE) scale is warranted at this time (*Table 4-7* of *GETP9*). An example of some verbal directions you could read to your client before asking him or her to use the RPE scale to give a general rating is: "Rate your feelings that are caused by exercise using this scale. The feelings should be general, about your whole body. We will

ask you to select one number that most accurately corresponds to your perception of your total body feeling. You can use the verbal qualifiers to help you select your RPE number. There is no right or wrong answer. Use any number that you think is appropriate."

5. Take the baseline or resting measures of heart rate and blood pressure with your client seated. If necessary, these seated measurements can be performed on the cycle ergometer.

6. Adjust seat height. The knee should be flexed at approximately 5–10 degrees in the pedal-down position with the foot held horizontally. Also, you can align the seat height with you client's greater trochanter, or hip, with your client standing next to the cycle. Most important is for your client to be comfortable with the seat height. Have your client turn the pedals to test for the seat height appropriateness. While pedaling, your client should be comfortable, and there should be no rocking of the hips (as viewed from behind). Also, be sure your client maintains an upright posture (by adjusting the handlebars, if necessary) and does not grip the handlebars tightly.

7. START THE TEST. Have your client begin pedaling without any resistance (0 kg) at a cadence of 50 rpm. Adjust the resistance to a low amount to begin a 2–3 min warm-up period. If using the YMCA protocol, the first stage has a resistance of 0.5 kp, which serves as both the warm-up and the first data collection stage. Maintaining 50 rpm throughout the test is essential. The rpm may vary between about 48 and 52 rpm; any more variance than this may invalidate the test.

classification (discussed earlier in this chapter and in *Chapter 20* of this *Resource Manual*). According to these guidelines, clients who are low risk are not recommended to have a maximal exercise test before starting an exercise program, regardless of the program's intensity. Clients who are moderate risk are not recommended to have a maximal test if they intend to begin a moderate-intensity exercise program, but they are for beginning a vigorous intensity program. Clients who are at a high risk for disease are recommended to have a maximal GXT with a medical examination before starting any exercise program.

Personnel Needs for Conducting the Maximal Graded Exercise Test

Research indicates that allied health personnel (*i.e.,* exercise physiologists or nurses) who have been adequately trained can safely perform maximal exercise testing (9). These personnel should be health care professionals who are certified at the basic life support (advanced life support preferred) level and have a professional certification (ACSM Certified Clinical Exercise Specialist [CES] or Registered Clinical Exercise Physiologist [RCEP]). Personnel should be skilled at monitoring HR, BP, and signs and symptoms suggesting

BOX 21-10 YMCA Submaximal Cycle Ergometer Protocol

1. Start the clock/timer. It may be best to think of timing each stage (*e.g.*, 3 min) rather than the entire test time. Therefore, you may wish to reset the time at the end of each stage. In reality, timing of this test is the most difficult part for individuals to learn. Suggested timing sequence for each stage of the test are included in the following steps.

2. Measure the heart rate (HR) near the end of the second minute into the first work rate or stage. Count HR for 10 or 15 s. Some suggest a 30-s count for more accuracy, but it may be impractical to spend a full 30 s of each minute counting the HR. The use of an HR monitor may be helpful; however, it should only be used as a teaching aid to check your results by palpation. Record the HR on the test form.

3. Measure and record the blood pressure (BP) one time during each stage; usually after having completed the 2-min HR of that stage. ACSM's GETP9 for test termination and BP is applicable:
   - BP >250/115 mm Hg
   - Significant drop (>10 mm Hg) in systolic blood pressure or a failure to rise with an increase in exercise intensity

4. Ask your client for the RPE for that stage. Choose either the 6–20 scale or the 0–11 scale. Be sure to monitor your client for general appearance and any symptoms that may develop.

5. Take another HR after the BP and RPE measurements, around 3 min into the stage. Record the HR on the appropriate testing data form.
   Compare minute 2 HR to minute 3 HR during each stage:

   A. If there is a difference of within 5 bpm, consider that work rate or stage finished. Steady state conditions apply.

   B. If there is a difference of >5 bpm, continue on for another minute (*i.e.*, minute 4 of that stage) and check HR again. Do not change to the next stage until you have a steady-state HR (HR_{SS}; difference within 5 bpm). If you fail to have your client achieve an HR_{SS} for a stage, then you may have to discontinue the test and plan to test again on another day. It has been noted that up to 10% of individuals who are tested with this protocol are unable to obtain HR_{SS} in a stage.

In summary:

HR_{SS} (within 5 bpm): Go to step 7

No HR_{SS} (>5 bpm) achieved: Continue stage until HR_{SS}

6. Regularly check the work output of the cycle ergometer using the pendulum resistance scale on the side of the ergometer and the rpm of your client. For the resistance, do not use the scale on the top front panel of the cycle ergometer for measurement. Adjust the work output if necessary. Regularly check your client's rpm and correct if necessary.

7. After completing the first stage of $150 \text{ kp} \cdot \text{m} \cdot \text{min}^{-1}$ compare your client's HR_{SS} to the protocol sheet. Adjust resistance appropriately for the second stage based on HR response to first stage. This is a multistage test; the client will typically perform three or four stages.
   - You need to obtain HR_{SS} from a stage (within 5 bpm).
   - The test requires completion of at least two separate stages with HR_{SS} at each stage.
   - Consider for the test results the third minute HR as the HR_{SS}, if it is a steady state (for plotting or calculations) for that stage.
   - These two stages must have HRs between 110 bpm and 85% of age-predicted maximum HR to be used in the plotting and calculation of $\dot{V}O_{2max}$.

8. Allow your client to cool down after the last stage of the protocol is complete. Have your client continue to pedal at 50 rpm, and adjust the resistance down to 0.5 to 1.0 kp for 3 min of cool-down or recovery. Take your client's HR and BP at the end of the 3-minute active recovery period. Next, allow him or her to sit quietly in a chair for 2 to 3 min to continue the recovery process. Be sure to check the HR and BP before allowing him or her to leave the lab. It is hoped that the HR and BP will approach the resting measures.

Reprinted with permission from American College of Sports Medicine. *Health-Related Physical Fitness Assessment Manual.* 3rd ed. Philadelphia (PA): Lippincott Williams & Wilkins; 2010.

BOX 21-11   Suggested Stage Procedures for YMCA Submaximal Cycle Ergometer Test

0:00–0:45	Monitor your client's work output (cadence and resistance)
0:45–1:00	Pulse count for 15 s (for practice)
1:00–1:45	Monitor your client's work output (cadence and resistance)
1:45–2:00	Pulse count for 15 s (2 min HR)
2:00–2:30	Stage BP check
2:30–2:45	Stage RPE check
2:45–3:00	Pulse count for 15 s (3 min HR)

Reprinted with permission from American College of Sports Medicine. *Health-Related Physical Fitness Assessment Manual.* 3rd ed. Philadelphia (PA): Lippincott Williams & Wilkins; 2010.

BOX 21-12   Astrand Submaximal Cycle Ergometer Test Procedures

In summary, the client performs a 6-min submaximal exercise session on the cycle ergometer. Thus, this is typically a single-stage test. The heart rate (HR) response to this session will determine the maximal aerobic capacity by plotting the HR response to this one stage on a nomogram.

The calibration of the cycle ergometer is the same as in the YMCA protocol:

1. Explain the test to your client: same as in the YMCA protocol.
2. Explain informed consent: same as in the YMCA protocol.
3. You should also discuss with your client the concept of your general preparedness to handle any emergencies: same as in the YMCA protocol.
4. Take the baseline or resting measures of HR and blood pressure (BP) with your client seated: same as in the YMCA protocol.
5. Adjust seat height: same as in the YMCA protocol.
6. START THE TEST. Have your patient freewheel, without any resistance (0 kg), at the pedaling cadence of 50 rpm. Maintaining 50 rpm throughout the test is essential.
7. Set the first stage's work output according to protocol *Table 21-1*.
8. Start the clock/timer.
9. Measure the HR after each minute starting at minute 2. Count the HR for 10 to 15 s. You may wish to use a HR monitor, only as a teaching tool. Record the HR on the test form.
10. Measure and record the BP after the 3-min HR; ACSM guidelines for test termination and BP are applicable.
11. The fifth and sixth minute HR will be used in the test determination of $\dot{V}O_{2max}$ as long as there is not more than a 6-beat difference between the two HRs.

    The following applies for steady-state HR (HR_{SS}):

    If there is a difference of ≤6 bpm, then consider the test finished.

If there is a difference of >6 bpm, then continue for another minute and check HR again.

12. Regularly check the work output of the cycle ergometer using the pendulum resistance scale on the side of the ergometer and the rpm of subject. For the resistance, do not use the scale on the top front panel for measurement. Adjust the work output if necessary.
13. Regularly check your client's rpm and correct if necessary.

    The Astrand protocol requires the following for test completion:

    You need to obtain HR_{SS} from the test with the fifth and sixth minute HR (within 6 bpm).

    For the best (most accurate) prediction of $\dot{V}O_{2max}$, the HR should be between 125 and 170 bpm.

    If the HR response to the initial work rate is not greater than 125 bpm after 6 min, then the test is continued for another 6-min interval by increasing the work rate by 300 kp · m · min^{-1} (0.5 kp).

    The HR at the fifth and sixth minutes, if acceptable to the criteria mentioned earlier, is averaged for the nomogram method.

14. Allow your client to cool down after the protocol is complete. Have your client continue to pedal at 50 rpm, and adjust the resistance down to 0.5 to 1 kp for 3 min of cool-down or recovery. Take your client's HR and BP at the end of the 3-min active recovery period. Next, allow your client to sit quietly in a chair for 2–3 min to continue the recovery process. Be sure to check your client's HR and BP before allowing your client to leave the lab. It is hoped that the HR and BP will approach the resting measures.

Reprinted with permission from American College of Sports Medicine. *Health-Related Physical Fitness Assessment Manual.* 3rd ed. Philadelphia (PA): Lippincott Williams & Wilkins; 2010.

TABLE 21-1. Åstrand Cycle Submaximal Cycle Ergometer Test Initial Workloads

This protocol table is designed as a guide. The protocol is designed to elicit an HR of between 125 and 170 bpm by 6 min. You can adjust the work output as necessary during the test (usually after the first 6 min) to achieve an HR in or near this range in your subject.

Individual	Work Output (kp · m · min⁻¹)
Men	
Unconditioned	300–600
Conditioned	600–900
Women	
Unconditioned	300–450
Conditioned	450–600
Poorly conditioned or older individuals	300

Reprinted with permission from American College of Sports Medicine. *Health-Related Physical Fitness Assessment Manual.* 3rd ed. Philadelphia (PA): Lippincott Williams & Wilkins; 2010.

the presence of disease or exercise intolerance. In addition, personnel should understand ECG interpretation and be able to recognize myocardial ischemia and rhythm disturbances (9).

Although those who are low risk may not need physician supervision for a maximal GXT, those at moderate or high risk are recommended to have a physician within close proximity to the testing area who will be readily available in the event of an emergency situation. Qualified personnel, independent of job title, should be aware of, and adhere to, the recommendations found in *GETP9* regarding test contraindications, test termination criteria, and emergency procedures.

Protocols for Maximal Exercise Testing

Traditionally, the treadmill has been the most utilized mode for graded exercise testing in the United States. Treadmill walking involves the use of a large muscle mass, enabling the subject to generally achieve a physiological maximum. Performing a maximal exercise test using a cycle ergometer, which is more reflective of localized quadriceps activity, results in a lower peak $\dot{V}O_2$ in subjects unaccustomed to that form of exercise. Various modes of testing and protocols are available and appropriate for special populations. A visual summary of common protocols used for maximal exercise testing can be found in *Figure 21-3*.

Measurements Taken during Exercise Testing

Common variables measured during maximal exercise testing include HR, BP, RPE, ECG, and subjective measurements of signs or symptoms related to coronary ischemia. In addition, direct measurements of ventilatory

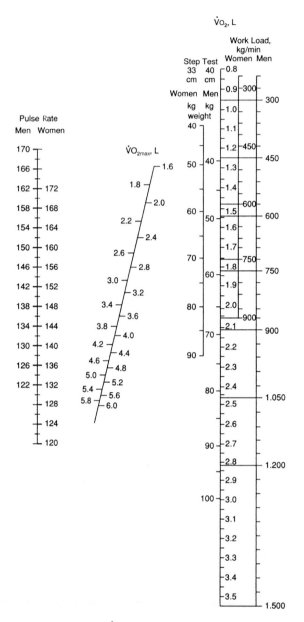

FIGURE 21-2. Modified Åstrand-Ryhming nomogram. (Reprinted with permission from Astrand PO, Ryhming I. A nomogram for calculation of aerobic capacity [physical fitness] from pulse rate during sub-maximal work. *J Appl Physiol.* 1954;7[2]:218–21.)

responses and expired gases can also be observed during maximal exercise testing. Typically, BP and HR are measured at rest, during each exercise stage, and during recovery. In addition, ECG measurements are observed during these same intervals.

During exercise, exercise-induced measurements, including RPE, gas exchange, and signs or symptoms related to cardiovascular or pulmonary disorders, should be observed. These measures should be obtained routinely throughout the examination and throughout recovery. *Box 21-13* provides the recommended sequence for measurement of HR, BP, RPE, and ECG during exercise testing.

FIGURE 21-3. Visual Summary of Protocols for Maximal Exercise Testing.

FUNCTIONAL CLASS	CLINICAL STATUS	O₂ COST ml/kg/min	METS	BICYCLE ERGOMETER (FOR 70 KG BODY WEIGHT Kpm/min (WATTS))	BRUCE 3 MIN STAGES (MPH / %AGR)	RAMP PER 30 SEC (MPH / %GR)	BRUCE RAMP PER MIN (MPH / %GR)	BALKE-WARE (%GRADE AT 3.3 MPH 1 MIN STAGES)	USAFSAM (MPH / %GR)	"SLOW" USAFSAM (MPH / %GR)	MODIFIED BALKE (MPH / %GR)	ACIP (MPH / %GR)	MOD. NAUGHTON (CHF)[a] (MPH / %GR)	METS
NORMAL AND I (HEALTHY, DEPENDENT ON AGE, ACTIVITY)		73.5	21				5.8 / 20							21
		70	20		5.5 / 20									20
		66.5	19				5.6 / 19							19
		63	18				5.3 / 18							18
		59.5	17		5.0 / 18		5.0 / 18	26						17
		56.0	16			3.0 / 25.0	4.8 / 17	25	3.3 / 25		3.0 / 25	3.4 / 24.0		16
		52.5	15			3.0 / 24.0; 3.0 / 23.0		24; 23			3.0 / 22.5	3.1 / 24.0		15
		49.0	14	1500 (246)	4.2 / 16	3.0 / 22.0; 3.0 / 21.0; 3.0 / 20.0	4.5 / 16; 4.2 / 16	22; 21	3.3 / 20		3.0 / 20	3.0 / 21.0	3.0 / 25	14
		45.5	13	1350 (221)		3.0 / 19.0; 3.0 / 18.0	4.1 / 15	20			3.0 / 17.5		3.0 / 22.5	13
		42.0	12	1200 (197)		3.0 / 17.0; 3.0 / 16.0	3.8 / 14	19; 18			3.0 / 15		3.0 / 20	12
		38.5	11			3.0 / 15.0; 3.0 / 14.0	3.4 / 14	17; 16			3.0 / 12.5			11
	SEDENTARY HEALTHY	35.0	10	1050 (172)	3.4 / 14	3.0 / 13.0; 3.0 / 12.0	3.1 / 13	15	3.3 / 15	2 / 25	3.0 / 10	3.0 / 17.5	3.0 / 17.5	10
		31.5	9	900 (148)		3.0 / 11.0; 3.0 / 10.0	2.8 / 12	14; 13		2 / 20	3.0 / 7.5		3.0 / 15	9
		28.0	8	750 (123)		3.0 / 9.0; 3.0 / 8.0	2.5 / 12	12; 11	3.3 / 10	2 / 15	3.0 / 5	3.0 / 14.0	3.0 / 12.5	8
		24.5	7		2.5 / 12	3.0 / 7.0; 3.0 / 6.0	2.3 / 11	10; 9		2 / 10	3.0 / 2.5		3.0 / 10	7
II	LIMITED	21.0	6	600 (98)		3.0 / 5.0; 3.0 / 4.0	2.1 / 10	8; 7	3.3 / 5	2 / 5	3.0 / 0	3.0 / 10.5	3.0 / 7.5	6
		17.5	5	450 (74)	1.7 / 10	3.0 / 3.0; 3.0 / 2.0	1.7 / 10	6; 5			2.0 / 0	3.0 / 7.0	2.0 / 10.5	5
III	SYMPTOMATIC	14.0	4	300 (49)		3.0 / 1.0; 3.0 / 0	1.3 / 5	4; 3	3.3 / 0	2 / 0		3.0 / 3.0	2.0 / 7.0	4
		10.5	3	150 (24)		2.5 / 0; 2.0 / 0	1.0 / 0	2; 1	2.0 / 0		2.0 / 0	2.5 / 2.0	2.0 / 3.5	3
		7.0	2			1.5 / 0; 1.0 / 0						2.0 / 0.0	1.5 / 0	2
IV		3.5	1			0.5 / 0							1.0 / 0	1

(Reprinted with permission from American College of Sports Medicine. *ACSM's Guidelines for Exercise Testing and Prescription.* 9th ed. Philadelphia [PA]: Wolters Kluwer Health Ltd; 2013.)

[a]There are multiple variations of the modified Naughton protocol.

BOX 21-13	Sequence of Measures for HR, BP, RPE, and Electrocardiogram (ECG) During Exercise Testing

PRETEST

1. 12-lead ECG in supine and exercise postures
2. Blood pressure measurements in supine and exercise postures

EXERCISE[a]

1. 12-lead ECG recorded during the last 15 s of every stage and at peak exercise (3-lead ECG observed/recorded every minute on monitor)
2. Blood pressure measurements should be obtained during the last minute of each stage[b]
3. Rating scales: RPE at the end of each stage, other scales if applicable

POSTTEST

1. 12-lead ECG immediately after exercise, then every 1–2 min for at least 5 min to allow any exercise-induced changes to return to baseline
2. Blood pressure measurements should be obtained immediately after exercise, then every 1–2 min until stabilized near baseline level.
3. Symptomatic ratings should be obtained using appropriate scales as long as symptoms persist after exercise

....

[a]In addition, these referenced variables should be assessed and recorded whenever adverse symptoms or abnormal ECG changes occur.

[b]Note: An unchanged or decreasing systolic blood pressure with increasing workloads should be retaken (*i.e.*, verified immediately)

Reprinted with permission from American College of Sports Medicine. *Health-Related Physical Fitness Assessment Manual.* 3rd ed. Philadelphia (PA): Lippincott Williams & Wilkins; 2010.

Test Termination Criteria

Graded exercise testing, whether maximal or submaximal, is considered safe when subjects are appropriately screened and testing guidelines are followed. Occasionally, the test may be terminated before the subject achieves $\dot{V}O_{2max}$ because of signs, symptoms, or a predetermined endpoint (*e.g.*, a designated target HR). Indications for terminating an exercise test in a clinical setting are listed in *Box 5.2* in *GETP9*. As mentioned previously, general indications for stopping a test in a nonclinical setting are listed in *Box 4.5* of *GETP9*.

CRITERION-REFERENCED STANDARDS VERSUS NORMATIVE DATA

Upon completion of an exercise test, the results should be interpreted by comparing the test results with established standards or norms. Traditionally, two sets of standards are used for comparisons: criterion-referenced standards and normative standards. Criterion-referenced standards are those that are considered desirable to achieve based on external criteria and may use adjectives such as "excellent" or "poor" in the data interpretation tables. Criterion-referenced standards exist mostly in CRF evaluations and in body fat analyses. These standards, however, are open to subjective interpretation, and disagreement is present among experts regarding what these results truly mean when used for interpretation.

Normative standards (norms) are based on previous performances by a similar group of individuals. Norms compare how the client performed versus other like individuals, and the data are presented using percentile values to assist in identifying level of fitness.

Evaluative decisions about a client's health-related physical fitness can be based on either criterion-referenced standards or normative standards.

INTERPRETATION OF RESULTS

When using submaximal exercise testing to establish a client's fitness status, the accuracy of the comparison with published norms depends on the similarities of the groups being compared and the testing methodology used. Although maximal exercise testing reduces some of the error involved in determining CRF, the use of submaximal exercise testing introduces some assumptions that can be easily met (*e.g.*, HR_{ss} can be verified) and others (*e.g.*, HR_{max}) that introduce errors into the prediction of $\dot{V}O_{2max}$. Regardless, it can be assumed that a reduction in HR response at a fixed work rate during repeated submaximal exercise tests over a period of weeks or months indicates an improved CRF. Therefore, despite the differences in test accuracy and various errors introduced with each methodology, virtually all evaluations can establish a baseline and be used to track progress relative to improvement in fitness.

MUSCULAR FITNESS ASSESSMENT

Muscular fitness encompasses muscular strength, muscular endurance, and flexibility, and is an integral portion of total health-related fitness (11,22). Testing for these components of fitness should be accomplished following a CRF assessment to allow the muscles to warm up and to reduce the risk for muscle injury during testing. The development and maintenance of muscular fitness contributes to health by increasing fat-free mass and resting metabolic rate, maintaining bone mass, stimulating modest improvements in cardiovascular fitness, and improving the ability to perform activities of daily living (ADL). Additional information on muscular fitness, including more in-depth information on muscular fitness assessment techniques, can be found in *Chapter 22* of this Resource Manual.

MUSCULAR STRENGTH

Muscular strength is defined as the maximal force (expressed in newtons or pounds) that can be generated by a specific muscle or muscle group (22). It is specific to the muscle group being tested, the type of contraction (static or dynamic, concentric or eccentric), the speed of the contraction, and the joint angle being tested (1). Because of the specificity of strength measurement, there is no single test for total body muscle strength.

The measurement of muscle force production is used for assessing muscular strength, identifying weaknesses in muscle groups, monitoring progress in the rehabilitation of muscles, and measuring the effectiveness of training (1).

Strength can be assessed either statically (no overt muscular movement or limb movement) or dynamically (movement of an external load or body part, in which the muscle changes length). Various devices are available to measure static strength, including cable tensiometers and handgrip dynamometers. These measures, however, cannot be generalized for total body strength because they are specific to both the muscle group and joint angle tested (7). The measure of the peak force development during these tests is referred to as the maximum voluntary contraction (MVC).

Common techniques/protocols for measuring muscular strength include the one-repetition maximum (1-RM) bench press test, the 1-RM leg press test, and isokinetic testing. The 1-RM test identifies the greatest weight that can be moved through the full range of motion (ROM) in a controlled manner and has traditionally been used as the standard measure of dynamic strength. Multiple RM tests, such as 4- or 8-RM, are also used as a measure of muscular strength to allow the participant to integrate evaluation into his or her training program (17). The 1-RM may be estimated from multiple RM tests. However, the number of lifts one can perform at a fixed percentage of 1-RM varies for different muscle groups (*e.g.*, leg press vs. bench press). Thus, care must be taken to account for these differences if estimating 1-RM (12,13). Traditional measures of upper-body strength use 1-RM values for the bench press or military press, whereas 1-RM indices of lower-body strength include leg press or leg extension. Norms — which are based on weight lifted divided by body mass — for the bench press and leg press are provided in *Tables 4.9* and *4.10* of *GETP9*. *Box 21-14* provides the basic steps in 1-RM testing.

Isokinetic testing differs from dynamic muscle testing in that it involves the assessment of constant-speed muscular contraction against accommodating resistance. The speed of angular movement is controlled and the amount of resistance is proportional to the amount of force produced throughout the full ROM. Commercial devices that will measure the peak force and torque at various joints (knee, hip, shoulder, elbow) are available, yet these pieces of equipment are limited by their cost.

BOX 21-14 1-RM Bench Press Test Procedures

1. For each lift, the subject keeps his or her buttocks, upper back, and head on the bench; both feet on the floor; and hands shoulder width apart with a pronated (overhand), closed (thumbs opposing fingers) grip. A spotter should be present for all lifts and assists the subject with liftoff. The subject starts the lift with the bar in the up position with arms fully extended, then lowers the bar to gently touch the chest and pushes it back up until the arms are locked. Encourage regular breathing and avoidance of breath holding during exertion.

2. The subject should warm up by completing several submaximal repetitions with a light weight (at 40%–60% of perceived maximum) without going to failure.

3. After 1 min of rest, the subject performs 3–5 repetitions with a moderate weight (70%–80% of perceived maximum).

4. After 2 min of rest, the subject attempts 1 repetition at an estimated near-maximum weight.

5. After 3–5 min of rest, the subject attempts 1 repetition with a heavier weight; if successful, additional attempts are made following 3–5 min rest periods with increasingly heavier weights until the 1-RM is obtained. This should occur in a total of three to five attempts.

6. Once an attempt is failed, an attempt may be made at a weight between the last two attempts.

Note: The aforementioned procedure can also be used for testing the 1-RM of other lifts.

MUSCULAR ENDURANCE

Muscular endurance is the ability of a muscle group to repeatedly perform muscular contractions over a period that is sufficient to cause muscular fatigue, or the ability to maintain a percentage of MVC for an extended period. Common assessments for muscular endurance include the YMCA Bench Press Test, push-up test, and the partial curl-up (crunch) test. Procedures for performing these tests, and norms for evaluating clients' results, are provided in *Chapter 4* of *GETP9*.

Special Considerations

Older Adults

Using muscular strength and muscular endurance assessments, in combination with other aspects of health-related physical fitness, for older adults can aid in the detection of deteriorating health while yielding important information that can be used to design an individualized exercise program to improve strength and functional independence. The Senior Fitness Test (SFT) was developed in response to a need for specialized tools that improved the overall assessment capabilities for older persons to assess the key physiologic parameters (*e.g.*, strength, endurance, agility, and balance) needed to perform activities that become increasingly difficult as one ages (19). The SFT meets scientific standards for reliability and validity, is an easy to administer field test, and has normative data for older men and women (19). Two specific tests included in the SFT, the 30-s chair stand and the single arm curl, can be used to safely and effectively assess muscular strength and muscular endurance in most older adults.

Coronary Heart Disease Patients

Moderate-intensity resistance training, when performed 2–3 d · wk^{-1}, has been shown to be safe and effective for improving muscular fitness, preventing and managing certain chronic medical conditions, modifying coronary risk factors, and enhancing psychosocial well-being in those with and without cardiovascular disease. Consequently, influential health organizations, including the American Heart Association and ACSM, support the inclusion of resistance training exercises as a beneficial adjunct to endurance exercises for individuals with cardiovascular disease (18).

Those cardiac patients deemed low-risk (*e.g.*, persons without resting or exercise-induced evidence of myocardial ischemia, severe left ventricular dysfunction, or complex ventricular dysrhythmias, and with normal or near-normal CRF) can perform moderate- to high-intensity (*e.g.*, 40%–80% 1-RM) resistance testing and training safely. Additionally, research does not support the occurrence of an abnormal cardiovascular "pressor response" in cardiac patients or those with controlled hypertension, indicating strength testing and training should be safe to include in comprehensive evaluation and training programs. However, data on the safety of muscular fitness testing in moderate- to high-risk cardiac patients, especially those with poor left ventricular function, are limited and require additional investigation (18).

Current guidelines suggest that the following contraindications be recognized when considering muscular strength and endurance testing: unstable angina, uncontrolled hypertension (systolic BP $\geq$160 mm Hg and/or diastolic BP $\geq$100 mm Hg), uncontrolled dysrhythmias, poorly managed or untreated heart failure, severe stenotic or regurgitant valvular disease, and hypertrophic cardiomyopathy (18). In addition, it is suggested that those with cardiac disease should also have well-preserved left ventricular function and CRF ($>$5 or 6 metabolic equivalents) without anginal symptoms or ischemic ST-segment changes to participate in traditional resistance training programs (10,18). Significant care should be taken during preparticipation screening, and proper supervision should be provided in an effort to reduce the risk of a serious cardiac event during muscular strength and endurance testing.

Children and Adolescents

As with other fitness parameters, muscular fitness is recognized as an important component of health-related fitness in children and adolescents. Enhancing muscular strength and muscular endurance in youth provides significant benefits, including the development of proper posture, reducing injury risk, enhancing body composition, and improving motor performance skills. Muscular strength and muscular endurance are typically assessed with push-up and abdominal curl-up tests and standardized testing procedures with normative comparison data are currently available to use with children and adolescents.

Strength and weakness can be assessed in children using various muscular fitness measures. Data derived from these tests can be used to develop an individualized fitness program, and to motivate participants to continue with and progress in their current exercise program. To enhance safety and to ensure adequate completion of each exercise, fitness professionals should demonstrate the proper skill techniques and ensure proper technique is being followed.

FLEXIBILITY

Flexibility is defined as the functional ability of a joint to move through its full ROM. *Functional ability* refers to movement through the ROM without incurring pain or a limit to performance. Flexibility is joint specific because it depends on the muscle and joint that is being evaluated. It also depends on the distensibility of the joint capsule, adequate warm-up, muscle viscosity, and the compliance of ligaments and tendons.

Assessment of flexibility is important because there is an associated decrease in performance of ADL with inadequate flexibility. No single test can characterize overall flexibility.

The sit-and-reach test is the most widely used test for flexibility assessment. The sit-and-reach test is a reflection of hamstring, hip, and lower-back flexibility, which is important to the prevention of chronic lower back pain and the promotion of a healthy lifestyle (15,16).

Procedures for performing the Canadian trunk flexion test and the YMCA sit-and-reach test are provided in *Box 4.7* of *GETP9*. Fitness categories by age groups and sex for the Canadian trunk forward flexion test are provided in *Table 4.16* of *GETP9*, and percentiles by age group and sex for the YMCA sit-and-reach test are presented in *Table 4.17*.

ROM at any joint can be measured. In addition, postural analysis and body alignment are also important to assess. ACSM's *Health-Related Physical Fitness Assessment Manual* (1) provides thorough step-by-step instructions for measuring these, which are outside of the scope of this chapter.

SUMMARY

The assessment of an individual's health-related physical fitness can provide valuable information to help develop a safe, effective, and individualized exercise program. The development of an exercise program requires careful consideration to the medical/health history, preactivity screening (including risk stratification), and the individual responses to the selected tests of health-related physical fitness. The following is a summary of chapter points:

- The first step in any assessment of health-related physical fitness is to perform a preactivity screening, including an informed consent, medical/health history, risk classification, and (possibly) a focused physical examination.
- Test procedures should be selected according to the population being tested, facilities and equipment available, and the qualifications of those performing the tests.
- There are various techniques available to assess body composition, including height/weight charts, BMI, anthropometric measurements, and percent body fat estimation.
- CRF can be assessed using several techniques that can be classified as either laboratory or field tests for the estimation and/or measurement of $\dot{V}O_{2max}$.
- Several submaximal cycle and treadmill protocols exist that can be used to estimate CRF.
- Maximal exercise testing using various treadmill or cycle ergometer protocols exist for determining CRF.

- The assessment of muscular strength, muscular endurance, and flexibility is often grouped together and can occur using several different testing measures.

REFERENCES

1. American College of Sports Medicine. *ACSM's Health-Related Physical Fitness Assessment Manual*. 3rd ed. Baltimore (MD): Lippincott Williams & Wilkins; 2010. 224 p.
2. Astrand PO, Ryhming I. A nomogram for calculation of aerobic capacity (physical fitness) from pulse rate during sub-maximal work. *J Appl Physiol*. 1954;7(2):218–21.
3. Balady GJ, Chaitman B, Driscoll D, et al. Recommendations for cardiovascular screening, staffing, and emergency policies at health/fitness facilities. *Circulation*. 1998;97(22):2283–93.
4. Blair SN, Kohl HW 3rd, Barlow CE, Paffenbarger RS Jr, Gibbons LW, Macera CA. Changes in physical fitness and all-cause mortality. A prospective study of healthy and unhealthy men. *JAMA*. 1995;273(14):1093–8.
5. Blair SN, Kohl HW 3rd, Paffenbarger RS Jr, Clark DG, Cooper KH, Gibbons LW. Physical fitness and all-cause mortality. A prospective study of healthy men and women. *JAMA*. 1989;262(17): 2395–401.
6. Caspersen CJ, Powell KE, Christenson GM. Physical activity, exercise, and physical fitness: definitions and distinctions for health-related research. *Public Health Rep*. 1985;100(2):126–31.
7. Clarkson HM, Gilewich GB. *Musculoskeletal Assessment: Joint Range of Motion and Manual Muscle Strength*. Baltimore (MD): Williams & Wilkins; 1989. 366 p.
8. Folsom AR, Kaye SA, Sellers TA, et al. Body fat distribution and 5-year risk of death in older women. *JAMA*. 1993;269(4):483–7.
9. Franklin BA, Gordon S, Timmis GC, O'Neill WW. Is direct physician supervision of exercise stress testing routinely necessary? *Chest*. 1997;111(2):262–5.
10. Franklin BA, Gordon NF. *Contemporary Diagnosis and Management in Cardiovascular Exercise*. Premiere ed. Newtown (PA): Handbooks in Health Care Co; 2005. 357 p.
11. Garber CE, Blissmer B, Deschenes MR, et al. Quantity and quality of exercise for developing and maintaining cardiorespiratory, musculoskeletal, and neuromotor fitness in apparently healthy adults: guidance for prescribing exercise. *Med Sci Sports Exerc*. 2011; 43(7):1334–59.
12. Hoeger WW, Barette SL, Hale DF, Hopkins DR. Relationship between repetitions and selected percentages of one repetition maximum. *J Appl Sport Sci Res*. 1987;1(1):11–3.
13. Hoeger WWK, Hopkins DR, Barette SL, Hale DF. Relationship between repetitions and selected percentages of one repetition maximum: a comparison between untrained and trained males and females. *J Appl Sport Sci Res*. 1990;4(2):47–54.
14. Leger L, Thivierge M. Heart rate monitors: validity, stability, and functionality. *Phys Sportsmed*. 1988;16(5):143,146;148–149;151.
15. Liemohn WP, Sharpe GL, Wasserman JF. Lumbosacral movement in the sit-and-reach and in Cailliet's protective-hamstring stretch. *Spine (Phila Pa 1976)*. 1994;19(18):2127–30.
16. Minkler S, Patterson P. The validity of the modified sit-and-reach test in college-age students. *Res Q Exerc Sport*. 1994;65(2):189–92.
17. Palmer ML, Epler ME. *Fundamentals of Musculoskeletal Assessment Techniques*. 2nd ed. Philadelphia (PA): Lippincott; 1998. 415 p.
18. Pollock ML, Franklin BA, Balady GJ, et al. Resistance exercise in individuals with and without cardiovascular disease: benefits, rationale, safety, and prescription: An advisory from the Committee on Exercise, Rehabilitation, and Prevention, Council on Clinical Cardiology, American Heart Association; Position paper endorsed by the American College of Sports Medicine. *Circulation*. 2000;101(7):828–33.
19. Rikli RE, Jones CJ. *Senior Fitness Test Manual*. Champaign (IL): Human Kinetics; 2001. 161 p.

20. Rimm EB, Stampfer MJ, Giovannucci E, et al. Body size and fat distribution as predictors of coronary heart disease among middle-aged and older US men. *Am J Epidemiol.* 1995;141(12):1117–27.

21. Shephard RJ, Thomas S, Weller I. The Canadian Home Fitness Test. 1991 update. *Sports Med.* 1991;11(6):358–66.

22. U.S. Department of Health and Human Services, Centers for Disease Control and Prevention, National Center for Chronic Disease Prevention and Health Promotion, The President's Council on Physical Fitness and Sports. *Physical Activity and Health: A Report of the Surgeon General.* Atlanta (GA): President's Council on Physical Fitness and Sports; 1996. 278 p.

SELECTED REFERENCES FOR FURTHER READING

Garber CE, Blissmer B, Deschenes MR, et al. Quantity and quality of exercise for developing and maintaining cardiorespiratory, musculoskeletal, and neuromotor fitness in apparently healthy adults: guidance for prescribing exercise. *Med Sci Sports Exerc.* 2011;43(7):1334–59.

Franklin BA, Gordon NF. *Contemporary Diagnosis and Management in Cardiovascular Exercise.* Premiere ed. Newtown (PA): Handbooks in Health Care Co; 2005.

American College of Sports Medicine. *ACSM's Health-Related Physical Fitness Assessment Manual.* 3rd ed. Baltimore (MD): Lippincott Williams & Wilkins; 2010.

INTERNET RESOURCES

- American College of Sports Medicine (ACSM): http://www.acsm.org
- American Council on Exercise (ACE): http://www.acefitness.org
- American Heart Association (AHA): http://www.heart.org
- National Heart, Lung, Blood Institute of the National Institutes of Health (NHLBI): http://www.nhlbi.nih.gov/guidelines/cholesterol
- National Strength and Conditioning Association (NSCA): http://www.nsca-lift.org

Muscular Fitness and Assessment

Skeletal muscle has several functions, including force generation, movement stimulation, joint stabilization, and caloric expenditure. Relative and absolute muscular assessment has relevance in athletics, general fitness, and clinical settings. Strength, endurance, power generation, physical work capacity, and flexibility are measurable components of muscular health and fitness. Muscular endurance is measured both for duration of sustained (*isometric/static*) muscle contraction, as well as repetitive skeletal motion (*dynamic*), and refers to a muscle's ability to resist or delay the onset of fatigue (32). Each of these measures is both clinically and practically relevant and may be used to assess functional capacity (107,116), joint stability (83,84), and performance (78). Flexibility, or *range of motion* (ROM), is another muscular fitness parameter for both performance enhancement and rehabilitation, and is commonly evaluated and employed when prescribing an exercise regimen (40,48). This chapter reviews characteristics of strength generation, assessment techniques for muscular strength and flexibility, and practical applications of each.

PRINCIPLES OF MUSCULAR FUNCTION

MUSCLE FIBER RECRUITMENT

Enhancement of musculoskeletal function (*i.e.*, strength, endurance, and flexibility) is an important goal and

outcome of all athletic development, physical fitness, and rehabilitation programs. Musculoskeletal assessment techniques used by coaches, rehabilitation specialists, and health/fitness professionals can help one develop and modify exercise programs for athletes, patients, and clients. Several musculoskeletal parameters should be assessed. Both testing and performance enhancement programs should address the concept of specificity (8). *Specificity* refers to the type of testing and training necessary to isolate and maximize performance of a given sport or physical activity (97). Conducting an activity-specific needs assessment can help exercise professionals identify the physiological parameters in most need of testing (8,116). Musculoskeletal assessments should address biomechanical, physiological, and functional factors considered essential to the performance of specific tasks or skills (8,116). Specificity also involves identifying realistic training goals for the client as well as limitations to participation. Other factors warranting consideration include baseline health status and muscular fitness, program progression, training modalities and techniques, and joint flexibility. Knowledge of various exercise modalities is required to meet specific goals and will assist the exercise professional in developing effective conditioning programs. Although this chapter briefly reviews some of the anatomical, biomechanical, and physiological determinants of musculoskeletal performance, more detailed reviews are provided in *Chapters 1–3* of this *Resource Manual*.

KEY TERMS

Atrophy: Loss of tissue; muscle atrophy is loss of skeletal muscle mass as a result of decreased protein synthesis/increased protein degradation.

Electromyography (EMG): The measurement of motor unit activity in skeletal muscle.

Flexibility: The joint's ability to pass through a given range of motion without significant impingement or restriction.

Hyperplasia: Increased number of cells; muscle hyperplasia is an increase in the number of muscle fibers.

Hypertrophy: Increased size of cells or of an entire tissue; muscle hypertrophy is an increase in the size of muscle fibers or of an entire muscle.

One-repetition maximum (1-RM): The greatest load that can be lifted through a full range of motion one time.

Valsalva maneuver: Contraction of the muscles of exhalation without allowing air to escape; this results in increased intra-thoracic pressure and (transiently) increased blood pressure.

As an example of applying specificity, a conditioning program to enhance performance in an endurance activity, such as cross-country skiing, should focus on aerobic metabolism and recruitment of appropriate muscle fiber types. Although training will include both aerobic and anaerobic activities, the program should be designed specifically for the muscular and cardiovascular demands of cross-country skiing. In such situations, cross-training, high-repetition sets, and other endurance training techniques should be considered before high-resistance, low-repetition exercises are primarily used for power training.

Specificity of training is designed to maximize metabolic adaptations of the specific skeletal muscle fiber types and thus enhance contractile characteristics. Type I muscle fibers are primarily used during sustained endurance activities. Muscle fibers classified as type II are generally recruited for higher-intensity, power-oriented resistance exercises and shorter bouts of work. *Table 1*-8 in this *Resource Manual* details the functional characteristics of type I (slow) and type II (fast) twitch muscle fiber types, including IIa and IIx sub-types. The relative exercise intensity and duration will largely determine the predominant type(s) and recruitment of motor units (39). Muscular fitness assessments test either for endurance, power, maximal force production, or combinations thereof, and can provide insight regarding a person's ability to recruit a predominant muscle fiber type. Techniques of assessment are fitness and performance parameter specific. Many factors, including safety, should be considered before testing. For example, muscular endurance may be evaluated with less risk of injury than the measurement of muscle strength as less acute strain is placed on the musculoskeletal system because of lower resistances and loads used (50). Maximal muscle force is accurately represented by use of the one repetition maximum (1-RM) for a given exercise (8,74). In some instances, multiple repetition maximum (*e.g.*, 8-RM) protocols, which require muscular endurance as well as strength, may be safer and also represent a reasonable predictor of maximal force production (51,61,78,104,127).

MUSCULAR FORCE DEVELOPMENT

Muscular contractions are stimulated by the central nervous system in response to release of acetylcholine at the neuromuscular junction. Cellular voltage changes (action potentials) lead to release of calcium ions into the sarcoplasm. Cross-bridge formation and a power stroke between actin and myosin filaments is then powered by intracellular adenosine triphosphate (ATP), thereby shortening the sarcomere. This process is repeated within individual muscle fibers to produce tension development. Additional fiber recruitment leads to more cross-bridge formations and greater relative force production, ultimately achieving the maximum voluntary contraction (MVC). The number of fibers recruited is related to the strength and frequency of neurologic stimulus from a motor neuron (39), termed *motor unit recruitment*. Although mitochondrial activity plays a significant role in longer duration fiber recruitment, during resistance exercises energy is supplied predominantly from phosphagen pools and glycolysis within the sarcoplasm. Motor unit recruitment depends on the intensity or amount of force and/or power required for the given movement and the level of motor control. Movement requiring a considerable power output will recruit more muscle fibers simultaneously (19,116); however, fine motor control will be sacrificed, and vice versa.

MECHANICS OF FORCE DEVELOPMENT

Biomechanical factors such as joint architecture, joint angle, point of muscle attachment, muscle angle of pull, muscle architecture, muscle length, type of muscle contraction, velocity of muscle contraction, muscle cross sectional area, and body size all influence the ability of muscles to generate force; display strength, power, and muscular endurance; and to control joint movements within a specific ROM (8,46,97). Human movement is based on a system involving three classes of levers. *Figure 22-1* illustrates classifications of levers with corresponding anatomical examples. As shown, each system combines three separate components: force application (muscular insertion), fulcrum or center of rotation (joint center), and resistance application (center of gravity or point of external load), all applied along a lever arm (bone). The relative positions of the fulcrum, point of force application, and resistance application determine the class of lever and the efficiency in which forces and torques are generated (46,93). Levers associated with human joints are primarily of the third-class, which are well designed for generating speed/velocity and ROM at the expense of maximal force generation and do not allow for a significant *mechanical advantage* (MA) (8,46). In third class levers, the muscle insertion is commonly distal to the joint center and proximal to the resistance application. The perpendicular distance measured between the joint center and muscle insertion, termed the *force arm*, provides the lever with mechanical torque required for movement. The force arm changes throughout the ROM as a function of both joint angle and muscle angle of pull (46). The changing force arm and length-tension in activated muscles control and modify the amount of internal force and torque a muscle or muscles can produce at any given point and time within the ROM (46,93). The distance measured from the joint center and the point of resistance application (often identified as the center of mass for the limb and any external resistance[s]) is termed the *resistance arm* (46). *Figure 22-2* uses the elbow joint to illustrate the force arm (distance from the elbow joint to the biceps brachii insertion) and two resistance arms (distance from the elbow

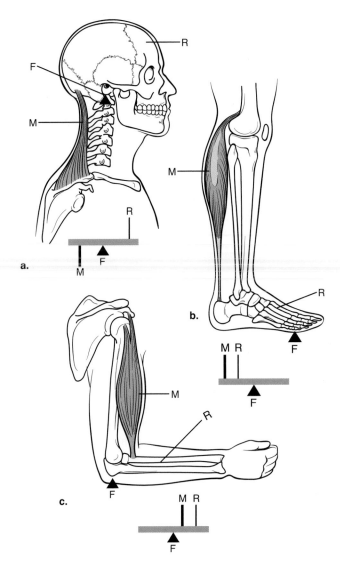

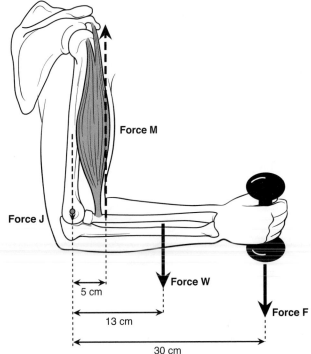

FIGURE 22-2. Mechanical representation of force and torque development in the elbow, where force *M* is muscular force generation in response to force *W* and force *F*. Distances indicated represent moments created by the bony lever of the forearm at various points relative to the joint fulcrum. Force *J* represents joint reaction force produced during muscular contraction.

FIGURE 22-1. Classes of Anatomical Levers. Class 1 **(A)**, class 2 **(B)**, and class 3 **(C)**. *F*, fulcrum (joint center); *M*, force generation (muscle); *R*, resistance (center of gravity, external load). Anatomic examples are illustrated. Recall most human examples are class 3. (Adapted with permission from Kreighbaum E, Barthals K. *Biomechanics: A Qualitative Approach for Studying Human Movement*. New York [NY]: Allyn and Bacon; 1996. 619 p.)

joint to center of mass of the forearm and the distance to the hand holding a dumbbell) in a third-class lever. Development of tension in the elbow flexors (force M) produces torque, causing movement against opposing resistance(s). Measures indicated are force and resistance movement arms; however, note that the distances in the figure will vary depending on body size and stature.

MA, maximal force, and torque generating capabilities do not occur uniformly throughout a joint's ROM. Peak force and torque generally occur at a point in the ROM where the joint's mechanical advantage (true force arm length) is greatest and where activated muscles are at an optimal length to produce high levels of tension or force (46). *Figure 2-7* of this *Resource Manual* provides a visual

representation of the changing force and torque generating capabilities (also known as strength curves) of muscles throughout the joint's ROM. The point of attachment of a tendon to bone is its *insertion*. At any given point in the joint's ROM, the tendon and bone create a constantly changing angle of insertion, or *angle of muscle pull* (the angle created at the point of insertion between the muscle's line of pull and the long axis of the bone in the proximal direction). Muscle force can be separated into two components: *turning* (rotary) and *stabilizing*. Acting concurrently, muscle tension creates both a torque (which moves the lever about the fulcrum) and a joint stabilizing effect. The changing muscle angle of pull determines which component of muscle force predominates at any given point in the joint's ROM. The turning force acts perpendicular to the lever (bone), and the stabilizing force acts parallel and toward the joint center. In *Figure 22-3*, the left panel shows the elbow extended to 135 degrees; thus, the angle of insertion for the biceps is 45 degrees. The applied muscle force is split into rotational and stabilizing components. As the joint angle decreases with flexion, muscle force becomes increasingly more rotary and the stabilizing force decreases, until the entire muscle force is rotary at a joint angle of 90 degrees (and an angle of insertion of 90 degrees), as seen in the center panel of the figure. As flexion continues and the joint angle decreases further

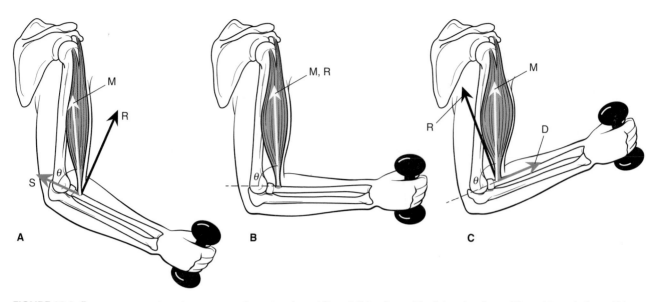

FIGURE 22-3. Force component vectors representing rotary force (*R*), stabilizing force (*S*), dislocating force (*D*), and muscle force (*M*). Note as muscle insertion angle (θ) changes from A (45 degrees) to B (90 degrees) to C (>90 degrees), force vectors shift properties from stabilizing/rotary, to purely rotary, and to dislocating/rotary, respectively.

(and the angle of insertion increases past 90 degrees), some of the muscle force is now directed outward along the axis of the insertion bone (radius), creating a dislocating force, as seen in the right panel of the figure. Maximal mechanical advantage occurs at exactly 90 degrees. Consequently, muscles display characteristics relative to their potential angles of muscle pull. Strength scores from maximal muscular strength tests performed with free weights reflect the maximal weight/load that can be moved at the weakest point in the joint ROM (50). Small angles of muscle pull contribute primarily to stabilization, and those that approach or exceed 90 degrees of pull can be considered primary movers for an ROM.

SKELETAL MUSCLE RESPONSE TO RESISTANCE EXERCISE

MUSCLE FIBER ADAPTATION

The acute and chronic responses to resistance exercise and *resistance training* (RT) have been previously reported (3,101,127). *Resistance exercise* refers to a single bout of resistance exercise, whereas RT describes a long-term program of progression and overload leading to many benefits as described in *Chapter 33* of this *Resource Manual*. A comparison with the adaptations observed following aerobic exercise training is provided in *Table 22-1*. Controversy exists about whether measurable strength gains associated with RT are the result of hyperplasia (additional fiber production) or hypertrophy (increased fiber size). Generally, strength gains after RT are attributable primarily to hypertrophy

(22,80) rather than hyperplasia. Unfortunately, cross-sections of muscle fibers large enough to analyze are difficult to obtain in human subjects for ethical and practical reasons. The relative contributions from neurological adaptations and muscular hypertrophy to strength enhancements are largely determined by age, training status, and genetic predisposition (17,19,41,68,98,111). The type of training stimuli employed will dictate the physiological responses underlying muscular improvements. Prolonged endurance training may stimulate metabolic and muscle morphology changes, including mitochondria biogenesis, type II to type I fiber-type transformation, and adjusted substrate metabolism (22,108). Likewise, heavy resistance exercise will augment contractile proteins that are responsible for hypertrophy and increased MVC (8,22). A transition in both the myosin adenosine triphosphatease and heavy chains occurs during resisitance training and leads to a transformation from IIx to IIax to IIa. Exercises that recruit type IIx muscle fibers initiate a shift toward type IIa fibers (8). Some highly advanced training techniques may lead to hyperplasia of skeletal muscle tissue (6). Hyperplasia has been reported as a result of both exercise and stretch overload of skeletal muscle using nitric acid digestion and cross-section techniques (6) (*Box 22-1*). However, it remains unclear whether this methodology and these findings, derived primarily from animal models, can be extrapolated to human physiology.

Loss of skeletal muscle (atrophy) is a natural physiological response to disuse as a result of injury, immobilization, sedentary lifestyle, and/or certain disease processes. Atrophy causes reduced muscle protein synthesis (98,116,125), usually first in type II fibers, and

TABLE 22-1. Comparison of the Effects of Aerobic and Resistance Training on Selected Physiologic Variables

Physiologic Variable	Aerobic Exercise	Resistance Exercise
Bone mineral density	↑↑	↑↑
Body composition		
% fat	↓↓	↓
Lean body mass	↔	↑↑
Muscular strength	↔	↑↑↑
Glucose metabolism		
Insulin response	↓↓	↓↓
Basal insulin levels	↓	↓
Insulin sensitivity	↑↑	↑↑
Serum lipids		
High-density lipoprotein	↑↔	↑↔
Low-density lipoprotein	↓↔	↓↔
Resting heart rate	↓↓	↔
Stroke volume, rest and maximal	↑↑	↔
Cardiovascular dynamics		
Resting systolic blood pressure	↓↔	↔
Resting diastolic blood pressure	↓↔	↓↔
Submaximal exercise RPP	↓↓↓	↓↓
Maximal oxygen uptake	↑↑↑	↑↔
Overall endurance time	↑↑↑	↑↑
Basal metabolism	↑	↑↑
Health-related quality of life	↑↔	↑↔

RPP, rate pressure product.

↑, values increase; ↓, values decrease; ↔, values remain unchanged; ↑ or ↓, small effect; ↑↑ or ↓↓, medium effect; ↑↑↑ or ↓↓↓, large effect.

Reprinted with permission from Williams M, Haskell W, Ades P, et al. Resistance exercise in individuals with and without cardiovascular disease: 2007 update: a scientific statement from the American Heart Association Council on Nutrition, Physical Activity, and Metabolism. *Circulation.* 2007;116:572–584.

BOX 22-1 Muscle Fiber Measurement Techniques

Histologic cross-sectioning methods extract muscle fiber, commonly from the belly of the muscle, and fibers are counted utilizing ATPase staining. ATPase staining allows for relatively accurate counting of total fiber number and percentage of each fiber type. Limitations to this technique make it difficult to know whether accurate counts are indeed obtained.

Nitric acid digestion is a more definitive method of isolating and counting muscle fibers accurately. Direct counts using this technique may result in an underestimation of total fiber number.

---

muscle protein degradation primarily in type I fibers. Force generation capacity diminishes as muscle atrophy occurs, contributing to generalized weakness. Atrophy occurs as a result of a change in balance between protein synthesis and degradation, during which there is a down-regulation of the former and enhancement of the latter. *Sarcopenia* is associated with "body wasting" and is common in elderly persons and patients suffering from chronic diseases or medical conditions, congestive heart failure, chronic obstructive pulmonary disease, and liver failure. It has also been considered a result of selective type IIx motor unit degradation in some elderly individuals and persons with clinical pathologies (17,31,68,85). Resistance training programs have obvious benefits for reversing atrophy, as well as sarcopenia, associated with varied clinical pathologies (4,17,68 98,116). Selective fiber-type atrophy associated with congestive heart failure, for example, has been shown to be reversible with participation in a RT program (101).

Initial strength gains when beginning an RT program may be attributable to neurological adaptations in the skeletal muscle motor units (44,111). Synchronization of motor units leading to more succinct recruitment of muscle fibers is believed to initiate considerable gains in strength and coordination, particularly early in training (19,111). Increases in microvascularization and capillary density serve to enhance oxygen delivery to skeletal muscle, thereby improving energy production and muscular endurance (80,123). Some research has demonstrated no change in capillary density per muscle fiber with high-intensity and eccentric RT (49). Others have reported little or no change or enhancements in muscle capillary density, depending on the training protocol used (80). Collectively, these data support the principle of training specificity and suggest that type I fibers demonstrate that vascular adaptations improve aerobic endurance.

Architectural changes in skeletal muscle after both concentric and eccentric RT affect torque production capabilities and fiber length and may contribute to improvements in MVC (13). Other adaptations associated with strength improvements include more actin/myosin cross-bridge formations (44,49). Microscopic increases are not only observed in actin and myosin proteins but also in connective tissue proteins like titin and nebulin, increases in the muscle cross-sectional area, and increased myofibril density. Functional adaptations to training are determined by the volume (*sets × reps × weight*), intensity, and frequency of exercise (3,22,40). It has been shown that muscle fiber number increases during fetal growth and that postnatal improvement in strength are caused by hypertrophy (81). Some evidence suggests that both hypertrophy and hyperplasia are responsible for strength gains early in life. For example, using nitric acid digestion measurement techniques (see *Box 22-1*), both exercise and stretch overload have been shown to result in significant increases in muscle fiber number, signifying hyperplasia (80).

Progressive overload is essential for promoting increases in muscular fitness (3,40,48). Plateaus often occur in novice exercisers because not enough emphasis is placed on progression early in training. Modest increments in exercise regimens will promote rapid improvements in muscular strength and endurance. Promoting adaptation without causing overuse injury is essential to successfully developing and executing training programs. Wolff's law illustrates progressive adaptation and remodeling of bony tissue to specific stresses and loading patterns, and may also be applied to connective and muscle tissue. This law also demonstrates how tissues can adapt negatively to under-utilization (atrophy) and overutilization (injury) (20). Progressive tissue adaptation is maximized within the "physiologic training zone," within which training intensity can be enhanced without causing tissue damage (*Fig. 22-4*). Periodization training programs may be used to avoid plateaus and ensure adequate progression. For example, a training program may incorporate seasonal cycles or advancing monthly intensity and modality changes throughout the year (3).

SPECIAL POPULATION AND SAFETY CONSIDERATIONS

Resistance training has been shown to elicit overall muscular strength and endurance improvements with an adequate dosage (3). Blood pressure, heart rate response, *rate pressure product* (RPP), body composition, and biochemical markers, such as lactic acid accumulation (45), nitric oxide (43), and creatine kinase (43) and ratings of perceived exertion (using the 10-Point OMNI Resistance training RPE Scale) may be monitored selectively during

RT and muscle testing (28,109,110). Ongoing research has consistently demonstrated the safety of using higher intensity RT programs in several special populations. Higher-intensity training (>80% 1-RM) regimens have been examined in healthy elderly men (44), women (121), patients with heart disease (2,11,12,81,121,127) and cancer (114,115), multiple sclerosis, and other clinical populations that may benefit from increases in muscular fitness (27,126). Collectively, these findings demonstrate cardioprotective and physical performance benefits from high-intensity resistance training in various populations. Traditionally, resistance training, specifically with higher intensities, has been contraindicated in CVD patients because of concerns regarding the potential for cardiovascular events. Extensive research has now shown RT to be safe and effective in achieving improvements in muscular strength in selected low-to-moderate risk cardiac and other chronically ill patients (100). In fact, cardiac demands during RT may be less than that of prescribed aerobic exercise training in these individuals, if it is executed following established guidelines (29,115). This area of investigation warrants future study because RT at both high and low intensities may benefit certain patient subsets (*e.g.*, stable coronary artery disease, congestive heart failure, peripheral vascular disease) (2,11,12).

Breath holding during exercise or daily lifting activities may allow for an increase in force generation; however, it is not recommended and may compromise safety (8). This technique, which is referred to as the Valsalva maneuver, may elicit a dramatic and potentially dangerous rise and subsequent fall in systolic blood pressure, resulting in dizziness, cardiac dysrhythmias, and related syncope. Cardiac and chronically debilitated patients have been cautioned against performing this maneuver and are instructed in proper lifting and breathing patterns (38). Exhalation during the concentric phase of lifting and inhalation during the eccentric phase is the recommended breathing pattern for individuals with and without heart disease (8).

MUSCULAR FITNESS ASSESSMENT

Muscular assessment is important for defining a baseline fitness level and tracking subsequent improvements. Muscular fitness testing can be conducted with persons of all ages, levels of physical conditioning, and training experience; however, protocols and techniques should be individualized to accommodate each client's levels of fitness and strength. The evaluation must consider various musculoskeletal fitness parameters and be age appropriate in order to ensure that valid and reliable measurements are obtained (9,33,34,57,58,105,106,116).

Muscular strength is defined as peak *force* (Newton) or *torque* (Newton-meters) developed during MVC under standardized or unique conditions (112). Muscular endurance is generally measured either statically (with

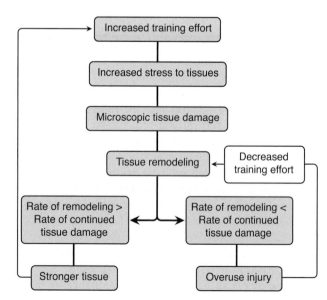

FIGURE 22-4. Tissue adaptation to training stimulus. Appropriate stress on muscle or connective tissue results in remodeling and stronger tissue. Overuse injury occurs when tissue continues to be trained and damaged without adequate remodeling time.

isometric dynamometers) or dynamically with either maximal-repetition calisthenic (body weight) tests (push-ups, sit-ups and abdominal crunches, pull-ups, chin-ups) or with tests of maximal repetitions using specific resistance exercises and with percentages of the 1-RM for that exercise (32,50,51). Strength, endurance, and power are assessed for four main purposes: to quantify fitness for athletic events and activities of daily living (57,58,94,105–107,116–118,120), to identify deficiencies in muscular function so that serial improvements might be monitored (strength diagnosis) (20,23), to evaluate the potential of individuals for particular athletic pursuits, and to assess the effects of training and rehabilitation programs (1).

Clinical exercise specialists, health fitness specialists, therapists, athletic trainers, and others each have differing interests in assessing musculoskeletal strength. Muscular strength is frequently difficult to assess because of the level of specificity and reproducibility of the parameter being measured. Crucial determinants of musculoskeletal testing include *reliability*, *reproducibility*, and *accuracy* of measurements and are enhanced by performing all testing functions consistently.

The general public may derive considerable benefits from an accurate musculoskeletal fitness assessment. Many health and fitness clubs offer initial fitness assessments to determine baseline measures and to assist in goal setting for their clients. Sessions often include both a cardiorespiratory fitness assessment and musculoskeletal strength/endurance and flexibility analysis. Two types of musculoskeletal assessments gaining popularity with the general public include trunk/spine stability tests (50,83,84) and movement screening test batteries (20,24). Allied health and medical professionals may use muscular strength, endurance, and ROM assessments before and after a course of rehabilitation to determine the effectiveness of treatments and modalities. Accuracy and standardization of measurements is crucial to deriving optimal clinical outcomes, reimbursement, and patient satisfaction. Lumbar spine instability can increase the risk of developing low back pain (50,82,83). Research indicates that muscular endurance, coordinated recruitment, and firing of trunk stabilizing muscles (multifidus, transverse abdominis, internal/external obliques, errector spinae, rectus abdominus, and quadratus lumborum) may be more protective than muscle strength for reducing the potential for low-back injuries (50,82,83). Poor trunk stability has also been considered a risk factor for lower extremity injuries (72,129). In addition, movement screens or functional movement screens are used to evaluate quality of human movements and to identify deficits in the body during dynamic tasks that potentially contribute to or cause injuries (20,24,94). McGill, Childs, and Liebenson (84) developed a 3-item isometric lumbar stabilization test requiring minimal equipment. Test procedures, scores and normative data are provided in other resources (50,82–84,103). Clark and Lucett (19)

and Cook (24) developed movement screening assessments that utilize overhead squat exercises as a primary test of musculoskeletal integrity.

Controversy exists however over the ability of trunk stability and movement screening measurements to predict (82) or fail to predict (94) successful athletic performance.

TECHNIQUES AND LIMITATIONS

Maximal *dynamic* strength has been reported in the scientific literature and may be assessed by various protocols and techniques; however, the 1-RM test remains the gold standard when evaluating MVC (36). The term "isotonic" contraction suggests that a constant resistance is applied throughout a given ROM, which, in the human body, does not occur. As previously discussed, joint and muscle insertion angles change the moment of inertia of the load being lifted and determine whether a muscle's role is primarily as a stabilizer or agonist. The angle of insertion and the mechanical advantage change throughout a joint's ROM, thereby altering the rotary force potential. A muscle's maximal force generating capacity occurs when muscle contractile protein filaments are optimally aligned. This generally occurs when the muscle is at its resting length (46). Muscle tension or contractile strength potential decreases as each muscle either shortens or lengthens beyond this position (46).

The 1-RM is defined as the highest load that can be lifted through full ROM one time (36). Reproducibility of the test may vary slightly depending on the technician and the equipment employed, and should be standardized for retesting. Commonly, the 1-RM is accepted as a muscle-group–specific measure of strength and is often expressed relatively to subject's body weight or mass. This enables strength comparisons between subjects of different body weights (8,36,42). For example, *Tables 4-10* and *4-11* in *GETP9* show normative data of 1-RM for the bench press and leg press, respectively. Heyward developed normative strength-to-body weight tables in college-aged men and women for six resistance exercises: the bench press, leg press, latissimus pulldown, leg extension, leg curl, and arm curl (50).

The measurement of 1-RM has been used safely to assess strength in many populations, including healthy adults (95), athletes (25), elderly persons (74,99), and those with chronic disease (2,11,43,45,81,121). Orthopedic limitations should always be considered and testing should be avoided or terminated if the loaded movement causes pain or exacerbates an existing medical condition. Accordingly, 1-RM evaluation may be contraindicated for persons with acute musculoskeletal injuries or symptoms. A 1-RM testing can be performed for muscle isolation exercises (*e.g.*, leg extension for quadriceps strength) or for multi-jointed and complex exercises (*e.g.*, bench press for pectorals, triceps brachii, and anterior deltoids). More dynamic movements, such as standing squats, may also be tested for strength (8,51); however, higher-repetition tests are recommended to lower the risk of injury because of excessive joint and connective tissue loading. *Box 21-14* describes the 1-RM protocol for bench press testing, which can be applied to other lifts as well. A similar process is used if testing a specific RM at a higher number of repetitions, such as the 5-RM. In such a case, after the initial warm-up, a conservative estimate of the 5-RM load would be made and the subject would attempt to complete 5 repetitions. If successful, the subject would rest 3–5 min and attempt 5 repetitions with a higher weight, and repeat the process until the subject fails to perform 5 repetitions with the selected weight, the 5-RM being the greatest weight for which 5 repetitions were properly completed.

The 1-RM can be estimated using repetitions to failure (RTF) performed with a submaximal load (16,30,61,78,79,104). Typically, the subject performs a warm-up set with a light weight, then a weight is chosen that is expected to be close to the 10-RM, and the subject performs as many repetitions as possible. As more repetitions are incorporated into the assessment (using a lighter load), the activated muscles will become increasingly reliant on muscular endurance and less on strength (3,50,51). If the RTF is more than 20, the test is repeated after a 5-min rest period with a higher weight. Generally, tests in which RTF is 10 or fewer repetitions provide an accurate estimation of 1-RM (16,30,78,79). Some of the available equations are linear and others non-linear (16,30,78,79). A recent study found that 1-RM bench press was accurately estimated in a variety of male athletes using the equation 1-RM = (weight lifted)/(1 − 0.02 × RTF) (30). The most accurate equation may vary with sex, training status and, especially, the muscle group and lift being tested.

Selecting ergonomically appropriate equipment will minimize extraneous muscle fatigue and difficulty in maintaining proper posture and body mechanics during 1-RM strength testing (102). For example, using thicker bars (Olympic vs. 2-in vs. 3-in bar) during the 1-RM bench press, bent-over-row, and deadlift tests can significantly reduce measured strength values in resistance-trained individuals (102). Calisthenic-type (body weight) tests provide a crude index of strength and endurance when other equipment is not available (50). The Maximum number of push-ups performed by males and females and pull-ups performed by males and maximum flexed-arm hang time performed by females are assessed in athletic populations, the military, and certain professions requiring high levels of upper body muscular strength and endurance (50,51,56,70,124,128). The pull-ups and flexed arm hang tests are often considered assessments of muscular strength as opposed to muscular endurance. LaChance and Hortobagyi published two equations to calculate average concentric work performed and power output produced during performance of a maximal set of

pull-ups and push-ups (70). Descriptions of these tests and proper exercise technique are provided elsewhere (32,51,56,70).

Dynamometry is a testing modality currently used to assess force-generation capability and performance associated with activities during which either the load or movement velocity remains constant. Various forms of dynamometry are useful for evaluating muscle strength, endurance, and power during dynamic (constant external load) and isokinetic (constant velocity) exercise, and for evaluating strength and endurance during static (isometric) exercise (50).

Power is defined as the rate at which mechanical work is performed under a defined set of conditions (3,8,40). This parameter is of particular interest to many athletes, professional trainers, health/fitness and rehabilitation professionals, and should be evaluated within the context of a given event (1). Although strength and power are closely related and are often considered in tandem, for optimal measures they should be evaluated independently. Dynamometric evaluation of strength and power is possible, although methodologically challenging. Athletic skills and activities of daily living often involve considerable variability, making the biomechanics difficult to isolate and evaluate independently and in real time. Signorile recently developed tests to measure power output during the performance of tasks simulating activities of daily living (116–118,120). Technology, such as digital movement analysis, has advanced dramatically and has allowed for these data to be routinely applied to training programs. Identifying the load for peak power output is often the variable to be quantified. However, assessment of maximal or near maximal power output is possible through incremental loading of working muscle (47). This recent finding diminishes the importance of identifying one load for maximal power output in athletes.

Isometric dynamometry measures MVC achieved at specific joint angles against a fixed object. Muscle tension is quantified by a device connected to a strain gauge, cable tensiometer, force platform, or force transducer. Static strength can be measured in 38 muscle groups using cable tensiometers (50). This information is subsequently conveyed to the client or trainer and provides a useful index of strength at a given joint angle (130). Isometric MVC varies as both joint angles and muscle angles of pull change; therefore, one must conduct serial muscle strength assessments at exactly the same joint angles. Test–retest reliability of isometric dynamometry depends on the consistency of the joint angle, among other parameters (59) (*Box 22-2*). During isometric training, muscular strength benefits may be realized at the joint angle maintained during contraction, with a potential carryover effect extending to ± 15 degrees from the training position. Isometric exercises may also be effective when training individuals for whom movement

BOX 22-2 Considerations for Test–Retest Reliability and Consistency (20)

SUBJECT-RELATED FACTORS

- Age
- Sex
- Weight
- Athletic conditioning
- Orthopedic disability
- Side dominance

TESTING-RELATED FACTORS

- Warm-up procedures
- Starting position and posture
- Joint stabilization
- Alignment of anatomic and dynamometer axis of rotation

- Lever arm length and position
- Muscle preloading and/or stretch reflex

DURING MOVEMENT

- Velocity of contraction
- Rest intervals
- Patient feedback
- Joint angle and ROM tested
- Mode of contraction (isometric, isokinetic, isodynamic)

POSTTESTING

- Type of data analyzed
- Data analysis

---

elicits pain, such as those with rheumatoid arthritis or orthopedic injuries. Initiating muscle contraction at a fixed angle may not provoke the magnitude of pain that occurs with dynamic exercise.

The *rate of force development* (RFD) is often used to assess athletic power; it represents how rapidly muscular force is generated immediately on the initiation of a contraction and is commonly measured using isometric dynamometry. Despite the lack of dynamic measures involved with this assessment, RFD has reliably predicted athletic performance requiring sudden bursts of muscular strength (55,86). A high jumper, for example, requires a sudden burst of strength from leg extensor muscles to clear the height of the bar. Immediate force development is crucial to overcome gravitational forces adequately to complete the jump successfully. Although the propelling movements may be difficult to assess, RFD provides a useful measure when evaluating a high jumper's potential performance.

When assessing the use of performing isometric dynamometry, consider the subject's posture, body mechanics, and how difficult the position might be to reproduce. Careful attention must be paid to such details to extrapolate these data to potential performance indicators. Isometric tests should mimic specific tasks as closely as possible. Accordingly, testing angles should approximate those at which peak force generation is required for a given movement or activity. Some authorities suggest testing should be done only at the angle of insertion capable of greatest force generation (for example, 90 degrees for the biceps brachii in elbow flexion), which would improve retest reliability (1).

Isoinertial dynamometry refers to continuous resistance to movement and accurately describes external loading through a ROM as in weight lifting or training. Although resistance training is often mischaracterized as isotonic, isoinertial reflects the change in load as joint angle varies, thereby increasing or decreasing the mechanical leverage of the joint. The 1-RM is a measure of maximum isoinertial force and represents the maximal weight that can be moved at the weakest point or point of least mechanical advantage within the ROM (50). Because of its dynamic nature, the 1-RM provides greater utility and practical application than isometric measure (51). Measurements of isoinertial force capability are performed using weighted systems (*e.g.*, weighted squat jump), machines with loading throughout the ROM, or hydraulic loading devices. The 1-RM testing offers excellent test–retest reliability for field studies and can be employed to assess maximal isoinertial force. However, regression equations that have been developed to predict 1-RM may often overestimate actual measured value (51). Overestimation of a person's strength may be potentially hazardous at high loads as orthopedic injuries and cardiovascular events are more likely to occur. Kim and Mayhew developed a prediction equation for 1-RM strength with the YMCA submaximal bench press test that has demonstrated high validity and reliability in novices (61). A description of the YMCA submaximal bench press test is provided in *Table 21.15* of this *Resource Manual* as well as in *GETP9*. Trainer intuition and progressive overloading should be employed when evaluating strength during each exercise, thereby reducing the potential for musculoskeletal injury and related complications.

Isokinetic dynamometry measures torque and power through the ROM when the joint angular velocity remains constant. Analysis of agonist/antagonist torque, power-velocity and torque-velocity curves, and comparisons between limbs are representative applications of such devices. Researchers commonly use isokinetic dynamometry because it has excellent reliability and consistency, while minimizing the effects of numerous extraneous variables. It might be difficult to extrapolate measurements into practical applications because isolation of individual movements is rarely seen in sports or activities of daily living. Isokinetic evaluations have been used extensively in endurance studies, physical rehabilitation, and biomechanical analysis, and to further clarify the intricacies of movement with good *internal validity*. Recommended muscle strength balance ratios for agonist and antagonist muscle groups have been established from isokinetic testing at low velocities of between 30 and 60 degrees per s and are available in a resource produced by Heyward (50). Generally, strength differences between contralateral (right vs. left sides) muscle groups should not exceed 10%–15% in healthy, uninjured persons (50). In addition to dynamometry, tensiometers are instruments commonly used for measuring isometric strength. Tensiometers include a steel cable, a testing table, wall hooks, and a goniometer. A strap is attached to the moving limb while the cable is fixed to an immovable object, placing the joint at the desired angle for measurement based on the goniometer reading (see flexibility assessment section for discussion of goniometers). The client is asked to exert as much force as possible against the strap (maximal contraction) and hold for a minimum of 5 s. The tensiometer can measure the maximum force exerted. Muscular strength at several joint angles can be measured during a testing session. Three trials should be completed, with the highest measure recorded as strength at a given joint angle. Normative strength scores for several muscle groups and tasks are provided elsewhere (50).

TESTING SAFETY AND EQUIPMENT CONSIDERATIONS

A gradual and progressive, pretest warm-up is recommended prior to resistance training and testing. The warm-up serves to increase blood flow to primary muscles and connective tissues and may reduce the risk of injury during testing (26,131,132). During the maximal lift, proper posture and mechanics must be maintained to maximize contractile force capabilities of agonist muscle(s). It is recommended that the eccentric phase of a lift be completed with half the velocity of the concentric phase. *Concentric* lifting time of 3–5 s is appropriate to achieve MVC for the lift and ensures volitional fatigue in muscle fibers; however, exercise intensity and overload is greater during the *eccentric* phase of movement. Initial weight can be accurately estimated based on previous training loads, self-reported lifting capability, or a practice set performed before the testing (37). Rest between successive attempts should be no less than 3 min to ensure full recovery of muscle fibers.

In addition to muscular strength assessment, 1-RM may also be used to estimate training levels for a given exercise. Once 1-RM is determined, considerable information can be extracted. As previously discussed, to stimulate appropriate muscle protein synthesis for hypertrophy, higher weights (60%–80% 1-RM) may be used during a particular exercise (3,22,40,127). For endurance improvements, a lighter load (up to 50% of 1-RM) is used for the same exercise, using more repetitions (3,22,40,127). These 1-RM percentages will vary with age, health status and muscle group. Knowledge of a person's 1-RM is crucial when attempting to maximize eccentric contraction using muscular overload during a particular exercise. Accordingly, loading with 110%–130% of 1-RM, eccentric contractions are maximized until muscle fiber failure occurs. Heavy eccentric training, however, should only be done with appropriate supervision (3).

Retesting provides measurable outcomes of the training program and should be done with consistency. To ensure the retest is valid, careful consideration to reproducing the baseline methodology should be used. If testing was initially done on resistance training equipment, the same equipment should be used for retesting (97). More complex movements, however, may be more difficult to recreate. For example, the environment during a vertical jump test should be carefully recorded initially and reconstructed using the same equipment, flooring, and footwear. Measured strength gains after a given training program provide useful feedback and motivation to the client and are valid if testing was done appropriately before, at given intervals, and after the physical conditioning regimen. Although regression equations may be used to predict 1-RM, some professionals have used isometric grip strength to predict overall muscle strength; however, this methodology has limitations for predicting 1-RM (112,113).

Although 1-RM is an excellent measure of force generation capabilities, functional performance is often of greater interest in athletics (24) and during activities of daily living. Strength is often a poor predictor of skill and performance during a given task (78). There appears to be no relationship between the relative improvement in 1-RM and functional performance in skilled athletes (91). Optimal performance in dynamic skills requires unique physical attributes; moreover, improvements in performance are not always paralleled by increases in muscular strength (91).

Although many athletic resistance training regimens emphasize strength and power improvements, training effectiveness should be evaluated beyond the MVC or 1-RM and include functional performance tests, such as the athlete's vertical jump or sprint times (90). Testing protocols specifically designed for a given sport or event are more accurate for evaluating performance of the skills involved, rather than for making predictions based on other parameters. For example, standard anthropometric, strength, and power assessments were shown to be inadequate predictors of sprint performance (69). Similarly, isometric testing of muscle activation and force development at various joint angles proved to be a poor predictor of dynamic performance (89,94), further demonstrating the need to measure performance variables beyond the MVC.

RELIABILITY OF ASSESSMENT

The test–retest reliability of isokinetic, isometric, and isoinertial dynamometry is normally high; however, one should consider all variables before reporting and applying data from any assessment. Factors influencing reliability during testing include the individual's athletic ability, instructions provided, recent bouts of exertion and fatigue, selected testing angles, postures, and, most importantly, a standardized testing environment. Although many of these variables are often controlled and/or explained with ease, one must consider them before investing time and effort in testing procedures. Consistency in performing assessment and reassessments is paramount to translating results into practice (59). Potentially confounding variables during comparisons include athletic history, subject age and anthropometrics, rest between tests, points of resistance application, joint axis alignment, specific equipment used during assessment, adherence to specific test protocols and standards, and whether positive/negative feedback was given to participants. Biomechanical torque production will vary based on joint angle measurements and the position in which neutral or zero angles are determined. For example, lack of consistency in strength and torque generation and measurement techniques during leg (knee) extension exist in the literature (46,59). Consistency in the velocity of muscular contraction within a given ROM is also necessary during retesting, as the force-velocity curve demonstrates (see the discussion of *Fig. 2-6* in this *Resource Manual*). Such an oversight can contribute to inconclusive data. *Box 22-2* summarizes some considerations during testing and retesting of muscular strength and performance.

Strength is often assessed by a physical therapist or athletic trainer using *manual muscle testing*. Relative unilateral strength is commonly used to establish a baseline or monitor progress during rehabilitation. The patient is asked to move through either a full ROM or to the pain threshold. At the end of the ROM, the therapist or trainer provides stationary resistance to the movement and requests an isometric contraction from the patient. Force production is interpreted and scored numerically by the therapist on a subjective scale ranging from 0 to 5. Zero represents no perceivable contraction, whereas 5 demonstrates complete ROM without difficulty resisting. Recently, several handheld dynamometers have been evaluated and determined to be reliable tools to manually test muscle strength (14,66,77). Their usefulness might be limited when applied to lower extremity testing in young, healthy adults (21,60,88). A subjective assessment such as this, although common, may be confounded by the examiner's ability to produce more force than the test subject through a given ROM (88). If, for

example, more torque force is produced by the patient than the therapist, weakness becomes difficult or impossible to detect. This scenario may be significantly limiting with a lower-extremity test (*e.g.*, knee extension) and an examiner with insufficient leverage, either from lower relative muscular strength or ineffective mechanical positioning (14,60,88). Although the reliability of manual muscle testing may be low, this methodology has proven to be useful for subjective assessment and field testing of varied movements and muscle groups and for reevaluations of strength (7,14,66,77).

As is the case with most objective measures, such as muscular strength and flexibility, assessments must be both *valid* and *reliable*. A reliable test will essentially replicate the same results under the same conditions, whereas a valid test will measure what it is intended to measure. Careful attention to ensuring testing validity can enhance the accuracy of reported responses. Conversely, an invalid test might still be repeatable, and therefore will still be reliable.

CLINICAL RELEVANCE AND APPLICATION

Strength and movement efficacy are measured using dynamometry and other methods that may be useful when attempting to predict a person's health and/or performance of activities of daily living or athletic skills. Testing should address specificity of each movement or physical challenge (*e.g.*, athletics, rehabilitation); however, the prognostic value of performance testing decreases with more complex sports or activities. For example, power generated during a vertical jump does not necessarily translate to speed during a 100-m sprint (89). Testing should be as performance and sports specific as possible in order to reliably predict athletic performance in a competitive environment.

Isokinetic and isometric test results are generally considered poor predictors of training-induced performance improvements because they lack specificity (87,89,130). Trainers should perform an activity needs assessment and closely match testing protocols with desired performance outcomes whenever possible (8).

As is the case with many testing protocols and procedures, normative or average data are desired for comparison of results and for measuring improvements in strength, function, and performance. Reliable data are often unavailable for accurate comparisons because of significant variability in testing procedures, equipment used, and individual parameters that are inadequately controlled for across study groups (*e.g.*, prior training, medical history, orthopedic limitations). There are, however, normative values for widely used and reproducible movements, such as the vertical jump, grip strength, curl-ups, and leg power production (watts), that can be used for comparison with other individuals of similar age and body weight (8,50,51,56,96).

Analysis or results from such testing can enhance goal setting, training program design, and individual motivation for initiating or modifying a training program. When adequate normative values for muscle strength are not available, relative comparisons may become necessary (70). Comparative pretraining and posttraining assessments are common among teams and small groups for movements or skills that do not have normative data available. Although not advised for widespread recommendation, such techniques may be used for motivation or to evaluate a given group of athletes or individuals. For example, bench press data may not be specific to football offensive linemen; however, upper-body strength has been identified as a measurement of interest by this cohort and the bench press is a good surrogate measure of upper body strength.

BODY STATURE AND TESTING

Strength measures are commonly normalized to body mass in order to make comparisons between individuals of different sizes. When considering individuals who are geometrically similar but different in size (*i.e.*, larger vs. smaller individuals whose body proportions are similar), larger individuals have greater mass and muscle mass. The larger muscles have greater cross-sectional area, which provides greater force generation capability (46,54). Larger individuals would also have longer limbs, which might be considered capable of greater velocity; however, in geometrically similar limbs both the force arm and resistance arm will be longer (see *Fig. 22-2*), with no difference in the ratio and, thus, no difference in torque producing potential based on length alone. It is the greater mass and cross-sectional area of the muscles that provide greater force production. Although it is common to normalize strength measures to body mass, the cross-sectional area of muscles scales with linear dimensions squared, while the volume (and thus mass) of the muscles (and entire body) scales with linear dimensions cubed. For this reason, some experts recommend normalizing strength to body mass raised to the 2/3 power, that is, dividing strength measures by this factor to compare individuals of different size (18,54).

As training programs progress from beginner to advanced levels, the sophistication of testing will necessarily advance. Exercise professionals must use assessment techniques and develop corresponding training and conditioning programs that address the specific physiologic needs, goals, current physical capabilities, and safety of their clients/athletes.

TECHNOLOGIC INSTRUMENTATION

Development of computerized equipment and instruments has increased dramatically over the past two decades. From video imaging to digital re-creation of the most complex athletic skills and movements, technology provides opportunity for creative exercise design, including training specificity. Dynamic force output is commonly measured using computer-aided isokinetic dynamometers. Through the application of force transducers, resistance is instantaneously modulated throughout each repetition to match the constantly changing internal force generated by the muscle and torque output, respectively.

Electromyography (EMG) is the measurement of motor unit activity in skeletal muscle. During movement, the EMG graphically records electrical activity stimulated by individual motor units. Isolating individual muscles involved in a given movement is achieved by proper placement of electrodes. From complex athletic movements to pathologic muscular conditions, EMG testing can provide valuable adjunctive analyses to a testing laboratory. A thorough and working knowledge of neuromuscular anatomy is critical for effective EMG testing. Development of treatment strategies and training programs can be greatly enhanced using EMG equipment, when available (67,73,83).

Computer-generated animations allow therapists and trainers to design physical conditioning programs specifically for complex, dynamic, and high-velocity movements. Segmentation of movements (*e.g.*, pitcher's arm during throwing motion) now permits a complete and thorough analysis, potentially identifying areas for performance improvement or potential injury. Digital analysis of the sport's movement patterns may provide this opportunity for sport-specific training.

Beyond movement analysis, technology is providing opportunities to study effects of training interventions on biological and physiologic markers. Skeletal muscle proteins, tissue adaptations, and early-response genes are being isolated and studied, which may lead to innovative training techniques and new concepts for musculoskeletal fitness (22). Knowledge of mechanisms and exercise-induced adaptation pathways in skeletal muscle is important for the understanding of disease processes, attenuation of the aging process, and peak performance in athletics (17,19,22,35,41,68,98).

As noted earlier, specificity of training remains an important factor in assessment techniques. Technologic advances may be paralleled by higher levels of performance. Training regimens and exercise program design must be modified according to new information and advancing technology to meet this objective. Similarly, in clinical settings, patients may be provided with enhanced specificity in their rehabilitation and regimens that potentially offer accelerated recoveries.

OLDER ADULTS

Helping to delay physical frailty and improve functional mobility are two important goals for fitness professionals who work with older adults (>60 yr of age) (57). *Table 8.4* in *GETP9* describes three common senior fitness testing batteries. Rikli and Jones (57,105–107) developed and validated the 7-item "Senior Fitness Test" (SFT) battery from a population of more than 7,000 older adults between the ages of 60 and 94 yr. The SFT measures muscular strength and endurance, cardiorespiratory endurance, flexibility, motor ability (power, speed, agility, and balance), body composition, and physical impairment(s) by using functional movement tasks, such as standing, bending, lifting, reaching, and walking (57). The 30-s chair stand and the arm curl tests assess muscular strength and endurance, while the back scratch and chair sit-and-reach tests assess upper and lower extremity and trunk flexibility, respectively (57,107). Specific descriptions, scoring directions and normative tables are available from the "Senior Fitness Test Manual" (57,107). In addition, Smith (120) developed an equation to predict lower body power during the 30-s chair rise test. Signorile and Sandler developed the ramp power test and the gallon jug shelf transfer test to assess power and evaluate deteriorating function in older adults, respectively. Full descriptions of testing and scoring are available (116–118).

FLEXIBILITY AND RANGE OF MOTION

ASSESSMENT

Every joint in the body has an acceptable ROM, which is dependent on various factors, including genetics, orthopedic health, surgeries of the articulating bones or joints, muscular tension, and strength. The joint's ability to pass through a given ROM without significant impingement or restriction is its *flexibility*. Measurement and assessment of flexibility and ROM is particularly useful in athletic training, rehabilitation, and conditioning settings; however, the measurements can be misleading if performed without standard procedures, calibration, and instruments. *Table 4.15* in *GETP9* provides normal ROM for most joints. Various measuring procedures exists that may contribute to modest variability of measurements.

The most common instrument used for measuring joint ROM is the two-arm *goniometer* (*Fig. 22-5*). This device is portable, relatively easy to use, and inexpensive; moreover, the measurements obtained are highly reproducible. The transparent plastic device includes two arms with a protractor for measuring degrees of joint displacement. One arm remains fixed to the proximal articulating segment (*e.g.*, upper arm), and the other adjusts through the ROM with the distal segment (*e.g.*, forearm), measuring the resulting degree of movement. The center of the protractor remains fixed at the joint's axis of rotation. Limitations of the conventional goniometer include difficulty stabilizing

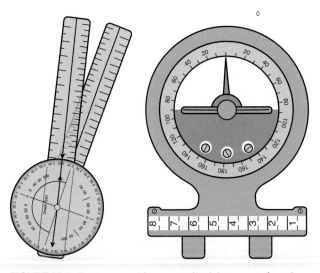

FIGURE 22-5. Devices used for measuring joint range of motion. *Left:* standard goniometer. *Right:* mechanical inclinometer.

moving segments and visually determining a vertical axis; however, higher validity and reliability are demonstrated when proper procedures are followed (71). Goniometers of various sizes and shapes have been developed to minimize limitations of the traditional design and allow for accurate measurement with small and larger joints (71).

Spinal and other complex movements, including supination, pronation, ankle inversion, and eversion, are difficult if not impossible to assess with a traditional goniometer. Such data are more accurately measured using an *inclinometer* (see *Fig. 22-5*). Inclinometers use a universal center of gravity to establish a starting point that remains constant from test to test. The pendulum-weighted inclinometer indicates degrees of motion using a weighted needle and protractor. Difficulties positioning and securing the device have led to its modification and alteration. This makes both electronic and mechanical inclinometers adaptable and reliable in various situations and environments (71).

The American Medical Association (5) suggests that ROM should be measured using three consecutive trials and averaged as the true value. ROM of the spine and other joints can be accurately evaluated using video motion analysis. Originally used in gait analysis by kinesiology laboratories, the technology has been adapted for measurement of ROM in given joints. Both postural angles and dynamic movement capabilities may be measured using these techniques. Dynamic rather than static studies more accurately measure naturally occurring movements. *Digitation* uses reflective markers placed on the skin as reference points. ROM is measured based on angular changes during movement. Validity and reliability of testing and retesting measurements can vary with reference reflector placement (71).

FACTORS INFLUENCING RELIABILITY AND VALIDITY

As with strength testing, consistency and accuracy during flexibility assessment are critical. Several factors that may compromise accuracy include anatomic landmark identification, positioning and stabilization of the body, application and stabilization of the measurement device, consistency in technique and protocol, appropriate recording of measures, and recognition of limiting factors or situations during recording. In order for a specific joint ROM to be compared with available norms, standardized landmarks for each measurement should be identified and used whenever possible. Several commonly measured joints have standard landmarks identified and should be used consistently when measuring ROM, including the knee, elbow, hip, and ankle. Inaccurate identification of bony or surface landmarks is a common source of error during assessment; therefore, knowledge of surface anatomy is required before accurate measurements can be recorded. Several authors have reported ROM measures and techniques that vary considerably from those of the American Medical Association (5) standards discussed in this chapter (5,15,50,51,71,93).

When using a goniometer, the proximal segment of the joint should be stabilized, and the distal segment remains freely moveable. Body position should be conducive to the movement being measured and comfortable for the subject. Joints can be measured in varied positions; however, reliability depends on reproducibility of the position. The client should be able to maintain the reference position without performing extraneous movement during the measurement. Careful consideration of the movement requirements and complexity should be made before selecting the appropriate assessment tool.

In addition to stabilizing body segments, the measurement device must also be properly positioned to ensure data accuracy. The technician should be familiar with the device being used, as well as the methodology and biomechanics. Inappropriate placement and use of the device represents a major source of error in many studies examining ROM (71). On the other hand, limitations based on equipment design are inevitable. Because of its size and shape, for example, the inclinometer is often more difficult to stabilize than a traditional goniometer, causing it to move or wobble during measurements. Mounting devices for inclinometers have been developed that may reduce the associated measurement error. In addition to device size and shape, stabilizing tools against limbs and joints with pathology and pain (such as in rheumatoid arthritis or scleroderma) may pose a challenge for assessors. Repeated adjustment of device position may be required in such cases (50,51).

ROM measurements are most accurately made using a universal starting point with the body in the *anatomical position*. Anatomical position is defined by a person standing upright, toes pointing forward, arms resting at their sides with palms facing forward (anterior) (15,50,51,71). Basic understanding of anatomy and the movement being measured is helpful during testing. The ROM being tested often involves complex movements or postures, and reproduction through several trials may be required for accurate measurement. Therefore, adequate instruction and practice by the client may be warranted. This will not only increase the reproducibility and reliability of the measurements but will also provide a warm-up for the joint(s) being measured. Some questions remain regarding the optimal number of repetitions required for accurate measurement; however, most authorities favor multiple repetitions and either a "best number" or average value recorded as the ROM (71,96). Using different devices for retesting is not advised because reliability is compromised. Likewise, measurements such as ROM and flexibility should be reevaluated by the same technician whenever possible. Moreover, accuracy of retesting is improved if initial procedures are well documented and the methodology and equipment are replicated in several studies.

SIT-AND-REACH EVALUATION

Hamstring and lower back flexibility are often measured using a *sit-and-reach test*. Done either with a sit-and-reach box, a properly placed tape measure or in a modified manner in a chair, this test is valid and reliable for evaluating flexibility. Detailed test instructions appear in *Box 4.9* of *GETP9*, and scoring results in *Tables 4.16* and *4.17* of *GETP9*.

STRETCHING

Along with resistance training and cardiovascular exercise, flexibility training is an important aspect of fitness development. Athletes, healthy and aging adults, and those with chronic disease affecting muscular performance may benefit from participation in a flexibility program (4,63–65,116). The primary goal of stretching is to alter tendon inflexibility and muscular resistance, which contributes to a reduced joint ROM; specifically, elasticity is improved acutely and chronically through stretching. This results in both a transient increase in musculotendon unit length resulting from actin-myosin complex relaxation (119) and chronic alteration of the extracellular matrix (122). Stretching should be incorporated into warm-up and cooldown phases of exercise (4,116).

Stretching programs will vary depending on specific goals: whether for improved athletic performance, injury rehabilitation, or general fitness. The volume of stretching required for a positive effect may vary. Three primary forms of stretching are presented: static, *proprioceptive neuromuscular facilitation* (PNF), and dynamic stretching. *Static*, as the term implies, is done with no movement either passively or actively. The muscle is first moved into position and then held for 10–30 s at the point of tightness is recommended (4,40). The stretch may be repeated for a total of 2–4 repetitions; however, research has not shown greater benefit with repeating beyond four cycles (122). PNF, also termed contract/relax or hold/relax, combines isometric and (in some cases) concentric contractions with passive, static stretching in series for a specific muscle. Isometric contraction for 6–10 s is followed with 10–30 s of passive stretching and repeated (116). *Dynamic* stretching involves movement of the targeted joint (132). Different from *ballistic*, dynamic stretching incorporates muscle tension development and is performed actively. This technique has been described as a sport- or function-specific warm-up (52). Ballistic stretching involves bouncing, or rapid movements, in an attempt to hold the motion at peak tension. For example, for the sit-and-reach test, correct form is a slow reach to maximal tension, a brief hold of the position, and a return to resting. This would be a static, active stretch. Trying to maximize the test by bouncing forward and pushing the limit would be considered ballistic.

Muscle groups isolated during exercise and/or muscles crossing major moving joints should be stretched two to three times each week or more (40). Although stretching may be done any time of the day for beneficial results, a warm-up or exercise stimulus should precede it (131). It had been thought that stretching before an athletic event would help with force production (131), performance, and reduced soreness associated with training. However, recent research suggests that acute bouts of stretching might have detrimental effects on performance parameters (26), such as sprinting (62), jumping ability (10,53), balance (67), reaction time, power (76,132), and torque-generation capabilities (40,48,75,92,116,131). Although stretching prior to engaging in an athletic event may be counterproductive, regular performance of stretching (either post-exercise or on its own) is an important component of exercise and should be incorporated into musculoskeletal analysis, fitness, and training.

SUMMARY

Proper assessment of musculoskeletal function is the key to any program designed to increase muscular strength, endurance and flexibility. Programs designed by qualified professionals must be specific to address the essential components of the performance, and additionally be safe and realistic for the client to achieve. Muscular fitness testing can be conducted with persons of all ages, levels of physical conditioning and training experience; however, protocols and techniques should be individualized to accommodate each client's level of fitness and strength. The evaluation must consider various musculoskeletal fitness parameters and be age appropriate in order to ensure that valid and reliable measurements are

obtained. Measurement and assessment of flexibility and ROM is particularly useful in athletic training, rehabilitation and conditioning settings. From these assessments, programs to improve flexibility can be developed for a variety of populations including athletes, healthy and aging adults, and those with chronic disease for whom muscular performance is affected.

REFERENCES

1. Abernethy P, Wilson G, Logan P. Strength and power assessment. Issues, controversies and challenges. *Sports Med.* 1995;19(6):401–17.
2. Adams KJ, Barnard KL, Swank AM, Mann E, Kushnick MR, Denny DM. Combined high-intensity strength and aerobic training in diverse phase II cardiac rehabilitation patients. *J Cardiopulm Rehabil.* 1999;19(4):209–15.
3. American College of Sports Medicine. American College of Sports Medicine position stand. Progression models in resistance training for healthy adults. *Med Sci Sports Exerc.* 2009;41(3):687–708.
4. American College of Sports Medicine Position Stand. The recommended quantity and quality of exercise for developing and maintaining cardiorespiratory and muscular fitness, and flexibility in healthy adults. *Med Sci Sports Exerc.* 1998;30(6):975–91.
5. American Medical Association. *Guides to the Evaluation of Permanent Impairment.* 4th ed. Chicago (IL): American Medical Association; 1993. 339 p.
6. Antonio J, Gonyea WJ. Skeletal muscle fiber hyperplasia. *Med Sci Sports Exerc.* 1993;25(12):1333–45.
7. Arnold CM, Warkentin KD, Chilibeck PD, Magnus CR. The reliability and validity of handheld dynamometry for the measurement of lower-extremity muscle strength in older adults. *J Strength Cond Res.* 2010;24(3):815–24.
8. Baechle TR, Earle RW, National Strength & Conditioning Association. *Essentials of Strength Training and Conditioning.* 3rd ed. Champaign (IL): Human Kinetics; 2008. 641 p.
9. Behm DG, Faigenbaum AD, Falk B, Klentrou P. Canadian Society for Exercise Physiology position paper: resistance training in children and adolescents. *Appl Physiol Nutr Metab.* 2008;33(3):547–61.
10. Behm DG, Kibele A. Effects of differing intensities of static stretching on jump performance. *Eur J Appl Physiol.* 2007;101(5):587–94.
11. Beniamini Y, Rubenstein JJ, Faigenbaum AD, Lichtenstein AH, Crim MC. High-intensity strength training of patients enrolled in an outpatient cardiac rehabilitation program. *J Cardiopulm Rehabil.* 1999;19(1):8–17.
12. Beniamini Y, Rubenstein JJ, Zaichkowsky LD, Crim MC. Effects of high-intensity strength training on quality-of-life parameters in cardiac rehabilitation patients. *Am J Cardiol.* 1997;80(7):841–6.
13. Blazevich AJ, Cannavan D, Coleman DR, Horne S. Influence of concentric and eccentric resistance training on architectural adaptation in human quadriceps muscles. *J Appl Physiol.* 2007;103(5):1565–75.
14. Bohannon RW. Reference values for extremity muscle strength obtained by hand-held dynamometry from adults aged 20 to 79 years. *Arch Phys Med Rehabil.* 1997;78(1):26–32.
15. Boone DC, Azen SP. Normal range of motion of joints in male subjects. *J Bone Joint Surg Am.* 1979;61(5):756–9.
16. Brzycki M. Strength testing. Predicting a one-rep max from reps-to-fatigue. *Journal of Physical Education, Recreation & Dance.* 1993;64(1):88–90.
17. Candow DG, Chilibeck PD, Abeysekara S, Zello GA. Short-term heavy resistance training eliminates age-related deficits in muscle mass and strength in healthy older males. *J Strength Cond Res.* 2011;25(2):326–33.
18. Challis JH. Methodological report: the appropriate scaling of weightlifting performance. *Journal of Strength & Conditioning Research (Allen Press Publishing Services Inc).* 1999;13(4):367–71.

19. Clark DJ, Patten C, Reid KF, Carabello RJ, Phillips EM, Fielding RA. Muscle performance and physical function are associated with voluntary rate of neuromuscular activation in older adults. *J Gerontol A Biol Sci Med Sci.* 2011;66(1):115–21.

20. Clark MA, Lucett SC. Movement assessments. In: Clark M, Lucett S, National Academy of Sports Medicine, editors. *NASM's Essentials of Corrective Exercise Training.* 1st ed. Philadelphia: Wolters Kluwer Health/Lippincott Williams & Wilkins; 2011. p. 105–141.

21. Click Fenter P, Bellew JW, Pitts TA, Kay RE. Reliability of stabilised commercial dynamometers for measuring hip abduction strength: a pilot study. *Br J Sports Med.* 2003;37(4):331–4.

22. Coffey VG, Hawley JA. The molecular bases of training adaptation. *Sports Med.* 2007;37(9):737–63.

23. Cook G. Baseline Sports-Fitness Testing. In: Foran B, editor. *High-Performance Sports Conditioning.* Champaign: Human Kinetics; 2001. p. 19–48.

24. Cook G. Mobility and Stability Testing. In: *Athletic Body in Balance: Optimal Movement Skills and Conditioning for Performance.* Champaign: Human Kinetics; 2003. p. 26–38.

25. Cronin JB, Jones JV, Hagstrom JT. Kinematics and kinetics of the seated row and implications for conditioning. *J Strength Cond Res.* 2007;21(4):1265–70.

26. Curry BS, Chengkalath D, Crouch GJ, Romance M, Manns PJ. Acute effects of dynamic stretching, static stretching, and light aerobic activity on muscular performance in women. *J Strength Cond Res.* 2009;23(6):1811–9.

27. Dalgas U, Stenager E, Jakobsen J, et al. Resistance training improves muscle strength and functional capacity in multiple sclerosis. *Neurology.* 2009;73(18):1478–84.

28. Day ML, McGuigan MR, Brice G, Foster C. Monitoring exercise intensity during resistance training using the session RPE scale. *J Strength Cond Res.* 2004;18(2):353–8.

29. DeGroot DW, Quinn TJ, Kertzer R, Vroman NB, Olney WB. Circuit weight training in cardiac patients: determining optimal workloads for safety and energy expenditure. *J Cardiopulm Rehabil.* 1998;18(2):145–52.

30. Desgorces FD, Berthelot G, Dietrich G, Testa MS. Local muscular endurance and prediction of 1 repetition maximum for bench in 4 athletic populations. *J Strength Cond Res.* 2010;24(2):394–400.

31. Estrada M, Kleppinger A, Judge JO, Walsh SJ, Kuchel GA. Functional impact of relative versus absolute sarcopenia in healthy older women. *J Am Geriatr Soc.* 2007;55(11):1712–9.

32. Fahey TD, Insel PM, Roth WT. *Fit & Well: Core Concepts and Labs in Physical Fitness and Wellness.* 9th ed. New York (NY): McGraw-Hill; 2011. 320 p.

33. Faigenbaum AD, Kraemer WJ, Blimkie CJ, et al. Youth resistance training: updated position statement paper from the national strength and conditioning association. *J Strength Cond Res.* 2009;23(5 Suppl):S60–79.

34. Faigenbaum AD, Milliken LA, Westcott WL. Maximal strength testing in healthy children. *J Strength Cond Res.* 2003;17(1):162–6.

35. Faulkner JA, Larkin LM, Claflin DR, Brooks SV. Age-related changes in the structure and function of skeletal muscles. *Proc Austr Physiol Soc.* 2007;38:69–75.

36. Fernandez R. One repetition maximum clarified [2]. *J Orthop Sports Phys Ther.* 2001;31(5):264.

37. Fleck SJ, Kraemer WJ. *Designing Resistance Training Programs.* Champaign (IL): Human Kinetics Books; 1987. 264 p.

38. Franklin BA, Bonzheim K, Gordon S, Timmis GC. Snow shoveling: a trigger for acute myocardial infarction and sudden coronary death. *Am J Cardiol.* 1996;77(10):855–8.

39. Fuglevand AJ, Segal SS. Simulation of motor unit recruitment and microvascular unit perfusion: spatial considerations. *J Appl Physiol.* 1997;83(4):1223–34.

40. Garber CE, Blissmer B, Deschenes MR, et al. Quantity and quality of exercise for developing and maintaining cardiorespiratory, musculoskeletal, and neuromotor fitness in apparently healthy adults: guidance for prescribing exercise. *Med Sci Sports Exerc.* 2011;43(7):1334–59.

41. Goodpaster BH, Park SW, Harris TB, et al. The loss of skeletal muscle strength, mass, and quality in older adults: the health, aging and body composition study. *J Gerontol A Biol Sci Med Sci.* 2006;61(10):1059–64.

42. Grimsby O. More on 1RM testing. *J Orthop Sports Phys Ther.* 2001; 31(5):264–5.

43. Güzel NA, Hazar S, Erbas D. Effects of different resistance exercise protocols on nitric oxide, lipid peroxidation and creatine kinase activity in sedentary males. *Journal of Sports Science and Medicine.* 2007;6(4):417–22.

44. Hagerman FC, Walsh SJ, Staron RS, et al. Effects of high-intensity resistance training on untrained older men. I. Strength, cardiovascular, and metabolic responses. *J Gerontol A Biol Sci Med Sci.* 2000;55(7):B336–46.

45. Hale T. History of developments in sport and exercise physiology: A. V. Hill, maximal oxygen uptake, and oxygen debt. *J Sports Sci.* 2008;26(4):365–400.

46. Harman E. Biomechanical factors in human strength. *Strength Cond J.* 1994;16(1):46–53.

47. Harris NK, Cronin JB, Hopkins WG. Power outputs of a machine squat-jump across a spectrum of loads. *J Strength Cond Res.* 2007; 21(4):1260–4.

48. Haskell WL, Lee IM, Pate RR, et al. Physical activity and public health: updated recommendation for adults from the American College of Sports Medicine and the American Heart Association. *Circulation.* 2007;116(9):1081–93.

49. Hather BM, Tesch PA, Buchanan P, Dudley GA. Influence of eccentric actions on skeletal muscle adaptations to resistance training. *Acta Physiol Scand.* 1991;143(2):177–85.

50. Heyward VH. *Advanced Fitness Assessment and Exercise Prescription.* 6th ed. Champaign (IL): Human Kinetics; 2010. 465 p.

51. Hoffman J. *Norms for Fitness, Performance, and Health.* Leeds (England): Human Kinetics; 2006. 221 p.

52. Holcomb WR. Stretching and warm up. In: Baechle TR, Earle RW, National Strength & Conditioning Association (U.S.), editors. *Essentials of Strength Training and Conditioning.* 2nd ed. Champaign: Human Kinetics; 2000. p. 321–342.

53. Hough PA, Ross EZ, Howatson G. Effects of dynamic and static stretching on vertical jump performance and electromyographic activity. *J Strength Cond Res.* 2009;23(2):507–12.

54. Jaric S. Muscle strength testing: use of normalisation for body size. *Sports Med.* 2002;32(10):615–31.

55. Jaric S, Ristanovic D, Corcos DM. The relationship between muscle kinetic parameters and kinematic variables in a complex movement. *Eur J Appl Physiol Occup Physiol.* 1989;59(5):370–6.

56. Johnson BL, Nelson JK. *Practical Measurements for Evaluation in Physical Education.* 4th ed. New York (NY): Macmillan; 1986. 475 p.

57. Jones CJ, Rikli RE. Measuring functional fitness of older adults. *The Journal on Active Aging.* 2002. p. 24–30.

58. Jones CJ, Rikli RE, Beam WC. A 30-s chair-stand test as a measure of lower body strength in community-residing older adults. *Res Q Exerc Sport.* 1999;70(2):113–9.

59. Keating JL, Matyas TA. The influence of subject and test design on dynamometric measurements of extremity muscles. *Phys Ther.* 1996;76(8):866–89.

60. Kelln BM, McKeon PO, Gontkof LM, Hertel J. Hand-held dynamometry: reliability of lower extremity muscle testing in healthy, physically active, young adults. *J Sport Rehabil.* 2008;17(2):160–70.

61. Kim PS, Mayhew JL, Peterson DF. A modified YMCA bench press test as a predictor of 1 repetition maximum bench press strength. *J Strength Cond Res.* 2002;16(3):440–5.

62. Kistler BM, Walsh MS, Horn TS, Cox RH. The acute effects of static stretching on the sprint performance of collegiate men in the 60- and 100-m dash after a dynamic warm-up. *J Strength Cond Res.* 2010;24(9):2280–4.

63. Knapik JJ, Bauman CL, Jones BH, Harris JM, Vaughan L. Preseason strength and flexibility imbalances associated with athletic injuries in female collegiate athletes. *Am J Sports Med.* 1991;19(1):76–81.

64. Knapik JJ, Jones BH, Bauman CL, Harris JM. Strength, flexibility and athletic injuries. *Sports Med.* 1992;14(5):277–88.

65. Kokkonen J, Nelson AG, Eldredge C, Winchester JB. Chronic static stretching improves exercise performance. *Med Sci Sports Exerc.* 2007;39(10):1825–31.

66. Kolber MJ, Beekhuizen K, Cheng MS, Fiebert IM. The reliability of hand-held dynamometry in measuring isometric strength of the shoulder internal and external rotator musculature using a stabilization device. *Physiother Theory Pract.* 2007;23(2):119–24.

67. Kreighbaum E, Barthels KM. *Biomechanics: A Qualitative Approach for Studying Human Movement.* 4th ed. Boston (MA): Allyn and Bacon; 1996. 619 p.

68. Kryger AI, Andersen JL. Resistance training in the oldest old: consequences for muscle strength, fiber types, fiber size, and MHC isoforms. *Scand J Med Sci Sports.* 2007;17(4):422–30.

69. Kukolj M, Ropret R, Ugarkovic D, Jaric S. Anthropometric, strength, and power predictors of sprinting performance. *J Sports Med Phys Fitness.* 1999;39(2):120–2.

70. LaChance PF, Hortobagyi T. Influence of cadence on muscular performance during push-up and pull-up exercise. *J Strength Cond Res.* 1994;8(2):76–9.

71. Lea RD, Gerhardt JJ. Range-of-motion measurements. *J Bone Joint Surg Am.* 1995;77(5):784–98.

72. Leetun DT, Ireland ML, Willson JD, Ballantyne BT, Davis IM. Core stability measures as risk factors for lower extremity injury in athletes. *Med Sci Sports Exerc.* 2004;36(6):926–34.

73. Levangie PK, Norkin CC. *Joint Structure and Function: A Comprehensive Analysis.* 4th ed. Philadelphia (PA): F.A. Davis Co; 2005. 588 p.

74. Levinger I, Goodman C, Hare DL, Jerums G, Toia D, Selig S. The reliability of the 1RM strength test for untrained middle-aged individuals. *J Sci Med Sport.* 2009;12(2):310–6.

75. Little T, Williams AG. Effects of differential stretching protocols during warm-ups on high-speed motor capacities in professional soccer players. *J Strength Cond Res.* 2006;20(1):203–7.

76. Manoel ME, Harris-Love MO, Danoff JV, Miller TA. Acute effects of static, dynamic, and proprioceptive neuromuscular facilitation stretching on muscle power in women. *J Strength Cond Res.* 2008;22(5):1528–34.

77. Martin HJ, Yule V, Syddall HE, Dennison EM, Cooper C, Aihie Sayer A. Is hand-held dynamometry useful for the measurement of quadriceps strength in older people? A comparison with the gold standard Bodex dynamometry. *Gerontology.* 2006;52(3):154–9.

78. Mayhew JL, Ball TE, Arnold MD, Bowen JC. Relative muscular endurance performance as a predictor of bench press strength in college men and women. *Journal of Applied Sport Science Research.* 1992;6(4):200–6.

79. Mayhew JL, Johnson BD, Lamonte MJ, Lauber D, Kemmler W. Accuracy of prediction equations for determining one repetition maximum bench press in women before and after resistance training. *J Strength Cond Res.* 2008;22(5):1570–7.

80. McCall GE, Byrnes WC, Dickinson A, Pattany PM, Fleck SJ. Muscle fiber hypertrophy, hyperplasia, and capillary density in college men after resistance training. J Appl Physiol. 1996;81(5):2004–12.

81. McCartney N, McKelvie RS, Haslam DR, Jones NL. Usefulness of weightlifting training in improving strength and maximal power output in coronary artery disease. Am J Cardiol. 1991;67(11):939–45.

82. McGill S. Core Training: Evidence Translating to Better Performance and Injury Prevention. Strength Cond J. 2010;32(3):33–46.

83. McGill S. Low Back Disorders: Evidence-Based Prevention and Rehabilitation. 2nd ed. Leeds: Human Kinetics; 2007. 210–212 p.

84. McGill SM, Childs A, Liebenson C. Endurance times for low back stabilization exercises: clinical targets for testing and training from a normal database. Arch Phys Med Rehabil. 1999;80(8):941–4.

85. Melton LJ 3rd, Khosla S, Crowson CS, O'Connor MK, O'Fallon WM, Riggs BL. Epidemiology of sarcopenia. J Am Geriatr Soc. 2000;48(6):625–30.

86. Mero A, Luhtanen P, Viitasalo JT, Komi PV. Relationships between the maximal running velocity, muscle fiber characteristics, force production and force relaxation of sprinters. Scandinavian Journal of Sports Sciences. 1981;3(1):16–22.

87. Mirkov DM, Nedeljkovic A, Milanovic S, Jaric S. Muscle strength testing: evaluation of tests of explosive force production. Eur J Appl Physiol. 2004;91(2–3):147–54.

88. Mulroy SJ, Lassen KD, Chambers SH, Perry J. The ability of male and female clinicians to effectively test knee extension strength using manual muscle testing. J Orthop Sports Phys Ther. 1997; 26(4):192–9.

89. Murphy AJ, Wilson GJ. The ability of tests of muscular function to reflect training-induced changes in performance. J Sports Sci. 1997;15(2):191–200.

90. Murphy AJ, Wilson GJ. The assessment of human dynamic muscular function: a comparison of isoinertial and isokinetic tests. J Sports Med Phys Fitness. 1996;36(3):169–77.

91. Murphy AJ, Wilson GJ. Poor correlations between isometric tests and dynamic performance: relationship to muscle activation. Eur J Appl Physiol Occup Physiol. 1996;73(3–4):353–7.

92. Nelson AG, Kokkonen J, Arnall DA. Acute muscle stretching inhibits muscle strength endurance performance. J Strength Cond Res. 2005;19(2):338–43.

93. Norkin CC, Levangie PK. Joint Structure & Function: A Comprehensive Analysis. 2nd ed. Philadelphia (PA): Davis; 1992. 512 p.

94. Okada T, Huxel KC, Nesser TW. Relationship between core stability, functional movement, and performance. J Strength Cond Res. 2011;25(1):252–61.

95. Okamoto T, Masuhara M, Ikuta K. Combined aerobic and resistance training and vascular function: effect of aerobic exercise before and after resistance training. J Appl Physiol. 2007; 103(5):1655–61.

96. Payne N, Gledhill N, Katzmarzyk PT, Jamnik VK, Keir PJ. Canadian musculoskeletal fitness norms. Can J Appl Physiol. 2000;25(6): 430–42.

97. Pearson DR, Costill DL. The effects of constant external resistance exercise and isokinetic exercise training on work-induced hypertrophy. J Appl Sport Sci Res. 1988;2:39–41.

98. Peterson MD, Sen A, Gordon PM. Influence of resistance exercise on lean body mass in aging adults: a meta-analysis. *Med Sci Sports Exerc.* 2011;43(2):249–58.

99. Phillips WT, Batterham AM, Valenzuela JE, Burkett LN. Reliability of maximal strength testing in older adults. *Arch Phys Med Rehabil.* 2004;85(2):329–34.

100. Pierson LM, Herbert WG, Norton HJ, et al. Effects of combined aerobic and resistance training versus aerobic training alone in cardiac rehabilitation. J Cardiopulm Rehabil. 2001;21(2):101–10.

101. Pollock ML, Franklin BA, Balady GJ, et al. AHA Science Advisory. Resistance exercise in individuals with and without cardiovascular disease: benefits, rationale, safety, and prescription: An advisory from the Committee on Exercise, Rehabilitation, and Prevention, Council on Clinical Cardiology, American Heart Association; Position paper endorsed by the American College of Sports Medicine. *Circulation.* 2000;101(7):828–33.

102. Ratamess NA, Faigenbaum AD, Mangine GT, Hoffman JR, Kang J. Acute muscular strength assessment using free weight bars of different thickness. *J Strength Cond Res.* 2007;21(1):240–4.

103. Reiman MP, Krier AD, Nelson JA, Rogers MA, Stuke ZO, Smith BS. Reliability of alternative trunk endurance testing procedures using clinician stabilization vs. traditional methods. *J Strength Cond Res.* 2010;24(3):730–6.

104. Reynolds JM, Gordon TJ, Robergs RA. Prediction of one repetition maximum strength from multiple repetition maximum testing and anthropometry. *J Strength Cond Res.* 2006;20(3):584–92.

105. Rikli RE, Jones CJ. Development and validation of a functional fitness test for community-residing older adults. *J Aging Phys Activity*. 1999;7(2):129–61.

106. Rikli RE, Jones CJ. Functional fitness normative scores for community-residing older adults, ages 60–94. *J Aging Phys Act*. 1999;7(2):162–81.

107. Rikli RE, Jones CJ. *Senior Fitness Test Manual*. Champaign (IL): Human Kinetics; 2001. 161 p.

108. Roberts MD, Kerksick CM, Dalbo VJ, Hassell SE, Tucker PS, Brown R. Molecular attributes of human skeletal muscle at rest and after unaccustomed exercise: an age comparison. *J Strength Cond Res*. 2010;24(5):1161–8.

109. Robertson RJ, Goss FL, Andreacci JL, et al. Validation of the Children's OMNI-Resistance Exercise Scale of perceived exertion. *Med Sci Sports Exerc*. 2005;37(5):819–26.

110. Robertson RJ, Goss FL, Rutkowski J, et al. Concurrent validation of the OMNI perceived exertion scale for resistance exercise. *Med Sci Sports Exerc*. 2003;35(2):333–41.

111. Sale DG. Neural adaptation to resistance training. *Med Sci Sports Exerc*. 1988;20(5 Suppl):S135–45.

112. Sale DG. Testing Strength and Power. In: MacDougall JD, Wenger HA, Green HJ, Canadian Association of Sports Sciences, editors. *Physiological Testing of the High-Performance Athlete*. 2nd ed. Champaign: Human Kinetics Books; 1991. p. 21–103.

113. Sale DG, Martin JE, Moroz DE. Hypertrophy without increased isometric strength after weight training. *Eur J Appl Physiol Occup Physiol*. 1992;64(1):51–5.

114. Schmitz KH, Ahmed RL, Troxel A, et al. Weight lifting in women with breast-cancer-related lymphedema. *N Engl J Med*. 2009;361(7):664–73.

115. Schneider CM, Hsieh CC, Sprod LK, Carter SD, Hayward R. Cancer treatment-induced alterations in muscular fitness and quality of life: the role of exercise training. *Ann Oncol*. 2007;18(12):1957–62.

116. Signorile JF. *Bending the Aging Curve: The Complete Exercise Guide for Older Adults*. Leeds (England): Human Kinetics; 2011. 328 p.

117. Signorile JF, Sandler D, Kempner L, Stanziano D, Ma F, Roos BA. The ramp power test: a power assessment during a functional task for older individuals. *J Gerontol A Biol Sci Med Sci*. 2007;62(11):1266–73.

118. Signorile JF, Sandler D, Ma F, et al. The gallon-jug shelf-transfer test: an instrument to evaluate deteriorating function in older adults. *J Aging Phys Act*. 2007;15(1):56–74.

119. Smith CA. The warm-up procedure: To stretch or not to stretch. A brief review. *J Orthop Sports Phys Ther*. 1994;19(1):12–7.

120. Smith WN, Del Rossi G, Adams JB, et al. Simple equations to predict concentric lower-body muscle power in older adults using the 30-second chair-rise test: a pilot study. *Clin Interv Aging*. 2010;5:173–80.

121. Taaffe DR, Pruitt L, Pyka G, Guido D, Marcus R. Comparative effects of high- and low-intensity resistance training on thigh muscle strength, fiber area, and tissue composition in elderly women. *Clin Physiol*. 1996;16(4):381–92.

122. Taylor DC, Dalton JD Jr, Seaber AV, Garrett WE Jr. Viscoelastic properties of muscle-tendon units. The biomechanical effects of stretching. *Am J Sports Med*. 1990;18(3):300–9.

123. Tesch PA, Thorsson A, Kaiser P. Muscle capillary supply and fiber type characteristics in weight and power lifters. *J Appl Physiol*. 1984;56(1):35–8.

124. Vanderburgh PM, Edmonds T. The effect of experimental alterations in excess mass on pull-up performance in fit young men. *J Strength Cond Res*. 1997;11(4):230–3.

125. Vescovo G, Ravara B, Dalla Libera L. Skeletal muscle myofibrillar protein oxidation and exercise capacity in heart failure. *Basic Res Cardiol*. 2008;103(3):285–90.

126. White LJ, McCoy SC, Castellano V, et al. Resistance training improves strength and functional capacity in persons with multiple sclerosis. *Mult Scler*. 2004;10(6):668–74.

127. Williams MA, Haskell WL, Ades PA, et al. Resistance exercise in individuals with and without cardiovascular disease: 2007 update: a scientific statement from the American Heart Association Council on Clinical Cardiology and Council on Nutrition, Physical Activity, and Metabolism. *Circulation*. 2007;116(5):572–84.

128. Williford HN, Duey WJ, Olson MS, Howard R, Wang N. Relationship between fire fighting suppression tasks and physical fitness. *Ergonomics*. 1999;42(9):1179–86.

129. Willson JD, Dougherty CP, Ireland ML, Davis IM. Core stability and its relationship to lower extremity function and injury. *J Am Acad Orthop Surg*. 2005;13(5):316–25.

130. Wilson GJ, Murphy AJ. The use of isometric tests of muscular function in athletic assessment. *Sports Med*. 1996;22(1):19–37.

131. Woods K, Bishop P, Jones E. Warm-up and stretching in the prevention of muscular injury. *Sports Med*. 2007;37(12):1089–99.

132. Yamaguchi T, Ishii K, Yamanaka M, Yasuda K. Acute effects of dynamic stretching exercise on power output during concentric dynamic constant external resistance leg extension. *J Strength Cond Res*. 2007;21(4):1238–44.

SELECTED REFERENCES FOR FURTHER READING

Abernethy PJ, Jurimae J, Logan PA, et al. Acute and chronic response of skeletal muscle to resistance exercise. *Sports Med*. 1994;17:22–38.

Bohanon RW, Bubela, DJ, Wang YC, et al. Adequacy of belt stabilized testing of knee extension strength. *J Strength Cond Res*. 2011;25(7):1963–7.

Gleim GW, McHugh MP. Flexibility and its effects on sports injury and performance. *Sports Med*. 1997;24:289–99.

Kraemer WJ, Ratamess NA. Fundamentals of resistance training: progression and exercise prescription. *Med Sci Sports Exerc*. 2004;36:674–88.

McDermott MM, Ades P, Guralnick JM, et al. Treadmill and Resistance training in patients with peripheral arterial disease with and without intermittent claudication: A randomized controlled trial. *JAMA*. 2009;301(2):165–174.

Naclerio F, Rodriguez-Romo G, Barriopedro-Moro MI, et al. Control of resistance training by the OMNI perceived exertion scale. *J Strength Cond Res*. 2011;25(7):1879–88.

McGuigan MR, Bronks R, Newton RU, et al. Resistance training in patients with peripheral arterial disease: Effects on myosin isoforms, fiber type distribution, and capillary supply to skeletal muscle. *J Gerentol Bio Sci*. 2001;56A(7):B302–10.

Stone MH, Fleck SJ, Triplett NT, Kraemer WJ. Health- and performance-related potential of resistance training. *Sports Med*. 1991;11:210–31.

Thacker SB, Gilchrist J, Stroup D, et al. The impact of stretching on sports injury risk: a systematic review of the literature. *Med Sci Sports Exerc*. 2004;36:371–8.

Winett RA, Carpinelli RN. Potential health-related benefits of resistance training. *Prev Med*. 2001;33:503–13.

INTERNET RESOURCES

- American College of Sports Medicine (ACSM): http://www.acsm.org
- American Council on Exercise (ACE): http://www.acefitness.org
- International Fitness Association: http://www.ifafitness.com/stretch/index.html
- National Strength and Conditioning Association (NSCA): http://www.nsca-lift.org
- Exercise Prescription on the Net (ExRx.net): http://exrx.net
- Military.comFitnessCenter: http://www.military.com/fitness-center/military-fitness/stew-smith/archive
- Functional Movement Screen: http://www.functionalmovement.com/site/index.php

Clinical Exercise Testing Procedures

Clinical exercise testing has been part of the **differential diagnosis** of patients with suspected coronary artery disease (CAD) for at least 50 yr. Although there are other indications for clinical exercise testing, such as assessing functional capacity or **prognosis**, clinical exercise testing has been and remains an initial step in the **diagnosis** of CAD; the primary diagnostic criteria for exertional myocardial ischemia due to obstructive CAD being ST-segment changes and their correlation with symptoms (*e.g.*, angina pectoris, shortness of breath).

During clinical exercise testing, patients are monitored while they perform increasing levels of exercise intensity, usually while walking on a treadmill or pedaling a stationary cycle ergometer. Such testing involves graded or incremental exercise and employs predefined and standardized protocols. Traditionally, patients are monitored until they reach a sign (*e.g.*, hypertensive blood pressure [BP] response) or symptom-limited (*e.g.*, fatigue, excessive shortness of breath) maximal level of exertion. The goal is to observe how the cardiovascular, pulmonary, and skeletal muscles collectively respond to increases in metabolic demand. For a thorough evidence-based review of indications for clinical exercise testing, the reader is referred to the Practice Guidelines published jointly by the American College of Cardiology (ACC) and the American Heart Association (AHA) (1). Other historical names for this test are a graded exercise test (GXT), stress test, and exercise tolerance test.

INDICATIONS FOR A CLINICAL EXERCISE TEST

Indications for clinical exercise testing fall into three general categories: (a) diagnosis, (b) prognosis, and (c) evaluation of functional capacity. The most common diagnostic indication is the assessment of symptoms suspected to be caused by obstructive CAD. The ACC/AHA recommends a logistic approach to determining the type of testing in the evaluation of stable chest pain. In this approach, a symptom-limited maximal GXT with electrocardiogram (ECG) only (without nuclear or echocardiographic imaging) should be considered in the evaluation of these patients when the diagnosis of CAD is not certain, the patient has an interpretable resting ECG, and the patient is able to exercise (1). This is true for the evaluation of both men and women. Data from the WOMEN trial (What is the Optimal Method for Ischemia Evaluation in Women) — a prospective randomized trial of symptomatic women with suspected CAD — showed there was no clinical advantage by initially performing a GXT with ECG and nuclear imaging versus a GXT with ECG alone (56). In addition, the total diagnostic costs to evaluate the presence of CAD among the women who

KEY TERMS

Chronotropic: Affecting the heart rate.

Diagnosis: The determination of the presence of a disease.

Differential diagnosis: A systematic method to identify the causal factor(s) of a presenting problem (or chief complaint) through the use of physical exam and diagnostic tests to rule out unlikely causes.

Hemodynamic: Referring to the mechanics of blood flow.

Ischemic: Temporary lack or inadequate circulation of blood to a tissue.

Prognosis: The probable outcome of a disease.

Sensitivity: The percentage of individuals with a disease who have a positive diagnostic test.

Specificity: The percentage of healthy individuals who have a negative diagnostic test.

were initially referred for a GXT using ECG only was less than half the cost of the group referred for GXT with nuclear imaging (56).

The evidence is insufficient to support the routine use of GXT (with or without imaging) for the screening (diagnosis) of CAD in asymptomatic individuals with a low pretest probability of CAD, as well as those with a high pretest probability of CAD based on age, sex, and symptoms (1). The evidence is also insufficient to support the use of GXT with ECG alone for the screening of CAD in individuals taking digoxin with <1 mm ST-segment depression on their resting ECG and those who meet the ECG criteria for left ventricular hypertrophy with <1 mm ST-segment depression on their resting ECG (1). Additionally, the GXT with ECG alone is not useful for the diagnosis of CAD in patients with Wolff-Parkinson-White, ventricular pacing, >1 mm of ST-segment depression on their resting ECG, or left bundle branch block (1). Beyond the diagnosis of CAD, other reasons that might warrant the use of a GXT for diagnostic purposes might include the assessment of syncope or near-syncope, unexplained dyspnea, exercise-induced asthma, exercise-induced arrhythmias, pacemaker or heart rate (HR) response to exercise, and preoperative clearance. Although the evidence supporting each of these indications is largely anecdotal, it is based on sound physiological and clinical principles.

Risk stratification is important to the physician when developing the management plan for a patient. Over the past several years, the application of exercise testing has been broadened in response to a better understanding of the considerable risk stratification (e.g., prognostic) information that is available from the exercise test, such as exercise capacity and chronotropic and BP responses during and after exercise (10,11,21,30,31,36,41,46,49). In particular is the use of test scores that combine multiple pieces of information derived from the exercise test. One example is the Duke Treadmill Nomogram (and the related Duke Treadmill Score), which provides an estimate of the annual and 5-yr mortality based on the magnitude of ST-segment depression, presence of angina, and peak exercise capacity (36). The use of multiple variables derived from the exercise test has been shown to be better than the evaluation of ST segments alone in the diagnosis of obstructive CAD (57).

Clinical exercise testing is also indicated for the measurement of exercise capacity and may assist with guiding recommendations for return to work after an injury or cardiac event, as well as help guide the exercise prescription in patients with known heart disease (1). In the past, many clinically supervised exercise programs performed an exercise test before and after program participation, as a means to document changes in exercise capacity and to provide positive reinforcement to the patient. However, this practice has diminished over time due partly to cost. In spite of this change, the symptom-limited GXT remains the best way to objectively measure exercise capacity. Although exercise time and/or peak workload achieved during a GXT can be used to estimate metabolic equivalents (METs), the best assessment of exercise capacity is obtained by measuring respiratory gas exchange using open-circuit indirect spirometry for the determination of peak oxygen uptake ($\dot{V}O_2$) (1).

PRETEST CONSIDERATIONS

Before conducting an exercise test, several things must be considered that will affect the information derived from the test. These include the contraindications to exercise testing, the mode of exercise, the protocol, the endpoint of the exercise test, safety considerations, and medication decisions.

There are both absolute and relative contraindications to exercise testing, which are presented in *GETP9, Box 3-5*. For the most part, contraindications are based on decisions designed to avoid unstable ischemic, rhythm, or hemodynamic conditions or other situations in which the risk associated with undergoing the exercise test is likely to exceed the information to be gained from it. The number of conditions considered to be absolute contraindications has decreased over the past 50 yr. At the same time, the general practice of exercise testing has become safer (19).

Patients should be educated regarding the purpose, expectations, and risks of the testing and then provide informed consent (see *GETP9, Fig. 3-1*). The extent and quality of data obtained from an exercise test depends on the patient's ability and willingness to provide a maximal exertion; therefore, it is important to educate the patient regarding signs and symptoms they are likely to experience during the test (*e.g.*, fatigue, shortness of breath, chest pain). Prior to performing a test, the patient's medical history, current medications, and indications for the test should be reviewed with the patient, along with current or recent changes in symptoms. Lastly, the resting ECG should be examined for recent changes that may preclude testing, such as new onset atrial fibrillation or new repolarization changes. Also, if the purpose of the test is the assessment of exercise-induced myocardial ischemia, then the resting ECG should allow for interpretation of any repolarization changes that might occur. If the resting ECG does not allow for such interpretation, consideration should be given to adjunctive imaging procedures such as nuclear or echocardiographic imaging. These additional imaging procedures are not necessary if the GXT is being conducted for reasons other than the assessment of myocardial ischemia.

The mode selected for the exercise test can impact the results. In the United States, treadmill walking is the most frequently used mode, whereas in Europe, a leg cycle ergometer is more common. With individuals unaccustomed to cycling exercise, the peak exercise capacity (*e.g.*, $\dot{V}O_2$) will be 10%–20% lower during a maximal exercise test performed on a leg cycle ergometer compared to a treadmill due to regional muscle fatigue (5). This is an important consideration when data from serial tests are compared, such as during a longitudinal research study or when tracking a patient's response to a new medical regimen. Other exercise testing modes can be considered as needed, such as an arm ergometer, a dual-action ergometer, or a seated stepping ergometer. These can be useful options for patients with difficulty walking due to balance issues, amputation, or extreme obesity.

PERSONNEL

Before about 1980, symptom-limited maximal exercise testing in a clinical setting was primarily (90%) supervised by a cardiologist. Since that time, they have been performed by many health care professionals, including registered clinical exercise physiologists and certified clinical exercise specialists. In their "Recommendations for Clinical Exercise Laboratories," the AHA states that nonphysician health care professionals, when appropriately trained and possessing specific performance skills (*e.g.*, American College of Sports Medicine clinical certification), can safely supervise maximal exercise tests when a qualified physician is immediately available and who later overreads the tests results (43).

The average morbidity and mortality rates in four studies of clinical exercise testing with physician supervision averaged 3.6 and 0.44 per 10,000 tests, respectively (6,54,55,58). In three studies involving nonphysician supervision, average morbidity and mortality rates of 2.4 and 0.77 per 10,000 tests were observed, respectively (20,28,32). These data suggest that there are no differences in morbidity and mortality rates between direct physician and allied health professionals (*e.g.*, clinical exercise physiologist) in the supervision of a GXT. In addition, when a test is performed on a high-risk patient (*e.g.*, with cardiomyopathy), nonphysician supervision has been observed to be safe when a physician is immediately available (55). In addition to the test supervisor, at least one support technician should assist with testing. This person should have knowledge and skills in obtaining informed consent and medical history, skin preparation and ECG electrode placement, equipment operation, the measurement of BP at rest and during exercise, and effective patient interaction skills (43).

PROTOCOL

The exercise protocol represents a convenient and repeatable way to conduct the exercise test for both the patient and the professional supervising the test. There are several general principles that can be applied to the selection of the exercise protocol. The initial level of exertion should be clearly submaximal, and the increments of work from one stage to the next should be relatively small and of consistent size. The protocol should allow easy estimation of the exercise capacity, and the test should be time efficient for both patient and clinician. The Bruce treadmill protocol is the most widely used exercise protocol in the United States (9,47). This will likely continue due to physician familiarity, availability of equations to predict functional capacity (17,38,44), and efficiency of time utilization for both the clinician and patient. The aerobic requirements (~5 METs) associated with the first stage of the Bruce protocol and the large increases (~3 METs) between stages may make it less than optimal for persons with a low functional capacity; as such, it encourages extensive handrail support, which results in over estimation of the patient's peak exercise capacity (24,38). In response to these limitations, modifications of the Bruce protocol and many other treadmill and cycle protocols have been developed, including patient-specific ramping protocols (15,24,26,44,51). A common recommendation is to choose a protocol that will result in test duration of 8–12 min (5). See *GETP9, Figure 5-3* for many popular protocols.

MONITORING AND TERMINATION

The ECG, HR, BP, patient symptoms, and perceived exertion (*e.g.*, Borg Scale) should be monitored and recorded throughout the test (1). Heart rate should be observed to increase with increasing workloads and should not be used as a criterion to stop a symptom-limited maximal exercise test. BP and perceived exertion should be assessed and an ECG recorded near the end of each stage (every 2–3 min during a ramped protocol), again at peak exercise, and regularly through at least 6 min of recovery. Throughout the test, the ECG should be monitored for ST-segment abnormalities and other electrocardiographic manifestations of myocardial ischemia and arrhythmias. Standard chest pain evaluation — and, if indicated, evaluation for dyspnea and claudication pain — should also be assessed at regular intervals during the test.

Termination criteria for exercise testing are well established (see *GETP9, Box 5-2*). In general, the test should be continued until the clinical question that prompted the exercise test to be ordered has been answered. When the goal is a symptom-limited maximal exercise test, a predetermined workload, percentage of the age-predicted maximal HR, or predetermined respiratory exchange ratio should not be used as a reason to end the test (1). The use of a predetermined endpoint tends to overly stress the more debilitated patients and suboptimally challenge healthy, well-conditioned patients. Additionally, given the strong relationship between peak exercise capacity and prognosis (46), failure to take the patient to either a maximal exertion or symptom/sign limitation (*e.g.*, significant ST-segment depression, moderate-to-severe angina) will result in an underestimation of the patient's peak exercise capacity and, therefore, negatively influence prognosis. Some clinicians view the achievement of 85% of the age-predicted maximal HR as adequate stress for revealing exertional ischemia. This practice is based on older observations that 50% of ischemic abnormalities were observed by the time 85% of age-predicted maximal HR was achieved. The sensitivity of GXT results is increased when the HR achieved is greater than 85% of predicted. In the context of interpreting a clinically indicated test with no abnormal findings, clinicians are compelled to ask themselves if they have really ruled out exertional ischemia or if something may have been missed. Given that strenuous exercise in a previously sedentary person is a well-established trigger of acute myocardial infarction (40,60) and the likelihood that patients who receive reassurance after a normal exercise test result might be more willing to engage in strenuous exercise, the risk of missing an abnormal finding by inadequately stressing the patient is clinically relevant. Accordingly, it seems reasonable to argue that the best place to provoke abnormal findings is in the clinical exercise laboratory, where complications can be more readily identified and addressed appropriately.

POSTEXERCISE

A laboratory's routine operating procedures should include some standardized process in the period immediately following the exercise test. Older studies suggest that the sensitivity of ST-segment changes to diagnose CAD can be maximized when the patient is placed in a sitting or supine position immediately following exercise (8,22,29). More recent data focusing on the prognostic value of exercise testing have demonstrated the important data derived from the pattern of HR and BP responses during the postexercise period (4,10,11,30,31,39,41). These data suggest that the gain in ST-segment associated sensitivity during seated or supine recovery is less than the HR and BP information that is gathered during an active exercise recovery period. Thus, it is probably best to perform a 2-min period of very low-intensity exercise during the initial postexercise period to document the recovery pattern of HR and BP. Further, because profound hypotension during recovery, resulting from a large drop in venous return, can itself cause significant ischemia by decreasing perfusion pressure into the myocardium, performing low-intensity exercise may support venous return and thus hemodynamic stability. As a side note, the recovery period following a GXT represents a unique opportunity

for "teachable moments" during which the clinician conducting the test can communicate with the patient about important lifestyle-related habits (*e.g.*, the value of habitual exercise, weight loss, stopping smoking, or the safety of resuming activities that the patient might fear).

SAFETY

Exercise testing is generally quite safe. The classic data of Rochmis and Blackburn (54) suggested that the risk of serious complications was on the order of 6 per 10,000 tests. More recent data suggest that the risk of serious complications is <2 per 10,000 tests (47). Most of these tests were in patients without established heart disease. Among 2,331 patients with New York Heart Association Class II–IV heart failure symptoms due to left ventricular systolic dysfunction who performed maximal exercise tests as part of a clinical trial, there were no deaths and the rate of nonfatal major cardiovascular events was 4.5 per 10,000 tests (27). Proper attention to contraindications for exercise testing, careful monitoring during the test, and recognizing criteria for terminating the exercise test all contribute to improved safety.

In tests that are performed to assess the likelihood of obstructive CAD, some physicians might request that isolated patients withhold medications that are known to limit the hemodynamic response to exercise (*e.g.*, β-adrenergic blocking agents) because they may limit test sensitivity. Most institutions encourage patients to continue to take their medications on the day of testing (1). When the exercise test is performed to evaluate the effectiveness of therapy (or exercise capacity), patients should not withhold their medications because the clinical question to be answered is how effectively the treatment protocol is working (1).

INTERPRETATIVE STRATEGY

Interpreting exercise test data should be done within the clinical context of the indication for the test. At least five factors must be considered during the interpretation of the exercise test. These include patient symptoms, ECG responses, exercise capacity, hemodynamic responses, and the integrated response, as reflected by exercise test scores.

Symptoms that are consistent with myocardial ischemia (*e.g.*, chest discomfort, shortness of breath) or hemodynamic instability (*e.g.*, light-headedness) should be reported. In the case of chest discomfort that may be angina pectoris, the timing, character, magnitude, and resolution should be described. It is also important to recognize that dyspnea can be an anginal equivalent. Ideally, the appearance of symptoms, if present, will be correlated with either ECG or hemodynamic abnormalities. However, these can be masked by baseline ECG abnormalities, arrhythmias, pacemaker activity, or medications. There is a tendency for fewer symptoms to be observed during exercise testing than during spontaneous activity, perhaps because of the influence of the warm-up afforded by the early stages during exercise testing (37).

Changes in the ST segments on the ECG are the traditional interpretative sign related to the presence of exertional ischemia (see *Chapter 29*). ST-segment depression that is >1 mm, is horizontal or downsloping in nature, and persists for at least 80 msec after the J-point is considered the minimal diagnostic threshold to support a diagnosis of exertional myocardial ischemia. Alternately, >1.5 mm of upsloping ST-segment depression 80 msec after the J-point is also considered a minimal threshold for exercise-induced myocardial ischemia. In the case of ST-segment depression (or elevation), there is usually a lead with the greatest magnitude of ST-segment deviation, surrounded by leads with progressively less deviation. Although it might appear intuitive to infer that the ECG leads in which the ST-segment depression is observed reflect the area of the heart that might be ischemic (*e.g.*, leads II, III and aVF for inferior ischemia) or that a particular coronary artery might have an obstructive lesion, this is not the case. Using the traditional criteria of a 70% narrowing of at least one epicardial artery, the sensitivity and specificity of ECG exercise testing is about 70%. However, there is likely a significant workup bias, and the true sensitivity may be as low as 40% (30). ST-segment changes that occur early during an exercise test, are evident in multiple leads, or persist into recovery are strong predictors of the presence of at least one coronary vessel with obstructive atherosclerosis.

Dysrhythmias, especially ventricular dysrhythmias, are particularly disturbing during exercise testing because they are widely thought to portend a catastrophic hemodynamic collapse. In general, dysrhythmias that increase in frequency or complexity with progressive exercise and are associated with ischemia or with hemodynamic instability are thought to be more malignant than isolated dysrhythmias. Evidence indicating that high-grade dysrhythmias occurring during exercise or recovery are associated with a poor long-term prognosis has served to reinforce the traditional concern about the ominous nature of dysrhythmias (21).

Exercise capacity has always been viewed as an important aspect of exercise testing. A high peak $\dot{V}O_2$ can be inferred to predict a relatively high cardiac output and, therefore, the absence of serious limitations of left ventricular function. Within the past decade, several studies have been published demonstrating the profound importance of exercise capacity relative to the prognosis of patients with heart failure or cardiovascular disease (3,5,7). Either absolute or age/sex normalized exercise capacity is highly related to survival. A significant issue relative to exercise capacity

is the imprecision of estimating exercise capacity from exercise performance (*e.g.*, based on exercise time or peak workload). The error in estimating exercise capacity from various published prediction equations is at least 1 MET (15,17,24,26,44,50). This may be relatively unimportant (<10% error) in young healthy individuals with a peak exercise capacity of 13–15 METs but is much more significant (15%–25% error) in individuals with reduced exercise capacities, typical of those observed in patients with cardiovascular disease (4–8 METs). In view of the prognostic importance of exercise capacity, the frequent custom of stopping the exercise test early because the subject has reached an arbitrary HR (or percentage of an assumed maximal HR) cannot be justified. Further, allowing patients to use the handrail for excessive support will result in an overestimation of their exercise capacity and will inaccurately imply a more favorable prognosis than is justified. Although some of the equations for predicting functional capacity from exercise performance account for handrail support, their relative prediction error is larger than when the patient is not allowed to use handrail support (38).

In addition to describing a patient's exercise capacity as estimated peak METs or measured peak $\dot{V}O_2$, exercise capacity is frequently expressed relative to age- and sex-predicted norms. This is especially true when peak $\dot{V}O_2$ is reported. Several equations exist to estimate peak $\dot{V}O_2$ based on select demographics (*e.g.*, sex, age, height, weight) (3). Reference tables are also available to provide a percentile ranking for an individual's measured exercise capacity by sex and age categories (see *GETP9, Table 4-8*). Most of these references are based on apparently healthy individuals. In order to provide a reference for patients entering cardiac rehabilitation, Ades et al. (2) developed nomograms stratified by age, sex, and diagnosis.

Hemodynamic responses have historically been used to identify high-risk situations during exercise testing. Abnormalities in either the pattern or magnitude of the systolic BP response have long been recognized for their prognostic significance. A decrease in systolic BP — especially below the preexercise level, particularly when linked with ECG abnormalities or symptoms — during the course of an exercise test is widely accepted as a marker of a decreasing cardiac output and has represented an unequivocal criterion to terminate an exercise test.

A relatively recent development in our understanding of exercise testing is in the data regarding the prognostic significance of hemodynamic responses during and immediately after exercise testing (3,8,9,24,25,33,42). Lauer (30) has presented evidence that patients who cannot achieve an adequate HR response to exercise (*i.e.*, chronotropic incompetence) have an unfavorable prognosis beyond that accounted for by symptoms or

ECG changes. The most widely accepted cut point is a failure to achieve 80% of the age-predicted maximal HR in patients with no pharmacologic reason to have a limitation in their HR response. The prognostic value of a poor HR response is as great as an exercise-induced myocardial perfusion deficit. An abnormal chronotropic response apparently provides information that is independent of myocardial perfusion because the combination of perfusion deficit and an abnormal chronotropic index suggests a worse prognosis than either abnormality alone (30). In a similar fashion, the failure of the HR to recover promptly after exercise provides independent information related to prognosis (30). A failure of the HR to decrease by at least 12 beats per minute (bpm) by the end of the first minute or 22 bpm by the end of the second minute of recovery are strongly associated with future mortality (30). The unfavorable prognosis conveyed by the failure of HR to recover may be related to the inability of the parasympathetic nervous system to reassert vagal control over HR, which is known to predispose an individual to arrhythmic heart conditions (30).

EXERCISE TEST SCORES

Within the past decade, the use of exercise test scores that combine information derived during the exercise test into a single prognostic estimate have gained popularity (34,36). The most widely accepted and used is the Duke Treadmill Score or the related Duke Treadmill Nomogram (36). Either would be appropriate for patients with known or suspected CAD being considered for coronary angiography without a history of a myocardial infarction or revascularization procedure. The Duke Score/Nomogram (see *GETP9*, Fig. 6-2) considers exercise capacity, the magnitude of ST-segment depression, and the presence and severity of angina pectoris. The calculated score has been shown to be related to annual and 5-yr survival rates and allows the categorization of patients into low-, moderate-, and high-risk subgroups. This categorization may guide the physician caring for the patient toward conservative or aggressive therapies, depending on their classification. Prognosis estimates based on the Duke Treadmill Score/ Nomogram can also be used in combination with other hemodynamic findings, such as an abnormal pattern of recovery of HR or the combination of an abnormal chronotropic index and an abnormal HR recovery (30). Each of these abnormalities of exercise testing contributes independent prognostic information. Although there is a general belief that physicians informally integrate much of this information without the specific calculation of an exercise test score, recent data suggest that estimates of the presence of CAD provided by scores are superior to physician estimates and analysis of ST-segment changes alone (34).

BLOOD PRESSURE RESPONSE

Systolic BP normally increases in a progressive manner during incremental exercise. The magnitude of increase approximates 10 mm Hg $\cdot$ MET^{-1} in the general population (see *GETP9*, Box 6-1). However, given that training increases $\dot{V}O_{2max}$ without increasing maximal systolic BP, the increase in systolic BP per MET decreases with training. For example, it is only 4 mm Hg $\cdot$ MET^{-1} in national-class marathon runners with a $\dot{V}O_{2max}$ of 22 METs (12). An absolute peak systolic pressure of >250 mm Hg or a relative increase of >140 mm Hg above resting levels is considered a hypertensive response and is predictive of future resting hypertension (50). In patients with limitations of cardiac output, there is either an inappropriately slow increase in BP or a decrease in systolic BP midway through the exercise test. A decrease of systolic BP to below the resting value, or by >10 mm Hg after a preliminary increase, particularly in the presence of other indices of ischemia, is grossly abnormal (see *GETP9*, Box 6-1). A systolic BP >250 mm Hg is a relative indication to stop a test (see *GETP9*, Box 5-2). There is typically no change or a slight decrease in diastolic BP during an exercise test. An increase by >10 mm Hg is generally considered to be an abnormal finding and may occur with exertional ischemia, as is an increase to >115 mm Hg (50). A diastolic BP >115 mm Hg is a relative indication to stop a test (see *GETP9*, Box 5-2).

During the postexercise period, systolic BP normally decreases promptly (4,39). Several recent investigators have demonstrated that a delay in the recovery of systolic BP is highly related both to ischemic abnormalities and to a poor prognosis (4,39). As a general principle, the 3-min postexercise systolic BP should be <90% of the systolic BP at peak exercise. If peak exercise BP was not available, the 3-min postexercise systolic BP should be less than the systolic BP measured 1 min after exercise.

RESPIRATORY GAS EXCHANGE

Although the majority of exercise testing is performed without direct measurements of respiratory gas exchange, such measurements have been shown to be clinically useful. A major advantage of measuring gas exchange is the more accurate measurement of exercise capacity. A complete review of this topic can be found in the American Thoracic Society/ American College of Chest Physicians statement on cardiopulmonary gas exchange methods (3). In addition to providing an accurate measurement of aerobic capacity, gas exchange data may be particularly useful in defining prognosis (and thus helping to define the timing of transplantation) in patients with heart failure (35,42,45,52) and may help to guide the differential diagnosis in patients with possible cardiovascular or respiratory disease (14,59). In addition to peak $\dot{V}O_2$, the slope of the change in minute ventilation ($\dot{V}_E$) to change in carbon dioxide ($\dot{V}CO_2$) production (i.e., $\dot{V}_E$-$\dot{V}CO_2$ slope) during an exercise test has been shown to be related to prognosis, especially in patients with heart failure (7). Other measurements that can be determined through the measurement of respiratory gas exchange include the ventilatory threshold, oxygen pulse, slope of the change in work rate to change in $\dot{V}O_2$, oxygen uptake efficiency slope, end-tidal partial pressure of CO_2, breathing reserve, and the respiratory exchange ratio (7). Respiratory gas exchange measurements are particularly useful in identifying whether the cause of unexplained dyspnea has a cardiac or pulmonary etiology.

ADJUNCTIVE IMAGING PROCEDURES

In patients with an abnormal resting ECG, exercise testing may be coupled with techniques designed to either augment the information provided by the ECG or to replace the ECG when resting abnormalities (e.g., left bundle branch block) make evaluation of changes during exercise impossible. Various radioisotopes can be used effectively either to evaluate the presence of perfusion abnormalities, which is the index event in exertional ischemia and the beginning of the "ischemic cascade" (23,25,48), or of abnormalities of ventricular function that often occur with myocardial infarction or exertional ischemia (13,16,18,53). When exercise testing is coupled with myocardial perfusion imaging or echocardiography, all other aspects of the exercise test should remain the same, including HR and BP monitoring during and after exercise, symptom evaluation, rhythm monitoring, and symptom-limited maximal exertion.

Myocardial perfusion imaging (e.g., nuclear stress test) can be performed with a variety of agents and imaging approaches, although the two most common isotopes are [201]Thallium or [199m]Technetium sestamibi (Cardiolyte). Delivery of the isotope is proportional to coronary flow, and these agents cross cell membranes of metabolically active tissue either actively (thallium) or passively (sestamibi). In the case of myocardial infarction, the necrotic tissue does not take up the isotope, and thus, a permanent reduction of tracer activity is observed on the image. This is called a nonreversible, or fixed, perfusion defect. In the case of exertional ischemia, the tissue uptake in the ischemic region is reduced during exercise by virtue of the relative reduction of blood flow (and thus isotope) to the ischemic tissue during exercise. This abnormality is reversed when the myocardial perfusion is evaluated at rest. This is called a reversible, or transient, perfusion defect and is diagnostic of exertional myocardial ischemia.

Echocardiography can also be used as an adjunct during an exercise test (i.e., stress echocardiography). Echocardiographic examination allows evaluation of wall motion, wall thickening, and valve function. Although it is theoretically possible to perform echocardiography during the course of upright cycle ergometer exercise, it is technically challenging. Typical practice is to have the patient lie down immediately following completion of the exercise test in the left lateral decubitus position. This allows optimization of the echocardiographic window to the heart. Regional wall motion of various segments of the left ventricle is assessed. Deterioration in regional wall motion with exercise (compared to rest) is a sign of myocardial ischemia. Left ventricular ejection fraction (LVEF) is also measured before and after exercise. Normally, postexercise imaging in the upright position gives a spuriously high LVEF and normalization of wall motion abnormalities (13). The volume loading associated with assuming a supine position allows for adequate resolution of left ventricular dysfunction associated with exercise.

Imaging techniques such as radionuclide perfusion and echocardiography allow localization of myocardial ischemia. In patients incapable of exercising, it is also possible to perform either myocardial perfusion imaging or stress echocardiography (e.g., ventricular function studies) with pharmacologic stress, but these techniques are beyond the scope of this chapter. Additional information is provided in *Chapter 24*.

SUMMARY

Recent evidence suggests that there is much more information in the relatively simple symptom-limited maximal GXT than formerly believed. However, these new data are more important in terms of defining prognosis than in making a specific diagnosis of obstructive CAD. Changes in the ST segments of the ECG are not the only feature of this contemporary approach to evaluating exercise test data. An extremely important feature is the exercise capacity, as this serves as a surrogate of peak cardiac output. The prognostic impression gained from the exercise capacity is typically balanced by either ECG or symptomatic evidence of exertional myocardial ischemia. This relationship is well expressed in exercise test scores, such as the Duke Treadmill Score. Lastly, hemodynamic responses during and following a GXT have also been shown to be very powerful prognostic markers. It is reasonable to suggest that if all of the components of the standard maximal exercise test are considered that clinical exercise testing may provide almost as much diagnostic information and possibly more prognostic information as exercise myocardial perfusion scans or exercise echocardiography, which have been the sine qua non of noninvasive diagnostics for more than two decades.

REFERENCES

1. *ACC/AHA 2002 Guideline Update for Exercise Testing: A Report of the American College of Cardiology/American Heart Association Task Force on Practice Guidelines (Committee on Exercise Testing)* [Internet]. Washington (DC): American College of Cardiology; [cited 2011 Feb 28]. Available from: http://www.americanheart.org/downloadable/heart/1032279013658exercise.pdf

2. Ades PA, Savage PD, Brawner CA, et al. Aerobic capacity in patients entering cardiac rehabilitation. *Circulation.* 2006;113(23):2706–12.

3. American Thoracic Society, American College of Chest Physicians. ATS/ACCP Statement on cardiopulmonary exercise testing. *Am J Respir Crit Care Med.* 2003;167(2):211–77.

4. Amon KW, Richards KL, Crawford MH. Usefulness of the postexercise response of systolic blood pressure in the diagnosis of coronary artery disease. *Circulation.* 1984;70(6):951–6.

5. Arena R, Myers J, Williams MA, et al. Assessment of functional capacity in clinical and research settings: a scientific statement from the American Heart Association Committee on Exercise, Rehabilitation, and Prevention of the Council on Clinical Cardiology and the Council on Cardiovascular Nursing. *Circulation.* 2007;116(3):329–43.

6. Atterhog JH, Jonsson B, Samuelsson R. Exercise testing: a prospective study of complication rates. *Am Heart J.* 1979;98(5):572–9.

7. Balady GJ, Arena R, Sietsema K, et al. Clinician's guide to cardiopulmonary exercise testing in adults: a scientific statement from the American Heart Association. *Circulation.* 2010;122(2):191–225.

8. Bigi R, Cortigiani L, Gregori D, De Chiara B, Fiorentini C. Exercise versus recovery electrocardiography in predicting mortality in patients with uncomplicated myocardial infarction. *Eur Heart J.* 2004;25(7):558–64.

9. Bruce RA, Kusumi F, Hosmer D. Maximal oxygen intake and nomographic assessment of functional aerobic impairment in cardiovascular disease. *Am Heart J.* 1973;85(4):546–62.

10. Cole CR, Blackstone EH, Pashkow FJ, Snader CE, Lauer MS. Heart-rate recovery immediately after exercise as a predictor of mortality. *N Engl J Med.* 1999;341(18):1351–7.

11. Cole CR, Foody JM, Blackstone EH, Lauer MS. Heart rate recovery after submaximal exercise testing as a predictor of mortality in a cardiovascularly healthy cohort. *Ann Intern Med.* 2000;132(7):552–5.

12. deJong AT, Bonzheim K, Franklin BA, Saltarelli W. Cardiorespiratory responses to maximal arm and leg exercise in national-class marathon runners. *Phys Sportsmed.* 2009;37(2):120–6.

13. Dymond DS, Foster C, Grenier RP, Carpenter J, Schmidt DH. Peak exercise and immediate postexercise imaging for the detection of left ventricular functional abnormalities in coronary artery disease. *Am J Cardiol.* 1984;53(11):1532–7.

14. Eschenbacher WL, Mannina A. An algorithm for the interpretation of cardiopulmonary exercise tests. *Chest.* 1990;97(2):263–7.

15. Foster C, Crowe AJ, Daines E, et al. Predicting functional capacity during treadmill testing independent of exercise protocol. *Med Sci Sports Exerc.* 1996;28(6):752–6.

16. Foster C, Georgakopoulos N, Meyer K. Physiological and pathological aspects of exercise left ventricular function. *Med Sci Sports Exerc.* 1998;30(10 Suppl):S379–86.

17. Foster C, Jackson AS, Pollock ML, et al. Generalized equations for predicting functional capacity from treadmill performance. *Am Heart J.* 1984;107(6):1229–34.

18. Foster C, Pollock ML, Anholm JD, et al. Work capacity and left ventricular function during rehabilitation after myocardial revascularization surgery. *Circulation.* 1984;69(4):748–55.

19. Foster C, Porcari JP. The risks of exercise training. *J Cardiopulm Rehabil.* 2001;21(6):347–52.

20. Franklin BA, Dressendorfer R, Bonzbeim K. Safety of exercise testing by non-physician health care providers: eighteen year experience [abstract]. *Circulation.* 1995;92(Suppl I):1–37.

21. Frolkis JP, Pothier CE, Blackstone EH, Lauer MS. Frequent ventricular ectopy after exercise as a predictor of death. *N Engl J Med.* 2003;348(9):781–90.

22. Gutman RA, Alexander ER, Li YB, et al. Delay of ST depression after maximal exercise by walking for 2 minutes. *Circulation.* 1970;42(2):229–33.

23. Hammond HK, Kelly TL, Froelicher VF. Noninvasive testing in the evaluation of myocardial ischemia: agreement among tests. *J Am Coll Cardiol.* 1985;5(1):59–69.

24. Haskell WL, Savin W, Oldridge N, DeBusk R. Factors influencing estimated oxygen uptake during exercise testing soon after myocardial infarction. *Am J Cardiol.* 1982;50(2):299–304.

25. Heller GV, Ahmed I, Tilkemeier PL, Barbour MM, Garber CE. Influence of exercise intensity on the presence, distribution, and size of thallium-201 defects. *Am Heart J.* 1992;123(4 Pt 1):909–16.

26. Kaminsky LA, Whaley MH. Evaluation of a new standardized ramp protocol: the BSU/Bruce Ramp protocol. *J Cardiopulm Rehabil.* 1998;18(6):438–44.

27. Keteyian SJ, Isaac D, Thadani U, Roy BA, et al. Safety of symptom-limited cardiopulmonary exercise testing in patients with chronic heart failure due to severe left ventricular systolic dysfunction. *Am Heart J.* 2009;158(4 Suppl):S72–7.

28. Knight JA, Laubach CA Jr, Butcher RJ, Menapace FJ. Supervision of clinical exercise testing by exercise physiologists. *Am J Cardiol.* 1995;75(5):390–1.

29. Lachterman B, Lehmann KG, Abrahamson D, Froelicher VF. "Recovery only" ST-segment depression and the predictive accuracy of the exercise test. *Ann Intern Med.* 1990;112(1):11–6.

30. Lauer MS. Exercise electrocardiogram testing and prognosis. Novel markers and predictive instruments. *Cardiol Clin.* 2001;19(3):401–14.

31. Lauer MS, Francis GS, Okin PM, Pashkow FJ, Snader CE, Marwick TH. Impaired chronotropic response to exercise stress testing as a predictor of mortality. *JAMA.* 1999;281(6):524–9.

32. Lem V, Krivokapich J, Child JS. A nurse-supervised exercise stress testing laboratory. *Heart Lung.* 1985;14(3):280–4.

33. Lepretre PM, Foster C, Koralsztein JP, Billat VL. Heart rate deflection point as a strategy to defend stroke volume during incremental exercise. *J Appl Physiol.* 2005;98(5):1660–5.

34. Lipinski M, Froelicher V, Atwood E, et al. Comparison of treadmill scores with physician estimates of diagnosis and prognosis in patients with coronary artery disease. *Am Heart J.* 2002;143(4):650–8.

35. Mancini DM, Eisen H, Kussmaul W, Mull R, Edmunds LH Jr, Wilson JR. Value of peak exercise oxygen consumption for optimal timing of cardiac transplantation in ambulatory patients with heart failure. *Circulation.* 1991;83(3):778–86.

36. Mark DB, Shaw L, Harrell FE Jr, et al. Prognostic value of a treadmill exercise score in outpatients with suspected coronary artery disease. *N Engl J Med.* 1991;325(12):849–53.

37. Maybaum S, Ilan M, Mogilevsky J, Tzivoni D. Improvement in ischemic parameters during repeated exercise testing: a possible model for myocardial preconditioning. *Am J Cardiol.* 1996;78(10):1087–91.

38. McConnell TR, Foster C, Conlin NC, Thompson NN. Prediction of functional capacity during treadmill testing: effect of handrail support. *J Cardiopulm Rehabil.* 1991;11(4):255–60.

39. McHam SA, Marwick TH, Pashkow FJ, Lauer MS. Delayed systolic blood pressure recovery after graded exercise: an independent correlate of angiographic coronary disease. *J Am Coll Cardiol.* 1999;34(3):754–9.

40. Mittleman MA, Maclure M, Tofler GH, Sherwood JB, Goldberg RJ, Muller JE. Triggering of acute myocardial infarction by heavy physical exertion. Protection against triggering by regular exertion. Determinants of myocardial infarction onset study investigators. *N Engl J Med.* 1993;329(23):1677–83.

41. Morshedi-Meibodi A, Larson MG, Levy D, O'Donnell CJ, Vasan RS. Heart rate recovery after treadmill exercise testing and risk of cardiovascular disease events (The Framingham Heart Study). *Am J Cardiol.* 2002;90(8):848–52.

42. Myers J. Effects of exercise training on abnormal ventilatory responses to exercise in patients with chronic heart failure. *Congest Heart Fail.* 2000;6(5):243–9.

43. Myers J, Arena R, Franklin B, et al. Recommendations for clinical exercise laboratories: a scientific statement from the American Heart Association. *Circulation.* 2009;119(24):3144–61.

44. Myers J, Bellin D. Ramp exercise protocols for clinical and cardiopulmonary exercise testing. *Sports Med.* 2000;30(1):23–9.

45. Myers J, Madhavan R. Exercise testing with gas exchange analysis. *Cardiol Clin.* 2001;19(3):433–45.

46. Myers J, Prakash M, Froelicher V, Do D, Partington S, Atwood JE. Exercise capacity and mortality among men referred for exercise testing. *N Engl J Med.* 2002;346(11):793–801.

47. Myers J, Voodi L, Umann T, Froelicher VF. A survey of exercise testing: methods, utilization, interpretation, and safety in the VAHCS. *J Cardiopulm Rehabil.* 2000;20(4):251–8.

48. Nesto RW, Kowalchuk GJ. The ischemic cascade: temporal sequence of hemodynamic, electrocardiographic and symptomatic expressions of ischemia. *Am J Cardiol.* 1987;59(7):23C–30C.

49. Nissinen SI, Makikallio TH, Seppanen T, et al. Heart rate recovery after exercise as a predictor of mortality among survivors of acute myocardial infarction. *Am J Cardiol.* 2003;91(6):711–4.

50. Pescatello LS, Franklin BA, Fagard R, et al. American College of Sports Medicine position stand. Exercise and hypertension. *Med Sci Sports Exerc.* 2004;36(3):533–53.

51. Peterson MJ, Pieper CF, Morey MC. Accuracy of VO2(max) prediction equations in older adults. *Med Sci Sports Exerc.* 2003;35(1):145–9.

52. Ramos-Barbon D, Fitchett D, Gibbons WJ, Latter DA, Levy RD. Maximal exercise testing for the selection of heart transplantation candidates: limitation of peak oxygen consumption. *Chest.* 1999;115(2):410–7.

53. Rerych SK, Scholz PM, Newman GE, Sabiston DC Jr, Jones RH. Cardiac function at rest and during exercise in normals and in patients with coronary heart disease: evaluation by radionuclide angiocardiography. *Ann Surg.* 1978;187(5):449–64.

54. Rochmis P, Blackburn H. Exercise tests. A survey of procedures, safety, and litigation experience in approximately 170,000 tests. *JAMA.* 1971;217(8):1061–6.

55. Rodgers GP, Ayanian JZ, Balady G, et al. A report of the American College of Cardiology/American Heart Association/American College of Physicians-American Society of Internal Medicine Task Force on clinical competence. *Circulation.* 2000;102(14):1726–38.

56. Shaw LJ, Mieres JH, Hendel RH, et al. Comparative effectiveness of exercise electrocardiography with or without myocardial perfusion single photon emission computed tomography in women with suspected coronary artery disease: results from the what is the optimal method for ischemia evaluation in women (WOMEN) Trial. *Circulation.* 2011;124(11):1239–49.

57. Shaw LJ, Peterson ED, Shaw LK, et al. Use of a prognostic treadmill score in identifying diagnostic coronary disease subgroups. *Circulation.* 1998;98(16):1622–30.

58. Squires RW, Allison TG, Johnson BD, Gau GT. Non-physician supervision of cardiopulmonary exercise testing in chronic heart failure: safety and results of a preliminary investigation. *J Cardiopulm Rehabil.* 1999;19(4):249–53.

59. Wasserman K. Diagnosing cardiovascular and lung pathophysiology from exercise gas exchange. *Chest.* 1997;112(4):1091–101.

60. Willich SN, Lewis M, Lowel H, Arntz HR, Schubert F, Schroder R. Physical exertion as a trigger of acute myocardial infarction. Triggers and Mechanisms of Myocardial Infarction Study Group. *N Engl J Med.* 1993;329(23):1684–90.

SELECTED REFERENCES FOR FURTHER READING

ACC/AHA 2002 Guideline Update for Exercise Testing: A Report of the American College of Cardiology/American Heart Association Task Force on Practice Guidelines (Committee on Exercise Testing) [Internet]. Washington (DC): American College of Cardiology; [cited 2011 Feb 28]. Available from: http://www.americanheart.org/downloadable/heart/1032279013658exercise.pdf

Balady GJ, R Arena, K Sietsema, et al. Clinician's guide to cardiopulmonary exercise testing in adults: a scientific statement from the American Heart Association. *Circulation.* 2010;122(2):191–225.

Myers J, R Arena, B Franklin, et al. Recommendations for clinical exercise laboratories: A scientific statement from the American Heart Association. *Circulation.* 2009;119(24):3144–61.

Wassermann K, Hansen JE, Sue DY, et al. *Principles of Exercise Testing and Interpretation: Including Pathophysiology and Clinical Applications.* 5th ed. Baltimore (MD): Lippincott Williams & Wilkins; 2011. 592 p.

INTERNET RESOURCES

- Guidelines and Quality Standards from the American College of Cardiology: http://www.cardiosource.org/Science-And-Quality/Practice-Guidelines-and-Quality-Standards.aspx
- Statements and Guidelines on Exercise Testing from the American Heart Association: http://my.americanheart.org/professional/StatementsGuidelines/ByTopic/TopicsD-H/Exercise-Testing_UCM_321540_Article.jsp

24

Diagnostic Procedures for Cardiovascular Disease

The diagnosis of cardiovascular disease is made using a medical history, physical examination, and various non-invasive and invasive tests. These tests are ordered by physicians (typically internists and cardiologists) or mid-level providers (nurse practitioners and physician assistants) and should follow the recommendations made by the American College of Cardiology (ACC) and the American Heart Association (AHA) Task Forces (1,10).

Current guidelines grade the strength of the evidence in the scientific literature for a given recommendation. The ACC/AHA Task Force applies a grade of A, B, or C based on data derived from multiple randomized clinical trials or meta-analyses (level A); data derived from a single randomized trial or nonrandomized studies (level B); and information derived only from consensus opinion of experts, case studies, or standard of care (level C). From this evidence, three levels or classes of recommendations for performing a certain diagnostic test or treatment are made. Class I indicates conditions for which there is evidence and/or general agreement that a given procedure or treatment is beneficial, useful, and effective, and in general suggests an action *should be done*; class II indicates conditions for which there is conflicting evidence and/or a divergence of opinion about the usefulness/efficacy

KEY TERMS

Akinesis: Absence of contraction of a myocardial segment.

Augmentation: Enhancement of contraction of a myocardial segment.

Bruits: A harsh or musical intermittent auscultatory sound, especially an abnormal one.

Differential diagnosis: The determination of which two or more diseases with similar symptoms is the one the patient suffers from by a systematic comparison and contrasting of the clinical findings.

Dyskinesis: Impaired contraction resulting in outward movement of a myocardial segment with systole.

Edema: An accumulation of an excessive amount of watery fluid in cells or intercellular tissues.

False negative: An initial negative diagnostic assessment that is ultimately untrue, that is, the diagnostic test failed to indicate the presence of disease, but the individual has the disease.

False positive: An initial positive diagnostic assessment that is ultimately untrue, that is, the diagnostic test indicated the presence of disease, but the individual does not have the disease.

Gold standard: The diagnostic test that serves as the comparison for all other tests evaluating the same condition, disease, or physiologic response.

Hypokinesis: Diminished or reduced contraction of a myocardial segment.

Predictive value: The probability of disease being present/absent in the setting of a positive/negative test.

Pretest likelihood: The probability that an individual has a given disease based on history and physical findings before the performance of a diagnostic test.

Prevalence: The number of cases of a disease existing in a given population at a specific time (*period prevalence*) or at a particular moment (*point prevalence*).

Sensitivity: The proportion of individuals with a given disease who have a positive test result for the disease.

Specificity: The proportion of individuals without a given disease who have a negative test result for the disease.

True negative: Denoting an initial negative diagnostic assessment that is ultimately true.

True positive: Denoting an initial positive diagnostic assessment that is ultimately true.

of a procedure or treatment (subdivided into class IIa, for which the weight of evidence/opinion is in favor of usefulness/efficacy, interpreted as "probably should do it," and class IIb, for which the usefulness/efficacy is less well established by evidence/opinion, interpreted as "can consider doing it"); and class III indicates conditions for which there is evidence and/or general agreement that a procedure/treatment is not useful/effective and in some cases may be harmful, and in general suggests that the action *should not* be done. An example of a guideline statement is the ACC/AHA 2009 guideline update for the management of patients with heart failure with the following, which is listed as a class IIa recommendation: "Maximal exercise testing with measurement of respiratory gas exchange is reasonable to identify high-risk patients presenting with HF [heart failure] who are candidates for cardiac transplantation or other advanced treatments (Level of Evidence: B)" (17).

Clinical exercise professionals should be familiar with both the general decision-making process of cardiovascular diagnosis and the specific diagnostic procedures used to make the diagnosis. Often in the cardiac rehabilitation setting, for instance, patients ask about diagnostic procedures and why a diagnostic assessment was or was not performed. Even though clinical exercise professionals would not be expected to provide a definitive answer to these types of questions, they can provide some insight during a teaching moment with the patient, provided they have the requested knowledge. Specific questions concerning diagnosis, prognosis, test results, and disease management should be referred to the patient's physician.

Additionally, there is an increasing role for the clinical exercise professional in the administration and preliminary interpretation of some cardiac diagnostic procedures. Often, noninvasive cardiology laboratories and other settings in which cardiac stress imaging is performed use these individuals to perform technical duties and supervise exercise testing or cardiac physiologic response to pharmacologic agents (adenosine, dipyridamole, regadenoson, or dobutamine).

This chapter focuses on common forms of cardiovascular testing that are relevant to the clinical exercise professional. It is important to keep in mind that testing serves many important clinical functions, including screening for disease, making a diagnosis when symptoms are present, indicating prognosis when disease status is known, and, finally, guiding the management of the patient.

HISTORY AND PHYSICAL EXAMINATION

The cornerstone of the evaluation and clinical workup of the patient with suspected heart disease is the history and physical examination. This is the basis of any subsequent cardiovascular testing that may be performed. The history and physical examination may be performed by a physician, midlevel provider or other qualified personnel (*e.g.*, clinical exercise physiologist) who is working with a patient during the clinical encounter.

When evaluating a patient for the first time, it is always best to perform a complete history and physical examination and obtain as many of the previous medical records as possible. Creation of a problem list and list of current medications and allergies to medications is essential. It is only with a complete knowledge of all of the patient's health and medical information that an accurate diagnosis and effective treatment plan can be designed. The major signs/symptoms common to patients with heart disease are listed in *Box 24-1*.

Each patient should be questioned regarding the presence of these symptoms at each visit. For each symptom, additional information needs to be obtained, such as how long ago it began, the duration of the symptom with each occurrence, any precipitating event, frequency of the symptoms, and how the patient relieves the discomfort. The most common symptom in those with cardiac disease is chest discomfort. With chest discomfort, the key components to assess include (a) location and type of sensation, especially substernal discomfort with possible radiation to the arms, upper back, or jaw; (b) if it occurs with myocardial stress, such as exertion or mental stress; and (c) if it is relieved by using nitroglycerin or rest and relaxation. If a patient has all of these components, it is considered "typical" or "definite" angina; if one of the components is missing, it is considered "atypical" angina (*GETP9, Chapter 6*). It should be noted that women can have more atypical chest pain that is ischemic in nature than men. It should also be noted that patients with

---

BOX 24-1 | **Major Signs/Symptoms of Heart, Lung, or Metabolic Disease**[a]

1. Anginal discomfort (in the chest, neck, jaw, arms, or upper back)
2. Shortness of breath at rest or with mild exertion
3. Dizziness or syncope (fainting)
4. Orthopnea or paroxysmal nocturnal dyspnea (waking at night short of breath)
5. Ankle edema
6. Palpitations or tachycardia
7. Intermittent claudication
8. Known heart murmur
9. Unusual fatigue or shortness of breath with usual activities

[a]Modified from *Table 2.2* in Pescatello LS, senior editor. *ACSM's Guidelines for Exercise Testing and Prescription*. 9th ed. Baltimore (MD): Lippincott Williams & Wilkins; 2014.

diabetes more commonly have atypical features or no ischemic symptoms despite the presence of significant coronary disease.

Angina typically presents as a dull pressure or burning discomfort (gripping, heavy, suffocating, or tightness are also used to describe the sensation) in the chest, jaw, shoulder, upper back, or arm. It usually occurs with physical exertion or emotional stress and is relieved with rest or nitroglycerin. It is incorrect to ask about chest "pain." Most patients do not experience sharp pain in their chest as a symptom of heart disease. Rather, they may describe the discomfort as "bothersome" rather than painful. By asking about chest pain, many patients with heart disease may be missed. Discomfort that persists for hours or days, is localized to a small area defined by a fingertip, or is sharp in nature, is less likely to be angina. The other symptoms listed in *Box 24-1* may occur in association with angina or with other types of cardiac disease (*e.g.*, valvular, nonischemic heart failure, arrhythmias). Associated symptoms such as lightheadedness, diaphoresis, angina at rest, and nausea are more suggestive of unstable angina or acute coronary syndrome (ACS), and further consideration regarding the appropriateness of exercise testing at that time should be pursued.

The history intake should also include an evaluation of the risk factors associated with cardiac disease: age (>45 yr for men, >55 yr for women), obesity (body mass index >30 kg · m^{-2}), sedentary lifestyle, hypertension (6), diabetes or prediabetes, dyslipidemia (15), smoking, and a family history of heart disease in a male/female parent or sibling younger than 55/65 yr of age. Any previous history of cardiovascular disease should also be noted, including myocardial infarction (MI), prior revascularization, stroke, or known peripheral arterial disease (*GETP9, Box 3.1*). All patients identified with risk factors should be counseled and educated about how lifestyle plays a central role in risk factor and disease development and should be treated accordingly. The clinician may also consider ordering laboratory tests for fasting blood lipids (total high- and low-density lipoprotein cholesterols [HDL-C and LDL-C], and triglycerides), thyroid function (if dyslipidemia is present), and fasting blood glucose (diabetes evaluation) (see *GETP9, Box 3.3*). In some instances, blood lipids and glucose may be assessed at the time of the clinic visit using point-of-care testing procedures.

The physical examination should include blood pressure, pulse, and body weight, including body mass index. The person who places the patient in the examination room typically determines vital signs. The general physical examination performed by the clinician is best approached by inspection, palpation, auscultation, and percussion.

Inspection includes assessment of the patient's general condition, such as the appearance of distress; color and texture of the skin; presence of cyanosis or edema of the extremities; and presence of skin lesions or jugular venous distention. Palpation involves feeling the major arteries — including the abdominal aorta, femoral, pedal, radial, and carotid arteries — to determine the presence and magnitude of the pulse, and in the case of the abdominal aorta, to estimate its size. The apex of the left ventricle (LV) can be palpated to determine if cardiac enlargement is present. Peripheral edema is assessed by palpation, first to determine its presence and second to grade its severity. Percussion of vital organs can also be performed but is of little value in the assessment for cardiac disease. The final step of the physical examination is auscultation. Each of the major arteries should be evaluated for bruits. The lungs are auscultated for signs of pneumonia, emphysema, or heart failure, and the heart is auscultated for regularity of rhythm, murmurs, and extra sounds (*GETP9, Box 3.2*).

For patients with symptoms that are potentially related to myocardial ischemia, a resting electrocardiogram (ECG) should be performed. It is useful as a baseline for future reference and as a screen for previous or current cardiac problems, including infarction, arrhythmia, and left ventricular hypertrophy (LVH). It is also an important aid for determining the type of diagnostic test to be performed next. For instance, any preexisting abnormality may suggest the need to add an imaging study to a graded exercise test to evaluate the patient with ischemic symptoms.

DETERMINING THE GOALS OF CARDIOVASCULAR TESTING

SCREENING FOR CORONARY ARTERY DISEASE

The clinician should estimate the coronary heart disease risk (MI or death) using the Framingham or other scoring scheme based on age, sex, total cholesterol or LDL-C or HDL-C, blood pressure, diabetes, and smoking (*Fig. 24-1*) (27). In general, when the coronary heart disease risk exceeds 20% over 10 yr (or 2% per year), a patient is considered at high risk, and current recommendations support the action of using exercise stress testing as a screening test for significant coronary artery disease (CAD) (19).

EVALUATION OF CHEST DISCOMFORT

There is a broad differential diagnosis for chest discomfort (*Box 24-2*). The Diamond and Forrester model uses age, sex, and symptoms to determine the probability of CAD (9). The scheme stratifies the patient's risk into a low-, intermediate-, or high-risk group, which is used to determine the next step in the evaluation process. In general, those in whom a low probability of CAD is suspected based on the history and physical examination should be

Estimate of 10-yr Risk for Men
(Framingham Point Scores)

A

Age, yr	Points
20–34	−9
35–39	−4
40–44	0
45–49	3
50–54	6
55–59	8
60–64	10
65–69	11
70–74	12
75–79	13

B

Total Cholesterol, mg·dL⁻¹	Points				
	Age 20–39	Age 40–49	Age 50–59	Age 60–69	Age (yr) 70–79
<160	0	0	0	0	0
160–199	4	3	2	1	0
200–239	7	5	3	1	0
240–279	9	6	4	2	1
≥280	11	8	5	3	1

C

	Points				
	Age 20–39	Age 40–49	Age 50–59	Age 60–69	Age (yr) 70–79
Nonsmoker	0	0	0	0	0
Smoker	8	5	3	1	1

D

HDL, mg·dL⁻¹	Points
≥60	−1
50–59	0
40–49	1
<40	2

E

Systolic BP, mmHg	If Untreated	If Treated
<120	0	0
120–129	0	1
130–139	1	2
140–159	1	2
≥160	2	3

F

Point Total	10-yr Risk, %
<0	<1
0	1
1	1
2	1
3	1
4	1
5	2
6	2
7	3
8	4
9	5
10	6
11	8
12	10
13	12
14	16
15	20
17	25
≥17	≥30

Estimate of 10-yr Risk for Women
(Framingham Point Scores)

A

Age, yr	Points
20–34	−7
35–39	−3
40–44	0
45–49	3
50–54	6
55–59	8
60–64	10
65–69	12
70–74	14
75–79	16

B

Total Cholesterol, mg·dL⁻¹	Points				
	Age 20–39	Age 40–49	Age 50–59	Age 60–69	Age (yr) 70–79
<160	0	0	0	0	0
160–199	4	3	2	1	1
200–239	8	6	4	2	1
240–279	11	8	5	3	2
≥280	13	10	7	4	2

C

	Points				
	Age 20–39	Age 40–49	Age 50–59	Age 60–69	Age (yr) 70–79
Nonsmoker	0	0	0	0	0
Smoker	9	7	4	2	1

D

HDL, mg·dL⁻¹	Points
≥60	−1
50–59	0
40–49	1
<40	2

E

Systolic BP, mmHg	If Untreated	If Treated
<120	0	0
120–129	1	3
130–139	2	4
140–159	3	5
≥160	4	6

F

Point Total	10-yr Risk, %
<9	<1
9	1
10	1
11	1
12	1
13	2
14	2
15	3
16	4
17	5
18	6
19	8
20	11
21	14
22	17
23	22
25	27
≥25	≥30

FIGURE 24-1. Estimation of coronary heart disease risk (nonfatal myocardial infarction or death) using the Framingham equation. HDL, high-density lipoprotein; BP, blood pressure. Add points accordingly for **A–E** and determine 10-yr risk percentage in **F**.

BOX 24-2	Differential Diagnosis of Chest Discomfort

CARDIAC

- Angina
- Acute coronary syndrome
- Mitral valve prolapse
- Pericarditis
- Aortic stenosis
- Aortic dissection

GASTROINTESTINAL

- Peptic ulcer disease
- Esophageal spasm or reflux disease
- Cholecystitis or cholelithiasis

PULMONARY

- Pneumonia
- Pleurisy
- Pulmonary embolism

MUSCULOSKELETAL

- Costochondritis

TRAUMA

- Cervical and thoracic spine disorders

considered for treatment of cardiac disease risk factors and assessed for a noncardiac cause of their symptoms (*e.g.*, referrals for gastrointestinal testing, pulmonary function testing, and musculoskeletal assessment). However, patients with risk stratified into the intermediate- or high-risk groups should be assessed using diagnostic tests for cardiac disease (14). Intermediate-risk patients who are appropriate candidates for a graded exercise test should undergo an ECG or an ECG plus imaging (radionuclide or echocardiography) stress test. Pharmacologic stress assessment is considered when a patient cannot perform exercise. Patients who are in the high-risk group may begin with an exercise test or directly undergo cardiac catheterization depending on their individual clinical situation. Cardiac catheterization is also appropriate for those who are initially categorized as intermediate risk and move into the high-risk group after stress testing. As a general rule of thumb, when a patient has a pretest probability of >80% for significant coronary disease, it is clinically more cost-effective to move directly to coronary angiography as the initial step (25).

DETERMINING PROGNOSIS

Conventional exercise stress testing gives considerable prognostic information concerning cardiovascular and all-cause mortality. There is a strong relationship between work capacity (as expressed in metabolic equivalents [METs]) and survival (19). The Duke Treadmill Score is an example of how METs, as well as other information, can be integrated to predict risk of future events (20). One important variable to report is the heart rate recovery. A heart rate recovery of <12 beats $\cdot$ min^{-1} after 1 min has been related to cardiovascular deconditioning and predicts an overall higher mortality that is independent from other information on the stress test (19). Importantly, directly measured peak oxygen consumption expressed in mL $\cdot$ kg^{-1} $\cdot$ min^{-1} is considered the best single predictor of survival among all of the diagnostic tests available in medicine today (11). Use of peak oxygen consumption has specific applications in determining prognosis in systolic heart failure and consideration of patients who may require heart transplant (peak oxygen consumption <10 mL $\cdot$ kg^{-1} $\cdot$ min^{-1}) (17). In addition, peak oxygen consumption has been shown to be predictive of complications in obese patients undergoing elective noncardiac surgery (21).

GUIDING MANAGEMENT

The most common application of stress testing in terms of management is the determination of ischemic threshold. In a patient with established CAD, irrespective of whether angioplasty or bypass surgery has been performed, there is atherosclerosis throughout the coronary tree and the exercise capacity and level of activity at which symptoms and/or signs of ischemia develop is critical. It is important to keep in mind that ischemia can manifest itself according to symptoms (chest discomfort, dyspnea), ST-segment elevation or depression, and, in some instances, ventricular arrhythmias. The clinician's counseling concerning job functions, leisure activity, exercise, and prescription of medications is dependent on the results of stress testing in the presence of known CAD. It is important for the clinical exercise professional to convey the important information discussed previously to give the clinician the clearest picture possible with respect to the patient's ischemic heart disease and response to exercise stress.

DECISION STATISTICS OF DIAGNOSTIC TESTS

The ability of a diagnostic test to accurately identify individuals with heart disease is dependent on the sensitivity and specificity of the test, as well as the prevalence of the disease in the population being tested. Bayes theorem clarifies the importance that these variables play in the selection of the appropriate test in the workup of patients for heart disease. Depending on the **pretest likelihood** (low, intermediate, or high) of the patient having heart disease, physicians have various clinical tests that can be performed. The following paragraphs define the terms used in the process of determining and understanding the accuracy of these diagnostic tests.

A positive test result is considered one in which the patient evaluated has an abnormality that was identified by the test. Likewise, a negative test result is one that did not find an abnormality — or in others words, the finding was normal. It must be understood that any clinical test, even if considered the gold standard, will not always correctly identify whether a person has or does not have an abnormality. When the test result is considered positive and the patient is later found to not have the abnormality, the test result is then considered a false positive result. On the other hand, if a test result is determined to be negative, and later the patient is found to have the abnormality or disease, the initial test is considered a false negative result. And likewise, tests that accurately assess a patient as positive or negative for an abnormality or disease are considered true positive and true negative results, respectively.

Based on this knowledge, the sensitivity and specificity of a type of clinical test can be determined (see *GETP9, Box 6.2* to determine how to calculate sensitivity and specificity). *Sensitivity* refers to how often the test uncovers an abnormality or disease in a population of individuals who all have the abnormality or disease. *Specificity* is the percentage of tests that are negative or normal in a population without the abnormality or disease. For any type of clinical test, the success of a test to uncover an abnormality, if it is present, is only as good as the technical performance of the test, the appropriateness of the test for the person being evaluated, and the interpretation or clinical judgment of the clinician who evaluates the test results. It is important to remember that sensitivity and specificity are terms applied to the performance of a diagnostic test in a population.

The predictive value of a clinical test provides insight into the ability of a test to accurately determine the presence or absence of an abnormality or disease in a single person. The predictive value relies on the test sensitivity and specificity and the prevalence of disease in the population being tested. Thus, the positive predictive value is the probability of disease being present in a person with a positive test. Conversely, the negative predictive value is the probability of disease being absent in a person with a negative test. Bayes theorem states that the predictive value of a positive test is high in a population with high prevalence of disease, but the predictive value is low in a population with a low prevalence of disease. In other words, when testing a large number of individuals who are at low risk of heart disease, most of the positive tests will be false positives. For this reason, diagnostic stress tests are not recommended as a general screening tool but should instead only be performed when heart disease is suspected. As such, it is important that the proper population, techniques, and interpretation be applied to any clinical test to enhance the predictive value. It is this criterion in which studies in the literature are evaluated and recommendations are made for diagnostic testing. *Table 24-1* provides an overview of the sensitivity, specificity, and predictive values of various cardiac tests that are presented in the next several sections.

There are two statistical methods used to evaluate the overall value of a diagnostic test. The **diagnostic accuracy** is the ability of the test to make the correct determination — that is, be positive when disease is present and be negative when disease is absent — and holds the test at a single cutpoint. Diagnostic accuracy is calculated as the sum of true positives and true negatives divided by the total number of tests. For example, if a test has 85% diagnostic accuracy, then in 85% of the cases the decision (whether that decision was positive or negative) was correct. The other statistical method used to evaluate diagnostic tests is the **receiver operating characteristic curve** (ROC curve). This is a plot of sensitivity (true positive rate) on the *y* axis and specificity (*i.e.*, false positive rate) on the *x* axis (*Fig. 24-2*).

TABLE 24-1. Comparison of Tests for Sensitivity, Specificity, and Predictive Accuracy

Grouping	Studies, *n*	Total Patients, *N*	Sensitivity, %	Specificity, %	Predictive Accuracy, %
Standard exercise test	147	24,047	68	77	73
Thallium scintigraphy	59	6,038	85	85	85
SPECT	30	5,272	88	72	80
Adenosine SPECT	14	2,137	89	80	85
Exercise echocardiography	58	5,000	84	75	80
Dobutamine echocardiography	5	<1,000	88	84	86
Dobutamine scintigraphy	20	1,014	88	74	81
Coronary calcium score	16	3,683	60	70	65

SPECT, single-photon emission computed tomography.

Adapted from http://www.cardiology.palo-alto.med.va.gov/slides/ExerciseTest.ppt.

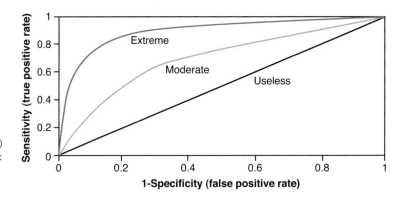

FIGURE 24-2. Receiver operating characteristic (ROC) curves. Three curves are shown illustrating diagnostic tests that are extremely, moderately, or not useful based on sensitivity and specificity.

The ROC curve is important because it gives information about the test performance through a range of values and allows one to determine the optimal cutpoint for a positive test. In general, an ROC curve with 50% of the area under the curve is considered useless (no different than tossing a coin), 70% is considered moderately useful, and >80% considered extremely useful.

HOW TO DECIDE WHICH DIAGNOSTIC TEST TO SELECT

As mentioned in the previous section, it is important to select the appropriate test for the patient and the indication (screening, diagnosis, prognosis, or management) (*Box 24-3*). The decision tree in *Figure 24-3* was developed by the ACC and the AHA (12). It can be used to illustrate to clinical exercise personnel how decisions are made during the diagnosis of CAD. The next several sections review the common diagnostic methods for CAD. These techniques are from the ACC/AHA guidelines for stable angina (10).

GRADED EXERCISE TESTING WITH ELECTROCARDIOGRAPHY

In-depth information regarding the performance and interpretation of graded exercise tests can be found in *Chapter 23* and in *GETP9 Chapters 5* and *6*. This section discusses only the decision-making process with respect to patient evaluation for ischemia. The decision to perform a graded exercise test should be made based on several criteria, including the pretest likelihood that the patient has CAD (see *GETP9, Table 5.1*), whether the patient can adequately exercise to symptom-limited maximum, and whether the ECG will be interpretable at peak exercise for possible ischemia.

Patients with repolarization abnormalities (*i.e.*, ST-T abnormalities, left bundle branch block [LBBB], LVH, using digoxin), are not appropriate candidates for graded exercise testing without imaging when the indication is screening or diagnosis of CAD. However, those with right bundle branch block or <1 mm ST-segment depression (not including V1–3) can be tested. *Box 24-4* lists the types of patients who are appropriate and inappropriate candidates for diagnostic testing using graded exercise testing without imaging. Those in the inappropriate category should be considered for stress testing with imaging, angiography if considered intermediate or high risk, or noncardiac testing or risk factor treatment if considered low risk. Depending on the interpretation of the graded exercise test (see *Chapter 23* and *GETP9 Chapter 6*), a recommendation for no further testing (negative test result) or for further testing (equivocal or positive test result) is made. When the indications are prognosis and management, information other than ECG findings becomes more valuable, and often testing without adjunctive imaging is performed.

There is a clinical workup "gap" between what is recommended by the ACC/AHA Guidelines for Exercise Testing and what is commonly practiced by the medical community when faced with making a decision about a patient requiring assessment for heart disease (1). The guidelines recommend that patients with chest discomfort, a normal resting ECG, and the ability to ambulate should be scheduled for an exercise test with ECG monitoring alone. In clinical practice, many physicians faced with this scenario begin with an imaging test. Instead, the guidelines recommend an exercise test with imaging as an initial diagnostic test for patients with an abnormal resting ECG, those who are unable to walk, and those

BOX 24-3	**Four Major Applications for Cardiovascular Testing**

Screening

Diagnosis

Prognosis

Management

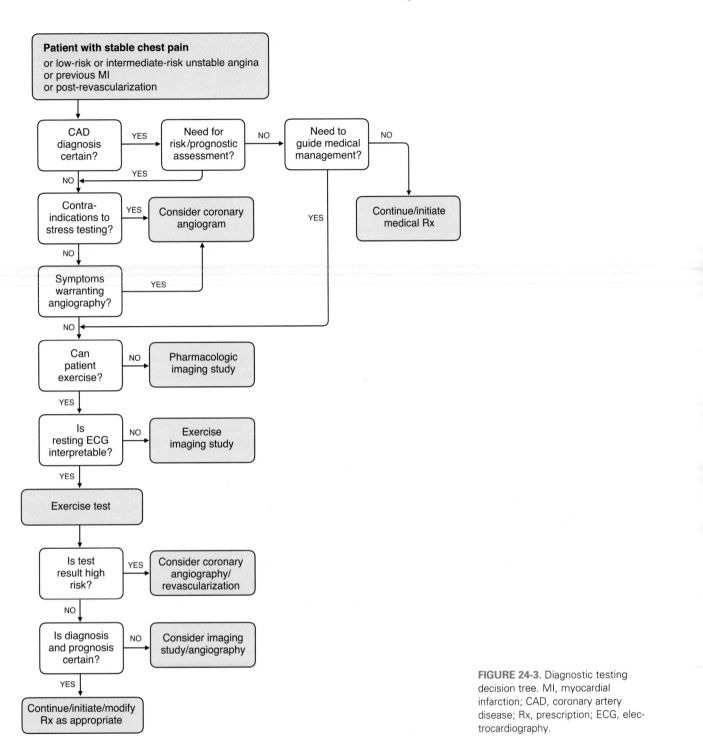

FIGURE 24-3. Diagnostic testing decision tree. MI, myocardial infarction; CAD, coronary artery disease; Rx, prescription; ECG, electrocardiography.

with a history of coronary bypass surgery. Although this strategy provides a slight improvement in predictive accuracy over the stress ECG combined with the Duke Treadmill Score (20) (see *GETP9, Figure 6.2*), it does so at a significantly increased cost. Many believe the one exception to this rule is women. Women commonly have exercise-induced ECG changes without ischemia resulting in lower sensitivity and specificity, thus, in women with chest discomfort, adjunctive imaging is commonly performed (22).

IMAGING METHODS

Imaging techniques for the diagnosis of CAD provide slightly higher sensitivity and specificity than exercise testing with ECG analysis. Candidates for imaging studies, versus stress ECG, are those with an uninterpretable ECG and those unable to exercise to a level high enough to produce an adequate myocardial stress. In general, imaging studies allow for the patient to be further risk stratified to either a low- or high-risk group. If the test

---

BOX 24-4 **Candidates for Exercise Electrocardiographic Assessment (Regular Stress Testing without Imaging)**

APPROPRIATE CANDIDATES/APPLICATIONS

Able to exercise to achieve adequate myocardial stress (*i.e.*, >85% of predicted peak heart rate or double product greater than ~24,000)

If repolarization abnormality is either right bundle branch block or <1 mm ST-segment depression not caused by digoxin use

Screening for significant coronary artery disease (CAD) when the 10-yr Framingham risk is >20%

Diagnosis of chest discomfort in intermediate-risk patients based on age, sex, and symptoms

Prognosis of patients with established CAD, heart failure, and for entry into cardiac rehabilitation

Guiding medical and revascularization therapy in patients with established CAD

INAPPROPRIATE CANDIDATES

Anyone, especially women, with baseline ST-T wave abnormalities

Low or high risk of ischemic heart disease, including asymptomatic patients with possible ischemia during ambulatory electrocardiographic monitoring or those with acute coronary syndromes

Preexisting repolarization abnormalities (left bundle branch block, left ventricular hypertrophy with strain, digoxin, ventricular pacing, nonspecific ST-segment depression >1 mm)

Preexcitation syndrome (Wolff-Parkinson-White syndrome)

Patients unable to exercise to an adequate myocardial stress level (*i.e.*, <85% of predicted peak heart rate or double product less than ~24,000) because of arthritis, pulmonary disease, or peripheral vascular disease

---

is equivocal, a different imaging test or coronary angiography may be suggested as a next step in the diagnostic process. These imaging techniques are categorized as echocardiography or myocardial perfusion imaging and are reviewed in the next several sections (also see *GETP9, Chapter 5*).

ECHOCARDIOGRAPHY

Over the past 25 yr, echocardiography has become the second most frequently ordered test in the evaluation of cardiac patients after the resting ECG. With its high resolution, echocardiography provides an accurate anatomic view of the heart. Doppler allows the evaluation of the heart physiology (*e.g.*, blood flow). Echocardiography and Doppler are almost always used in combination and provide an assessment of the pathophysiology of cardiac disease processes. The principle of cardiac ultrasound is that high-frequency sound waves bouncing off cardiac structures and returning to the transducer provide information regarding that structure. The time it takes for the sound wave to return to the transducer is twice the time (which can be converted to distance) that it takes to travel from the transducer to the structure, such as a wall of the LV or a valve. By analyzing all of the returning sound waves with computers, it is possible to identify multiple structures and their relationships to each other. This allows the measurement of chamber size and wall motion, as well as identifying valvular structures and pericardial effusions.

Cardiac Doppler assessment uses the principle of Doppler shift to evaluate intracardiac blood flow. The frequency of the returning sound wave varies depending on whether the object is moving toward or away from the transducer. For example, objects moving toward the transducer reflect a sound wave with a higher frequency than the emitted sound wave, whereas objects traveling away from the transducer have a lower frequency. Therefore, blood flow toward the transducer can be distinguished from blood flow away from the transducer. Using Doppler, blood velocity and volumetric flow can be measured to determine intracardiac gradients, valve areas, valvular regurgitation, and intracardiac pressures. The addition of color to Doppler created much excitement in the world of echocardiography. The two dimensional (2D) display is enhanced with easier identification of velocity and direction of flow. Two colors are used: blue represents flow away from the transducer; red indicates flow shifts toward it. Velocity is demonstrated by the shade of the color: the lighter the color, the higher the velocity; the darker colors indicate slower velocities. Turbulent flow created by stenosis or regurgitation is represented by a mosaic pattern of color, whereas laminar or streamlined flow has a solid color that looks smooth. Three dimensional (3D) echocardiography is now being used in a small number of facilities, especially research and teaching hospitals. Although more costly, 3D echocardiograms provide higher quality images and can be used in place of conventional 2D in exercise echocardiography. However, despite the better images, a study that is "technically difficult" in 2D will also be "technically difficult" in 3D. At this time, the clinical significance of differences between these two types of echocardiographic imaging is minimal.

Exercise echocardiography combines surface echocardiography and graded exercise testing (2,23). The echocardiographic images are obtained at rest and within 90 s after exercise. These images are then viewed using a side-by-side digital display format that allows the visualization of cardiac function both at rest and during exercise. Exercise echocardiography allows assessment of wall motion abnormalities, ejection fraction, and systolic and diastolic function. The normal response to exercise is for the LV to decrease in size, ejection fraction to increase, and augmentation of LV wall motion to occur. Patients with ischemia frequently have normal wall motion at rest, and during exercise develop hypokinesis or akinesis of the LV wall(s) being supplied by an artery with a stenonis of 70% or more. Patients with a previous MI may have hypokinesis, akinesis, or possibly dyskinesis of the infarcted wall at rest as well as with exercise. Dilation of the LV with exercise is a sign of triple-vessel disease.

It is ideal to use exercise to deliver the increased myocardial oxygen demand because this best replicates the physiologic processes leading to ischemia. However, some patients may not be able to perform exercise. Intravenous dobutamine, a β-adrenergic–stimulating agent, offers a pharmacologic alternative for patients who are unable to exercise. Infusion of an incremental dose of dobutamine evokes a positive inotropic and chronotropic response. Unlike dipyridamole, regadenoson, and adenosine, dobutamine closely parallels the exercise response by creating an oxygen supply and demand imbalance. In cases in which a patient who is scheduled for a "nonexercise" stress test is actually able to perform an adequate amount of exercise, an alternate plan using graded exercise testing should be discussed. Dobutamine echocardiography has a special value in the detection of myocardial viability. In a hypokinetic segment at rest that is viable but served by a critically diseased vessel, low-dose dobutamine will increase augmentation in this segment that will degrade to hypokinesis and then akinesis at higher levels. This so-called triple-phase response has a high predictive value for myocardial viability and response to revascularization.

When to Use Echocardiography

Echocardiography is useful at *rest* in patients who present with symptoms suggestive of valvular disorders, pericardial disease, or LV dysfunction. *Exercise* echocardiography is useful for those with suspected ischemic heart disease and improves the predictive accuracy of the graded exercise test from 75% to 85%. This improved predictive accuracy remains even after excluding normal submaximal stress tests and nondiagnostic exercise ECGs. An increased test predictive accuracy, compared with exercise ECG assessment alone, has also been observed in a population with a high prevalence of

| BOX 24-5 | Candidates for Experience Echocardiography (Stress-Echo) |

APPROPRIATE CANDIDATES

Those with uninterpretable resting ECG including baseline ST-T wave abnormalities

Intermediate pretest probability of coronary artery disease

Coronary calcium score ≥400

INAPPROPRIATE CANDIDATES

Patients with multiple myocardial infarctions

Those with complex wall motion abnormalities (such as those seen in LBBB and paced rhythms)

Coronary calcium score <100

Those with a poor imaging window (e.g., obese patients and patients with chronic obstructive pulmonary disease)

Patients with a history or high risk of serious arrhythmias and/or AICDs, use of dobutamine is contraindicated

Candidates for revascularization with questions concerning myocardial viability (may be more suitable to perform a radionuclide test)

LBBB, left bundle branch block; AICDs, automatic implantable cardioverter defibrillators.

symptomatic CAD (2). Specificity is also enhanced by exercise echocardiography (2).

Box 24-5 identifies candidates for exercise echocardiographic testing and those for whom testing would be inappropriate. In addition, stress echocardiography is useful in patients with a high likelihood of false positive test results, such as women, and in patients with concurrent valvular or primary myocardial disease. Stress echocardiography is less useful in patients with multiple MIs, complex wall motion abnormalities, or a poor imaging window (*e.g.*, obese individuals or those with chronic obstructive pulmonary disease).

MYOCARDIAL PERFUSION IMAGING

Radionuclide imaging, in combination with exercise or pharmacologic stress, is a commonly applied means for diagnosing CAD. Use of radionuclide imaging is indicated in follow-up of patients with abnormal ECG test findings and in the diagnostic evaluation of women, patients taking digitalis, and those with an abnormal resting ECG (*i.e.*, LBBB, LVH, Wolff-Parkinson-White syndrome, intraventricular conduction defects, and resting ST-T wave abnormalities) (3). It is also useful for the assessment of myocardial perfusion in patients with angiographically documented CAD and to study myocardial viability.

Thallium 201 (^{201}Tl) and technetium 99m (^{99m}Tc) injected at peak exercise and at rest are proportionally distributed within the myocardium in relation to regional myocardial blood flow and muscle viability. Newer ^{99m}Tc-based radiopharmaceutical flow tracers, such as sestamibi, provide diagnostic benefits over ^{201}Tl on the basis of their physical and biological attributes. ^{99m}Tc sestamibi has a higher energy output and a shorter half-life than ^{201}Tl. This allows administration of a larger dose, providing superior images (3). Also, the traditional stress–rest ^{201}Tl scan can be replaced with a protocol in which the rest images are acquired before stress, reducing the time required for the study and allowing acquisition of ECG-gated functional images.

In a normal myocardium, rest and stress images show accumulation of the isotope throughout the LV, reflecting integrity of regional blood supply. In areas of decreased perfusion, there is delayed uptake and slower washout. The presence of a perfusion defect on the stress images that was not present on the rest images suggests ischemia. Areas of scar from previous infarction characteristically show no uptake, either at rest or with stress. In addition to uniformity of isotopic uptake, ventricular size, wall motion, ejection fraction, and wall thickness can be assessed.

The diagnostic accuracy of ^{201}Tl and ^{99m}Tc are similar (7). Recent advances in radionuclide imaging, such as quantification of radionuclide data, tomographic imaging, and single-photon emission computed tomography (SPECT) have enhanced the sensitivity and specificity beyond that provided by planar imaging. A review of studies using SPECT analysis indicated an overall sensitivity of 89% and a specificity of 75% (18).

As stated previously, it is always best to use exercise to deliver the myocardial stress in patients. However, some patients may not be able to exercise. In these cases, pharmacologic techniques, including the use of dipyridamole, regadenoson, or adenosine, which are coronary artery selective vasodilators, can be used. With exercise, the myocardial oxygen demand is increased, and after it exceeds the ability of oxygen delivery by the blood, ischemia can be detected, if present. Use of the coronary artery vasodilators results in a mismatch of blood flow increase between the normal and diseased coronary arteries that can be detected on the perfusion imaging studies. It is important for the clinical personnel to realize that when monitoring the ECG during radionuclide stress tests with these vasodilators, if ischemic ST changes do occur, they have a high positive predictive value for significant CAD and should always be flagged (7).

When to Use Myocardial Perfusion Imaging

Myocardial perfusion imaging is most useful in patients who are intermediate or high risk for CAD, have abnormal ECG findings (LBBB, paced rhythm), or have poor echocardiographic images (*Box 24-6*). Additionally, those who cannot exercise are candidates for pharmacologic imaging studies using dipyridamole, regadenoson, adenosine, or dobutamine. However, adenosine and dipyridamole should not be used in patients with reactive airway disease because severe bronchospasm may occur. Additionally, these vasodilators plus regadenoson should not be used in those with sinus node dysfunction or second or third degree AV block unless the patient has

---

| BOX 24-6 | **Candidates for Radionuclear Imaging (Stress-Nuclear)** |

APPROPRIATE CANDIDATES

Those with baseline ST-T wave abnormalities

Those who have an uninterpretable resting electrocardiogram (*i.e.*, left bundle branch block, paced rhythms, left ventricular hypertrophy, digoxin, >1 mm ST-segment depression) or preexcitation syndrome (Wolff-Parkinson-White syndrome)

Use in conjunction with pharmacologic modes if patient cannot exercise to achieve adequate/diagnostic heart rate or systolic blood pressure

Intermediate pretest probability of CAD

Those with a poor imaging window for echocardiogram

Coronary calcium score ≥400

INAPPROPRIATE CANDIDATES

In those patients with a history of bronchospasm or reactive airway disease, use of adenosine or dipyridamole is contraindicated

In those patients with a history of a high-degree AV block without a permanent pacemaker, use of regadenoson, adenosine, and dipyridamole is contraindicated

Coronary calcium score <100

....

AV, atrioventricular; CAD, coronary artery disease.

a functioning artificial pacemaker. Also, dobutamine in certain cases should not be used because of the risks of serious arrhythmias.

POSITRON EMISSION TOMOGRAPHY

Positron emission tomography (PET) scanning is one of the most accurate methods for noninvasively identifying and assessing the severity of CAD. There are two specific clinical applications for PET scanning in patients with suspected CAD. The first is the noninvasive detection of coronary artery stenosis. This is performed using a PET perfusion agent at rest and during pharmacologic vasodilation similar to that done for pharmacologic nuclear scintigraphy (4). Radionuclide tracers used to diagnose coronary artery stenosis are nitrogen-13, ammonia, and rubidium-82. Reviews of PET indicate higher sensitivity and specificity (~93%) than with SPECT. In institutions with both SPECT and PET scanning, PET scanning is typically reserved for patients with equivocal SPECT scans. Recent data suggest PET scanning generates superior imaging in the obese compared with nuclear scintigraphy because of the higher energy of the radiotracers used and less attenuation of the nuclear image data with PET acquisition. The second and more frequent clinical application of PET is the assessment of myocardial viability in patients with CAD and LV impairment, which is useful in determining if revascularization would be beneficial. Hibernating myocardium can be differentiated from scar using fluorine-18 fluorodeoxyglucose. In a summary of three studies that included 313 patients, if PET scanning demonstrated myocardial viability, mortality was reduced from 41% in a medically treated population to 8% in the surgically revascularized group (24). However, more recent data has demonstrated no significant reduction in cardiac events in those with severe LV dysfunction who received care based on PET results versus those who received standard care (5).

CARDIAC MAGNETIC RESONANCE IMAGING

Magnetic resonance imaging (MRI) provides an anatomic view of the heart by measuring the emitted electromagnetic waves from resonating nuclei and locating these nuclei in space. Because of a natural high contrast that exists between blood and cardiac tissue, no contrast agent is needed to identify the blood pool. In cardiology, MRI is used primarily to evaluate the patient for structural heart disease. The most frequent uses are to (a) assess the extent of damage to the LV as a complication of ischemic heart disease; (b) assess the type of cardiomyopathy and quantify physiologic parameters, such as wall stress and LV volume; (c) visualize the pericardium and assess its thickness in pericardial disease; (d) evaluate intracardiac and pericardial neoplastic disease; (e) provide information regarding morphology, size of

shunts, and valvular function in congenital heart disease; and (f) evaluate the thoracic aorta for dissection, false lumens, periaortic disease, and abnormalities of the thoracic aortic arch (16).

Cardiac MRI can be used as the imaging method for pharmacologic stress with adenosine, dipyridamole, or dobutamine. Like echocardiography, wall motion can be evaluated. In addition, the degree of perfusion and late enhancement of the myocardium can be seen, giving the clinician an idea of how much ventricular damage is present.

CORONARY COMPUTED TOMOGRAPHY ANGIOGRAPHY

Computed tomography (CT) has been used for decades to image motionless solid organs, such as the brain, abdominal organs, etc. However, CT of the heart has only recently been mastered, using technology that acquires images very rapidly and timed (gated) to the cardiac cycle. This technology is called multidetector-row cardiac CT angiography (CTA). This form of imaging supplanted earlier forms of electron-beam computed tomography (EBCT), which could only evaluate the coronaries for the presence of calcium. Modern CTA gives a full evaluation of the degree of coronary calcium and generates a calcium score. Anatomic studies indicate that all human atheroma become calcified, beginning at the necrotic core of the lesion. Thus, the presence of coronary calcification represents the presence of atherosclerosis. The U.S. Centers for Medicare and Medicaid Services (CMS) approved reimbursement for CTA in 2006, however, reimbursement from other carriers is still regionally determined. CTA generates images of the coronary arteries that are comparable to conventional angiography. A randomized trial by Goldstein et al. demonstrated that CTA was superior to conventional chest pain and stress test evaluations done in emergency department patients with acute chest discomfort (13). Given the much lower cost of CTA compared with some forms of stress imaging, a growing number of patients are expected to be referred for this form of testing. The circumstances that are considered appropriate for use of CTA include intermediate pretest probability of CAD, uninterpretable baseline ECG, inability to exercise, or uninterpretable/equivocal completed stress test with or without imaging (26) (*Box 24-7*). Now, clinicians are witnessing the integration of information from multiple imaging modalities. A common scenario is the discovery of moderate CAD by CTA. The next question is whether the lesion is hemodynamically significant, calling for a form of stress imaging. The most sophisticated approach thus far is CTA-PET, in which patients in the same scanner undergo anatomic CTA with pharmacologic stress imaging using PET (8). Computer algorithms then attempt to match up coronary anatomy with perfusion territories seen on PET.

BOX 24-7	Candidates for Coronary Computed Tomographic Angiography

APPROPRIATE CANDIDATES	INAPPROPRIATE CANDIDATES
Suspected coronary artery disease (CAD) based on history and physical (chest discomfort)	Asymptomatic patients
Intermediate pretest probability of CAD	Significant chronic kidney disease or allergic reaction to iodinated contrast
Uninterpretable baseline electrocardiogram, inability to exercise	Hyperparathyroidism or known disorders of calcium/phosphate metabolism
Uninterpretable/equivocal completed stress test with or without imaging	Medically unstable patients (noncardiac medical problems)

CORONARY ANGIOGRAPHY

Coronary angiography using the cardiac catheterization technique is considered the gold standard for assessing the presence of CAD. Given the time, expense, and invasive nature of the test, it is often considered a last resort for diagnostic testing among the large menu of tests currently available.

The technique requires the placement of a catheter through an incision in the common femoral artery (done in >95% of cases), radial artery, or brachial artery. The catheter is then guided through the artery to the aortic arch and the openings of the coronary arteries. Iodinated contrast media is injected during radiographic fluoroscopy, which allows for its visualization while flowing through the coronary tree. An area of narrowing can then be identified, located with respect to the coronary artery anatomy, and quantified for the amount of stenosis within a given artery. Angiography cannot determine if a coronary artery lesion is flow limiting and causing ischemia during stress, and, therefore, most patients undergoing this test are previously symptomatic. However, the assumption can be made that an identified lesion is causing ischemia. Generally, coronary artery stenosis of 70% or more is required to cause ischemia. Those lesions between 50% and 70% of lumen diameter are considered borderline significant and are only considered clinically important if they correspond to abnormalities seen on the stress imaging test, or the patient is experiencing typical angina. Lesions ≤50% of lumen diameter are not generally thought to cause ischemia.

When to Use Angiography

Referral for angiography is appropriate when noninvasive assessment cannot be made because of contraindications, test inadequacy, or in symptomatic patients who are considered to be at high risk for CAD either before or after noninvasive testing. Additionally, patients who have an equivocal noninvasive test, and thus an uncertain diagnosis, are also potential candidates for coronary angiography. Most commonly, coronary angiography is appropriate for patients with acute symptoms (acute coronary syndromes) in the hospital and for those outpatients with positive noninvasive studies discussed previously. *Box 24-8* presents appropriate and inappropriate patients for angiography referral. A trend is to combine the diagnostic and therapeutic parts of the procedure with the aim in most patients to perform angiography and move to coronary angioplasty with stenting during the same procedural setting.

INTRAVASCULAR ULTRASOUND

In addition to the standard cardiac catheterization assessments commonly performed, many laboratories also offer intracoronary diagnostic procedures to evaluate

BOX 24-8	Cardiac Catheterization and Coronary Angiography

APPROPRIATE CANDIDATES	INAPPROPRIATE CANDIDATES
Positive stress testing with or without imaging	Asymptomatic patients
Very high pretest probability of coronary artery disease (CAD) based on clinical evaluation	Patients who are deemed not candidates for revascularization
Known CAD in the setting of acute coronary syndrome	Significant chronic kidney disease or allergic reaction to iodinated contrast (relative contraindications)

the severity of coronary artery stenosis. Atherosclerotic plaque development in the wall of the coronary artery results in a remodeling process of the entire blood vessel, which helps to maintain the lumen diameter. Traditional coronary angiography allows only for the visualization of the lumen of the coronary artery and thus may underestimate the size of a plaque in a remodeled artery. Also, coronary angiographic evaluation of coronary artery stenosis frequently identifies a lesion that appears "borderline significant" (*i.e.*, stenoses of 50%–70%). Further evaluation of these lesions using intravascular ultrasound (IVUS), intravascular Doppler (coronary flow velocity), and fractional flow reserve helps to determine which of these stenoses requires revascularization with either percutaneous coronary intervention (PCI) or coronary bypass surgery.

During diagnostic evaluation, IVUS provides the visualization of the lumen and wall of the vessel as well as the size of the plaque. During interventional angiography, IVUS can be used after angioplasty to evaluate vessel patency and to look for complications such as coronary artery dissection. Additionally, IVUS is used in coronary stenting to provide information about the deployment of the stent. The most common use of IVUS at this time is to assess the severity and significance of left main coronary lesions, which are found incidentally. These lesions may not have been suggested by noninvasive imaging but, when present, can lead to higher rates of sudden death.

Intravascular Doppler techniques provide information about the amount of obstruction to blood flow from an individual plaque within a coronary artery. By measuring the velocity of blood flow at the level of the lesion and determining the vessel's cross-sectional area, an estimate of coronary blood flow distal to the coronary stenosis can be made. Adenosine, a vasodilator that is infused into the coronary artery, is used to assess coronary artery vasodilation. Normal coronary arteries increase blood flow by 250% or more in response to the adenosine challenge. Increases of <250% suggest that the distal vasculature is maximally dilated and that the coronary stenosis is limiting vasodilation and thus negatively affecting blood flow.

Fractional flow reserve is a measure of the pressure across a section of a coronary artery. It is performed using small guide wires capable of measuring pressure. A decrease in pressure across a coronary artery stenosis indicates a reduction in blood flow. Fractional flow reserve of <0.75 suggests that the lesion is significantly affecting blood flow and is likely resulting in ischemia.

These adjunctive techniques require the coronary arteries to be instrumented with wires and equipment, which runs the risk of inducing coronary ischemia or infarction. Thus, they are infrequently done and are reserved for the most difficult cases in the catheterization laboratory.

SUMMARY

Diagnostic testing in cardiovascular disease is done for screening, diagnosing, assessing prognosis, and guiding therapy. Exercise capacity is the most important prognostic variable for cardiac and all-cause mortality. Graded exercise testing, with or without imaging (echocardiography or radionuclide methods), CTA, and coronary angiography are the primary methods to detect CAD. Cardiac MRI has emerged as the test of choice for structural and congenital heart disease, particularly when it involves the great vessels and aorta. In the future, screening CTA to identify preclinical disease or the status of existing disease composition and structure may become main stream and is likely to change the practice of preventive cardiology. The concept of reduction in cardiac risk to treatment of known and proven CAD by CTA is likely to gain popularity among clinicians and patients alike.

REFERENCES

1. *ACC/AHA 2002 Guideline Update for Exercise Testing A Report of the American College of Cardiology/American Heart Association Task Force on Practice Guidelines (Committee on Exercise Testing)* [Internet]. Dallas (TX): American College of Cardiology/American Heart Association; [cited 2011 Mar 14]. Available from: http://www.americanheart.org/downloadable/heart/1032279013658exercise.pdf

2. Armstrong WF, Pellikka PA, Ryan T, Crouse L, Zoghbi WA. Stress echocardiography: recommendations for performance and interpretation of stress echocardiography. Stress Echocardiography Task Force of the Nomenclature and Standards Committee of the American Society of Echocardiography. *J Am Soc Echocardiogr.* 1998;11(1):97–104.

3. *ASNC Imaging Guidelines for Nuclear Cardiology Procedures: Stress Protocols and Tracers* [Internet]. Bethesda (MD): American Society of Nuclear Cardiology; [cited 2011 Jul 12]. Available from: http://www.snc.org/imageuploads/ImagingGuidelinesStressProtocols021109.pdf

4. Bateman TM. Cardiac positron emission tomography and the role of adenosine pharmacologic stress. *Am J Cardiol.* 2004;94(2A):19D–24D; discussion 24D–5D.

5. Beanlands RS, Nichol G, Huszti E, et al. F-18-fluorodeoxyglucose positron emission tomography imaging-assisted management of patients with severe left ventricular dysfunction and suspected coronary disease: a randomized, controlled trial (PARR-2). *J Am Coll Cardiol.* 2007;50(20):2002–12.

6. Chobanian AV, Bakris GL, Black HR, et al. The Seventh Report of the Joint National Committee on Prevention, Detection, Evaluation, and Treatment of High Blood Pressure: the JNC 7 report. *JAMA.* 2003;289(19):2560–72.

7. Cortigiani L, Lombardi M, Michelassi C, Paolini EA, Nannini E. Significance of myocardial ischemic electrocardiographic changes during dipyridamole stress echocardiography. *Am J Cardiol.* 1998;82(9):1008–12.

8. Di Carli MF, Dorbala S, Hachamovitch R. Integrated cardiac PET-CT for the diagnosis and management of CAD. *J Nucl Cardiol.* 2006;13(2):139–44.

9. Diamond GA, Forrester JS. Analysis of probability as an aid in the clinical diagnosis of coronary-artery disease. *N Engl J Med.* 1979;300(24):1350–8.

10. Fraker TD Jr, Fihn SD, Gibbons RJ, et al. 2007 chronic angina focused update of the ACC/AHA 2002 Guidelines for the management of patients with chronic stable angina: a report of the

American College of Cardiology/American Heart Association Task Force on Practice Guidelines Writing Group to develop the focused update of the 2002 Guidelines for the management of patients with chronic stable angina. *Circulation.* 2007;116(23):2762–72.

11. Franklin BA. Survival of the fittest: evidence for high-risk and cardioprotective fitness levels. *Curr Sports Med Rep.* 2002;1(5):257–9.

12. Gibbons RJ, Balady GJ, Beasley JW, et al. ACC/AHA Guidelines for Exercise Testing. A report of the American College of Cardiology/American Heart Association Task Force on Practice Guidelines (Committee on Exercise Testing). *J Am Coll Cardiol.* 1997;30(1):260–311.

13. Goldstein JA, Gallagher MJ, O'Neill WW, Ross MA, O'Neil BJ, Raff GL. A randomized controlled trial of multi-slice coronary computed tomography for evaluation of acute chest pain. *J Am Coll Cardiol.* 2007;49(8):863–71.

14. Greenland P, Alpert JS, Beller GA, et al. 2010 ACCF/AHA guideline for assessment of cardiovascular risk in asymptomatic adults: a report of the American College of Cardiology Foundation/American Heart Association Task Force on Practice Guidelines. *Circulation.* 2010;122(25):e584–636.

15. Grundy SM, Cleeman JI, Merz CN, et al. Implications of recent clinical trials for the National Cholesterol Education Program Adult Treatment Panel III guidelines. *Circulation.* 2004;110(2):227–39.

16. Hendel RC, Patel MR, Kramer CM, et al. ACCF/ACR/SCCT/SCMR/ASNC/NASCI/SCAI/SIR 2006 appropriateness criteria for cardiac computed tomography and cardiac magnetic resonance imaging: a report of the American College of Cardiology Foundation Quality Strategic Directions Committee Appropriateness Criteria Working Group, American College of Radiology, Society of Cardiovascular Computed Tomography, Society for Cardiovascular Magnetic Resonance, American Society of Nuclear Cardiology, North American Society for Cardiac Imaging, Society for Cardiovascular Angiography and Interventions, and Society of Interventional Radiology. *J Am Coll Cardiol.* 2006;48(7):1475–97.

17. Jessup M, Abraham WT, Casey DE, et al. 2009 focused update: ACCF/AHA Guidelines for the Diagnosis and Management of Heart Failure in Adults: a report of the American College of Cardiology Foundation/American Heart Association Task Force on Practice Guidelines: developed in collaboration with the International Society for Heart and Lung Transplantation. *Circulation.* 2009;119(14):1977–2016.

18. Klocke FJ, Baird MG, Lorell BH, et al. ACC/AHA/ASNC guidelines for the clinical use of cardiac radionuclide imaging—executive summary: a report of the American College of Cardiology/American Heart Association Task Force on Practice Guidelines (ACC/AHA/ASNC Committee to Revise the 1995 Guidelines for the Clinical Use of Cardiac Radionuclide Imaging). *J Am Coll Cardiol.* 2003;42(7):1318–33.

19. Lauer M, Froelicher ES, Williams M, Kligfield P, American Heart Association Council on Clinical Cardiology, Subcommittee on Exercise, Cardiac Rehabilitation, and Prevention. Exercise testing in asymptomatic adults: a statement for professionals from the American Heart Association Council on Clinical Cardiology, Subcommittee on Exercise, Cardiac Rehabilitation, and Prevention. *Circulation.* 2005;112(5):771–6.

20. Mark DB, Shaw L, Harrell FE Jr, et al. Prognostic value of a treadmill exercise score in outpatients with suspected coronary artery disease. *N Engl J Med.* 1991;325(12):849–53.

21. McCullough PA, Gallagher MJ, Dejong AT, et al. Cardiorespiratory fitness and short-term complications after bariatric surgery. *Chest.* 2006;130(2):517–25.

22. Mieres JH, Shaw LJ, Arai A, et al. Role of noninvasive testing in the clinical evaluation of women with suspected coronary artery disease: Consensus statement from the Cardiac Imaging Committee, Council on Clinical Cardiology, and the Cardiovascular Imaging and Intervention Committee, Council on Cardiovascular Radiology and Intervention, American Heart Association. *Circulation.* 2005;111(5):682–96.

23. Quinones MA, Douglas PS, Foster E, et al. American College of Cardiology/American Heart Association clinical competence statement on echocardiography: a report of the American College of Cardiology/American Heart Association/American College of Physicians—American Society of Internal Medicine Task Force on Clinical Competence. *Circulation.* 2003;107(7):1068–89.

24. Schelbert HR. 18F-deoxyglucose and the assessment of myocardial viability. *Semin Nucl Med.* 2002;32(1):60–9.

25. Sox HC Jr, Hickam DH, Marton KI, et al. Using the patient's history to estimate the probability of coronary artery disease: a comparison of primary care and referral practices. *Am J Med.* 1990;89(1):7–14.

26. Taylor AJ, Cerqueira M, Hodgson JM, et al. ACCF/SCCT/ACR/AHA/ASE/ASNC/NASCI/SCAI/SCMR 2010 appropriate use criteria for cardiac computed tomography. A report of the American College of Cardiology Foundation Appropriate Use Criteria Task Force, the Society of Cardiovascular Computed Tomography, the American College of Radiology, the American Heart Association, the American Society of Echocardiography, the American Society of Nuclear Cardiology, the North American Society for Cardiovascular Imaging, the Society for Cardiovascular Angiography and Interventions, and the Society for Cardiovascular Magnetic Resonance. *J Am Coll Cardiol.* 2010;56(22):1864–94.

27. Wilson PW, D'Agostino RB, Levy D, Belanger AM, Silbershatz H, Kannel WB. Prediction of coronary heart disease using risk factor categories. *Circulation.* 1998;97(18):1837–47.

SELECTED REFERENCES FOR FURTHER READING

Cheitlin MD, Armstrong WF, Aurigemma GP, et al. ACC/AHA/ASE 2003 guideline update for the clinical application of echocardiography: a report of the American College of Cardiology/American Heart Association Task Force on Practice Guidelines (ACC/AHA/ASE Committee to Update the 1997 Guidelines for the Clinical Application of Echocardiography); 2003. Available from: http://www.acc.org/clinical/guidelines/echo/index.pdf

Ehrman JK, Gordon PM, Visich PS, Keteyian SJ. *Clinical Exercise Physiology.* 2nd ed. Champaign (IL): Human Kinetics; 2008. 691 p.

Myers J, Arena R, Franklin B, et al. Recommendations for clinical exercise laboratories: a scientific statement from the American Heart Association. *Circulation.* 2009;119(24):3144–3161.

INTERNET RESOURCES

- American College of Cardiology: http://www.acc.org
- American Heart Association: Scientific statements and practice guidelines topic list: http://www.my.americanheart.org/professional/StatementsGuidelines/Statements-Guidelines_UCM_316885_SubHomePage.jsp
- International Atherosclerosis Society: http://www.athero.org

CHAPTER 25

Diagnostic Procedures in Patients with Pulmonary Diseases

Lung disease can generally be classified into one of the three following categories: obstructive, restrictive, or vascular. Patients with lung disease often develop shortness of breath precipitated by exercise or strenuous conditions as the first symptom regardless of the type of disease process that is present. Although this presenting symptom is the same, the pathophysiology associated with the development of such symptomatology is varied depending on the underlying disease process. This chapter addresses the pathophysiology and associated limitations of each of these disease processes and the clinical assessment of patients with lung disease.

NORMAL VENTILATORY MECHANICS

During normal inhalation, the diaphragm contracts and moves downward, and the rib cage moves upward and outward. Pressure within the thorax decreases, and atmospheric pressure drives air through the nose/mouth and into the lungs. During normal exhalation, the diaphragm relaxes and moves upward, and the rib cage moves inward, increasing intrathoracic pressure to drive air from the lungs to the mouth. Exhalation is assisted by the elastic recoil of the lung parenchyma.

The larger airways remain open during inhalation and exhalation because they are supported by cartilage in their walls. As the size of the airway decreases, the amount of cartilage present in the airway wall is reduced. The smallest airways have no cartilage and are tethered open by the surrounding meshwork of the lung, which includes the alveoli. During inhalation, these smaller airways are pulled open by the expansion of the lungs, resulting in traction of the airways. During exhalation, these airways may collapse because of the positive intrathoracic pressure causing a reduction in the lung volume and traction over the smaller airways (*Fig. 25-1*).

OBSTRUCTIVE AIRWAY DISEASES

CHRONIC OBSTRUCTIVE PULMONARY DISEASE

Chronic obstructive pulmonary disease (COPD) is a common disorder characterized by progressive and persistent airflow limitation that is usually associated with chronic inflammation of the airways (26). Symptoms develop insidiously over many years and include dyspnea

KEY TERMS

Asthma: A continuum of disease processes characterized by inflammation of the airway wall.

Chronic bronchitis: A clinical diagnosis for patients who have chronic cough and sputum production.

Chronic obstructive pulmonary disease (COPD): A group of lung diseases (*e.g.*, emphysema, chronic bronchitis) that result in airflow obstruction.

Dyspnea: The perception of shortness of breath.

Emphysema: A pathologic or anatomic description marked by abnormal permanent enlargement of the respiratory bronchioles and alveoli accompanied by destruction of the lung parenchyma.

Hypercapnia: Excess carbon dioxide in the blood.

Hypoxemia: Deficient oxygenation of the blood.

Polycythemia: Excess red blood cells often secondary to hypoxemia.

Pulmonary hypertension: An elevation in the blood pressure within the arteries of the lung.

Restrictive lung disease: A group of diseases characterized by the inability to normally inflate the lungs.

Timed walk test: One of various tests (*e.g.*, 6-min walk test, shuttle walk test, endurance shuttle walk test) used to assess functional status. The distance walked over a certain period of time is measured during these tests.

Vascular lung disease: A group of diseases that affect the vascular supply (pulmonary arteries, capillaries, and veins) of the lungs.

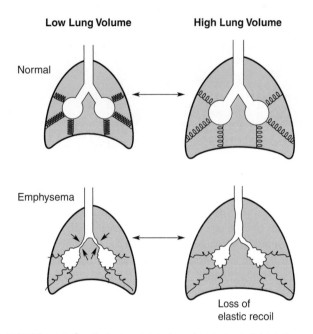

FIGURE 25-1. Small airways are tethered open by radial traction of lung tissue. Airway caliber depends on recoil of the lung, which is greater at high lung volume; hence, airway caliber is also greater at a high lung volume. In diseases in which elastic recoil is lost, small airways are prone to dynamic collapse when pressure outside the airway becomes more positive, as during forced exhalation.

at rest and with exertion, cough, and sputum production. Two obstructive airway diseases include emphysema and chronic bronchitis. Although these are often considered to be distinct entities, their physiologic and clinical features often overlap in individual patients.

COPD is characterized by nonuniform narrowing of airways secondary to inflammation. The airway narrowing increases resistance to airflow and results in uneven distribution of ventilation and expiratory flow limitation (*Fig. 25-2*). Loss of elastic recoil of the lungs occurs, causing the small airways to close at an abnormally high lung volume, resulting in an increase in residual volume (RV) at the end of a forced exhalation (also known as air trapping). Air trapping causes an increase in the total lung capacity (TLC) and causes the diaphragm to flatten, ultimately causing a mechanical disadvantage for contraction (*Fig. 25-3*). All of these mechanisms lead to an increase in the work of breathing, which results in dyspnea for the patient.

Emphysema

Emphysema is a type of COPD in which destruction of lung parenchyma and smaller airways occurs. Various mechanisms are responsible for this lung tissue destruction: protease–antiprotease imbalance, chronic inflammation, and pulmonary vascular wall thickening and smooth muscle proliferation (27,33,65). The inflammation is a result of exposure to cigarette smoke (44,58) or, in undeveloped countries, the use of biofuels for cooking

and heating (48) and is mediated by various inflammatory cell types (macrophages, lymphocytes, and neutrophils). For example, cigarette smoke stimulates alveolar macrophages to release tumor necrosis factor (TNF)-α, which leads to nuclear factor-kappaB (NF-kB) protein production and subsequently interleukin 8 (IL-8), which then activates neutrophils. IL-8 activates the gene for matrix metalloproteinase-9 (MMP9), which is an enzyme that destroys elastin. Transforming growth factor (TGF)-β is also released and causes fibrosis of the small airways. Other mechanisms (*e.g.*, reduced histone deacetylation) are being uncovered that contribute to this inflammatory response (6,49,55). Genetic factors are also being uncovered as an important reason why some people who smoke develop COPD, and how such individuals may respond to treatment (35,41,54).

As a result of these pathologic processes, the lung loses its elasticity and its elastic recoil pressure. Small airways lose traction with the surrounding alveolar walls and become easily collapsible during exhalation. Distribution of ventilation is nonuniform, and alterations in perfusion occur. Ventilation occurs in areas in which the capillary bed has been destroyed, and an increase in dead space ventilation occurs, resulting in an increased ratio of dead space volume (V_D) to tidal volume (V_T).

In an attempt to overcome this elevation in V_D/V_T and alteration of the normal ventilation–perfusion balance, a patient with emphysema must maintain a high minute ventilation (by initially increasing the V_T and, once this is maximized, by then increasing the ventilation rate). With all of these physiologic changes, an increase in the work of breathing occurs. A larger-than-normal supply of oxygen is needed by the ventilatory muscles to maintain a stable ventilatory process. Oxygen supply is then diverted from the gut toward the ventilatory muscles. An increase in overall metabolism occurs, resulting in malnutrition. Functional skeletal muscle (in terms of strength and endurance) is lost, and severe muscular deconditioning occurs.

Patients with emphysema alter their pattern of breathing in an attempt to reduce the work of breathing. Air trapping can be decreased by breathing through pursed lips. This causes external resistance to flow and maintains a more positive intra-airway pressure during exhalation, minimizing compression of the small airways.

Patients with pure emphysema have been characterized as "pink puffers." They report significant dyspnea, are barrel chested because of the marked lung hyperinflation, and have little cough or sputum production. They are typically thin with general muscle wasting. With mild-to-moderate emphysema, the arterial oxygen and carbon dioxide tensions are relatively normal. As the disease progresses, arterial oxygen tension may decrease (first during exercise and then while at rest). Progressive elevation in pulmonary artery pressure may eventually develop and be followed by right heart failure

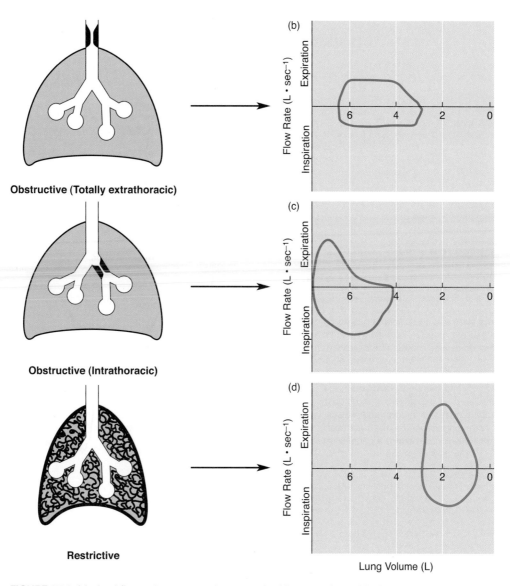

FIGURE 25-2. Maximal flow-volume curves in a normal subject, a patient with obstructive airways disease, and a patient with restrictive lung disease.

(*Fig. 25-4*) (36). The diagnosis of emphysema is based on the patient's history and abnormal pulmonary function tests showing a reduced forced expiratory volume in 1 s ($FEV_{1.0}$)/forced vital capacity (FVC) ratio, elevated TLC, and a reduced diffusing capacity for carbon monoxide.

Chronic Bronchitis

Chronic bronchitis is another type of COPD and is characterized by chronic cough and mucous production. Unlike emphysema, which primarily involves abnormalities within the lung parenchyma and smaller airways, chronic bronchitis primarily involves the large airways. The intrathoracic pressure generated by muscular effort and lung elastic recoil is normal in patients with chronic bronchitis. Airway wall injury occurs because of the effects of infiltration of inflammatory cells and mucous

gland enlargement. As the body attempts to repair the inflamed areas, structural remodeling occurs, with an increase in the deposition of collagen in the airway walls (58). Such bronchial and peribronchiolar inflammation results in further airway narrowing, ultimately resulting in an increase in airway resistance (42,43). Those areas of the lung that have an elevation in airway resistance receive little ventilation. The blood flow to these areas remains unchanged or decreased to a lesser extent than the ventilation, causing underventilation and overperfusion. This ventilation–perfusion imbalance leads to arterial hypoxemia, which, in turn, may lead to increased pulmonary vascular resistance and pulmonary arterial hypertension. Eventually, right ventricular failure (cor pulmonale) may develop (*Fig. 25-5*). Hypoxemia stimulates the production of erythropoietin, resulting in excess red blood cell production (also known as secondary

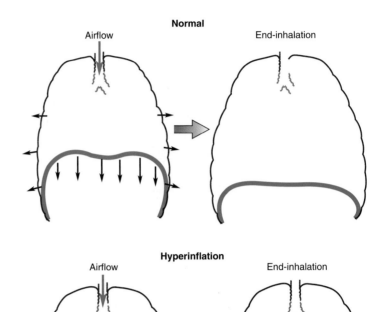

FIGURE 25-3. Top: Normally, the diaphragm is dome shaped, with most of the muscle fibers nearly vertical. Diaphragm contraction causes muscle fibers to shorten and the dome to descend, simultaneously expanding the rib cage. These actions reduce pressure inside the thorax, causing airflow into the lungs. **Bottom:** In the lung that is hyperinflated (as in a patient with chronic obstructive pulmonary disease), the diaphragm loses its dome shape. With contraction, the diaphragm cannot descend normally, which can create a paradoxical inward movement of the lower rib cage.

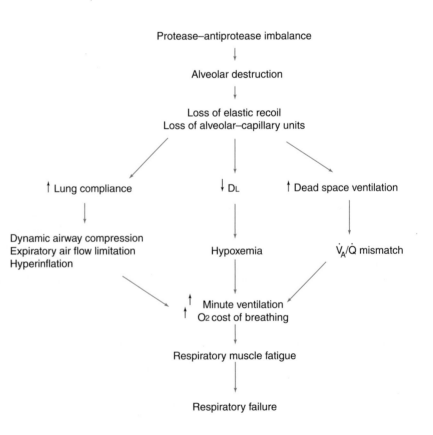

FIGURE 25-4. Progression of emphysema. $\dot{V}_A/\dot{Q}$ ventilation–perfusion ratio. DL, lung diffusion capacity.

Chronic cough and sputum production

↓

Expiratory airflow limitation
progressive dyspnea on exertion

↓

Progressive $\dot{V}_A/\dot{Q}$ mismatch
↓ Arterial pO_2
↑ Arterial pCO_2

↓

Pulmonary hypertension
Right heart strain
Polycythemia

↓

Right heart failure

FIGURE 25-5. Progression of chronic bronchitis.

polycythemia). Polycythemia may lead to a high blood viscosity, increasing flow resistance in blood vessels and further compromising blood flow.

Patients with chronic bronchitis have been characterized as "blue bloaters" because they exhibit a stocky habitus with central and peripheral cyanosis. Reduced airflow rate is associated with only mildly increased lung volumes and a relatively normal rate of oxygen transfer across the alveolar–capillary membrane (normal diffusing capacity for carbon monoxide). Secondary derangements in ventilatory control may develop, resulting in an elevation in the arterial carbon dioxide tension. Patients with chronic bronchitis tend to maintain low minute ventilation, which may further decrease during sleep and may result in nocturnal hypoxemia. The diagnosis of chronic bronchitis is based on the patient's history and abnormal pulmonary function tests (showing a reduced $FEV_{1.0}/FVC$ ratio without a response to bronchodilators, mildly increased TLC, and a normal diffusing capacity). These characterizations are of limited application. Many, if not most, patients with COPD cannot be fully "characterized" into one of these two categories. Many of the clinical findings from either type can be seen in an individual patient (or may not been seen at all). There is often significant overlap in symptoms and signs in an individual patient. In order to truly determine whether a patient has COPD, a high index of clinical suspicion in the determination of a patient who is at risk for the disease followed by confirmation of the diagnosis by spirometry should be performed.

Asthma

Asthma is another type of obstructive pulmonary disease that is complex in nature, characterized by airflow obstruction, bronchial hyperreactivity, and inflammation (19). Its episodic nature and reversibility are important features that separate it from COPD. The airway reactivity is often in response to one of various stimuli. Although a precipitating factor often cannot be accurately identified in most instances, it is possible to identify a specific agent (*e.g.*, pollens, dust mites, chemical, animal dander, drugs, exposure to cold, and exercise). In such instances, appropriate avoidance of the precipitating agent is recommended.

Such as other obstructive lung diseases, the pathophysiology of asthma is related to an underlying inflammatory response. An antigen presented to the airway often initiates asthma. An antibody to that antigen is produced, ultimately resulting in the release of various chemical mediators from mast cells and eosinophils. This response promotes ongoing inflammation of the airway walls and airway smooth muscle (3,32). The airway lumen becomes structurally changed and becomes occluded by a combination of mucus and denuded epithelium. Abnormal collagen deposition in the airways and subepithelial fibrosis subsequently develops and results in persistent airway narrowing (57).

The clinical symptoms of asthma are similar to other obstructive lung diseases. Shortness of breath and wheezing are commonly present, as can be episodes of coughing (particularly in the morning) and chest tightness (19). The diagnosis is made by using a combination of the patient's history, clinical examination, and pulmonary function tests. Reduced maximal expiratory flow rates, increased expiratory airway resistance, and elevated RV and TLC, which are corrected with the administration of a bronchodilator, are hallmarks of this disease. Bronchial hyperresponsiveness to methacholine (a medication that causes airway irritation) or eucapnic voluntary hyperventilation may be seen in those patients who have asthma and have normal pulmonary function tests. In some patients, asthma is only present during or after exercise and can be diagnosed based on the clinical history and measurement of pulmonary function tests following an exercise challenge (39).

Some patients with asthma may develop an acute worsening of symptoms. During this acute exacerbation, the lung units distal to the areas of airway narrowing are underventilated, resulting in ventilation perfusion imbalance. Initially, hyperventilation occurs, and the arterial oxygen tension remains normal, and the arterial carbon dioxide tension decreases. As the exacerbation worsens, the distribution of ventilation and perfusion becomes more imbalanced, resulting in a decrease in the arterial oxygen tension and an increase in the arterial carbon dioxide tension. This can ultimately lead to respiratory failure.

CLINICAL FEATURES AND LABORATORY ASSESSMENT OF PATIENTS WITH OBSTRUCTIVE PULMONARY DISEASES

Most patients with COPD are current or former smokers. The development of symptoms may lag up to 20 yr after the initiation of cigarette smoking. Many factors appear to play a role in the development of COPD. The amount and duration of cigarette use, a family history of lung disease (*e.g.*, α-1-antitrypsin deficiency), childhood illnesses such as asthma, viral infections and allergies, air pollution, obesity, and a complete work history are important to know in an attempt to help determine the underlying basis for the COPD. Interestingly, sex also appears to play an important role in the development of lung disease, with women being more prone to developing lung disease at an earlier age than men (12,23,26,27,48). Finally, genetic factors are now being uncovered that are being associated with the development of COPD in smokers (35,54).

It is important to determine if a patient is at risk for underlying COPD. As noted before, the clinical presentation may not be initially helpful in this determination. Several questionnaires have been developed (38,70) that assist in this determination and can be easily answered by the patient in a very brief period of time. If the results of the questionnaire were positive, then that person would be considered to be at risk for COPD and should have further testing to confirm the diagnosis.

Early in the course of the disease, there are no physical examination abnormalities. As the disease progresses, wheezing may be noted only on a forced exhalation maneuver, and hyperinflation of the lung and chest wall occurs. A decrease in breath sounds with a decrease in movement of the diaphragm and a decrease in heart sounds become noticeable. A prolongation of the time for a forced exhalation (>3 s) is seen. With ongoing progression, the patient may use techniques that are more effective to reduce the work of breathing, such as leaning forward with the arms outstretched and weight supported by the palms or breathing using pursed lips. If cor pulmonale develops, neck vein distention, enlarged liver, and peripheral edema may be seen.

Routine laboratory testing supplements the patient's history and physical examination. A chest radiograph is essential to confirm the presence of COPD (*e.g.*, through the presence of lung hyperinflation, increase in the retrosternal airspace, flattening of the diaphragm, and enlargement of the pulmonary artery) and also to determine whether there may be another cause for dyspnea (*e.g.*, pleural effusion, lung cancer, congestive heart failure).

An electrocardiogram (ECG) is helpful to determine whether cardiac disease may be present. Measurement of oxyhemoglobin saturation by cutaneous pulse oximetry or arterial blood gas analysis will help determine the presence of hypoxemia. With the blood gas analysis, arterial carbon dioxide tension can also be determined. Measurement of hemoglobin will help to determine the duration of hypoxemia, particularly in the instance in which the hematocrit is >50%, suggesting hypoxemia of longstanding duration. Computed tomography (CT) scanning of the chest will help to assess the lung parenchyma and to evaluate for other intrathoracic pathology (*e.g.*, masses, pleural disease).

Measurement of pulmonary function should be performed on all patients suspected of having lung disease. Pulmonary function testing in the form of simple spirometry should be performed for all smokers older than the age of 45 yr and for any smoker who has pulmonary symptoms (*e.g.*, cough, sputum production, dyspnea), regardless of age, or for those who have been determined to be at risk following completion of one of the screening questionnaires (21,38,66,70). The pulmonary function testing should include measurement of TLC, RV, vital capacity (VC), inspiratory capacity (IC), $FEV_{1.0}$, forced expiratory volume in 6 s ($FEV_{6.0}$), FVC, peak expiratory flow rate (PEFR), and diffusing capacity for carbon monoxide (D_{LCO}). Although some of the measures (*e.g.*, TLC, VC, RV, D_{LCO}, fractional concentration of nitrogen in expired gas [F_{EN_2}]) require the use of sophisticated equipment, many (*e.g.*, $FEV_{1.0}$, $FEV_{6.0}$, FVC) can be performed using very simple equipment. Pulmonary function testing will often help in the determination of the type of lung disease process that is present (*Table 25-1*).

Pulmonary function testing is helpful not only with the diagnosis of the disease but also with determination of the severity of the disease process. The $FEV_{1.0}$ is the best correlate with morbidity and mortality in these patients, and several proposals for staging have been developed using the $FEV_{1.0}$. Since 2004, The American Thoracic Society suggests staging based on the severity of airflow obstruction, and they mirror the spirometric classification used by the Global Initiative for Chronic Obstructive Lung Disease (GOLD) (26). The GOLD guidelines base the severity of the disease on spirometry. Mild COPD is characterized by a patient who has mild airflow limitation ($FEV_{1.0}$/FVC <70% but $FEV_{1.0}$ ≥80%

TABLE 25-1. Pulmonary Function Testing: Interpretation for Various Disease States

	Obstructive	Restrictive	Vascular
$FEV_{1.0}$ (L)	↓	↓	↔
FVC (L)	↓	↓	↔
$FEV_{1.0}$/FVC	↓	↔ or ↓	↔
($FEV_{1.0}$/$FEV_{6.0}$)			
TLC (L)	↑	↓	↔
VC (L)	↓	↓	↔
FRC (L)	↑	↓	↔
RV (L)	↑	↓	↔
D_{LCO}	↔ or ↓	↔ or ↓	↓

↔, no change; ↑, increased; ↓, decreased; ↔ or ↑, no change early in disease process, increase late in disease; ↔ or ↓, no change early in disease process, decrease late in disease; $FEV_{1.0}$, forced expiratory volume in 1 s; FVC, forced vital capacity; $FEV_{6.0}$, forced expiratory volume in 6 s; TLC, total lung capacity; VC, vital capacity; FRC, functional residual capacity; RV, residual volume; D_{LCO}, diffusing capacity for carbon monoxide.

predicted) and usually, but not always, has symptoms. Moderate COPD is characterized by a patient who has worsening airflow limitation ($FEV_{1.0}$ between 50% and 80% predicted) and who has progression of symptoms to include dyspnea with exertion. Severe COPD is characterized by a patient who has severe airflow limitation ($FEV_{1.0}$ between 30% and 50% predicted), further designated as very severe with the presence of respiratory failure or if $FEV_{1.0}$ is less than 30% of predicted. This staging system is becoming the more widely accepted severity staging system for patients with COPD but is not without its own pitfalls. Misclassification of patients can still occur particularly with patients of extreme age (48).

EXERCISE LIMITATIONS IN CHRONIC OBSTRUCTIVE PULMONARY DISEASE

Exercise intolerance (either through the development of shortness of breath or easy fatigability) is invariably present in a patient with COPD. As the disease progresses, dyspnea and fatigability at even minimal levels of exercise can occur. Various factors are involved in exercise intolerance for patients with COPD: ventilatory abnormalities (impaired pulmonary system mechanics and ventilatory muscle dysfunction), metabolic and gas exchange abnormalities, peripheral muscle dysfunction, and cardiovascular abnormalities (*Box 25-1*).

Ventilatory abnormalities are the primary cause for exercise limitation in patients with COPD. Airflow limitation, prominent on maximal expiratory efforts, occurs secondary to loss of elastic recoil of the lung parenchyma, airway inflammation, and airway collapse. As exercise effort increases (*e.g.*, during exercise), expiratory flow increases to a point beyond which further

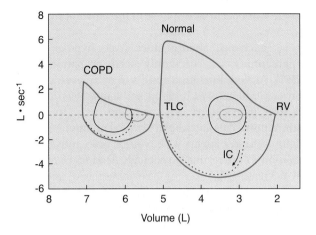

FIGURE 25-6. Flow volume curve for a patient with chronic obstructive pulmonary disease (COPD) (rest and exercise). TLC, total lung capacity; RV, residual volume; IC, inspiratory capacity.

effort produces no further increase in expiratory flow (*Fig. 25-6*) and results in exercise limitation. In patients with normal ventilatory mechanics, only a small fraction of the expiratory flow is used during tidal breathing, and airflow limitation is never reached, either at exercise or during rest. In patients with COPD, the anatomic and physiologic processes causing expiratory flow limitation (noted as scalloping of the expiratory portion of the flow volume curve) may be so severe in some that even during tidal breathing, expiratory limitation is reached. Patients with expiratory airflow limitation cannot reach the increased demands placed on the ventilatory system during exercise by increasing their expiratory flow as would occur in normal individuals.

As expiratory flow limitation occurs, the lung cannot fully empty during resting breathing. This is particularly worsened during exercise. As a result of this expiratory flow limitation, end-expiratory lung volume remains elevated, and *dynamic hyperinflation* of the respiratory system occurs. Dynamic hyperinflation results in a decrease in the inspiratory capacity and places severe mechanical constraints on V_T expansion during exercise despite an increase in the respiratory drive (15,46). The reduction in resting inspiratory capacity and resting expiratory flow limitation results in poorer exercise performance (9,45).

Dynamic hyperinflation also causes an increased elastic loading of the inspiratory muscles. Alterations of the normal length-tension relationship of the inspiratory muscles (*e.g.*, the diaphragm, sternomastoids, and scalenes) compromise the ability of these muscle groups to function efficiently. As exercise increases, progressive limitation of the normal increase in V_T despite maximal inspiratory efforts occurs because of this dynamic hyperinflation. In fact, dyspnea is likely more related to the effects of dynamic hyperinflation than it is to airflow obstruction. An increase in muscle oxygen use and

BOX 25-1	**Common Abnormalities Noted During Exercise in Patients with Chronic Obstructive Pulmonary Disease**

Dyspnea

Leg discomfort

Reduced peak oxygen consumption

Reduced peak work rate

High dead space ventilation (V_D/V_T)

Decreased V_T response with increased ventilation rate

Reduced inspiratory capacity with exercise (*i.e.*, dynamic hyperinflation)

Variable arterial oxyhemoglobin desaturation

V_D, dead space; V_T, tidal volume.

muscle work occur in response to these pathophysiologic processes.

Gas exchange abnormalities (*e.g.*, hypoxemia and hypercapnia) are commonly seen in patients with COPD. Airflow limitation results in an uneven distribution of ventilation with blood perfusion. Destruction of the lung parenchyma (*e.g.*, as might occur in patients with emphysema), alveolar hypoventilation (*e.g.*, as might occur in patients with chronic bronchitis), and an elevation in the resting physiologic dead space that does not decrease with exercise also may play a role in the gas exchange abnormalities. As patients exercise, the gas exchange abnormalities become more prominent, resulting in worsening hypoxemia.

Ventilatory and peripheral muscle dysfunction (both structural and functional) are also present in these patients (10,14). Strength and endurance (the primary characteristics of muscle performance) of the muscles of ventilation are significantly reduced. The work of breathing increases significantly for a given level of ventilation as the disease progresses (*Fig. 25-7*). However, the ventilatory and peripheral muscle groups are affected differently. Endurance limitation (fatigue) is noted with the peripheral muscles, and strength limitation is noted with the ventilatory muscles. Muscle biopsy of the peripheral muscles of a patient with COPD shows a consistent reduction in type I (slow-twitch, low-tension, fatigue-resistant) fibers and an increase in type II (fast-twitch, high-tension) fibers. At a microscopic level, these muscles show increased oxidative stress, increased apoptosis, and inflammatory changes. The systemic inflammatory state that is present in patients with COPD is only now being more fully understood as a causative mechanism for the local and systemic complications associated with the disease (7,51,62,71).

The skeletal muscle dysfunction results from various pathophysiologic mechanisms. Hypoxia and oxidative stress (caused by reactive oxygen species and oxygen free radicals), disuse atrophy (deconditioning), malnutrition, skeletal muscle myopathy, and weight loss with altered substrate (*e.g.*, amino acid, anabolic steroids, leptin) metabolism have all been shown to be associated with muscle dysfunction in patients with COPD. Current evidence also suggests an alteration of the oxidative capacity (reduction in citrate synthase and hydroxyacyl-coenzyme A dehydrogenase activities and increase in glycolytic activities) of both the peripheral skeletal muscles and the ventilatory muscles, along with a reduction in the capillary density in patients with COPD (37).

RESTRICTIVE LUNG DISEASE

Restrictive lung diseases reduce lung volume through their involvement of the lung parenchyma or thoracic cage. There are more than 200 disorders that can affect the pleural space (*e.g.*, hemothorax, pleural effusion), alveoli (*e.g.*, pulmonary alveolar proteinosis, pneumonia), interstitial space (*e.g.*, interstitial lung disease), neuromuscular system (*e.g.*, myasthenia gravis, spinal cord injury), immune system (rheumatoid arthritis and other autoimmune diseases), thoracic cage (*e.g.*, kyphoscoliosis, ankylosing spondylitis), and obesity, all can result in a restrictive lung process (16). A patient with restrictive lung disease develops dyspnea (often first noted during exertion) that is related to the reduction in lung volume caused by the underlying disease process. Prognosis for patients with restrictive lung disease is often poor and depends on the extent and severity of tissue involvement. Early diagnosis and treatment are essential.

CLINICAL EVALUATION AND LABORATORY ASSESSMENT OF PATIENTS WITH RESTRICTIVE LUNG DISEASE

The initial evaluation of the patient should include a complete history and physical examination. The patient often seeks medical attention because of progressive shortness of breath (particularly with exertion) or a nonproductive cough. The history is helpful to elicit clues to the diagnosis, particularly when interstitial lung disease is being considered as a potential cause (*Box 25-2*). Attention should be paid to the patient's occupational history, environmental exposure history, medication history, family history, and smoking history. In the individual who is obese, shortness of breath and reduced lung compliance increase the work of breathing irrespective of underlying pulmonary disease (4). Pulmonary function values will vary depending on the severity and type of lung disease that coexists.

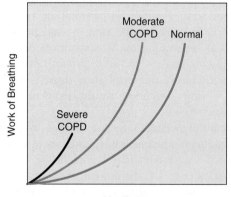

FIGURE 25-7. Work of the ventilatory muscles increases as ventilation increases. As chronic obstructive pulmonary disease (COPD) progresses, the work of breathing is higher than normal at any given level of ventilation. In addition, the maximum work that can be generated by the ventilatory muscles is diminished as the disease progresses.

BOX 25-2	Causes of Interstitial Lung Disease

1. Occupational and environmental exposures to inorganic dusts (silica, asbestos, tin, coal, hard metals)
   Organic (hypersensitivity pneumonitis caused by bacteria, fungi, animal proteins)
2. Drugs or medications (chemotherapy agents, radiation exposure, oxygen)
3. Collagen vascular diseases (scleroderma, systemic lupus erythematosus, rheumatoid arthritis, polymyositis)
4. Neoplasm (bronchoalveolar carcinoma, lymphoma)
5. Unknown causes (interstitial pulmonary fibrosis, sarcoidosis, lymphangioleiomyomatosis, eosinophilic granuloma, nonspecific interstitial pneumonia, bronchiolitis obliterans organizing pneumonia)

Dyspnea is defined as the "subjective experience of breathing discomfort that consists of qualitatively distinct sensations that vary in intensity" (48). The shortness of breath develops insidiously because a patient will often decrease his or her level of activity to compensate for the impairment. As the shortness of breath progresses and interferes with the patient's activities of daily living (ADLs), medical attention is then sought. The most accurate gauge for dyspnea comes from the patient (48). The duration of shortness of breath is helpful in the evaluation process. A short, rapid onset of symptoms is suggestive of hypersensitivity pneumonitis, eosinophilic pneumonia, or alveolar hemorrhage syndrome. A more prolonged course, with the development of symptoms over years or longer, is more characteristic of the interstitial lung diseases (particularly idiopathic pulmonary fibrosis) (16).

The physical examination may be helpful but often not until the patient has developed significant symptoms. A thorough examination of the patient, with particular attention to the chest and neuromuscular systems, is important. A decrease in excursion of the chest with an increase in respiratory rate at rest is often present. A decrease in breath sounds over one side of the chest is seen in patients with pleural disease; an anatomic deformity of the chest and thoracic cage is seen in patients with kyphoscoliosis; and fine-end inspiratory rales (Velcro crackles) are seen in patients with interstitial fibrosis. Weakness of the extremities is present in patients with neuromuscular disease (*e.g.*, myasthenia gravis). Arthritis can be associated with collagen vascular diseases or sarcoid. Integration of the history and physical findings should then prompt further diagnostic testing.

A chest radiograph should be performed during the initial evaluation. This helps to assess the lung volume, structure of the chest wall and thorax, and presence or absence of pleural, interstitial, or alveolar abnormalities. CT scanning (particularly high-resolution scanning) can assess for the presence of interstitial changes. Pulse oximetry and arterial blood gases are helpful to determine the degree of gas exchange abnormalities that may be present. Pulmonary function tests reveal a decrease in the $FEV_{1.0}$, FVC, and TLC with maintenance (or an increase) in the $FEV_{1.0}$/FVC ratio. A low diffusing capacity may be seen late in the disease course, particularly for patients with interstitial fibrosis. A reduction in the maximal expiratory and inspiratory pressures may be seen in patients with neuromuscular diseases. To determine the effects of the restrictive process during exertion, exercise testing must be performed. Measurements of pulse oximetry and expired gases can help assess the effects of the restrictive process. An abnormal response to exercise is noted in most patients with restrictive lung disease (28). The type of response may help determine the type of restrictive disease present. For example, a patient with interstitial fibrosis might be expected to primarily have gas exchange abnormalities, whereas a patient with neuromuscular weakness might be expected to primarily have abnormalities in the ability to increase ventilation with exercise.

EXERCISE LIMITATIONS ASSOCIATED WITH PATIENTS WITH RESTRICTIVE LUNG DISEASE

The abnormality common to all of the restrictive lung diseases is a reduction in the TLC and FVC. This reduction in lung volume may lead to collapse of the smaller airway units with subsequent decrease in the functional alveolar–capillary interface and may lead to impaired gas exchange. A decrease in the diffusing capacity of the lungs may result in those who have disruption of this alveolar–capillary unit.

Interstitial lung diseases are the best studied of the restrictive lung processes. Although there are various causes for interstitial lung disease, they share some pathophysiologic and clinical characteristics. Chronic inflammation of the interstitium and alveoli results in fibrosis of these structures. These changes reduce lung compliance and increase lung stiffness (29). A stiff lung requires more energy to stretch, requiring an increase in the transpulmonary pressure to achieve a given VT. Not only are there changes in the lung capacity and stiffness but also the alveolar–capillary units are altered as well as being replaced with fibrous tissue.

Gas exchange is often disrupted as a result of these pathologic changes and is the major factor in exercise limitation. In the early stages of the disease process, the resting arterial oxygen tension is normal but decreases during exercise, and the alveolar–arterial oxygen gradient increases (*Box 25-3*). As the disease progresses, resting hypoxemia with widening of the alveolar–arterial oxygen gradient occurs. Imbalances of ventilation and perfusion, shunting, and impaired oxygen diffusion all play a role in the development of the hypoxemia (14).

A characteristic ventilatory response to exercise occurs in patients with interstitial lung disease. The V_T is functionally limited because of the interstitial process, and an increase in minute ventilation occurs through an increase in the respiratory rate rather than the expected increase in V_T. Because of the constraints noted, the patient breathes with very rapid, shallow breaths in an attempt to reduce the work of breathing. This results in an increase in V_D/V_T because of the decrease in V_T. Normally during exercise, V_D/V_T decreases because of the increase in V_T, but in patients with interstitial lung disease, the V_D/V_T remains constant or increases.

An increase in elastic recoil of the lung at functional residual capacity is present in patients with interstitial lung disease. In combination with the reduction in lung volumes, an adverse impact occurs on the ability of the respiratory system to adapt to the increasing ventilatory demands required during exercise.

Pulmonary hypertension may develop because of hypoxic vasoconstriction and obliteration of the pulmonary vascular bed by the underlying interstitial process. Most patients with significant interstitial lung disease develop significant pulmonary hypertension with exercise (71), and nearly all patients with interstitial lung disease have right ventricular hypertrophy. Pulmonary

hypertension has been shown to significantly correlate with hypoxemia during exercise. Hypoxemia plays a more important role than does the abnormal ventilatory mechanics in the exercise limitation found in these patients. In fact, it has been suggested that the gas exchange abnormalities (secondary to this circulatory pathophysiology) are perhaps the most important factors in exercise limitation in patients with interstitial lung disease (14).

There are several other types of restrictive lung disease (*e.g.*, neuromuscular, pleural, thoracic cage abnormality, or alveolar), and in each, a different pathophysiology regarding the response to exercise occurs. For a patient with neuromuscular disease (*e.g.*, myasthenia gravis), the ventilation and perfusion units of the lungs are normal. In such an instance, the gas exchange of the lungs is normal. Patients with neuromuscular disease will have limitation to exercise based on muscular limitations. Patients will not be able to increase V_T with exercise and will have a rapid increase in the ventilatory rate. Once the ventilation is limited by the underlying neuromuscular process, exercise will end. Patients with pleural disease or thoracic cage abnormalities will have a similar response to exercise. Patients with alveolar processes will have impairment in gas exchange, and exercise limitation is often secondary to hypoxemia.

In all of the various types of restrictive lung disease, gas exchange abnormalities can eventually occur secondary to loss of effective matching of ventilation and perfusion and diffusing abnormalities. As the diseases progress, hypoxemia and carbon dioxide retention results, and exercise limitation occurs.

VASCULAR LUNG DISEASE

Various etiologies can result in **vascular lung disease**. These include diseases that involve the pulmonary veins and arteries and are generally characterized by obstruction of the pulmonary circulation and or disruption of the alveolar–capillary membrane. Both cause a decrease of the effective vascular bed, resulting in impairment of diffusion and gas exchange. Pulmonary hypertension and right ventricular failure ultimately develop.

Pulmonary hypertension is a mean pulmonary artery pressure at rest of >25 mm Hg or >30 mm Hg with exercise. It is often characterized as idiopathic or secondary. Idiopathic pulmonary hypertension is a disease, by definition, of uncertain etiology (7). Secondary pulmonary hypertension is a result of a specific disease process (*e.g.*, severe COPD, interstitial lung disease, left ventricular [LV] dysfunction, mitral valvular stenosis, chronic thromboembolic disease [51], HIV infection [50]), sleep-disordered breathing, connective tissue disease, medications, and portopulmonary hypertension).

BOX 25-3	**Abnormalities Noted During Exercise in Patients with Interstitial Lung Disease**

Dyspnea

Reduced peak oxygen consumption

Reduced peak rate

Reduced V_T with increased ventilation rate at sub-maximal work rates

Increased dead space ventilation (V_D/V_T)

Arterial oxyhemoglobin desaturation during exercise

Unchanged $PaCO_2$ during exercise

V_D, dead space; V_T, tidal volume; $PaCO_2$, partial pressure of arterial carbon dioxide.

CLINICAL ASSESSMENT AND LABORATORY EVALUATION OF PATIENTS WITH VASCULAR LUNG DISEASE

Patients with vascular lung disease present with the symptom of shortness of breath, often first noted during exercise. Typically, very few historical clues are present as to the cause of the patient's pulmonary hypertension. The clinical examination of the patient is often normal, with clear lung fields and normal mechanical movement of the chest and abdominal walls during inspiration and expiration. A cardiac murmur, heard best at the base of the heart, may suggest mitral stenosis. A gallop is suggestive of LV systolic dysfunction. A loud second heart sound, heard best over the second left intercostal space, can be present and is secondary to the accentuated closure of the pulmonary valve. With longstanding disease, right-sided heart failure may develop, and hepatomegaly, peripheral edema, and jugular venous distention may be seen. Clubbing of the fingers can also be seen.

The laboratory evaluation of a patient with pulmonary hypertension should include a chest radiograph and ECG. The radiograph will show clear lung fields and an enlargement of the cardiac silhouette. An ECG will show a right ventricular strain pattern. Pulse oximetry determination of oxyhemoglobin saturation and arterial blood gas analysis are helpful to determine the presence of gas exchange abnormalities. The diagnosis is often first noted following an echocardiogram. Valvular heart abnormalities, LV systolic dysfunction, and right ventricular dysfunction can be determined via echocardiography. An estimation of the systolic pulmonary artery pressure can be made. Ventilation perfusion scanning is helpful to determine the presence of chronic thromboembolic pulmonary hypertension. CT scanning and pulmonary angiography can help to assess the pulmonary parenchyma and the pulmonary vascular bed. Right heart catheterization with measurement of the right atrial, right ventricular, pulmonary artery, and left atrial pressures is necessary to confirm the diagnosis and to help direct therapy.

EXERCISE LIMITATION OF PATIENTS WITH VASCULAR LUNG DISEASE

The pulmonary circulation is normally able to experience a fivefold to sixfold increase in blood flow with only a minimal increase in pressure. Although pulmonary artery pressure increases during exercise, right atrial pressure increases only minimally. The pressure gradient increase across the pulmonary vascular bed occurring during exercise is less than the increase in cardiac output. This is caused by a decrease in the pulmonary vascular resistance and is felt to occur because of recruitment and distention of pulmonary capillaries. At peak exercise, improved efficiency of ventilation and

BOX 25-4	**Abnormalities Noted During Exercise in Patients with Pulmonary Vascular Disease (Pulmonary Hypertension)**

Reduced peak oxygen consumption

Reduced peak rate

Decreased ventilatory threshold

Arterial oxyhemoglobin desaturation

Elevation in pulmonary artery wedge pressure (>30 mm Hg)

Elevation in right atrial pressure (>14 mm Hg)

perfusion and a decrease in the alveolar dead space occur (resulting in an increase in the V_D/V_T ratio).

The exercise limitation associated with pulmonary hypertension is primarily caused by cardiac dysfunction (*Box 25-4*). Pulmonary vasoconstriction and remodeling of the vascular bed increase right ventricle afterload and limit stroke volume in response to exercise. As the right ventricle dilates over the course of the disease, a decrease in LV compliance and diastolic filling occurs. With exercise, an abnormal increase in right atrial and mean pulmonary artery pressure with a relatively normal pulmonary capillary wedge pressure is present. A decrease in the maximal cardiac output and arterial oxyhemoglobin desaturation occur, resulting in the production of lactic acidosis at a lower level of exercise. Underperfused and well-ventilated lung units cause an increase in V_D/V_T and the ventilatory requirements for exercise. These factors result in the production of lactic acidosis at a lower level of exercise (reduced anaerobic threshold) and a decrease in the maximal oxygen consumption. A normal breathing reserve is usually found because the ventilatory mechanisms themselves are usually intact (53,64).

EXERCISE ASSESSMENT IN DIAGNOSIS AND MONITORING OF LUNG DISEASE

Exercise testing is an important component of the evaluation and management of most patients with pulmonary disease (*Box 25-5*). It is important to determine the patient's ability to undergo exercise testing. Contraindications to exercise testing (also see *GETP9, Box 3-5*) include an unstable cardiac condition (*e.g.*, unstable angina), severe hypoxemia, orthopedic impairment, neurologic impairment, psychiatric disorders, poor motivation, or inability to perform the test. Neither carbon dioxide retention nor age are contraindications to the performance of exercise testing.

Indications for Exercise Testing in Patients with Lung Disease

Evaluation of exercise tolerance

Evaluation of undiagnosed exercise intolerance

Evaluation of patients with pulmonary symptoms

Exercise evaluation and prescription for pulmonary rehabilitation

Evaluation of impairment or disability

Evaluation for lung transplantation

Evaluation for oxyhemoglobin desaturation

MODE OF EXERCISE TESTING

The assessment of exercise capacity is an important component of the overall evaluation and management of patients with lung disease (also see *GETP9, Chapter 10*). Various exercise testing modalities are available to help with this evaluation. The selection of the exercise testing modality depends on the clinical question being asked and available equipment and facilities (*Box 25-6*). Exercise testing should be performed when further information (*e.g.*, in addition to the history and physical examination, chest radiograph, pulmonary function tests, and ECG) is necessary regarding the patient's underlying disease process (40). Exercise testing plays a very important role in patients undergoing lung transplantation, no matter what the disease process is. Exercise testing is used not only to evaluate the candidate for their appropriateness to be listed for transplantation but also for ongoing medical surveillance and evaluation of yearly progress (17).

Stair Climbing

Stair climbing is a simple and inexpensive test that has been primarily used to assess postoperative risk for patients undergoing thoracic or upper abdominal

BOX 25-6 **Modalities of Clinical Exercise Testing for Patients with Lung Disease**

Stair climbing

Timed walk tests (6- or 12-min walk)

Shuttle walk tests

Graded exercise tests

Cardiopulmonary exercise test

surgery and is currently being used to assess functional capacity in patients with COPD (68). Although there is no standardized testing procedure, the patient is asked to climb as many stairs as possible until needing to stop for symptoms (*e.g.*, dizziness, shortness of breath, fatigue, chest pain). Measurements made during the test include the number of stairs walked, oxyhemoglobin saturation, level of dyspnea, and heart rate (HR). Variable reporting of the pace of the stair climbing and the actual number of stairs climbed (often referred to as "flights of stairs") adds to the nonuniform nature of the testing procedure. The inability to walk two flights of stairs has been reported to result in a significant increase in the number of postoperative complications (20,68). This test can provide a general assessment of the postoperative risk for patients with lung disease in a simple and low-cost manner (25,31,52). It is a useful measure for the patient's lower limb muscular power and provides a closer examination of functional performance, including fall risk (59).

Timed Walk Tests

The timed walk tests (6-min walk [6-MWT], shuttle walk) are practical and simple to perform (40). They do not require advanced training or specialized equipment and provide an objective assessment of exercise tolerance or functional capacity in a manner that is comfortable for most patients to perform. The 6-MWT is the most commonly used test. A standardized protocol for the performance of the test exists (2), and guidelines have been recently developed to include a track size and length, patient preparation, monitoring, protocol, measurements, and practice testing. The track should be 30 m in length and clearly marked every 3 m. Comfortable shoes should be worn by the patient, and the test should be performed each time at the same time of the day with the patient taking his or her usual medication regimen. Monitoring equipment should include a stopwatch, a pulse oximeter, and a sphygmomanometer. Before beginning the test, baseline HR and blood pressure (BP) measurements should be made as well as a measure of the patient's level of dyspnea (see *GETP9, Figure 5-4*) and oxyhemoglobin saturation. Standardized instructions should be read to the patient, and the words for encouragement and notification of time elapsed should be consistent for all patients. At the end of the testing, immediate measurements of oxyhemoglobin saturation, pulse, BP, perceived exertion (*e.g.*, using a Borg Scale) (5), level of dyspnea (ACSM dyspnea scale [*GETP9, Figure 5-4*]), and length of walk should be made. Because there may be a training effect noted with such testing, it is important to perform several tests (up to three) on the same day (with 1 h of rest in between tests), with reporting of the longest distance walked. Reference values for healthy adults have been reported (18).

The 6-MWT has good reproducibility and correlation with other measures of functional capacity and, thus, has been used in lieu of cardiopulmonary exercise test (CPET) when this testing modality is not available. A good correlation between the 6-MWT and maximal oxygen consumption ($r = 0.73$) has been shown in patients with COPD (8). The 6-MWT represents a submaximal and motivational alternative compared with the CPET. It also represents a test for which patients are familiar with the testing modality (i.e., walking). A prediction equation developed by Hill (2008) estimates maximal work rate for patients with moderate-to-severe COPD based on the results of the 6-MWT and measures of body height (30). This may be a useful tool for developing exercise prescription guidelines for these patients.

The 6-MWT has been usefully applied to the evaluation of functional capacity (e.g., patients with COPD [65], interstitial lung disease [11], medical interventions [47], response to pulmonary rehabilitation [13], and prediction of morbidity [34]). It has also been used successfully in the evaluation and management of patients with congestive heart failure (8,60). A recent addition to the Lung Allocation Score (LAS), the 6-MWT does not provide reliable information to replace more traditional indicators of functional capacity. Rather, it serves to assist in the decision-making process regarding transplantation and provides a clearer picture of the ability to perform ADLs and predicting survival (17).

There are some concerns about the actual performance of the test and the comparisons that are made from one testing site to another, but the 6-MWT has been used in large multicenter trials (22). There is a statistically significant improvement (averaging 7%) in distance walked when the test is repeated on a second day. The shape of the walking course (continuous vs. straight) appears to be more a determinant of the distance walked than does the length of a straight course (61). The minimally clinically important difference (MCID) for the 6-MWT is estimated to be 54 m (69).

Shuttle Walk Tests

The incremental shuttle walk test (ISWT) is a symptom-limited, maximal exercise test (63). Subjects are instructed to walk around a 10-m course at a speed indicated by beeps played from a CD player. The speed increases incrementally until the patient is unable to continue or maintain the required speed. The total time walked is recorded. Performance in the ISWT is predictive of peak oxygen consumption, and the test is reproducible after a single practice walk.

The endurance shuttle walk test (ESWT) is a constant work rate exercise test. After a 2-min warm up period, the subject is asked to walk around a 10-m course. The speed is constant and is set at an equivalent of 85% of the predicted peak maximal oxygen consumption achieved during the ISWT. The total time walked is recorded (56). These tests are externally paced tests of maximal and submaximal exercise performance, respectively. Each may be used to compare the distance walked before and after an intervention (e.g., response to pulmonary rehabilitation). There are no established minimal clinically important distances for either the shuttle walk test or the ESWT (69).

Cardiopulmonary Exercise Test

CPET is a traditional symptom-limited graded exercise test with the addition of a metabolic cart that collects and analyzes expired gases, thereby assessing the integration of the cardiovascular, pulmonary, and muscular systems during exercise performance. This type of testing allows an evaluation of the patient's ability to perform exercise and of the system responsible for the exercise impairment. Modalities for CPET can include the treadmill or cycle ergometer and are performed in a continuous ramp-type protocol until fatigue, dyspnea, or other indications for stopping an exercise test are evident (*GETP9*, Chapter 5). Expired gases from the patient are collected using a metabolic cart that has the capability to determine the V_T, ventilatory rate, rate of oxygen consumption, and rate of carbon dioxide production. Measurements of HR and oxyhemoglobin saturation (via pulse oximetry or arterial blood gas analysis) are also made. All measurements are on a continuous basis, thus allowing for interpretation at various levels of exercise.

Interpretation of CPET involves a significant amount of information obtained with each study (1,67,72). The use of gas collection spirometry and pulse oximetry provides for a comprehensive interpretation of CPET data. To organize the data to make functional and diagnostic assessments, several questions need to be evaluated (67,72).

1. Is exercise capacity normal? Peak oxygen consumption, peak work rate, functional aerobic impairment, and respiratory exchange ratio can be used to assess exercise capacity.
2. Is cardiovascular function normal? ECG responses, rate pressure product, oxygen pulse, and ventilatory threshold can be used to evaluate cardiovascular function.
3. Is ventilatory function normal? Maximal ventilation rate and ventilatory reserve can assess ventilatory function.
4. Is gas exchange normal? Oxygen saturation and V_D/V_T can evaluate gas exchange.

The various disease states discussed in this chapter have major distinguishing features regarding the measurements obtained during CPET. Patients with COPD have a reduced exercise capacity (reduced peak oxygen consumption), ventilatory limitation (reduced

TABLE 25-2. Distinguishing Features Noted at End of Exercise

Disease	COPD	Interstitial Lung Disease	Vascular Lung Disease
Exercise capacity	↓	↓	↓
Oxygen consumption	↓	↓	↓
Ventilatory limitation	Yes	Yes	No
Cardiovascular response	Normal	Normal	Abnormal

COPD, chronic obstructive pulmonary disease; ↓, decreased.

or absent ventilatory reserve, hypercapnia, hypoxemia), and a normal cardiovascular response (normal oxygen pulse), with exercise (24). However, the HR response may be blunted secondary to pulmonary limitations and dyspnea. Patients with interstitial lung disease have a reduced exercise capacity (reduced peak oxygen consumption), ventilatory limitation (high maximum ventilation rate and low V_T at end exercise, elevated V_D/V_T with an abnormal reduction during exercise), and a normal cardiovascular response with exercise. Patients with vascular lung disease have a reduced exercise capacity (reduced peak oxygen consumption), no ventilatory limitation, and an abnormal cardiovascular response (early onset of ventilatory threshold, early plateau of the oxygen pulse with a low maximum value) with exercise (*Table 25-2*). Although CPET is an applicable tool for evaluating the exercise capacity for the different types of lung diseases, its specific usefulness in the diverse pulmonary transplantation population is limited (17).

During any type of exercise testing, a complete knowledge of the patient's comorbid illnesses and medication usage are of vital importance. The effects of various types of medications on the response to exercise must also be considered. Although most medications will not limit exercise endurance *per se* over the limitations associated with the disease state itself, in some instances (*e.g.*, β-blocker use), the exercise response may be limited.

Maintenance of an adequate level of oxyhemoglobin saturation during exercise is important. Oxyhemogloblin desaturation (usually below a level of 90%) will limit exercise performance. During all exercise testing, measurement of the oxyhemoglobin saturation by pulse oximetry should be made. If the oxyhemoglobin saturation falls below 88%, the administration of supplemental oxygen (usually via a nasal cannula) should be afforded to the patient. An oxyhemoglobin level >88% should be maintained throughout the exercise with an increase in the level of oxygen delivery as so needed. Correct interpretation of oxyhemogloblin values is important as accurate results may be obscured in patients with vascular disease.

SUMMARY

Shortness of breath is a common presenting symptom for a patient with lung disease. There are three general types of lung disease: obstructive, restrictive, and vascular. Patients with obstructive lung disease have airflow limitation, primarily during exhalation. Those with restrictive lung disease have reduction in lung volumes, and those with vascular lung disease have alterations of the pulmonary vascular bed. Each disease process has a specific pathophysiology, both at rest and during exercise. Appropriate assessment of patients with lung disease includes performance of a thorough history and physical examination, laboratory studies (including chest radiograph, ECG, arterial blood gas, pulse oximetry, complete blood count, and pulmonary function tests), and, in some instances, a CT scan of the chest or a ventilation-perfusion scan. Exercise testing is helpful to confirm the disease's pathophysiology and to help direct treatment.

REFERENCES

1. American Thoracic Society, American College of Chest Physicians. ATS/ACCP Statement on cardiopulmonary exercise testing. *Am J Respir Crit Care Med*. 2003;167(2):211–77.
2. ATS Committee on Proficiency Standards for Clinical Pulmonary Function Laboratories. ATS statement: guidelines for the six-minute walk test. *Am J Respir Crit Care Med*. 2002;166(1):111–7.
3. Barnes PJ, Chung KF, Page CP. Inflammatory mediators of asthma: an update. *Pharmacol Rev*. 1998;50(4):515–96.
4. Bautista J, Ehsan M, Normandin E, Zuwallack R, Lahiri B. Physiologic responses during the six minute walk test in obese and non-obese COPD patients. *Respir Med*. 2011;105(8):1189–94.
5. Borg GA. Psychophysical bases of perceived exertion. *Med Sci Sports Exerc*. 1982;14(5):377–81.
6. Brines R, Thorne M. Clinical consensus on COPD. *Respir Med: COPD Update*. 2007;3(2):42–8.
7. Broekhuizen R, Wouters EF, Creutzberg EC, Schols AM. Raised CRP levels mark metabolic and functional impairment in advanced COPD. *Thorax*. 2006;61(1):17–22.
8. Cahalin LP, Mathier MA, Semigran MJ, Dec GW, DiSalvo TG. The six-minute walk test predicts peak oxygen uptake and survival in patients with advanced heart failure. *Chest*. 1996;110(2):325–32.
9. Calverley PMA. Exercise and dyspnea in COPD. *European Respiratory Review*. 2006;15(100):72–9.
10. Casaburi R. Skeletal muscle dysfunction in chronic obstructive pulmonary disease. *Med Sci Sports Exerc*. 2001;33(7 Suppl):S662–70.
11. Chang JA, Curtis JR, Patrick DL, Raghu G. Assessment of health-related quality of life in patients with interstitial lung disease. *Chest*. 1999;116(5):1175–82.
12. Chen Y, Horne SL, Dosman JA. Increased susceptibility to lung dysfunction in female smokers. *Am Rev Respir Dis*. 1991;143(6): 1224–30.
13. De Torres JP, Pinto-Plata V, Ingenito E, et al. Power of outcome measurements to detect clinically significant changes in pulmonary rehabilitation of patients with COPD. *Chest*. 2002;121(4):1092–8.
14. Debigare R, Cote CH, Maltais F. Peripheral muscle wasting in chronic obstructive pulmonary disease. Clinical relevance and mechanisms. *Am J Respir Crit Care Med*. 2001;164(9):1712–7.
15. Diaz O, Villafranca C, Ghezzo H, et al. Role of inspiratory capacity on exercise tolerance in COPD patients with and without tidal expiratory flow limitation at rest. *Eur Respir J*. 2000;16(2):269–75.

16. Dixon AE, Holguin F, Sood A, et al. An official American Thoracic Society Workshop report: obesity and asthma. *Proc Am Thorac Soc.* 2010;7(5):325–35.

17. Dudley KA, El-Chemaly S. Cardiopulmonary exercise testing in lung transplantation: a review. *Pulm Med.* 2012;2012:237852.

18. Enright PL, Sherrill DL. Reference equations for the six-minute walk in healthy adults. *Am J Respir Crit Care Med.* 1998;158(5 Pt 1): 1384–7.

19. *Expert Panel Report 3: Guidelines for the Diagnosis and Management of Asthma* [Internet]. Bethesda (MD): National Heart, Lung, and Blood Institute National Asthma Education and Prevention Program; [cited 2011 Mar 15]. Available from: http://www.nhlbi .nih.gov/guidelines/asthma/asthgdln.pdf

20. Fedullo PF, Auger WR, Channick RN, Kerr KM, Rubin LJ. Chronic thromboembolic pulmonary hypertension. *Clin Chest Med.* 2001;22(3):561–81.

21. Ferguson GT, Enright PL, Buist AS, Higgins MW. Office spirometry for lung health assessment in adults: A consensus statement from the National Lung Health Education Program. *Chest.* 2000;117(4):1146–61.

22. Fishman A, Martinez F, Naunheim K, et al. A randomized trial comparing lung-volume-reduction surgery with medical therapy for severe emphysema. *N Engl J Med.* 2003;348(21):2059–73.

23. Foreman MG, Zhang L, Murphy J, et al. Early-onset chronic obstructive pulmonary disease is associated with female sex, maternal factors, and African American race in the COPDGene Study. *Am J Respir Crit Care Med.* 2011;184(4):414–20.

24. Ganju AA, Fuladi AB, Tayade BO, Ganju NA. Cardiopulmonary exercise testing in evaluation of patients of chronic obstructive pulmonary disease. *Indian J Chest Dis Allied Sci.* 2011;53(2): 87–91.

25. Girish M, Trayner E,Jr, Dammann O, Pinto-Plata V, Celli B. Symptom-limited stair climbing as a predictor of postoperative cardiopulmonary complications after high-risk surgery. *Chest.* 2001;120(4):1147–51.

26. *Global Strategy for the Diagnosis, Management, and Prevention of COPD, Global Initiative for Chronic Obstructive Lung Disease (GOLD) 2011* [Internet]: Global Initiative for Chronic Obstructive Lung Disease (Gold); [cited 2012 Jul 1]. Available from: http:// www.goldcopd.org

27. Gold DR, Wang X, Wypij D, Speizer FE, Ware JH, Dockery DW. Effects of cigarette smoking on lung function in adolescent boys and girls. *N Engl J Med.* 1996;335(13):931–7.

28. Hansen JE, Wasserman K. Pathophysiology of activity limitation in patients with interstitial lung disease. *Chest.* 1996;109(6): 1566–76.

29. Hill AT, Bayley D, Stockley RA. The interrelationship of sputum inflammatory markers in patients with chronic bronchitis. *Am J Respir Crit Care Med.* 1999;160(3):893–8.

30. Hill K, Jenkins SC, Cecins N, Philippe DL, Hillman DR, Eastwood PR. Estimating maximum work rate during incremental cycle ergometry testing from six-minute walk distance in patients with chronic obstructive pulmonary disease. *Arch Phys Med Rehabil.* 2008;89(9):1782–7.

31. Holden DA, Rice TW, Stelmach K, Meeker DP. Exercise testing, 6-min walk, and stair climb in the evaluation of patients at high risk for pulmonary resection. *Chest.* 1992;102(6):1774–9.

32. Holgate ST. The cellular and mediator basis of asthma in relation to natural history. *Lancet.* 1997;350:5–9.

33. Keatings VM, Collins PD, Scott DM, Barnes PJ. Differences in interleukin-8 and tumor necrosis factor-alpha in induced sputum from patients with chronic obstructive pulmonary disease or asthma. *Am J Respir Crit Care Med.* 1996;153(2):530–4.

34. Kessler R, Faller M, Fourgaut G, Mennecier B, Weitzenblum E. Predictive factors of hospitalization for acute exacerbation in a series of 64 patients with chronic obstructive pulmonary disease. *Am J Respir Crit Care Med.* 1999;159(1):158–64.

35. Kim V, Han MK, Vance GB, et al. The chronic bronchitic phenotype of COPD: an analysis of the COPDGene study. *Chest.* 2011;140(3):626–33.

36. MacNee W. Pathophysiology of cor pulmonale in chronic obstructive pulmonary disease. Part two. *Am J Respir Crit Care Med.* 1994;150(4):1158–68.

37. Maltais F, Simard AA, Simard C, Jobin J, Desgagnes P, LeBlanc P. Oxidative capacity of the skeletal muscle and lactic acid kinetics during exercise in normal subjects and in patients with COPD. *Am J Respir Crit Care Med.* 1996;153(1):288–93.

38. Markovitz GH, Cooper CB. Exercise and interstitial lung disease. *Curr Opin Pulm Med.* 1998;4(5):272–80.

39. Martinez FJ, Raczek AE, Seifer FD, et al. Development and initial validation of a self-scored COPD Population Screener Questionnaire (COPD-PS). *COPD.* 2008;5(2):85–95.

40. Miller MR, Quanjer PH, Swanney MP, Ruppel G, Enright PL. Interpreting lung function data using 80% predicted and fixed thresholds misclassifies more than 20% of patients. *Chest.* 2011;139(1):52–9.

41. Molfino NA. Genetics of COPD. *Chest.* 2004;125(5):1929–40.

42. Montes de Oca M, Ortega Balza M, Lezama J, Lopez JM. Chronic obstructive pulmonary disease: evaluation of exercise tolerance using three different exercise tests. *Arch Bronconeumol.* 2001;37(2):69–74.

43. Mueller R, Chanez P, Campbell AM, Bousquet J, Heusser C, Bullock GR. Different cytokine patterns in bronchial biopsies in asthma and chronic bronchitis. *Respir Med.* 1996;90(2):79–85.

44. Mullen JB, Wright JL, Wiggs BR, Pare PD, Hogg JC. Reassessment of inflammation of airways in chronic bronchitis. *Br Med J (Clin Res Ed).* 1985;291(6504):1235–9.

45. Niewoehner DE, Kleinerman J, Rice DB. Pathologic changes in the peripheral airways of young cigarette smokers. *N Engl J Med.* 1974;291(15):755–8.

46. O'Donnell DE, Laveneziana P. Physiology and consequences of lung hyperinflation in COPD. *European Respiratory Review.* 2006;15(100):61–7.

47. O'Donnell DE, Revill SM, Webb KA. Dynamic hyperinflation and exercise intolerance in chronic obstructive pulmonary disease. *Am J Respir Crit Care Med.* 2001;164(5):770–7.

48. *An Official American Thoracic Society Statement: Update on the Mechanisms, Assessment, and Management of Dyspnea* [Internet]. New York (NY): American Thoracic Society; [cited 2012 Jul 1]. Available from: http://www.thoracic.org/statements/resources/ respiratory-disease-adults/update-on-mamd.pdf

49. Pauwels RA, Buist AS, Calverley PM, Jenkins CR, Hurd SS, GOLD Scientific Committee. Global strategy for the diagnosis, management, and prevention of chronic obstructive pulmonary disease. NHLBI/WHO Global Initiative for Chronic Obstructive Lung Disease (GOLD) Workshop summary. *Am J Respir Crit Care Med.* 2001;163(5):1256–76.

50. Pellicelli AM, Barbaro G, Palmieri F, et al. Primary pulmonary hypertension in HIV patients: a systematic review. *Angiology.* 2001;52(1):31–41.

51. Petty TL, Weinmann GG. Building a national strategy for the prevention and management of and research in chronic obstructive pulmonary disease. National Heart, Lung, and Blood Institute Workshop Summary. Bethesda, Maryland, August 29–31, 1995. *JAMA.* 1997;277(3):246–53.

52. Pinto-Plata VM, Mullerova H, Toso JF, et al. C-reactive protein in patients with COPD, control smokers and non-smokers. *Thorax.* 2006;61(1):23–8.

53. Pollock M, Roa J, Benditt J, Celli B. Estimation of ventilatory reserve by stair climbing. A study in patients with chronic airflow obstruction. *Chest.* 1993;104(5):1378–83.

54. Raeside DA, Smith A, Brown A, et al. Pulmonary artery pressure measurement during exercise testing in patients with suspected pulmonary hypertension. *Eur Respir J.* 2000;16(2):282–7.

55. Regan EA, Hokanson JE, Murphy JR, et al. Genetic epidemiology of COPD (COPDGene) study design. *COPD.* 2010;7(1):32–43.

56. Repine JE, Bast A, Lankhorst I. Oxidative stress in chronic obstructive pulmonary disease. Oxidative Stress Study Group. *Am J Respir Crit Care Med.* 1997;156(2 Pt 1):341–57.

57. Revill SM, Morgan MD, Singh SJ, Williams J, Hardman AE. The endurance shuttle walk: a new field test for the assessment of endurance capacity in chronic obstructive pulmonary disease. *Thorax.* 1999;54(3):213–22.

58. Roche WR, Beasley R, Williams JH, Holgate ST. Subepithelial fibrosis in the bronchi of asthmatics. *Lancet.* 1989;1(8637):520–4.

59. Roig M, Eng JJ, MacIntyre DL, Road JD, Reid WD. Associations of the Stair Climb Power Test with muscle strength and functional performance in people with chronic obstructive pulmonary disease: A cross-sectional study. *Phys Ther.* 2010;90(12):1774–82.

60. Ross RM, Murthy JN, Wollak ID, Jackson AS. The six minute walk test accurately estimates mean peak oxygen uptake. *BMC Pulm Med.* 2010;10:31.

61. Rubin LJ. Primary pulmonary hypertension. *N Engl J Med.* 1997;336(2):111–7.

62. Sciurba F, Criner GJ, Lee SM, et al. Six-minute walk distance in chronic obstructive pulmonary disease: reproducibility and effect of walking course layout and length. *Am J Respir Crit Care Med.* 2003;167(11):1522–7.

63. Seshadri N, Gildea TR, McCarthy K, Pothier C, Kavuru MS, Lauer MS. Association of an abnormal exercise heart rate recovery with pulmonary function abnormalities. *Chest.* 2004;125(4):1286–91.

64. Sin DD, Man SF. Skeletal muscle weakness, reduced exercise tolerance, and COPD: is systemic inflammation the missing link? *Thorax.* 2006;61(1):1–3.

65. Singh SJ, Morgan MD, Hardman AE, Rowe C, Bardsley PA. Comparison of oxygen uptake during a conventional treadmill test and the shuttle walking test in chronic airflow limitation. *Eur Respir J.* 1994;7(11):2016–20.

66. Strategies in preserving lung health and preventing COPD and associated diseases: National Lung Health Education Program (NLHEP). *Chest.* 1998;113(Suppl 2):123S–63S.

67. Sun XG, Hansen JE, Oudiz RJ, Wasserman K. Exercise pathophysiology in patients with primary pulmonary hypertension. *Circulation.* 2001;104(4):429–35.

68. Vernooy JH, Kucukaycan M, Jacobs JA, et al. Local and systemic inflammation in patients with chronic obstructive pulmonary disease: soluble tumor necrosis factor receptors are increased in sputum. *Am J Respir Crit Care Med.* 2002;166(9):1218–24.

69. Weisman IM, Zeballos RJ. Clinical exercise testing. *Clin Chest Med.* 1994;15:173–451.

70. Widimsky J, Riedel M, Stanek V. Central haemodynamics during exercise in patients with restrictive pulmonary disease. *Bull Eur Physiopathol Respir.* 1977;13(3):369–79.

71. Wise RA, Brown CD. Minimal clinically important differences in the six-minute walk test and the incremental shuttle walking test. *COPD.* 2005;2(1):125–9.

72. Yawn BP, Mapel DW, Mannino DM, et al. Development of the Lung Function Questionnaire (LFQ) to identify airflow obstruction. *Int J Chron Obstruct Pulmon Dis.* 2010;5:1–10.

SELECTED REFERENCES FOR FURTHER READING

Arena R. Exercise testing and training in chronic lung disease and pulmonary arterial hypertension. *Prog Cardiovascular Dis.* 2011;53:454–63.

Swank AM, Berry MS, Woodward CM. Chronic obstructive pulmonary disease. In: Ehrman JK, Gordon PM, Visich PS, Keteyian SJ, editors. *Clinical Exercise Physiology.* 2nd ed. Champaign: Human Kinetics; 2008. p. 371–90.

Wasserman K, Hansen JE, Sue DY, Stringer WW. *Principles of Exercise Testing and Interpretation.* 5th ed. Baltimore (MD): Lippincott, Williams & Wilkins; 2012. 592 p.

Weisman IM, Zeballos RJ. *Clinical Exercise Testing.* Basel (Switzerland): Karger; 2002. 329 p.

INTERNET RESOURCES

- AACVPR: American Association of Cardiovascular and Pulmonary Rehabilitation: http://www.aacvpr.org
- American College of Chest Physicians: http://www.chestnet.org
- American Thoracic Society: http://www.thoracic.org
- COPD Alliance: http://www.copd.org
- Global Initiative for Lung Disease (GOLD): http://www.goldcopd.org
- National Lung Health Education Program: http://www.nlhep.org

26

Diagnostic Procedures in Patients with Metabolic Disease

EPIDEMIOLOGY

The 2011 National Diabetes Fact Sheet (Centers for Disease Control and Prevention) reports that 8.5% of the U.S. population has diabetes, including 25.8 million children and adults (38). It is estimated that approximately 7 million of these individuals have not been diagnosed. Type 1 diabetes (T1D) accounts for 5%–10% of diagnosed cases, whereas Type 2 diabetes (T2D) accounts for 90%–95% of diagnosed cases. In addition, an estimated 79 million American adults older than the age of 20 yr have prediabetes as determined by fasting glucose or hemoglobin A1c levels. This report also revealed 215,000 Americans younger than the age of 20 yr, or 0.26% have diabetes; the great majority of those with diabetes in this age group have T1D (38).

KEY TERMS

Autonomic neuropathy: Abnormal function of the nerve fibers that belong or relate to the autonomic nervous system.

Blood glucose (sugar): *Blood sugar* is a common term used to refer to the amount of glucose in the blood plasma.

Compensatory hyperinsulinemia: As a result of insulin resistance, the pancreas may compensate by producing more insulin, leading to excessive blood insulin levels.

Diabetic neuropathy: A generic term for diabetes-related disorder of the peripheral or autonomic nervous system and some cranial nerves.

Fasting blood glucose: Measurement of blood glucose after at least 8 h with no caloric intake.

Glycosylated hemoglobin (HbA1C): Glycosylation (or glycation) is the process or result of the addition of sugars (*i.e.*, saccharides) to proteins and lipids. This test is used as a tool to monitor long-term control of blood glucose.

Hyperglycemia: High levels of glucose in the blood.

Insulin: Insulin is an anabolic hormone with a primary action to control (promote) carbohydrate metabolism and blood glucose disposal that acts to lower blood glucose levels.

Insulin resistance: Inadequate glucose uptake following normal insulin secretion; clinically determined when glucose uptake to a given concentration of insulin is less than expected.

Oral glucose tolerance test (OGTT): Specific test to assess the ability to regulate blood glucose and to screen or diagnose patients for diabetes mellitus.

Pancreatic β-cells: Cells that respond to elevations in blood glucose by producing and releasing insulin.

Radionuclide ventriculography: The display, by means of a stationary scintillation camera device, of the passage of a bolus of a rapidly injected radiopharmaceutical through the ventricles of the heart.

Silent ischemia: Ischemia of the myocardium that does not result in angina-like symptoms. In diabetes, this may result from the dysfunction of the peripheral nerves (neuropathy — see "function" stated previously).

Individuals with diabetes have a higher incidence and prevalence of symptomatic as well as asymptomatic coronary artery disease (CAD) than those without diabetes. Patients with diabetes have more diffuse and more severe atherosclerotic disease than other populations and are at higher risk for cardiovascular (CV) events and mortality from those events (38). Women with diabetes are at greater risk for CV events compared with women without diabetes (32,50), especially if other risk factors are present (16). Asymptomatic individuals with diabetes have a higher prevalence of silent myocardial ischemia and associated autonomic nerve dysfunction than those without diabetes (24).

In addition, patients on insulin therapy or who have microalbuminuria have a significantly higher prevalence of silent myocardial ischemia compared with those not taking insulin or without retinopathy (37). Wackers et al. reported that 22% of asymptomatic patients with diabetes demonstrated silent ischemia through positive myocardial perfusion imaging scan (63). These results could also be predicted by an abnormal Valsalva maneuver and diabetes duration but not by prothrombotic or inflammatory markers or traditional risk factors (62,63).

Routine exercise testing is an important diagnostic and prognostic procedure for individuals with diabetes (2). Because of the risk of exercise-related sudden death, it is recommended that adults with a long history of diabetes and those with one or more additional CV risk factors undergo exercise testing before beginning a vigorous exercise program (54).

The metabolic syndrome (MetS) not only predicts a future diagnosis of diabetes but is also shown to cause significant increases in risk for premature cardiovascular disease (CVD). Insulin resistance is a primary pathophysiology of MetS (22). Hyperglycemia is initially controlled by insulin but at the cost of hyperinsulinemia. The pancreas usually responds with excessive pancreatic β-cell production of insulin, resulting in compensatory hyperinsulinemia in an attempt to successfully control blood glucose (48). In addition, insulin resistance within adipose tissue is thought to inhibit lipid metabolism, be associated with elevated cholesterol levels, and increase the risk of T2D. Hyperglycemia, altered lipoproteins, and hyperinsulinemia are associated with increases in various inflammatory markers and cytokines known to promote vascular inflammation and atherosclerosis (61). A more detailed and complete discussion of MetS is found subsequently.

This chapter will address the diagnostic procedures for T1D, T2D and gestational diabetes mellitus. Currently, there is a debate whether MetS should be considered a disease in its own entity independent of its individual risk factors, or should be used in addition to T1D and/or T2D (28). In this section, MetS will be examined as an emerging condition that precedes T2D, has a very high prevalence, and displays significant elevations in CV risk.

BOX 26-1 Risk Factors for Metabolic Syndrome

Waist circumference: $\geq$102 cm ($\geq$40 in) in men or $\geq$88 cm ($\geq$35 in) in women

Triglycerides: $\geq$150 mg · dL^{-1}

HDL-C: <40 mg · dL^{-1} in men or <50 mg · dL^{-1} in women

Blood pressure: $\geq$130/85 mm Hg

Blood glucose: $\geq$100 mg · dL^{-1}

DIAGNOSIS OF METABOLIC SYNDROME

Throughout the last several decades, there has been much revision as well as increasing interest in the constellation of conditions that make up MetS. MetS is reviewed in *Chapter 8* of this *Resource Manual*.

The most current diagnostic guidelines are set forth in the Adult Treatment Panel III criteria (22). The presence of three out of five risk factors for MetS determines the diagnosis. See *Box 26-1* for risk factors for MetS and *Table 26-1* for definitions of MetS.

If a diagnosis of MetS is made, the individual should be assessed for safety for exercise before beginning any moderate-to-high intensity exercise training program (54). Treatment as well as assessment for CAD is important because of the higher risk of atherosclerosis that accompanies MetS. This is often initially assessed by radionuclide stress testing, as discussed later in this chapter.

DIAGNOSIS OF DIABETES MELLITUS

The diagnostic criteria for the diagnosis of diabetes mellitus and prediabetes are found in *Table 26-2*. Positive test results must be confirmed by repeating the fasting plasma glucose (FPG), glycosylated hemoglobin (HbA1C) testing, or the oral glucose tolerance test (OGTT) on a different day.

Gestational diabetes is also diagnosed using plasma glucose values measured during the OGTT, although the criteria differ. For women with no diabetes who are pregnant, at 24–28 wk of gestation, the blood glucose levels are checked three times following the ingestion of a known amount of glucose (100 g), at fasting, 1 and 2 h. If blood glucose levels are above normal (>92, 180, and 153 mg · dL^{-1}, respectively) at any time point during the test, the patient is considered to have gestational diabetes (see *Table 26-3*) (3).

TABLE 26-1. A Comparison of the Various Organizational Definitions for Metabolic Syndrome (22)

Clinical Measure	WHO (1998)	EGIR	ATP III (2001)	AACE (2003)	IDF (2005)
Insulin resistance	IGT, IFG, T2DM, or lowered insulin sensitivity[a] plus any two of the following	Plasma insulin >75th percentile plus any two of the following	None, but any three of the following five features	IGT or IFG plus any of the following based on clinical judgment	None
Body weight	Men: waist-to-hip ratio >0.90; women: waist-to-hip ratio >0.85 and/or BMI >30 kg · m^{-2}	WC ≥94 cm in men or ≥80 cm in women	WC ≥102 cm in men[b] or ≥88 cm in women	BMI ≥25 kg · m^{-2}	Increased WC (population specific) plus any two of the following
Lipid	TG ≥150 mg · dL^{-1} and/or HDL-C <35 mg · dL^{-1} in men or <39 mg · dL^{-1} in women	TG ≥150 mg · dL^{-1} and/or HDL-C <39 mg · dL^{-1} in men or women	TG ≥150 mg · dL^{-1} HDL-C <40 mg · dL^{-1} in men or <50 mg · dL^{-1} in women	TG ≥150 mg · dL^{-1} and HDL-C <40 mg · dL^{-1} in men or <50 mg · dL^{-1} in women	TG ≥150 mg · dL^{-1} or on TG Rx, HDL-C <40 mg · dL^{-1} in men or <50 mg · dL^{-1} in women or on HDL-C Rx
Blood pressure	≥140/90 mm Hg	≥140/90 mm Hg or on hypertension Rx	≥130/85 mm Hg	≥130/85 mm Hg	≥130/85 mm Hg or on hypertension Rx
Glucose	IGT, IFG, or T2DM	IGT or IFG (but not diabetes)	>110 mg · dL^{-1} (includes diabetes)[c]	IGT or IFG (but not diabetes)	≥100 mg · dL^{-1} (includes diabetes)
Other	Microalbuminuria			Other features of insulin resistance[d]	

WHO, World Health Organization; EGIR, European Group for the Study of Insulin Resistance; ATP, Adult Treatment Panel; AACE, American Association of Clinical Endocrinologists; IDF, International Diabetes Federation; IGT, impaired glucose tolerance; IFG, impaired fasting glucose; T2DM, Type 2 diabetes mellitus; BMI, body mass index; WC, waist circumference; TG, triglycerides; HDL-C, high-density lipoprotein cholesterol; Rx, prescription. All other abbreviations as in text.

[a]Insulin sensitivity measured under hyperinsulinemic euglycemic conditions, glucose uptake below lowest quartile for background population under investigation.

[b]Some male patients can develop multiple metabolic risk factors when the waist circumference is only marginally increased (i.e., 94–102 cm [37–39 in]). Such patients may have a strong genetic contribution to insulin resistance. They should benefit from changes in lifestyle habits, similar to men with categorical increases in waist circumference.

[c]The 2001 definition identified fasting plasma glucose of ≥110 mg · dL^{-1} (6.1 mmol · L^{-1}) as elevated. This was modified in 2004 to ≥100 mg · dL^{-1} (5.6 mmol · L^{-1}), in accordance with the American Diabetes Association's updated definition of impaired fasting glucose (IFG) (3).

[d]Includes family history of Type 2 diabetes mellitus, polycystic ovary syndrome, sedentary lifestyle, advancing age, and ethnic groups susceptible to Type 2 diabetes mellitus.

WHO SHOULD BE TESTED FOR DIABETES MELLITUS?

The initial "diagnosis" of diabetes is often made through ordinary health screening and/or through new signs and symptoms that result from the diabetes, such as vision changes or unexplainable fatigue. The diagnosis of T1D and many cases of T2D is prompted by recent-onset symptoms of excessive urination (polyuria) and excessive thirst (polydipsia), often accompanied by weight loss. These symptoms typically worsen over days to weeks. Diabetes screening is recommended for many

TABLE 26-2. Diagnostic Criteria for Diabetes Mellitus (4)

	Prediabetes	Diabetes
Hb$_{A1c}$	≥5.7%–6.4%	≥6.5%
Fasting plasma glucose (FPG)	100–125 mg · dL^{-1} (5.6–6.9 mmol · L^{-1}) (fasting is defined as no caloric intake for at least 8 h)	≥126 mg · dL^{-1} (7.0 mmol · L^{-1})
Random plasma glucose		≥200 mg · dL^{-1} (with symptoms of hyperglycemia or hyperglycemic crisis)
Oral glucose tolerance test (OGTT) (After fasting, a beverage of 75 g of glucose is consumed and blood glucose is measured 2 h later. The OGTT is more sensitive than the FBG test for diagnosing diabetes but is less convenient to administer.)	140–199 mg · dL^{-1} (7.8–11.0 mmol · L^{-1}) at 2-h point	≥200 mg · dL^{-1} (11.1 mmol · L^{-1}) at 2-h point"

Hb$_{A1c}$, glycosylated hemoglobin.

TABLE 26-3. Gestational Diabetes: Above-Normal Results for the Oral Glucose Tolerance Test

When	Plasma Glucose Result (mg · dL^{-1})
Fasting	92 or higher
At 1 h	180 or higher
At 2 h	153 or higher

people at various stages of life as well as for those with CV risk factors such as hypertension, obesity, and abnormal lipid values. Generally, adults who are overweight (body mass index [BMI] $\geq$25 kg · m^{-2}) or 45 yr of age or older should be considered for initial and routine diabetes testing, especially if they have the aforementioned risk factors or overt CAD (3,11,12). Assessment for diabetes is especially important not only in those who have the general risks for diabetes but also for those who wish to begin an exercise training program, in particular to one that is of moderate or high intensity (12).

CLINICAL EVALUATION

The American Diabetes Association (ADA) recommends assessment of CV risk factors on an annual basis, including dyslipidemia, hypertension, smoking, family history, and microalbuminuria or macroalbuminuria for those with established diabetes (3). Patients with diabetes should undergo both a detailed history and a thorough physical examination with a focus on determining the presence of macrovascular and microvascular disease, a neuropathic assessment for both peripheral and autonomic dysfunction, and, if appropriate, diagnostic studies before embarking on an exercise program (3). The 1998 Consensus Development Conference of the ADA proposed that patients with multiple risk factors for CVD might have the highest yield of positive results from cardiac testing, and this is a basis for criteria for selection of patients who should undergo routine and preexercise stress testing (12). However, more recent studies have shown that the burden of traditional risk factors do not predict inducible ischemia with myocardial perfusion imaging and also demonstrate similar rates of ischemia in asymptomatic patients with diabetes, with or without traditional risk factors (62,63).

In the absence of symptomatic CAD, clinical features that help to identify the patient at increased risk for myocardial infarction (MI) or sudden cardiac death include evidence of other atherosclerotic vascular disease (e.g., heart, carotid, peripheral); renal disease; abnormal resting electrocardiogram (ECG); and diabetes complications, including autonomic neuropathy, retinopathy, hypertension, and dyslipidemia. Although these factors do not indicate the presence or absence of inducible ischemia, they still warrant careful consideration for identifying patients at risk for events.

A resting 12-lead ECG may be useful to identify evidence of ischemic heart disease, a previous MI, or even an unknown cardiac rhythm disturbance (7,50). These may include the presence of nonspecific ST-T wave changes, which may be a predictor of inducible ischemia in asymptomatic patients with diabetes (46). However, a resting ECG is insufficient for diagnosing ischemic cardiac conditions that often require a high degree of myocardial work, as during exercise, to invoke an ischemic response (36,56). Thus, there is a need for exercise testing in these individuals before beginning exercise training.

Microalbuminuria is predictive for vascular disease complications as well as progression to overt nephropathy (52). Patients with T2D and chronic kidney disease as a result of diabetic nephropathy display a high risk for acute MI and sudden cardiac death. This is reported to be as high as 40% over a 5-yr period and, thus, indicates another marker of vascular disease in this population (31).

Autonomic neuropathy is associated with a poor overall prognosis in patients with T1D and T2D. The mechanisms that confer the high risk are poorly understood but may include impairment in ischemia awareness, delaying the diagnosis of CAD, or hemodynamic dysfunction as a result of blunted parasympathetic activation. Autonomic neuropathy was a major predictor of inducible ischemia in the DIAD (Detection of Ischemia in Asymptomatic Diabetics) study and is associated with abnormal cardiac test findings in other studies (7,63). See *Table 26-4* for some abnormal CV responses to exercise testing in individuals with diabetes-related autonomic neuropathy.

The ADA recently recommended a screening for autonomic neuropathy for patients with indications of autonomic dysfunction, beginning at the diagnosis of T2D and 5 yr after the diagnosis of T1D (3). The possibility of cardiac autonomic neuropathy should be considered in the presence of unexplained resting tachycardia, exercise intolerance, orthostatic hypotension and/or hypotension, constipation, gastroparesis, erectile dysfunction, sudomotor dysfunction, impaired neurovascular function, and the chance for autonomic failure in hypoglycemic conditions. Autonomic dysfunction may affect the ability to regulate blood pressure during exercise and make it difficult to use heart rate (HR) to guide exercise intensity (12).

Retinopathy is a manifestation of microvascular disease and a risk for CAD in both T1D and T2D. Risk factors for retinopathy include the duration of diabetes, chronic hyperglycemia, nephropathy, and hypertension. In clinical studies, retinopathy is associated with inducible ischemia in some, but not all, screenings (27). However, diabetic retinopathy in patients with T1D and T2D is associated with increased mortality from all causes as well as risk for CV event (28). Patients with diabetes should be regularly screened for retinopathy, and when present, limitations in lifting (i.e., resistance training) and any other activity that increases intraocular pressure may be indicated.

TABLE 26-4. Abnormal Exercise-Induced Cardiovascular Parameters in Patients with Diabetes Having Autonomic Neuropathy

Parameters	Potential Abnormalities or Etiologies
Nervous system	Impaired sympathetic Impaired parasympathetic
Electrocardiogram	Resting tachycardia (>100 bpm) Reduced resting heart rate variability Prolonged QT intervals Attenuated chronotropic response ST-T wave abnormalities
Arrhythmia	Potentially secondary to exercise-induced hypoglycemia and its stimulation of the sympathetic nervous system
Diastolic function	Abnormal
Left ventricular ejection fraction	Impaired, both at rest and with exercise
Rate-pressure product	Higher resting; lower at maximum exercise
Blood pressure	Hypertension or hypotension during or postexercise
Orthostasis ($\downarrow$SBP >20 mm Hg upon standing)	Decreased release of catecholamines with increased vasoconstrictive effect
Silent ischemia	Advanced coronary artery disease

bpm, beats per minute; SBP, systolic blood pressure.

A consistently elevated and uncontrolled blood glucose value, as indicated by an A1c value >7.0%, is a strong predictor of microvascular disease (3). Interventions to improve glycemic control are shown to reduce coronary events in populations with T1D and T2D. Hence, chronic uncontrolled hyperglycemia is a risk factor for CVD. Patients with diabetes are also at risk of hypoglycemia associated with exercise. This is especially true for those who use insulin. It is prudent to assess blood glucose values before and after exercise, including exercise testing, in patients who use insulin.

Given these comorbid circumstances, routine stress testing with standard ECG is valuable to assess the CV status of the patient with diabetes and to prescribe exercise training. Additionally, several important developments in CV imaging technology have evolved to assist in detecting CAD in asymptomatic patients with risk factors, including diabetes. Professional societies have updated their recommendations for the use of computed tomography imaging (1).

PRACTICAL CONSIDERATIONS OF ROUTINE EXERCISE TESTING

Because CAD is the major cause of morbidity, mortality, and medical costs in population with diabetes, early detection and intervention have significant prognostic appeal. More than 10 yr ago, the ADA convened an expert panel and developed the consensus statement on the diagnosis of coronary heart disease in patients with diabetes (14). This document focused on the burden of

risk factors and the duration of diabetes to determine the need for stress testing. Since that time, new technologies of noninvasive cardiac imaging have demonstrated a high incidence of unknown cardiac ischemia in patients with diabetes who do not have the traditional risk factors indicated in the 1998 consensus statement. The DIAD study reported that silent ischemia was found by single-photon emission computed tomography (SPECT) in 22% of asymptomatic subjects with diabetes. It was determined that if the 1998 guidelines were applied, that CAD would have remained undetected in as many as 41% of patients with T2D (63).

The decreased sensitivity and specificity of exercise testing in an asymptomatic individual may result in a minimal diagnostic value depending on many variables, including the type, severity, and duration of the diabetes. One major concern is that exercise testing can be costly for routine screening, and with the significant number of individuals with T2D, exercise testing such a large cohort would place a large financial burden on the health care system. Furthermore, in an asymptomatic population, exercise testing may result in a false-positive diagnosis and may be a poor predictor for major cardiac events (54). See *Chapter 23* in this *Resource Manual* for a more detailed discussion of clinical exercise testing.

Diagnostic cardiac stress testing is suggested by the ADA for those with typical or atypical cardiac symptoms or an abnormal resting ECG (3). Screening stress testing is suggested by the ADA for those with (a) history of peripheral or carotid occlusive disease, (b) sedentary lifestyle (<35 yr of age with plans to start a vigorous exercise program), or (c) two or more risk factors

BOX 26-2	Guidelines for Determining the Need for Exercise Testing in Individuals with Diabetes (12)

1. >45 yr of age, with BMI >25 kg · m^{-2} without other CVD risk factors or <45 yr of age, with BMI >25 kg · m^{-2} and additional CVD risk factors
2. Age >35 yr

   T2DM >10-yr duration

   T1DM >15-yr duration

   Any additional atherosclerotic CVD risk factor

   Microvascular disease evidenced by proliferative retinopathy or nephropathy including microalbuminuria

3. Autonomic dysfunction
4. Any of the following at any age:
   - Suspected or known CAD, cerebrovascular disease, and/or peripheral artery disease
   - Autonomic neuropathy
   - Advanced nephropathy with renal failure

BMI, body mass index; CAD, coronary artery disease; CVD, cardiovascular disease; T1DM, Type 1 diabetes mellitus; T2DM, Type 2 diabetes mellitus.

(dyslipidemia, hypertension, smoking, family history of premature coronary disease, and microalbuminuria or macroalbuminuria) (3).

Prior to an exercise test, patients with diabetes should be evaluated for absolute and relative contraindications (see *GETP9* for more information) to determine appropriateness and safety of testing (12,54). *Box 26-2* summarizes clinical guidelines to help determine if an individual with diabetes should undergo a graded exercise test to evaluate CV health status before beginning a moderate- to high-intensity exercise program (12). Clinical judgment is needed to determine if an individual with diabetes should have an exercise test prior to beginning a light-intensity exercise program. Generally, for patients planning to participate in no more than moderate-intensity exercise, particularly in those without medical conditions that are contraindicative to regular exercise, an exercise test may not be warranted before starting an exercise program (12). However, it is recommended that an individual with typical or atypical cardiac symptoms or an abnormal resting ECG result have a diagnostic exercise test, even when beginning light exercise (54).

It is recommended that individuals with diabetes undergo an exercise test before engaging in vigorous-intensity ($\geq$60% $\dot{V}O_2$ reserve, 77% HR$_{max}$) exercise (12). Individuals with diabetes and advanced disease states, even those diseases not commonly associated with risks for CAD, should undergo exercise testing because microvascular and neuropathic complications (*e.g.*, diabetic retinopathy, nephropathy, and autonomic neuropathy) are often seen in these individuals, and they are associated with increased prevalence of sudden death (63).

To date, there are no recommendations relative to exercise testing for individuals with MetS. On a case-by-case basis, it may be indicated to assess those with MetS or CAD by exercise testing. The following recommendations pertain to those with diabetes only.

CARDIAC COMPLICATIONS SPECIFIC TO INDIVIDUALS WITH DIABETES

Silent myocardial ischemia in asymptomatic men with diabetes occurs frequently (39,40,63), especially in those on long-term insulin treatment and/or with long-term uncontrolled hyperglycemia. These individuals often have autonomic neuropathy (33), which is associated with an increased risk of sudden death (18). Individuals with diabetes often demonstrate early loss of parasympathetic function with later progression to sympathetic dysfunction. Additionally, cardiac autonomic control is frequently altered with diabetes, resulting in reduced HR variability (51), a condition related to chronic hyperglycemia (55), an elevated resting HR, and a reduced exercise HR response. *Table 26-4* summarizes clinical issues during exercise in patients with diabetes and autonomic dysfunction.

EXERCISE TESTING MODALITIES

Different testing modalities may be used in individuals with diabetes for detecting underlying CAD. Certain exercise testing modalities may be suited for persons with diabetes who may have peripheral artery disease or peripheral neuropathy. Specifically, those with foot ulcerations or a tendency for ulceration may consider avoiding exercise that involves foot impact, such as walking. Supportive shoes should be used for stability and for protection, especially in those with peripheral neuropathy and loss of sensation in their feet (29). The room should be kept at a comfortable, cool temperature, and adequate hydration should be given during and after the test because some patients may have inhibited ability to regulate body temperature secondary to autonomic dysfunction. Before testing, vision and neurologic problems should be assessed because these complications may interfere with exercise testing protocols.

EXERCISE TESTING WITH ELECTROCARDIOGRAPHY

A standard method to evaluate CV status in response to exercise is through observation of their ECG response during and after progressive stages of exercise. This type of exercise test is relatively easy to administer and less costly than other stress testing modalities using echocardiography or radionuclide imaging. Symptom-limited, rather than HR-limited testing procedures, provides the best prognostic value, although test administrators should be aware of the increased possibility of chronotropic incompetence in individuals with diabetes (23). The addition of cardiac imaging modalities, especially in asymptomatic individuals, is being increasingly used to more accurately diagnose myocardial ischemia and assess myocardial function during physical exertion. It is highly recommended in patients with longstanding diabetes or other CVD risk factors (see *GETP9* for complete guidelines on exercise testing).

Stress testing with cardiac imaging is a common modality for diagnosing underlying CAD, and it may be especially important for women with diabetes (32). Women demonstrate an increased frequency of false-positive exercise stress tests and because of their lower pretest likelihood of having advanced CAD compared with men, the increased diagnostic specificity and sensitivity is clinically significant (58). The diagnostic accuracy obtained from a meta-analysis using exercise stress ECG testing results from patients without a prior MI showed the mean sensitivity to be 68% and the mean specificity of 77% for detecting underlying CAD (21).

STRESS ECHOCARDIOGRAPHIC TESTING

Patients with diabetes who have an abnormal resting ECG result or a slightly positive ECG response to exercise stress (1.0–1.5 mm ST-segment depression at a moderate-to-high exercise-induced HR) or who are asymptomatic for CAD may be further evaluated using other tests, such as stress echocardiography. A stress echocardiography assessment identifies positive findings in 12%–31% of asymptomatic patients with diabetes and is an effective prognostic tool in patients with diabetes with known or suspected CAD (44,45). Dobutamine stress echocardiography is equivalent to ^{201}Thallium SPECT in detecting asymptomatic CAD in patients with diabetes, making it a good testing modality for facilities without nuclear scanning equipment (42).

RADIONUCLIDE STRESS IMAGING

Radionuclide Ventriculography

Patients with diabetes who have an abnormal resting ECG result or a slightly positive ECG response to exercise stress may be further evaluated using stress SPECT myocardial perfusion imaging. Those with non-specific ST-segment and T-wave changes on a resting ECG or who have exercise-induced nonspecific ECG changes may need further assessment using radionuclide or radiotracer imaging. Radionuclide ventriculography studies are also useful in patients needing an evaluation for exercise-induced ischemia who have abnormalities such as resting ST-segment depression >1 mm, left bundle branch block (LBBB), or electronically paced rhythm. Of the different noninvasive imaging tests used to diagnose occlusive coronary disease, stress nuclear imaging has established itself as one of the most reliable and informative tools (15,25).

A myocardial perfusion image showing a small fixed defect should not restrict an individual with diabetes from exercising. However, imaging suggesting a large perfusion abnormality in a patient with diabetes with symptomatic or silent ischemia indicates significant risk for cardiac event (42).

Radionuclide Imaging in Combination with Pharmacologic Stress

Individuals who are unable to undergo exercise testing may be assessed via pharmacologic stress testing using dobutamine, adenosine, or dipyridamole (Persantine) to cause myocardial hyperemia when performing ^{201}Thallium myocardial perfusion imaging. This is covered in more detail in *Chapter 23* of this *Resource Manual*.

OTHER EXERCISE TESTING CONSIDERATIONS

A review of diabetes medications should be completed before stress testing. This is important for anticipating the blood glucose changes to an upcoming exercise bout or stress test. An excessive insulin level during exercise is the primary cause of reduced blood glucose after exercise. Patients taking supplemental (exogenous) insulin are at risk of exercise-induced hypoglycemia (EIH) as are patients who are taking oral antiglycemic drugs that cause the pancreas to produce more insulin. These drugs are referred to as *insulin secretagogues* and are found in the sulfonylurea and meglitinide drug classes. Patients taking other oral antihyperglycemic drugs (biguinide or thiazolidinediones, dipeptidyl peptidase (DPP)-IV inhibitors) are not at great risk for EIH, and supplemental feedings may not be required.

Ideally, the time of day individuals with diabetes undergo an exercise test should coincide with the time they would normally exercise if they plan to begin an exercise program, and the time should be coordinated with meals and insulin or oral antihyperglycemic agent doses. These individuals should be tested while taking their usual medications if test results are to be used for planning a systematic, individualized exercise program.

Testing should be avoided if the glucose levels are >250 mg · dL^{-1} and ketosis is present, or if glucose levels are >300 mg · dL^{-1} with or without ketosis. If glucose levels are <100 mg · dL^{-1} and the patient is taking insulin or oral insulin secretogogue drugs, then glucose (~20–30 g) should be ingested before exercise testing to prevent a hypoglycemic response. It is helpful to have patients monitor their blood glucose levels before and after exercise testing, especially those patients taking insulin or oral insulin secretogogue drugs because these drugs cause the risk of EIH. Guidance during the exercise test can include beneficial information for the patients about maintaining glycemic control while balancing medications, meals, and exercise. Having patients self-monitor their blood glucose also provides the health care team the opportunity to ensure that patients are correct in their glucose monitoring methods. Some clinic facilities, however, may have their own testing equipment and require any testing performed for the purpose of guiding treatment to be performed using that equipment.

Patients taking medications that cause vasodilation may be at risk for postexercise hypotension and may require an extended cool-down period, during which they should be closely monitored. This is especially true in patients with autonomic neuropathy because sympathetic control may be impaired. Those undergoing exercise testing while using an insulin pump should be advised to reduce or stop their insulin infusion rate, as indicated, during the exercise test to prevent EIH.

SENSITIVITY AND SPECIFICITY OF STRESS TESTS

The most effective method of stress testing for detecting underlying CAD depends on good clinical judgment. One consideration to determine an appropriate diagnostic testing modality depends on the pretest probability of CAD, which is influenced by factors such as age, sex, symptoms, and medical history. Examples regarding the sensitivity and specificity values for diagnosing CAD using different myocardial testing modalities can be found in *Chapter 23* of this *Resource Manual*. Pooled data of different patient populations or single laboratory studies are provided (5,10,19,20,49) and, when indicated, reports for individuals with diabetes (7,8,10,40,58) are available (5,6,8,40,57).

PROGNOSTIC ASSESSMENT WITH EXERCISE TESTING

Both the resting and exercise ECG can help predict mortality in individuals with diabetes. Resting ECG shows HR, QT interval, and right bundle branch blocks (RBBB) and LBBB, which may predict future adverse conditions. A prolonged QT interval (corrected for HR [QTc] and calculated as QT/QTc) may lengthen over time in patients with diabetes (17). Patients with either T1D or T2D have a high prevalence of QT prolongation, which is associated with ischemic heart disease in population-based studies (30,59,60). Along with associated cardiac ischemia, those with T2D and a prolonged QT dispersion may have other complications, such as left ventricular hypertrophy or autonomic dysfunction (47). This abnormal electrophysiologic finding is also an independent predictor of mortality in those with T1D (43). Independent of the QT interval, HR variability has also been associated with mortality. RBBB and LBBB have both been associated with heart failure (43). Another independent predictor of mortality for older patients (including those with diabetes) is impaired functional capacity (34).

Individuals with diabetes are more likely to experience impaired chronotropic response (failure of HR to increase normally with exercise). Individuals who experience impaired chronotropic response are at an increased risk for all-cause mortality, MI, or future coronary revascularization procedures (23). Abnormal HR recovery after exercise testing is an independent predictor of silent myocardial ischemia, CV, and all-cause death (11). Attenuated HR recovery after exercise (<12 beats per minute [bpm] at 1-min postexercise) is associated with increased mortality. Patients with diabetes and/or hyperglycemia may demonstrate attenuated HR recovery after exercise (13,41,53). The clinical value of close monitoring during the postexercise period in individuals with diabetes is emphasized by these data.

In patients with T2D with known or suspected CAD, abnormal dobutamine stress echocardiography results were independent predictors of death. In this population, myocardial ischemia proved to be an independent predictor of mortality, incremental to the clinical risks for CAD and left ventricular dysfunction (32). Even with a negative stress echocardiogram, patients with diabetes are at higher risk for major cardiac events secondary to a higher prevalence of CAD (22).

Cardiac death rates in 6,173 patients (2,677 men; 2,656 women) with diabetes undergoing rest ^{201}Thallium/ stress ^{99m}Technetium sestamibi scanning dual-isotope myocardial perfusion SPECT with exercise or adenosine pharmacologic testing have been reported (9). This study indicates increased cardiac deaths in all individuals with diabetes (including women) compared with those without diabetes for any test result (see *Table 26-5*).

CORONARY ARTERY CALCIFICATION IMAGING

Those with diabetes tend to have larger amounts of coronary artery calcium (CAC) deposits than patients with no diabetes (35). Asymptomatic patients with diabetes

TABLE 26-5. Annual Rates for Cardiac Death for Men and Women with Diabetes (9)

	Cardiac Death Rates	
Nuclide Scan Results	**Men**	**Women**
Normal	0.6%	0.9%
Mildly abnormal	1.8%	1.4%
Moderate to abnormal	3.8%	3.8%
Severely abnormal	5.5%	7.0%

have similar CAC scores to patients with symptomatic CAD but without diabetes. There are no differences in CAC scores between men and women with diabetes (26). A CAC score of >400 has been shown in one-third of asymptomatic patients with diabetes (4). In subjects with diabetes, mortality increases in proportion to CAC score more so than those with no diabetes (47). Recent evidence suggests that prevalence of CAC is a better predictor of myocardial ischemia and short-term CV events than traditional risk factors (4).

SUMMARY

Individuals at risk for or with diagnosed diabetes should be routinely screened for CVD. The risk of CVD increases significantly once a diagnosis of diabetes has been established. The use of exercise testing for the diagnosis of underlying CAD is clinically important for individuals with diabetes. Because regular exercise is an important component in the management of diabetes, exercise testing can assist with the identification of ischemia during increased myocardial demands, such as those associated with exercise training. Although exercise test results can be used for diagnostic and prognostic purposes, an additional important use of test results is to produce a systematic, individualized exercise prescription. *Chapter 40* reviews the development and implementation of the exercise prescription in people with diabetes.

REFERENCES

1. American College of Cardiology Foundation Task Force on Expert Consensus Documents, Mark DB, Berman DS, et al. ACCF/ACR/AHA/NASCI/SAIP/SCAI/SCCT 2010 expert consensus document on coronary computed tomographic angiography: a report of the American College of Cardiology Foundation Task Force on Expert Consensus Documents. *J Am Coll Cardiol*. 2010;55(23):2663–99.
2. American Diabetes Association. Diabetes mellitus and exercise (position statement). *Diabet Care*. 2001;24(Suppl 1):S51–5.
3. American Diabetes Association. Standards of medical care in diabetes—2011. *Diabetes Care*. 2011;34 Suppl 1:S11–61.
4. Anand DV, Lim E, Hopkins D, et al. Risk stratification in uncomplicated type 2 diabetes: prospective evaluation of the combined use of coronary artery calcium imaging and selective myocardial perfusion scintigraphy. *Eur Heart J*. 2006;27(6):713–21.
5. Bacci S, Villella M, Villella A, et al. Screening for silent myocardial ischaemia in type 2 diabetic patients with additional atherogenic risk factors: applicability and accuracy of the exercise stress test. *Eur J Endocrinol*. 2002;147(5):649–54.
6. Bar-Or O, Rowland TW. *Pediatric Exercise Medicine: From Physiologic Principles to Health Care Application*. Leeds (United Kingdom): Human Kinetics; 2004. 520 p.
7. Bax JJ, Young LH, Frye RL, Bonow RO, Steinberg HO, Barrett EJ, ADA. Screening for coronary artery disease in patients with diabetes. *Diabetes Care*. 2007;30(10):2729–36.
8. Bell DS, Yumuk VD. Low incidence of false-positive exercise thallium 201 scintigraphy in a diabetic population. *Diabetes Care*. 1996;19(2):185–6.
9. Berman DS, Kang X, Hayes SW, et al. Adenosine myocardial perfusion single-photon emission computed tomography in women compared with men. Impact of diabetes mellitus on incremental prognostic value and effect on patient management. *J Am Coll Cardiol*. 2003;41(7):1125–33.
10. Cheitlin MD, Alpert JS, Armstrong WF, et al. ACC/AHA Guidelines for the Clinical Application of Echocardiography. A report of the American College of Cardiology/American Heart Association Task Force on Practice Guidelines (Committee on Clinical Application of Echocardiography). Developed in collaboration with the American Society of Echocardiography. *Circulation*. 1997;95(6):1686–744.
11. Cheng YJ, Lauer MS, Earnest CP, et al. Heart rate recovery following maximal exercise testing as a predictor of cardiovascular disease and all-cause mortality in men with diabetes. *Diabetes Care*. 2003;26(7):2052–7.
12. Colberg SR, Albright AL, Blissmer BJ, et al. Exercise and type 2 diabetes: American College of Sports Medicine and the American Diabetes Association: joint position statement. Exercise and type 2 diabetes. *Med Sci Sports Exerc*. 2010;42(12):2282–303.
13. Cole CR, Blackstone EH, Pashkow FJ, Snader CE, Lauer MS. Heart-rate recovery immediately after exercise as a predictor of mortality. *N Engl J Med*. 1999;341(18):1351–7.
14. Consensus development conference on the diagnosis of coronary heart disease in people with diabetes: 10–11 February 1998, Miami, Florida. American Diabetes Association. *Diabetes Care*. 1998;21(9):1551–9.
15. De Lorenzo A, Lima RS, Siqueira-Filho AG, Pantoja MR. Prevalence and prognostic value of perfusion defects detected by stress technetium-99m sestamibi myocardial perfusion single-photon emission computed tomography in asymptomatic patients with diabetes mellitus and no known coronary artery disease. *Am J Cardiol*. 2002;90(8):827–32.
16. De S, Searles G, Haddad H. The prevalence of cardiac risk factors in women 45 years of age or younger undergoing angiography for evaluation of undiagnosed chest pain. *Can J Cardiol*. 2002;18(9):945–8.
17. Elming H, Brendorp B, Kober L, Sahebzadah N, Torp-Petersen C. QTc interval in the assessment of cardiac risk. *Card Electrophysiol Rev*. 2002;6(3):289–94.
18. Ewing DJ, Campbell IW, Clarke BF. The natural history of diabetic autonomic neuropathy. *Q J Med*. 1980;49(193):95–108.
19. Fleg JL. Stress testing in the elderly. *Am J Geriatr Cardiol*. 2001;10(6):308–15.
20. Fleischmann KE, Hunink MG, Kuntz KM, Douglas PS. Exercise echocardiography or exercise SPECT imaging? A meta-analysis of diagnostic test performance. *JAMA*. 1998;280(10):913–20.
21. Gibbons RJ, Smith SC Jr, Antman E, American College of Cardiology, American Heart Association. American College of Cardiology/American Heart Association clinical practice guidelines: Part II: evolutionary changes in a continuous quality improvement project. *Circulation*. 2003;107(24):3101–7.
22. Grundy SM, Cleeman JI, Daniels SR, et al. Diagnosis and management of the metabolic syndrome: an American Heart Association/National Heart, Lung, and Blood Institute Scientific Statement. *Circulation*. 2005;112(17):2735–52.
23. Ho PM, Maddox TM, Ross C, Rumsfeld JS, Magid DJ. Impaired chronotropic response to exercise stress testing in patients with

diabetes predicts future cardiovascular events. *Diabetes Care.* 2008;31(8):1531–3.

24. Huxley R, Barzi F, Woodward M. Excess risk of fatal coronary heart disease associated with diabetes in men and women: meta-analysis of 37 prospective cohort studies. *BMJ.* 2006;332(7533):73–8.

25. Kang X, Berman DS, Lewin HC, et al. Incremental prognostic value of myocardial perfusion single photon emission computed tomography in patients with diabetes mellitus. *Am Heart J.* 1999;138(6 Pt 1):1025–32.

26. Khaleeli E, Peters SR, Bobrowsky K, Oudiz RJ, Ko JY, Budoff MJ. Diabetes and the associated incidence of subclinical atherosclerosis and coronary artery disease: implications for management. *Am Heart J.* 2001;141(4):637–44.

27. Kramer CK, Rodrigues TC, Canani LH, Gross JL, Azevedo MJ. Diabetic retinopathy predicts all-cause mortality and cardiovascular events in both type 1 and 2 diabetes: meta-analysis of observational studies. *Diabetes Care.* 2011;34(5):1238–44.

28. Kurth T, Logroscino G. The metabolic syndrome: more than the sum of its components? *Stroke.* 2008;39(4):1068–9.

29. Lampman RM. Musculoskeletal disorders and sports injuries. In: Ruderman N, Devlin JT, Schneider SH, Kriska AM, American Diabetes Association, editors. *Handbook of Exercise in Diabetes.* 2nd ed., rev., and expanded ed. Alexandria: American Diabetes Association; 2002. p. 497–507.

30. Linnemann B, Janka HU. Prolonged QTc interval and elevated heart rate identify the type 2 diabetic patient at high risk for cardiovascular death. The Bremen Diabetes Study. *Exp Clin Endocrinol Diabetes.* 2003;111(4):215–22.

31. Mann JF, Gerstein HC, Pogue J, Bosch J, Yusuf S. Renal insufficiency as a predictor of cardiovascular outcomes and the impact of ramipril: the HOPE randomized trial. *Ann Intern Med.* 2001;134(8):629–36.

32. Manson JE, Colditz GA, Stampfer MJ, et al. A prospective study of maturity-onset diabetes mellitus and risk of coronary heart disease and stroke in women. *Arch Intern Med.* 1991;151(6):1141–7.

33. May O, Arildsen H, Damsgaard EM, Mickley H. Cardiovascular autonomic neuropathy in insulin-dependent diabetes mellitus: prevalence and estimated risk of coronary heart disease in the general population. *J Intern Med.* 2000;248(6):483–91.

34. Messinger-Rapport B, Pothier Snader CE, Blackstone EH, Yu D, Lauer MS. Value of exercise capacity and heart rate recovery in older people. *J Am Geriatr Soc.* 2003;51(1):63–8.

35. Mielke CH, Shields JP, Broemeling LD. Coronary artery calcium, coronary artery disease, and diabetes. *Diabetes Res Clin Pract.* 2001;53(1):55–61.

36. Nabel EG, Rocco MB, Selwyn AB. Characteristics and significance of ischemia detected by ambulatory electrocardiographic monitoring. *Circulation.* 1987;75(6 Pt 2):V74–83.

37. Naka M, Hiramatsu K, Aizawa T, et al. Silent myocardial ischemia in patients with non-insulin-dependent diabetes mellitus as judged by treadmill exercise testing and coronary angiography. *Am Heart J.* 1992;123(1):46–53.

38. *National Diabetes Fact Sheet, 2011: National Estimates and General Information on Diabetes and Prediabetes in the United States* [Internet]. Atlanta (GA): Centers for Disease Control and Prevention; [cited 2011 Sep 13]. 12 p. Available from: http://www.cdc.gov/diabetes/pubs/factsheet11.htm

39. Nesto RW, Phillips RT, Kett KG, et al. Angina and exertional myocardial ischemia in diabetic and nondiabetic patients: assessment by exercise thallium scintigraphy. *Ann Intern Med.* 1988;108(2):170–5.

40. Nesto RW, Watson FS, Kowalchuk GJ, et al. Silent myocardial ischemia and infarction in diabetics with peripheral vascular disease: assessment by dipyridamole thallium-201 scintigraphy. *Am Heart J.* 1990;120(5):1073–7.

41. Nishime EO, Cole CR, Blackstone EH, Pashkow FJ, Lauer MS. Heart rate recovery and treadmill exercise score as predictors of mortality in patients referred for exercise ECG. *JAMA.* 2000;284(11):1392–8.

42. Penfornis A, Zimmermann C, Boumal D, et al. Use of dobutamine stress echocardiography in detecting silent myocardial ischaemia in asymptomatic diabetic patients: a comparison with thallium scintigraphy and exercise testing. *Diabet Med.* 2001;18(11):900–5.

43. Pfister R, Cairns R, Erdmann E, Schneider CA, on behalf of the PROactive investigators. Prognostic impact of electrocardiographic signs in patients with Type 2 diabetes and cardiovascular disease: results from the PROactive study. *Diabet Med.* 2011;28(10):1206–12.

44. Raggi P, Bellasi A, Ratti C. Ischemia imaging and plaque imaging in diabetes: complementary tools to improve cardiovascular risk management. *Diabetes Care.* 2005;28(11):2787–94.

45. Raggi P, Shaw LJ, Berman DS, Callister TQ. Prognostic value of coronary artery calcium screening in subjects with and without diabetes. *J Am Coll Cardiol.* 2004;43(9):1663–9.

46. Rajagopalan N, Miller TD, Hodge DO, Frye RL, Gibbons RJ. Identifying high-risk asymptomatic diabetic patients who are candidates for screening stress single-photon emission computed tomography imaging. *J Am Coll Cardiol.* 2005;45(1):43–9.

47. Rana J, Gransar H, Shaw L, et al. Diabetes mellitus, coronary artery calcification and all-cause mortality among asymptomatic men and women. *J Am Coll Cardiol.* 2010;55(10A).

48. Reaven G. The metabolic syndrome or the insulin resistance syndrome? Different names, different concepts, and different goals. *Endocrinol Metab Clin North Am.* 2004;33(2):283–303.

49. Ritchie JL, Bateman TM, Bonow RO, et al. Guidelines for clinical use of cardiac radionuclide imaging. Report of the American College of Cardiology/American Heart Association Task Force on Assessment of Diagnostic and Therapeutic Cardiovascular Procedures (Committee on Radionuclide Imaging), developed in collaboration with the American Society of Nuclear Cardiology. *J Am Coll Cardiol.* 1995;25(2):521–47.

50. Scheidt-Nave C, Barrett-Connor E, Wingard DL. Resting electrocardiographic abnormalities suggestive of asymptomatic ischemic heart disease associated with non-insulin-dependent diabetes mellitus in a defined population. *Circulation.* 1990;81(3):899–906.

51. Schneider SH, Khachadurian AK, Amorosa LF, Clemow L, Ruderman NB. Ten-year experience with an exercise-based outpatient life-style modification program in the treatment of diabetes mellitus. *Diabetes Care.* 1992;15(11):1800–10.

52. Schuijf JD, Pundziute G, Jukema JW, et al. Diagnostic accuracy of 64-slice multislice computed tomography in the noninvasive evaluation of significant coronary artery disease. *Am J Cardiol.* 2006;98(2):145–8.

53. Seshadri N, Acharya N, Lauer MS. Association of diabetes mellitus with abnormal heart rate recovery in patients without known coronary artery disease. *Am J Cardiol.* 2003;91(1):108–11.

54. Sigal RJ, Kenny GP, Wasserman DH, Castaneda-Sceppa C, White RD. Physical activity/exercise and type 2 diabetes: a consensus statement from the American Diabetes Association. *Diabetes Care.* 2006;29(6):1433–8.

55. Singh JP, Larson MG, O'Donnell CJ, et al. Association of hyperglycemia with reduced heart rate variability (The Framingham Heart Study). *Am J Cardiol.* 2000;86(3):309–12.

56. Siscovick DS, Ekelund LG, Johnson JL, Truong Y, Adler A. Sensitivity of exercise electrocardiography for acute cardiac events during moderate and strenuous physical activity. The Lipid Research Clinics Coronary Primary Prevention Trial. *Arch Intern Med.* 1991;151(2):325–30.

57. Tomassoni TL. Conducting the pediatric exercise test. In: Rowland TW, editor. *Pediatric Laboratory Exercise Testing: Clinical Guidelines.* Champaign: Human Kinetics; 1993. p. 1–17.

58. Vanzetto G, Halimi S, Hammoud T, et al. Prediction of cardiovascular events in clinically selected high-risk NIDDM

patients. Prognostic value of exercise stress test and thallium-201 single-photon emission computed tomography. *Diabetes Care.* 1999;22(1):19–26.

59. Veglio M, Bruno G, Borra M, et al. Prevalence of increased QT interval duration and dispersion in type 2 diabetic patients and its relationship with coronary heart disease: a population-based cohort. *J Intern Med.* 2002;251(4):317–24.

60. Veglio M, Sivieri R, Chinaglia A, Scaglione L, Cavallo-Perin P. QT interval prolongation and mortality in type 1 diabetic patients: a 5-year cohort prospective study. Neuropathy Study Group of the Italian Society of the Study of Diabetes, Piemonte Affiliate. *Diabetes Care.* 2000;23(9):1381–3.

61. Vykoukal D, Davies MG. Vascular biology of metabolic syndrome. *J Vasc Surg.* 2011;54(3):819–31.

62. Wackers FJ, Chyun DA, Young LH, et al. Resolution of asymptomatic myocardial ischemia in patients with type 2 diabetes in the Detection of Ischemia in Asymptomatic Diabetics (DIAD) study. *Diabetes Care.* 2007;30(11):2892–8.

63. Wackers FJ, Young LH, Inzucchi SE, et al. Detection of silent myocardial ischemia in asymptomatic diabetic subjects: the DIAD study. *Diabetes Care.* 2004;27(8):1954–61.

SELECTED REFERENCES FOR FURTHER READING

American Diabetes Association. Standards of medical care in diabetes—2011. *Diabetes Care.* 2011;34:S11–61.

Colberg SR, Albright AL, Blissmer BJ, et al. Exercise and type 2 diabetes: American College of Sports Medicine and the American Diabetes Association: joint position statement. Exercise and type 2 diabetes. *Med Sci Sports Exerc.* 2010;42(12):2282–303.

INTERNET RESOURCES

- American Diabetes Association: http://www.diabetes.org
- CDC Diabetes Public Health Resource: http://www.cdc.gov/diabetes
- National Institute of Diabetes and Digestive and Kidney Disease: http://www.niddk.nih.gov

Occupational and Functional Assessments

Health care professionals can play an important role in optimizing vocational and nonvocational activity-related decisions for many patients, especially during the early recovery period after a major cardiac event. The focus of this chapter is on assessment and rehabilitative procedures that may promote optimal short-term as well as long-term activity decisions for those with known heart disease.

OCCUPATIONAL ASSESSMENT

Employment-related decisions in patients with heart disease can be complex. In addition to the patient and employer, work-related decisions involve various professional agencies, including medical, disability, insurance, or legal (43,50). Several factors may influence the return-to-work process, including the patient's desire to return to work, job satisfaction, perception of disability, previous employment record, age, education level, work tolerance in relation to job demands, disease severity, family concerns, coworkers, supervisor's attitudes or restrictions, support mechanisms, psychological variables, available financial resources (*e.g.*, disability income, insurance, savings), or other work incentives/disincentives (5,11,12,15,24,29,43,44,50,53). For those who resume work, employment can produce positive psychosocial, physical, and material benefits.

Because of the various factors that can influence work-related decisions, a significant percentage of patients do not resume work after a cardiac event, or do not remain employed until a normal retirement age (5,12,31,50). Some of these individuals are granted disability benefits despite relatively good functional work reserve. In a study of 175 men who were receiving Social Security

Disability Insurance (SSDI) secondary to ischemic heart disease, 65% were found to have a work capacity of ≥5 metabolic equivalents (METs) and 12% a work capacity of ≥7 METs (44). In this study, peak MET levels were determined with measurement of oxygen uptake. Based on their responses to an activity questionnaire, these men were fairly active with home or leisure-time physical activities, with approximately 20%–30% of them performing relatively demanding home tasks, such as gardening, mowing (walking), and snow removal (blowing or shoveling). It is possible that greater reliance on functional work reserve in relation to expected job demands may lead to more optimal decisions regarding return to work and granting of disability benefits.

Premature loss of employment has significant societal economic implications and may also affect the social well-being of patients. In the United States, coronary heart disease (CHD) is a leading cause of disability under the Social Security Administration (SSA) program (11). In Canada, a Health Canada report indicated that cardiovascular disease (CVD) is the highest cost in terms of burden of illness, equaling $18.5 billion annually, with long-term disability costs being $3.1 billion per year (26,63). Procedures that may help to optimize work resumption are reviewed in this chapter. Primary topics include clinical assessment, early intervention, job analysis, work tolerance testing, counseling, and early rehabilitation.

CLINICAL ASSESSMENT

Information gathered from several sources can be used to assess a patient's current medical status and future prognosis in terms of morbidity and mortality secondary

---

KEY TERMS

Job analysis: Assessment of key job requirements and work conditions.

Metabolic equivalents (METs): Unit used to estimate the metabolic cost or energy requirements of physical activity, with 1 MET defined as the average resting

oxygen uptake of 3.5 mL of oxygen per kilogram body mass per minute.

Simulated work testing: An evaluation of an individual undertaking a test that is designed to represent a specific type of work task and/or work condition.

to heart disease. Risk classification of patients with heart disease into low-, moderate-, and high-risk categories for future events can be helpful in counseling patients on resuming physical activity (3) (see *GETP9, Boxes 2-2 and 2-3*). Most jobs today are not physically demanding, so unnecessary delays in work resumption beyond the normal convalescent period should be avoided. This includes avoiding delays specifically to permit completion of a cardiac rehabilitation program or waiting for results from nonessential diagnostic tests before providing medical clearance for work resumption. Individuals who have physically demanding jobs, especially those in moderate and high clinical risk categories, may require further diagnostic evaluation or intervention before work resumption. Identification of signs of depression and other psychological disorders may be beneficial because psychological issues can have a negative influence on work-related decisions in some patients (11,53). Lewin indicated that 40%–50% of individuals who do not return to work have reasons other than physical illness (32). An easily administered brief depression scale, the depression subscale, part of the Hospital Anxiety and Depression Scale, can help identify patients with depression who are less likely to return to work (35). Various methods can be used to help identify and treat psychological disorders (4).

EARLY INTERVENTION AND COUNSELING

Return to work should be discussed as early as possible with patients. In some situations, work resumption can be discussed while the patient is in hospital. Some possible factors to consider in discussing work-related issues with patients are listed in *Box 27-1*. Ignoring work-related matters early in the recovery process may cause patients to inappropriately perceive their event as leading to an inability to resume work. Patients can generally be given a positive message regarding work resumption along with a tentative timetable for resuming work before discharge. For some patients, particularly women, it is important to receive positive affirmations about domestic and social responsibilities (27). The actual timing for return to work can vary with several factors, such as the cardiac event, disease severity, prognosis, job requirements, safety regulations, and employer attitudes or concerns. Most individuals can resume their jobs within 1–12 wk after a major cardiac event. A study conducted by Kovoor et al. showed that patients following an acute myocardial infarction (MI) and stratified as low risk were able to safely return to full normal activities, including work, at 2 wk postevent (28). Early return can be especially useful for individuals who are self-employed or lack the financial resources to remain off work. Some, especially those who work in jobs that may place coworkers and/or the public at risk, such as firefighters, commercial drivers, and airline pilots, may have greater delays or restrictions on returning to work, including meeting specific medical criteria to maintain a license to work (9,23,52).

JOB ANALYSIS

A job analysis performed soon after a major cardiac event can serve as a basis for (a) delineating expected physical and psychological demands of the patient's job, thus determining if an individual will be safe on the job; (b) identifying the patient's concerns regarding work resumption; (c) establishing a tentative timeline for work resumption; and (d) individualizing assessment or rehabilitation procedures that may be undertaken during the early recovery period to optimize return-to-work decisions and capability (50,56). Generally, job titles provide little or, in some cases, misleading information about the work demands. Some of the factors that can be assessed in a job analysis include determination of specific job tasks from which expected energy cost requirements can be estimated: weight lifting, stacking, carrying, pushing, and pulling requirements; environmental conditions,

---

BOX 27-1	Checklist for Possible Work Return Interventions

- Assess disease severity and prognosis of patient after event.
- Ask the patient about preadmission employment status.
- Discuss expected recovery course with the patient, including return to work.
- Establish a tentative timetable for work resumption, when appropriate.
- Ask the patient about any work return concerns.
- Be prepared to discuss qualifying criteria for disability benefits.

- Determine if a job analysis, including an employer contact/work site visit, is warranted.
- Suggest that the patient contact the employer to maintain contact and, if appropriate, discuss return to work.
- Encourage participation in a progressive exercise program to enhance work resumption potential.
- Consider referrals for procedures or treatments that may assist patients in returning to work.

including exposure to potentially hazardous materials; and psychological stressors. This information can be obtained by interviewing the patient, and with the patient's permission, an employer contact and work site visit can provide a wealth of information. The work demands from the employer's perspective, the employer's expectations, the return-to-work policy, sick leave, worker's compensation, the possibilities for a gradual return to work in terms of hours and duties or modifications, and specific job/union regulations (31,39,50,56,57,64,66) can be obtained using a standard questionnaire, such as the job analysis questionnaire designed by Sheldahl et al. (50).

In estimating the average and peak physical demands of work for patients, various resources can be used. Employers may be able to provide specific work requirements that relate directly to their work sites. Increasingly, written physical demands analyses are available. If the employer cannot be contacted, then *The Dictionary of Occupational Titles* (57) and the *Occupational Outlook Handbook* (39) provide general information regarding work requirements under specific job titles. MET tables (see *GETP9, Table 1-1*) provide approximations for average energy demands of various job and other activity tasks in units of multiples of resting energy expenditure (2). It should be emphasized that the values listed in MET tables are only approximations and that expected energy demands listed for some activities are estimated based on their similarity to other types of activities. The actual MET demands can vary with pace of work, worker efficiency, orthopedic disabilities, automation, assistive devices, protective equipment, body size, terrain, and temperature. A study on lawn mowing, for example, showed that the mean MET levels for lawn mowing using a walk-behind mower varied from 3–10 METs, depending on the type of mower (push, power push, or self-propelled), walking speed, lawn terrain, and subject characteristics (49). Sheldahl, Wilke, and others performed several energy expenditure studies in work simulation settings and at occupational work sites (18,47,60–62). In the job site studies (47), oxygen uptake was measured for 20 min with a portable device in workers at various physical labor work settings. The on-the-job studies indicated that the average energy expenditure of most jobs requiring physical labor corresponds to <4 METs. Higher demands were required in some tasks, such as chainsawing or chipping, power push mowing, barn cleaning, air hammering, drywall and masonry, and weight carrying and repetitive lifting tasks. In addition to the influence of energy expenditure on myocardial oxygen requirements, it is important to assess whether other work-related conditions (*e.g.*, adverse temperature stress, psychological stress, awkward body positioning, static work, etc.) may increase myocardial oxygen demands (50). The influence of selected environmental factors on myocardial oxygen requirements is discussed later in the chapter.

TRADITIONAL EXERCISE TESTING

The traditional symptom-limited graded exercise test (GXT) on a treadmill or cycle ergometer can be very helpful in providing realistic vocational recommendations (16). Information on work tolerance along with submaximal and maximal exercise-induced hemodynamic responses, electrocardiographic (ECG) responses, and possible symptoms can help assess the ability of patients to resume work within a reasonable period and identify areas that need better management or further assessment. Exercise testing may also reassure the patient, patient's family, and employer regarding the patient's ability to safely handle the job demands (see *GETP9, Chapter 5*).

An important exercise test measurement is determination of functional MET capacity. In the clinical setting, functional MET capacity is typically estimated based on the peak workload achieved. GXTs using protocols with smaller increments, such as the Naughton or Balke, are more useful (see *GETP9, Chapter 5*). The patient should undergo the GXT while on usual medications to evaluate functional capacity in his or her "normal state." Ideally, oxygen uptake can be measured with a cardiopulmonary exercise (stress) test using a metabolic cart, which assesses if a maximal effort has been made while determining if any respiratory problems occur and the workload equivalent to the ventilatory threshold (12). After functional MET capacity is determined, it can be compared with the estimated average and peak METs of the individual's job. The noninvasive measurement of the degree of cardiac output impairment during the recovery phase following exercise testing may also be useful to estimate exercise capacity (37). Work requirements should not induce myocardial ischemia or produce excessive fatigue. Over an 8-h day, fatigue is more likely to occur when the average energy expenditure rate exceeds 50% of the individual's peak aerobic capacity. The appropriate upper intensity level to recommend for short-term (*e.g.*, <60 min) occupational work tasks should be individualized based on patient characteristics (*e.g.*, severity of disease, serious arrhythmias, etc.), tolerance for physical work, type of work performed, duration and frequency of work tasks, and work environment. Most patients should be able to use the same physical activity guidelines that are individualized for them for home and leisure-time physical activities or for an unsupervised exercise program.

SIMULATED WORK TESTING

For most people with heart disease, the only exercise test needed to assess functional tolerance for work resumption is the traditional GXT. There are limitations in advising some on work resumption based only on graded dynamic exercise testing. One limitation is that although the traditional GXT evaluates dynamic exercise tolerance, certain jobs may require a significant static workload (*e.g.*, lift, carry, push, pull, etc.). This can result in questions regarding the patient's ability to tolerate the greater myocardial afterload stress expected with static work, along with potential questions regarding the appropriate upper static load to recommend. For some patients who have performed work that has mainly involved arm work (*e.g.*, operating heavy equipment), their arms may be better conditioned than their legs. Thus, the exercise test results would underestimate their ability to perform upper extremity work. Another limitation is that in contrast to the traditional exercise test, work sites may have less-than-ideal work conditions (*e.g.*, hot or cold climates, air pollution, and intermittent heavy work tasks) (25).

It is impractical and unnecessary to evaluate workers under all the various stressors encountered in the course of a typical work routine, although some of the more demanding work tasks can be evaluated in select patients using work simulation testing. Patients most likely to benefit from simulated work testing are those whose ability to return to work remain in question despite traditional exercise testing, perhaps because of lower aerobic capacity (<7 METs), left ventricular dysfunction, ischemia at submaximal levels, significant arrhythmias, or apprehension about resuming a physically demanding job (50,59). Simple and inexpensive work simulation tests can be set up. In terms of protocols, a weight-carrying test protocol and a repetitive weight-lifting test protocol have been published for evaluating tolerance for static work combined with light-to-moderate dynamic work (50). Both of these test protocols are graded and designed to be applicable to several types of work tasks requiring a static component. In some instances — for example, when there are sudden high demands on the job, it is preferable to design the test to simulate the work demands more closely, perhaps having an individual immediately lift the required weight without a warm-up.

The weight-carrying test protocol (*Table 27-1*) is designed to evaluate tolerance for light-to-heavy static effort combined with light dynamic work. In one protocol, the patient walks on a treadmill at a slow pace while carrying specified weight loads (*e.g.*, dumbbell weights) in one or both hands. The repetitive weight-lifting test protocol (see *Table 27-1*) is designed to evaluate tolerance for intermittent static work combined with a dynamic work component. In this protocol, the patient repetitively lifts specified weight loads, typically from the floor or pallet to a table or bench for a set period. Patients can be instructed to lift at a set pace or select a rate that simulates or somewhat exceeds their job requirement.

In assessing blood pressure (BP) responses to static or static–dynamic work, it is important to measure the

TABLE 27-1. Dynamic-Static Work Simulation Test Protocols

Weight-Carrying Test Example[a] **Protocol**

Stage[b]	Duration (min)	Speed (mph)	Load[c] (lb)	Predicted METs[d]
1	3	2.0	0	2.4
2	3	2.0	20	3.0
3	3	2.0	30	4.2
4	3	2.0	40	5.0
5	2	2.0	50	4.8[e]

Repetitive Lifting Test Example[a] **Protocol**

Stage[b]	Duration (min)	Lift Rate	Load[c] (lb)	Predicted METs[d]
1	6	Self-paced	30	3.8
2	6	Self-paced	40	4.2
3	6	Self-paced	50	4.5
4	6	Self-paced	30, 40, 50	4.2

METs, metabolic equivalents with 1 MET = oxygen uptake of 3.5 mL · kg^{-1} · min^{-1}.

[a]Test protocols can be modified to meet specific work conditions.

[b]A seated rest period of 1–3 min follows each stage.

[c]Weight load in weight-carrying test (*e.g.*, dumbbell) can be carried in one or both hands; weight load in repetitive test can be lifted from floor or pallet to work bench.

[d]METs are based on tests using the specific protocol listed.

[e]The slightly lower MET level for carrying 50 lbs versus 40 lbs is likely because of the shorter walk time and the inability to achieve steady-state conditions.

BP in the nonexercising arm just before lifting and just before releasing the weight. BP decreases rapidly upon release of the static load. ECG monitoring can be the same as for the traditional exercise test, or telemetry can be used if ischemia is not expected based on prior traditional exercise testing. Specialized work simulators (*e.g.*, Baltimore Therapeutic and Valpar work simulators) are available for simulating various tasks, although the energy cost with some stations may be less than when performing tasks in the work setting (62).

ON-THE-JOB MONITORING

Ambulatory ECG monitoring can be considered for patients in whom concerns exist regarding potential for serious arrhythmias or ischemia on the job despite laboratory testing. Heart rate (HR) responses to work can also be evaluated with this procedure, although inexpensive HR monitors can be used or patients can be instructed to check their pulse rates during their more demanding work tasks. Some of the HR monitors can be programmed to emit a sound when a preprogrammed HR is exceeded or to provide average and peak HR information over a period of time. On-the-job HR monitoring can help evaluate the combined effects of the physical work and work-related factors (*e.g.*, environmental) or work conditions that can increase myocardial demands. Patients may also be assured that their jobs are not causing an excessive myocardial demand by simply checking their pulse rate.

EARLY REHABILITATION

Participation in cardiac rehabilitation-supervised exercise programs after a cardiac event (see *GETP9, Chapter 9*) has shown mixed results in terms of enhancing work resumption outcomes (11). Failure to find a positive impact in several studies may stem from the complexity of factors reported to influence work-related decisions. Tailoring of cardiac rehabilitation programs in the early phase of recovery to address the work-related concerns of patients resuming work may enhance work resumption potential (35,50). Recovery goals including return to work seem to be gender specific and should be taken into consideration when planning an intervention (22). There may be a benefit from early intervention focusing on improving psychological parameters, as previously discussed, and encouraging use of exercise modes designed to enhance resumption of specific types of work (*e.g.*, arm exercise, resistive exercise) (see *GETP9, Chapter 9* and *Box 9-9*). Early rehabilitation should also consider the underestimated cardiovascular impact of routine daily tasks after returning home (21). Performing real-life domestic obligations when considering the individual's environment could be beneficial during rehabilitation. Enrollment in a multidisciplinary stress management program increased the return-to-work rate in persons with work-related stress (38) and may improve the confidence for return to work in this population as well. For patients who will need to resume work in a hot environment, a gradual exposure to outdoor exercise may be more beneficial than only exercising in a climate-controlled facility.

DISABILITY

A small percentage of patients with heart disease, who were previously working, will not be able to resume paid employment because of the severity of their disease. These patients may qualify for disability income through programs such as SSDI in the United States and Canada Pension Plan Disability (CPP-D) benefits in Canada, private long-term disability insurance, or Veterans Administration service- and nonservice-related pensions. Some patients may inappropriately think they will qualify for disability income. If they are not informed about the stringent qualifying criteria, some of them may unnecessarily go through the long process of applying for SSDI or CPP-D only to be rejected. In discussing return-to-work matters with patients, it is helpful to have a good understanding of the rules and regulations regarding common disability plans such as SSDI (58) and CPP-D (7).

In the SSDI program, Social Security pays benefits for individuals who cannot work because they have a medical condition that is expected to last at least 1 yr or could result in death. The patient needs to have worked enough years to qualify (58). Eligibility for CPP-D is similar, requiring that an individual be between ages 18 and 65 yr has made contributions to CPP-D for a minimum qualifying period and has a disability that is prolonged and severe. Thus, the person is incapable regularly of pursuing any substantially gainful occupation.

In some states, uniformed police officers or firefighters are covered under "accidental disability" (often referred to as "Heart Laws") (33,43,50). Under these programs, workers may be able to establish the existence of a disabling cardiac disease or hypertension without proving that the job caused the disabling condition. Considerable variability exists among states in terms of the coverage provided under "accidental disability." Contacting the public employee state retirement agency may help to inform/advise patients. In Canada, if the cardiac event can be directly attributed to the job, there may be eligibility for compensation through the Worker's Safety and Insurance Board (65). An example is an individual with no known coronary artery disease (CAD) who is chopping ice at work and suffering an MI while working.

NEW EMPLOYMENT

Some patients may need to find employment after a cardiac event because they are unemployed or cannot return to their previous employment. The Americans with Disabilities Act (ADA) "prohibits private sector employers who employ 15 or more individuals and all State and local government employers from discriminating against qualified individuals with disabilities in all aspects of employment" (56). The Canadian Human Rights Commission ensures that the principles of equal opportunity and nondiscrimination are followed in all areas of federal jurisdiction (8). State or provincial vocational services may be available for individuals who need retraining for employment. The extent of vocational services varies widely.

NONVOCATIONAL ACTIVITIES

An important goal after a cardiac event is for patients to maintain as active a lifestyle as possible considering the magnitude of the disease, which includes encouraging patients to participate in appropriate home and leisure-time activities. Maintaining an active daily routine with home and leisure-time activities can help those with heart disease meet secondary prevention guidelines as recommended by The American Heart Association (AHA)/American College of Cardiology (ACC) in 2006 (51). These guidelines suggest 30–60 min of moderate-intensity aerobic activity on most or preferably all days of the week, supplemented by an increase in daily lifestyle activities. Leisure-time activities that raise the HR into an aerobic zone can provide some individuals with an enjoyable way to participate in a regular aerobic-type exercise program. It is important to note that regular exercise and good physical fitness provide many benefits in terms of prevention of disease progression and quality of life (30). Maintaining physical fitness may help to reduce cardiac events stemming from strenuous activity (54). Investigators (36,63) have shown that the risk of an acute MI is temporarily increased during high-intensity physical activity, especially in those who are habitually sedentary. People who exercise regularly have a much lower relative risk associated with strenuous exercise. They also have the protective preventative effect associated with a regular program of exercise. A position statement from AHA discusses potential exercise-related cardiovascular events and how to reduce them. Both AHA and American College of Sports Medicine (ACSM) have addressed the importance of exercise testing. Their recommendation is clear: Individuals who appear to be at greater risk for having underlying CAD should be considered for exercise testing before beginning a vigorous ($\geq$60% $\dot{V}O_2$ reserve) exercise training program. In addition to preparticipation screening, several other strategies to reduce events appear necessary, such as excluding high-risk patients from some activities, preparing fitness personnel and facilities for cardiovascular emergencies, and recommending prudent exercise activities (54).

Most of the same procedures used for optimizing occupational work decisions are also applicable to advising patients on resumption of home and leisure-time activities, including medical assessment, early intervention, activity analysis, counseling, work tolerance testing, and exercise conditioning.

A major risk factor for CHD is age. Therefore, CHD is more common in elderly persons than within other age groups. Just as resumption of occupational work can have important individual and societal ramifications, so can resumption of independent living in the elderly population. In addition to the economic cost associated with assisted living, maintenance of an independent lifestyle affects the quality of life in elderly individuals. In a study of people >65 yr of age with CHD, peak aerobic capacity and depression were shown to be predictors of physical functioning (1). Encouraging elderly patients to participate in supervised exercise programs, as well as resuming their home and leisure-time activities after a cardiac event, may promote greater tolerance and confidence among the elderly in performing activities important for independence. Because of the comorbidities common in elderly individuals, their exercise programs may need special tailoring to meet specific needs. Psychosocial counseling may help those with depression maintain a more positive outlook on life and, thus, engage in a more active lifestyle.

INFLUENCE OF ENVIRONMENTAL CONDITIONS

Many home, leisure-time, and job activities are performed in less-than-ideal environmental conditions, which can alter myocardial oxygen uptake requirements and work tolerance.

HEAT STRESS

During sustained work in a hot environment, circulatory demand typically is increased to meet the dual blood flow demands for metabolism (muscle) and thermoregulation (skin) (17,46). A common characteristic of work combined with heat stress is a more progressive drift upward in HR and drift downward in stroke volume with work time compared with the same type of work performed in a thermoneutral environment. The addition of a humid environment produces an even greater drift. This cardiovascular drift represents an increase in myocardial oxygen requirements.

Most studies involving exercise in a hot environment have been performed on healthy individuals. In a study of asymptomatic men with heart disease, a similar cardiovascular drift response was seen with sustained moderate-intensity work (45). Left ventricular ejection fraction (LVEF) and cardiac output were maintained, and the incidence of arrhythmias was not increased with heat stress. The effect of work or exercise, combined with heat stress in symptomatic patients or those at high risk, is unknown.

Encouraging individuals to monitor their pulse rate during work in a hot environment provides a useful means for adjusting work rate downward to avoid excessive myocardial demand. Individuals should also be informed about the importance of gradual exposure to exercise combined with heat stress after a period of cool or cold weather exposure to permit heat acclimation. Heat acclimation results in improved capacity to dissipate heat, which, in turn, reduces the magnitude of the cardiovascular drift and, thereby, myocardial oxygen demands. Heat acclimation can occur within a few days (3–10 d) of undertaking mild, sustained (up to 90 min) physical activity in a warm environment (see *GETP9*, *Chapter 8* for guidelines).

COLD STRESS

Work in a cold environment may add to myocardial oxygen requirements by increasing myocardial afterload (*e.g.*, BP, vascular resistance) and/or energy expenditure as a result of wearing heavier clothing, walking through snow, and perhaps shivering (15,45,48). Some patients with CHD report angina at a lower work level in a cold environment (11). Meyer et al. reported that the ischemic threshold was reduced in patients with CAD during treadmill exercise testing at extremely cold temperature (−20° C) (34). Cardiovascular mortality has shown a significant negative correlation with daily mean temperature (55) and it is increased in the winter months.

One of the more demanding wintertime physical activities is snow removal (15,48). In a study (19) of younger men shoveling wet snow, mean relative work intensity corresponded to 97% of peak HR. A large number of sudden cardiac deaths were reported and associated with snow removal (10), raising questions regarding the ability of patients with CHD to safely perform static–dynamic work tasks in a cold environment. Moderate- and high-risk patients with CHD and those with a work capacity of <6.5 METs should be advised not to exert themselves in a cold environment.

ALTITUDE

Those traveling to the mountains for skiing or other physical activities should understand that hypoxia at altitude can significantly lower their work tolerance (40,67). The impact on work tolerance is greatest during the first few days at a high altitude. Over a few days (5–10) of altitude exposure, tolerance for physical activities improves through acclimatization. Wyss et al. (67) reported that patients with CAD showed a significant decrease in coronary flow reserve (CFR) when evaluated immediately after supine cycle exercise under acute hypoxic conditions comparable to 2,500-m altitude. These patients also showed greater ECG and symptomatic evidence of exercise-induced ischemia with simulated altitude. In contrast, healthy control subjects did not show an exercise-induced decrease in CFR with hypoxic conditions at altitude simulations of 2,500 m and 4,500 m. The investigators concluded that patients with CAD with reduced CFR should be cautioned about performing physical activity at moderate or higher altitudes. De Vries et al. (13) reported that a small number of low-risk patients with CAD (ejection fraction >45%) showed similar decreases in exercise capacity and maximum heart rate compared to healthy controls at 4,200-m altitude. However, there is a lack of data concerning exercise tolerance in high-risk patients with CAD at high altitudes.

Another environment factor that needs to be considered at altitude is exposure to less-than-ideal temperature conditions (see *GETP9, Chapter 8* for guidelines). Recently practical recommendations were published regarding how to counsel patients with CHD traveling to high-altitude locations (42).

POLLUTANTS

Air pollutants should be taken into consideration in advising those on resuming work in certain affected communities or work sites, especially those who have cardiopulmonary disease or are expected to work at relatively high work intensities. Reports indicate that both short- and long-term exposure to air pollutants results in an increased risk for cardiopulmonary events (6,14,17,25,26,41). A recent review summarizes the relationship between air pollutants and CVD and explores the underlying biologic mechanisms in the population of the Multi-Ethnic Study of Atherosclerosis (MESA) (20).

SUMMARY

Enabling patients with heart disease to resume as active and productive a lifestyle as possible for their disease state is an important goal. This includes helping patients resume employment, when appropriate, as well as home and leisure-time activities. Various techniques can be used to help optimize work and activity resumption for patients, including a job or activity analysis, exercise testing, simulated work testing, and activity monitoring. Exercise training programs can also be tailored to enhance the potential of patients to resume specific types of work. To help optimize the return-to-work process for patients, health care professionals should have a basic understanding of job requirements and governmental policies and procedures that can influence work resumption and work conditions for patients.

REFERENCES

1. Ades PA, Savage PD, Tischler MD, Poehlman ET, Dee J, Niggel J. Determinants of disability in older coronary patients. *Am Heart J.* 2002;143(1):151–6.
2. Ainsworth BE, Haskell WL, Whitt MC, et al. Compendium of physical activities: an update of activity codes and MET intensities. *Med Sci Sports Exerc.* 2000;32(9 Suppl):S498–504.
3. American Association of Cardiovascular & Pulmonary Rehabilitation. *Guidelines for Cardiac Rehabilitation and Secondary Prevention Programs.* 4th ed. Champaign (IL): Human Kinetics; 2004. 280 p.
4. Blumenthal JA, Babyak MA, Carney RM, et al. Exercise, depression, and mortality after myocardial infarction in the ENRICHD trial. *Med Sci Sports Exerc.* 2004;36(5):746–55.
5. Boudrez H, De Backer G. Recent findings on return to work after an acute myocardial infarction or coronary artery bypass grafting. *Acta Cardiol.* 2000;55(6):341–9.
6. Brook RD, Franklin B, Cascio W, et al. Air pollution and cardiovascular disease: a statement for healthcare professionals from the Expert Panel on Population and Prevention Science of the American Heart Association. *Circulation.* 2004;109(21):2655–71.
7. *Canada Pension Plan: Disability* [Internet]. Ottawa (Ontario): Service Canada; [cited 2011 Mar 14]. Available from: http://www.servicecanada.gc.ca/eng/sc/cpp/disability/disabilitypension.shtml
8. *Canadian Human Rights Act* [Internet]. Ottawa (Ontario): Canadian Human Rights Commission; [cited 2011 Mar 14]. Available from: http://www.chrc-ccdp.gc.ca
9. *Cardiovascular Advisory Panel Guidelines for the Medical Examination of Commercial Motor Vehicle Drivers* [Internet]. Washington (DC): U.S. Department of Transportation, Federal Motor Carrier Safety Administration; [cited 2011 Mar 14]. Available from: http://www.fmcsa.dot.gov/facts-research/research-technology/publications/cardio.htm
10. Chowdhury PS, Franklin BA, Boura JA, et al. Sudden cardiac death after manual or automated snow removal. *Am J Cardiol.* 2003;92(7):833–5.

11. *Clinical Practice Guideline, No. 17* [Internet]. Bethesda (MD): National Center for Biotechnology Information, U.S. National Library of Medicine; [cited 2011 Mar 14]. Available from: http://purl.access.gpo.gov/GPO/LPS48035

12. Dafoe W. Employment and insurability. In: Crawford MH, DiMarco JP, editors. *Cardiology*. 2nd ed. London: Mosby; 2003. p. 1625–1634.

13. De Vries ST, Komdeur P, Aalbersberg S, van Enst GC, Breeman A, van 't Hof AW. Effects of altitude on exercise level and heart rate in patients with coronary artery disease and healthy controls. *Neth Heart J.* 2010;18(3):118–21.

14. Delfino RJ, Gillen DL, Tjoa T, et al. Electrocardiographic ST-segment depression and exposure to traffic-related aerosols in elderly subjects with coronary artery disease. *Environ Health Perspect.* 2011;119(2):196–202.

15. Dougherty CM. The natural history of recovery following sudden cardiac arrest and internal cardioverter-defibrillator implantation. *Prog Cardiovasc Nurs.* 2001;16(4):163–8.

16. Fletcher GF, Balady G, Froelicher VF, Hartley LH, Haskell WL, Pollock ML. Exercise standards. A statement for healthcare professionals from the American Heart Association. Writing Group. *Circulation.* 1995;91(2):580–615.

17. Folinsbee LJ. Heat and air pollution. In: Pollock ML, Schmidt DH, editors. *Heart Disease and Rehabilitation*. 3rd ed. Champaign: Human Kinetics; 1995. p. 327–342.

18. Foss-Campbell B, Sheldahl L, Wilke N. Effects of upper extremity load distribution on weight-carrying in men with ischemic heart disease. *J Cardiopulm Rehabil.* 1993;13(1):37–42.

19. Franklin BA, Hogan P, Bonzheim K, et al. Cardiac demands of heavy snow shoveling. *JAMA.* 1995;273(11):880–2.

20. Gill EA, Curl CL, Adar SD, et al. Air pollution and cardiovascular disease in the multi-ethnic study of atherosclerosis. *Prog Cardiovasc Dis.* 2011;53(5):353–60.

21. Gosse S, Fischbach M, Gosse P. Domestic activities after myocardial infarction. Their impact is underestimated. *Eur J Phys Rehabil Med.* 2011;47(1):1–8.

22. Grande G, Romppel M. Gender differences in recovery goals in patients after acute myocardial infarction. *J Cardiopulm Rehabil Prev.* 2011;31(3):164–72.

23. *Guidelines for the Assessment of Cardiovascular Fitness in Licensed Aviation Personnel 2003* [Internet]. Ottawa (Ontario): Transport Canada; [cited 2011 Mar 14]. Available from: http://www.tc.gc.ca/eng/civilaviation/publications/tp13312-2-cardiovascular-menu-2356.htm

24. Gutmann MC, Sheldahl LM, Tristani FE, Wilke NA. Returning the patient to work. In: Pollock ML, Schmidt DH, editors. *Heart Disease and Rehabilitation*. 3rd ed. Champaign: Human Kinetics; 1995. p. 405–22.

25. Henrotin JB, Zeller M, Lorgis L, Cottin Y, Giroud M, Bejot Y. Evidence of the role of short-term exposure to ozone on ischaemic cerebral and cardiac events: the Dijon Vascular Project (DIVA). *Heart.* 2010;96(24):1990–6.

26. Johnson RL Jr. Relative effects of air pollution on lungs and heart. *Circulation.* 2004;109(1):5–7.

27. King KM, Collins-Nakai RL. Short-term recovery from cardiac surgery in women: suggestions for practice. *Can J Cardiol.* 1998;14(11):1367–71.

28. Kovoor P, Lee AK, Carrozzi F, et al. Return to full normal activities including work at two weeks after acute myocardial infarction. *Am J Cardiol.* 2006;97(7):952–8.

29. Kushnir T, Luria O. Supervisors' attitudes toward return to work after myocardial infarction or coronary artery bypass graft. *J Occup Environ Med.* 2002;44(4):331–7.

30. Lakka TA, Venalainen JM, Rauramaa R, Salonen R, Tuomilehto J, Salonen JT. Relation of leisure-time physical activity and cardiorespiratory fitness to the risk of acute myocardial infarction. *N Engl J Med.* 1994;330(22):1549–54.

31. Leopold RS. *A Year in the Life of a Million American Workers*. New York (NY): Metlife Group Disability; 2003. 206 p.

32. Lewin R. Return to work after MI, the roles of depression, health beliefs and rehabilitation. *Int J Cardiol.* 1999;72(1):49–51.

33. Massachusetts Public Employee Retirement Administration Commission Web site [Internet]. Somerville (MA): Massachusetts Public Employee Retirement Administration Commission; [cited 2011 Mar 14]. Available from: http://www.mass.gov/perac

34. Meyer P, Guiraud T, Curnier D, et al. Exposure to extreme cold lowers the ischemic threshold in coronary artery disease patients. *Can J Cardiol.* 2010;26(2):e50–3.

35. Mital A, Shrey DE, Govindaraju M, Broderick TM, Colon-Brown K, Gustin BW. Accelerating the return to work (RTW) chances of coronary heart disease (CHD) patients: part 1—development and validation of a training programme. *Disabil Rehabil.* 2000; 22(13–14):604–20.

36. Mittleman MA, Maclure M, Tofler GH, Sherwood JB, Goldberg RJ, Muller JE. Triggering of acute myocardial infarction by heavy physical exertion. Protection against triggering by regular exertion. Determinants of Myocardial Infarction Onset Study Investigators. *N Engl J Med.* 1993;329(23):1677–83.

37. Myers JN, Gujja P, Neelagaru S, Hsu L, Burkhoff D. Noninvasive measurement of cardiac performance in recovery from exercise in heart failure patients. *Clinics (Sao Paulo).* 2011;66(4):649–56.

38. Netterstrom B, Bech P. Effect of a multidisciplinary stress treatment programme on the return to work rate for persons with work-related stress. A non-randomized controlled study from a stress clinic. *BMC Public Health.* 2010;10:658.

39. *Occupational Outlook Handbook, 2006–07 Edition* [Internet]. Washington (DC): U.S. Department of Labor, Bureau of Labor Statistics; [cited 2007 May 30]. Available from: http://www.bls.gov/oco/home.htm

40. Pandolf KB, Young AJ. Altitude and cold. In: Pollock ML, Schmidt DH, editors. *Heart Disease and Rehabilitation*. 3rd ed. Champaign: Human Kinetics; 1995. p. 309–326.

41. Pope CA 3rd, Burnett RT, Thurston GD, et al. Cardiovascular mortality and long-term exposure to particulate air pollution: epidemiological evidence of general pathophysiological pathways of disease. *Circulation.* 2004;109(1):71–7.

42. Rimoldi SF, Sartori C, Seiler C, et al. High-altitude exposure in patients with cardiovascular disease: risk assessment and practical recommendations. *Prog Cardiovasc Dis.* 2010;52(6):512–24.

43. Sagall EL, Nash IS. Cardiac evaluations for legal purposes. In: O'Rourke RA, Hurst JW, editors. *Hurst's the Heart Manual of Cardiology*. 10th ed. New York: McGraw-Hill, Health Professions Division; 2001. p. 2519–32.

44. Sheldahl LM, Wilke NA, Dougherty SM. Work capacity of men on disability for heart disease [abstract]. *Circulation.* 1992;86 (Suppl I):400.

45. Sheldahl LM, Wilke NA, Dougherty SM, Levandoski SG, Hoffman MD, Tristani FE. Effect of age and coronary artery disease on response to snow shoveling. *J Am Coll Cardiol.* 1992;20(5):1111–7.

46. Sheldahl LM, Wilke NA, Dougherty S, Tristani FE. Cardiac response to combined moderate heat and exercise in men with coronary artery disease. *Am J Cardiol.* 1992;70(2):186–91.

47. Sheldahl LM, Wilke NA, Dougherty SM, Tristani FE. Energy cost of occupational work [abstract]. *J Am Coll Cardiol.* 1995;25(2, Suppl 1):173A.

48. Sheldahl LM, Wilke NA, Dougherty S, Tristani FE. Snow blowing and shoveling in normal and asymptomatic coronary artery diseased men. *Int J Cardiol.* 1994;43(3):233–8.

49. Sheldahl LM, Wilke NA, Hanna RD, Dougherty SM, Tristani FE. Responses of people with coronary artery disease to common lawn-care tasks. *Eur J Appl Physiol Occup Physiol.* 1996;72(4): 357–64.

50. Sheldahl LM, Wilke NA, Tristani FE. Evaluation and training for resumption of occupational and leisure-time physical activities

in patients after a major cardiac event. *Med Exerc Nutr Health.* 1995;4:273–89.

51. Smith SC Jr, Allen J, Blair SN, et al. AHA/ACC guidelines for secondary prevention for patients with coronary and other atherosclerotic vascular disease: 2006 update: endorsed by the National Heart, Lung, and Blood Institute. *Circulation.* 2006;113(19):2363–72.

52. Smith TW. Driving after ventricular arrhythmias. *N Engl J Med.* 2001;345(6):451–2.

53. Soderman E, Lisspers J, Sundin O. Depression as a predictor of return to work in patients with coronary artery disease. *Soc Sci Med.* 2003;56(1):193–202.

54. Thompson PD, Franklin BA, Balady GJ, et al. Exercise and acute cardiovascular events placing the risks into perspective: a scientific statement from the American Heart Association Council on Nutrition, Physical Activity, and Metabolism and the Council on Clinical Cardiology. *Circulation.* 2007;115(17):2358–68.

55. Toro K, Bartholy J, Pongracz R, Kis Z, Keller E, Dunay G. Evaluation of meteorological factors on sudden cardiovascular death. *J Forensic Leg Med.* 2010;17(5):236–42.

56. U.S. Department of Labor, Office of Disability Employment Policy Web site [Internet]. Washington (DC): U.S. Department of Labor, Office of Disability Employment Policy; [cited 2011 Mar 14]. Available from: http://www.dol.gov/odep

57. United States, Employment and Training Administration, United States Employment Service. *Dictionary of Occupational Titles.* 4th ed. Indianapolis (IN): JIST Works; 1991. 1404 p.

58. U.S. Social Security Administration Web site [Internet]. Baltimore (MD): U.S. Social Security Administration; [cited 2011 Mar 14]. Available from: http://www.ssa.gov

59. Vona M, Capodaglio P, Iannessa A, et al. The role of work simulation tests in a comprehensive cardiac rehabilitation program. *Monaldi Arch Chest Dis.* 2002;58(1):26–34.

60. Wilke NA, Sheldahl LM, Dougherty SM, Hanna RD, Nickele GA, Tristani FE. Energy expenditure during household tasks in women with coronary artery disease. *Am J Cardiol.* 1995;75(10):670–4.

61. Wilke NA, Sheldahl LM, Dougherty SM, Levandoski SG, Tristani FE. Baltimore Therapeutic Equipment work simulator: energy expenditure of work activities in cardiac patients. *Arch Phys Med Rehabil.* 1993;74(4):419–24.

62. Wilke NA, Sheldahl LM, Dougherty SM. Metabolic cost of wood splitting in men with and without ischemic heart disease [abstract]. *J Cardiopulm Rehabil.* 1990;10(10):382.

63. Willich SN, Lewis M, Lowel H, Arntz HR, Schubert F, Schroder R. Physical exertion as a trigger of acute myocardial infarction. Triggers and Mechanisms of Myocardial Infarction Study Group. *N Engl J Med.* 1993;329(23):1684–90.

64. *Workers' Compensation* [Internet]. Washington, DC: U.S. Department of Labor, Bureau of Labor Statistics; [cited 2011 Mar 14]. Available from: http://www.dol.gov/dol/topic/workcomp/index.htm

65. Workplace Safety and Insurance Board Ontario Web site [Internet]. Toronto (Ontario): Workplace Safety and Insurance Board Ontario; [cited 2011 Mar 14]. Available from: http://www.wsib.on.ca/en/community/WSIB

66. Wyman DO. Evaluating patients for return to work. *Am Fam Physician.* 1999;59(4):844–8.

67. Wyss CA, Koepfli P, Fretz G, Seebauer M, Schirlo C, Kaufmann PA. Influence of altitude exposure on coronary flow reserve. *Circulation.* 2003;108(10):1202–7.

SELECTED REFERENCES FOR FURTHER READING

Leopold RS. *A Year in the Life of a Million American Workers.* New York (NY): Metlife Group Disability; 2003. 206 p.

Ranavaya MI, LeFevre P, Denniston PL Jr. Evidence-based disability duration guidelines. *J Disabil Med.* 2002;2:75–78.

Sagall EL, Nash IS. Cardiac evaluations for legal purposes. In: Fuster V, Alexander RW, O'Rourke RA, et al., editors. *Hurst's The Heart.* 10th ed. New York: McGraw-Hill; 2001. p. 2519–2532.

Sheldahl LM, Wilke NA, Tristani FE. Evaluation and training for resumption of occupational and leisure-time physical activities in patients after a major cardiac event. *Med Exerc Nutr Health.* 1995;4:273–289.

Wyman DO. Evaluating patients for return to work. *Am Fam Physician.* 1999;59:844–848.

INTERNET RESOURCES

- Social Security Online: Employment Support for People with Disabilities: http://www.ssa.gov/work
- Social Security Online: Medical/Professional Relations: http://www.socialsecurity.gov/disability/professionals/bluebook
- U.S. Department of Labor: Occupational Outlook Handbook, 2010–11 Edition: http://www.bls.gov/oco
- U.S. Department of Labor, Office of Disability Employment Policy: http://www.dol.gov/odep

Exercise Assessment in Special Populations

General principles of exercise testing apply to all individuals, but in some special populations, additional factors may need to be considered. The focus of this chapter will be to provide additional information on how the general principles of exercise testing, as described in *Chapters 20–23*, may be applied. Specifically, this chapter will include considerations in exercise testing for pregnant women, the elderly, and children.

PREGNANCY

The safety of physical activity during pregnancy is a significant question for clinicians and researchers. In addition to maternal safety, fetal responses to strenuous maternal exercise are of concern. Fetal heart rates (HR) have been examined with no changes suggestive of fetal distress or changes in behavior during maternal exercise (64). Investigations regarding compromise of uterine blood flow if blood flow is redistributed to working skeletal muscle have not been conclusive (76,77), although uterine contractions have been found to increase in frequency during exercise, with rapid recovery after exercise (64). In general, it appears that the physiologic reserve of mother and fetus allow for short periods of exercise to be tolerated (77).

The American College of Obstetricians and Gynecologists (ACOG) suggests that pregnant women without medical or obstetric complications can follow the American College of Sports Medicine (ACSM) and Surgeon General's recommendation to accumulate 30 or more minutes of moderate exercise on most, if not all, days of the week (1). However, these recommendations pertain to pregnant women of normal weight participating in primarily aerobic exercise programs. The potential benefits of exercise for previously sedentary, obese women in this population are of increased importance, and more specific guidelines regarding exercise should be provided. For example, a recent study identified a target heart rate (THR) of 101–124 beats per minute (bpm) (20%–39% oxygen uptake reserve [$\dot{V}O_2R$]) for this population, which represents the lower threshold of the ACSM's recommended training stimulus (16). The benefits of physical activity during pregnancy as they relate to chronic disease risk have been outlined in a round table consensus statement (54), recent literature review (75), and current sports medicine report (46). Physical activity may reduce the risk of developing preeclampsia, gestational diabetes (GDM), excess weight gain, and delivery complications (*i.e.*, shorter labor duration, less risk for cesarean delivery) while improving overall mental health (11,17,33,80). Although research is still needed to determine the optimal exercise program to prevent GDM, resistance exercise (RE) programs have reduced the development of GDM in overweight women (8). More recently, RE has been shown to be safe not only in women who were active pregravid but also for those who were sedentary until gravidae, with greater benefits observed in overweight women (5,7,46,79). Light-to-moderate intensity RE programs may be better tolerated than aerobic activities during later stages of pregnancy because of the stationary nature of the activity, providing not only musculoskeletal benefits (improved posture, prevention of low back pain) but also increased exercise adherence (7,8,46). For more detailed information on these issues, as well as the relationship of physical activity to postpartum musculoskeletal conditions, breastfeeding, postpartum weight loss, and offspring health, please refer to the published statements (17,46,54,75).

KEY TERMS

Oscillometric: Relating to the oscillometer, which is an apparatus for measuring oscillations of any kind, especially those of the bloodstream in sphygmomanometry.

Postpartum: Immediate period following childbirth.

Preeclampsia: A condition of hypertension occurring in pregnancy, typically accompanied by edema and proteinuria.

Volitional: A choice or decision made by will.

As outlined in the ACSM's *Guidelines for Exercise Testing and Prescription*, many physiologic changes occur during pregnancy that result in increased cardiopulmonary responses to a given submaximal intensity of exercise. Guidelines set forth by ACOG (1) as well as the Joint Committee of the Society of Obstetricians and Gynecologists of Canada and the Canadian Society for Exercise Physiology (18) are endorsed by ACSM and will serve as the foundation for the recommendations in this section.

PRETESTING SCREENING

Before beginning an exercise program, overall health and obstetric and medical risks should be reviewed (4). The Physical Activity Readiness Questionnaire (PAR-Q) is a frequently used instrument to determine an individual's readiness to start an exercise program. The Canadian Society for Exercise Physiology has taken a step beyond the PAR-Q for pregnant women with their development of the Physical Activity Readiness Medical Examination, termed as the PARmed-X for Pregnancy (49). This instrument includes a preexercise health checklist as well as contraindications for exercise. As stated within the instrument:

> The safety of prenatal exercise programs depends on an adequate level of maternal-fetal physiological reserve. PARmed-X for Pregnancy is a convenient checklist and prescription for use by healthcare providers to evaluate pregnant patients who want to enter a prenatal fitness program and for ongoing medical surveillance of exercising pregnant patients (see PARmed-X for Pregnancy in *Fig. 28-1*).

EXERCISE TESTING

In general, physician clearance is recommended for women who have been sedentary before pregnancy or who have a medical condition. In any exercise situation, which would include exercise testing, ACOG highlights warning signs to terminate exercise (see *Box 28-1*).

Typically, maximal exercise testing is not recommended for pregnant women. If a maximal exercise test is warranted because of a medical situation, the test should only be performed with physician supervision. Maximal responses for weight-supported activity (*i.e.*, cycle ergometer) have been found to be similar between a matched group of pregnant and nonpregnant women, although carbohydrate use appeared to be blunted at maximal exercise levels (28). The lower respiratory exchange ratio observed in pregnant women may be a protective mechanism regarding glucose sparing for the fetus or to resist changes in pH (28). Fetal responses to maximal exercise are an ongoing area of research interest. Brief maximal exertion, as done during a maximal exercise test, has been suggested to be safe in active women with uncomplicated pregnancies (76,77). Pregnant women who exercised on a cycle ergometer had minor electrocardiographic changes (*e.g.*, T-wave inversion in V2, shorter onset to maximal ST depression) at rest and during exercise compared with a control group of nonpregnant women, although the changes were considered normal unless symptoms were reported (72).

When a metabolic cart is not available, it is possible to predict $\dot{V}O_{2peak}$. Recently, the following equation was developed using a modified Balke protocol (to **volitional** fatigue) to predict $\dot{V}O_{2peak}$ for those without access to a metabolic cart (NOTE: Peak HR is in bpm, incline is in percent, speed is in mph, body mass index [BMI] is in $kg \cdot m^{-2}$) (44):

$$\dot{V}O_{2peak} \text{ (predicted)} = (0.055 \times \text{peak HR}) \\ + (0.381 \times \text{incline}) \\ + (5.541 \times \text{speed}) \\ + (-0.090 \times \text{BMI}) - 6.846$$

In place of a maximal test, typically, a submaximal exercise test (*i.e.*, <75% HR reserve) is used to predict $\dot{V}O_{2peak}$. Most research studies have selected cycle ergometry for testing. Given the changes in posture and center of gravity during pregnancy, cycle ergometry would appear to provide a safe and secure exercise mode. Information on submaximal testing is found in the *GETP9* and, although not specific for pregnant women, provides guidance on testing procedures.

SUMMARY

Benefits of physical activity during pregnancy have been well documented. Exercise, even brief maximal exercise, appears safe for women with uncomplicated pregnancy. Maximal exercise testing during pregnancy is not routinely recommended unless a medical condition warrants. In such situations, a physician should be present. More commonly, submaximal testing is conducted. Contraindications to exercise as well as warning signs to terminate exercise should be considered to ensure safety of mother and fetus (1).

ELDERLY

The term *older adult* includes individuals at least 65 yr of age and those between 50 and 64 yr of age with clinically significant chronic conditions or physical limitations that affect movement, physical fitness, or physical activity (51). Because of many factors, differences between chronologic age and physiologic age exist. As a result, exercise testing for this group must be individualized.

The 2008 U.S. Census has identified that 12% of the total population (almost 35 million people) are older than age 65 yr. This number is projected to increase

PARmed-X for PREGNANCY
PHYSICAL ACTIVITY READINESS MEDICAL EXAMINATION

PARmed-X for PREGNANCY is a guideline for health screening prior to participation in a prenatal fitness class or other exercise.

Healthy women with uncomplicated pregnancies can integrate physical activity into their daily living and can participate without significant risks either to themselves or to their unborn child. Postulated benefits of such programs include improved aerobic and muscular fitness, promotion of appropriate weight gain, and facilitation of labour. Regular exercise may also help to prevent gestational glucose intolerance and pregnancy-induced hypertension.

The safety of prenatal exercise programs depends on an adequate level of maternal-fetal physiological reserve. PARmed-X for PREGNANCY is a convenient checklist and prescription for use by health care providers to evaluate pregnant patients who want to enter a prenatal fitness program and for ongoing medical surveillance of exercising pregnant patients.

Instructions for use of the 4-page PARmed-X for PREGNANCY are the following:

1. The patient should fill out the section on PATIENT INFORMATION and the PRE-EXERCISE HEALTH CHECKLIST (PART 1, 2, 3, and 4 on p. 1) and give the form to the health care provider monitoring her pregnancy.

2. The health care provider should check the information provided by the patient for accuracy and fill out SECTION C on CONTRAINDICATIONS (p. 2) based on current medical information.

3. If no exercise contraindications exist, the HEALTH EVALUATION FORM (p. 3) should be completed, signed by the health care provider, and given by the patient to her prenatal fitness professional.

In addition to prudent medical care, participation in appropriate types, intensities and amounts of exercise is recommended to increase the likelihood of a beneficial pregnancy outcome. PARmed-X for PREGNANCY provides recommendations for individualized exercise prescription (p. 3) and program safety (p. 4).

NOTE: Sections A and B should be completed by the patient before the appointment with the health care provider.

A PATIENT INFORMATION

NAME _____

ADDRESS _____

TELEPHONE _____ BIRTHDATE _____ HEALTH INSURANCE No. _____

NAME OF
PRENATAL FITNESS PROFESSIONAL _____

PRENATAL FITNESS
PROFESSIONAL S PHONE NUMBER _____

B PRE-EXERCISE HEALTH CHECKLIST

PART 1: GENERAL HEALTH STATUS

In the past, have you experienced (check YES or NO):

		YES	NO
1.	Miscarriage in an earlier pregnacy?	❏	❏
2.	Other pregnancy complications?	❏	❏
3.	I have completed a PAR-Q within the last 30 days.	❏	❏

If you answered YES to question 1 or 2, please explain:

_____

Number of previous pregnancies? _____

PART 2: STATUS OF CURRENT PREGNANCY

Due Date: _____

During this pregnancy, have you experienced:

		YES	NO
1.	Marked fatigue?	❏	❏
2.	Bleeding from the vagina ("spotting")?	❏	❏
3.	Unexplained faintness or dizziness?	❏	❏
4.	Unexplained abdominal pain?	❏	❏
5.	Sudden swelling of ankles, hands or face?	❏	❏
6.	Persistent headaches or problems with headaches?	❏	❏
7.	Swelling, pain or redness in the calf of one leg?	❏	❏
8.	Absence of fetal movement after 6th month?	❏	❏
9.	Failure to gain weight after 5th month?	❏	❏

If you answered YES to any of the above questions, please explain:

_____

PART 3: ACTIVITY HABITS DURING THE PAST MONTH

1. List only regular fitness/recreational activities:

_____

_____

INTENSITY	FREQUENCY (times/week)			TIME (minutes/day)		
	1-2	2-4	4+	<20	20-40	40+
Heavy	—	—	—	—	—	—
Medium	—	—	—	—	—	—
Light	—	—	—	—	—	—

2. Does your regular occupation (job/home) activity involve:

	YES	NO
Heavy Lifting?	❏	❏
Frequent walking/stair climbing?	❏	❏
Occasional walking (>once/hr)?	❏	❏
Prolonged standing?	❏	❏
Mainly sitting?	❏	❏
Normal daily activity?	❏	❏

		YES	NO
3.	Do you currently smoke tobacco?*	❏	❏
4.	Do you consume alcohol?*	❏	❏

PART 4: PHYSICAL ACTIVITY INTENTIONS

What physical activity do you intend to do?

_____

Is this a change from what you currently do?   ❏ YES   ❏ NO

*NOTE: PREGNANT WOMEN ARE STRONGLY ADVISED NOT TO SMOKE OR CONSUME ALCOHOL DURING PREGNANCY AND DURING LACTATION.

C CONTRAINDICATIONS TO EXERCISE: to be completed by your health care provider

Absolute Contraindications

Does the patient have:

		YES	NO
1.	Ruptured membranes, premature labour?	❏	❏
2.	Persistent second or third trimester bleeding/placenta previa?	❏	❏
3.	Pregnancy-induced hypertension or pre-eclampsia?	❏	❏
4.	Incompetent cervix?	❏	❏
5.	Evidence of intrauterine growth restriction?	❏	❏
6.	High-order pregnancy (e.g., triplets)?	❏	❏
7.	Uncontrolled Type I diabetes, hypertension or thyroid disease, other serious cardiovascular, respiratory or systemic disorder?	❏	❏

Relative Contraindications

Does the patient have:

		YES	NO
1.	History of spontaneous abortion or premature labour in previous pregnancies?	❏	❏
2.	Mild/moderate cardiovascular or respiratory disease (e.g., chronic hypertension, asthma)?	❏	❏
3.	Anemia or iron deficiency? (Hb < 100 g/L)?	❏	❏
4.	Malnutrition or eating disorder (anorexia, bulimia)?	❏	❏
5.	Twin pregnancy after 28th week?	❏	❏
6.	Other significant medical condition?	❏	❏

Please specify: _____

NOTE: Risk may exceed benefits of regular physical activity. The decision to be physically active or not should be made with qualified medical advice.

PHYSICAL ACTIVITY RECOMMENDATION: ❏ Recommended/Approved   ❏ Contraindicated

FIGURE 28-1. PARmed-X for Pregnancy. Source: Physical Activity Readiness Medical Examination for Pregnancy (PARmed-X for Pregnancy), 2002. (Reprinted with permission from the Canadian Society for Exercise Physiology, http://www.csep.ca.)

BOX 28-1	Exercise and Pregnancy: Medical and Safety Concerns for the Mother and Fetus

MOTHER		FETUS	
Concern	**Solution**	**Concern**	**Solution or Effect**
Poor balance while running or jogging because of shifts in weight distribution and center of gravity.	Slow down, run cautiously, and never alone.	Direct fetal trauma. Tissue and fluid surrounding fetus provides protection.	No scientific data.
Overheating and dehydration. Pregnancy elevates body core temperature by approximately 0.5°C, elevating resting metabolic rate by 15%–20%. Excessive sweating might reduce blood volume.	Drink plenty of fluids before, during, and after exercise. Use appropriate exercise clothing and/or avoid exercise during extremely hot and humid weather.	Hyperthermia and reduced fetal blood flow.	Might cause neural tube defects, growth retardation, reduced birth weight, and/or fetal abnormalities.
Leg, hip, and abdominal pain. Reduced circulation to lower extremities during late pregnancy, extra weight to carry.	Never forget to stretch and warm up before any exercise session. Wear cushioned and comfortable shoes.	Reduced fetal blood flow.	No scientific data.
Nutrient availability. Pregnancy increases energy requirements by approximately 300 kcal/day.	It is expected for pregnant women to gain 25–40 lbs.	Substrate availability and hypoxia: reduced fetal glucose and oxygen availability.	Might cause growth retardation, reduced birth weight, and/or fetal abnormalities.
Reduced oxygen availability for aerobic exercise. Cardiovascular drift: added blood circulation to placenta.	Modify exercise intensity. Never exercise to the point of fatigue or exhaustion. Avoid intense and prolonged exercise. Monitor heart rate and rates of perceived exertion.	Reduced fetal blood flow. Intense exercise causes a redistribution of blood flow. More to muscles, less to other areas, including the placenta.	Light to moderate physical activities are considered safe for mother and fetus.
Musculoskeletal injury. Ballistic movements, sudden postural changes can increase the risk of injury. However, the risk of injury for fit pregnant women should be lower.	Continuous/aerobic exercises are more acceptable than intermittent/anaerobic exercises.	Umbilical cord entanglement. Can cause reduced blood flow to important fetal organs.	No scientific data.

Note: A physician with background in exercise physiology should be consulted before any exercise program is considered during pregnancy. Ask about contraindications to exercise and a list of "high risk" sports to avoid during pregnancy.

Reprinted with permission from American College of Obstetricians and Gynecologists. Exercise during pregnancy and the postpartum period. ACOG Committee Opinion No. 267. *Obstet Gynecol.* 2002;99:171–3.

rapidly with the aging baby boomer population. In 2020, the number of individuals in this group is projected to be 20.8% of the total population (68). Understanding the age-associated changes in cardiovascular response to exercise allows clinicians and researchers to fully understand and appreciate stress test results (19). Between the ages of 20 and 80 yr, reductions have been observed in the following peak values: oxygen consumption (50%), arteriovenous (AV) oxygen difference (25%), cardiac output (25%), HR (25%), stroke volume (0%–15%),

and ejection fraction (15%) (19). Other changes include increases in end-diastolic volume (30%) and end-systolic volume (150%) (19).

CLINICAL EVALUATION

The ACSM guidelines consider age as a positive risk factor for atherosclerotic cardiovascular disease (CVD), specifically ≥45 yr of age for men and ≥55 yr of age for women. Despite age-related risk, exercise testing prior to engaging in a physical activity program is not routinely recommended except for individuals classified as high risk or those individuals at moderate risk who wish to engage in vigorous intensity exercise (see *GETP9, Tables 2-2* and *2-4*). Although asymptomatic individuals of moderate risk require a medical exam prior to beginning a vigorous-intensity exercise program, they may begin a moderate-intensity exercise program, such as walking, without physician clearance.

PRACTICAL CONSIDERATIONS OF ROUTINE EXERCISE TESTING

The use of exercise testing has value for both diagnosis and prognosis in the elderly (38). The sensitivity and specificity of exercise testing in asymptomatic individuals has been reviewed (21). The pretest probability of coronary artery disease (CAD) has been reported for men and women in the 60–69 yr age range and indicates a high probability (>90%) for those with typical/definite angina pectoris, intermediate pretest probability (10%–90%) for those with atypical/probable angina pectoris as well as nonanginal chest pain, and low probability (<10%) for those who are asymptomatic (21). No data are available for individuals beyond 69 yr of age, although the assumption is that CAD risk increases with age (21).

EXERCISE TESTING CONSIDERATIONS

Understanding potential compromise of functional capacity in the elderly is important when selecting an appropriate stress test (*i.e.*, exercise or pharmacologic) (21,71). Many test protocols result in fatigue within the first or second stage before maximal effort is achieved (71). Use of tests with shorter intervals and increased treadmill grade may be a viable alternative for those who cannot walk briskly (71). If steady state is desired during each stage, longer intervals may be warranted (62).

Test modality appears to be an important factor to consider regarding prognostic markers, as suggested by a recent study of patients with known or suspected CAD (55). Patients in this study had a higher peak HR but slower drop in HR in recovery with a treadmill exercise test compared with a bicycle test. Duke treadmill scores were significantly higher on the treadmill than bicycle because of the higher sensitivity in determining ST-segment deviations that result from exercise (55). Additionally, the Duke treadmill score is not valid in those individuals older than 75 yr of age. (Note: The Duke treadmill score is determined by the following calculation: exercise time − [5 × ST deviation] − [4 × angina index]. Time is in minutes on the Bruce protocol, ST deviation is in mm, and angina index is coded 0–2 [40]). Bicycle ergometry could result in a low-risk classification when a treadmill test may result in a higher risk classification. Thus, it is not recommended to use chronotropic index or Duke treadmill scores for risk classification with bicycle exercise tests (55).

Selection of exercise mode must be made considering the benefits and potential shortcoming of each. Although bicycle exercise may be preferred to accommodate for gait or coordination concerns (71), many elderly are not familiar with cycle ergometry because mainly, leg muscles are used, systolic blood pressure (SBP) tends to be higher (55), and localized leg fatigue may be an impediment to achieving maximal effort (42). Cycle ergometry does, however, allow for better stability, and thus electrocardiogram (ECG) tracings may be of better quality (42), although most current systems produce high-quality tracings regardless of modality (62). When a treadmill is used, the stress placed on the cardiovascular system will be greater because of the use of a larger muscle mass (71). Arm ergometry is typically used for those with severe orthopedic, neurologic, or peripheral vascular disease (71).

Several factors can influence exercise testing in the elderly and may warrant a modification of the test to produce an optimal evaluation. *Table 28-1* outlines some common characteristics of the elderly, along with suggested test adaptations (47,62).

PROGNOSTIC ASSESSMENT WITH EXERCISE TESTING

Exercise ECG and exercise echocardiogram have been found to be superior to resting tests for predicting cardiac death and cardiac events and there appears to be no differences observed between genders (3,13,14). Of particular interest is the value of workload achieved in predicting both cardiac events and cardiac death (13,57). The Duke treadmill score has been found to be an independent predictor of cardiac mortality in a group of asymptomatic women because of the exercise capacity component of the score (25). The prognostic value of workload achieved on a treadmill exercise test was found to be similar between individuals <65 yr of age compared with those ≥65 yr of age (24,63).

For those with intermediate Duke treadmill scores, the use of exercise echocardiogram may be helpful in predicting mortality (43). Similarly, exercise echocardiography was found to be helpful in stratifying those with intermediate, as well as low, Duke treadmill scores into risk categories, although the cost-effectiveness of the low-score subgroup is questionable because of low absolute risk (52). The use of multiple tests (Duke treadmill score, first-pass radionuclide angiography with ejection fraction calculation, and perfusion single-photon emission computed tomography [SPECT]) resulted in optimal risk stratification, as each was a significant predictor of cardiovascular events in a group of high-risk patients with a median age of 60 yr (39). Dobutamine stress [99m]Technitium-tetrofosmin SPECT provided

TABLE 28-1. Exercise Testing for the Elderly

Characteristic	Suggested Test Modification
Low $\dot{V}O_{2max}$	Start at a low intensity (2–3 METs)
More time required to reach a steady state	Long warm-up (3+ min); small rise in power output (0.5–1 MET) and/or 2–3 min at each stage
Increased fatigability	Reduce total test time to 12–15 min or use an intermittent protocol
Increased need to monitor ECG, BP, and HR	Bike > treadmill > step test
Poor balance	Bike > treadmill > step test; use treadmill built into the floor
Poor strength (especially upper thighs)	Treadmill > bike or step test
Less ambulatory ability	Increase treadmill grade rather than speed (maximum of 3–3.5 mph)
Poor neuromuscular coordination	Increase amount of practice; may require more than one test
Difficulty holding mouthpiece with dentures	Add support or use face mask to measure $\dot{V}O_2$
Impaired vision	Bike > treadmill or step test
Impaired hearing	Treadmill > bike or step test, if person needs to follow a cadence; difficulty understanding and responding in a noisy environment (use electronic bike)
Senile gait patterns and foot problems (*e.g.,* bunions and calluses)	Bike > treadmill or step test

$\dot{V}O_{2max}$, maximal volume of oxygen consumed per unit time; METs, metabolic equivalents; ECG, electrocardiogram; BP, blood pressure; HR, heart rate; $\dot{V}O_2$, volume of oxygen consumed per unit time.

Reprinted with permission from Tanner CS, Heise CT, Barber G. Correlation of the physiologic parameters of a continuous ramp versus an incremental James exercise protocol in normal children. *Am J Cardiol.* 1991;67:309–12.

incremental prognostic information for prediction of all-cause mortality and cardiac events in a group of elderly patients (61).

In older men (>75 yr of age), neither exercise test responses were found to be predictive of either all-cause or cardiovascular death (78) nor was the Duke treadmill score (37), although high cycling power was strongly and independently associated with decreased death risk for 75-yr-old men and women in a population-based study (32). Other more sophisticated tests, such as the exercise SPECT, may provide additional ability to accurately predict risk level as found in an older (>75 yr of age) population capable of exercise (70).

EXERCISE PROTOCOLS

Specific protocols for testing are outlined in *GETP9.* Considerations for protocol selection include the following:

- The purpose of the evaluation
- The specific outcomes desired
- The characteristics of the individual being tested

Realize that additional practice may be needed to allow individuals to feel comfortable with the testing protocol.

Treadmill testing requires some special considerations because older individuals will often have poor balance and muscular strength. Allowing individuals to hold the treadmill handrail may allow them to feel more comfortable but can also alter the energy cost of the activity. If $\dot{V}O_{2max}$ is being measured rather than predicted

from work capacity or HR, this may not be an issue. Conversely, if prediction of maximal work capacity or $\dot{V}O_2$ is made from HR responses during such testing, error will be introduced (62).

Although the Bruce treadmill test remains one of the most commonly used protocols, it may not be appropriate for all elderly patients because of its longer stages (3 min) and relatively large and unequal workload increases with each stage (2–3 metabolic equivalents [METs]). Older individuals may benefit from protocols such as the Naughton or Balke-Ware, in which workload increments between stages are smaller (≤1 MET). Consider protocols in which the grade increases rather than speed. The initial workload should be low (*i.e.,* ≤3 METs). Increases in treadmill grade of 1%–3% · min^{-1} with constant belt speeds of 1.5–2.5 mph (2.4–4.0 kph) have been recommended for older populations (51). Ramp protocols are another option in which work rate increases in a series of small but constant increments. Ramp protocols are most common for cycle ergometry testing, but many treadmills now also have this capacity.

Cycle ergometry may be preferred over a treadmill for those with poor balance, poor neuromuscular coordination, impaired vision, impaired gait patterns, weight-bearing limitations, and/or foot problems (62). However, a lack of familiarity with cycling activity may be a limitation in this population (21). Increments of 10–15 W · min^{-1} (1 W = 6.12 kg · m · min^{-1}) can be used on the cycle ergometer for elderly persons (51).

Although fatigue may become an issue when conducting exercise testing with the elderly, no unique test termination criteria for older individuals have been published. Recommended termination criteria established for adults should be used (see *GETP9, Chapter 5*).

Special Considerations for Those Older Than 75 Years

In those older than 75 yr, potential chronic medical conditions, increased physical limitations, and higher prevalence of asymptomatic CAD may necessitate a different approach (22). Exercise testing in this age group will often require pharmacologic stress testing with radionuclide imaging to detect myocardial ischemia in asymptomatic patients because of the inability of most to achieve maximal effort on an exercise test (22). In a community-based study including individuals >75 yr with no known CVD or other medical contraindications, only 12.2% were able to achieve a maximal effort on a treadmill test (defined as a respiratory exchange ratio of >1.10 and at least 2 min on the Cornell treadmill protocol) in the 75–79-yr-old group. The ability to attain maximal effort continued to decrease with advancing age (7.1% in the 80–84-yr-old age group and 1.7% in the >85-yr-old age group) (30).

In addition, individuals in older than 75 age range are unlikely to engage in vigorous exercise (one indication for an exercise test). Promoting physical activity should be encouraged, and the benefits of physical activity should not be lost because of the expense or fear of exercise testing. Thus, a complete medical history and physical examination may be sufficient to identify potential cardiac issues related to exercise (22).

Those with CVD or overt symptoms should be treated according to published guidelines (see *GETP9, Chapter 2*) prior to beginning in exercise program, whereas those without symptoms or disease should be able to initiate a low-intensity (≤3 METs) exercise program without undue risk. Functional fitness testing examining aspects related to health (including body composition, endurance, strength, flexibility, and balance) have been highlighted for emphasis in the elderly (62), and specific suggestions are available for those older than age 75 yr (10).

MEDICATION USE

Commonly, elderly individuals will be taking medication(s), both over-the-counter (OTC) and prescribed. In the Slone Survey, 91% of men and 94% of women >65 yr of age reported using a medication and/or supplement (prescription, OTC, vitamin/mineral, herbal/supplement) in the previous week (35). When only prescription medications were considered, 71% of men and 81% of women reported usage, whereas 19% of men and 23% of women reported taking more than five prescription medications (35). Many medications influence the ECG, blood pressure (BP), or HR

responses to exercise. Understanding the influence of medications is vital in any testing situation, especially with the elderly.

SUMMARY

Stress testing in the elderly has both a diagnostic and prognostic value. Understanding the potential benefits and limitations of various testing methods will allow for optimal test outcomes and appropriate test interpretation. Physiologic limitations and medication use must also be considered with this population.

CHILDREN

Indications for exercise testing of children have been described and include the following: (a) evaluating cardiac and pulmonary functional capacity, (b) detecting myocardial ischemia, (c) evaluating cardiac rhythm and rate, (d) determining BP response, (e) assessing symptoms with exercise, (f) detecting and managing exercise-induced asthma, (g) assessing physical fitness, (h) charting the course of a progressive disease and evaluating therapy, and (i) assessing the success of rehabilitation programs (58,59). Although this list could apply to other populations, the following section will focus on aspects unique to pediatric exercise testing.

Children present a greater challenge in exercise testing because of their smaller body size (when compared with testing equipment), relatively poor peak performance (in contrast to the work rate increments possible with exercise equipment), potentially shorter attention span, and reduced motivation (26). Hemodynamic and respiratory characteristics of children's responses to exercise are shown in *Table 28-2* (27).

EXERCISE TESTING CONSIDERATIONS

Whether to allow a parent(s) or guardian(s) into the room during testing should be determined on an individual basis with consideration for the relationship between the adult and the child and also the child's temperament (67). If a parent/guardian is allowed into the testing room, the person must not distract the child or interfere with the test (67). Maintaining a space at the back of the testing room for the parent is suggested (48).

The testing procedure must be explained clearly to both the parent/guardian and the child. All questions must be answered completely but in simple terms. The child must understand what is being asked of him or her, so he or she can communicate with the tester when he or she is unable to continue. Once both parent/guardian and the child are comfortable with the testing procedure, the informed consent should be signed by the parent (67), and verbal assent should be obtained from the child if older than 7 yr of age (48).

TABLE 28-2. Hemodynamic and Pulmonary Characteristics of Children's Responses to Exercise

Function	Typical for Children (Compared with Adults)
HR at submaximal intensity	Higher, especially at first decade
HR_{max}	Higher
Stroke volume (submax and max)	Lower
$\dot{Q}$ at given $\dot{V}O_2$	Somewhat lower
AV difference for O_2 at given $\dot{V}O_2$	Somewhat higher
Blood flow to active muscle	Higher
SBP, DBP submax and max	Lower
$\dot{V}E$ at given $\dot{V}O_2$	Higher
Ventilatory threshold	Similar
Ventilation rate	Higher
Vt/VC	Lower

HR, heart rate; HR_{max}, maximal heart rate; $\dot{Q}$, cardiac output; $\dot{V}O_2$, volume of oxygen consumed per unit time; AV, arteriovenous; SBP, systolic blood pressure; DBP, diastolic blood pressure; $\dot{V}E$, ventilation; Vt, tidal volume; VC, vital capacity.

Reprinted with permission from James FW, Kaplan S, Glueck CJ, Tsay JY, Knight MJ, Sarwar CJ. Responses of normal children and young adults to controlled bicycle exercise. *Circulation.* 1980;61:902–12.

Primary oversight of the exercise test should be by a physician trained in exercise testing and exercise physiology (48). The presence of the physician for direct supervision of the test depends on the risk to the patient (48). Laboratory personnel should include at least two trained individuals, at least one of whom should be trained in pediatric advanced life support (48).

EQUIPMENT USED IN TESTING

The American Heart Association (AHA) notes three purposes of ECG recording for children, including (a) to accurately assess HR as related to exercise effort and test end point; (b) to diagnose and evaluate arrhythmia; and (c) to assess conduction abnormalities, ST segment, and T-wave changes consistent with myocardial ischemia

and QT interval (48). AHA recommendations for ECG recording equipment are listed in *Box 28-2.*

BP is another important variable. AHA recommends that the BP be measured before the exercise test (rest), during the exercise test, and in recovery (48). Typically, the exercise and recovery measures are taken every 3 min (48). Various devices are available (*e.g.*, aneroid, automated), each with limitations. Because mercury-based devices are no longer commonly used, it is important to realize the importance of frequent calibration of aneroid devices. Automated (oscillometric) devices are sensitive to movement and vibration and, thus, may be problematic in exercise testing. The cuff must completely surround the arm, and the width of the cuff bladder should be least 40% of the arm circumference (48). Potentially, the most important factor in attaining accurate and reliable BP measures is the person taking the measurement, and thus periodic retraining and technique evaluation is recommended (48).

The metabolic cart is another piece of valuable equipment when testing children. Various carts are available and have been reviewed elsewhere (48). No matter the particular metabolic system used, collection of expired air must be made with care to avoid leaks. For children who do not easily handle a mouthpiece and nose clip, the use of a mask with sealant gel may be more appropriate (48).

Other devices potentially used in testing include echocardiography, nuclear myocardial blood flow imaging, and spirometry (48). Equipment related to safety should include a defibrillator, oxygen, suction system, and emergency drugs (48).

EXERCISE EQUIPMENT

Cycle ergometers and treadmills are the two most common exercise modes used in pediatric exercise testing (6). The equipment used must be appropriate for the child's age and size (48). Treadmills should have side and front handrails at appropriate heights (48). Ideally, cycle ergometers used in testing will have adjustable leg cranks and handlebars. If not available, use of blocks to increase pedal height may be necessary for smaller children to allow for 10–15 degrees

---

BOX 28-2 **Equipment Recommendations for Electrocardiogram (ECG) Recording Equipment (American Heart Association)**

- Real-time display screen of adequate size to see easily during testing
- Display at least three leads
- Printer to create copies
- Able to print immediate copies of real-time ECG and continuous ECG rhythm strips
- Helpful to print median ECG complexes at each stage

- Analogue recording is acceptable but digital is preferred
- Computer-based recording system can provide review of tracings at a later time

Reprinted with permission from Paridon SM, Alpert BS, Boas SR, et al. Clinical stress testing in the pediatric age group: a statement from the American Heart Associate Council on Cardiovascular Disease in the Young, Committee on Atherosclerosis, Hypertension, and Obesity in Youth. *Circulation.* 2006;113:1905–20.

TABLE 28-3. Comparison of Treadmill Versus Cycle Ergometer for Pediatric Exercise Testing

Variable	Treadmill	Cycle Ergometer
Expense	More expensive	Less expensive
Noise	Louder	Quieter
Safety	More dangerous	Less dangerous
Workload adjustments	Easy to adjust workload by speed and grade changes	Easy to adjust work rate
Determination of work efficiency	More difficult to quantify work rate because of influence of body size, weight, gait, and stride length	Electronically braked ergometers provide a more accurate measurement of mechanical power output than mechanically braked ergometers
Measurement ease	More difficult to obtain blood pressure because of movement artifact	Easier to obtain blood pressure and measures of gas exchange
Space	Require more laboratory space	Require less laboratory space
Other	Easier to calibrate than either mechanically braked or electronically braked cycle ergometers	More difficult to maintain workload as younger children may not maintain a steady cadence

Reprinted with permission from Paridon SM, Alpert BS, Boas SR, et al. Clinical stress testing in the pediatric age group: a statement from the American Heart Associate Council on Cardiovascular Disease in the Young, Committee on Atherosclerosis, Hypertension, and Obesity in Youth. *Circulation.* 2006;113:1905–20.

of knee flexion at the bottom of the pedal stroke (48). Realize that with both exercise modes, however, children may need additional time to practice (48). Treadmill exercise is typically preferred, especially for younger children, to avoid limitations because of undeveloped thigh musculature, resulting in early fatigue when cycling (27). Additionally, treadmill exercise involves a greater muscle mass and, thus, allows for higher $\dot{V}O_{2max}$ (6).

Advantages and disadvantages of each mode of exercise are shown in *Table 28-3* as adapted from the 2006 statement from the AHA on Clinical Stress Testing in the Pediatric Age Group (48).

MAXIMAL EFFORT CRITERIA AND OTHER MEASURES

Criteria commonly used to verify maximal effort in children include (a) respiratory exchange ratio of >1.1, (b) peak HR approaching 200 bpm, and (c) subjective observation by experienced testers of extreme effort (48). Attainment of a plateau in $\dot{V}O_2$ despite increasing workload (an adult criterion) is not typically observed in children (48,59).

Use of rating of perceived exertion (RPE) scales is possible in children, in particular, the children's OMNI Scale of perceived exertion, which has been validated for cycling exercise and walking/running (56,69). See *Figure 28-2* for these two visual scales.

INDICATIONS AND CONTRAINDICATIONS FOR STRESS TESTING

Generally, children with acute myocardial or pericardial inflammatory disease or those with severe outflow obstruction requiring surgery should not be tested.

Other than these situations, general safety of testing has been established. Understanding the risk level helps to ensure safety and minimizes risk. *Table 28-4* includes relative risks for exercise testing (48). Recent discussion has surrounded the appropriateness of including an ECG to the preparticipation screening procedure, which currently involves a preparticipation evaluation (PPE) (*i.e.*, medical history and physical examination). The PPE is used specifically to assess children and young adults prior to engaging in sport. However, those children not participating in sport may be excluded from the opportunity to receive such an evaluation (9). The recent release of the updated AHA's recommendations and considerations related to participation screening for cardiovascular abnormalities in competitive athletes does not support the motion to mandate 12-lead ECGs as part of the preparticipation screening process (41). Inconsistencies in the literature, largely attributed to the number of false positives, make it difficult to support the inclusion of an ECG in the preparticipation procedure (29). Despite noted inconsistencies, some professionals regard the PPE as limited screening tool to identify important and serious cardiovascular abnormalities that can contribute to sudden cardiac arrest (SCA) or even sudden cardiac death (9,53). A recent pilot study of 400 healthy children was conducted to determine the feasibility of heart screening for SCA. ECG screening revealed 23 (5.8%) cases of previously undiagnosed abnormalities and an additional 10 potential serious cases of which no case reported a positive family history (73). Researchers observed that the ECG was three times more likely than the history and physical examination to identify cardiac abnormalities and increased evaluation screening time by less than 10 min (73).

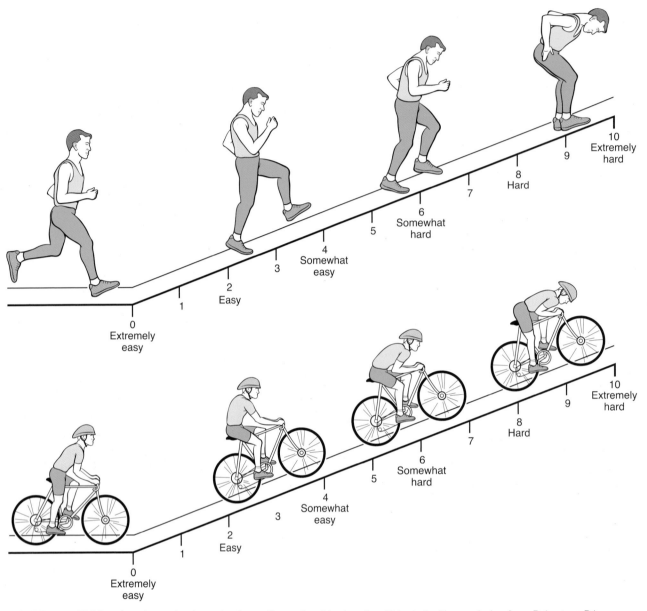

FIGURE 28-2. OMNI scales of perceived exertion for cycling and walking/running. (Adapted with permission from Robertson RJ, Goss FL, Boer NR, et al. Children's OMNI Scale of Perceived Exertion: mixed gender and race validation. *Med Sci Sports Exerc.* 2000;32[3]:452–8 and Utter AC, Roberston RJ, Nieman DC, Kang J. Children's OMNI Scale of Perceived Exertion: walking/running evaluation. *Med Sci Sports Exerc.* 2002;34[1]:139–44.)

The American College of Cardiology (ACC) and AHA also do not recommend the use of exercise testing to screen healthy children and adolescents prior to sport involvement, supporting the use of exercise testing only when evaluating children who present exercise-related symptoms (20).

Because the goal of most stress testing is to elicit symptoms and access cardiopulmonary reserves, maximal effort is desired. Test termination is typically indicated when diagnostic findings are established, monitoring equipment fails, or when signs/symptoms indicate a compromise to the child's well-being (48). Specifically, see *Box 28-3* for a listing of usual

indications for test termination made in light of clinical judgment (these should not be seen as rigid guidelines) (48).

EXERCISE PROTOCOLS

Protocol selection is based on the individual being tested and the purpose of the test (65). In general, to obtain $\dot{V}O_{2max}$, the child should reach his or her tolerance limit in 10 ± 2 min (48). In the United States, treadmills are more frequently used than cycle ergometers (12). Multistage incremental protocols commonly used include the Bruce and Balke treadmill protocols and

TABLE 28-4. Relative Risks for Stress Testing

Lower Risk	Higher Risk
Symptoms during exercise in an otherwise healthy child who has a normal cardiovascular exam and ECG	Patients with pulmonary hypertension
Exercise-induced bronchospasm studies in the absence of severe resting airway obstruction	Patients with documented long-QTc syndrome
Asymptomatic patients undergoing evaluation for possible long-QTc> syndrome	Patients with dilated/restrictive cardiomyopathy with congestive heart failure or arrhythmia
Asymptomatic ventricular ectopy in patients with structurally normal hearts	Patients with a history of hemodynamically unstable arrhythmia
Patients with unrepaired or residual congenital lesions who are asymptomatic at rest (including left to right shunts, obstructive right heart lesions without severe resting obstruction, obstructive left heart lesions with severe resting obstruction, regurgitation lesions regardless of severity)	Patients with hypertrophic cardiomyopathy who have symptoms, greater than mild left ventricular outflow tract obstruction, and documented arrhythmia
Routine follow-up of asymptomatic patients at risk for myocardial ischemia, including Kawasaki disease without giant aneurysm or known coronary stenosis, after repair of anomalous left coronary artery, after arterial switch procedure	Patients with greater than moderate airway obstruction on baseline pulmonary function tests
Routine monitoring in cardiac transplant patients not currently experiencing rejection	Patients with Marfan syndrome and activity-related chest pain in whom a noncardiac cause of chest pain is suspected
Patients with palliated cardiac lesions without uncompensated congestive heart failure, arrhythmia, or extreme cyanosis	Patients suspected to have myocardial ischemia with exertion
Patients with a history of hemodynamically stable supraventricular tachycardia	Routine testing of patients with Marfan syndrome
Patients with stable dilated cardiomyopathy without uncompensated congestive heart failure or documented arrhythmia	Unexplained syncope with exercise

ECG, electrocardiogram.

Reprinted with permission from Paridon SM, Alpert BS, Boas SR, et al. Clinical stress testing in the pediatric age group: a statement from the American Heart Associate Council on cardiovascular disease in the young. Committee on Atherosclerosis, Hypertension, and Obesity in Youth. *Circulation*. 2006;113:1905–20.

the James and McMaster cycle protocols. Incremental protocols (ramps and 1-min stages), such as the Godfrey test, have been used as well. Individualized protocols (based on predicted $\dot{V}O_{2max}$ and basal $\dot{V}O_2$) are also well tolerated by children (34).

The Bruce protocol has been used on subjects of all ages, and normative data are available for children (15). Advantages of the Bruce protocol include the ability to track a person over time and that $\dot{V}O_{2max}$ can be estimated from test duration (48). Disadvantages of the Bruce

---

BOX 28-3   Usual Indications for Test Termination

1. Decrease in ventricular rate with increasing workload associated with extreme fatigue, dizziness, or other symptoms suggestive of insufficient cardiac output
2. Failure of heart rate to increase with exercise and extreme fatigue, dizziness, or other symptoms suggestive of insufficient cardiac output
3. Progressive fall in systolic blood pressure with increasing workload
4. Severe hypertension, >250 mm Hg systolic or 115 mm Hg diastolic, or blood pressures higher than can be measured by laboratory equipment
5. Dyspnea that the patient finds intolerable
6. Symptomatic tachycardia that the patient finds intolerable
7. Progressive fall in oxygen saturation to <90% or a 10-point drop from resting saturation in a patient who is symptomatic
8. Presence of ≥3 mm flat or downward sloping ST-segment depression
9. Increasing ventricular ectopy with increasing workload, including a >3-beat run
10. Patient requests termination of the study

Reprinted with permission from Paridon SM, Alpert BS, Boas SR, et al. Clinical stress testing in the pediatric age group: a statement from the American Heart Associate Council on cardiovascular disease in the young. Committee on Atherosclerosis, Hypertension, and Obesity in Youth. *Circulation*. 2006;113:1905–20.

protocol include the larger work increments leading to potential premature termination within the first minute of the stage, boredom with the initial low-intensity stages, boredom with the 3-min stages, and steep grades that encourage excessive handrail holding (48).

The Balke protocol involves a constant speed with increasing grade. The Balke protocol has been modified in various ways, including use of a faster speed and starting at a higher grade (2,58–60). Faster speeds (jogging, running) compared with slower (walking) have been found to be appropriate for $\dot{V}O_{2max}$ determination (50).

The James cycle ergometer protocol includes three exercise protocols (predetermined work rates based on body surface area) using three 3-min stages followed by work rate increase each minute until volitional fatigue (31). An advantage of this protocol is the availability of normative data (31,74). A disadvantage is the possibility of early test termination by younger or less fit children. Another cycle testing protocol, the McMaster cycle ergometer protocol, also includes three predetermined work rates (based on height). This protocol, however, uses 2-min stages (6).

The Godfrey test is a 1-min incremental test that includes three protocols (predetermined by height) in which the work rate increments are 10–20 W. Normative data are available for this protocol (23). Ramp protocols have also been used in this patient population with similar maximal responses (45,66,81). Although selection of work rate increment is made on a case-by-case basis, typical increases of 20–25 W · min^{-1} are appropriate for fit children and 10 W · min^{-1} for younger and unfit children (48).

PHARMACOLOGIC STRESS TESTING

In situations in which exercise testing is inappropriate, pharmacologic stress testing may be used (*e.g.*, patients who are too young or are unable to perform exercise or when exercise may interfere with data collection, including some echocardiographic studies) (48). The two main types of pharmacologic agents include those that increase oxygen consumption of the heart (*e.g.*, dobutamine, isoproterenol) and those that cause vasodilatation of the coronary arteries (*e.g.*, adenosine, dipyridamole) (48). The rate of adverse reactions to pharmacologic stress testing in children is unknown, although it appears low (48).

ECHOCARDIOGRAPHY

Echocardiography allows for assessment of regional wall motion abnormalities when evaluating myocardial perfusion or gradients and/or function when assessing issues related to the coronary arteries (34,36). Conditions related to coronary artery pathology for which echocardiography are appropriate include Kawasaki disease, transplant graft vasculopathy, arterial switch operation

for transposition of the great arteries, anomalous coronary artery origins or pathways, pulmonary atresia with intact ventricular septum, hyperlipidemia, insulin-dependent diabetes mellitus, and supravalvular aortic stenosis (36). Other aspects, which can be examined under stress, include gradients (*e.g.*, for conditions such as hypertrophic cardiomyopathy or aortic and pulmonic stenosis), cardiac pressures (*e.g.*, in pulmonary hypertension), and ventricular function (*e.g.*, in dilated cardiomyopathy or mitral and aortic regurgitation) (34).

Pharmacologic or exercise stress can be used with echocardiography. Typically, with treadmill exercise and upright cycling, echocardiography is done before and immediately after the exercise. With supine cycling, echocardiography is done before and then during each stage of the test (48). Pharmacologic stressors include dobutamine, isoproterenol, adenosine, and dipyridamole (the latter two for ischemic evaluation only) (34).

SUMMARY

Exercise testing in children can present unique challenges related to ensuring complete understanding of the stress test, adaptability of equipment for smaller size, protocol selection to avoid boredom and elicit maximal effort, and exercise modality selection to ensure patient comfort with the activity. Staffing of pediatric testing requires individuals with an appropriate knowledge base as well as the experience and skill to work with children.

REFERENCES

1. ACOG Committee Obstetric Practice. ACOG Committee opinion. Number 267, January 2002: exercise during pregnancy and the postpartum period. *Obstet Gynecol.* 2002;99(1):171–3.
2. Armstrong N, Balding J, Gentle P, Williams J, Kirby B. Peak oxygen uptake and physical activity in 11- to 16-year-olds. *Pediatric Exercise Science.* 1990;2(4):349–58.
3. Arruda AM, Das MK, Roger VL, Klarich KW, Mahoney DW, Pellikka PA. Prognostic value of exercise echocardiography in 2,632 patients > or = 65 years of age. *J Am Coll Cardiol.* 2001;37(4):1036–41.
4. Artal R, O'Toole M. Guidelines of the American College of Obstetricians and Gynecologists for exercise during pregnancy and the postpartum period. *Br J Sports Med.* 2003;37(1):6–12; discussion 12.
5. Barakat R, Lucia A, Ruiz JR. Resistance exercise training during pregnancy and newborn's birth size: a randomised controlled trial. *Int J Obes (Lond).* 2009;33(9):1048–57.
6. Bar-Or O, Rowland TW. *Pediatric Exercise Medicine: From Physiologic Principles to Health Care Application.* Leeds (United Kingdom): Human Kinetics; 2004. 501 p.
7. Benton MJ, Swan PD, Whyte M. Progressive resistance training during pregnancy: a case study. *PM R.* 2010;2(7):681–4.
8. Brankston GN, Mitchell BF, Ryan EA, Okun NB. Resistance exercise decreases the need for insulin in overweight women with gestational diabetes mellitus. *Am J Obstet Gynecol.* 2004;190(1):188–93.
9. Campbell RM. Preparticipation screening and preparticipation forms. *Pacing Clin Electrophysiol.* 2009;32 Suppl 2:S15–8.
10. Carr K, Emes C, Rogerson M. Exercise testing protocols for different abilities in the older population. *Act Adapt Aging.* 2003;28(1):49–66.

11. Cedergren MI. Non-elective caesarean delivery due to ineffective uterine contractility or due to obstructed labour in relation to maternal body mass index. *Eur J Obstet Gynecol Reprod Biol.* 2009;145(2):163–6.

12. Chang RK, Gurvitz M, Rodriguez S, Hong E, Klitzner TS. Current practice of exercise stress testing among pediatric cardiology and pulmonology centers in the United States. *Pediatr Cardiol.* 2006;27(1):110–6.

13. Chuah SC, Pellikka PA, Roger VL, McCully RB, Seward JB. Role of dobutamine stress echocardiography in predicting outcome in 860 patients with known or suspected coronary artery disease. *Circulation.* 1998;97(15):1474–80.

14. Cortigiani L, Sicari R, Bigi R, Landi P, Bovenzi F, Picano E. Impact of gender on risk stratification by stress echocardiography. *Am J Med.* 2009;122(3):301–9.

15. Cumming GR, Everatt D, Hastman L. Bruce treadmill test in children: normal values in a clinic population. *Am J Cardiol.* 1978; 41(1):69–75.

16. Davenport MH, Charlesworth S, Vanderspank D, Sopper MM, Mottola MF. Development and validation of exercise target heart rate zones for overweight and obese pregnant women. *Appl Physiol Nutr Metab.* 2008;33(5):984–9.

17. Davies GA, Maxwell C, McLeod L, et al. SOGC Clinical Practice Guidelines: Obesity in pregnancy. No. 239, February 2010. *Int J Gynaecol Obstet.* 2010;110(2):167–73.

18. Davies GA, Wolfe LA, Mottola MF, MacKinnon C, Society of Obstetricians and gynecologists of Canada, SOGC Clinical Practice Obstetrics Committee. Joint SOGC/CSEP clinical practice guideline: exercise in pregnancy and the postpartum period. *Can J Appl Physiol.* 2003;28(3):330–41.

19. Fleg JL. Stress testing in the elderly. *Am J Geriatr Cardiol.* 2001;10(6): 308–15.

20. Gibbons RJ, Balady GJ, Beasley JW, et al. ACC/AHA guidelines for exercise testing: executive summary. A report of the American College of Cardiology/American Heart Association Task Force on Practice Guidelines (Committee on Exercise Testing). *Circulation.* 1997;96(1):345–54.

21. Gibbons RJ, Balady GJ, Bricker JT, et al. ACC/AHA 2002 guideline update for exercise testing: summary article: a report of the American College of Cardiology/American Heart Association Task Force on Practice Guidelines (Committee to Update the 1997 Exercise Testing Guidelines). *Circulation.* 2002;106(14):1883–92.

22. Gill TM, DiPietro L, Krumholz HM. Role of exercise stress testing and safety monitoring for older persons starting an exercise program. *JAMA.* 2000;284(3):342–9.

23. Godfrey S, Davies CT, Wozniak E, Barnes CA. Cardio-respiratory response to exercise in normal children. *Clin Sci.* 1971;40(5): 419–31.

24. Goraya TY, Jacobsen SJ, Pellikka PA, et al. Prognostic value of treadmill exercise testing in elderly persons. *Ann Intern Med.* 2000;132(11):862–70.

25. Gulati M, Arnsdorf MF, Shaw LJ, et al. Prognostic value of the duke treadmill score in asymptomatic women. *Am J Cardiol.* 2005;96(3):369–75.

26. Hebestreit H. Exercise testing in children—what works, what doesn't, and where to go? *Paediatr Respir Rev.* 2004;5 Suppl A: S11–4.

27. Hebestreit HU, Bar-Or O. Differences between children and adults for exercise testing and exercise prescription. In: Skinner JS, editor. *Exercise Testing and Exercise Prescription for Special Cases: Theoretical Basis and Clinical Application.* 3rd ed. Philadelphia: Lippincott Williams & Wilkins; 2005. p. 68–84.

28. Heenan AP, Wolfe LA, Davies GA. Maximal exercise testing in late gestation: maternal responses. *Obstet Gynecol.* 2001;97(1):127–34.

29. Hill AC, Miyake CY, Grady S, Dubin AM. Accuracy of interpretation of preparticipation screening electrocardiograms. *J Pediatr.* 2011;159(5):783–8.

30. Hollenberg M, Ngo LH, Turner D, Tager IB. Treadmill exercise testing in an epidemiologic study of elderly subjects. *J Gerontol A Biol Sci Med Sci.* 1998;53(4):B259–67.

31. James FW, Kaplan S, Glueck CJ, Tsay JY, Knight MJ, Sarwar CJ. Responses of normal children and young adults to controlled bicycle exercise. *Circulation.* 1980;61(5):902–12.

32. Kallinen M, Kauppinen M, Era P, Heikkinen E. The predictive value of exercise testing for survival among 75-year-old men and women. *Scand J Med Sci Sports.* 2006;16(4):237–44.

33. Kardel KR, Johansen B, Voldner N, Iversen PO, Henriksen T. Association between aerobic fitness in late pregnancy and duration of labor in nulliparous women. *Acta Obstet Gynecol Scand.* 2009;88(8):948–52.

34. Karila C, de Blic J, Waernessyckle S, Benoist MR, Scheinmann P. Cardiopulmonary exercise testing in children: an individualized protocol for workload increase. *Chest.* 2001;120(1):81–7.

35. Kaufman DW, Kelly JP, Rosenberg L, Anderson TE, Mitchell AA. Recent patterns of medication use in the ambulatory adult population of the United States: the Slone survey. *JAMA.* 2002;287(3): 337–44.

36. Kimball TR. Pediatric stress echocardiography. *Pediatr Cardiol.* 2002;23(3):347–57.

37. Kwok JM, Miller TD, Hodge DO, Gibbons RJ. Prognostic value of the Duke treadmill score in the elderly. *J Am Coll Cardiol.* 2002;39(9):1475–81.

38. Lai S, Kaykha A, Yamazaki T, et al. Treadmill scores in elderly men. *J Am Coll Cardiol.* 2004;43(4):606–15.

39. Liao L, Smith WT 4th, Tuttle RH, Shaw LK, Coleman RE, Borges-Neto S. Prediction of death and nonfatal myocardial infarction in high-risk patients: a comparison between the Duke treadmill score, peak exercise radionuclide angiography, and SPECT perfusion imaging. *J Nucl Med.* 2005;46(1):5–11.

40. Mark DB, Shaw L, Harrell FE Jr, et al. Prognostic value of a treadmill exercise score in outpatients with suspected coronary artery disease. *N Engl J Med.* 1991;325(12):849–53.

41. Maron BJ, Thompson PD, Ackerman MJ, et al. Recommendations and considerations related to preparticipation screening for cardiovascular abnormalities in competitive athletes: 2007 update: a scientific statement from the American Heart Association Council on Nutrition, Physical Activity, and Metabolism: endorsed by the American College of Cardiology Foundation. *Circulation.* 2007;115(12):1643–455.

42. Martinez-Caro D, Alegria E, Lorente D, Azpilicueta J, Calabuig J, Ancin R. Diagnostic value of stress testing in the elderly. *Eur Heart J.* 1984;5 Suppl E:63–7.

43. Marwick TH, Case C, Vasey C, Allen S, Short L, Thomas JD. Prediction of mortality by exercise echocardiography: a strategy for combination with the duke treadmill score. *Circulation.* 2001;103(21):2566–71.

44. Mottola MF, Davenport MH, Brun CR, Inglis SD, Charlesworth S, Sopper MM. VO2peak prediction and exercise prescription for pregnant women. *Med Sci Sports Exerc.* 2006;38(8):1389–95.

45. Myers J, Buchanan N, Walsh D, et al. Comparison of the ramp versus standard exercise protocols. *J Am Coll Cardiol.* 1991;17(6):1334–42.

46. Olson D, Sikka RS, Hayman J, Novak M, Stavig C. Exercise in pregnancy. *Curr Sports Med Rep.* 2009;8(3):147–53.

47. Paillole C, Ruiz J, Juliard JM, Leblanc H, Gourgon R, Passa P. Detection of coronary artery disease in diabetic patients. *Diabetologia.* 1995;38(6):726–31.

48. Paridon SM, Alpert BS, Boas SR, et al. Clinical stress testing in the pediatric age group: a statement from the American Heart Association Council on Cardiovascular Disease in the Young, Committee on Atherosclerosis, Hypertension, and Obesity in Youth. *Circulation.* 2006;113(15):1905–20.

49. *PARmed-X for Pregnancy* [Internet]. Gloucester (Ontario): Canadian Society for Exercise Physiology; [cited 2011 Feb 24]. Available from: http://www.csep.ca/english/view.asp?x=698

50. Paterson DH, Cunningham DA, Donner A. The effect of different treadmill speeds on the variability of VO2 max in children. *Eur J Appl Physiol Occup Physiol*. 1981;47(2):113–22.

51. Pescatello LS, Arena R, Riebe D, American College of Sports Medicine. *ACSM's Guidelines for Exercise Testing and Prescription*. 9th ed. Philadelphia (PA): Lippincott Williams & Wilkins; 2012. 380 p.

52. Peteiro J, Monserrrat L, Pineiro M, et al. Comparison of exercise echocardiography and the Duke treadmill score for risk stratification in patients with known or suspected coronary artery disease and normal resting electrocardiogram. *Am Heart J*. 2006;151(6):1324.e1–e10.

53. Peterson AR, Bernhardt DT. The preparticipation sports evaluation. *Pediatr Rev*. 2011;32(5):e53–65.

54. Pivarnik JM, Chambliss HO, Clapp JF, et al. Impact of physical activity during pregnancy and postpartum on chronic disease risk. *Med Sci Sports Exerc*. 2006;38(5):989–1006.

55. Rahimi K, Thomas A, Adam M, Hayerizadeh BF, Schuler G, Secknus MA. Implications of exercise test modality on modern prognostic markers in patients with known or suspected coronary artery disease: treadmill versus bicycle. *Eur J Cardiovasc Prev Rehabil*. 2006;13(1):45–50.

56. Robertson RJ, Goss FL, Boer NF, et al. Children's OMNI scale of perceived exertion: mixed gender and race validation. *Med Sci Sports Exerc*. 2000;32(2):452–8.

57. Roger VL, Jacobsen SJ, Pellikka PA, Miller TD, Bailey KR, Gersh BJ. Prognostic value of treadmill exercise testing: a population-based study in Olmsted County, Minnesota. *Circulation*. 1998;98(25):2836–41.

58. Rowland TW. Aerobic exercise testing protocols. In: Rowland TW, editor. *Pediatric Laboratory Exercise Testing: Clinical Guidelines*. Champaign: Human Kinetics; 1993. p. 19–42.

59. Rowland TW. Does peak VO2 reflect VO2max in children?: evidence from supramaximal testing. *Med Sci Sports Exerc*. 1993; 25(6):689–93.

60. Rowland TW, Varzeas MR, Walsh CA. Aerobic responses to walking training in sedentary adolescents. *J Adolesc Health*. 1991;12(1): 30–4.

61. Schinkel AF, Elhendy A, Biagini E, et al. Prognostic stratification using dobutamine stress 99mTc-tetrofosmin myocardial perfusion SPECT in elderly patients unable to perform exercise testing. *J Nucl Med*. 2005;46(1):12–8.

62. Skinner JS. Aging for exercise testing and prescription. In: Skinner JS, editor. *Exercise Testing and Exercise Prescription for Special Cases: Theoretical Basis and Clinical Application*. 3rd ed. Philadelphia: Lippincott Williams & Wilkins; 2005. p. 385–99.

63. Spin JM, Prakash M, Froelicher VF, et al. The prognostic value of exercise testing in elderly men. *Am J Med*. 2002;112(6):453–9.

64. Spinnewijn WE, Lotgering FK, Struijk PC, Wallenburg HC. Fetal heart rate and uterine contractility during maternal exercise at term. *Am J Obstet Gynecol*. 1996;174(1 Pt 1):43–8.

65. Stephens P Jr, Paridon SM. Exercise testing in pediatrics. *Pediatr Clin North Am*. 2004;51(6):1569–87, viii.

66. Tanner CS, Heise CT, Barber G. Correlation of the physiologic parameters of a continuous ramp versus an incremental James exercise protocol in normal children. *Am J Cardiol*. 1991;67(4):309–12.

67. Tomassoni TL. Conducting the pediatric exercise test. In: Rowland TW, editor. *Pediatric Laboratory Exercise Testing: Clinical Guidelines*. Champaign: Human Kinetics; 1993. p. 1–17.

68. U.S. Census Bureau Web site [Internet]. Suitland (MD): U.S. Census Bureau; [cited 2011 Feb 24]. Available from: http://www.census.gov

69. Utter AC, Robertson RJ, Nieman DC, Kang J. Children's OMNI Scale of Perceived Exertion: walking/running evaluation. *Med Sci Sports Exerc*. 2002;34(1):139–44.

70. Valeti US, Miller TD, Hodge DO, Gibbons RJ. Exercise single-photon emission computed tomography provides effective risk stratification of elderly men and elderly women. *Circulation*. 2005;111(14):1771–6.

71. Vasilomanolakis EC. Geriatric cardiology: when exercise stress testing is justified. *Geriatrics*. 1985;40(12):47–50, 53–4, 57.

72. Veille JC, Kitzman DW, Bacevice AE. Effects of pregnancy on the electrocardiogram in healthy subjects during strenuous exercise. *Am J Obstet Gynecol*. 1996;175(5):1360–4.

73. Vetter VL, Dugan N, Guo R, et al. A pilot study of the feasibility of heart screening for sudden cardiac arrest in healthy children. *Am Heart J*. 2011;161(5):1000–6.e3.

74. Washington RL, van Gundy JC, Cohen C, Sondheimer HM, Wolfe RR. Normal aerobic and anaerobic exercise data for North American school-age children. *J Pediatr*. 1988;112(2):223–33.

75. Weissgerber TL, Wolfe LA, Davies GA, Mottola MF. Exercise in the prevention and treatment of maternal-fetal disease: a review of the literature. *Appl Physiol Nutr Metab*. 2006;31(6):661–74.

76. Wolfe LA. Pregnancy. In: Skinner JS, editor. *Exercise Testing and Exercise Prescription for Special Cases: Theoretical Basis and Clinical Application*. 3rd ed. Philadelphia: Lippincott Williams & Wilkins; 2005. p. 377–391.

77. Wolfe LA, Charlesworth SA, Glenn NM, Heenan AP, Davies GA. Effects of pregnancy on maternal work tolerance. *Can J Appl Physiol*. 2005;30(2):212–32.

78. Yamazaki T, Myers J, Froelicher VF. Effect of age and end point on the prognostic value of the exercise test. *Chest*. 2004;125(5): 1920–8.

79. Zavorsky GS, Longo LD. Adding strength training, exercise intensity, and caloric expenditure to exercise guidelines in pregnancy. *Obstet Gynecol*. 2011;117(6):1399–402.

80. Zhang J, Bricker L, Wray S, Quenby S. Poor uterine contractility in obese women. *BJOG*. 2007;114(3):343–8.

81. Zhang YY, Johnson MC,2nd, Chow N, Wasserman K. Effect of exercise testing protocol on parameters of aerobic function. *Med Sci Sports Exerc*. 1991;23(5):625–30.

SELECTED REFERENCES FOR FURTHER READING

Carr K, Emes C, Rogerson M. Exercise testing protocols for different abilities in the older population. *Act Adapt Aging*. 2003;28(1): 49–66.

Davies GA, Maxwell C, McLeod L, et al. SOGC Clinical Practice Guidelines: Obesity in pregnancy. No. 239, February 2010. *Int J Gynaecol Obstet*. 2010;110(2):167–73.

Hill AC, Miyake CY, Grady S, Dubin AM. Accuracy of interpretation of preparticipation screening electrocardiograms. *J Pediatr*. 2011;159(5):783–8.

INTERNET RESOURCES

AHA Scientific Statement. Exercise Standards for Testing and Training: http://circ.ahajournals.org/content/104/14/1694.full

American Congress of Obstetricians and Gynecologists: http://www.acog.org

PARmed-X for Pregnancy: http://www.csep.ca/english/view.asp?x=698

29

Electrocardiography

Electrocardiography is the clinical representation and study of the electrical activity of the myocardium. The electrocardiogram (ECG) gives basic information about rate, rhythm, impulse conduction through the myocardium, pathology of the myocardium, and previous heart disease and/or damage as well as yielding information about current physiologic status of the myocardium.

The ECG is one of the most basic, commonly used tools in diagnostic cardiology. Careful interpretation of the ECG is necessary because abnormal ECGs are not uncommon in healthy individuals, and they may be present in the

KEY TERMS

Acute pericarditis: Infected or inflamed pericardium.

Antiarrhythmic agent: A pharmacologic agent that acts physiologically to decrease dysrhythmias. These agents are subdivided into classes (I through V) by mechanism of action.

Atrioventricular block: An obstruction or delay in electrical conduction that occurs in the normal conduction pathways between the sinus node and the Purkinje fibers.

Automaticity: The ability of specialized cells in the heart (normally in the sinus node) to spontaneously depolarize and initiate a new electrical impulse.

Bigeminy: A conduction pattern in which a premature beat (either supraventricular or ventricular) follows every normal sinus beat.

Bundle branch blocks: Conduction block in either the left or right bundle branch; results in a wider (>0.10 s) than normal QRS complex. The QRS configuration is different for a left versus a right bundle branch block.

Digitalis: A drug in a class called *cardiac glycosides* that increases the force of myocardial contraction and decreases heart rate.

Dysrhythmia: Any cardiac rhythm that is not a regular sinus rhythm; it may be a single beat or a sustained rhythm.

Fascicular block: A conduction block that occurs in one or more of the fascicles of the intraventricular Purkinje system.

False positive: A test result that indicates the presence of disease when no disease is present.

Left ventricular hypertrophy: An increase in thickness of the left ventricular wall that results in increased amplitude of the R wave in leads over the left ventricle (V5, V6) and increased amplitude in the S wave in leads over the right ventricle (V1, V2).

P wave: The wave or deflection on the ECG caused by atrial depolarization.

Pathologic Q waves: Q waves that have a longer duration (>0.04 s) than normal and greater amplitude (≥one-fourth the amplitude of the R wave in the same QRS complex).

Q wave: A downward deflection associated with ventricular depolarization that occurs prior to an R wave.

QRS complex: A deflection or group of deflections on the ECG caused by ventricular depolarization.

R wave: An upward deflection in the QRS complex.

S wave: A downward deflection associated with ventricular depolarization that occurs after an R wave.

ST segment: The line in the ECG connecting the end of the QRS to the beginning of the T wave; a measure of time from the end of ventricular depolarization to the start of ventricular repolarization.

T wave: The wave or deflection on the ECG that reflects repolarization of the ventricles.

U wave: The inconstant, rounded, and upward deflection that is sometimes seen following the T wave.

Ventricular aneurysm: Thinning of the ventricular wall, resulting in a paradoxical bulging in that area during ventricular contraction.

absence of heart disease. Use of the ECG for diagnostic testing has changed considerably, with less reliance placed on the ECG and more on an adjunctive imaging modality for diagnostic purposes. The most common modalities include nuclear or echocardiographic imaging, in combination with pharmacologic or exercise testing, all of which significantly improve both specificity and sensitivity of the test.

Depolarization of myocardial cells is normally a very orderly process. The *normal* ECG is consistent and relatively easy to discern because there are predictable waveforms as well as established normal time intervals for those waveforms. Abnormalities of myocardial anatomy and physiology, various cardiovascular diseases (CVDs), and many other influences can result in abnormal waveforms and/or rhythms. The normal ECG and many of the most common abnormal ECGs will be discussed in this chapter.

BASIC ELECTROCARDIOGRAPHY

EQUIPMENT

All equipment used in both resting and exercise electrocardiography must be maintained and calibrated on a regular basis. Ongoing maintenance of such equipment should include electronic and mechanical checks by qualified biomedical engineers or technicians. ECG equipment is standardized with respect to paper speed and waveform deflection, and normally the documentation of this standardization should be part of the warm-up routines on all ECG equipment. Treadmill calibration with respect to

both speed and elevation should be checked on a regular basis. Other equipment used in exercise and resting electrocardiography must be regularly maintained and checked at least quarterly. All such quality checks must be documented and records must be retained. Equipment that does not meet standards and that cannot be brought to standard calibration and operation should be discarded.

LEAD PLACEMENT AND PREPARATION FOR THE ELECTROCARDIOGRAM

Surface electrodes are placed on the chest, wrists, and ankles for a standard 12-lead ECG. The limb leads, one on each wrist and ankle, are modified for exercise testing (the Mason-Likar lead system) by placing these leads in the subclavicular and suprailiac areas. See *Box 29-1* and *Figure 29-1* for details on lead placement in the Mason-Likar leads.

The ECG gives electrical views of the heart from all three planes: horizontal, frontal, and vertical. *Figure 29-2* shows the anatomy of the heart along with the conduction system. *Figure 29-3* shows a normal ECG complex with associated representation of the anatomic correlates for each wave. The six chest leads (V1–V6) show the heart in a horizontal plane. A view of the heart in the vertical plane is derived from information received from the limb electrodes, which produce the six limb leads (I, II, III, aVR, aVL, aVF). Lead II, III, and aVF view the inferior surface of the heart; leads V1–V4 view the anterior surface of the heart; and leads I, aVL, V5, and V6 view the lateral surface of the heart. By examining the ECG in more than one plane and lead, normal and

---

BOX 29-1   Mason-Likar 12-Lead System

The Mason-Likar 10 electrode placement allows for conventional 12-lead exercise ECG tracings. The location of these electrodes are described as follows:

Right arm: upper right arm-chest region immediately below the midpoint of the clavicle

Left arm: upper left arm-chest region immediately below the midpoint of the clavicle

Right leg: lower right abdominal region, at the midclavicular line, at the level of the last rib

Left leg: lower left abdominal region, at the midclavicular line, at the level of the last rib

V1: on the right sternal border in the fourth intercostal space

NOTE: The fourth intercostal space can be found by locating the sternoclavicular joint and by placing the index finger in the space immediately below the first

rib. This is the first intercostal space. Proceed down the sternum until the fourth space is found.

V2: on the left sternal border in the fourth intercostal space

V3: at the midpoint on a straight line between V2 and V4

V4: on the fifth intercostal space at the midclavicular line

V5: on the anterior axillary line, horizontal to V4

V6: on the midaxillary line, horizontal to both V4 and V5

The leg electrodes may also be placed at the level of the navel. However, there may be excessive motion artifact with this placement. Placement on the last rib at the midclavicular line tends to be more stable with no effect on the ECG tracing.

ECG, electrocardiogram.

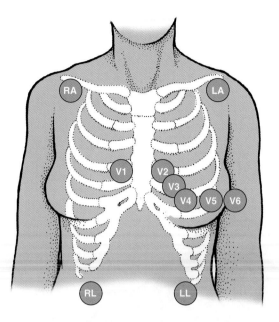

FIGURE 29-1. The Mason-Likar simulated 12-lead ECG electrode placement for exercise testing. For females, the V4-6 electrodes are typically placed on the chest wall underneath the lower portion of the breast.

abnormal function of the myocardium can be determined. *Table 29-1* shows the ECG wave associated with the corresponding electrical event in the myocardium.

Artifacts from movement, electrical interference, and poor skin preparation can significantly affect both resting and exercise ECG quality. It is extremely important to minimize all artifacts through proper skin preparation, precise electrode placement, and standardized operating conditions within ECG and exercise testing facilities.

THE CONDUCTION SYSTEM

The anatomy of the conduction system is depicted in *Figure 29-2*. Electrical depolarization originates in the sinoatrial (SA) node, located in the right atrium near the superior vena cava. The wave of depolarization subsequently spreads through the right atrium into the left atrium and to the atrioventricular (AV) node. The impulse next proceeds through the AV node and depolarizes the bundle of His, which extends into the intraventricular septum, then into the right and left bundle branches. The right bundle branch travels down the right side of the septum and into the right ventricle (RV). The left bundle branch divides into anterior and posterior branches as it proceeds through the left ventricle (LV). The bundle branches terminate in Purkinje fibers, which are diffuse throughout the LV.

The SA node is responsible for initiating depolarization of the myocardium. However, in people with both normal and abnormal hearts, abnormal depolarization sequences may occur. These abnormalities result in dysrhythmias and/or blocks. Dysrhythmias are often classified as bradydysrhythmias or tachydysrhythmias (slow or fast).

SINUS RHYTHMS

"Normal sinus rhythm" is indicative of a normal rhythm originating at the SA node with a rate between 60 and 100 beats per minute (bpm). Rates slower than 60 bpm are termed **bradycardia**, and rates faster than 100 bpm are termed **tachycardia**, with the normality of these two conditions dependent on the situation and the individual. For example, sinus tachycardia at rates in excess of 150–200 bpm may be entirely normal in the context of exercise but not in an individual with coronary artery disease (CAD) who is at rest. Likewise, bradycardia at rates lower than 50 bpm — and even less than 40 bpm in some cases — may occur asymptomatically and without problem in highly trained endurance athletes; however, in an individual with significant myocardial pathology, bradycardia may indicate beta-blockade therapy, the presence of a rhythm disturbance, or other clinical condition.

BRADYCARDIAS

Most bradycardia is related to physiologic or neurogenic factors, including increased vagal tone related to physical fitness (*e.g.*, the slow resting heart rate of many endurance athletes) or to other mechanisms that affect parasympathetic/sympathetic tone. Sinus bradycardia is defined as having a sinus rate <60 bpm. These bradycardias are rarely clinically significant in the absence of heart disease or other myocardial pathology.

Bradycardias related to sinus or other pacemaker (PM) nodal dysfunction, vasovagal reactions, or other pathologic entities can be more problematic. Pathologic PM failure (sometimes called "sick sinus syndrome"), for example, usually requires the implantation of a PM. AV nodal block and frequent sinus pauses are other examples of potential pathologic bradycardias that may or may not require therapeutic intervention.

Sinus bradycardia occurs when the impulse originates from the sinus node at a rate <60 bpm. This may be present in trained individuals with high parasympathetic (vagal) tone, in patients who are receiving drugs that slow the heart rate (*e.g.*, β-blockers), or in individuals who have disease of the sinus node (*e.g.*, sick sinus syndrome).

SINUS TACHYCARDIA

Sinus tachycardia is defined by a rate >100 bpm and is the result of an enhanced firing rate of the sinus node. Sinus tachycardia results when increased activity of the sympathetic nervous system is present, including during times of fear, exercise, fever, hypovolemia, bleeding, hypoxia, or other acute illness. Decreased stroke volume related to severe LV dysfunction may also result in sinus

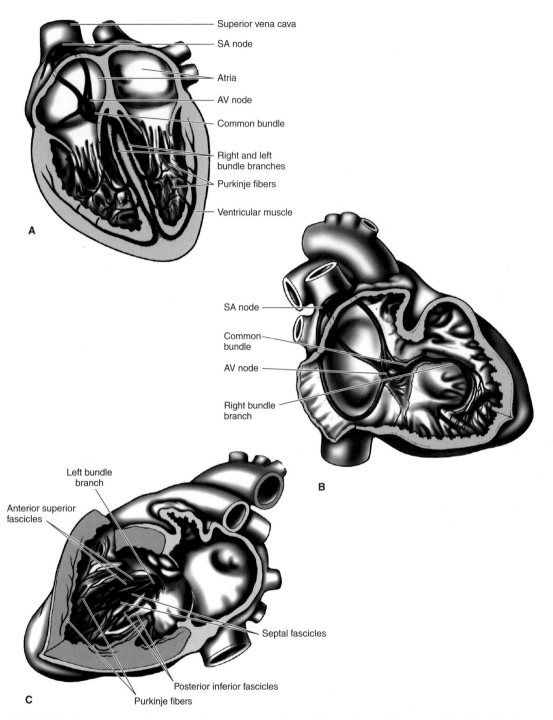

FIGURE 29-2. The anatomy of the conduction system from three different views: **(A)** anterior, **(B)** right, **(C)** left. SA, sinoatrial; AV, atrioventricular.

tachycardia due to sympathetic nervous system activation in an attempt to preserve adequate cardiac output.

Three key features of sinus tachycardia are important. First, patients typically exhibit a gradual increase in heart rate (*e.g.*, sudden acceleration from 80 to 150 bpm does not occur). Second, although exceptions occur, the sinus rate typically does not exceed the maximum heart rate. Finally, the P wave must be normal.

MECHANISMS OF TACHYDYSRHYTHMIAS

Three mechanisms are primarily responsible for most cardiac tachydysrhythmias: (a) circus reentry, (b) enhanced automaticity, and (c) triggered activity. Brief explanations of these appear in *Box 29-2*, but the interested reader is referred to additional recommended reading for more complete explanations.

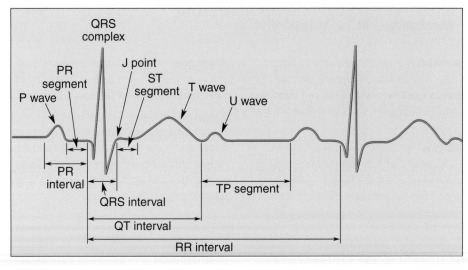

FIGURE 29-3. A normal ECG waveform.

ATRIAL DYSRHYTHMIAS

PREMATURE ATRIAL COMPLEXES

Many people experience premature atrial complexes (PACs) or premature ventricular complexes (PVCs) during exercise or other periods when catecholamine levels are increased. PACs occur when an atrial site outside of the sinus node depolarizes prematurely. The impulse proceeds through the AV node and the ventricles (in the absence of bundle branch block or myocardial disease) to generate a normal, narrow QRS complex. A single PAC on an ECG is recognized as an early QRS complex preceded by a P wave that is abnormally shaped (although this may be difficult to discern). A series of normal sinus beats alternating with PACs is called atrial bigeminy.

ATRIAL TACHYCARDIA

Atrial tachycardia may be the result of rapid firing of an automatic or triggered atrial focus or reentry within the atrium (*Box 29-2*). The ventricular rate depends on the

atrial rate and the refractory period of the AV node. The P wave has altered waveform shape, and the PR interval is often short.

ATRIAL FIBRILLATION

Atrial fibrillation (*Fig. 29-4*) is a relatively common dysrhythmia that results from multiple reentrant waves of depolarization in the atria. These waves are not organized and do not cause contraction of the atria. Causes of atrial fibrillation are varied, with many cases being idiopathic. The characteristics of atrial fibrillation are an irregular ventricular rate and rhythm, which is often tachycardic, with an ECG baseline composed of multiple, small, indistinct P waves. This rhythm may have important consequences, including decreased cardiac output, which can be clinically significant in the presence of compromised left ventricular function, often impairing one's ability to perform physical activities and causing symptoms. Atrial fibrillation increases the risk of developing atrial thrombus, which may cause stroke or other embolic events.

Treatment of atrial fibrillation centers on normalizing the ventricular rate. This can often be done with pharmacologic agents, such as digitalis, calcium channel blockers, β-blockers, and antiarrhythmic agents. Anticoagulation is often also necessary. Synchronized electrical cardioversion (delivery of a timed electrical shock to the myocardium) may be required if the rhythm persists beyond pharmacologic therapy. Most patients with atrial fibrillation have underlying cardiac disease.

ATRIAL FLUTTER

Atrial flutter (*Fig. 29-5*) results from a reentrant circuit in the atria that generates flutter waves, usually at a rate of 250–350 per minute. The atrial waves are best visualized

TABLE 29-1. Normal Sequence of Depolarization and the Electrocardiographic Correlation

Sinoatrial Node	Flat
Atrial depolarization	P wave
Atrioventricular node	PR interval
His bundle	PR interval
Purkinje fibers	PR interval
Ventricular muscle depolarization	QRS complex
Ventricular isoelectric period	ST segment
Ventricular muscle repolarization	T wave

BOX 29-2   Mechanisms of Tachydysrhythmias

Enhanced automaticity: An increased rate of depolarization of a single myocardial cell occurs, and the threshold potential is reached rapidly. The cell depolarizes, and that impulse depolarizes the remainder of the myocardium.

Reentry: The substrate for reentry requires two pathways. If an impulse arrives at a time when the slow pathway has recovered but the fast pathway is refractory (not recovered from the previous depolarization),

the impulse conducts over the slow pathway. If the slow pathway has recovered, depolarization of the slow path occurs, and a reentrant loop occurs.

Triggered activity: Triggered activity exhibits features of both reentry and automaticity. After-depolarization or increases in the membrane potential occur during the repolarization phase of the action potential. If the magnitude of these after-depolarizations is great enough, depolarization may be triggered.

---

in inferior leads (II, III, aVF) or lead V1. The ventricular rate may or may not be accelerated during atrial flutter, and rhythm may be regular or irregular. Flutter waves typically have a classic "sawtooth" appearance in inferior leads. Commonly, there is a 2:1 block (two flutter waves for each ventricular complex) configuration in atrial flutter, resulting in a ventricular rate near 150 bpm. This rhythm may convert back to sinus rhythm but more often degenerates into atrial fibrillation. Treatment may include pharmacologic agents or radiofrequency catheter ablation.

SUPRAVENTRICULAR TACHYCARDIA

Supraventricular tachycardia (SVT) is any tachydysrhythmia that originates at or above the AV node. Atrial fibrillation and atrial flutter are types of SVTs. However, there are other mechanisms of SVT including AV node reentrant tachycardias, Wolf-Parkinson-White syndrome (W-P-W), and concealed accessory pathways. SVTs often result in an accelerated heart rate and can be symptomatic, requiring pharmacologic or therapeutic intervention.

VENTRICULAR DYSRHYTHMIAS

Unlike many of the atrial dysrhythmias, ventricular dysrhythmias can be serious and even life threatening. Recognition and understanding of these ventricular

dysrhythmias is essential to patient safety in ECG interpretation, both at rest and during exercise testing. The exercise professional must be prepared for emergencies, and the presence of ventricular dysrhythmias can be precursors for such emergent situations.

PREMATURE VENTRICULAR COMPLEXES

PVCs (*Fig. 29-6*) occur when a site in the ventricle fires before the next wave of depolarization from the sinus node reaches the ventricle. PVCs are usually wide QRS complexes and may occur singly, in groups, in runs, or even alternating with sinus beats. A single PVC is recognized as an early QRS complex that is wide and abnormally shaped and is not preceded by a P wave. The various combinations are defined and named in *Box 29-3*.

VENTRICULAR TACHYCARDIA

Ventricular tachycardia (*Figs. 29-7 and 29-8*) is typically seen in patients with underlying heart disease, most commonly CAD or cardiomyopathy. Ventricular tachycardia is defined as three or more consecutive ventricular beats at 100 bpm or faster. Nonsustained ventricular tachycardia lasts <30 s, and sustained ventricular tachycardia is generally said to last >30 s.

People with ventricular tachycardia can have normal blood pressure and few symptoms if the hemodynamics

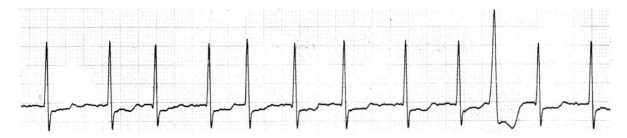

FIGURE 29-4. Atrial fibrillation with rapid ventricular response along with a single PVC.

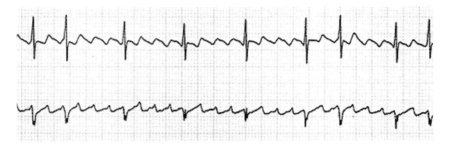

FIGURE 29-5. Atrial flutter with variable atrioventricular conduction.

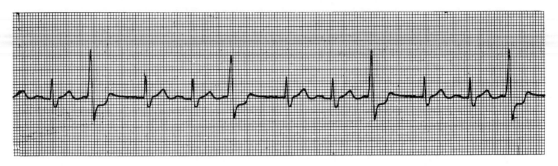

FIGURE 29-6. Normal sinus rhythm with premature ventricular complexes (trigeminy).

BOX 29-3	Types of Dysrhythmic Premature Ventricular Complexes

Couplet: Two consecutive PVCs without intervening sinus beats.

Triplet: Three consecutive PVCs without intervening sinus beats.

Multiform: The PVC waveform is not consistent in all instances, indicating that the PVC may emanate from more than one foci in the ventricle or may be the result of more than a single physiologic or pathologic process.

Bigeminy: A single PVC alternating with single sinus beats.

Trigeminy: Single PVCs alternating with two consecutive sinus beats.

PVC, premature ventricular complex.

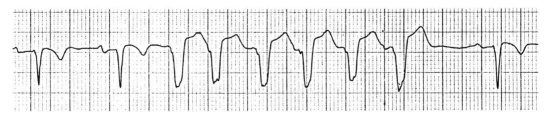

FIGURE 29-7. Normal sinus rhythm with a run of nonsustained ventricular tachycardia.

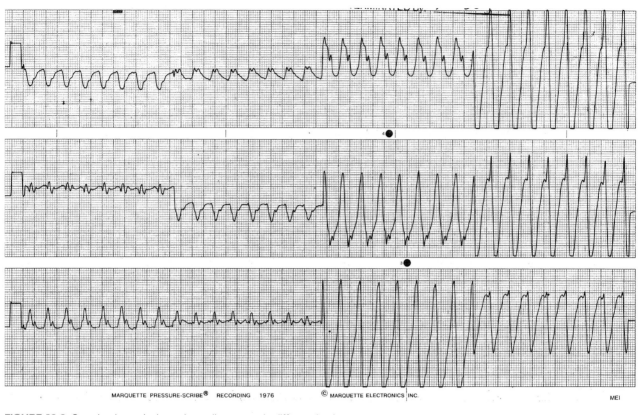

MARQUETTE PRESSURE-SCRIBE® RECORDING 1976   © MARQUETTE ELECTRONICS INC.   MEI

FIGURE 29-8. Sustained ventricular tachycardia as seen in different leads.

of the LV remain relatively normal and the ventricular rate is not excessively high. More commonly, ventricular tachycardia compromises hemodynamic status because of poor ventricular filling between rapid beats. Ventricular tachycardia may lead to cardiac arrest and sudden death. Sustained ventricular tachycardia usually requires emergency measures in the form of pharmacologic administration and/or defibrillation to resolve.

TORSADE DE POINTES

Torsade de pointes is a type of ventricular tachycardia in which the appearance of the complexes are somewhat "twisted" — thus the name *torsade*. This rhythm is also usually lethal and requires immediate emergent measures to resolve and ensure patient safety.

VENTRICULAR FIBRILLATION

Ventricular fibrillation (*Fig. 29-9*) is a condition in which multiple, reentrant depolarizations of the ventricles occurs, and the resulting contraction is uncoordinated. This uncoordinated contraction results in a quivering of the ventricles, preventing adequate cardiac output. Ventricular fibrillation is a life-threatening rhythm that must be treated with immediate electrical defibrillation per advanced cardiac life support (ACLS) protocol; if left untreated, it will likely degenerate into asystole and cardiac death.

ATRIOVENTRICULAR BLOCKS

There are generally three accepted classifications of AV block. **First-degree** AV block is a prolongation of the PR interval. This may be the result of intraatrial or interatrial conduction delay, delayed conduction through the AV node, impaired conduction through the His-Purkinje system, or a combination thereof.

Second-degree AV block (*Figs. 29-10* and *29-11*) may be divided into type I and type II. Type I is also known as Wenckebach. The PR interval progressively lengthens on consecutive beats until a P wave is not conducted to the ventricles. Type II is characterized by a fixed PR interval until a P wave is not conducted. Type II block is often associated with a wide QRS complex. A rhythm disorder that may cause interpretive confusion is called *2:1 AV block*. Typically, in AV block, the pathology is present below the AV node.

Third-degree or complete heart block (*Figure 29-12*) occurs when no atrial activity is conducted through the AV junction to generate a QRS complex, thus atrial and ventricular depolarizations (and, therefore, contractions) are unrelated. The atrial rate is faster than the ventricular rate, and the P waves have no influence on the QRS complexes (therefore, the PR interval will be neither gradually increasing nor constant but random). QRS complexes may be narrow (if depolarizations of the ventricles are initiated from

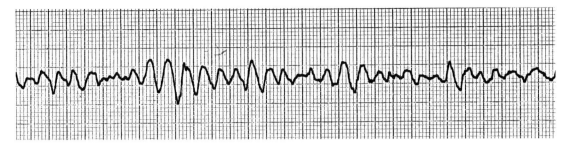

FIGURE 29-9. Ventricular fibrillation (coarse).

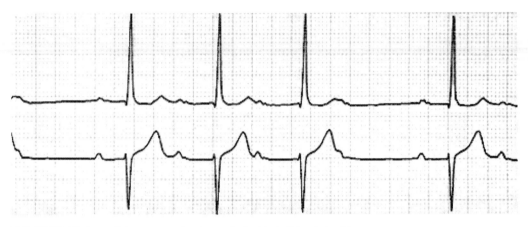

FIGURE 29-10. Second-degree, type I atrioventricular block (Wenckebach).

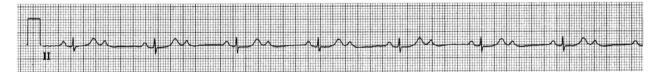

FIGURE 29-11. Second-degree, type II atrioventricular block.

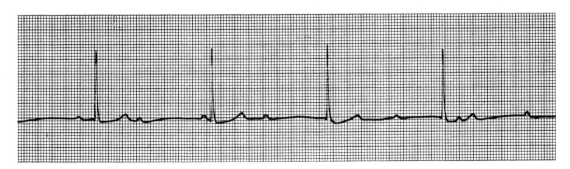

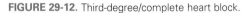

FIGURE 29-12. Third-degree/complete heart block.

the AV node or high in the bundle of His) or wide (if depolarizations of the ventricles are initiated within the ventricles).

BUNDLE BRANCH BLOCKS

Bundle branch blocks are characterized by a wide QRS complex (>0.10 s). Wide QRS complexes usually result from disease in the bundle branches or ventricular abnormalities but may also be related to the effects of drugs, electrolytes, or metabolic disorders. These blocks are classified as right bundle branch block (RBBB), left bundle branch block (LBBB), or nonspecific intraventricular conduction delays (IVCDs), which occur when a QRS >0.10 s does not display the morphology of RBBB or LBBB.

In RBBB (*Fig. 29-13*), activation of the LV occurs before that of the RV. After the septum is depolarized, the impulse travels through the LV, generating the initial portion of the QRS complex. After the LV has been partially depolarized, the RV depolarizes, resulting in a triphasic complex in lead V1, (and often also in lead V2) sometimes described as having a "rabbit ears" appearance or an RSR' complex. RBBB does not prohibit ECG interpretation of ST changes in leads other than V1, V2, and V3.

In LBBB (*Fig. 29-14*), the initial force travels across the septum from right to left, altering the initial QRS deflection. This results in an initial negative deflection in lead V1 and an initial upright deflection in lead V6. The depolarization of the RV is obscured by the LV. The repolarization pattern is altered in LBBB, thus the ECG may not be used to ascertain ischemic ST-T changes during exercise.

FASCICULAR BLOCKS

Fascicular block, also known as *hemiblocks*, are recognized by their effects on the frontal plane axis. Disease in the left bundle branch results in minimal prolongation of the QRS complex. Left anterior fascicular block causes significant left axis deviation, resulting in small Q waves in lead I and aVL and small R waves in leads II, III, and aVF. Left posterior fascicular block produces right axis deviation with small Q waves in leads II, III, and aVF and small R waves in leads I and aVL. Unlike left bundle branch, these entities have no adverse effect on the ability to interpret ECG changes during exercise testing. A fascicular block plus a bundle branch block is known as a bifascicular block.

MYOCARDIAL ISCHEMIA

Myocardial ischemia is an inadequate supply of blood to the myocardium, thus resulting in inadequate delivery of oxygen. Myocardial ischemia is typically a reversible phenomenon. Myocardial infarction (MI) occurs when a portion of the myocardium receives inadequate oxygen supply for several minutes or longer, resulting in the death of myocardial cells in the affected area. ECG changes are associated with both myocardial ischemia and MI.

Myocardial ischemia is typically reflected by ST-segment depression or inversion or flattening of the T waves. In addition, tall T waves may be seen in the anterior leads, which can be an early indication of an acute MI, particularly of the posterior wall of the left ventricle. These ECG changes should be considered as part of the entire clinical picture when diagnosing myocardial

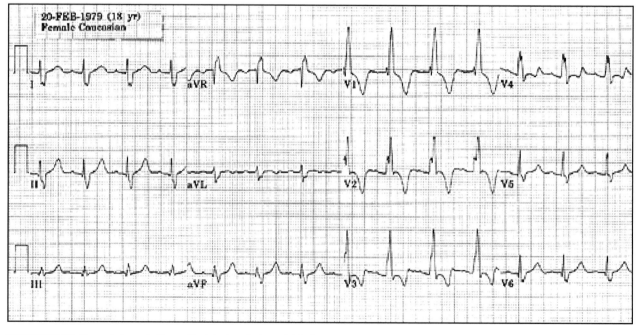

FIGURE 29-13. Normal sinus rhythm with right bundle branch block.

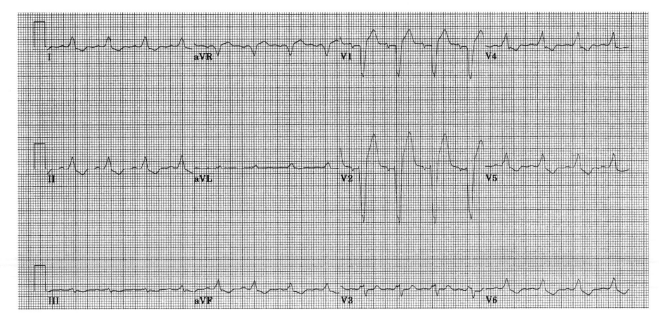

FIGURE 29-14. Normal sinus rhythm with left bundle branch block.

ischemia. In particular, when abnormalities occur in association with chest pain, but in the absence of an MI, prognostic significance can be assumed. The magnitude of ischemia is usually considered to be proportional to the degree of ST-segment depression, the shape of the depressed ST segment (upsloping is less significant than flat, which is less significant than downsloping), the number of ECG leads involved, and the duration of ST-segment depression in recovery (*Figs. 29-15 and 29-16*). Resting ST-T segment changes, especially ST

segment elevation, are associated with transmural myocardial ischemia, are termed as *current of injury*, and are associated with acute MI.

MYOCARDIAL INFARCTION

MI results from the near total or total occlusion of a coronary artery, which blocks blood flow to an area of the myocardium. The use of the ECG as an adjunct to

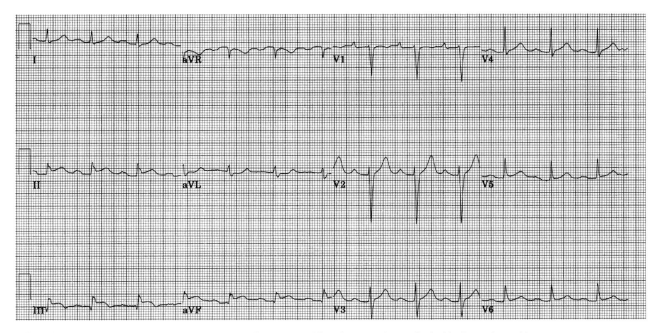

FIGURE 29-15. Acute inferior wall injury. Abnormal P waves and first-degree atrioventricular block are also evident.

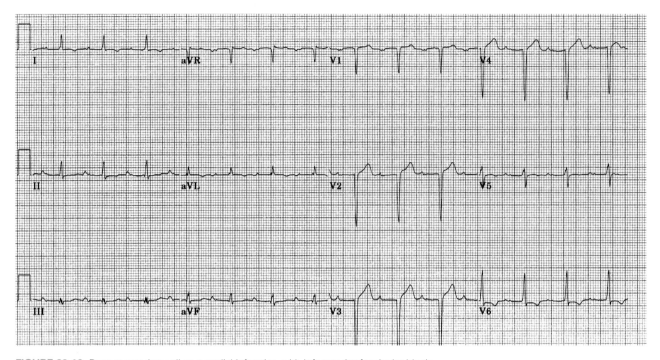

FIGURE 29-16. Recent anterior wall myocardial infarction with left anterior fascicular block.

clinical history and physical examination to assist in the accurate diagnosis of an acute MI is vital.

Acute MI is often diagnosed by the presence of ST elevation or hyperacute T waves. Reciprocal horizontal or downsloping ST-segment depression may also be seen in leads of the ECG remote from the site of the acute MI. Typically, pathologic Q waves, baseline ST segments, and inverted T waves indicate recent MI (2 wk–1 yr), often read as "of indeterminate age" or "subacute." In ECGs containing pathologic Q waves that are not associated with ST- or T-wave changes, the infarction is considered "remote" or "old." Specific combinations or configurations of leads with abnormalities (Q waves, loss of R wave amplitude, etc.) indicate the region of the injury and infarction (*Table 29-2*). In the days and weeks following an MI, T waves often invert, and ST segments gradually return to baseline. Depending on the location and extent of myocardial damage, pathologic Q waves and/or loss of R waves may also develop. MIs that are not accompanied by pathologic Q waves or ST-segment elevation are called non-ST elevation myocardial infarction (non-STEMI), whereas MIs that are accompanied by the aforementioned ST-T changes are called ST elevation myocardial infarction (STEMI). Patients with non-STEMI infarcts have a better short-term but a worse long-term prognosis than patients with STEMI (1).

Specific causes of ST-segment elevation other than myocardial injury and infarction are common. Acute pericarditis (*Fig. 29-17*) causes generalized ST-segment elevation (usually a concave appearance) in all ECG leads. This differs from acute injury and infarction caused by CAD, which usually affects adjacent leads.

Benign or early repolarization variants are another common cause of ST-segment elevation. These variants are most commonly seen in young African American men but may be seen in others as well. In this situation, elevation of the J point is present, and the ST segments are elevated but exhibit a concave upward appearance (*Fig. 29-18*).

PACEMAKERS AND INTERNAL DEFIBRILLATORS

PMs, implantable cardioverter defibrillators (ICDs), and other electronic devices used for therapy of dysrhythmias exhibit ECG "signatures" that indicate their presence. They

TABLE 29-2. Locations of Myocardial Infarction and Injury

Location	Leads Affected
Anteroseptal	V1, V2
Anterior	V1–V4
Extensive anterior	V1–V6, I, aVL
Anterolateral	V3–V6, I, aVL
High lateral	I, aVL
Inferior	II, III, aVF
Posterior	V1, V2 (ST depression, tall R waves noted)

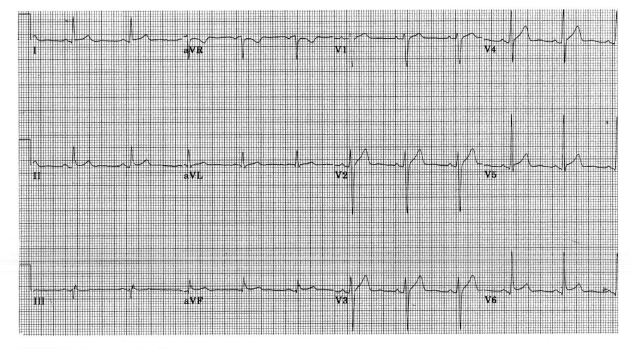

FIGURE 29-17. Acute pericarditis.

are implanted for treatment of sudden death and dangerous ventricular dysrhythmias, sinus node dysfunction, certain AV blocks, severe bradycardias associated with diseases of the conduction system, and chronic congestive heart failure (CHF). These biventricular PMs deliver an innovative therapy called cardiac resynchronization therapy, which, in specific subpopulations of people with CHF, is very effective at decreasing symptoms and increasing functional capacity.

The usual indicator of such devices is a "pacemaker" spike that precedes in either the P wave or the QRS complex, depending on the type and role of the implanted PM. The ECG is not necessarily abnormal or altered by the PM, other than the presence of the spike, but may be abnormal because of the inherent pathology that resulted in PM implantation. *Figure 29-19* is an example of a 12-lead ECG with PM spikes. Pacemakers are "coded"

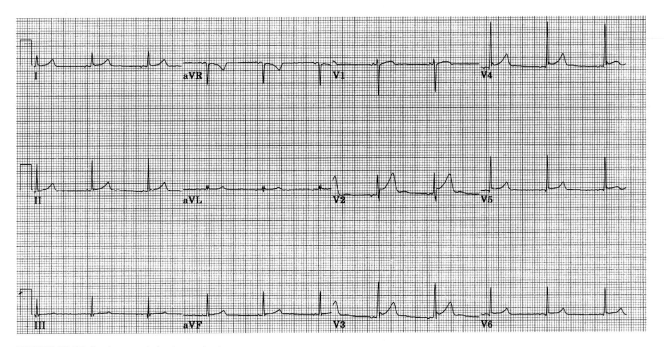

FIGURE 29-18. Benign repolarization variant.

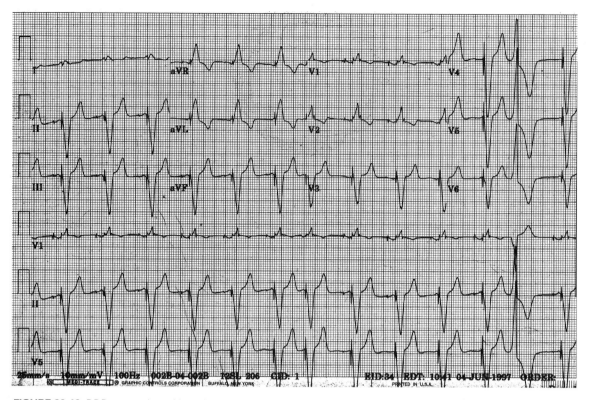

FIGURE 29-19. DDD pacemaker with pacing spikes present before the P waves and QRS complexes.

according to a five-letter system. The convention for the system is, in the order of the letter:

1. Chamber paced (A = atrium; V = ventricle; D = dual or A + V)
2. Chamber sensed (A = atrium; V = ventricle; D = dual or A + V)
3. Response to sensing (T = triggered; I = inhibited; D = dual)
4. Rate modulation (R = rate modulation)
5. Multisite pacing (A = atrium; V = ventricle; D = dual or A + V)

A pacemaker-coded *DDDV* would, therefore, be one that paces both atria and ventricles, that senses both, that responds to both chambers, and that paces only ventricles.

EXERCISE ELECTROCARDIOGRAPHY

MYOCARDIAL ISCHEMIA

Exercise testing that incorporates ECG monitoring can detect dysrhythmias and ischemic changes precipitated by or associated with exercise, but in the absence of additional diagnostic tools, such as echocardiography or nuclear imaging, it may be less sensitive and specific than necessary for proper diagnosis of CAD. Dysrhythmias, discussed earlier, can be elicited and appear during exercise

or recovery. Professionals performing exercise testing, particularly on individuals who are at moderate to high risk for CVD, should be skilled with interpretation of dysrhythmias and with ACLS.

Ischemia may induce ST-segment depression during exercise testing, but if baseline ST-T changes are present, the test becomes less specific. Both the magnitude and the character of the ST depression are important. Horizontal or downsloping ST depression is more specific for CAD than upsloping ST depression. Also, as the subendocardial area of the left ventricular apex is most often rendered ischemic during exercise, ST-segment shifts in V4, V5, and V6 are the most sensitive for detection of ischemia.

Persistent ST-segment elevation after an infarction may suggest ventricular aneurysm formation. This typically involves the anterior wall of the LV and typically occurs after large infarcts. The presence of Q waves in the involved leads in a patient after MI suggests this diagnosis.

FACTORS AFFECTING INTERPRETATION OF THE ST SEGMENT

Digitalis is a medication that interferes with the interpretation of ST-T segment changes for myocardial ischemia. Digitalis is often used to treat patients with CHF or atrial dysrhythmias. Digitalis may cause false-positive exercise or pharmacologic ECG findings by depressing the ST segment (*Fig. 29-20*). Additional imaging modalities should be used to increase the specificity of the study.

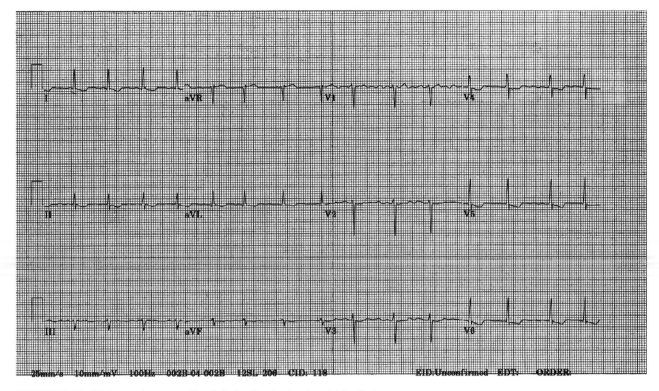

FIGURE 29-20. ST depression caused by digitalis. The rhythm is atrial fibrillation.

Electrolyte disorders can also be associated with ECG changes that interfere with ST-T interpretation. Hyperkalemia can cause a prolonged QRS interval, peaked T waves, and even disappearance of P waves. Hypokalemia can be associated with diminished T waves, prolonged QT interval, and prominent U waves. Hypocalcemia can prolong the QT interval, whereas hypercalcemia can shorten the QT interval. Note that prolonged QT interval can predispose individuals to malignant ventricular tachycardias. Those individuals with prolonged QT should be referred to a cardiologist or an electrophysiologist for further assessment before exercise testing.

CHAMBER ENLARGEMENT

VENTRICULAR HYPERTROPHY

All four chambers can be physiologically enlarged as a result of several common pathologic conditions, including pulmonary disease, valvular disease, ischemic disease, and congenital heart disease. The ECG can be used as one diagnostic tool for evaluating chamber enlargement, but other diagnostic tools, including echocardiography and angiography, are considered gold standards for these diagnoses. Although some specific criteria for chamber enlargement exist, they should be considered within the entire clinical picture and should direct further diagnostic assessment.

Ventricular hypertrophy (right or left) can be either hypertrophic (increased ventricular mass and wall thickness) or dilated (enlarged chamber size with decreased ventricular mass and wall thickness).

Increased voltages in R waves across the myocardium are usual indicators of left ventricular hypertrophy (LVH). There are several ECG scoring systems that assist in this diagnosis. One of these systems, Estes criteria for LVH, is illustrated in *Table 29-3*. LVH

TABLE 29-3. Estes Electrocardiogram Criteria for the Determination of Left Ventricular Enlargement

	Points

1. Any of the following:
   R or S in limb lead ≥20 mm
   S wave in V1–V3, ≥25 mm
   R wave in V4–V6 ≥25 mm
	3

2. Any ST shift Typical strain ST-T changes	3 1
3. LAD >15 degrees	2
4. QRS interval >0.09 s	1
5. Intrinsicoid deflection >0.04 s	1
6. P-terminal force V1 >0.04 s	3
Total (LVH >5 points, probable LVH >4 points)	13

LAD, left axis deviation; LVH, left ventricular hypertrophy.

Adapted with permission from Wagner GS. *Marriott's Practical Electrocardiography*. 9th ed. Baltimore (MD): Williams & Wilkins; 1994. 365 p.

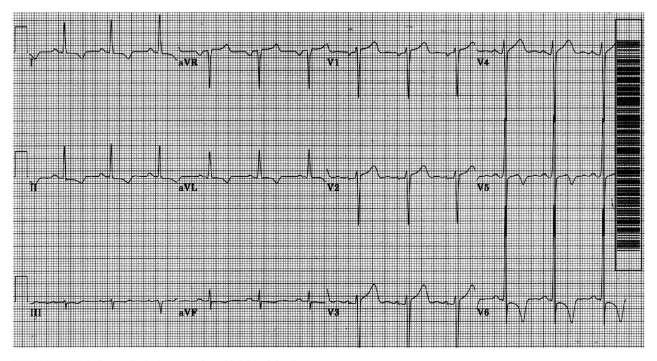

FIGURE 29-21. Left ventricular hypertrophy with left atrial enlargement.

(*Fig. 29-21*) can be a cause of ST-segment changes without the presence of ischemia. Longstanding hypertension, especially if untreated, is often associated with LVH. The presence of LVH on the baseline tracing may result in an indeterminate or false-positive stress ECG result. **Right ventricular hypertrophy** (RVH) is less common than LVH and is usually associated with pulmonary disease. *Table 29-4* outlines the requisites for ECG manifestations of RVH.

ATRIAL ENLARGEMENT

Atrial enlargement may or may not be associated with ventricular hypertrophy. Atrial hypertrophy (both right and left) is associated with changes in P-wave morphology. Features such as notching of P waves; biphasic P waves; and/or tall, peaked P waves are often seen in atrial enlargement.

METABOLIC DISORDERS

Metabolic disorders, such as thyroid disorders and obesity, as well as other conditions, such as hypothermia, are associated with ECG changes. See *Table 29-5* for examples of those changes.

SUMMARY

Electrocardiography and exercise electrocardiography, as well as associated diagnostic procedures, are basic and fundamental methods of evaluation in CVD and health assessment. To provide safe and effective care for patients, exercise professionals must have knowledge of both normal and abnormal cardiovascular physiology and pathophysiology that can lead to changes in the ECG, as well as the waveforms and patterns that are associated with the pathophysiology.

TABLE 29-4. Electrocardiographic Manifestations of Right Ventricular Hypertrophy

Right axis deviation
R wave in V1 >7 mm
R in V1 + 5 in V5 or V6 >10 mm
R:S ratio in V1 >.0
S:R in V6 >.0
Right intraventricular conduction delay
Right ventricular strain pattern in V1, V2, or II, III, and aVF

Adapted with permission from Wagner GS. *Marriott's Practical Electrocardiography.* 9th ed. Baltimore (MD): Williams & Wilkins; 1994. 365 p.

TABLE 29-5. Metabolic Disease and Electrocardiogram

Metabolic Disorders and Electrocardiogram Changes	
Thyroid conditions	
Hypothyroid	• Decreased sinus rate
Hyperthyroid	• Increased sinus rate
Obesity	• Increased sinus rate • Increased PR, QRS, and QTc interval
Hypothermia	• Lengthened PR, RR, QRS, and QT intervals • J point deflection (called *Osborn waves*)

REFERENCES

1. Garcia S, Henry TD, Wang YL, et al. Long-term follow-up of patients undergoing postconditioning during ST-elevation myocardial infarction. *J Cardiovasc Transl Res.* 2011;4(1):92–8.

SELECTED REFERENCES FOR FURTHER READING

Atwood S, Stanton C, Storey-Davenport J. *Introduction to Basic Dysrhythmias.* 4th ed. St. Louis (MO): Mosby; 2008. 416 p.

Dubin D. *Rapid Interpretation of EKGs: An Interactive Course.* Tampa (FL): Cover Publishing Company; 2000. 368 p.

ECG Interpretation: An Incredibly Easy! Pocket Guide. 4th ed. Philadelphia (PA): Lippincott/Springhouse Nursing Collection; 2007. 288 p.

Ellenbogen KA, Kay GN, Lau C, Wilkoff BL. *Clinical Cardiac Pacing, Defibrillation and Resynchronization Therapy.* 4th ed. Philadelphia (PA): Saunders-Elsevier; 2011. 1104 p.

Huff J. *ECG Workout: Exercises in Arrhythmia Interpretation.* 6th ed. Philadelphia (PA): JB Lippincott; 2011. 384 p.

Huzar RJ. *Basic Dysrhythmias: Interpretation and Management.* 3rd ed. St. Louis (MO): Mosby; 2002. 544 p.

Lip GYH, Godtfredsen J. *Cardiac Arrhythmias.* St. Louis (MO): Mosby; 2003. 512 p.

Thaler MS. *The Only EKG Book You'll Ever Need.* 7th ed. Philadelphia (PA): Lippincott Williams & Wilkins; 2012. 305 p.

Wagner GS. *Marriott's Practical Electrocardiography.* 11th ed. Philadelphia (PA): Lippincott Williams & Wilkins; 2007. 488 p.

INTERNET RESOURCES

- The Alan E. Lindsay ECG Learning Center: http://medstat.med.utah.edu/kw/ecg
- ECG Library: http://www.ecglibrary.com

Exercise Prescription for Healthy Populations

DAVID P. SWAIN, PhD, FACSM, ACSM-CES, ACSM-PD, *Section Editor*

Cardiorespiratory Exercise Prescription

Cardiorespiratory capacity is the maximum ability to perform large muscle, dynamic exercise through the use of oxygen — that is, maximum oxygen consumption ($\dot{V}O_{2max}$). Cardiorespiratory capacity is the best indicator of the fitness of the heart, vasculature, and pulmonary system. Attaining a high level of cardiorespiratory capacity requires the development of a large cardiac output (via a large stroke volume), vascular adaptations to deliver blood flow to the working muscles without excessive increases in systemic arterial blood pressure, tissue adaptations to increase the utilization of oxygen, and sufficient alveolar ventilation and gas exchange to support the body's demand for oxygen. Cardiorespiratory endurance is the ability to perform a given intensity of large muscle, dynamic exercise — that is, aerobic exercise — for prolonged periods of time. Cardiorespiratory endurance is related, in part, to the ability to effectively process substrates for energy while avoiding or postponing glycogen depletion and also avoiding an excessive build up of lactic acid in the blood. The lactate and ventilatory thresholds are useful, although not complete, indicators of cardiorespiratory endurance. Cardiorespiratory capacity and endurance, along with muscle strength, muscle endurance, flexibility, body composition, balance, and agility, are components of physical fitness. Both physical activity (36,55) and

cardiorespiratory capacity (4) have been found to produce significant health benefits. However, cardiorespiratory capacity is more strongly correlated with a reduced risk of heart disease than physical activity (59). Physical activity is defined as any bodily movement produced by skeletal muscles that results in energy expenditure (EE) (55). The physiologic adaptations resulting from cardiorespiratory exercise are described in *Chapter 32*, and the health benefits from physical activity and exercise are summarized in *GETP9, Chapter 1*. This chapter addresses the prescription of cardiorespiratory exercise to achieve health and physical fitness benefits for apparently healthy adults, as presented in *GETP9, Chapter 7* and the American College of Sports Medicine's (ACSM) 2011 position stand on exercise prescription (13). Cardiorespiratory exercise prescription to treat or rehabilitate individuals with chronic disease, and for other special populations, is covered in other chapters of this *Resource Manual*.

PRINCIPLES OF TRAINING

Exercise training is defined as planned, structured, and repetitive bodily movement done to improve or maintain one or more components of physical fitness. The principles of training apply more to exercise training and

KEY TERMS

Cardiorespiratory capacity: The maximum ability to perform aerobic exercise ($\dot{V}O_{2max}$).

Cardiorespiratory endurance: The ability to perform submaximal aerobic exercise for prolonged periods of time.

Exercise prescription: Individualized exercise design based on specific assessment information.

Exercise training: Planned, structured, and repetitive bodily movement done to improve or maintain one or more components of physical fitness.

FITT principle: A method of prescribing exercise that incorporates frequency, intensity, time (duration), and type (mode).

Heart rate reserve (HRR): The range of heart rate from rest to maximum; a percentage of this range is typically used to establish target heart rates in training, as %HRR provides similar intensities as equivalent values of %$\dot{V}O_2R$.

Oxygen consumption reserve ($\dot{V}O_2R$): The range of oxygen consumption from rest to maximum; a percentage of this range is used to establish cardiorespiratory exercise intensity.

Physical activity: Any bodily movement produced by skeletal muscles that results in energy expenditure.

exercise therapy than to physical activity. A basic assumption in exercise programming is that something useful or beneficial occurs as a result of repeated bouts of exercise. This assumption is predicated on several physiologic principles. The most central of these is the *principle of adaptation*, which states that if a specific physiologic capacity is taxed by a physical training stimulus within a certain range and on a regular basis, this physiologic capacity usually expands. Adaptation also depends on two correlated physiologic principles: *threshold* and *overload*. To elicit an adaptation, the physiologic capacity must be challenged beyond a certain minimal intensity called the *training threshold*. If the training stimulus exceeds this threshold, it is a training *overload*, and the process of physiologic adaptation will occur. As the physiologic capacities of the body expand, the initial training stimulus may be rendered subthreshold, and the workload must increase (*progression*) to maintain overload. The concept of progression also encompasses the practice of using very modest intensities of work during the initial sessions of an exercise program. *Detraining* refers to a cessation or diminution of training that results in a decrease in physiologic capacity — that is, the loss of previous adaptations. *Overtraining* is when the overload is excessive relative to the amount of time allotted for recovery, resulting in a chronic overtaxing of physiologic systems and a decrease in performance. The term *overreaching* is sometimes used to refer to a brief period of excessive overload that may overtax the body but does not result in overt decreases in ability.

A final principle of central importance in exercise programming is the concept of *specificity*. Specific physiologic capacities expand only if they are stressed in the course of an exercise program. For example, swimmers have an 11% increase in swim ergometry performance over the course of a training season but show no change in run time to exhaustion on a treadmill (29).

Each of these principles guides the design of an exercise program. In exercise training, the mode of exercise — as well as the frequency, duration, and intensity of training — are critical in achieving fitness, athletic, or health outcomes. The mode must be specific to the targeted component of fitness; and the frequency, duration, and intensity must be combined in a systematic overload that will result in physiologic adaptations.

DESIGNING AN EXERCISE PRESCRIPTION

The process of exercise prescription can be divided into three steps. The first step is assessing health and fitness information. The second step is to interpret that information. The third step is to formulate an exercise prescription based on the interpreted information and the goals of the client.

Exercise training spans a broad continuum from improving and maintaining physical fitness, including athletic performance, to disease prevention, treatment, and rehabilitation. Exercise prescription is a means of using the principles of training along with assessment to provide an effective exercise training regimen. The nature of the assessments (see *Chapter 13*) may vary by setting (clinical vs. health or fitness), program goals (weight loss vs. athletic performance), and clientele (low fit vs. high fit).

An example of exercise prescription in the commercial health and fitness industry is when an exercise professional uses information from a health and medical history, anthropometric estimation of body fat, one-repetition maximum, and submaximal cycle ergometer test with heart rate (HR) monitoring to develop an exercise program for a client. On the opposite end of the spectrum, for exercise prescription in the clinical setting, medical records, blood reports, pulmonary function tests, and symptom-limited maximal exercise testing with the analysis of expired gases and electrocardiography (ECG) may be incorporated to develop an exercise prescription to treat a patient with chronic obstructive pulmonary disease.

One of the most common uses of exercise training in the health and fitness setting has been to improve physical fitness. As stated earlier, the mode is selected specific to the targeted fitness component, whether it is muscle strength, muscle endurance, cardiorespiratory capacity, cardiorespiratory endurance, or flexibility. Intensity, duration, and frequency combine to create the overload. After a desired level of fitness is achieved, exercise training can be modified to maintain physical fitness. Most often, the overload duration or frequency can be reduced for maintenance purposes. Athletic performance requires similar but more intensive exercise training. In addition to the higher levels of physical fitness, skill practice and strategic development combine to develop athletic performance. Exercise therapy is the use of exercise training to treat modern chronic diseases and associated comorbidities. Certain health benefits, including a reduced risk of coronary heart disease (CHD), accrue from a general increase in physical activity. The U.S. Department of Health and Human Services presented guidelines in 2008 that recommend a minimum of 150 min of moderate-intensity (or 75 min of vigorous intensity) physical activity per week to obtain these benefits (1). The guidelines also state that twice this level of physical activity result in additional health benefits (1). In 2011, Sattelmair et al. published a meta-analysis of prospective epidemiological studies that compared the amount of physical activity with the incidence of CHD (44). With no physical activity as baseline, people who performed either the recommended amount or half the recommended amount of physical activity had a 14% reduced risk of CHD. However, those who performed two times or five times the recommended amount had a 20% or 25% reduction, respectively. Thus, a greater quantity is desirable when it comes to the prevention of heart disease. Moreover, the quality of the physical activity is an important factor, as evidence suggests that the best reductions in cardiovascular risk occur when exercise training is aimed at improving cardiorespiratory fitness (50).

ELEMENTS OF THE EXERCISE PRESCRIPTION

Whether the purpose of exercise is to train athletes or treat disease, the exercise prescription can be expressed with the FITT principle, incorporating frequency, intensity, time (*i.e.*, duration), and type (*i.e.*, mode). Of these four elements, the type, or mode of exercise, should be selected first using the specificity principle of training to choose a type of exercise that will stimulate the desired outcome. *Frequency* is typically the number of exercise sessions per week or, in some cases, per day. *Intensity* is the level of effort, which may be expressed relative to the client's maximum ability, specifically as a percentage of oxygen consumption reserve ($\dot{V}O_2R$), the difference between resting $\dot{V}O_2$ and maximum $\dot{V}O_2$. Once selected, the intensity can be translated to a HR, workload, or subjective level of perceived exertion. *Time* is the duration of each session, not including warm-up and cool-down, generally expressed in minutes. As stated earlier, frequency, intensity, and time combine to produce an overload.

Further considerations in implementing the FITT principle are the volume of exercise and progression over time — *FITT-VP*. The total *volume* of exercise is determined by the product of frequency, intensity, and duration. If the $\dot{V}O_2$ or workload of the exercise is known, then this volume can be expressed as the number of kilocalories expended per week through exercise (*i.e.*, the net value above resting EE; see the following text for calculations). This net EE can be used to estimate expected fat weight loss. From an epidemiological perspective, volume is often expressed as metabolic equivalent (MET) per minute per week, in which the exercise intensity is expressed in METs (1 MET = resting metabolism or $3.5 \text{ mL} \cdot \text{min}^{-1} \cdot \text{kg}^{-1}$), and this value is multiplied by the number of minutes that the activity is performed. If the gross MET level is used (such as the values obtained in the Compendium of Physical Activities [2]), then the volume is being expressed in gross units as well. The net MET level (gross value — 1) should be used in order to determine net volume.

Progression of the absolute intensity must occur as the client's fitness improves to maintain an overload. However, the relative intensity may remain the same. For example, if a client initially walks at 3 mph (4.8 kph) to achieve 50% HRR, in a few weeks, the client may need to walk at 4 mph (5.4 kph) to attain the same HR. Of course, the relative intensity can also be increased.

For example, a new target of 60% HRR may be prescribed to further develop the client's aerobic capacity. Although progression of intensity is important, progression is also applied to duration and frequency, especially in the case of weight loss prescription.

Precautions for exercise are the modifications in the prescription or the additional concerns that must be addressed for each disease process, comorbidity, or disability to make exercise safe (see *Chapters 37–43*). For example, individuals with diabetes who exercise should be given several precautions for the timing of meals, insulin injections, and glucose monitoring that are not given to individuals without diabetes who exercise (see *Chapter 40* and *GETP9, Chapter 10*). Precautions given to individuals with angina are not the same as those given to individuals with low back pain. Each chronic disease and disability has a specific set of precautions.

DEVELOPING CARDIORESPIRATORY FITNESS

The 2011 ACSM position stand on the recommended quantity and quality of exercise (13) and *Chapter 7* of *GETP9* provide the following recommendations for developing cardiorespiratory fitness:

- **Frequency** of 5–7 d · wk^{-1} at a moderate **intensity** (40%–59% $\dot{V}O_2R$) for a **time** (duration) of 30–60 min each day.
- **Frequency** of 3–5 d · wk^{-1} at a vigorous **intensity** (60%–89% $\dot{V}O_2R$) for a **time** (duration) of 20–60 min each day.
- A combination of moderate-intensity exercise sessions and vigorous-intensity exercise sessions to achieve a similar total volume of exercise.
- The **type** (mode) of exercise is continuous and rhythmic using large muscle groups in order to sufficiently elevate oxygen consumption.
- The **volume** of exercise should be a total duration ≥150 min · wk^{-1} of moderate intensity or ≥75 min · wk^{-1} of vigorous intensity, resulting in >1,000 kcal · wk^{-1}. This is the minimum volume recommended, with twice this volume providing greater health benefits (1). As noted earlier, five times the minimum has been shown to provide even greater health benefits (44). A volume of 1,000 kcal · wk^{-1} is approximately 500–1,000 MET · min · wk^{-1}.

An exercise program that follows these guidelines will result in an increase in both cardiorespiratory capacity and cardiorespiratory endurance. Higher intensity training places more emphasis on the development of capacity, whereas longer duration training places more emphasis on the development of endurance and also allows one to accumulate a large volume of EE for purposes of weight loss.

PRESCRIBING MODE

In accordance with the principle of specificity, cardiorespiratory (*i.e.*, aerobic) exercises should be used to improve cardiorespiratory fitness. Cardiorespiratory exercises are continuous, rhythmic exercises that use a large amount of muscle mass and require aerobic metabolic pathways to sustain the activity. The requirement of a large amount of muscle mass is to cause a sufficient increase in total body oxygen consumption to result in adaptations of the central cardiopulmonary system, not just adaptations in the locally active muscle. Examples of these exercises include walking, jogging, cycling, swimming, rowing, dancing, in-line skating, and cross-country skiing.

Some modes of exercise provide predictable levels of EE that are not significantly affected by age, sex, or skill; and the effect of body weight is highly predictable. For example, walking at any given speed requires the same relative oxygen consumption (expressed in $mL \cdot kg^{-1} \cdot min^{-1}$) from individuals of different sizes. The same is true of running (although at a higher $\dot{V}O_2$ than walking). The absolute oxygen consumption ($L \cdot min^{-1}$) of stationary cycling is largely unaffected by body weight (except for a small effect of moving the mass of the legs, as described later in this chapter). Exercises with predictable levels of $\dot{V}O_2$ are commonly used with beginners so that their intensity can be closely controlled. Similarly, such exercises are used in rehabilitation programs in which the control of exercise intensity is vital to the safety of the exercise program.

Other forms of exercise have widely variable levels of $\dot{V}O_2$ because of the effect of skill on the economy of motion (*e.g.*, swimming) or because of frequent changes in intensity (tennis, soccer, etc.). These forms of exercise may provide more variation in the types of activities that a person chooses to engage in while meeting fitness goals. To determine the intensity of exercise when performing such activities, one relies on the HR response or subjective ratings of perceived exertion. Alternatively, a rough estimate of the metabolic demand of the activities can be obtained from the Compendium of Physical Activities (2). However, it should be noted that MET values (where 1 MET is equivalent to oxygen consumption at rest — *i.e.*, $3.5 \, mL \cdot kg^{-1} \cdot min^{-1}$) for many of the activities in the compendium vary not only with skill but also with an individual's chosen level of effort.

Classifying cardiovascular exercise by body-weight dependency is a different classification system than by skill and EE. Weight-dependent exercises, or weight-bearing activities, are those in which the body weight is moved throughout the exercise. Examples of weight-bearing exercise are walking, jogging, running, and hiking. On the other hand, in weight-independent exercise, or non–weight-bearing activity, the body weight is supported by the implement or media and may contribute minimally to the energy demand. Examples of non–weight-bearing exercise are cycling and swimming. (Note that larger individuals do require more energy to swim or to cycle outdoors than smaller individuals, but the difference is proportional to surface area, which varies less between individuals than body mass) (49). Non–weight-bearing exercise may be more effective in preventing lower limb overuse injuries associated with exercise, but this advantage must be balanced by the lack of bone stimulation. Non–weight-bearing exercise is good for minimizing orthopedic stress but not for reducing the risk of osteoporosis.

The mode of exercise that is effective in producing the desired outcome must be the first consideration in choosing the mode of exercise. However, modifications and variations can be made in mode to promote adherence if needed. Varying the mode of exercise among the weekly workouts and substituting recreational activities may be strategies that promote a higher adherence to the program.

PRESCRIBING FREQUENCY AND DURATION

Frequency is prescribed in sessions per day and in days per week. To improve cardiorespiratory fitness for apparently healthy adults, the range of frequency is from 3 to 7 $d \cdot wk^{-1}$. If only moderate-intensity exercise (40%–59% $\dot{V}O_2R$) is being performed, then the frequency should be fairly high: 5–7 $d \cdot wk^{-1}$. If only vigorous-intensity exercise (60%–89% $\dot{V}O_2R$) is being performed, it should be done 3–5 $d \cdot wk^{-1}$. Depending on the orthopedic stress of the mode of exercise chosen, vigorous exercise should be performed on alternate days, not on consecutive days. For many clients, the best approach is to do moderate-intensity exercise on some days and vigorous-intensity exercise on others, for a total of 3–5 $d \cdot wk^{-1}$. When sedentary individuals begin an exercise program, the intensity should be moderate and the frequency should be 3 alternating $d \cdot wk^{-1}$. As the client adapts to the stress of the exercise, and as the client's fitness increases, greater frequency and duration of exercise and the addition of vigorous intensity may be incorporated to reach the client's goals for weekly EE and increased aerobic capacity. In some rehabilitation settings, patients with very low initial fitness may be prescribed a frequency as high as several times per day (*e.g.*, in phase I cardiac rehabilitation). However, the intensity and the duration will be very low.

Exercise duration typically ranges from 20 to 60 min. A minimum duration of 20 min is recommended to achieve improvement in cardiorespiratory fitness (13). Sedentary clients should begin with 20 min per session and increase gradually. It is not necessary that the entire duration for a given day be completed in one session. Multiple, shorter sessions performed throughout the day may be added to attain the desired duration, but each minisession should entail at least 10 min of exercise at the prescribed intensity (although shorter bouts may be used in rehabilitation for specific patient groups). Prescribed exercise duration rarely exceeds 60 min. However, for weight loss, a duration of up to 90 min may be needed to achieve the necessary total volume of exercise per week (17,20); that is, the combination of frequency, duration, and intensity should be at least 2,000 kcal $\cdot$ wk^{-1} for weight loss (17,20). Overweight individuals, who may not be capable of vigorous-intensity exercise, will need to gradually increase duration up to 90 min to achieve this targeted volume of EE. Endurance athletes often exercise for longer than 90 min in a given session, but the guidelines presented in *GETP9* and here are aimed primarily at the general public.

The combination of exercise frequency and duration should be viewed with caution. Pollock et al. exercised six groups of men with various combinations of frequency and duration (39). Intensity was the same for all groups. Three groups exercised for 15, 30, or 45 min per session for 3 d $\cdot$ wk^{-1}. Three other groups exercised for 30 min per session but with frequencies of one, three, or five times per week. As expected, the improvements in fitness were related to the overload (*Fig. 30-1*). However, high overloads were also related to higher injury rates. The group with the highest duration and the group with the highest frequency experienced the highest injury rates. Therefore, caution should be taken in determining the optimal duration and frequency to improve fitness without causing overuse injuries.

PRESCRIBING INTENSITY

Intensity of cardiorespiratory exercise is measured as a percent of maximal capacity or, more specifically, as a percent of $\dot{V}O_2$ reserve (%$\dot{V}O_2$R). Two steps are involved

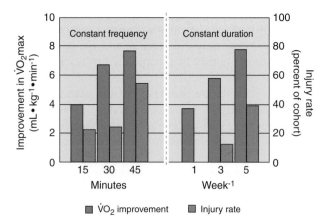

FIGURE 30-1. The influence of overload on improvement in $\dot{V}O_{2max}$ and subsequent injury rates. (Adapted from Pollock ML, Gettman LR, Milesis CA, Bah MD, Durstine L. Effects of frequency and duration of training on attrition and incidence of injury. *Med Sci Sports.* 1977;9[1]:31–6.)

in prescribing exercise intensity for cardiorespiratory exercise:

- Select a target intensity range based on %$\dot{V}O_2$R.
- Provide the client with a means of monitoring the intensity, such as by HR, workload, or a subjective rating of perceived exertion.

The translation of intensity into HR, workload, or perceived exertion will be presented in a later section. First, the selection of a target intensity will be discussed.

Threshold Intensity for Improving Cardiorespiratory Fitness

The classic study of Karvonen et al. in 1957 is well known for introducing the use of heart rate reserve (HRR) as a means of prescribing exercise intensity (21). The study's purpose, however, was to determine if a threshold intensity was required to improve aerobic fitness, that is, is there a minimum intensity of exercise below which no improvement in aerobic fitness will occur? Karvonen et al. studied six young adult men and found that an intensity of 60% HRR was not sufficient to increase aerobic fitness, but an intensity of 71%–75% HRR was. Since 1957, other studies provided further insight on a possible threshold, and in its 1998 position stand, ACSM concluded that deconditioned individuals need to use an intensity of at least 40% $\dot{V}O_2$R or HRR, whereas more active individuals needed an intensity of at least 50% $\dot{V}O_2$R or HRR (38). In 2002, Swain and Franklin (51) did an extensive review of past training studies and found that studies using subjects with mean initial $\dot{V}O_{2max}$ values lower than 40 mL $\cdot$ kg^{-1} $\cdot$ min^{-1} (range is 13–39 mL $\cdot$ kg^{-1} $\cdot$ min^{-1}) were always successful in increasing $\dot{V}O_{2max}$, with intensities ranging as low as 30% $\dot{V}O_2$R. However, subjects with mean initial $\dot{V}O_{2max}$ values of 41–51 mL $\cdot$ kg^{-1} $\cdot$ min^{-1} demonstrated a threshold. These moderately fit subjects failed to achieve any increase in $\dot{V}O_{2max}$ when using intensities of approximately 45% $\dot{V}O_2$R or less but always succeeded in raising $\dot{V}O_{2max}$ in studies using intensities higher than approximately 45% $\dot{V}O_2$R. In the study of Karvonen et al., $\dot{V}O_{2max}$ was not measured, but HR and workload data provided about the subjects allows one to estimate their mean initial $\dot{V}O_{2max}$ as 54 mL $\cdot$ kg^{-1} $\cdot$ min^{-1}. They had a threshold at approximately 70% HRR or $\dot{V}O_2$R. A study by Helgerud et al. (18) failed to obtain increases in $\dot{V}O_{2max}$ using either 70% or 85% maximal heart rate (HR$_{max}$) (approximately 47% and 72% of $\dot{V}O_2$R) in subjects with an initial mean $\dot{V}O_{2max}$ of 58 mL $\cdot$ kg^{-1} $\cdot$ min^{-1} but did increase in $\dot{V}O_{2max}$ using intervals at approximately 85% of $\dot{V}O_2$R (90%–95% HR$_{max}$). As the upper limit of one's genetic potential is reached, as in highly trained athletes, training with aerobic intervals may be the only means of obtaining any remaining available improvement in $\dot{V}O_{2max}$. Smith et al. (45) obtained

TABLE 30-1. Threshold Intensities for Increasing $\dot{V}O_{2max}$ Based on Initial Fitness

Initial Fitness	Initial $\dot{V}O_{2max}$ (mL · kg^{-1} · min^{-1})	Recommended Minimum Intensity[a]
Low to moderate	<40	30% $\dot{V}O_2R$ or HRR
Average to good	40–51	45% $\dot{V}O_2R$ or HRR
High	52–59	75% $\dot{V}O_2R$ or HRR
Very high	≥60	90%–100% $\dot{V}O_2R$ or HRR

$\dot{V}O_{2max}$, maximum oxygen consumption; $\dot{V}O_2R$, oxygen uptake reserve; HRR, heart rate reserve.

[a]These intensities are the minimum for obtaining further increases in $\dot{V}O_{2max}$. Other benefits, such as caloric expenditure for weight loss, may be obtained at lower intensities.

a 5% increase in $\dot{V}O_{2max}$ of runners with a mean initial value of 62 mL · kg^{-1} · min^{-1}, whereas Billat et al. (3) obtained no increase with athletes starting at 71 mL · kg^{-1} · min^{-1}.

Therefore, when selecting an exercise intensity for clients, knowledge of their initial fitness is important. The higher the initial aerobic capacity, the higher is the minimum intensity required to further increase that capacity (*Table 30-1*). Current ACSM guidelines, as presented in the 2011 position stand (13) and *Chapter 7* of *GETP9* state that most adults should be prescribed an intensity within the range of 40%–89% $\dot{V}O_2R$ for exercise of a continuous nature, with 40%–59% $\dot{V}O_2R$ representing a moderate intensity and 60%–89% $\dot{V}O_2R$ for a vigorous intensity. Deconditioned individuals may begin with intensities as low as 30% of $\dot{V}O_2R$. The exercise professional must use sound judgment in choosing a specific range of intensity for a given client using light (30%–40% $\dot{V}O_2R$) to moderate (40%–59% $\dot{V}O_2R$) in the early weeks of a training program for those unaccustomed to exercise and employing vigorous (60%–89% $\dot{V}O_2R$) as part of the weekly activity after an individual has become accustomed. As discussed later in this chapter, near-maximal intensities (90%–100% $\dot{V}O_2R$) may be judiciously used for interval training.

The Value of Higher Intensities

Although the previous section described the *minimum* intensity needed to increase cardiorespiratory fitness, intensities above the threshold are more effective at increasing fitness — that is, $\dot{V}O_{2max}$ — and may also be more effective for reducing the risk of CHD (50). Several research studies have compared two or more groups of subjects who trained at different intensities while the total volume of exercise (*i.e.*, EE) was held constant across groups. Of nine such studies identified in an earlier review (51), all nine found a greater increase in $\dot{V}O_{2max}$ in the higher intensity versus lower intensity groups, with three of the nine studies reaching statistical significance. Given the generally low sample size in the individual studies, the combined evidence points to greater increases in $\dot{V}O_{2max}$ with higher intensity training. The initial fitness of the subjects plays a role in the

training response, as illustrated in *Figure 30-2* (48). More recently, a study by Gormley et al. compared continuous training at a moderate intensity (50% $\dot{V}O_2R$), continuous training at a vigorous intensity (75% $\dot{V}O_2R$), and interval training at near maximal intensity (95% $\dot{V}O_2R$) (16). The final intensities were maintained for the last 4 wk of the study, with interval training performed three times per week and continuous training four times per week, and with total volume of exercise equalized between groups. $\dot{V}O_{2max}$ increased significantly by 10%, 14%, and 21% in the three groups, respectively, with the vigorous group's increase significantly greater than the moderate group's, and the interval group's increase significantly greater than the vigorous group's.

Interval training, once confined to the training of athletes, has been increasingly studied in other populations. Gormley et al.'s subjects were young adult women and men with a mean initial $\dot{V}O_{2max}$ of 35 mL · kg^{-1} · min^{-1} (16). They performed five sets of 5-min intervals three times per week for 4 wk. Helgerud et al.'s subjects were young adult men with a mean initial $\dot{V}O_{2max}$ of 58 mL · kg^{-1} · min^{-1} (18). They performed four sets of 4-min intervals three times per week for 8 wk. In 2005, Warburton et al. looked at male patients with heart disease with an average age of 56 yr and mean initial $\dot{V}O_{2max}$ of 32 mL · kg^{-1} · min^{-1} to compare continuous training at 65% $\dot{V}O_2R$ 5 d · wk^{-1} for 16 wk, with an isocaloric program that combined 3 d of continuous

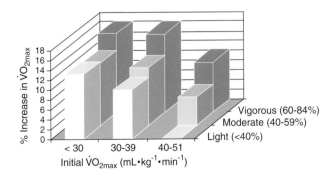

FIGURE 30-2. Influence of initial fitness and intensity of training on increase in $\dot{V}O_{2max}$. (Reprinted with permission from Swain DP. Moderate or vigorous intensity exercise: which is better for improving aerobic fitness? *Prev Cardiol*. 2005;8[1]:55–8.)

training with 2 d of interval training at 90% $\dot{V}O_2R$ (58). Seven 2-min intervals were performed in each training session. The combination group increased $\dot{V}O_{2max}$ by 18% compared with 13% in the continuous training only group. Although the increases in $\dot{V}O_{2max}$ were not statistically different from each other, the combination group did have significantly greater increases in ventilatory threshold and time to exhaustion. In 2007, Wisloff et al. trained male and female patients with congestive heart failure with an average age of 76 yr and mean initial $\dot{V}O_{2max}$ of 13 mL $\cdot$ kg^{-1} $\cdot$ min^{-1} (60). One group performed continuous training at 70% of peak HR (~47% $\dot{V}O_2R$), whereas another group performed isocaloric interval training at 95% peak HR (~90% $\dot{V}O_2R$), using four 4-min intervals per session. Both groups trained 3 d $\cdot$ wk^{-1} for 12 wk. The interval group had a significantly greater increase in $\dot{V}O_{2max}$ (46% vs. 14%), and only the interval group demonstrated significant improvements in left ventricular function.

These studies of interval training using near-maximal aerobic intensity demonstrate that such training can be safely and effectively used in a wide range of clients, and that it results in greater improvements in fitness than does lower intensity training using the same volume of EE. Therefore, such training should be considered as an adjunct to continuous training at moderate or vigorous intensities. For example, sedentary individuals who begin a training program using moderate intensity (40%–59% $\dot{V}O_2R$ for 20–30 min three times per week will normally be progressed in duration and frequency for a period of 2–3 mo. During this time, intensity may be progressed within the 40%–59% $\dot{V}O_2R$ window. After this initial training period, the incorporation of continuous vigorous training and/or aerobic interval training two to three times per week into the overall program should be considered to maximize gains in both fitness and health.

Interval training is typically done in the following manner. A 10-min warm-up is performed, then a near-maximal effort (≥90% $\dot{V}O_2R$ for 2–5 min, which is immediately followed by an equal period at a low-to-moderate intensity. The work/recovery periods are repeated for a total of four to six intervals. Although interval training has been successfully used for as long as 12–16 wk at a time (58,60), one should consider using this high-intensity exercise training intermittently in a program to avoid excessive orthopedic stress.

One additional caution with the use of vigorous-intensity exercise and near-maximal intensity interval training is the elevated risk of cardiac events in those with underlying disease (32). Although interval training has been used safely with patients with heart disease (58,60), the patients must be medically stable. Vigorous and higher intensities should not be used in the fitness setting with moderate-risk or high-risk clients, even though they may have no *known* disease, unless clearance is obtained by a physician (see *Chapter 2* of *GETP9*).

Figure 30-3 illustrates the full range of intensities of which humans are capable. The power levels are derived from elite athletes, and thus would be much less in average individuals, yet they illustrate the comparative power that can be sustained for very brief periods (less than 1 s) to extremely long durations (24 h of continuous exercise). "Maximal" intensity in cardiorespiratory exercise refers to the highest intensity that can be supported aerobically, but humans can exercise much more intensely for brief periods of time anaerobically. In *Figure 30-3*, the highest power output sustained for 4 min in a $\dot{V}O_{2max}$ test is 572 W (35), but three times this value can be sustained for 5 s in a Wingate bike test (46), and more than seven times can be produced for nearly 1 s during a power clean (14). The decline in power from $\dot{V}O_{2max}$ when engaging in endurance activities is much less, with 89% of $\dot{V}O_{2max}$ power sustained for 1 h in an elite cyclist (35) and a little more than 50% for 24 h (calculated from the 24-h bicycling record of 840 km [56]). Note that these values come from different athletes (other than the 4-min and 1-h values), and thus the comparisons may not hold for a given individual, especially if the individual is untrained (*e.g.*, percent of $\dot{V}O_{2max}$ sustained for 1 h would be much less than 89% in anyone but aerobic athletes). Interval training performed at supra-aerobic power levels is used by athletes

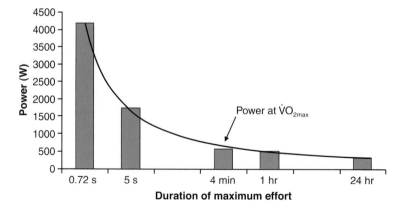

FIGURE 30-3. Range of maximum power generated by humans over given durations.

to improve anaerobic ability. Such training has been used experimentally to induce aerobic benefits. Typically, four to six all-out 30-s sprints are separated by 4 min of recovery, and this training is performed three times per week. Improvements have been reported in $\dot{V}O_{2max}$ (7,28), oxidative enzymes (7,28), and vascular function (40) despite minimal EE. The safety and utility of this training for use with the general public has not been established at this time and is not currently being recommended by the ACSM. Moreover, the very low EE would not be effective for weight loss.

TRANSLATING INTENSITY INTO PRACTICAL TERMS

After assessing a client, the fitness professional chooses a range of exercise intensity based on the client's goals and current level of fitness. For example, a sedentary client interested in improving fitness and reducing risk of heart disease might begin with 30%–45% $\dot{V}O_2R$. However, unless the client is going to perform his or her training while attached to a metabolic cart, this intensity range must be translated into practical indicators that the client and professional can monitor. This is done in one of the following ways:

- Target HR, based on either %HRR or %HR$_{max}$
- Target workload, calculated from %$\dot{V}O_2R$ or %$\dot{V}O_{2max}$, or from MET tables
- Subjective rating, based on the talk test or a rating scale

TARGET HEART RATE USING PERCENTAGE OF HEART RATE RESERVE

The HRR method (also known as the Karvonen method) is the most accurate way of establishing a target HR for two reasons. First, percentages of HRR have been shown to accurately reflect the same percentages of $\dot{V}O_2R$. This was first demonstrated by Swain and Leutholtz in 1997 (52), prompting the ACSM to adopt $\dot{V}O_2R$ and HRR as the primary means of establishing exercise intensity in its 1998 position stand (38). Swain and Leutholtz studied young adults who performed cycle ergometry and confirmed the finding in young adults performing treadmill exercise (53). The one-to-one relationship of %$\dot{V}O_2R$ and %HRR has subsequently been confirmed in various studies in a wide range of populations, including patients with heart disease with or without β-blocker medication (6), patients with diabetes with or without autonomic neuropathy (9), individuals who are obese (8), young adults exercising on an elliptical machine (10), and elite competitive cyclists (27).

The second advantage of using %HRR is that it takes into account the resting heart rate (HR$_{rest}$) of different clients, which can vary over a wide range. If HR$_{rest}$ is

not accounted for, as in prescriptions calculated from %HR$_{max}$, two individuals prescribed the same intensity may actually be exercising at different relative levels of effort (see the following text).

To prescribe exercise intensity using %HRR, select the desired intensity based on %$\dot{V}O_2R$ and express this value as a fraction in the Karvonen equation:

Target HR = (fractional intensity)(HR$_{max}$ − HR$_{rest}$) + HR$_{rest}$

For example, what is the target HR at 60%–75% of $\dot{V}O_2R$ for a client with an HR$_{max}$ of 175 beats per minute (bpm) and an HR$_{rest}$ of 64 bpm? At the lower limit (60%):

Target HR = 0.60 (175 − 64) + 64
Target HR = 0.60 (111) + 64
Target HR = 67 + 64 = 131 bpm

Repeating the process at the upper limit (75%) yields 147 bpm.

HR$_{rest}$ should be measured after at least 5 min of quiet rest, preferably with the client in a similar position as in the prescribed exercise mode. HR$_{max}$ would best be obtained from an incremental exercise test. If that information is not available, it may be estimated from the following equation:

Estimated HR$_{max}$ = 220 − age

A more accurate equation, especially for older clients is 208 − 0.7 (age), based on cross-sectional research by Tanaka et al. (54) and longitudinal research by Gellish et al. (15). Regardless of which equation is used to estimated HR$_{max}$, one must recognize that true HR$_{max}$ varies widely among individuals of a given age and that the resulting target HRs are also only estimates.

TARGET HEART RATE USING PERCENTAGE OF MAXIMAL HEART RATE

As mentioned earlier, the %HR$_{max}$ method is less accurate than the %HRR method because of variation of HR$_{rest}$ within the population. For example, consider two clients who have the same HR$_{max}$ of 160 bpm but have HR$_{rest}$ of 55 and 85 bpm. If both are placed at an intensity of 64% HR$_{max}$, they would both be instructed to exercise at 102 bpm. However, the client with the lower HR$_{rest}$ would be raising his or her HR by 47 bpm (to 45% of HRR or $\dot{V}O_2R$, whereas the other raises his or her HR by only 17 bpm (to 23% of HRR or $\dot{V}O_2R$. The relative intensity is actually twice as great for one client.

Another consideration with the %HR$_{max}$ method is that the desired percentages of $\dot{V}O_2R$ must be adjusted upward to obtain relatively appropriate intensities, as seen in *Table 30-2*. Nonetheless, %HR$_{max}$ is a simpler calculation than %HRR, does not require the measurement of HR$_{rest}$, and is convenient for use in group exercise classes when individual prescriptions for each client are not feasible. To use this method, first, select a desired intensity range

TABLE 30-2. Cardiorespiratory Exercise Intensity: Comparison of Methods

Intensity	Relative Intensity				Intensity (%$\dot{V}O_{2max}$) Relative to Maximal Exercise Capacity in MET			Absolute Intensity	Absolute Intensity (MET) by Age		
	%HRR or %$\dot{V}O_2$R	%HR_{max}	%$\dot{V}O_{2max}$	Perceived Exertion (Rating on 6–20 RPE scale)	20 MET %$\dot{V}O_{2max}$	10 MET %$\dot{V}O_{2max}$	5 MET %$\dot{V}O_{2max}$	MET	Young (20–39 yr)	Middle Aged (40–64 yr)	Older (≥65 yr)
Very low (light)	≤30	≤57	≤37	≤Very light (RPE ≤9)	≤34	≤37	≤44	≤2	≤2.4	≤2	≤1.6
Low (light)	30–40	57–64	37–45	Very light–fairly light (RPE 9–11)	34–43	37–46	44–52	2–2.9	<4.8	<4	<3.2
Moderate	40–59	64–76	46–63	Fairly light to somewhat hard (RPE 12–13)	43–61	46–63	52–67	3–5.9	4.8–7.1	4–5.9	3.2–4.7
Vigorous	60–89	77–95	64–90	Somewhat hard to very hard (RPE 14–17)	62–90	64–90	68–91	6–8.7	7.2–10.1	6–8.4	4.8–6.7
Near maximal to maximal	≥90	≥96	≥91	≥Very hard (RPE ≥18)	≥91	≥91	≥92	≥8.8	≥10.2	≥8.5	≥6.8

$\dot{V}O_{2max}$, maximum oxygen consumption; MET, metabolic energy equivalent; HRR, heart rate reserve; $\dot{V}O_2$R = oxygen uptake reserve; HR_{max}, maximum heart rate; RPE = rating of perceived exertion.

Adapted from Garber CE, Blissmer B, Deschenes MR, et al. Quantity and quality of exercise for developing and maintaining cardiorespiratory, musculoskeletal, and neuromotor fitness in apparently healthy adults: guidance for prescribing exercise. *Med Sci Sports Exerc.* 2011;43(7):1334–59.

in %$\dot{V}O_2$R units and then identify the appropriate intensity in %HR_{max} units from *Table 30-2*. Then enter that value as a fraction in the following equation:

$$\text{Target HR} = (\text{intensity fraction})\, HR_{max}$$

For example, what is the target HR at 50% $\dot{V}O_2$R for a 62-yr-old client? From *Table 30-2*, 50% $\dot{V}O_2$R corresponds to approximately 70% HR_{max}. From the Tanaka equation, HR_{max} is calculated as:

$$HR_{max} = 208 - 0.7\,(62) = 165\ \text{bpm}$$

Therefore,

$$\text{Target HR} = 0.70\,(165) = 116\ \text{bpm}$$

TARGET WORKLOAD USING PERCENTAGE OF OXYGEN CONSUMPTION RESERVE

The intensity of exercise may be expressed as an absolute workload, such as a running speed outdoors, a treadmill walking speed and grade, or a power setting on a cycle ergometer. This method is especially useful for individuals whose HR is affected by medications or who find monitoring of HR difficult. In the case of β-blocker medication, if a stress test is performed while the patient is on the medication, the test results can still be used to establish intensity with HR (6); however, daily variations in the HR response to the medication may be problematic.

There are three steps in establishing the target workload:

- Select the desired intensity in %$\dot{V}O_2$R units.
- Calculate the target $\dot{V}O_2$.
- Convert the target $\dot{V}O_2$ to a workload using the ACSM metabolic equations.

To calculate the target $\dot{V}O_2$, use the $\dot{V}O_2$R formula, which is similar to the HRR formula.

$$\text{Target } \dot{V}O_2 = (\text{intensity fraction})(\dot{V}O_{2max} - \dot{V}O_{2rest}) + \dot{V}O_{2rest}$$

Substituting 3.5 mL · kg^{-1} · min^{-1} for resting $\dot{V}O_2$, this becomes

$$\text{Target } \dot{V}O_2 = (\text{intensity fraction})(\dot{V}O_{2max} - 3.5) + 3.5$$

For example, what is the target $\dot{V}O_2$ at 40% $\dot{V}O_2$R for a client with a $\dot{V}O_{2max}$ of 26 mL · kg^{-1} · min^{-1}?

$$\text{Target } \dot{V}O_2 = (0.40)(26 - 3.5) + 3.5$$
$$\text{Target } \dot{V}O_2 = (0.40)(22.5) + 3.5$$
$$\text{Target } \dot{V}O_2 = 9.0 + 3.5 = 12.5\ \text{mL} \cdot kg^{-1} \cdot min^{-1}$$

This $\dot{V}O_2$ would then be entered into a metabolic equation to determine the workload for a desired mode of exercise, as described in the following text.

TARGET WORKLOAD USING PERCENTAGE OF MAXIMUM OXYGEN CONSUMPTION

Before the publication of the ACSM's 1998 position stand (38), the primary basis for establishing exercise intensity was %$\dot{V}O_{2max}$, not %$\dot{V}O_2R$. The %$\dot{V}O_2R$ is a viable means of prescribing intensity that some practitioners may still use. However, %$\dot{V}O_{2max}$ has two drawbacks. First, it does not translate directly into %HRR units. A discrepancy exists between %HRR and %$\dot{V}O_{2max}$ units that is most noticeable with low-fit clients exercising at low intensities (52). However, even elite athletes obtain more accurate prescriptions using %$\dot{V}O_2R$ than %$\dot{V}O_{2max}$ (27). The second shortcoming using %$\dot{V}O_{2max}$ is that it does not provide equivalent relative intensities for individuals with different fitness levels. Consider a prescribed intensity of 40% $\dot{V}O_{2max}$ in three clients, one deconditioned (5 MET capacity; 17.5 mL $\cdot$ kg^{-1} $\cdot$ min^{-1}), one average (10 METs; 35 mL $\cdot$ kg^{-1} $\cdot$ min^{-1}), and one highly trained (20 METs; 70 mL $\cdot$ kg^{-1} $\cdot$ min^{-1}). An intensity of 40% $\dot{V}O_{2max}$ yields target $\dot{V}O_2$s of 7, 14, and 28 mL $\cdot$ kg^{-1} $\cdot$ min^{-1}, respectively. As percentages of $\dot{V}O_2R$, these translate to 25%, 33%, and 37%, respectively. Therefore, the deconditioned client would be asked to use a much smaller portion of his or her exercise capacity than the other clients. To accurately establish relative intensities, %$\dot{V}O_2R$ is preferred.

For those choosing to use %$\dot{V}O_{2max}$, the calculation is simpler than for %$\dot{V}O_2R$:

$$\text{Target } \dot{V}O_2 = (\text{intensity fraction}) \, \dot{V}O_{2max}$$

As a starting point, the same intensity fractions designated for %$\dot{V}O_2R$ may be selected, but these should be adjusted upward. The amount of adjustment is greater for lower intensities versus higher intensities of prescribed exercise and is greater for low-fit clients than for higher fit clients (see *Table 30-2*). As with the %$\dot{V}O_2R$ method, the resulting target $\dot{V}O_2$ would then be converted to a workload using the ACSM metabolic equations. Note that %$\dot{V}O_{2max}$ values do not match up with %HRR values, so one should not attempt to use a target HR based on %$\dot{V}O_{2max}$.

TARGET WORKLOAD USING METABOLIC EQUIVALENTS

As mentioned previously, the Compendium of Physical Activities provides rough intensity ranges for various activities in METs (2). First, select the desired intensity in %$\dot{V}O_2R$ units, then determine the target intensity using a modified Karvonen equation for METs:

$$\text{Target METs} = (\text{intensity fraction}) \, [(\dot{V}O_{2max} \text{ in METs}) - 1] + 1$$

$\dot{V}O_{2max}$ in METs is found by dividing the value in mL $\cdot$ kg^{-1} $\cdot$ min^{-1} by 3.5. For example, what is the target MET level at 60% of $\dot{V}O_2R$ for a client with a $\dot{V}O_{2max}$ of 22 mL $\cdot$ kg^{-1} $\cdot$ min^{-1}?

$$\text{Maximum MET value} = (22 \text{ mL} \cdot \text{kg}^{-1} \cdot \text{min}^{-1})/$$
$$(3.5 \text{ mL} \cdot \text{kg}^{-1} \cdot \text{min}^{-1} \text{ per MET}) = 6.3 \text{ METs}$$
$$\text{Target METs} = (0.60)(6.3 - 1) + 1$$
$$\text{Target METs} = (0.60)(5.3) + 1$$
$$\text{Target METs} = 3.2 + 1 = 4.2 \text{ METs}$$

Then, the compendium is consulted to identify activities with an appropriate MET intensity range. However, caution must be used to discuss the appropriate subjective level of effort that the client will use during the activity.

TARGET INTENSITY USING PERCEIVED EXERTION

Many individuals are able to regulate the intensity of exercise based on how hard it feels. Well-trained athletes can easily establish a pace that they feel is light or moderate or hard and pace themselves for a given distance or duration. Novice exercisers may be taught to subjectively regulate their intensity through various methods, including the talk test and various scales for rating one's perceived level of exertion.

The Talk Test

The talk test can establish a moderate exercise intensity. The client is asked to work at a level that causes a sensation of increased breathing but that still allows comfortable speaking in complete sentences. When asked "Can you still speak comfortably?" answering "yes" is consistently associated with an intensity below the ventilatory threshold (37). The intensity when a client provides an equivocal answer is approximately at the ventilatory threshold, whereas intensities at which the client says "no" are above the ventilatory threshold.

Ratings of Perceived Exertion

The original, linear, Borg Scale (see *GETP9, Table 4-7*) is mostly widely used (5), although a newer "category-ratio" Borg Scale is also available (34). The original Borg Scale ranges from 6 to 20, with 6 being rest and 20 being maximal effort. Descriptors such as "very light" and "somewhat hard" are associated with every other number. The scale was designed to correspond to HRs of 60–200 bpm in young adults but may be used by individuals of any age to subjectively rate their level of effort. Clients should be instructed to report the overall sensation of effort and not to localize their rating onto how the legs feel or how difficult the breathing is.

The OMNI Scale has been recently reported (41,57), which uses pictures illustrating varying levels of exertion along with short descriptors and numbers from 0 to 10 and has been used to differentiate feelings of exertion in the legs and chest. The Borg (5,34) and OMNI scales (19,41,57) have been validated against physiologic measures, such as $\dot{V}O_{2max}$, HR, and serum lactate concentration during incremental exercise. However, when a client is asked to report increasing numbers on a scale as the intensity of exercise is increased, strong correlations with physiologic measures that also increase must occur. The ability of subjective scales to place a client at a desired intensity during a prescribed exercise session is less certain. To maximize the use of these scales, clients should be familiarized with them during an incremental exercise test, and the levels corresponding to desired exercise intensity should be pointed out.

DETERMINING WORKLOAD FROM THE ACSM METABOLIC EQUATIONS

When using the %$\dot{V}O_2$R method to establish the exercise intensity as a target $\dot{V}O_2$, the $\dot{V}O_2$ must be translated into a workload with a given mode of exercise. *Table 7-3* in *GETP9* provides the equations for determining $\dot{V}O_2$ (in mL $\cdot$ kg^{-1} $\cdot$ min^{-1}) during walking, running, leg cycle ergometry, arm cycle ergometry, and stepping. The derivations of the equations are discussed briefly in the following text (47). The values are gross, including both the $\dot{V}O_2$ needed for rest (*i.e.*, 3.5 mL $\cdot$ kg^{-1} $\cdot$ min^{-1}) and the net value needed to perform the exercise.

The equations may be used to prescribe a workload and may also be used to determine the $\dot{V}O_2$ and EE associated with a self-selected workload. To convert oxygen consumption to EE, the $\dot{V}O_2$ must first be expressed in absolute terms, L $\cdot$ min^{-1}. This is done by multiplying the relative $\dot{V}O_2$, in mL $\cdot$ kg^{-1} $\cdot$ min^{-1}, by the client's body mass and then dividing by 1,000 (*i.e.*, 1,000 mL $\cdot$ L^{-1}). Approximately 5 kcal of energy are expended when 1 L of O_2 is consumed (slightly more when using only carbohydrates, slightly less when using only fats). When determining the EE for weight loss purposes, it is essential that the net value, not the gross value, be used (see the following text).

OXYGEN CONSUMPTION OF WALKING

Walking requires 0.1 mL of O_2 for each meter of horizontal motion for each kilogram of body mass — that is, 0.1 mL $\cdot$ kg^{-1} $\cdot$ min^{-1} (11). Vertical ascent requires 1.8 mL of O_2 for each meter climbed for each kilogram of mass raised, that is, 1.8 mL $\cdot$ kg^{-1} $\cdot$ min^{-1} (11). The oxygen demand of downhill walking is complex, as it decreases as the slope becomes steeper up to a point (−10% grade), and then increases with greater steepness, surpassing the cost of level walking at grades steeper than −20% (31). Therefore, the ACSM equation

is not valid for downhill walking. The gross $\dot{V}O_2$ of level or uphill walking can be expressed as

$$\dot{V}O_2 \text{ of walking} = 3.5 + 0.1 \text{ (speed)} + 1.8 \text{ (speed)(grade)}$$

where speed is in m $\cdot$ min^{-1}, and grade is expressed as a fraction.

For example, what is the gross $\dot{V}O_2$ and net EE of a 70-kg client walking at 3 mph up to a 5% grade? The conversion factor for speed is 1 mph = 26.8 m $\cdot$ min^{-1}. Therefore, speed is (3 mph)(26.8 m $\cdot$ min^{-1} $\cdot$ mph^{-1}) = 80.4 m $\cdot$ min^{-1}.

$$\dot{V}O_2 = 3.5 + 0.1 \text{ (80.4)} + 1.8 \text{ (80.4)(0.05)}$$
$$\dot{V}O_2 = 3.5 + 8.04 + 7.236 = 18.8 \text{ mL} \cdot \text{kg}^{-1} \cdot \text{min}^{-1}$$

The gross $\dot{V}O_2$ is 18.8 mL $\cdot$ kg^{-1} $\cdot$ min^{-1}, whereas the net $\dot{V}O_2$ is 3.5 less — that is, 15.3 mL $\cdot$ kg^{-1} $\cdot$ min^{-1}. To determine the net EE, first, convert the net $\dot{V}O_2$ from relative units to absolute units: (15.3 mL $\cdot$ kg^{-1} $\cdot$ min^{-1}) (70 kg)/(1,000 mL $\cdot$ L^{-1}) = approximately 1.1 L $\cdot$ min^{-1}.

Now, convert the L $\cdot$ min^{-1} of $\dot{V}O_2$ to kcal $\cdot$ min^{-1} of EE: (1.1 L $\cdot$ min^{-1})(5 kcal $\cdot$ L^{-1}) = 5.5 kcal $\cdot$ min^{-1}.

OXYGEN CONSUMPTION OF RUNNING

Running requires exactly twice as much oxygen or energy for horizontal movement as does walking — that is, 0.2 mL $\cdot$ kg^{-1} $\cdot$ min^{-1} (11,30) — because of the work of jumping off the ground between steps. When running uphill, some of the vertical work of jumping between steps can be applied to the ascent, and the coefficient for uphill running is reduced from that of walking (*i.e.*, 0.9 mL $\cdot$ kg^{-1} $\cdot$ min^{-1}) (11,30). As with walking, the energy cost of downhill running is complex (31) and not covered in the ACSM equation:

$$\dot{V}O_2 \text{ of running} = 3.5 + 0.2 \text{ (speed)} + 0.9 \text{ (speed)(grade)}$$

For example, if a client runs comfortably at 6 mph (161 m $\cdot$ min^{-1}), what treadmill grade would be needed to exercise at a target $\dot{V}O_2$ of 50 mL $\cdot$ kg^{-1} $\cdot$ min^{-1}? Enter the known values into the running equation and solve for the unknown grade.

$$50 = 3.5 + 0.2 \text{ (161)} + 0.9 \text{ (161)(grade)}$$
$$50 = 3.5 + 32.2 + 144.9 \text{ (grade)}$$
$$50 = 35.7 + 144.9 \text{ (grade)}$$
$$50 - 35.7 = 144.9 \text{ (grade)}$$
$$14.3 = 144.9 \text{ (grade)}$$
$$14.3/144.9 = \text{grade}$$
$$0.099 = \text{grade, or approximately 10\%}$$

What is the net EE of walking or running 1 mile on level ground for a 136-lb (62-kg) client? One mile is 1,609 m. The oxygen cost of horizontal walking is 0.1 mL $\cdot$ kg^{-1} $\cdot$ min^{-1}, thus the oxygen consumed over 1 mile (above resting needs) would be (0.1 mL $\cdot$ kg^{-1} $\cdot$ min^{-1}) (1,609 m)(62 kg) = approximately 10,000 mL or 10 L.

The oxygen cost of running would be $(0.2 \text{ mL} \cdot \text{kg}^{-1} \cdot \text{min}^{-1})(1{,}609 \text{ m})(62 \text{ kg}) = 20{,}000 \text{ mL}$ or 20 L. Given $5 \text{ kcal} \cdot \text{L}^{-1}$ of O_2, the EE would be $10 \text{ L} \times 5 \text{ kcal} \cdot \text{L}^{-1} = 50$ kcal for walking, and $20 \text{ L} \times 5 \text{ kcal} \cdot \text{L}^{-1} = 100$ kcal for running. This is the derivation of the often cited "100 kcal for running a mile." However, the energy cost of walking a mile is exactly half of that. Clients who are heavier (or lighter) than 62 kg would have proportionally more (or less) EE.

OXYGEN CONSUMPTION OF LEG CYCLING

In addition to the resting component, stationary cycling requires approximately $3.5 \text{ mL} \cdot \text{kg}^{-1} \cdot \text{min}^{-1}$ just to spin the legs at 50–60 revolutions per minute (rpm) without any resistance (47). To overcome resistance, an additional 1.8 mL of O_2 is needed for each $\text{kg}^{-1} \cdot \text{m}^{-1}$ of work (as in the vertical component of the walking equation) (22,23,26). Thus, the leg cycling equation is

$$\dot{V}O_2 \text{ of leg cycling} = 3.5 + 3.5 + 1.8 \text{ (workload)/(body mass)}$$

where the workload is expressed in $\text{kg} \cdot \text{m} \cdot \text{min}^{-1}$. If power is measured in watts, note that 1 W equals approximately $6 \text{ kg} \cdot \text{m} \cdot \text{min}^{-1}$ (if greater accuracy is desired, use 6.12).

For example, what is the gross $\dot{V}O_2$ of a 62-kg client cycling at 100 W? First, convert the power to workload as $(100 \text{ W})(6 \text{ kg} \cdot \text{m} \cdot \text{min}^{-1} \cdot \text{W}^{-1}) = 600 \text{ kg} \cdot \text{m} \cdot \text{min}^{-1}$. Then use the leg cycling equation:

$$\dot{V}O_2 = 3.5 + 3.5 + 1.8 \, (600)/62$$
$$\dot{V}O_2 = 7 + 17.4 = 24.4 \text{ mL} \cdot \text{kg}^{-1} \cdot \text{min}^{-1}$$

OXYGEN CONSUMPTION OF ARM CYCLING

The arm cycling equation includes the resting component and a component to account for the resistance of the ergometer. The latter is $3 \text{ mL of } O_2 \cdot \text{kg}^{-1} \cdot \text{m}^{-1}$, as opposed to 1.8 for the legs (12). The higher value is apparently because of lower efficiency with the smaller muscle mass of the arms and also because the oxygen cost of unloaded cycling is incorporated within the term.

$$\dot{V}O_2 \text{ of arm cycling} = 3.5 + 3 \text{ (workload)/(body mass)}$$

OXYGEN CONSUMPTION OF STEPPING

In addition to the resting component, stepping requires a term for the forward and backward motion of the person as well as a term for raising and then lowering the body on and off the step. The horizontal term is 0.2 mL of O_2 times the stepping rate. The vertical term is $1.8 \text{ mL} \cdot \text{kg}^{-1} \cdot \text{min}^{-1}$ (as in the walking and leg cycling equations), plus one-third of that for lowering the body back down (33).

$$\dot{V}O_2 \text{ of stepping} = 3.5 + 0.2 \text{ (rate)} + 2.4 \text{ (rate)(H)}$$

where the stepping rate is in complete four-cycle steps per minute, and H is the height of the step in meter.

A complete four-cycle step involves (a) lifting the first leg and placing the foot on the step; (b) extending the first leg to raise the body, placing the foot of the second leg on the step; (c) moving the foot of the first leg back to the floor by lowering the body with the second leg; and (d) placing the foot of the second leg on the floor. In this sequence, the first leg does virtually all of the concentric work, and the second leg does virtually all of the eccentric work. The client should vary this by occasionally switching legs on the fourth beat. This is done by tapping the foot of the second leg on the ground and lifting it on the first beat of the next cycle.

THE CALORIC COST OF EXERCISE

The caloric cost of exercise can be determined from the metabolic equations mentioned previously, as illustrated in the walking example. This is best expressed in net terms and must be for weight-loss calculations. Resting oxygen consumption of $3.5 \text{ mL} \cdot \text{kg}^{-1} \cdot \text{min}^{-1}$ (i.e., 1 MET) translates to $1 \text{ kcal} \cdot \text{kg}^{-1} \cdot \text{hr}^{-1}$. Consider a 75-kg client with a resting EE of $(1 \text{ kcal} \cdot \text{kg}^{-1} \cdot \text{hr}^{-1})(75 \text{ kg})(24 \text{ h}) = 1{,}800 \text{ kcal} \cdot \text{d}^{-1}$. If the client walks 2 miles in 60 min or runs 2 miles in 15 min, the EE can be calculated from the metabolic equations. As displayed in *Table 30-3*, the client's gross EE would be 200 kcal during the 2-mile walk and 260 kcal during the 2-mile run. However, given the longer duration of the walk, a significant proportion of the gross EE is due to ongoing resting metabolism (80 kcal or 40%), whereas a much smaller fraction of the gross EE during the run is caused by resting metabolism (20 kcal, ~8%). The net EE caused by the exercise is only half of that for the walk (120 kcal) as for the run (240 kcal). It is incorrect to say that the walker has added 200 kcal to the day's total EE, as the 80 kcal of resting metabolism would have occurred even if the client did not walk. The total EE for the day is $1{,}800 + 120 = 1{,}920$ kcal for the day with

TABLE 30-3. Caloric Expenditure of a 75-kg Client During a 2-mile Walk or Run

	Duration	EE due to exercise (net)	EE due to resting metabolism	Gross EE
Walk 2 miles (at 2 mph)	60 min	120 kcal	80 kcal	200 kcal
Run 2 miles (at 8 mph)	15 min	240 kcal	20 kcal	260 kcal

EE, energy expenditure.

walking and is 1,800 + 240 = 2,040 kcal for the day with running. Whenever EE during exercise is expressed in gross terms, it overestimates the actual effect of the exercise. This overestimation is much worse for lower intensity exercise than for higher intensity exercise (40% vs. 8% in this example).

If the client did 1 h of walking 5 d · wk^{-1}, how much fat weight loss could be expected, assuming this is a new program for the client and diet is not changed? Five h · wk^{-1} times the net EE of 120 kcal · hr^{-1} = 600 kcal · wk^{-1} expended above rest. One lb (0.45 kg) of fat contains 3,500 kcal. Thus, 600/3,500 = 0.17 lb. The client would lose only 1/6 lb · wk^{-1}. Thus, a greater volume of exercise and a reduction in caloric intake would be needed to reach a weight loss of 1–2 lb weekly.

The ACSM recommends that a minimum of 1,000 kcal be expended per week in physical activity and exercise, which is associated with a significant 20%–30% reduction in risk of all-cause mortality (17,24), and this should be the initial goal for previously sedentary individuals. Based on the dose–response relationships between physical activity and health and fitness, individuals should be encouraged to move toward attainment of 2,000–4,000 kcal · wk^{-1} as their fitness improves during the training program. For the purposes of weight loss, the minimum exercise dose should reach 2,000 kcal · wk^{-1} (20). EE in excess of 2,000 kcal · wk^{-1} have been successful for both short- and long-term weight control (42,43).

An alternative to calculating the EE of exercise from the metabolic equations is to use the following equation based on the MET level of the activity:

$$(METs \times 3.5 \times body\ mass\ in\ kg)/200 = kcal \cdot min^{-1}$$

This formula (derived from conversions listed previously) helps an individual understand the components of the exercise prescription and the volume of exercise necessary to achieve the caloric goals of the program.

Consider the following example. The weekly goal of the exercise program has been set at 1,000 kcal for an individual who weighs 70 kg, and the MET level of a prescribed activity is 6 METs. In this example, the *net* caloric expenditure from the exercise would be 5 METs because 1 MET of the activity represents resting metabolic rate. Therefore, the net caloric expenditure from the exercise is (5 × 3.5 × 70)/200 = 6.1 kcal · min^{-1}, which requires 164 min · wk^{-1} to attain the 1,000 kcal threshold. Given a 4-d · wk^{-1} program, the individual would require approximately 41 min · d^{-1} to achieve the 1,000 kcal goal (or 33 min · d^{-1}, 5 d · wk^{-1}). Working backward from the caloric goal to determine the volume of exercise needed to reach the goal is useful in determining the appropriate exercise prescription components. If the goal was a more aggressive 2,000 kcal · wk^{-1}, the net caloric expenditure of 6.1 kcal · min^{-1} would require 328 min · wk^{-1} or approximately 47 min · d^{-1} on all days of the week.

EXERCISE PROGRESSION

The rate of progression of exercise depends on $\dot{V}O_2$, health status, age, activity preferences, and goals as well as the tolerance to training. Exercise progression is essential for sedentary individuals beginning exercise programs and is important for all populations. Most training programs feature three progressive stages: initiation, improvement, and maintenance.

INITIATION STAGE

The goal of the initial stage of training is to allow time to begin the adaptive process. Typically, this is accomplished by working at a lower intensity and shorter duration and with careful attention to signs of intolerance, particularly musculoskeletal or cardiopulmonary. The initial stage is the time to develop the habit of exercise with minimal discomfort and soreness. It is also a time to allow the exercise professional to instruct the individual as to proper exercise form. Every cardiorespiratory exercise session should be preceded by a 5- to 10-min warm-up, performing the mode of exercise prescribed for the work phase at a low intensity to allow the cardiopulmonary system to adjust to the new demand and to allow the temperature of the muscles to increase. Stretching may be performed at the end of the warm-up if desired and should be performed at the end of the cool-down. Following the work phase, the low-intensity cool-down is performed for 5–10 min to prevent blood pooling and to promote the clearance of lactic acid. If resistance training is to be performed in the same exercise session, it is best performed at the conclusion of the aerobic cool-down and before the stretching. See *Chapter 31* for additional information on resistance and flexibility exercise.

Suitable initial intensities may range from 30% $\dot{V}O_2R$ for very deconditioned individuals, 40% of $\dot{V}O_2R$ for other beginners, to more than 50% of $\dot{V}O_2R$ for individuals with higher aerobic capacities or experienced exercisers returning from time off regular exercise. Appropriate initial duration of exercise ranges from 20 to 30 min per session. Individuals who are older, obese, and profoundly sedentary may start with as little as 10 min of continuous exercise. In such situations, intermittent exercise or multiple daily sessions may be helpful. If intensity is kept low to moderate, sedentary but otherwise healthy adults may be able to start with sessions of 20–30 min.

The exercise session itself may be modified during the initial stage of training by expanding the warm-up period, using it to inventory possible signs of injury or soreness, providing information, and answering questions. The initial stage of training generally lasts for 4 wk but may be expanded for those requiring additional time to adapt. Monitoring exercise HRs may also be an indication for progression. If exercise or recovery HRs are lower for the same amount of work, the intensity or duration can be increased.

IMPROVEMENT STAGE

The goal of this stage of training is to provide a gradual increase in the overall exercise stimulus to allow for significant improvements in cardiorespiratory fitness. In the improvement stage, expanding physiologic capacities are further challenged. This stage is typified by the phrase *progressive overload*. Small increments in intensity and duration may occur nearly every week. The challenge of the improvement stage is to increase training at a rate that continues to stimulate further advancement without causing overtraining.

Failure to complete an exercise session, lack of normal interest in training, increased HR or rating of perceived exertion at the same rate of external work, and an increase in minor aches and pains are all signs that progression may be too rapid (25). In an appropriately incremented improvement stage, interest and appetite for exercise normally increase in tandem with the subjective and objective impressions that progress is being made. In general, frequency, intensity, and duration should not be increased together in any single week, and total weekly training volume should not be advanced by more than 10%. Increasing duration by 5–10 min per session on a weekly basis is usually well tolerated, as is building intensity gradually through the range of 40%–59% of aerobic capacity and eventually adding sessions of more vigorous intensity. Progression of both intensity and duration in a single session is not recommended.

Competitive athletes who train intensively and those encountering musculoskeletal or other physical obstacles impeding progress may benefit from the early incorporation of techniques such as cross-training, which are more typical of the maintenance stage.

The adaptive potential of physiologic function is finite, and large increments in fitness, typical in the improvement stage, always taper at some point. Aerobic capacity can be expected to expand by approximately 10%–30% in the course of a program following ACSM guidelines. Improvements of more than 30% rarely occur unless accompanied by a large reduction in body weight and fat. If training is discontinued, gains in fitness regress by approximately 50% within 4–12 wk (38). After approximately 6 mo of training, most individuals make the transition from improvement to maintenance.

MAINTENANCE STAGE

The goal of this stage of training is the long-term maintenance of cardiorespiratory fitness developed in the previous stage. The maintenance stage is typified by diversification of the training program and purposeful attempts to rotate and reduce the stresses of continued training. Diversification may take the form of using several modes of exercise to maintain enjoyment and explore new capabilities. This may be particularly important to lifelong programs with goals such as weight management and general health.

For those using the maintenance phase as a sustained period of performance or competition, diversification may be used as a means of reducing the potential for overuse injuries, particularly in programs with high training volumes or for participants with musculoskeletal limitations. *Cross-training*, as this approach is often called, refers to using various modes of cardiorespiratory endurance exercise (*e.g.*, swimming, running, biking) to maintain a high training stimulus for central aerobic adaptations, such as enhanced stroke volume and expanded blood volume. This approach allows rotation of local fatigue and musculoskeletal stresses across a range of muscle groups.

Cognitively, the maintenance stage is a time for enjoyment, surveillance, and reappraisal. It is a time for enjoying the fruits of labor by competing, engaging in new activities, or reducing the demands of weekly training. Surveillance for overuse injury must continue during the maintenance phase. Equipment and footwear should be reevaluated. Finally, the goals of the program may be reexamined, physiologic or performance testing may be repeated, and new goals may be established, triggering the start of a new improvement stage. Further advancing performance and cardiorespiratory fitness often requires special techniques such as periodization, in which volume and intensity of exercise are varied in a systematic way over several months.

SUMMARY

The proper application of frequency, intensity, time (duration), and type (mode) in an exercise prescription will result in improved cardiorespiratory fitness, reduced risk of CVD, and weight loss or maintenance. Intensity of exercise should be prescribed judiciously. Low-to-moderate intensities are appropriate for beginners. Higher intensities should be considered as fitness improves, provided the client is not at risk for cardiovascular events. Care should be taken in all programs to avoid excessive orthopedic stress and overtraining.

REFERENCES

1. *2008 Physical Activity Guidelines for Americans* [Internet]. Washington (DC): U.S. Department of Health and Human Services; [cited 2011 Sep 2]. Available from: http://www.health.gov/paguidelines/pdf/paguide.pdf
2. Ainsworth BE, Haskell WL, Whitt MC, et al. Compendium of physical activities: an update of activity codes and MET intensities. *Med Sci Sports Exerc*. 2000;32(9 Suppl):S498–504.
3. Billat VL, Flechet B, Petit B, Muriaux G, Koralsztein JP. Interval training at $\dot{V}O_{2max}$: effects on aerobic performance and overtraining markers. *Med Sci Sports Exerc*. 1999;31(1):156–63.

4. Blair SN, Kohl HW,3rd, Paffenbarger RS,Jr, Clark DG, Cooper KH, Gibbons LW. Physical fitness and all-cause mortality. A prospective study of healthy men and women. *JAMA.* 1989;262(17): 2395–401.

5. Borg GA. Perceived exertion. *Exerc Sport Sci Rev.* 1974;2:131–53.

6. Brawner CA, Keteyian SJ, Ehrman JK. The relationship of heart rate reserve to $\dot{V}O_2$ reserve in patients with heart disease. *Med Sci Sports Exerc.* 2002;34(3):418–22.

7. Burgomaster KA, Howarth KR, Phillips SM, et al. Similar metabolic adaptations during exercise after low volume sprint interval and traditional endurance training in humans. *J Physiol.* 2008;586(1):151–60.

8. Byrne NM, Hills AP. Relationships between HR and (.)VO(2) in the obese. *Med Sci Sports Exerc.* 2002;34(9):1419–27.

9. Colberg SR, Swain DP, Vinik AI. Use of heart rate reserve and rating of perceived exertion to prescribe exercise intensity in diabetic autonomic neuropathy. *Diabetes Care.* 2003;26(4):986–90.

10. Dalleck LC, Kravitz L. Relationship between %heart rate reserve and %$\dot{V}O_2$ reserve during elliptical crosstrainer exercise. *J Sports Sci Med.* 2006;5(4):662–71.

11. Dill DB. Oxygen cost of horizontal and grade walking and running on the treadmill. *J Appl Physiol.* 1965;20:19–22.

12. Franklin BA. Exercise testing, training and arm ergometry. *Sports Med.* 1985;2(2):100–19.

13. Garber CE, Blissmer B, Deschenes MR, et al. Quantity and quality of exercise for developing and maintaining cardiorespiratory, musculoskeletal, and neuromotor fitness in apparently healthy adults: guidance for prescribing exercise. *Med Sci Sports Exerc.* 2011;43(7):1334–59.

14. Garhammer J. A review of power output studies of Olympic and powerlifting: methodology, performance predecition, and evaluation tests. *Journal of Strength & Conditioning Research (Allen Press Publishing Services Inc).* 1993;7(2):76–89.

15. Gellish RL, Goslin BR, Olson RE, McDonald A, Russi GD, Moudgil VK. Longitudinal modeling of the relationship between age and maximal heart rate. *Med Sci Sports Exerc.* 2007;39(5):822–9.

16. Gormley SE, Swain DP, High R, et al. Effect of intensity of aerobic training on $\dot{V}O_{2max}$. *Med Sci Sports Exerc.* 2008;40(7):1336–43.

17. Haskell WL, Lee IM, Pate RR, et al. Physical activity and public health: updated recommendation for adults from the American College of Sports Medicine and the American Heart Association. *Med Sci Sports Exerc.* 2007;39(8):1423–34.

18. Helgerud J, Hoydal K, Wang E, et al Aerobic high-intensity intervals improve $\dot{V}O_{2max}$ more than moderate training. *Med Sci Sports Exerc.* 2007;39(4):665–71.

19. Irving BA, Rutkowski J, Brock DW, et al. Comparison of Borg- and OMNI-RPE as markers of the blood lactate response to exercise. *Med Sci Sports Exerc.* 2006;38(7):1348–52.

20. Jakicic JM, Clark K, Coleman E, et al. American College of Sports Medicine position stand. Appropriate intervention strategies for weight loss and prevention of weight regain for adults. *Med Sci Sports Exerc.* 2001;33(12):2145–56.

21. Karvonen MJ, Kentala E, Mustala O. The effects of training on heart rate; a longitudinal study. *Ann Med Exp Biol Fenn.* 1957;35(3): 307–15.

22. Lang PB, Latin RW, Berg KE, Mellion MB. The accuracy of the ACSM cycle ergometry equation. *Med Sci Sports Exerc.* 1992;24(2):272–6.

23. Latin RW, Berg KE. The accuracy of the ACSM and a new cycle ergometry equation for young women. *Med Sci Sports Exerc.* 1994;26(5):642–6.

24. Lee IM, Skerrett PJ. Physical activity and all-cause mortality: what is the dose-response relation? *Med Sci Sports Exerc.* 2001;33(6): S459–71.

25. Lehmann MJ, Lormes W, Opitz-Gress A, et al. Training and overtraining: an overview and experimental results in endurance sports. *J Sports Med Phys Fitness.* 1997;37(1):7–17.

26. Londeree BR, Moffitt-Gerstenberger J, Padfield JA, Lottmann D. Oxygen consumption of cycle ergometry is nonlinearly related to work rate and pedal rate. *Med Sci Sports Exerc.* 1997;29(6): 775–80.

27. Lounana J, Campion F, Noakes TD, Medelli J. Relationship between %HRmax, %HR reserve, %$\dot{V}O_{2max}$, and %$\dot{V}O_2$ reserve in elite cyclists. *Med Sci Sports Exerc.* 2007;39(2):350–7.

28. MacDougall JD, Hicks AL, MacDonald JR, McKelvie RS, Green HJ, Smith KM. Muscle performance and enzymatic adaptations to sprint interval training. *J Appl Physiol.* 1998;84(6):2138–42.

29. Magel JR, Foglia GF, McArdle WD, Gutin B, Pechar GS, Katch FI. Specificity of swim training on maximum oxygen uptake. *J Appl Physiol.* 1975;38(1):151–5.

30. Margaria R, Cerretelli P, Aghemo P, Sassi G. Energy cost of running. *J Appl Physiol.* 1963;18:367–70.

31. Minetti AE, Moia C, Roi GS, Susta D, Ferretti G. Energy cost of walking and running at extreme uphill and downhill slopes. *J Appl Physiol.* 2002;93(3):1039–46.

32. Mittleman MA, Maclure M, Tofler GH, Sherwood JB, Goldberg RJ, Muller JE. Triggering of acute myocardial infarction by heavy physical exertion. Protection against triggering by regular exertion. Determinants of Myocardial Infarction Onset Study Investigators. *N Engl J Med.* 1993;329(23):1677–83.

33. Nagle FJ, Balke B, Naughton JP. Gradational step tests for assessing work capacity. *J Appl Physiol.* 1965;20(4):745–8.

34. Noble BJ, Borg GA, Jacobs I, Ceci R, Kaiser P. A category-ratio perceived exertion scale: relationship to blood and muscle lactates and heart rate. *Med Sci Sports Exerc.* 1983;15(6):523–8.

35. Padilla S, Mujika I, Angulo F, Goiriena JJ. Scientific approach to the 1-h cycling world record: a case study. *J Appl Physiol.* 2000;89(4):1522–7.

36. Pate RR, Pratt M, Blair SN, et al Physical activity and public health. A recommendation from the Centers for Disease Control and Prevention and the American College of Sports Medicine. *JAMA.* 1995;273(5):402–7.

37. Persinger R, Foster C, Gibson M, Fater DC, Porcari JP. Consistency of the talk test for exercise prescription. *Med Sci Sports Exerc.* 2004;36(9):1632–6.

38. Pollock ML, Gaesser GA, Butcher JD, et al. American College of Sports Medicine position stand: the recommended quantity and quality of exercise for developing and maintaining cardiorespiratory and muscular fitness, and flexibility in healthy adults. *Med Sci Sports Exerc.* 1998;30(6):975–91.

39. Pollock ML, Gettman LR, Milesis CA, Bah MD, Durstine L. Effects of frequency and duration of training on attrition and incidence of injury. *Med Sci Sports.* 1977;9(1):31–6.

40. Rakobowchuk M, Tanguay S, Burgomaster KA, Howarth KR, Gibala MJ, MacDonald MJ. Sprint interval and traditional endurance training induce similar improvements in peripheral arterial stiffness and flow-mediated dilation in healthy humans. *Am J Physiol Regul Integr Comp Physiol.* 2008;295(1):R236–42.

41. Robertson RJ, Goss FL, Dube J, et al. Validation of the adult OMNI scale of perceived exertion for cycle ergometer exercise. *Med Sci Sports Exerc.* 2004;36(1):102–8.

42. Ross R, Janssen I. Physical activity, total and regional obesity: dose-response considerations. *Med Sci Sports Exerc.* 2001;33(6 Suppl):S521–7; discussion S528–9.

43. Saris WH, Blair SN, van Baak MA, et al. How much physical activity is enough to prevent unhealthy weight gain? Outcome of the IASO 1st Stock Conference and consensus statement. *Obes Rev.* 2003;4(2):101–14.

44. Sattelmair J, Pertman J, Ding EL, Kohl HW,3rd, Haskell W, Lee IM. Dose response between physical activity and risk of coronary heart disease: a meta-analysis. *Circulation.* 2011;124(7):789–95.

45. Smith TP, McNaughton LR, Marshall KJ. Effects of 4-wk training using Vmax/Tmax on $\dot{V}O_{2max}$ and performance in athletes. *Med Sci Sports Exerc.* 1999;31(6):892–6.

46. Stone MH, Sands WA, Carlock J, et al. The importance of isometric maximum strength and peak rate-of-force development in sprint cycling. *J Strength Cond Res.* 2004;18(4):878–84.

47. Swain DP. Energy cost calculations for exercise prescription: an update. *Sports Med.* 2000;30(1):17–22.

48. Swain DP. Moderate or vigorous intensity exercise: which is better for improving aerobic fitness? *Prev Cardiol.* 2005;8(1):55–8.

49. Swain DP, Coast JR, Clifford PS, Milliken MC, Stray-Gundersen J. Influence of body size on oxygen consumption during bicycling. *J Appl Physiol.* 1987;62(2):668–72.

50. Swain DP, Franklin BA. Comparison of cardioprotective benefits of vigorous versus moderate intensity aerobic exercise. *Am J Cardiol.* 2006;97(1):141–7.

51. Swain DP, Franklin BA. $\dot{V}O_2$ reserve and the minimal intensity for improving cardiorespiratory fitness. *Med Sci Sports Exerc.* 2002;34(1):152–7.

52. Swain DP, Leutholtz BC. Heart rate reserve is equivalent to $\%\dot{V}O_2$ reserve, not to $\%\dot{V}O_{2max}$. *Med Sci Sports Exerc.* 1997;29(3):410–4.

53. Swain DP, Leutholtz BC, King ME, Haas LA, Branch JD. Relationship between %heart rate reserve and $\%\dot{V}O_2$ reserve in treadmill exercise. *Med Sci Sports Exerc.* 1998;30(2):318–21.

54. Tanaka H, Monahan KD, Seals DR. Age-predicted maximal heart rate revisited. *J Am Coll Cardiol.* 2001;37(1):153–6.

55. U.S. Department of Health and Human Services, Centers for Disease Control and Prevention, National Center for Chronic Disease Prevention and Health Promotion, The President's Council on Physical Fitness and Sports. *Physical Activity and Health: A Report of the Surgeon General.* Atlanta (GA): President's Council on Physical Fitness and Sports; 1996. 278 p.

56. UltraMarathon Cycling Association. Timed Records [Internet]: UltraMarathon Cycling Association; [cited 2012 Feb 13]. Available from: http://www.ultracycling.com/sections/records/stats/timed

57. Utter AC, Robertson RJ, Green JM, Suminski RR, McAnulty SR, Nieman DC. Validation of the Adult OMNI Scale of perceived exertion for walking/running exercise. *Med Sci Sports Exerc.* 2004;36(10):1776–80.

58. Warburton DE, McKenzie DC, Haykowsky MJ, et al. Effectiveness of high-intensity interval training for the rehabilitation of patients with coronary artery disease. *Am J Cardiol.* 2005;95(9):1080–4.

59. Williams PT. Physical fitness and activity as separate heart disease risk factors: a meta-analysis. *Med Sci Sports Exerc.* 2001;33(5):754–61.

60. Wisloff U, Stoylen A, Loennechen JP, et al. Superior cardiovascular effect of aerobic interval training versus moderate continuous training in heart failure patients: a randomized study. *Circulation.* 2007;115(24):3086–94.

SELECTED REFERENCES FOR FURTHER READING

Garber CE, Blissmer B, Deschenes MR, et al. American College of Sports Medicine position stand. Quantity and quality of exercise for developing and maintaining cardiorespiratory, musculoskeletal, and neuromotor fitness in apparently healthy adults: guidance for prescribing exercise. *Med Sci Sports Exerc.* 2011;43(7):1334–59.

Haskell WL, Lee I-M, Pate RR, et al. Physical activity and public health: updated recommendations from the American College of Sports Medicine and the American Heart Association. *Med Sci Sports Exerc.* 2007;39:1423–34.

U.S. Department of Health and Human Services. *Physical Activity and Health: A Report of the Surgeon General.* Washington (DC): U.S. Department of Health and Human Services, Centers for Disease Control and Prevention, National Center for Chronic Disease Prevention and Health Promotion; 1996. 278 p.

INTERNET RESOURCES

- American College of Sports Medicine: http://www.acsm.org
- Centers for Disease Control and Prevention: http://www.cdc.gov
- United States Department of Health and Human Services Physical Activity Guidelines for Americans: http://www.health.gov/PAGuidlines/pdf/paguide.pdf

Musculoskeletal Exercise Prescription

Individualization and proper exercise prescription of resistance training are the most important features of a program for gaining needed physiologic adaptations (18). Perhaps the most well-known benefit of resistance training is increased strength, although increases in power and local muscular endurance are also very important characteristics of a resistance training program. Along with this comes an increase in muscle size, which is vital for men and women to offset any sarcopenia — significant muscular **atrophy** with disease or the aging process. Increased strength is important to athletes for performance improvement, but it is also important to everyone for the perfor-

mance of many activities of daily living (ADLs), such as doing the laundry or climbing stairs. As individuals age, a lack of strength may eventually impair many basic ADLs needed for independence, from walking to getting out of a chair (36). Lack of strength may also preclude performing recreational activities at a level that is safe and enjoyable, such as basketball, softball, downhill skiing, golf, or hiking. Resistance training brings about strength increases in both men and women no matter what their age is. It is important to increase or maintain strength as one ages so that recreational activities and ADLs may continue to be comfortably performed.

KEY TERMS

Accommodating resistance: Maximum resistance throughout the whole range of motion is maintained by controlling the speed of the movement.

Atrophy: The wasting or loss of muscle tissue resulting from disease or lack of use.

Classic (linear) periodization: A type of periodization using a systematic increase in the intensity and decrease in the volume of training over the course of a training program.

Concentric: A muscular action in which a muscle develops force and shortens, creating movement at a joint.

Constant resistance: Absolute (external) resistance remains constant throughout the range of motion.

Eccentric: A muscular action in which a muscle develops force but is lengthened by a greater opposing force.

Hypertrophy: Growth of individual muscle fibers and of whole muscle.

Isometric: A muscular action in which a muscle develops force against a fixed resistance and no limb or joint angle movement occurs.

Isotonic: A muscular action in which muscular force is constant throughout the movement; this term technically applies to the contractions of isolated muscles in laboratory experiments. Although sometimes used to denote dynamic (concentric and eccentric) contractions, normal movements are not isotonic, as intact muscles vary their force throughout the range of motion to compensate for changes in joint angle.

Nonlinear periodization: A type of periodization employing variation in the intensity and volume of training within each week over the course of the training program.

Periodization: Systematic manipulation of acute program variables over time with planned rest periods used to provide recovery.

Progressive resistance: A principle of training in which the stress on the muscle is increased over time as it becomes capable of producing greater force (a specific example of the overload principle).

Valsalva maneuver: Contracting the muscles of exhalation but not allowing air to escape. Performed as breath holding during muscular effort.

Variable resistance: Absolute (external) resistance changes during the range of motion.

HISTORY OF RESISTANCE TRAINING

Resistance training can be traced through much of recorded history for more than 5,000 yr. Interestingly, the training practices of the twentieth century were shaped by the three competitive sports of weightlifting, power lifting, and bodybuilding. In the twentieth century, Bob Hoffman at York Barbell Company in York, Pennsylvania, promoted weightlifting and was the epicenter for some of the world's strongest men well into the 1950s, dominating world weightlifting competitions. He also promoted weight training for bodybuilding and physical development for health. In the famous meeting in 1940 of Peter Karpovich, a founder of the *American College of Sports Medicine* (ACSM), and Bob Hoffman at Springfield College, one of Hoffman's body builders, John Grimek, demonstrated with feats of flexibility that bodybuilders and weightlifters did not have to be inflexible or muscle bound. This changed the minds of many that there was some merit in weight training beyond that of a spectacle. Also part of the development of weight-training programs in the twentieth century was Joe Weider, who promoted bodybuilding with such notables as Arnold Schwarzenegger.

Thomas Delorme might be considered the father of modern resistance training from the perspective of his study in medicine and science. His research as a captain in the U.S. Army and then as an orthopedic surgeon at the Massachusetts General Hospital in Boston provided medical evidence that resistance training could improve not only strength but also performance in the rehabilitation of injured soldiers from World War II (7). In a conversation with his wife over dinner one night, she came up with the term progressive resistance *training* to describe his use of different percentage loads of the 10-repetition maximum (RM) Delorme Method to elicit changes in muscular strength with resistance training (personal communication, Dr. Terry Todd). By the late 1970s into the early 1980s, the use of an expanded arsenal of laboratory techniques quickly extended our understanding of resistance exercise. During the 1980s, there was an exponential rise in the number of investigations on resistance training and on the multitude of physiologic systems studied: dramatic discoveries in the areas of muscle fiber subtype transitions, sex differences in adaptations, training compatibility (*i.e.*, simultaneous heavy resistance training and high-intensity endurance training), as well as opening up a whole new venue for resistance training with the elderly in combating sarcopenia (1). The exponential increase in the study of resistance exercise continued during the 1990s, culminating with a progressions model position stand by the ACSM in 2002 (16) and then a revision in 2009 (2).

BASIC PRINCIPLES OF RESISTANCE TRAINING

It is important to understand some of the basic principles of resistance training to optimize the exercise prescription and the programs developed. When undertaking a needs analysis for a training program, there are a few underlying principles to consider.

PROGRESSIVE OVERLOAD

Progressive overload is a universal training principle stipulating that one needs to continually increase the exercise demands to see progression in a performance variable, as defined within the construct of the variable being trained (*i.e.*, strength, power, or local muscular endurance). As a muscle becomes capable of producing greater force or greater power, or has more local muscular endurance, the stress needs to be increased to maintain an overload and have further gains. Consider an individual whose 3-RM (the maximum amount of weight that can be lifted three times without rest) for the bench press is 100 kg. Training with this weight is a sufficient stimulus to produce an increase in strength. Later in the training program, if the individual's strength has increased, 100 kg is no longer the 3-RM or a sufficient stimulus to further increase strength. If the training stimulus is not increased at this point, no further gains in strength will occur.

Several methods can be used to progressively overload the muscle (2). The resistance (amount of weight used) to perform a certain number of repetitions can be increased. The use of RMs automatically provides progressive overload because as the muscle's strength increases, the amount of resistance necessary to perform a true RM also increases. For example, a 3-RM may increase from 100 kg to 110 kg after several weeks of training. Another method of progressively overloading the muscle is to increase the volume of training performed (*i.e.*, the number of sets and repetitions of a particular exercise) or decrease the rest period between sets. (However, if increasing strength, *per se*, is the goal, then increasing the resistance appears to be the most important variable.) An important corollary is that progression must be varied as directed by the periodization principle of resistance training (see the following text) so that overtraining (see *Chapter 33*) is minimized or eliminated in an exercise prescription.

SPECIFICITY OF TRAINING

Specificity is very much the underlying principle of any exercise program. Adaptation is specific to the type of training program used, and only those muscles that are trained will adapt and change in response to a resistance training program. For example, light resistance will not activate many motor units; therefore, the muscle fibers contained in other motor units will neither be trained nor adapt to the loading (8). In addition, training the upper body only will not influence the lower-body muscle fibers or the whole muscle (21,23,24). Thus, resistance training is specific to the motor units that are activated and their influence on physiologic systems to support their homeostasis, repair, and remodeling.

SAID PRINCIPLE

SAID is the acronym for specific adaptations to imposed demands. The SAID principle states that the adaptations to resistance exercise are specific to the demands of the program (which, in turn, are determined by the acute program variables). This principle is an extension of the concept of specificity and underscores the importance of the exercise prescription in targeting those features of adaptation that are influenced by a specific resistance training program. These adaptations depend on the exercise range of motion and specific mode. For instance, isometric exercise may increase strength but only at the specific angle the exercise is performed.

PERIODIZATION OF TRAINING

Overtraining is a decrease in performance despite continued training. To eliminate the potential for overtraining and boredom in resistance training, variation in the exercise stimuli is vital. Periodization of training involves the systematic manipulation of the acute program variables over time with planned rest periods used to provide recovery, as opposed to the standard progressive overload method, in which the repetition range remains constant for several weeks while the weight is increased as strength allows. Unloading or lighter cycles of workouts also provide the body with recovery periods needed for optimal training. Both the classical linear periodization program (which manipulates workout protocols over each week within 4-wk microcycles) and the nonlinear method (which manipulates intensity, volume, and other acute program variables within a week) have been shown superior to standard progression programs (17,20,38,40).

PRIORITIZATION OF TRAINING

With any total conditioning program, one has to prioritize the training goals. Even within a periodized program, the trainable goals for resistance training are maximal strength, power, local muscular endurance, and muscle hypertrophy. As discussed in *Chapter 33*, many of the other systems adapt as well in support of these training goals (*e.g.*, connective tissue). Thus, each training cycle needs to have a training priority based on the goals of the individual.

NEEDS ANALYSIS

Before designing a resistance training program, a thorough needs analysis must take place (16). To ensure that the program is individualized, assessment should focus on goals and needs, such as the intended time frame for achieving these goals, targeted areas or muscle groups, health issues (*e.g.*, hypertension, asthma, diabetes), musculoskeletal limitations, recent surgeries, chronic injuries, and sites of pain. The needs analysis will dictate the prescription of the acute program variables and determine what energy systems and muscle actions are to be trained. Baseline fitness assessment, consisting of anthropometric measurements (*e.g.*, height, weight, circumferences), body composition, and tests of muscular strength and endurance, may assist in this by determining the level of the different fitness variables. In addition, follow-up assessments using these tools will provide feedback on progress. Designing an optimal resistance training program depends heavily on the individual strengths, weaknesses, and goals of the client (8).

METABOLIC DEMANDS

Each resistance training workout can be designed to give a very different metabolic response, ranging from short rest period workouts that are physiologically very demanding to heavy resistance workouts with long rest periods that focus on maximal force development (19,22). The metabolic demands of a resistance training program should match the goals of the individual. For example, short-rest, circuit-type programs help to develop acid–base tolerance and local muscular endurance, whereas heavy resistance training programs enhance maximal force production with little impact on local muscular endurance.

BIOMECHANICAL ACTIONS

Because of the principles of training specificity and SAID, fitness professionals must first conduct a thorough analysis of the movements performed by their clients during sports and ADLs before commencing with resistance training program design. Most training programs will include whole-body exercises to promote intramuscular coordination, exercises inclusive to both the upper and lower body musculature, and exercises that use all the muscles around each joint. Including these integral movements will ensure proper muscular development and transferability to the desired activity(s) performed by the client. Like acute program variables, the biomechanical portion of the needs analysis will be helpful in prescribing exercises and resistance levels that will best transfer to the primary sport or activity for which an individual trains.

INJURY POTENTIAL

Resistance exercises chosen should not predispose participants to injury. Rather, careful planning of the resistance training program can efficiently address the concept of "prehabilitation," or prevention of injury through planned, progressive improvements in strength and motor control of that strength. Further, exercises that address prior sites of injury are also important to eliminate the potential for tissue weakness and vulnerability in sport or recreational activities. For example, a client with a unilateral, injury-induced strength deficit may benefit from exercises that emphasize unilateral movements using dumbbells as opposed to bilateral movements using a barbell. With unilateral movements, the stronger, uninjured muscle group is unable to assist the weaker muscle group.

ACUTE PROGRAM VARIABLES

Once the needs analysis is completed, resistance training program design can occur (18). In program design, one has specific "tools" to work with, referred to as acute program variables. Examples of acute program variables include choice of exercises, order of exercises, split routines, number of sets, intensity of exercise, and the rest periods between sets and between exercises. Without an appreciation of how to properly implement and manipulate acute program variables, two fundamental flaws will occur: (a) all programs will look the same and, thus, not meet the specific needs of the individual and (b) the individual will not progress and training plateaus will ensue. Therefore, understanding the acute program variables and their influence on the effectiveness of a resistance training program is vital to optimal exercise prescription.

CHOICE OF EXERCISES

The choice of exercise is related to the biomechanical characteristics of the goals targeted for improvement. The number of possible joint angles and exercises are virtually limitless. Because muscle tissue that is not activated will not benefit from resistance training, the exercises should be selected so that they stress the muscles, joints, and joint angles specified by the client's needs analysis.

Exercises are designated as primary or assistance exercises. Primary exercises train the prime movers in a particular movement and are typically major muscle group exercises (*e.g.*, leg press, bench press, hang pulls). Assistance exercises train predominantly a single muscle group (*e.g.*, triceps press, bicep curls) that aid (synergists) in the movement produced by the prime movers.

Exercises may also be classified as multijoint or single-joint exercises. Multijoint exercises require the coordinated action of several muscle groups and joints.

Power cleans, hang power cleans, power snatches, dead lifts, and squats are good examples of whole-body multijoint exercises. The bench press, which involves movement of both the elbow and shoulder joints, is also a multijoint, multimuscle group exercise, although it only involves movement in the upper body. Other examples of multijoint exercises are the latissimus pulldown and military press.

Exercises that attempt to isolate the particular muscle group movement of a single joint are single-joint and/or single-muscle group exercises. Bicep curls, knee extensions, and knee curls are examples of isolated single-joint, single-muscle group exercises. Many assistance exercises are classified as single-muscle group or single-joint exercises.

Multijoint exercises require neural coordination to control several muscles working in concert. Multijoint exercises require a longer initial learning or neural phase compared with single-joint exercises; however, it is very important to include multijoint exercises in a resistance training program because most sports and functional activities in everyday life (*e.g.*, climbing stairs) depend on structural multijoint movements. For most sports, whole-body strength/power movements are the basis for success. Running and jumping — as well as activities such as tackling in American football, a takedown in wrestling, or hitting a baseball — all depend on whole-body strength/power movements. Thus, incorporating multijoint exercises in a resistance training program is important for both athletes and nonathletes. A basic program will include 8–10 different exercises (primarily multijoint) that work all the major muscle groups.

Many multijoint exercises, especially those with an explosive component, involve the need for advanced lifting techniques (*e.g.*, power cleans, power snatches). An important advantage to multijoint exercises is that they are time efficient, because several different muscle groups are activated in a single exercise. In addition, they allow for intramuscular coordination between joints. Multijoint exercises — in terms of muscle tissue activated, hormonal response, and metabolic demands — far outweigh the benefits of single-joint exercises, and most workouts should revolve around these exercises. Of course, because they involve more complex movements and larger muscle groups, the fitness professional must incorporate multijoint exercises into a training program judiciously and always with the abilities and disabilities of the client in focus.

ORDER OF EXERCISES

Sequencing of specific exercises within a session significantly affects force production and fatigue rate during a resistance exercise session (10). As already discussed (Choice of Exercises), multijoint exercises are more effective for increasing muscular strength than single-joint exercises. Therefore, these exercises should be given priority within the training session (*i.e.*, placed early in the training sessions when fatigue is minimal). Experts have made the following recommendations regarding exercise order (16):

When training all major muscle groups in a workout:

- Perform large muscle group exercises before small muscle group exercises.
- Perform multijoint exercises before single-joint exercises.
- Rotate upper- and lower-body exercises.

Also, for power training, perform total-body exercises (from most to least complex) before basic exercises. For example, perform power cleans before back squats (24). This is especially important when teaching new exercises.

When training individual muscle groups:

- Perform multijoint exercises before single-joint exercises.
- Perform higher intensity exercises (*i.e.*, those that require a greater percentage of one's 1-RM) before lower intensity exercises.
- An alternative technique sometimes used by bodybuilders is to perform single-joint exercises (*e.g.*, triceps extension) before multijoint exercises (bench press) to prefatigue the assistance muscles, thus increasing the overload on the primary muscles.

It is especially important to check for proper exercise technique anytime a change is made in the program design (*e.g.*, changing the order of exercise, changing the rest period lengths). This is especially important when rest period lengths are shortened because of metabolic fatigue or when resistances are increased. Changes in the program design could have an impact on the skills of a particular lift. Complex multijoint exercises (*e.g.*, power cleans) are more sensitive to such program alterations because of the higher technique demands.

Split Routines

Advanced lifters often use split routines, in which a portion of the body is trained two or three nonconsecutive days per week and a separate portion is trained on alternate days. This practice allows the lifter to perform a greater total volume of training without becoming overly fatigued in a given lifting session. Guidelines for the order of exercises are similar as for training the entire body in one workout. For example, when training upper-body exercises on 1 d and lower body exercises on a separate day:

- Perform large muscle group exercises before small muscle group exercises.

- Perform multijoint exercises before single-joint exercises.
- Rotate opposing (agonist and antagonist) exercises.

NUMBER OF SETS

This variable has received much attention, as the number of sets for an exercise is part of the total work equation for both fitness clients and elite athletes (34,35). When progression is desired for a given exercise, more work is needed (2,34,35,39). One to two sets of an exercise is a starting point for beginners because of limited tolerance of the exercise stress, whereas two to four sets is recommended for most adults to improve strength and power following the initial conditioning phase (9).

The number of sets performed for each exercise is a factor in the *volume* of exercise (*i.e.*, sets × repetitions × resistance). As such, one of the major roles of the number of sets performed is to regulate the volume performed during a particular exercise protocol or training program. In studies examining resistance-trained individuals, multiple-set programs have been found to be superior for strength, power, hypertrophy, and high-intensity endurance improvements (25). Continued recommendations by the ACSM is for the use of periodized multiple-set programs when long-term progression (not maintenance) is the goal (2). No study has shown single-set training superior to multiple-set training in either trained or untrained individuals. Thus, it appears that both single-set and multiset programs can be effective in increasing strength in untrained clients during short-term training periods (*i.e.*, 6–12 wk). However, meta-analysis of studies done on this topic support the contention that the greater training stimulus associated with the higher volume from multiple sets is needed to create further improvement and progression in physical adaptation and performance (26,39,40).

Variation in training stimuli, as will be discussed in detail later in this chapter, is also critical for continued improvement, and this variation often includes a reduction in training volume during certain phases of the overall training program. The determining factor here is in the "periodization" of training volume rather than in the number of sets, as sets is only one of the components in volume. Once initial fitness has been achieved, a multiple presentation of the exercise stimulus (typically two to four sets but as many as six in the training of athletes), with specific rest periods between sets allowing for the use of the desired resistance, is superior to a single presentation of the training stimulus (7,35). Some advocates of single-set programs believe that a muscle or muscle group can only perform maximal exercise for a single set; however, this has not been demonstrated. On the contrary, studies have found that with sufficient rest between sets, trained individuals can produce the same maximal effort during multiple sets (16).

Exercise volume is a vital concept in resistance training progression, especially for those who have already achieved a basic level of training or strength fitness. As mentioned earlier, the principle of variation in training — or, more specifically, "periodized training" — involves the number of sets and repetitions performed. Because the use of a constant volume program can lead to staleness and lack of adherence to training, variations in training volume (*i.e.*, both low- and high-volume exercise protocols) are important during a long-term training program to provide adequate rest and recovery periods. This concept is addressed later in the chapter under "Periodization."

INTENSITY OF EXERCISE

The amount of resistance used for a specific exercise is one of the key variables in any resistance training program (44). It is the major stimulus related to changes observed in measures of strength and local muscular endurance. When designing a resistance training program, the resistance for each exercise must be chosen in accordance with the abilities, disabilities, and goals of the participant. The **RM** is often used to designate intensity, defined as the greatest weight that can be lifted for a given number of repetitions with proper form. For example, the 10-RM is a weight that can be lifted 10 times, but not 11 times. Typically, a single training RM target (*e.g.*, 10-RM) or an RM target range (*e.g.*, 3- to 5-RM) is used. Throughout the training program, the absolute resistance is then adjusted to match the changes in strength, so the RM target (or RM target resistance range) continues to be used. Performing every set until failure occurs can be stressful on the joints, but it is important to ensure that the resistance used corresponds to the targeted number of repetitions. This is because performing four to five repetitions with a resistance that allows for only four to five repetitions compared with a resistance that would allow 14 or 15 repetitions produces quite different training results.

Another method of determining resistances for an exercise involves using a percentage of the 1-RM (*e.g.*, 70% or 85% of the 1-RM). If the client's 1-RM for an exercise is 200 lb (90.9 kg), a 70% resistance would be 140 lb (63.6 kg). This method requires that the maximal strength in all exercises used in the training program be evaluated regularly. Without regular 1-RM testing (*e.g.*, each week initially, or each month later in a program), the percentage of the true 1-RM used during training will decrease as the individual becomes stronger, and the relative training intensity will consequently fall. This is especially true at the beginning of a program when strength gains may be rapid. From a practical perspective, use of percentages of 1-RM as the resistance for many exercises may not be administratively effective because of the amount of testing time

required. In addition, for beginners, the reliability of a 1-RM test can be poor. It is therefore recommended that the RM target or RM target range be used as it allows the trainer to alter the resistance in response to changes in the number of repetitions that can be performed at a given absolute resistance. For general conditioning, lifting to the point of muscular fatigue (not complete failure) in 8–12 repetitions is recommended (corresponding to approximately 60%–80% of the 1-RM) (16) for most adults and 10–15 repetitions for older adults. Lifting to the point of muscular fatigue may be described as stopping the set when the lifter feels that he or she is unlikely to complete an additional repetition, whereas lifting to the point of complete failure refers to continuing to attempt additional repetitions until the lifter is unable to move through the full range of motion and must be spotted.

As is the case for all the acute program variables, the loading intensity should depend on the goal and training status of the client. The intensity of the loading (as a percentage of 1-RM) has an effect on the number of repetitions that can be performed and vice versa. It is ultimately the number of repetitions that can be performed at a given intensity that will determine the effects of training on strength development (13,14). If a given absolute resistance allows for a specific number of repetitions (defined as the RM), then any reductions in the number of repetitions without an increase in the resistance will cause a change in the training stimulus. In this case, the change in the stimulus will lead to a change in the motor units recruited to perform the exercise and, thus, the neuromuscular adaptations.

Specific neuromuscular adaptations to resistance training depend in large part on the resistance used. These adaptations follow the principle of specificity presented earlier in this chapter. Heavier resistances will produce lower numbers of repetitions (one to six) and have been found to lead to greater improvements in maximal strength (2,44). Thus, if development of maximal strength is desired, higher loads should be used. Alternately, if muscular endurance is the goal, a lower load should be used, which will in turn allow a greater number of repetitions (*e.g.*, 15–20) to be performed. Muscular hypertrophy requires that motor units are recruited, but for lower threshold motor units containing type I fibers, heavier loads (*e.g.*, 10-RM and heavier) are needed to stimulate muscle fiber hypertrophy (optimized by moderate loading and a moderate repetition range (4).

REST BETWEEN SETS AND EXERCISES

The rest periods play an important role in dictating the metabolic stress of the workout and influence the amount of resistance that can be used during each set or exercise. It also can affect proper technique and, with the popularity of "extreme exercise programs" commercially, care must be taken not to overshoot a client's physiological toleration (3). A major reason for this is that the primary energy system used during resistance exercise, the adenosine triphosphate (ATP)-creatine phosphate system, needs to be replenished, and this process takes time. Therefore, the duration of the rest period significantly influences the metabolic, hormonal, and cardiovascular responses to an acute bout of resistance exercise as well as the performance of subsequent sets. For advanced training emphasizing absolute strength or power (few repetitions and maximal or near-maximal resistance), rest periods of 3–5 min are recommended for large muscle mass, multijoint exercises (such as squat, power clean, or dead lift), whereas shorter rest periods (1–2 min) may be sufficient for smaller muscle mass exercises or single-joint movements (2). For a novice-to-intermediate resistance exercise protocol, rest periods of 2–3 min may suffice for large muscle mass, multijoint exercises because the lower absolute resistance used at this training level seems to be less stressful to the neuromuscular system. Performance of maximal resistance exercises requires maximal energy substrate availability at the onset of the exercise and a minimum fatigue level and, thus, requires relatively long rest periods between sets and exercises. Resistance training that stresses both the glycolytic and ATP-creatine phosphate energy systems appears to be superior in enhancing muscle hypertrophy (e.g., bodybuilding), thus less rest (1–2 min) between sets appears to be more effective in promoting local muscular endurance.

However, short-rest resistance training programs can cause greater psychological anxiety and fatigue (45), potentially because of the greater discomfort, muscle fatigue, and high metabolic demands of the program. Therefore, psychological ramifications of using short-rest workouts must be carefully considered and potentially discussed with the client before the training program is designed. The increase in anxiety appears to be associated with the high metabolic demands found with short-rest exercise protocols (i.e., 1 min or less of rest between sets). Despite the high psychological demands, the changes in mood states do not constitute abnormal psychological changes and may be a part of the normal arousal process before a demanding workout. The most important factor is physiological toleration because, in some clients, this type of short-rest workout might be contraindicated (e.g., clients with sickle-cell trait) (6). Dizziness, nausea, and vomiting are not indications of a "good workout," but rather indicate that the client has taken on too demanding of a workout or is showing signs of an emergency medical event. It is important for every professional in the field to know basic aspects of preventing sudden death in exercise and sports (5).

CHRONIC PROGRAMMING

Progressive resistance training programs often increase the absolute resistance over time (i.e., the weight increases), whereas the relative resistance (the RM range) does not vary. Such programs are considered constant in their approach to progression. However, greater variation in resistance training variables over time is vital for optimal results and has been shown to be superior to training programs that progress in a constant manner (2,44). Periodization is a type of chronic programming that allows for optimal variation of training.

PERIODIZATION OF TRAINING

Periodization of training has evolved into two specific models: classic (or linear) and nonlinear periodization. Classic periodization typically involves 2- to 4-wk periods called *microcycles*, in which the workouts within each microcycle are similar, and intensity is increased from one microcycle to the next. Nonlinear periodization uses great variation within each microcycle, such as having four or five distinct workouts in a 7- to 10-d period (17,37). Both are effective and are superior to constant relative resistance training programs (e.g., three sets of 8–10-RM) (20,28,47).

Classic (Linear) Periodization

Classic periodization methods use a progressive increase in the intensity with only small variations in each 2- to 4-wk microcycle (30,37). An example of a classic four-cycle linear periodized program (using 4 wk for each cycle) is given in *Box 31-1*. The group of four microcycles is termed a *mesocycle*. A long-term training program consisting of several mesocycles is termed a *macrocycle* (e.g., a 1-yr training plan).

BOX 31-1	**Sample Classic (Linear) Periodized Program**
Microcycle 1	**Microcycle 2**
3–5 sets of 12- to 15-RM	4–5 sets of 8- to 10-RM
Microcycle 3	**Microcycle 4**
3–4 sets of 4- to 6-RM	3–5 sets of 1- to 3-RM

Each microcycle lasts for 4 wk in this example. The group of four microcycles is a mesocycle. The next mesocycle would repeat the pattern with higher absolute resistance.

RM, repetition maximum.

There is some variation within each microcycle as the lifter progresses from the low end to the high end of the designated repetition range (and then increases the absolute resistance to return to the lower end of the repetition range). Still, the general trend for this example 16-wk program is a steady linear increase in the intensity of the training program (lower RM range in each succeeding microcycle) with a decrease in the volume of exercise (lower combination of sets × repetitions × weight in each microcycle, despite the increase in weight). Because of the straight-line increase in the intensity of the program, it has been termed as *linear periodized training*.

It is important to point out that one must be careful not to progress too quickly to train with high volumes of heavy weights. Pushing too hard can potentially lead to a serious overtraining syndrome. Overtraining can compromise progress for months. Although it takes a great deal of excessive work to produce such an overtraining effect, highly motivated trainees can easily make the mistake out of sheer desire to make gains and see progress in their training. Thus, it is important to monitor for signs of overtraining, such as decreased performance and undue fatigue.

High volume exercise in the early microcycles has been thought to promote the muscle hypertrophy needed to eventually enhance strength in the later phases of training (43). Thus, the late cycles of training are linked to the early cycles of training and enhance each other, as strength gains are related to size changes in the muscle. Programs that attempt to gain strength without increasing muscle tissue are limited in their potential.

The increases in the intensity of the periodized program develop the needed nervous system adaptations for enhanced motor unit recruitment. This happens as the program progresses and heavier resistances are used. Heavier weights demand high threshold motor units to become involved in the force production process. The associated increase in muscle protein in the muscles from the early cycle training enhances the force production of the motor units. Here again, one sees an integration of the different parts of the 16-wk training program.

The 16-wk program in the example provided is the mesocycle; a 1-yr training program, the macrocycle, is made up of several mesocycles (8). In classic periodization, each mesocycle in a single macrocycle uses the same pattern of sets and RM ranges, but the absolute resistance increases as the lifter improves. Each mesocycle attempts to progress the body's muscle hypertrophy, strength, and/or power upward toward one's theoretical genetic maximum. Thus, the theoretical basis for a linear method of periodization consists of developing hypertrophy followed by improved nerve function and strength (37). This is then repeated with each mesocycle, with a new resistance for each RM load, and progress is made in the training program.

Nonlinear Periodization

More recently, the concept of nonlinear periodized training programs has been developed to maintain variation in the training stimulus (17). The nonlinear program allows for variation in the intensity and volume within each microcycle (typically 7–10 d) over the course of the training program (*e.g.*, a 16-wk mesocycle). An example of a nonlinear periodized training program is given in *Box 31-2*.

In the nonlinear example, variation in training is much greater within the 7- to 10-d microcycle than in the 4-wk microcycle in the linear example described earlier. One can easily see that intensity spans over a large RM range (1-RM sets vs. 15-RM sets in the 1-wk cycle). This span in training variation appears to be as effective as linear programs. One can also add a "power" training day when loads may be from 30%–45% of 1-RM, and the light resistance allows for explosive movement (46). Training the entire force velocity curve is important in the variation in training (29). Exercise choice is vital as only power-type exercises should be used (*e.g.*, squat jumps, bench throws, hang power cleans, hang pulls). Exercises in which one holds onto the mass have a great deal of joint deceleration (*e.g.*, bench press) because of the mass not being released at the end of the range of motion to protect the joint (33). In essence, muscle activation in such situations is also inhibited; thus, they are not optimal exercises for increasing power output.

Different from the linear methods, nonlinear programs attempt to train both the hypertrophy and neural aspects of strength within the same week. Thus, one is working on two different physiologic adaptations within

---

BOX 31-2 **Sample Nonlinear Periodized Program**

Monday (Day 1)
4 sets of 12- to 15-RM

Wednesday (Day 2)
3–4 sets of 4- to 6-RM

Friday (Day 3)
4 sets of 8- to 10-RM

Monday (Day 4)
4–5 sets of 1- to 3-RM

Wednesday (Day 5)
Power day: 3–5 sets of 3 at 30%–45% of 1-RM or plyometrics

This protocol uses a 5-d rotation with 1 d of rest between each workout to create a 10-d microcycle. A mesocycle of, for example, 16 wk could be completed by increasing the absolute resistance in subsequent microcycles.

RM, repetition maximum.

the same 7- to 10-d period of the 16-wk mesocycle. This appears possible and may be more conducive to many individuals' schedules, especially when competitions, travels, or other schedule conflicts can make the traditional linear method difficult to adhere to.

In the nonlinear program, one rotates through the different protocols. The workout rotates between very heavy, heavy, moderate, power, and/or light training sessions. If one misses a given workout, the rotation order is just pushed forward, meaning one performs the missed workout on the next training day. For example, if the light (12- to 15-RM) workout was scheduled for Monday and it is missed, the lifter performs it on Wednesday and continues with the rotation sequence. In this way, no workout stimulus is missed in the training program. One can also say that a mesocycle will be completed when a certain number of workouts are completed (*e.g.*, 48) and not use training weeks to set the program length.

Again, the primary exercises are typically periodized, but one can also use a two-cycle program to vary the small muscle group exercises. For example, in the triceps pushdown, one could rotate between the moderate (8- to 10-RM) and the heavy (4- to 6-RM) cycle intensities. This would not only provide the hypertrophy needed for such isolated muscles of a joint but also provide the strength needed to support heavier workouts of the large muscle groups.

In conclusion, two different approaches can be used to periodize a training program: linear and nonlinear. The programs appear to produce similar benefits but are superior to constant training programs (4). It appears that this is accomplished by training either the hypertrophy component first and the neural strength component second in the linear method, or both components within a 7- to 10-d period in the nonlinear method. The key to workout success is variation, and different approaches can be used over the year to accomplish this training need.

BASIC TECHNIQUES IN RESISTANCE TRAINING

Basic understanding of various aspects of resistance training is vital to provide a safe environment for training. These techniques can include breathing, range of motion, repetition speed, and warm-up.

BREATHING

The lifter should inhale just before and during the eccentric (ECC) (lowering) phase of the repetition and exhale during the concentric (CON) (lifting) phase. During isometric training, the lifter should breathe throughout the muscular contraction. Although there is a tendency for lifters to hold breath during the last repetition of a set or during heavy lifts (*e.g.*, 1- to 6-RM), one should not allow breath holding throughout a complete repetition. When a

lifter holds his or her breath during effort and contracts the muscles of exhalation without allowing air to escape, intrathoracic pressure rises, resulting in a large increase in systemic arterial blood pressure. This is known as the Valsalva maneuver, and the increased arterial blood pressure can pose a hazard to individuals with underlying cardiovascular disease and may also result in damage to blood vessels (*e.g.*, in the eye, resulting in Valsalva retinopathy). The increased intrathoracic pressure limits venous return to the heart. If the Valsalva maneuver is held for several seconds (as during a maximal effort lift), the decreased venous return reduces cardiac output, arterial pressure falls, and blood flow to the brain is reduced. This can cause light-headedness and even fainting, which can result in loss of control of the weight and possible injury. This problem is especially true during maximal lifting and when going to failure in a set. One can limit the negative effects by using an RM zone and lifting to the point of muscular fatigue versus complete failure. If one exhales continuously through the CON phase of the lift, the problem can be avoided.

FULL RANGE OF MOVEMENT

Each exercise should be performed through a full range of motion in order for each part of the muscle to gain the benefits of the resistance used. With some resistance training machines, range of motion can be a concern if the machine poorly fits individual users. Many machines are designed to fit adult men. In smaller individuals, including prepubescent children, the limbs are too short for a proper fit, which makes correct technique and full range of motion of the exercise virtually impossible.

With some machines, simple alterations can be made to allow a child to safely use the machine, for example, use additional seat pads on a knee extension machine or use blocks under a bench for the child to place his or her feet. Simply adjusting the seat height often is not enough to make a machine fit the child. One may also need to adjust for proper positioning of the arms and legs on the contact points of the machine. In addition, raising the seat height may make it impossible for the child's feet to reach the floor. In many exercises, the feet need to touch the floor to aid in balance. Therefore, if the seat is raised, one may also need to place blocks under the child's feet.

MOVEMENT SPEED

When using maximal loads, movement speed will necessarily be slow. With submaximal loads, a lifter can choose to move the weight at various speeds. Maximal speed is used to move the weight explosively for power training. Slower speeds provide greater control over the weight. The speed of movement will often become slower during a set as fatigue occurs. This phenomenon was demonstrated in a study examining repetition velocity during a 5-RM bench press set. It was shown that the first three repetitions were 1.2–1.6 s in duration, whereas the last two repetitions were 2.5 and 3.3 s in duration, respectively (31).

Intentional use of a very slow velocity (10-s CON; 5-s ECC) compared with a slow velocity (2-s CON; 4-s ECC) has been shown to result in significantly less strength gains over a 10-wk training program (15). Compared with slow velocities, moderate and fast velocities have been shown to be more effective for increasing the number of repetitions performed, work and power output, and total volume of training (27,32) and for increasing the rate of strength gains (12).

WARM-UP

At the beginning of a resistance training session, a period of time should be devoted to warming up the muscles and preparing them for the intensity of the upcoming exercise. This may be accomplished by first performing 5–10 min of a general cardiorespiratory warm-up through such exercises as treadmill walking or stationary cycling. The general warm-up is followed by 5–10 min of specifically warming up the muscles to be targeted in the resistance-training session. This may involve dynamic stretching movements (see the following text) and the use of a light load on a preliminary set of each resistance exercise.

MACHINE AND FREE-WEIGHT EXERCISES

The use of free-weight versus machine resistance exercises is a topic of debate. The following are some points of comparison between the two modalities:

1. Machines are not always designed to fit the proportions of all individuals. Individuals who are obese have special physical considerations or disabilities, or are shorter, taller, or wider than the norm may not be able to fit comfortably in the machines and use them with ease. Free-weight exercises can easily be adapted to fit most clients' physical size or special requirements.
2. Machines use a fixed range of motion, thus the individual must conform to the movement limitations of the machine. Often, these movements do not mimic functional or athletic movements. Free weights allow for full range of motion, and the transfer to real-world movements is greater than for machines.
3. Most machines isolate a muscle or muscle group, thus negating the need for other muscles to act as assistant movers and stabilizers. Free-weight exercises almost always involve assisting and stabilizing muscles. On the other hand, if the goal is to isolate a specific muscle or muscle group, as in some rehabilitation settings or because of physical disabilities, machine exercises can more easily accomplish this.
4. Although it is never advisable to perform resistance exercise alone, machines do allow for greater independence as the need for a spotter or helper is usually diminished once the individual has learned the technique of the exercise. Moreover, it is simpler and easier to change the weight between sets when using machines. However, the perception of extra safety may lead to a lack of attention being paid to the exercise. It is still possible to become injured when using machines.
5. Machine exercises may be more useful than free-weight exercises in some special populations. One reason for this is that machines are often perceived to be less intimidating to a beginner. As the resistance training skill and experience level increases, free-weight exercise can gradually be introduced if desired. However, it is important to inform clients of the benefits that free weights have compared with machines (*e.g.*, increased musculoskeletal loading that reduces risk of developing osteoporosis) (16).
6. Some muscle groups can more easily be trained with specialized machines than with free weights (*e.g.*, training the latissimus dorsi with a pulldown machine).
7. Free-weights and many machines provide constant resistance, in that the external force (the weight being lifted) does not change. Some machines are designed to provide a variable resistance through the range of motion, providing less resistance when the joint angle is disadvantageous and more resistance when the joint angle is optimal. These variable resistance machines may be useful for providing a more consistent training stimulus through the range of motion. Some machines provide an accommodating resistance, in which the resistance is varied, typically by computer control, to force the joint to move at a constant angular velocity. The applicability of variable and accommodating resistance machines to real-world movements is limited compared to free weights.

From the comparison stated earlier, it is clear that there are advantages and disadvantages to both machines and free weights. In many cases, free weights are a superior training tool, but machine exercises can still be useful in resistance training when used appropriately. For midlevel and advanced clients and athletes, machines are best used as an adjunct to free-weight training. However, for beginners and some special populations, the ease of use may be an advantage when introducing an individual to resistance training. *Table 31-1* lists the common weight-training modalities and gives some examples and advantages and disadvantages of each.

SPOTTING REQUIREMENTS

Good spotting technique is vital for a safe resistance training program. Spotters should be cognizant of the following points:

1. Know proper exercise technique.
2. Know proper spotting technique for free weights or machines.

TABLE 31-1. Weight-Training Modalities

Modality	Definition	Examples	Advantages	Disadvantages
Variable resistance devices	Absolute resistance changes during the range of motion	– Machines with a cam or roll bar – Elastic bands	Increase the absolute resistance at the point in the range of motion where the musculoskeletal system is at a biomechanical advantage	At the beginning of a muscle contraction, the resistance is low and not offering a maximal tissue stimulus
Constant resistance devices	Absolute resistance remains constant throughout the range of motion	– Dumbbells – Barbells – Machines with a fixed pivot point or that use cables and pulleys – Medicine balls	Low or no limitation in the range of motion allowed Exercise can easily be adapted to accommodate for the size of an individual	Does not stimulate the neuromuscular systems involved maximally throughout the entire range of motion
Static resistance devices	Involve isometric muscle action	– Pushing against an immovable object, such as a wall	May be used for an athlete to overcome a sticking point	Not practical for most sports or for everyday functioning
Accommodating resistance devices	Maximum resistance throughout the whole range of motion is maintained by controlling the speed of the movement	– Hydraulic machines – Isokinetic devices	No real advantage over variable or constant resistive devices outside of a rehabilitation setting	Hydraulic machines typically have no eccentric movement Impractical Expensive

3. Be strong enough to assist the lifter with the resistance that he or she is using in a free-weight exercise.
4. Know how many repetitions the lifter intends to do.
5. Be attentive to the lifter at all times.
6. Stop the exercise if a movement technique is wrong. Have the lifter practice the exercise with little or no resistance.
7. Know the plan of action if a serious injury occurs.
8. Be prepared to assist the lifter with racking and unracking of the weights.
9. Do not assist the lifter with each repetition; rather, be prepared to assist if the lifter loses control or is unable to complete a repetition.
10. Use proper body mechanics as the spotter.

The goal of correct spotting is to prevent injury. A lifter should always have access to a spotter.

SUPPLEMENTAL EQUIPMENT

The three most commonly used strength-training accessories are a weight-training belt, gloves, and shoes. Although not absolutely necessary for a safe and effective strength-training program, all three do offer some benefits.

Weight-Training Belts

A weight-training belt has a wide back and is designed to help support the lower back. Although weight-training belts come in many sizes, a belt small enough to fit small children is not commonly available. A belt is not necessary for resistance training but is merely an aid to counteract a lack of strong abdominal and lower-back musculature.

Weight-training belts do help support the lower spine but not from the back as is commonly thought. The belt gives the abdominal muscles an object to push against, allowing a buildup of intra-abdominal pressure, which pushes against the lower spine from the front.

Wearing a tightly cinched belt during activity causes a higher blood pressure than if the activity is performed without a belt (11,38). This makes the pumping of blood by the heart more difficult and may cause undue cardiovascular stress. Thus, wearing a belt during resistance exercises in which the lower back is not heavily involved is not recommended. A belt can be worn during lifts involving the lower back, particularly when maximal or near-maximal loads are used, but it should not be used to alleviate technique problems that are caused by weak lower-back and abdominal muscles. Rather than allowing a lifter to rely on a belt, incorporate exercises into the program to strengthen the abdominal and lower-back muscles. This can help eliminate chronic lower-back weakness, which could otherwise lead to poor exercise technique. In addition, strong abdominals and lower-back muscles can help prevent injury to the lower back during all physical activity.

Weight-Training Gloves and Shoes

Specially designed resistance training gloves do not cover the fingers but only the palms. They protect the palms somewhat from such things as the knurling on many barbells, dumbbells, and equipment handles, and they may help prevent the formation of blisters or the ripping of calluses on the hands. However, gloves are typically not necessary for safe resistance training.

Weight-training shoes are mainly designed to provide good arch support, a tight fit, and a nonskid surface on the sole. In addition, weight-training shoes offer little or no shock absorbance in the soles; thus, any force or power that the lifter develops by extending the leg or hip is not used to compress the sole of the shoe and is available to lift the weight in such exercises as the squat or clean. A lifter should wear a shoe with a nonskid surface on the sole and good arch support, but it does not have to be a shoe specifically designed for power or Olympic weightlifting.

FLEXIBILITY TRAINING

Flexibility training can be done as part of the total conditioning program. Resistance training itself will help with this, but as one ages, additional flexibility training can cause greater augmentation. Flexibility is an important component of physical fitness and needs to be addressed in the context of both resistance and cardiorespiratory training programs.

TYPES OF FLEXIBILITY

Stretching can be performed in both the warm-up and cool-down phases of a training session. Dynamic stretching is recommended in the warm-up phase before resistance training because of possible negative influences of static stretching on muscle contractile forces (41). There are four basic types of stretching techniques:

- Static stretching
- Ballistic stretching
- Dynamic or slow movement stretching
- Proprioceptive neuromuscular facilitation (PNF) techniques

Static Stretching

The most common type of stretching is the static stretching technique. Use of this form of stretching typically involves a voluntary passive relaxation of the muscle while it is elongated. This technique has become popular because it is easy to learn, effective, and accompanied by minimal incidence of soreness. Static stretching is still one of the most effective and desirable techniques to use when comfort and limited training time are major factors in the implementation of a stretching program. In this technique, an opposing muscle or other external force is used to elongate the target muscle, and then the position of stretch is held for the desired time frame, typically 10–30 s. For example, in the figure-four hamstring stretch, a client sits with one leg fully extended along the floor and with the other leg bent such that the sole of that foot is against the knee or thigh of the extended leg. Using contraction of the hip flexors combined with the weight of the torso, the client leans forward to extend the

hamstrings (and gluteus maximus) of the extended leg. The stretch can be extended by the client pulling with the hands on the foot of the extended leg or by a partner or trainer applying pressure against the client's back. Two to four repetitions of the stretch are performed. The intensity of the stretch is usually defined as a feeling of tightness or slight discomfort.

Static stretches may also be performed with the target muscle in a state of contraction — an "active" as opposed to "passive" static stretch. Some yoga poses use this technique.

Ballistic Stretching

Ballistic stretching involves a swinging, bouncing, or bobbing movement during the stretch as the final position in the movement is not held. Ballistic stretching has become popular before maximal effort events or training, as this type of stretching has no negative effects on performance. Delayed muscle soreness in beginners who have no prior resistance training experience is possible with ballistic stretching.

Dynamic, Slow Movement Stretching

Slow movements of a muscle(s) — such as neck rotations, arm rotations, and trunk rotations — are a type of dynamic stretching activity. The value of using this type of stretching technique may be more important to warm-up activities than to achieving increases in flexibility.

Proprioceptive Neuromuscular Facilitation Techniques

PNF stretching techniques have increased in popularity as a method of improving flexibility. There are several variations of PNF techniques described in research literature and, unfortunately, the terminology is often overlapping or contradictory. Two basic techniques will be described here (42).

- Hold-relax (sometimes called contract-relax): After an initial passive stretch, the muscle that is being stretched is isometrically contracted for 3–6 s against resistance, subsequently relaxed, and passively moved into a greater stretch that is held for 10–30 s. For example, a client lies supine, and a trainer lifts one extended leg until the hamstrings are put in a position of stretch. Then the client forcefully contracts the hamstrings as if to return the leg to the floor, but no movement occurs as the trainer applies resistance. Following 3–6 s of this isometric contraction, the client relaxes the hamstrings, the trainer slowly moves the leg into a greater position of stretch, and this new position is held for up to 30 s.
- Agonist contract-relax: The procedure is the same as the hold-relax, with one addition. During the second stretch of the targeted muscle (e.g., hamstrings as

described earlier), the client contracts the opposing muscle group (quadriceps and hip flexors in this case; termed as the *agonist* as this muscle contracts concentrically) to assist the trainer in creating a greater range of motion.

The theoretic basis of these techniques is twofold (42). First, the isometric contraction of the muscle being stretched stimulates its own Golgi tendon organs, resulting in an autogenic inhibition of the stretched muscle, potentially increasing its subsequent stretch. Second, if the opposing muscle is contracted, this results in reciprocal inhibition of the muscle being stretched.

WHEN TO TRAIN FLEXIBILITY

Stretching to improve range of motion is typically performed after a cardiorespiratory or resistance training session and as a part of the cool-down. This has the advantage of exercising a neuromuscular system that is warm and physiologically more pliable to changes in the range of motion because of prior activity. A flexibility regimen of at least 10 min should be performed after other training sessions, with a minimum frequency of twice per week. Daily stretching is most effective for improving flexibility.

SUMMARY

Program design should be specific to training goals, but the potential for creating new resistance training programs is nearly unlimited. Via manipulation of acute program variables, it is easy to design many distinctly different programs. Further, any training systems, especially popular or faddish ones, should be evaluated in terms of their acute program variables and their ability to address the needs of an individual or sport. Determining which training system or systems to use depends on the goals of the program, time constraints, available training tools, and how the goals of the resistance training program relate to the goals of the individual's entire fitness program. However, the major goal of any program is to bring about physiologic adaptations (see *Chapter 33*) while providing the needed rest and recovery to avoid overtraining.

REFERENCES

1. Aagaard P, Suetta C, Caserotti P, Magnusson SP, Kjaer M. Role of the nervous system in sarcopenia and muscle atrophy with aging: strength training as a countermeasure. *Scand J Med Sci Sports*. 2010; 20(1):49–64.
2. American College of Sports Medicine. American College of Sports Medicine position stand. Progression models in resistance training for healthy adults. *Med Sci Sports Exerc*. 2009;41(3):687–708.
3. Bergeron MF, Nindl BC, Deuster PA, et al. Consortium for Health and Military Performance and American College of Sports Medicine consensus paper on extreme conditioning programs in military personnel. *Curr Sports Med Rep*. 2011;10(6):383–9.
4. Campos GE, Luecke TJ, Wendeln HK, et al. Muscular adaptations in response to three different resistance-training regimens: specificity of repetition maximum training zones. *Eur J Appl Physiol*. 2002;88(1–2):50–60.
5. Casa DJ. *Preventing Sudden Death in Sport and Physical Activity*. Sudbury (MA): Jones & Bartlett Learning; 2012. 367 p.
6. Casa DJ, Guskiewicz KM, Anderson SA, et al. National Athletic Trainers' Association position statement: Preventing sudden death in sports. *J Athl Training*. 2012;47(1):96–118.
7. Delorme TL, Watkins AL. Technics of progressive resistance exercise. *Arch Phys Med Rehabil*. 1948;29(5):263–73.
8. Fleck SJ, Kraemer WJ. *Designing Resistance Training Programs*. 3rd ed. Champaign (IL): Human Kinetics; 2004. 377 p.
9. Garber CE, Blissmer B, Deschenes MR, et al. Quantity and quality of exercise for developing and maintaining cardiorespiratory, musculoskeletal, and neuromotor fitness in apparently healthy adults: guidance for prescribing exercise. *Med Sci Sports Exerc*. 2011; 43(7):1334–59.
10. Hakkinen K, Komi PV, Alen M. Effect of explosive type strength training on isometric force- and relaxation-time, electromyographic and muscle fibre characteristics of leg extensor muscles. *Acta Physiol Scand*. 1985;125(4):587–600.
11. Harman EA, Rosenstein RM, Frykman PN, Nigro GA. Effects of a belt on intra-abdominal pressure during weight lifting. *Med Sci Sports Exerc*. 1989;21(2):186–90.
12. Hay JG, Andrews JG, Vaughan CL. Effects of lifting rate on elbow torques exerted during arm curl exercises. *Med Sci Sports Exerc*. 1983;15(1):63–71.
13. Hoeger WW, Barette SL, Hale DF, Hopkins DR. Relationship between repetitions and selected percentages of one repetition maximum. *J Appl Sport Sci Res*. 1987;1(1):11–3.
14. Hoeger WWK, Hopkins DR, Barette SL, Hale DF. Relationship between repetitions and selected percentages of one repetition maximum: a comparison between untrained and trained males and females. *J Appl Sport Sci Res*. 1990;4(2):47–54.
15. Keeler LK, Finkelstein LH, Miller W, Fernhall B. Early-phase adaptations of traditional-speed vs. superslow resistance training on strength and aerobic capacity in sedentary individuals. *J Strength Cond Res*. 2001;15(3):309–14.
16. Kraemer WJ, Adams K, Cafarelli E, et al. American College of Sports Medicine position stand. Progression models in resistance training for healthy adults. *Med Sci Sports Exerc*. 2002;34(2):364–80.
17. Kraemer WJ, Fleck SJ. *Optimizing Strength Training: Designing Nonlinear Periodization Workouts*. Champaign (IL): Human Kinetics; 2007. 245 p.
18. Kraemer WJ, Fragala MS. Personalize it: Program design in resistance training. *ACSM's Health & Fitness Journal*. 2006;10(4):7–17.
19. Kraemer WJ, Marchitelli L, Gordon SE, et al. Hormonal and growth factor responses to heavy resistance exercise protocols. *J Appl Physiol*. 1990;69(4):1442–50.
20. Kraemer WJ, Mazzetti SA, Nindl BC, et al. Effect of resistance training on women's strength/power and occupational performances. *Med Sci Sports Exerc*. 2001;33(6):1011–25.
21. Kraemer WJ, Nindl BC, Ratamess NA, et al. Changes in muscle hypertrophy in women with periodized resistance training. *Med Sci Sports Exerc*. 2004;36(4):697–708.
22. Kraemer WJ, Noble BJ, Clark MJ, Culver BW. Physiologic responses to heavy-resistance exercise with very short rest periods. *Int J Sports Med*. 1987;8(4):247–52.
23. Kraemer WJ, Patton JF, Gordon SE, et al. Compatibility of high-intensity strength and endurance training on hormonal and skeletal muscle adaptations. *J Appl Physiol*. 1995;78(3):976–89.
24. Kraemer WJ, Ratamess NA. Fundamentals of resistance training: progression and exercise prescription. *Med Sci Sports Exerc*. 2004; 36(4):674–88.
25. Kraemer WJ, Ratamess N, Fry AC, et al. Influence of resistance training volume and periodization on physiological and performance

adaptations in collegiate women tennis players. *Am J Sports Med.* 2000;28(5):626–33.

26. Krieger JW. Single vs. multiple sets of resistance exercise for muscle hypertrophy: a meta-analysis. *J Strength Cond Res.* 2010;24(4):1150–9.

27. Lachance PF, Hortobagyi T. Influence of cadence on muscular performance during push-up and pull-up exercises. *J Strength Cond Res.* 1994;8(2):76–9.

28. Marx JO, Ratamess NA, Nindl BC, et al. Low-volume circuit versus high-volume periodized resistance training in women. *Med Sci Sports Exerc.* 2001;33(4):635–43.

29. McBride JM, Haines TL, Kirby TJ. Effect of loading on peak power of the bar, body, and system during power cleans, squats, and jump squats. *J Sports Sci.* 2011;29(11):1215–21.

30. Medvedyev AS. Several bases on the methodics of training weightlifters. *Soviet Sports Rev.* 1987;22(4):203–6.

31. Mookerjee S, Ratamess N. Comparison of strength differences and joint action durations between full and partial range-of-motion bench press exercise. *J Strength Cond Res.* 1999;13(1):76–81.

32. Morrissey MC, Harman EA, Frykman PN, Han KH. Early phase differential effects of slow and fast barbell squat training. *Am J Sports Med.* 1998;26(2):221–30.

33. Newton RU, Murphy AJ, Humphries BJ, Wilson GJ, Kraemer WJ, Hakkinen K. Influence de la charge et du cycle etirement-raccourcissement sur l ' activation cinematique, cinetique et musculaire qui intervient lors d ' un mouvement explosif de la partie superieure du corps [Influence of load and stretch shortening cycle on the kinematics, kinetics and muscle activation that occurs during explosive upper-body movements]. *Eur J Appl Physiol Occ Physiol.* 1997;75(4):333–42.

34. Peterson MD, Rhea MR, Alvar BA. Applications of the dose-response for muscular strength development: a review of meta-analytic efficacy and reliability for designing training prescription. *J Strength Cond Res.* 2005;19(4):950–8.

35. Peterson MD, Rhea MR, Alvar BA. Maximizing strength development in athletes: a meta-analysis to determine the dose-response relationship. *J Strength Cond Res.* 2004;18(2):377–82.

36. Peterson MD, Rhea MR, Sen A, Gordon PM. Resistance exercise for muscular strength in older adults: a meta-analysis. *Ageing Res Rev.* 2010;9(3):226–37.

37. Plisk SS, Stone MH. Periodization strategies. *Strength Cond J.* 2003; 25:19–37.

38. Rhea MR, Alderman BL. A meta-analysis of periodized versus nonperiodized strength and power training programs. *Res Q Exerc Sport.* 2004;75(4):413–22.

39. Rhea MR, Alvar BA, Burkett LN. Single versus multiple sets for strength: a meta-analysis to address the controversy. *Res Q Exerc Sport.* 2002;73(4):485–8.

40. Rhea MR, Phillips WT, Burkett LN, et al. A comparison of linear and daily undulating periodized programs with equated volume and intensity for local muscular endurance. *J Strength Cond Res.* 2003; 17(1):82–7.

41. Rubini EC, Costa AL, Gomes PS. The effects of stretching on strength performance. *Sports Med.* 2007;37(3):213–24.

42. Sharman MJ, Cresswell AG, Riek S. Proprioceptive neuromuscular facilitation stretching : mechanisms and clinical implications. *Sports Med.* 2006;36(11):929–39.

43. Stone MH, O'Bryant H, Garhammer J. A hypothetical model for strength training. *J Sports Med Phys Fitness.* 1981;21(4):342–51.

44. Tan B. Manipulating resistance training program variables to optimize maximum strength in men: a review. *J Strength Cond Res.* 1999;13(3):289–304.

45. Tharion W, Harman E, Kraemer WJ, Rauch T. Effects of different weight training routines on mood states. *J Strength Cond Res.* 1991; 5(2):60–5.

46. Thomas GA, Kraemer WJ, Spiering BA, Volek JS, Anderson JM, Maresh CM. Maximal power at different percentages of one repetition maximum: influence of resistance and gender. *J Strength Cond Res.* 2007;21(2):336–42.

47. Willoughby D. The effects of mesocycle-length weight training programs involving periodization and partially equated volumes on upper and lower body strength. *J Strength Cond Res.* 1993;7(1):2–8.

SELECTED REFERENCES FOR FURTHER READING

Fleck SJ, Kraemer WJ. *Designing Resistance Training Programs.* 3rd ed. Champaign (IL): Human Kinetics; 2004. 377 p.

Kraemer WJ, Fleck SJ. *Optimizing Strength: Designing Non-Linear Periodization Workouts.* Champaign (IL): Human Kinetics; 2007. 245 p.

Kraemer WJ, Häkkinen K, editors. *Handbook of Sports Medicine and Science: Strength Training for Sport.* IOC Medical Commission Publication. Oxford (UK): Blackwell Science; 2002. 186 p.

Ratamess NA, editor. *ACSM's Foundations of Strength Training and Conditioning.* Baltimore (MD): Lippincott Williams & Wilkins; 2011. 560 p.

Zatsiorsky VM, Kraemer WJ. *Science and Practice of Strength Training.* 2nd ed. Champaign (IL): Human Kinetics; 2006. 251 p.

INTERNET RESOURCES

- American College of Sports Medicine: http://www.acsm.org
- National Strength and Conditioning Association: http://www.nsca-lift.org

Adaptations to Cardiorespiratory Exercise Training

Each day we engage in various types and intensities of physical activity. It may be carrying groceries, going for a 3-mile walk, playing soccer, or running an 800-m race. In each case, the cardiovascular, endocrine, pulmonary, blood (hematologic), and skeletal muscle systems must alter their function in a manner that allows the body to complete the activity. Additionally, repeated and regular exposure to physical activity or sports stimulates the body to develop long-term adaptations. It does this in a manner that is favorable for both exercise performance and health.

This chapter summarizes the chronic adaptations (training effects) that develop in the cardiovascular and pulmonary systems (collectively referred to as the cardiopulmonary system) when an individual participates in cardiorespiratory (aerobic) exercise training. It also describes the loss of these training adaptations that occurs when an individual stops training. Whenever possible, this chapter provides examples and data comparing healthy but untrained (sedentary) individuals with well-trained athletes to demonstrate how the cardiopulmonary system adjusts to exercise training.

CARDIORESPIRATORY FITNESS

Physical inactivity is a major contributing risk factor for cardiovascular disease, with an overall independent risk that is similar to dyslipidemia, cigarette smoking, and hypertension (1). Furthermore, longitudinal studies show that higher levels of aerobic or cardiorespiratory fitness, as well as physical activity, are associated with a lower rate of mortality from heart disease, even after statistical adjustments for other disease-related risk factors (5). This holds true for those with known heart disease (42,53). Given these findings, physical activity recommendations for exercise training have been established for both regular and older adults (24,29,33,52) and patients with existing cardiovascular disease, including coronary artery disease and heart failure (12,43,58,68).

Cardiorespiratory fitness is best described by maximal oxygen consumption ($\dot{V}O_{2max}$). Cardiorespiratory fitness is the maximal ability of the body to transport and use oxygen. It relies on the effective integration of the cardiovascular, pulmonary, hematologic, and skeletal muscle systems. To appreciate the effect of exercise training on $\dot{V}O_{2max}$, it is important to understand the factors that contribute to $\dot{V}O_{2max}$. Physiologically, it can be defined by rearranging the Fick equation (Adolph Fick, circa 1870):

$$\dot{V}O_2 = \dot{Q} \times a - \bar{v}O_2 \text{ (Also note that } \dot{Q} = HR \times SV)$$

Where: $\dot{V}O_2$ = oxygen consumption; volume of oxygen consumed per minute

$\dot{Q}$ = cardiac output; volume of blood ejected from the left ventricle per minute

---

KEY TERMS

Cardiac hypertrophy: Increase in the size of the heart; this may be an increase in the size of the ventricular chambers or an increase in the ventricular wall thickness; may occur following chronic cardiorespiratory training or as a result of cardiovascular disease.

Cardiorespiratory fitness: The ability to engage in physical activities that rely on oxygen consumption as the primary source of energy; best indicated by the body's ability to transport and use oxygen, that is, maximal oxygen consumption ($\dot{V}O_{2max}$).

Detraining: Changes in body structure or function caused by reduction or cessation of regular physical training.

Dyspnea: Labored breathing; shortness of breath disproportionate to the work being performed.

Overtraining: State in which there is altered mood and reduced exercise performance despite ongoing exercise training.

Rate–pressure product: Product of heart rate and systolic blood pressure; serves as an estimate of myocardial oxygen demand.

SV = stroke volume; volume of blood ejected from the left ventricle per heart beat

HR = heart rate; cardiac contractions per minute

$a - \bar{v}O_2$ = arteriovenous oxygen difference; volume of oxygen extracted per liter of blood

Based on the Fick equation, it should be clear that cardiorespiratory fitness (i.e., $\dot{V}O_{2max}$) is the product of the body's ability to transport oxygen (i.e., cardiac output [$\dot{Q}$], stroke volume [SV], heart rate [HR], blood volume, hemoglobin) and to use oxygen (i.e., myoglobin, aerobic capacity of muscle, arteriovenous oxygen difference [$a - \bar{v}O_2$]). Each of these components can affect the magnitude of $\dot{V}O_{2max}$ and can be influenced by age, sex, genetics, the volume and intensity of physical activity or inactivity, the environment (e.g., hypobaria, microgravity), medications, and illness. For example, someone with chronic heart failure has a reduced peak $\dot{Q}$, which results in a lower $\dot{V}O_{2max}$ (<50% of normal). On the other hand, a healthy person will have a lower $\dot{V}O_{2max}$ at 14,000 ft (4,300 m) than at sea level because of the reduced ambient pressure that reduces the diffusion gradient for oxygen from the alveoli to hemoglobin in the blood. In each example, $\dot{V}O_{2max}$ is reduced for different reasons, but the end result is a lower cardiorespiratory reserve (peak exercise minus rest) and increased physiologic responses (e.g., HR, ventilation rate) and, therefore, greater perceived effort at submaximal exercise.

PHYSIOLOGIC ADAPTATIONS TO CARDIORESPIRATORY (AEROBIC) EXERCISE TRAINING

OXYGEN CONSUMPTION

$$\dot{V}O_2 = \dot{Q} \times a - \bar{v}O_2$$

Improving cardiorespiratory fitness depends, in part, on the ability of the cardiovascular and pulmonary systems to adapt to a stimulus of regular bouts of physical activity. Many exercise studies involving healthy people demonstrate 10%–30% increase in $\dot{V}O_{2max}$ following 12–24 wk of exercise training, with the greatest percentage improvement from baseline occurring among the least fit (56). The upper limit of $\dot{V}O_{2max}$ in humans is likely ~85 mL · kg^{-1} · min^{-1} in men and ~75 mL · kg^{-1} · min^{-1} in women but may be <15 mL · kg^{-1} · min^{-1} in patients with congestive heart failure.

Factors contributing to the exercise training response of $\dot{V}O_{2max}$ have been elucidated through several reports from data obtained in the Heritage Family Study. The Heritage Family Study is a consortium of five institutions that have studied the variability in responses to 20 wk of exercise training among a heterogeneous group of more than 700 subjects (http://www.pbrc.edu/Heritage/index .html). Based on these data, researchers have concluded

that there are high, medium, and low responders to exercise training and that the *absolute change* in $\dot{V}O_{2max}$ is not related to age, sex, race, or initial fitness level. In general, initial fitness level is related to *percent change* in $\dot{V}O_{2max}$, in that those with initially low $\dot{V}O_{2max}$ experience greater proportional increases in $\dot{V}O_{2max}$ following training (67). In addition, data from the Heritage Family Study have also shown hereditary factors (e.g., genetic contribution) account for approximately 50% of the training response in $\dot{V}O_{2max}$ (7).

An absolute submaximal work rate, such as walking at 3 mph (4.8 kph), requires a fixed aerobic or oxygen requirement that is similar between humans. Activities like this will be perceived as easier and require less relative effort for individuals with higher cardiorespiratory fitness. A greater cardiorespiratory reserve allows individuals with a higher fitness level to work at a lower percentage of $\dot{V}O_{2max}$. On the other hand, activities of daily living, such as vacuuming, are perceived more difficult by those with lower $\dot{V}O_{2max}$ and therefore decrease cardiorespiratory reserve.

Enhanced oxygen transport, particularly increased maximal SV and $\dot{Q}$, is the primary mechanism underlying the increase in $\dot{V}O_{2max}$ with training. Other exercise training responses during submaximal or peak exercise that reflect improved cardiorespiratory fitness include changes in HR, $a - \bar{v}O_2$, peripheral resistance, blood volume, blood lactate, and ventilation. *Tables 32-1* and *32-2* summarize the physiologic responses to cardiorespiratory exercise training and provide common numerical values associated with those changes in previously unconditioned persons. Similar changes occur among moderately trained individuals who increase their exercise training, but the greatest relative changes occur in those that are initially sedentary.

TABLE 32-1. Normal Physiologic Adaptations to Cardiorespiratory Exercise Training

Variable	Rest	Submaximal Exercise[a]	Maximal Exercise
Workload	—	—	↑
Oxygen consumption	↔	↔	↑
Cardiac output	↔	↔	↑
Stroke volume	↑	↑	↑
Heart rate	↓	↓	↔ (or slight ↓)
Blood pressure	↓	↓	↔
$a - \bar{v}O_2$	↔	↔	↑
Minute ventilation	↔	↓ or ↔	↑
Blood volume	↑	—	—
Blood lactate	↔	↓	↑

↑, increase; ↓, decrease; ↔, no change; —, not applicable.

[a]Submaximal exercise refers to a standardized submaximal work rate, such as 100 W or walking at 2 mph (3.2 kph).

TABLE 32-2. Changes in Cardiovascular and Pulmonary Function as a Result of Endurance-Type Physical Training[a]

Measurement	Resting			Upright Submaximal "Steady-State" Exercise			Upright Maximal Exercise		
	Pre		Post	Pre		Post	Pre		Post
Heart rate (beats · min⁻¹)	70	$\bar{0}$	63	150	−	130	185	$\bar{0}$	182
Stroke volume (mL · beat⁻¹)	72	+	80	90	+	102	90	+	105
Cardiac output (liters · min⁻¹)	5.0	$\bar{0}$	5.0	13.5	$\bar{0}$	13.2	16.6	+	19.1
a − $\bar{v}O_2$ (arteriovenous oxygen difference) (vol %)	5.6	$\overset{+}{0}$	5.6	11.0	+	11.3	16.2	$\overset{+}{0}$	16.5
O_2 uptake (liters · min⁻¹)	0.280	0	0.280	1.485	$\bar{0}$	1.485	2.685	+	3.150
(mL · kg⁻¹ · min⁻¹)	3.7	0	3.7	19.8	$\bar{0}$	19.8	35.8	+	42.0
(METs)[b]	1.0	0	1.0	5.7	$\bar{0}$	5.7	10.2	+	12.0
Work load (kg · m · min⁻¹)	—		—	600	0	600	1050	+	1050
Blood pressure (mm Hg)									
Systematic arterial systolic BP	120	$\bar{0}$	114	156	$\bar{0}$	140	200	$\bar{0}$	200
Systematic arterial diastolic BP	75	$\bar{0}$	70	80	$\bar{0}$	75	85	$\bar{0}$	75
Systematic arterial mean	90	$\bar{0}$	88	126	$\bar{0}$	118	155	$\bar{0}$	152
Total peripheral resistance									
(dyne · s · cm⁻⁵)	1250	0	1250	750	$\bar{0}$	750	450	$\bar{0}$	390
Blood flow (mL · min⁻¹)									
Coronary	260	−	250	600	−	560	900	$\overset{+}{0}$	940
Brain	750	0	740	740	0	740	740	0	740
Viscera	2400	0	2500	900	$\overset{+}{0}$	1000	500	$\bar{0}$	500
Inactive muscle	600	±	555	500	0	500	300	0	300
Active muscle	600	−	555	10,360	$\bar{0}$	10,000	13,760	+	16,220
Skin	400	0	400	400	0	400	400	0	400
Total	5000		5000	13,500		13,200	16,600		19,100
Blood volume (liters)	5.1	$\overset{+}{0}$	5.3						
Plasma volume (liters)	2.8	$\overset{+}{0}$	3.0						
Red cell mass (liters)	2.3	$\overset{+}{0}$	2.3						
Heart volume (mL)	730	$\overset{+}{0}$	785						
Pulmonary ventilation (liters · min⁻¹)	10.2	0	10.3	44.8	$\bar{0}$	38.2	129	+	145
Ventilation rate (breaths · min⁻¹)	12	$\bar{0}$	12	30	−	24	43	±	52
Tidal volume	850	$\bar{0}$	855	1.5	$\overset{+}{0}$	1.6	3.0	$\bar{0}$	2.8
Lung diffusion capacity (D_L) (mL at STPD)[c]	34.1	0	35.2	40.6	$\overset{+}{0}$	42.8	48.2	+	50.6
Pulmonary capillary blood volume (mL)	90.1	+	97.2	129.3	+	141.2	124.5	+	220.0
Vital capacity (liters)	5.1	$\overset{+}{0}$	5.2						
Blood lactic acid (mM)	0.7	0	0.7	3.9	−	3.0	11.0	$\overset{+}{0}$	12.4
Blood pH	7.43	0	7.43	7.41	$\overset{+}{0}$	7.43	7.33	$\bar{0}$	7.29
Recovery rate					+			+	

[a]Estimated for a healthy man, age 45, body mass of 75 kg. Pre = pretraining; post = posttraining; minus (−) sign usually means a decrease in value with training; plus (+) sign usually means an increase in value with training; zero (0) sign usually means no change in value with training.

[b]A MET is equal to the O_2 cost at rest. One MET is equal to 3.5 mL · kg⁻¹ of body mass per minute of O_2 uptake or 1.2 kcal · min⁻¹.

[c]STPD is standard temperature (0°C), pressure 760 mm Hg, and dry.

Source: Data courtesy of W. Haskell.

Reprinted with permission from Brooks G, Fahey T, Baldwin K. *Exercise Physiology: Human Bioenergetics and Its Applications.* 4th ed. New York (NY): McGraw-Hill; 2005.

It is important to point out that the aforementioned increases in $\dot{V}O_{2max}$ are associated with repeated participation in an aerobic or large motor activity, such as walking/jogging, swimming, cycling, skating, or Nordic skiing. Resistance training, both dynamic (sometimes erroneously referred to as *isotonic*) and isometric, can have a small effect on improving cardiorespiratory fitness, but the magnitude of change is small compared with aerobic exercise training. This is not to say resistance-exercise training is not important. A balanced conditioning program that incorporates both aerobic and resistance training is preferred to help clients improve all aspects of fitness.

Regular aerobic exercise training in previously sedentary, apparently healthy people is associated with improved stamina, an improved ability to tolerate routine activities of daily living, and less fatigue during the day, often occurring within just weeks after starting a program. These changes in healthy people are largely caused by an improved cardiac or central response to exercise.

Modest levels of exercise volume (the product of intensity, duration, and frequency per week) can increase $\dot{V}O_{2max}$. This is illustrated in the study by Church et al. (9), in which they reported on more than 460 sedentary, low-fit, overweight/obese, postmenopausal women during 6 mo of aerobic exercise training of different exercise volumes. The lowest volume group exercised at just 50% of their peak $\dot{V}O_2$ for about 72 min $\cdot$ wk^{-1}, yet showed a 4% increase in peak $\dot{V}O_2$. Study groups assigned to increased duration of exercise, but also at 50% peak $\dot{V}O_2$, incrementally showed larger increases in peak $\dot{V}O_2$.

Patients with coronary artery disease who undergo aerobic training also experience improved function, and those who are symptomatic often experience a decrease in angina symptoms (65). In fact, until the late 1980s, when evidence was presented that regular exercise in these patients improved clinical outcomes (*e.g.*, mortality), the primary reasons for referring these patients to cardiac rehabilitation programs were symptom management and improved exercise tolerance. These reasons, along with the fact that most patients with clinically manifest coronary artery disease have cardiorespiratory fitness levels that are markedly below normal (50%–70% of age and sex predicted) (2), support the use of cardiac rehabilitation.

Aerobic exercise training has also been shown to improve peak $\dot{V}O_2$ in patients with heart failure, a population which typically exhibits very low aerobic capacity (<15 mL $\cdot$ kg^{-1} $\cdot$ min^{-1}). Although aerobic exercise training was widely considered to be a pathological stressor with the potential to worsen left ventricular characteristics for patients with heart failure until the late 1980s, considerable evidence now exists that regular aerobic exercise increases the oxidative capacity of these patients. Increases in $\dot{V}O_{2max}$ ranging from approximately 15%–45% have been observed following as little as 8 wk of cardiorespiratory exercise (12,43). Given the significant exercise

intolerance displayed by the this subgroup of patients, it is important to note that increased $\dot{V}O_2$ levels were found following aerobic training protocols using very low training intensities and frequencies ($\geq 40\%$ of $\dot{V}O_{2max}$; ≥ 3 d $\cdot$ wk^{-1}) (12). There is also evidence that interval training may be more effective than continuous aerobic training in patients with heart failure, allowing them to exercise at higher intensities using brief intervals of increased work, thus, providing a greater exercise stimulus while taking into account the exercise intolerance prevalent in this patient population (70).

CARDIAC OUTPUT

$$\dot{V}O_2 = \dot{Q} \times a - \bar{v}O_2$$

Maximum $\dot{Q}$ is significantly higher in trained than in untrained individuals, primarily because of the ability to increase SV (25,60). Among endurance-trained male subjects, maximal $\dot{Q}$ can exceed 30 L $\cdot$ min^{-1}, which represents a fivefold to sixfold increase over resting values. Among elite class endurance athletes, it is not uncommon to observe maximal $\dot{Q}$s near 40 L $\cdot$ min^{-1} (eightfold increase). Generally, the higher the maximal $\dot{Q}$, the higher the maximal aerobic power or $\dot{V}O_{2max}$. However, $\dot{Q}$ is essentially the same at any fixed submaximal work rate in both conditioned and unconditioned individuals (60). Among well-conditioned athletes, a small decrease may be observed, along with a decrease in $\dot{V}O_2$, because of improved economy of effort; however, these changes may not be observed in the average person. Although $\dot{Q}$ during submaximal exercise may not change following the exercise training, the ability to increase maximal $\dot{Q}$ does, which results in improved exercise capacity and $\dot{V}O_{2max}$.

STROKE VOLUME

$$\dot{V}O_2 = HR \times SV \times a - \bar{v}O_2$$

HR and SV both contribute to increases in $\dot{Q}$ during an acute exercise. SV increases during exercise secondary to (a) increased venous return (Frank-Starling mechanism), which allows left ventricular end-diastolic volume to remain unchanged or increase slightly, and (b) increased contractile state (perhaps by neurohormonal influences) (4,45,46). Regular aerobic exercise training also leads to cardiac hypertrophy, characterized by an enlarged ventricular chamber that does not exceed the upper limits of normal (<56 mm) and a proportionally increased wall thickness; considered together, the ratio of wall thickness to chamber diameter remains constant. For example, left ventricular end-diastolic diameter may approach 55 mm in highly trained endurance athletes versus <45 mm in inactive, age-matched unconditioned people (25). One important factor contributing to this adaptation of the left ventricle is the 10%–15% increase in blood volume that develops soon (days) after starting an exercise training program. Intensive exercise training usually results in blood volume increasing by approximately 500 mL through the expansion of plasma volume (13,31). Finally, another contributing factor induced by training is that it likely strengthens myocardial tissue and enables more forceful contractions (23,50,60,66). The result is an augmented ejection of end-diastolic volume (*i.e.*, increased ejection fraction). Cardiac hypertrophy may also develop in diseases such as hypertension or heart failure. Pathological hypertrophy, in contrast to the physiological hypertrophy developed following aerobic exercise training, is characterized by disproportionate increases in wall thickness or ventricular chamber that lead to either concentric (extensive wall thickening and decreased ventricular chamber) or eccentric (wall thinning with an extensive increase in ventricular chamber) hypertrophy. In either case, SV is often reduced as a result of either ventricular stiffening (concentric hypertrophy) leading to a decrease in the Frank-Starling mechanism or ventricular dysfunction (eccentric hypertrophy) caused by a decrease in the ventricular contractile state. Aerobic exercise training can also improve SV and $\dot{Q}$ in patients with heart disease. Improvements in exercise capacity are largely considered to be mediated by peripheral adaptations including improved skeletal muscle oxygen use (discussed later in this chapter), improved vascular endothelial function, and decreased sympathetic tone. However, an increasing amount of accumulating evidence in patients with heart failure indicates that increases in SV, ejection fraction, and $\dot{Q}$ are probable benefits of regular aerobic exercise (34,43,70). Additionally, some studies have shown increases in SV following exercise training in patients with heart disease using exercise intensities that exceed current recommendations (22).

As a result of aerobic exercise training, conditioned individuals are able to increase ejection fraction to a greater degree than their sedentary counterparts; hence, SV is higher in conditioned individuals at any fixed or relative submaximal work rate. The increased SV caused by training allows conditioned individuals to exercise at similar absolute work rates with a lower heart rate, thus decreasing the myocardial oxygen demand of submaximal exercise (45,46). The increase in ejection fraction is generally quite modest — approximately 5%–10% during maximal exercise. The aforementioned cardiovascular morphologic characteristics, along with increases in central blood volume and total hemoglobin, are closely correlated with $\dot{V}O_{2max}$.

HEART RATE

$$\dot{V}O_2 = HR \times SV \times a - \bar{v}O_2$$

HR is the second factor contributing to $\dot{Q}$. Among deconditioned persons, exercise causes a proportionally greater increase in HR from rest to any fixed submaximal work rate compared with better conditioned persons. Therefore, because of an attenuated SV response in untrained persons, HR plays a greater role in increasing $\dot{Q}$ during exercise of increasing intensity (62), such as during an exercise stress test.

In a meta-analysis by Cornelissen and Fagard (14), among 72 studies, exercise training resulted in an average reduction in resting HR of 7 beats $\cdot$ min^{-1}. The reduced HR may be caused by altered autonomic function (reduced sympathetic drive and increased parasympathetic drive) and an increase in blood volume. The increased blood volume results in a greater SV via the Frank-Starling mechanism. Maximal heart rate (HR_{max}) is unchanged or slightly decreased (3–10 beats $\cdot$ min^{-1}) after aerobic exercise training (25).

Although $\dot{Q}$ at rest or at a given submaximal intensity of exercise (*e.g.*, walking at 2 mph) does not change after an exercise training program, the $\dot{Q}$ is attained with a lower HR and greater SV. A lower heart rate (and, therefore, lower rate-pressure product; see discussion later in this chapter) requires less myocardial oxygen demand, which may mean delayed onset of angina for the person with exercise-induced angina or less shortness of breath during submaximal activities, such as typical activities of daily living.

ARTERIOVENOUS OXYGEN DIFFERENCE

$$\dot{V}O_2 = \dot{Q} \times a - \bar{v}O_2$$

A final major contributor to the training-induced increase in $\dot{V}O_{2max}$ is an improved $a - \bar{v}O_2$. The difference between arterial and venous content of oxygen in blood reflects the ability of skeletal muscle tissue to extract and use oxygen (55,60). Regular aerobic exercise training increases the number of capillaries surrounding each muscle fiber (25) and enhances the activity of mitochondrial enzymes used in aerobic metabolism, thereby enhancing the ability to extract and use the oxygen that is transported in circulating blood. This increased ability to transport oxygen to the working skeletal muscle and to remove and use it to generate energy is a hallmark adaptation of aerobic exercise training and occurs in both healthy and diseased individuals.

As was the case for $\dot{Q}$, $a - \bar{v}O_2$ is similar in trained and untrained persons at submaximal levels of exercise. However, at $\dot{V}O_{2max}$, $a - \bar{v}O_2$ difference is greater in trained than untrained persons (*e.g.*, 155 mL $\cdot$ L^{-1} vs. 135 mL $\cdot$ L^{-1}, respectively). Regular aerobic exercise training enhances the ability to increase $a - \bar{v}O_2$, which contributes to increased exercise capacity.

BLOOD PRESSURE AND BLOOD FLOW

Mean arterial blood pressure (BP) (P_{mean}) is relatively constant during exercise at intensities below 50% of $\dot{V}O_{2max}$ but increases in a relatively linear fashion at exercise intensities above 60% of $\dot{V}O_{2max}$ (*Fig. 32-1*). (51). P_{mean} can be expressed as follows:

$$P_{mean} = 1/3 \text{ (systolic BP} - \text{diastolic BP)} + \text{diastolic BP}$$

Note: At higher heart rates,

$$P_{mean} = 1/2 \text{ (systolic BP} - \text{diastolic BP)} + \text{diastolic BP}$$

$$P_{mean} = \dot{Q} \times T_SP_R$$

Where: $\dot{Q}$ = cardiac output
BP = blood pressure
T_SP_R = total systemic peripheral resistance

Primary control of BP is regulated by alterations in total systemic peripheral resistance (T_SP_R), which is accomplished by (a) neural mechanisms affecting peripheral arterioles, (b) locally released substances called endothelial-derived relaxing factors (the most studied is nitric oxide), and (c) changes in local chemistry (*e.g.*, temperature, hydrogen and potassium ions, adenosine) within the metabolically more active skeletal muscles (40,48). There is vasoconstriction in some areas (*e.g.*, splanchnic areas) during exercise and vasodilation in others (*e.g.*, skeletal muscle and myocardium). The overall effect is a decreased total peripheral resistance (25,66). These changes in vasomotor tone allow for a 15-fold or more increase in blood flow to the metabolically active skeletal muscles, a reduction of blood flow to the splanchnic areas, an increase in blood flow to the heart, and maintenance of blood flow to the central nervous system.

P_{mean} increases during an acute bout of progressively increasing exercise (such as during an exercise stress test) in healthy individuals because the magnitude of the increase in $\dot{Q}$ is greater than the decrease in T_SP_R. Because diastolic BP remains constant or may decrease slightly in both conditioned and unconditioned individuals, the increase in P_{mean} is mostly because of increased systolic BP.

Relative to pretraining, after an exercise training program, P_{mean} mean arterial and systolic BP at a fixed submaximal work rate (*e.g.*, walking at 2 mph) will be reduced, with no change in maximum BP. The greater maximum $\dot{Q}$ following training despite no change in maximum BP indicates that training increases the maximum vasodilatory capacity of the trained muscles. Greater vasodilation leads to a greater reduction in T_SP_R, allowing a greater volume of blood to be pumped without requiring a higher BP. Systolic BP at rest and at a fixed work rate is generally lower in trained than untrained people. In individuals with known mild or moderate hypertension, regular exercise training lowers resting systolic BP by 4–9 mm Hg (8). In a meta-analysis involving 72 studies of exercise training, Cornelissen and Fagard (14) concluded that exercise training among persons without hypertension lowered resting BP by 3.0 and 2.4 mm Hg for systolic and diastolic BP, respectively. The training effect was greater among those with hypertension, where resting systolic and diastolic BP were reduced by 6.9 and 4.9 mm Hg, respectively. Proposed mechanisms responsible for this decrease include neurohumoral, vascular, and structural adaptations. A decrease in plasma catecholamines, improved insulin sensitivity, and favorable changes in endogenous vasoconstricting and vasodilating agents have also been postulated as responsible for the antihypertensive effects of regular exercise training.

After a single bout of exercise, resting systolic BP will be reduced and will remain below preexercise values for up to 24 h. However, although instructive for patients, it is important to understand that this effect is likely a result of reduced T_SP_R that occurs during exercise and not a result of permanent biologic adaptations that occur following a program of aerobic exercise training.

RATE–PRESSURE PRODUCT

At rest, the heart consumes about 70% of the oxygen it receives from blood flowing through the coronary arteries, which is almost three times that of skeletal muscle. As a result, the heart responds to increased demand for oxygen by increasing blood flow. In fact, coronary blood flow can increase fourfold from rest to maximal exercise in an adult without coronary artery disease from 250 mL $\cdot$ min^{-1} to approximately 1,000 mL $\cdot$ min^{-1}.

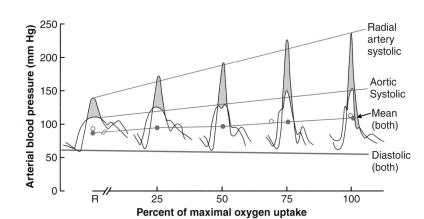

FIGURE 32-1. Simultaneously measured systolic, diastolic, and mean arterial pressures at rest and during upright exercise in the radial artery and aorta. (Adapted with permission from Rowell LB, Brengelmann GL, Blackmon JR, Bruce RA, Murray JA. Disparities between aortic and peripheral pulse pressures induced by upright exercise and vasomotor changes in man. *Circulation.* 1968;37[6]:954–64; and Rowell LB. *Human Circulation: Regulation During Physical Stress.* New York [NY]: Oxford University Press; 1986. 416 p.)

The main factors that influence **myocardial oxygen demand** are HR, left ventricular size, myocardial contractility, and type of work being performed (pressure vs. volume, *e.g.*, snow shoveling vs. jogging, respectively). However, except for HR, it is difficult to gather these measures in most exercise physiology laboratories. The product of HR and systolic BP provides a reasonable estimate of myocardial oxygen demand, called the rate–pressure product (RPP) (also known as double product). RPP is defined as:

$$RPP = HR \times SBP$$

Where: RPP = rate–pressure product
HR = heart rate
SBP = systolic blood pressure

After a program of aerobic exercise training, the magnitude of increase in RPP from rest to a given submaximal work rate is less compared with pretraining values. This attenuated increase is attributable to the previously mentioned adaptations in HR and BP, both of which increase less after training and translate to a lesser increase in RPP and myocardial oxygen demand. Collectively, this translates into a reduced oxygen demand for a given cardiac workload, resulting in improved efficiency of the heart.

PULMONARY FUNCTION

Because of the pulmonary system's ability to respond quickly to acute exercise and the fact that it does not normally limit maximal exercise, the demand for pulmonary system adaptations to exercise training is less than other systems (*e.g.*, cardiovascular, skeletal muscle). However, there are several pulmonary-related adaptations that result from a program of aerobic exercise training.

Before discussing these adaptations, it is important to point out that among patients with pulmonary diseases —such as those with chronic bronchitis, emphysema, or asthma—limitations in pulmonary function caused by the disease often minimize expected physiologic gains attributable to exercise training. Also, the dyspnea or labored breathing that is associated with most pulmonary disorders often causes individuals to avoid being active, which leads to a vicious circle of further self-imposed activity restriction. This does not mean that these patients do not improve exercise tolerance as a result of participating in an exercise or pulmonary rehabilitation program. Both submaximal endurance and total walking time are usually improved but typically with little change in $\dot{V}O_{2max}$.

MINUTE VENTILATION

Minute ventilation ($\dot{V}_E$) during exercise is augmented by increasing tidal volume (V_T) and breathing frequency. Ventilation is controlled by neural and chemical factors and by sensory mechanisms within the lungs and ventilatory muscles. Although ventilation generally does not limit exercise performance in apparently healthy individuals, the limits of ventilation may be reached at maximal exercise in elite aerobic trained athletes (25). $\dot{V}_E$ can be defined as:

$$\dot{V}_E = V_T \times f_B$$

Where: $\dot{V}_E$ = minute ventilation; volume of air expired per minute
V_T = tidal volume; volume of air expired per breath
f_B = breathing frequency; breaths per minute

Following a program of exercise training, $\dot{V}_E$ is unchanged at rest ($\sim$6 L · min^{-1}; V_T is $\sim$500 mL · breath^{-1}; breathing frequency [f_B] is $\sim$12 breaths · min^{-1}). However, $\dot{V}_E$ at maximal exercise is increased after training, with the increase attributable to increases in both maximal V_T and f_B. V_T and f_B may approach 3,000 mL · breath^{-1} and 55 breaths · min^{-1}, respectively.

Whereas untrained college-aged individuals may achieve a peak ventilation of 120 L · min^{-1}, a 60-yr-old patient with heart disease might only achieve a peak value of 60–80 L · min^{-1}. In both cases, it is reasonable to assume that an aerobic exercise training program will increase peak minute ventilation by 15%–25%. In contrast, well-conditioned male and female athletes may achieve peak ventilation that approaches 200 L · min^{-1} and 150 L · min^{-1}, respectively. Although exercise training may increase maximal ventilatory capacity, it is unclear that this provides any advantage except at peak exercise. Higher ventilatory capacity might increase the buffering capacity for lactate (via increased expiration of CO_2) and allow the partial pressure of oxygen in the alveoli to be maintained in the face of increased pulmonary blood flow to keep hemoglobin saturated. Because ventilation does not limit the ability to perform maximal exercise in apparently healthy persons, increased maximal ventilation following exercise training is likely a consequence of the increased peak workload and $\dot{V}O_{2max}$.

$\dot{V}_E$ at a standardized submaximal work rate decreases or is unchanged following exercise training. This is likely because of improved pulmonary diffusion. Ventilation changes in tandem with CO_2 because of neural feedback mechanisms that control ventilation in response to changes in blood pH (*i.e.*, hydrogen ion concentrations). Therefore, if following exercise training lactate threshold is delayed (*e.g.*, occurs at a higher work rate), then ventilation will also be lower. This will also be seen in an increased ventilatory efficiency, as evidenced by a reduced ventilatory equivalent for oxygen ($\dot{V}_E/\dot{V}O_2$) in trained, compared with untrained, individuals. Individuals with heart disease in which abnormal ventilatory control is frequently present, such as congestive heart failure, also exhibit reductions in $\dot{V}_E$ and improved ventilatory efficiency following aerobic exercise training, possibly resulting from increased lung alveolar diffusion capacity (12).

PULMONARY DIFFUSION CAPACITY

Diffusion capacity is defined as the volume of gas that diffuses through a membrane each minute for a partial pressure difference (*i.e.*, gas concentration difference) of 1 mm Hg. During exercise, diffusion capacity increases in a near linear manner before leveling off near peak exercise. This pattern is observed in trained and untrained individuals, regardless of sex.

At rest and during submaximal and peak exercise, diffusion capacity is greater in endurance-trained individuals. Functionally, this means that O_2 and CO_2 will pass between blood and alveoli more easily in trained persons. Among untrained and trained individuals, maximal diffusion capacity may approach 54 and 74 mL $O_2 \cdot min^{-1} \cdot mm\ Hg^{-1}$, respectively (25). It is common to note that the resting diffusion capacity of well-trained runners may approach the values observed at maximal exercise in unconditioned individuals, which may contribute to decreased ventilation at rest and submaximal exercise. The precise mechanism responsible for the increase in diffusion capacity with exercise training is unknown.

LACTATE AND VENTILATORY THRESHOLDS

The lactate threshold is the exercise intensity or oxygen consumption during incremental exercise when the blood lactate concentration rises abruptly (see *Chapter 3*). Blood lactate concentrations throughout submaximal exercise are reduced as a result of exercise training (*Fig. 32-2*). Conversely, following exercise training, the intensity of exercise (*e.g.*, speed of running, swimming, cycling) at the lactate threshold is increased, reflecting an improved ability to perform at a higher absolute workload (and $\dot{V}O_2$). Among athletes, it is common to guide training intensity using lactate threshold. For example, among elite male rowers, swimmers, and cyclists, the HR or work rate

corresponding to their individual lactate threshold is identified and then used to guide training intensity at below or above their lactate threshold.

Although the precise physiologic adaptations responsible for the aforementioned decrease in blood lactate during submaximal exercise are unknown, there are several possibilities. These include a smaller oxygen deficit incurred at the beginning of exercise attributable to a faster adjustment of oxygen uptake (oxygen kinetics) relative to energy demand; a greater clearance of lactate from the blood produced during exercise, as it is metabolized via the Cori cycle in the liver and also used as an energy source by other organs; and exercise training–induced increases in the size of skeletal muscle mitochondria and in the concentration of enzymes involved in fatty acid oxidation. Concerning the last point, the net result is an improved ability of the skeletal muscle to use fatty acids and to operate aerobically during prolonged exercise versus having to rely as much on anaerobic glycolysis to generate adenosine trisphosphate (ATP).

As discussed in *Chapter 3*, lactate threshold can be noninvasively identified using ventilatory gas exchange data (*i.e.*, ventilatory threshold) collected during a progressive exercise test. Changes in ventilatory threshold will parallel expected changes in lactate threshold.

DETRAINING AND BED REST

Although exercise training promotes various physiologic adaptations, long periods of inactivity (*i.e.*, **detraining**) are associated with a reversal of many of these favorable chronic changes. This detraining concept implies that when physical training is stopped or reduced, the organ systems readjust in accordance with the diminished physiologic stimuli.

An extreme example of detraining is bed rest, such as when a person suffers a myocardial infarction and is then confined to bed rest while in the hospital. In the 1960s, such a person may have been ordered to bed rest for up to 3 wk in the hospital. Upon arriving home, these people often reported being easily fatigued and having a loss of stamina throughout the day, much of it are caused by the marked effect that occurred during bed rest (63). Bed rest results in significant deconditioning and also causes central circulatory changes associated with remaining horizontal for a prolonged period of time (*e.g.*, orthostatic hypotension will occur when attempting to become upright).

Today, patients who suffer from an uncomplicated myocardial infarction are encouraged to ambulate within 48–72 h of their event and usually find themselves discharged for home within 3–5 d. People who suffer from a myocardial infarction today spend much less time in bed, which means much less detraining and preserved exercise tolerance and $\dot{V}O_{2max}$.

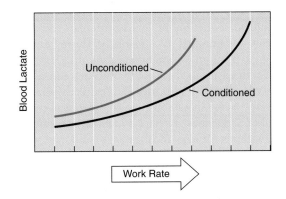

FIGURE 32-2. Blood lactate at increasing exercise intensities in conditioned versus unconditioned persons. The conditioned person typically exhibits lower lactate concentrations at any given work rate than the unconditioned person but reaches a higher maximum lactate.

MAXIMAL OXYGEN CONSUMPTION

Moderate endurance training increases $\dot{V}O_{2max}$ by 10%–30%, mostly attributable to increases in $\dot{Q}$ and SV (6,62). Conversely, prolonged detraining (8–10 wk or more) has been reported to result in a complete return of $\dot{V}O_{2max}$ to pretraining levels (54). Generally, $\dot{V}O_{2max}$ values decline rapidly during the first month of inactivity, with a slower decline to untrained levels occurring during the second and third months of detraining (21,25,28,44). Therefore, the available evidence suggests that increases in $\dot{V}O_{2max}$ produced by endurance training involving exercise of low-to-moderate intensities and durations are totally reversed after several months of detraining and adoption of a more sedentary lifestyle.

Whether an extended history of intensive endurance training results in a more persistent maintenance of $\dot{V}O_{2max}$ after subsequent inactivity than shorter periods of less intensive training has also been studied (18). *Figure 32-3* illustrates the time course of the decline in $\dot{V}O_{2max}$ and related variables (SV, HR, and a $-$ $\bar{v}O_2$) when subjects become sedentary after training intensively for approximately 10 yr (17). Note the rapid decline in $\dot{V}O_{2max}$ in the first 12–21 d and its association with a marked decline in maximal SV. *Table 32-3* compares a sedentary group with an athletic group and the changes associated with detraining at the central and peripheral levels (15,17,18).

STROKE VOLUME

Whereas prolonged intensive endurance training promotes increased heart mass (*i.e.*, cardiac hypertrophy), detraining typically results in decreased heart mass (23,37,48), although not all studies report a decrease (19,57). It is not clear whether training-induced increases

TABLE 32-3. Data for Sedentary Subjects ($n = 8$) Compared with Highly Trained Athletes ($n = 6$) Before and After 3 Months of Detraining

	Sedentary Group	Athlete Group	
		Trained	Detrained
$\dot{V}O_{2max}$ (mL $\cdot$ kg^{-1} $\cdot$ min^{-1})	43.3	62.1*	50.8*,†
Maximum stroke volume (mL $\cdot$ beat^{-1})	128	148*	129†
Maximum a $-$ $\bar{v}O_2$ (mL O_2 $\cdot$ L blood^{-1})	12.6	15.1*	14.1*,†
$\dot{V}O_2$ at lactate threshold (mL $\cdot$ kg^{-1} $\cdot$ min^{-1})	26.9	49.2*	37.6*,†
Submaximal $\dot{V}_E$ (L $\cdot$ min^{-1})	—	70.5	90.0†
Submaximal heart rate (beats $\cdot$ min^{-1})	—	158	184†

$\dot{V}O_{2max}$, maximal oxygen consumption; a $-$ $\bar{v}O_2$, arteriovenous oxygen difference; $\dot{V}O_2$, oxygen consumption; $\dot{V}_E$, minute ventilation.

*$p < 0.05$ for trained athletes or detrained athletes versus sedentary group.

†$p < 0.05$ for trained athletes versus detrained athletes.

Adapted from Coyle EF, Martin WH 3rd, Bloomfield SA, Lowry OH, Holloszy JO. Effects of detraining on responses to submaximal exercise. *J Appl Physiol.* 1985; 59(3):853–9; and Coyle EF, Martin WH 3rd, Sinacore DR, Joyner MJ, Hagberg JM, Holloszy JO. Time course of loss of adaptations after stopping prolonged intense endurance training. *J Appl Physiol.* 1984;57(6):1857–64.

in left ventricular dimension and myocardial contractility regress totally with inactivity. Athletes who become sedentary have larger hearts and higher $\dot{V}O_{2max}$ than those of people who have never trained (64).

One of the most striking effects of detraining in endurance-trained individuals is the rapid decline in SV. Martin et al. (47) measured SV during exercise in trained subjects in both the upright and supine positions and again after 21 and 56 d of inactivity (*Fig. 32-4*). The large decline in SV during upright cycling was associated with parallel reductions in left ventricular end-diastolic diameter. However, when the subjects exercised in the supine position, which usually augments ventricular filling because of increased venous return from elevated lower extremities, reduction in left ventricular end-diastolic diameter was minimal. As a result, SV during exercise in the supine position was maintained within a few percentage of trained levels during the 56-d detraining period. These observations indicate that cardiac filling is an important factor in establishing SV during exercise and that when it declines, perhaps as a result of reductions in blood volume, SV also declines.

BLOOD VOLUME

It appears that the rapid detraining-induced reduction of SV during exercise in the upright position is related to a decrease in blood volume (16). Blood volume increases within the first few days of an exercise training program but quickly reverses when training ceases. Therefore, the

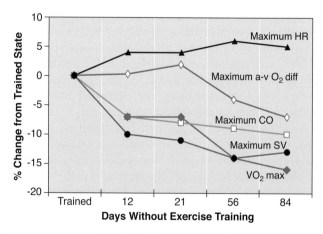

FIGURE 32-3. Effects of detraining on changes in heart rate (HR), arteriovenous oxygen difference (a $-$ $\bar{v}O_2$), stroke volume (SV), and oxygen consumption ($\dot{V}O_2$) at maximum exercise. (Adapted from Coyle EF, Martin WH 3rd, Sinacore DR, Joyner MJ, Hagberg JM, Holloszy JO. Time course of loss of adaptations after stopping prolonged intense endurance training. *J Appl Physiol.* 1984;57[6]:1857–64.)

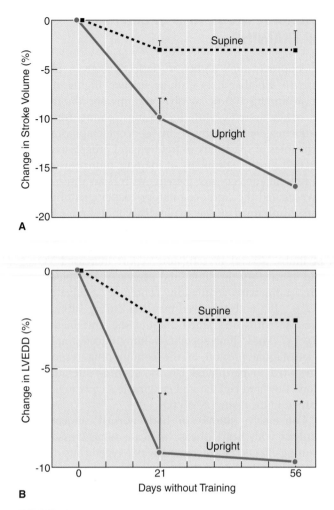

FIGURE 32-4. Percentage decline in exercise stroke volume **(A)** and left ventricular end-diastolic diameter (LVEDD) **(B)** during exercise in the upright and supine positions when trained and after 21 and 56 d of inactivity (solid line indicates upright, dashed line indicates supine). *Responses in upright position are significantly ($p < .05$) lower than in supine position and lower than when trained. (Reprinted with permission from Costill DL, Fink WJ, Hargreaves M, et al. Metabolic characteristics of skeletal muscle during detraining from competitive swimming. *Med Sci Sports Exerc.* 1985;17:339–43.)

decline in SV and the increase in HR during submaximal exercise, which normally accompany several weeks of detraining, can be reversed, returning to near-trained levels when the blood volume is artificially expanded to a level similar to that of trained subjects (16).

Because SV during exercise is maintained close to trained levels when blood volume is high, the ability of the heart to fill with blood is not significantly altered by detraining. If ventricular mass does decrease, then the thinning of ventricular walls, not decreased left ventricle end-diastole diameter, may be responsible (47). Thus, decreased intrinsic cardiovascular function, at least during submaximal exercise, is apparently minimal after several weeks of inactivity in men who had been training intensively for several years (16). The large reduction in SV

during exercise in the upright position is largely a result of reduced blood volume, not deterioration of heart function.

HEART RATE

HR_{max} may increase slightly with detraining, reflecting compensation by the cardiovascular system to offset the large reductions in blood volume and SV. Coyle et al. (18) observed 4% and 6% increases in HR_{max} after 3 and 12 wk of inactivity, respectively (*Fig. 32-3*). These results agree with the findings of others (19,41). During the course of detraining, HR also increases significantly at a given submaximal work rate. For example, 12 d of inactivity was shown to increase HR from 158 to 170 beats · min^{-1} at the same absolute intensity, then to 184 beats · min^{-1} after 84 d of detraining (17).

CARDIAC OUTPUT

Despite the detraining-related increase in HR that occurs at rest and during submaximal exercise, there is no appreciable change in Q̇ because of the aforementioned and offsetting decrease in SV that occurs both at rest and during exercise. At peak exercise, however, Q̇ is lower because of the decrease in peak SV.

RETRAINING

No discussion of detraining would be complete without at least mentioning the concept of retraining. Popular belief once held that the training effects one achieved via endurance training could be increased if the athlete had previously undergone training and detraining periods. However, scientific evidence does not support this concept. We now know that prior endurance training does not, in itself, positively influence the gains made through a subsequent retraining period (25). What is more important to remember is that a relatively brief layoff can significantly decrease exercise capacity.

MAINTENANCE OF TRAINING EFFECT

Discussion thus far has primarily focused on adaptations to both high-level endurance training and inactivity. However, most humans live the majority of life somewhere in between these two extremes, and it is unlikely one can be in "race shape" all of the time. Therefore, one would want to preserve, as much as possible, previously obtained fitness gains during the off-season or those periods of time associated with a reduced amount of exercise training. This begs the question: What level of exercise is required to maintain cardiorespiratory fitness once achieved by a high level of endurance training?

A series of papers by Hickson and Rosenkoetter provides insight into this question. In one study, $\dot{V}O_{2max}$ was maintained following a 15-wk period of decreased training frequency (from 6 to 2 d · wk^{-1}) by keeping intensity and duration constant (39). In a subsequent study (38), $\dot{V}O_{2max}$ was maintained following a 15-wk period of decreased training duration (from 40 to both 26 and 13 min per session) by keeping intensity and frequency constant. However, endurance performance (time of exhaustion at 80% $\dot{V}O_{2max}$) was reduced 10% in the 13 min per session group. In yet a third study (36), $\dot{V}O_{2max}$ and endurance performance were significantly reduced by 5%–10% and 20%–30%, respectively, following a 15-wk period of decreased training intensity (by both one-third and two-thirds of initial intensity), even though frequency and duration remained constant. Collectively, these studies suggest that after periods of intensive training, $\dot{V}O_{2max}$ can be maintained for up to 15 wk of reduced training frequency or duration as long as intensity is maintained.

Over a shorter period (4 wk), McConell et al. (49) showed that $\dot{V}O_{2max}$ was maintained despite reductions in training intensity, frequency, and time; however, endurance performance (5-km run time) was reduced. This suggests that $\dot{V}O_{2max}$ can be maintained for a shortened period (4 wk vs. 15 wk) despite a reduction in all training parameters (intensity, frequency, and time).

EXERCISE TRAINING WITH ARM ERGOMETRY

Upper-body exercise modes, such as arm ergometry, are widely accepted as an integral part of a comprehensive exercise training program in persons with and without heart disease. Franklin et al. (27) reported the effects of a 6-wk training program involving upper- and lower-extremity exercise devices in patients with a history of myocardial infarction. Following exercise training, RPP (an indicator of myocardial oxygen demand) during submaximal arm and leg exercise were similarly decreased, and exercise capacity measured during arm and leg ergometry increased 13% and 11%, respectively (*Fig. 32-5*). These findings indicated that the upper extremities respond to aerobic exercise training in a similar manner as the lower extremities.

EXERCISE MODE AND SPECIFICITY OF TRAINING

To improve one's ability to perform a given physical activity, whether it is walking up two flights of stairs or swimming 100 m, involves training specific muscles or organ systems with increasing volume (duration, frequency, or intensity). This concept emphasizes the principles of specificity of training and progressive overload. Regarding specificity of training, numerous studies of normal subjects and patients with heart disease have investigated the cardiorespiratory adaptations of trained versus untrained muscle to physical conditioning. Results generally demonstrate little or no crossover of arm and leg training. After endurance training of one limb or set of limbs, several investigators report increased $\dot{V}O_{2max}$ and ventilatory threshold and decreased HR, blood lactate, pulmonary ventilation, ventilatory equivalent for $\dot{V}O_{2max}$, BP, and perceived exertion during submaximal exercise with the trained but not the untrained limbs (11,59). These limb-specific training effects imply that a substantial portion of the conditioning response is attributed to peripheral factors, such as alterations in blood flow and cellular and enzymatic adaptations in the trained limbs alone (20,35,63).

Conversely, studies in both normal subjects and patients with heart disease indicate some crossover of training effects (*i.e.*, increased peak oxygen consumption [$\dot{V}O_{2peak}$] or reduced submaximal exercise HR in untrained limbs), providing evidence for central circulatory adaptations to endurance training (10,69). Although the conditions under which the crossover between arm and leg training may vary, evidence suggests that the initial fitness level — as well as the intensity, frequency, and duration of training — may be important variables in determining the extent of cross-training benefits from arms to legs and vice versa.

The limited degree of cardiorespiratory and metabolic crossover from one set of limbs to another appears to discount the general practice of restricting aerobic conditioning to the lower extremities. Several recreational

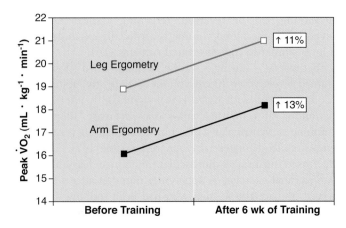

FIGURE 32-5. Peak $\dot{V}O_2$ during arm and leg ergometry before and after exercise training in men (*n* = 13) with previous myocardial infarction. (Adapted from Franklin BA, Vander L, Wrisley D, Rubenfire M. Trainability of arms versus legs in men previous myocardial infarction. *Chest.* 1994;105[1]:262–4.)

TABLE 32-4. Factors Influencing the Physiologic Adaptations to Cardiorespiratory Exercise Training

Variables(s)	Comments
Age, habitual physical activity, and initial $\dot{V}O_{2max}$	Improvement generally demonstrates an inverse relationship with these variables; however, recent studies suggest that older and younger adults demonstrate similar response.
Genetics	Hereditary contributions may account for 50%.
Volume of training (combination of intensity, frequency, and duration)	Improvement in aerobic capacity generally demonstrates a positive correlation to training volume.
Intensity of training	Improvement in aerobic capacity is positively correlated with intensity, even with total volume held constant.
Adherence to the exercise prescription	Parallels the magnitude of improvement in cardiorespiratory function
Detraining and prolonged bed rest	When physical conditioning is stopped or reduced, training-induced cardiorespiratory adaptations are reversed over time.
Beta-adrenergic blockade therapy	Despite an attenuated heart rate response, patients on β-blockers can derive similar adaptations from exercise training.
Heart disease, including coronary artery disease or chronic heart failure	Exercise training is generally safe and effective in improving cardiorespiratory function. The disease type and severity of each patient should be considered on an individual basis in designing an appropriate cardiorespiratory training program.

$\dot{V}O_{2max}$, maximal oxygen consumption.

activities and many occupational tasks require sustained arm work to a greater extent than legwork. Consequently, individuals who rely on their upper extremities for vocational or leisure-time pursuits should train their arms as well as their legs, with the expectation of improved cardiorespiratory, hemodynamic, and perceived exertion responses to both forms of effort. Arm ergometers or combined arm–leg ergometers are particularly beneficial for upper-extremity training. Other various factors affecting the response to exercise training are summarized in *Table 32-4*.

SEX-SPECIFIC IMPROVEMENT AND TRAINABILITY

For many years, most studies on the effects of aerobic exercise training involved men. However, numerous studies also provide ample data on $\dot{V}O_{2max}$, cardiovascular hemodynamics, body composition, and serum lipids in younger, middle-aged, and older women who undergo exercise training. The results demonstrate that women respond to aerobic exercise training in much the same way as men when subjected to comparable programs in terms of frequency, intensity, and duration of exercise (3,30) (*Fig. 32-6*). Improvement in cardiorespiratory fitness is inversely correlated with age, habitual physical activity, and initial $\dot{V}O_{2max}$ (which is generally lower in women than men), and positively correlated with exercise frequency, intensity, and duration (26). It is important to note that when comparing similar groups of athletes or apparently healthy persons, $\dot{V}O_{2max}$ expressed per kilogram of body weight is generally 15%–25% lower in women than men. This difference is caused by sex-specific biologic differences, including a slightly greater amount of essential body fat, a smaller peak SV attributable to smaller left ventricular dimension, and a lower hemoglobin concentration (25).

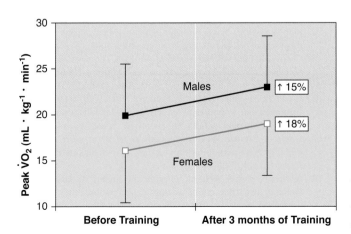

FIGURE 32-6. Peak $\dot{V}O_2$ before and after 20 wk of exercise training in men (*n* = 287) and women (*n* = 346). (Adapted from Skinner JS, Jaskolski A, Jaskolska A, et al. Age, sex, race, initial fitness, and response to training: the HERITAGE Family Study. *J Appl Physiol.* 2001;90[5]:1770–6.)

In general, an average increase in $\dot{V}O_{2max}$ of between 10% and 30% is anticipated for college-age men and women after an 8- to 12-wk endurance training program. When gain in $\dot{V}O_{2max}$ is expressed per kilogram of body mass, the values achieved for men and women are similar. However, because the initial $\dot{V}O_{2max}$ of women is generally lower than men, the percentage increase is often greater among women.

OVERTRAINING

As discussed in this chapter, regular exercise training can lead to adaptations in the cardiorespiratory system, which has a positive impact on exercise performance. A minimal training stimulus (*e.g.*, intensity or minutes per week) is likely to elicit minimal benefits. Similarly, a maximal training level or stimulus will potentially lead to maximal improvements in performance. It is widely believed that there is a point at which chronic exposure to high volumes of intense exercise training with insufficient recovery can lead to overtraining.

Overtraining, as described by athletes and coaches, is an altered mood state and a reduction in performance despite ongoing training. This condition may require weeks to months and maybe years to resolve. However, as discussed by Halson and Jeukendrup (32), researchers have had difficulty describing and detecting overtraining. This is, in part, because of a lack of consistent terminology, differences in diagnostic tools, differences in performance measures and training regimens, and individual differences in athletes and sporting activities. Overtraining is generally a diagnosis by exclusion of other causes for decreased performance and altered mood. The cause of overtraining is not fully understood but is likely related to both training (*e.g.*, exercise volume, recovery) and nontraining (*e.g.*, psychological stress, sleep, nutrition) factors (61). Several markers of overtraining have been investigated, including performance, mood state, cardiovascular physiology (*e.g.*, SV, HR), lactate, glycogen depletion, immune system function, hormone imbalances, and changes in autonomic nervous system function. Currently, there is no agreed-upon constellation of signs or symptoms characterizing overtraining.

SUMMARY

When exposed to repeated bouts of exercise (*i.e.*, exercise training), both the cardiac and pulmonary systems show measurable changes (adaptations) consistent with a training effect. Generally, these changes are associated with improved exercise performance and health and occur in both healthy individuals and those with preexisting cardiovascular disease. The adaptations that take place are organ system or tissue specific and generally occur similarly in men and women. Consistent with the earlier discussion, periods of detraining, lesser training, and bed rest are associated with loss of exercise performance, and many, if not all, of the previously attained training effects.

REFERENCES

1. *2008 Physical Activity Guidelines for Americans* [Internet]. Washington (DC): U.S. Department of Health and Human Services; [cited 2011 Sep 2]. Available from: http://www.health.gov/paguidelines/pdf/paguide.pdf
2. Ades PA, Savage PD, Brawner CA, et al. Aerobic capacity in patients entering cardiac rehabilitation. *Circulation.* 2006;113(23):2706–12.
3. Ades PA, Waldmann ML, Polk DM, Coflesky JT. Referral patterns and exercise response in the rehabilitation of female coronary patients aged greater than or equal to 62 years. *Am J Cardiol.* 1992;69(17):1422–5.
4. Bevegard BS, Shepherd JT. Regulation of the circulation during exercise in man. *Physiol Rev.* 1967;47(2):178–213.
5. Blair SN, Kohl HW,3rd, Paffenbarger RS,Jr, Clark DG, Cooper KH, Gibbons LW. Physical fitness and all-cause mortality. A prospective study of healthy men and women. *JAMA.* 1989;262(17):2395–401.
6. Blomqvist CG, Saltin B. Cardiovascular adaptations to physical training. *Annu Rev Physiol.* 1983;45:169–89.
7. Bouchard C, Daw EW, Rice T, et al. Familial resemblance for VO2max in the sedentary state: the HERITAGE family study. *Med Sci Sports Exerc.* 1998;30(2):252–8.
8. Chobanian AV, Bakris GL, Black HR, et al. The Seventh Report of the Joint National Committee on Prevention, Detection, Evaluation, and Treatment of High Blood Pressure: the JNC 7 report. *JAMA.* 2003;289(19):2560–72.
9. Church TS, Earnest CP, Skinner JS, Blair SN. Effects of different doses of physical activity on cardiorespiratory fitness among sedentary, overweight or obese postmenopausal women with elevated blood pressure: a randomized controlled trial. *JAMA.* 2007;297(19):2081–91.
10. Clausen JP, Klausen K, Rasmussen B, Trap-Jensen J. Central and peripheral circulatory changes after training of the arms or legs. *Am J Physiol.* 1973;225(3):675–82.
11. Clausen JP, Trap-Jensen J, Lassen NA. The effects of training on the heart rate during arm and leg exercise. *Scand J Clin Lab Invest.* 1970;26(3):295–301.
12. Coats AJ. Clinical utility of exercise training in chronic systolic heart failure. *Nat Rev Cardiol.* 2011;8(7):380–92.
13. Convertino VA, Brock PJ, Keil LC, Bernauer EM, Greenleaf JE. Exercise training-induced hypervolemia: role of plasma albumin, renin, and vasopressin. *J Appl Physiol.* 1980;48(4):665–9.
14. Cornelissen VA, Fagard RH. Effects of endurance training on blood pressure, blood pressure-regulating mechanisms, and cardiovascular risk factors. *Hypertension.* 2005;46(4):667–75.
15. Costill DL, Fink WJ, Hargreaves M, King DS, Thomas R, Fielding R. Metabolic characteristics of skeletal muscle during detraining from competitive swimming. *Med Sci Sports Exerc.* 1985;17(3):339–43.
16. Coyle EF, Hemmert MK, Coggan AR. Effects of detraining on cardiovascular responses to exercise: role of blood volume. *J Appl Physiol.* 1986;60(1):95–9.
17. Coyle EF, Martin WH,3rd, Bloomfield SA, Lowry OH, Holloszy JO. Effects of detraining on responses to submaximal exercise. *J Appl Physiol.* 1985;59(3):853–9.
18. Coyle EF, Martin WH,3rd, Sinacore DR, Joyner MJ, Hagberg JM, Holloszy JO. Time course of loss of adaptations after stopping prolonged intense endurance training. *J Appl Physiol.* 1984;57(6):1857–64.

19. Cullinane EM, Sady SP, Vadeboncoeur L, Burke M, Thompson PD. Cardiac size and VO2max do not decrease after short-term exercise cessation. *Med Sci Sports Exerc.* 1986;18(4):420–4.

20. Davies CT, Sargeant AJ. Effects of training on the physiological responses to one- and two-leg work. *J Appl Physiol.* 1975;38(3): 377–5.

21. Drinkwater BL. Physical exercise and bone health. *J Am Med Womens Assoc.* 1990;45(3):91–7.

22. Ehrman JK. Myocardial Infarction. In: Ehrman JK, editor *Clinical Exercise Physiology.* Champaign: Human Kinetics; 2003. p. 201–226.

23. Ehsani AA, Hagberg JM, Hickson RC. Rapid changes in left ventricular dimensions and mass in response to physical conditioning and deconditioning. *Am J Cardiol.* 1978;42(1):52–6.

24. Fletcher GF, Balady GJ, Amsterdam EA, et al. Exercise standards for testing and training: a statement for healthcare professionals from the American Heart Association. *Circulation.* 2001;104(14): 1694–740.

25. Foss ML, Keteyian SJ. *Fox's Physiological Basis for Exercise and Sport.* 6th ed. Boston (MA): McGraw-Hill; 1998. 620 p.

26. Franklin BA, Bonzheim K, Berg T. Gender differences in rehabilitation. In: Julian DG, Wenger NK, editors. *Women and Heart Disease.* London: Martin Dunitz; 1997. p. 151–171.

27. Franklin BA, Vander L, Wrisley D, Rubenfire M. Trainability of arms versus legs in men previous myocardial infarction. *Chest.* 1994;105(1):262–4.

28. Fringer MN, Stull GA. Changes in cardiorespiratory parameters during periods of training and detraining in young adult females. *Med Sci Sports.* 1974;6(1):20–5.

29. Garber CE, Blissmer B, Deschenes MR, et al. Quantity and quality of exercise for developing and maintaining cardiorespiratory, musculoskeletal, and neuromotor fitness in apparently healthy adults: guidance for prescribing exercise. *Med Sci Sports Exerc.* 2011;43(7):1334–59.

30. Getchell LH, Moore JC. Physical training: comparative responses of middle-aged adults. *Arch Phys Med Rehabil.* 1975;56(6):250–4.

31. Green HJ, Thomson JA, Ball ME, Hughson RL, Houston ME, Sharratt MT. Alterations in blood volume following short-term supramaximal exercise. *J Appl Physiol.* 1984;56(1):145–9.

32. Halson SL, Jeukendrup AE. Does overtraining exist? An analysis of overreaching and overtraining research. *Sports Med.* 2004;34(14): 967–81.

33. Haskell WL, Lee IM, Pate RR, et al. Physical activity and public health: updated recommendation for adults from the American College of Sports Medicine and the American Heart Association. *Med Sci Sports Exerc.* 2007;39(8):1423–34.

34. Haykowsky MJ, Liang Y, Pechter D, Jones LW, McAlister FA, Clark AM. A meta-analysis of the effect of exercise training on left ventricular remodeling in heart failure patients: the benefit depends on the type of training performed. *J Am Coll Cardiol.* 2007; 49(24):2329–36.

35. Henriksson J, Reitman JS. Time course of changes in human skeletal muscle succinate dehydrogenase and cytochrome oxidase activities and maximal oxygen uptake with physical activity and inactivity. *Acta Physiol Scand.* 1977;99(1):91–7.

36. Hickson RC, Foster C, Pollock ML, Galassi TM, Rich S. Reduced training intensities and loss of aerobic power, endurance, and cardiac growth. *J Appl Physiol.* 1985;58(2):492–9.

37. Hickson RC, Hammons GT, Holoszy JO. Development and regression of exercise-induced cardiac hypertrophy in rats. *Am J Physiol.* 1979;236(2):H268–72.

38. Hickson RC, Kanakis C,Jr, Davis JR, Moore AM, Rich S. Reduced training duration effects on aerobic power, endurance, and cardiac growth. *J Appl Physiol.* 1982;53(1):225–9.

39. Hickson RC, Rosenkoetter MA. Reduced training frequencies and maintenance of increased aerobic power. *Med Sci Sports Exerc.* 1981;13(1):13–6.

40. Holloszy JO. Adaptation of skeletal muscle to endurance exercise. *Med Sci Sports.* 1975;7(3):155–64.

41. Houston ME, Bentzen H, Larsen H. Interrelationships between skeletal muscle adaptations and performance as studied by detraining and retraining. *Acta Physiol Scand.* 1979;105(2):163–70.

42. Keteyian SJ, Brawner CA, Savage PD, et al. Peak aerobic capacity predicts prognosis in patients with coronary heart disease. *Am Heart J.* 2008;156(2):292–300.

43. Keteyian SJ, Pina IL, Hibner BA, Fleg JL. Clinical role of exercise training in the management of patients with chronic heart failure. *J Cardiopulm Rehabil Prev.* 2010;30(2):67–76.

44. Klausen K, Andersen LB, Pelle I. Adaptive changes in work capacity, skeletal muscle capillarization and enzyme levels during training and detraining. *Acta Physiol Scand.* 1981;113(1):9–16.

45. Levine BD, Lane LD, Buckey JC, Friedman DB, Blomqvist CG. Left ventricular pressure-volume and Frank-Starling relations in endurance athletes. Implications for orthostatic tolerance and exercise performance. *Circulation.* 1991;84(3):1016–23.

46. Longhurst JC, Kelly AR, Gonyea WJ, Mitchell JH. Chronic training with static and dynamic exercise: cardiovascular adaptation, and response to exercise. *Circ Res.* 1981;48(6 Pt 2):I171–8.

47. Martin WH,3rd, Coyle EF, Bloomfield SA, Ehsani AA. Effects of physical deconditioning after intense endurance training on left ventricular dimensions and stroke volume. *J Am Coll Cardiol.* 1986;7(5):982–9.

48. McAllister RM. Endothelial-mediated control of coronary and skeletal muscle blood flow during exercise: introduction. *Med Sci Sports Exerc.* 1995;27(8):1122–4.

49. McConell GK, Costill DL, Widrick JJ, Hickey MS, Tanaka H, Gastin PB. Reduced training volume and intensity maintain aerobic capacity but not performance in distance runners. *Int J Sports Med.* 1993;14(1):33–7.

50. Michielli DW, Stein RA, Krasnow N, Diamond JR, Horwitz B. Effects of exercise training on ventricular dimensions at rest and during exercise. *Med Sci Sports.* 1979;11:82.

51. Mortensen SP, Dawson EA, Yoshiga CC, et al. Limitations to systemic and locomotor limb muscle oxygen delivery and uptake during maximal exercise in humans. *J Physiol.* 2005;566(Pt 1): 273–85.

52. Nelson ME, Rejeski WJ, Blair SN, et al. Physical activity and public health in older adults: recommendation from the American College of Sports Medicine and the American Heart Association. *Circulation.* 2007;116(9):1094–105.

53. O'Connor CM, Whellan DJ, Lee KL, et al. Efficacy and safety of exercise training in patients with chronic heart failure: HF-ACTION randomized controlled trial. *JAMA.* 2009;301(14):1439–50.

54. Orlander J, Kiessling KH, Karlsson J, Ekblom B. Low intensity training, inactivity and resumed training in sedentary men. *Acta Physiol Scand.* 1977;101(3):351–62.

55. Oscai LB, Williams BT, Hertig BA. Effect of exercise on blood volume. *J Appl Physiol.* 1968;24(5):622–4.

56. Pate RR, Pratt M, Blair SN, et al. Physical activity and public health. A recommendation from the Centers for Disease Control and Prevention and the American College of Sports Medicine. *JAMA.* 1995;273(5):402–7.

57. Pavlik G, Bachl N, Wollein W, Langfy G, Prokop L. Resting echocardiographic parameters after cessation of regular endurance training. *Int J Sports Med.* 1986;7(4):226–31.

58. Pina IL, Apstein CS, Balady GJ, et al. Exercise and heart failure: A statement from the American Heart Association Committee on exercise, rehabilitation, and prevention. *Circulation.* 2003;107(8): 1210–25.

59. Rasmussen B, Klausen K, Clausen JP, Trap-Jensen J. Pulmonary ventilation, blood gases, and blood pH after training of the arms or the legs. *J Appl Physiol.* 1975;38(2):250–6.

60. Rerych SK, Scholz PM, Sabiston DC,Jr, Jones RH. Effects of exercise training on left ventricular function in normal subjects: a longitudinal study by radionuclide angiography. *Am J Cardiol.* 1980;45(2):244–52.

61. Robergs RA, Keteyian SJ. *Fundamentals of Exercise Physiology: For Fitness, Performance, and Health*. 2nd ed. Boston (MA): McGraw-Hill; 2002. 512 p.

62. Rowell LB. Human cardiovascular adjustments to exercise and thermal stress. *Physiol Rev*. 1974;54(1):75–159.

63. Saltin B, Blomqvist G, Mitchell JH, Johnson RL,Jr, Wildenthal K, Chapman CB. Response to exercise after bed rest and after training. *Circulation*. 1968;38(5 Suppl):VII1–78.

64. Saltin B, Nazar K, Costill DL, et al. The nature of the training response; peripheral and central adaptations of one-legged exercise. *Acta Physiol Scand*. 1976;96(3):289–305.

65. Schairer JR, Keteyian SJ. Exercise in patients with cardiovascular disease. In: Kraus WE, Keteyian SJ, editors. *Cardiac Rehabilitation*. Totowa: Humana Press; 2007. p. 169–183.

66. Schairer JR, Stein PD, Keteyian S, et al. Left ventricular response to submaximal exercise in endurance-trained athletes and sedentary adults. *Am J Cardiol*. 1992;70(9):930–3.

67. Skinner JS, Jaskolski A, Jaskolska A, et al. Age, sex, race, initial fitness, and response to training: the HERITAGE Family Study. *J Appl Physiol*. 2001;90(5):1770–6.

68. Thompson PD, Buchner D, Pina IL, et al. Exercise and physical activity in the prevention and treatment of atherosclerotic cardiovascular disease: a statement from the Council on Clinical Cardiology (Subcommittee on Exercise, Rehabilitation, and Prevention) and the Council on Nutrition, Physical Activity, and Metabolism (Subcommittee on Physical Activity). *Circulation*. 2003;107(24):3109–16.

69. Thompson PD, Cullinane E, Lazarus B, Carleton RA. Effect of exercise training on the untrained limb exercise performance of men with angina pectoris. *Am J Cardiol*. 1981;48(5):844–50.

70. Wisloff U, Stoylen A, Loennechen JP, et al. Superior cardiovascular effect of aerobic interval training versus moderate continuous training in heart failure patients: a randomized study. *Circulation*. 2007;115(24):3086–94.

SELECTED REFERENCES FOR FURTHER READING

Brooks G, Fahey T, Baldwin K. *Exercise Physiology: Human Bioenergetics and Its Applications*. 4th ed. New York (NY): McGraw-Hill; 2004. 905 p.

Rowell LB. *Human Circulation: Regulation During Physical Stress*. New York (NY): Oxford University Press; 1986. 416 p.

Rowell LB, Shephard JT. *Handbook of Physiology. Exercise: Regulation and Integration of Multiple Organ Systems*. New York (NY): Oxford University Press; 1996. 1224 p.

INTERNET RESOURCES

- Centers for Disease Control and Prevention, Division of Nutrition and Physical Activity: http://www.cdc.gov/nccdphp/dnpa/index.htm
- Exercise performance and training adaptations: http://www.home.hia.no/~stephens/exphys.htm
- HERITAGE Family Study: http://www.pbrc.edu/Heritage/index.html
- SPORTSCIENCE: http://www.sportsci.org

Adaptations to Resistance Training

Adaptations in resistance training are specific to the design of the program. A key factor in resistance exercise and its subsequent repeated exposure with resistance training is the activation of motor units (the alpha motor neuron and its associated muscle fibers). If muscle tissue is not activated, then it will not adapt. Thus, the resistance training program design is crucial to this process (43,97). The amount of muscle tissue activated dictates the magnitude of the support systems needed to maintain homeostasis during and after exercise. Progressive overloading of the musculoskeletal system is needed for subsequent adaptations to take place beyond the initial phase of training (105,106,108). The human body will only adapt to the specific stimulus created by the workout program configuration. Thus, challenging workouts are needed for progression to take place (10,106,108,175).

Although much research remains to be done and many questions remain to be answered, one principle that has been translated into an applied concept is the size principle that allows a general understanding of muscle tissue activation (37). The size principle conceptually developed by Henneman hypothesized that motor units are recruited in order by different "sizing factors" (*e.g.*, the size of the soma of motor neurons located within the spinal cord; those associated with type I slow-twitch

muscle fibers being smaller than those associated with type II fast-twitch muscle fibers) to produce the needed amount of force to meet the external demands or to lift a weight (69). For example, low-threshold motor units produce low levels of force. As the activation stimulus increases, higher threshold motor units are recruited, and more force is produced. Higher threshold motor units may contain larger muscle fibers, a higher number of muscle fibers, or type II (fast-twitch) muscle fibers. Essentially, some "sizing factor" will mediate greater force capabilities until the maximal amount of force is produced when all available motor units are recruited in a specific movement (31).

Organizing the order of resistance training loads may, in some cases, help produce a more optimal force or power output in the second exercise performed. This principle has been called *complex training* (27). Activated fast-twitch motor units may be better facilitated following a prior resistance loading, thereby enabling enhanced power performance, that is, *postactivation potentiation* (11,29,38,138,171). The use of this concept has been found to be successful in optimizing power development in certain individuals, but individualization is crucial as to the loading and rest period used (115,132). Not all individuals have the same complement of motor units in a specific muscle nor does every muscle in a given

KEY TERMS

Delayed Onset Muscle Soreness (DOMS): Delayed onset muscle soreness that typically occurs 24–48 h following resistance training, particularly when eccentric actions are emphasized.

Hyperplasia: An increase in the number of muscle fibers within a given muscle.

Hypertrophy: An increase in the size of individual muscle fibers; also, an increase in the size of an entire muscle.

Motor unit: A motor neuron and the muscle fibers that it innervates; the basic unit of muscular contraction.

Neuromuscular junction: The site where a motor neuron axon terminal connects with the sarcolemma of a muscle fiber (separated by a small space, the synaptic cleft); also known as a *motor endplate*.

Overtraining: A decrease in performance despite a maintenance or progressive increase in training.

Size principle: The concept by which motor units with smaller motor neuron somas (cell bodies located in the spinal cord) are more easily recruited by central motor command than are motor units with larger motor neuron somas. Type I (slow-twitch) motor units have smaller motor neuron somas than type II (fast-twitch) motor units individual have the same complement of motor units. Finally, the joint angle of a resistance exercise will dictate a different combination of motor units needed for movement. Exercise choices, resistance loading, metabolic demands, and fatigue state of the muscle all influence what muscle tissue is activated and what adaptations will occur.

Finally, although the activation of muscle is the key event in resistance training, the specific resistance exercise stimulus or the type of workout performed will determine the number of physiologic systems that are needed to support the exercise stress and allow for recovery, repair, and remodeling of tissue after the workout. The basis of any adaptation is the exercise stimulus created by the workout. The quality of the exercise stimulus is governed by the principles of *specificity*, *progressive overload*, and *variation* (105,106,108). How the workout is designed and changed over time (manipulation of intensity, volume, exercise selection and order, rest intervals, frequency, and velocity of muscle action) dictates the success in achieving a targeted training goal and the level of adaptations attained (see *Chapter 31*). For example, a whole-body workout will demand more physiologic system involvement and support than one set of an arm curl exercise using 50% of a one repetition maximum (1-RM) load. Thus, adaptations in the musculoskeletal system can carry over to other physiologic systems depending on the specific demands of the exercise protocol.

RESISTANCE TRAINING

Resistance training can encompass a wide range of workout protocols. A single workout may entail exercises only for the upper body, or for the lower body, or for the total body. This typically ranges from 8 to 10 exercises for a whole-body workout. Resistances can range from light to very heavy and are varied over time (periodized) to effectively stimulate the neuromuscular system and provide for recovery. Adaptations are then related to the principle of specificity and are dictated by the type of workouts used to address program goals and requirements of the individual. *Chapter 31* addresses the basic techniques and programming in resistance training.

RESPONSES VERSUS ADAPTATIONS

Training is typically thought of as repeated and systematic exposure of the body to an exercise stimulus. Some adaptations take place within one or two workouts. A *response* is the human body's acute change in physiologic function to the stress of resistance exercise. Thus, training adaptations may be viewed as the quantification of consistent individual responses to the stress of resistance exercise. The human body may adapt to resistance

exercise and training by altering its homeostatic balance or by modifying the acute responses to a workout. If one looks at it from a temporal perspective, or as adaptations taking place on a time continuum, the changes can range from early- and late-phase adaptations up to (potentially) an individual's genetic maximum for the phenotypic expression of a trait. For example, when a resistance exercise workout is performed over the first week, changes occur within two to four workouts for the type of myosin protein, yet few changes have been observed for many other morphologic characteristics, such as muscle fiber size, until a few weeks later (182). Thus, neurologic adaptations and changes in the "quality of muscle proteins" dominate the early-phase adaptations in skeletal muscle and are part of the adaptational continuum. If training is stopped, then detraining occurs, and over time phenotypic expression of the change reverts back to near-baseline physiologic status. The physiologic adaptations to critical bodily systems — such as the neuromuscular, connective tissue, endocrine, metabolic, cardiovascular, and immune systems — are discussed in this chapter and summarized in *Table 33-1*.

NEUROMUSCULAR ADAPTATIONS

Several neural mechanisms are responsible for the adaptations in strength and power observed with resistance training. Resistance training may elicit adaptations along the neuromuscular chain, initiating in the higher brain centers and continuing down to the level of individual muscle fibers. Interestingly, not all mechanisms are operational in every muscle or exercise; therefore, the mediators of neural adaptations are a complex set of mechanisms working to produce greater force. These include increased neural drive, in which the amount of electromyographic (EMG) activity is lower for a given resistance lifted; increased synchronization, in which a greater number of motor units are activated nearly simultaneously for a given lifting effort; increased time of neural activation, which might allow more higher threshold motor units to become activated; and reduction in central and local inhibitory reflexes, which limit neural activation (170). The combinations of mechanisms that can mediate such changes are debatable, but changes in force production occur rapidly with no changes in the cross-sectional area (CSA) of muscle, arguing for a strong neural component in the adaptational effects.

EARLY-PHASE ADAPTATIONS

The ability to increase neural drive begins in the motor cortex with the intent to produce maximal levels of muscular force and power. A substantial proportion of the neural changes that occur during resistance training take place in the spinal cord along the descending corticospinal tracts. A classic study by Moritani and

TABLE 33-1. Adaptations to Resistance Training

Adaptation	Significance
Neural Adaptations	
↑ Motor cortex activity ↑ Motor unit recruitment ↑ Motor unit firing rate ↑ Motor unit synchronization ↑ Fast-twitch fiber selective recruitment ↑ Postactivation potentiation ↑ Reflex potentiation ↓ Golgi tendon organ inhibition ↓ Antagonist muscle coactivation	↑ Muscle force production, rate of force development, power, "cross education," improved resistance exercise technique, and reduced bilateral deficit
Neuromuscular Junction	
↑ Terminal branching, asymmetry, area	↑ Neurotransmitter release, force, and power production
Muscle Adaptations	
↑ Muscle cross sectional area — mostly in type II fibers ↑ Hyperplasia (primarily because of neural sprouting) ↑ Upregulation of factors in myogenesis (MyoD, myogenin) ↓ Myostatin ↑ Expression of ~70 genes ↑ Net protein accretion via multiple pathways (contractile and noncontractile proteins) ↑ Myofibrillar volume ↑ SR- and T-tubule volume ↑ Na^+/K^+ ATPase activity ↑ Upregulation (transient) of muscle growth factors (*e.g.*, mechano-growth factor and calcineurin) ↑ Pennation angle and fascicle length ↑ Fiber type and myosin heavy chain transitions IIX–IIAX–IIA ↓ Muscle damage with repeated RE exposure ↑ Buffer capacity	↑ Muscle growth, strength, power, recovery, and endurance
Metabolic Adaptations	
↑, ↓, ↔ ATP–CP, glycolytic enzymes ↑ ATP, CP, and glycogen storage ↓ Capillary density (↑ # capillaries) ↓ Mitochondrial density (↑ # mitochondria) ↓ Myoglobin	↑ Energy liberation, force, and power ↓ Oxidative capacity
Endocrine Adaptations	
Hormonal response (see *Table 33-2*) ↑ Upregulation of androgen receptors	↑ Acute and chronic force, power, and endurance enhancement, muscle hypertrophy
Connective Tissue Adaptations	
↑ Bone mineral density ↑ Blood markers of bone osteogenesis ↑ Tendon and ligament cross-sectional area ↑ Tendon stiffness ↑ Collagen synthesis	↑ Skeletal strength, force transmission, and ability to sustain muscle hypertrophy
Cardiovascular Adaptations	
↑ Stroke volume ↑ Left ventricular wall thickness ↑ Septal wall thickness ↓, ↔ Resting heart rate ↓, ↔ Blood pressure ↓ Cardiovascular response to acute exercise of similar workload or intensity, low-density lipoproteins ↑, ↔ Blood high-density lipoproteins	Improved cardiovascular disease risk factors and health, ↑ tolerance to pressure overload, ↓ cardiovascular demand to submaximal exercise
Immune Adaptations	
↑ Leukocyte and cytokine response to resistance exercise ↔ Resting immune cell concentrations	Tissue remodeling, inflammation, and repair

(Continued)

TABLE 33-1. Adaptations to Resistance Training (*Continued*)

Adaptation	Significance
Performance Adaptations	
↑ Muscle strength ↑ Muscle power ↑ Balance and coordination ↑, ↔ Flexibility ↑ Lean tissue mass ↑ Muscle endurance ↑ Motor performance ↑, ↔ VO$_{2max}$	↑ Performance
Health and Fitness Adaptations	
↓ Percent body fat ↑ Insulin sensitivity ↓ Insulin concentrations and response to glucose challenge ↓ Sarcopenia and osteoporosis ↓ Low back pain ↑ Basal metabolic rate	↑ Health and wellness

↑, increase; ↓, decrease; ↔, no change; MyoD, myogenic differentiation antigen; SR, sarcoplasmic reticulum; T-tubule, transverse tubule; ATPase, adenosine triphosphatase; RE, resistance exercise; ATP–CP, adenosine triphosphate–creatine phosphate; VO$_{2max}$, maximal oxygen consumption.

deVries demonstrated the quintessential early-phase adaptations of the neural system (139). In examining an 8-wk resistance training program, they found that for a given level of force, less EMG activity was required following training. This indicated that a greater neural drive with training apparently mediated the adaptations in strength, and such early-phase improvements could not be accounted for by muscle **hypertrophy**. This and other subsequent research supports the idea that an increase in neural drive to a muscle results in greater strength. Neural factors related to strength gain include increased neural drive (*i.e.*, recruitment and rate of firing) to the muscle, increased synchronization of the motor units, increased activation of agonists, decreased activation of antagonists, coordination of motor units and muscle(s) involved in a movement, and inhibition of the protective mechanisms of the muscle (*i.e.*, Golgi tendon organs) (170). This is evident in untrained or moderately trained individuals, for whom it has been shown that untrained individuals may only activate 71% of their muscle CSA during maximal effort (4). However, training reduces this deficit greatly, thereby demonstrating a greater potential to recruit fast-twitch motor units during the early phase of training adaptation (2).

Studies have revealed some other interesting neural adaptations/responses to resistance exercise and training. Resistance training may enhance the reflex (*i.e.*, muscle spindle or stretch reflex) response by 15%–55%, thereby enhancing the magnitude and rate of force development (2,72,172). In fact, positive correlations have been shown between enhanced stretch reflex and increased rate of force development during resistance training (72). In untrained individuals, the force produced when both limbs are contracting together is less than the sum of each limb contracting unilaterally (*bilateral deficit*).

Research has shown that the corresponding EMG is lower during bilateral contractions, and the bilateral deficit is reduced with bilateral training (55). *Cross education*, training one limb only, can result in an increase in strength in the untrained limb up to 22%, with the average strength increase about 8% (140). The increase in strength in the untrained limb is accompanied by greater EMG activity. Lastly, the level of tissue activation that takes place during resistance training when muscle hypertrophy takes place is important. A larger muscle does not require as much neural activation to lift a standard weight as it did before the growth took place, thereby demonstrating the importance of progressive overload during resistance training to continually recruit an optimal amount of muscle tissue (153).

Neural factors and quality of protein changes (*e.g.*, alterations in the type of myosin heavy chains [MHC] and type of myosin adenosine triphosphatase [ATPase] enzymes) may explain some part of early (2–8 wk) strength gains. It is during this time that strength gains are much greater than what can be explained by muscle hypertrophy. The specific type of program used may be one of the most important factors in initial strength gains as a result of neural factors because programs that are of high to very high intensity (80%–90% of 1-RM) are needed to elicit muscle fiber hypertrophy in all of the muscle fiber types (19). Therefore, strength gains are dependent on resistance loading and are mediated by a combination of neural and hypertrophic factors over time (170,175). Neural adaptations are also prominent during power training, when moderate-to-heavy loads are lifted at maximal velocities (106). In general, from a time perspective, muscle fiber hypertrophy has been shown to require more than 16 workouts to show significant increases (182). Thus, it may be possible that various types of training might be able to more quickly enhance the hypertrophy of muscle in the early phases (1–8 wk) of training, thereby enhancing the hypertrophic contribution to strength and power gains (20,21,175). Most studies have demonstrated that in the early phases of a heavy resistance training program, increased voluntary activation of muscle is the largest contributor to strength increases (170). After this period, muscle hypertrophy becomes the predominant factor in strength increases, especially for younger men. On the basis of this kind of evidence, scientists have concluded that neural factors have a profound influence on muscular force production.

LATE-PHASE ADAPTATIONS

The classic curve developed by Sale shows that neural factors predominate in the early phase of strength-training adaptations until muscle protein accretion catches up with the process after about 2–3 mo (170). A theoretical interaction of neural and muscle fiber hypertrophic components is presented in *Figure 33-1*. Neural factors (most likely the eccentric phase of the normal repetition) mediate the strength-training adaptations in the early phase. As training time continues, a larger amount of the strength increase is explained by increases in muscle hypertrophy or the accretion of myofibril proteins (175). Thus, with advancing training, there appears to be an interaction of neural and hypertrophic mechanisms mediating strength and power gains depending on the manipulation of the acute program variables. For example, training phases characterized by heavy loading (low volume) or explosive, ballistic repetitions may stimulate the nervous system to a higher degree, whereas moderate-to-high intensity protocols with higher volumes may stimulate greater muscle growth (106). If one's current level of muscle size is capable of withstanding the training stimulus, then there is little need for neural adaptations to take place as well. As Ploutz et al.

have shown, less fiber recruitment is needed to lift a given load when hypertrophy occurs (153). Progressive overload during consistent resistance training is critical for neural adaptations to continue to take place, and it has been suggested that neural adaptations may precede hypertrophy in advanced training (106). This might be best seen in advanced competitive weightlifters, in whom little or no hypertrophy may take place. In a classic study by Häkkinen et al., minimal changes in muscle fiber size were observed in competitive Olympic weightlifters, but strength and power increased over 2 yr of training (66). EMG data demonstrated that voluntary activation of muscle was enhanced over the training period. Thus, even in advanced resistance-trained athletes, the mechanisms of strength and power improvement may be related to neural factors. It must be kept in mind that competitive weightlifters who compete in body mass classification groups were studied, and gains in muscle mass may not necessarily enhance their competitive advantage. Furthermore, the types of programs used by Olympic weightlifters are primarily related to strength and power development (100). Other types of programs for bodybuilders or other athletes may have some similar characteristics related to power development but must also be designed to meet muscle mass and/or specific sport performance needs. Thus, training goals and specific protocols play a key role in the neural adaptations to resistance training.

ADAPTATIONS IN SKELETAL MUSCLE

The primary target of resistance exercise is skeletal muscle. Resistance training is one of the important upper regulatory variables that will ultimately dictate what happens on the cellular and gene level of expression (165,179). In addition, connective tissue will be stimulated as well as the many physiologic systems needed to support tissue repair and recovery. Skeletal muscle is a heterogeneous mixture of several types of muscle fibers that potentially grow in size. The process of hypertrophy involves a proportionate increase in the net accretion of the contractile proteins, actin and myosin, as well as other noncontractile structural proteins (118,175). Mechanical loading leads to a series of intracellular signaling processes that ultimately regulate gene expression and subsequent protein synthesis. Several proteins have recently been identified that are responsive to mechanical stress and increase in activity before hypertrophy (87). Studies have shown that resistance training has the potential to alter the activity of nearly 70 genes, upregulate factors involved with *myogenesis* (*e.g.*, myogenin, myogenic differentiation antigen [MyoD]), and downregulate inhibitory growth factors (*e.g.*, myostatin) (91,167,168). It has been proposed that muscle progenitor cell (MPC) activity is very responsive to exercise stress and that following resistance-exercise changes in

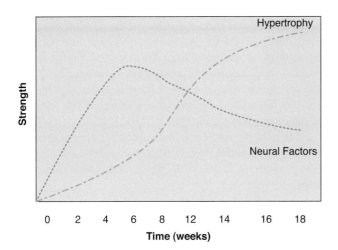

FIGURE 33-1. The theoretical interplay of the neural factors and hypertrophic factors over time with resistance training.

myogenic messenger ribonucleic acids (mRNAs) may initiate these hypertrophic events (165).

Skeletal muscle is multinucleated, with each nucleus governing a domain of protein (80). It has been postulated that the number of nuclei in part limit the amount of muscle hypertrophy and, after about a 26% increase in fiber size, the addition of more myonuclei are needed to mediate effective sizes of nuclear domains. A major adaptation in skeletal muscle fibers is the increase in the number of myonuclei through mitotic division of activated satellite cells stimulated in the damage-repair cycle (80,121). Optimal muscle growth may comprise maximizing the combination of mechanical (use of heavy weights, inclusion of eccentric muscle actions, and low-to-moderate volume) and metabolic (metabolite formation) stimuli via training periodization (106). Thus, one must consider a host of different mechanisms that may have regulatory control of function and adaptational abilities.

MUSCLE FIBER TYPES AND ADAPTATIONS

Quantification of different biochemical and physical characteristics of different muscle fibers has led to the development of several muscle fiber histochemical classifications (152). Most scientists use the myosin ATPase or MHC analyses to classify muscle fiber types of a given muscle. The major fiber types in humans are types I (slow-twitch) and II (fast-twitch), with each having muscle fiber subtypes: type I, IC, IIC, IIAC, IIA, IIAX, and IIX. Although genetics predominantly determines proportions of type I and II fibers in the human body, transitions within each fiber type may occur. Heavy resistance training (i.e., loads >80%–85% of the 1-RM) is needed to activate high-threshold motor units (IIX) because these fibers appear to be "reservoir" fibers and are mostly activated when high levels of force or power are needed (104). With such progressive programs, as stipulated in the American College of Sports Medicine (ACSM) position stand on progression, there is a transition in the percentage distribution from type IIX to IIA with little or no movement to IIC, with concomitant changes in MHC content (5,10,104). Thus, a major training adaptation is a shift to the more oxidative type IIA fiber type via an upregulation of type IIA protein synthesis and downregulation of type IIX protein synthesis. Further, an early study compared kayakers with runners and found that type I predominated in the arms of the kayakers (but not legs) and the legs of the runners (but not arms), suggesting some training effect on type I and II conversion (188).

There is a progressive increase in muscle fiber CSA via the addition of myofibrillar proteins to the periphery during resistance training. Fiber CSA increases in both type I and II fibers but to a greater extent in type II fibers (126). Muscle activation translates to whole-muscle hypertrophy. Interestingly, simultaneous use of high-intensity aerobic training with heavy resistance training can create some incompatibility of adaptation. Minimal or no hypertrophy may occur in type I fibers, with most taking place in type II fibers (15,62,104,156). This is caused by the need for high-force stimuli to be used in a resistance training program if type I fibers are to be stimulated to grow (19). In addition, concurrent training of both high-oxidative and high-force programs will limit type I muscle hypertrophy as high intensity aerobic training results in decreases in type I fiber size (104). Thus, care must be taken at the higher levels of simultaneous training with both endurance and resistance training, and some prioritization of training is needed to optimize each element over the entire training cycle. *Figure 33-2* shows the different muscle fiber types and the MHC in humans.

HYPERTROPHY VERSUS HYPERPLASIA

Whole-muscle growth occurs predominantly because of an increase in the net amount of protein deposition within muscle fibers, or *hypertrophy*. Resistance training results in an increase in protein synthesis rate, a decrease in protein breakdown rate, or both, resulting in a net increase in muscle proteins. Muscle fiber **hyperplasia** or an increase in the number of muscle fibers has also been one possible mechanism for increasing the size of muscle. The mechanism for hyperplasia appears to be related to satellite cell involvement in myogenesis (i.e., creating new fibers) or longitudinal splitting of existing fibers when a ceiling limit of cell size is reached. Although shown in animals, the concept of hyperplasia following resistance training in humans has not been directly proven because of methodological difficulties (e.g., one cannot take out the whole muscle for examination). Cross-sectional studies of strength-trained athletes show greater muscle fiber number compared with untrained individuals; however, genetics cannot be ruled out as an explanation. In a 12-wk training study of men, McCall et al. used both magnetic resonance imaging and biopsy techniques to examine hypertrophy, and the possible increase in cell number after a heavy resistance program showed some evidence for hyperplasia in the biceps muscle despite hypertrophy accounting for the greatest portion of muscle enlargement (131). It can be postulated that hyperplasia might account for approximately 3%–5% of the adaptational response to resistance training, possibly in response to fibers reaching a theoretic upper limit in size.

Neuromuscular Junction

Neural sprouting may occur where new fibers are added to motor units. At the **neuromuscular junction** (NMJ), high-intensity training has been shown to produce more dispersed, irregularly shaped synapses, high terminal branching, increased endplate perimeter length and area, and greater dispersion of acetylcholine receptors within the endplate region (32,34). Thus, changes in the NMJ with larger surface areas, higher amounts of neurotransmitters, and neuronal sprouting all may affect the adaptations to resistance training.

MUSCLE ARCHITECTURE

Muscle architecture refers to the geometric arrangement of muscle fibers in *pennate* muscles (1). Changes in muscle architecture occur during resistance training, accommodating muscle hypertrophy (46,75). Resistance training increases the angle of pennation in pennate muscles. Although during acute muscle contraction, an increase in pennation angle may result in force loss, the additional packing of contractile tissue with hypertrophy is compensatory, thereby allowing the muscle to produce more force and power. In addition, fascicle length has been shown to increase in some studies but not all (8,82,83,176). These architectural changes affect the manner in which force is transmitted to tendons and bones.

ENZYMATIC ADAPTATIONS

Increases in energy enzyme activity can lead to a greater adenosine triphosphate (ATP) production and increases in physical performance. However, there have been conflicting reports regarding enzymatic changes during resistance training. Enzyme activity of the adenosine energy source (*e.g.*, creatine phosphokinase and myokinase) has been shown to increase in humans during isokinetic and traditional resistance training (28,89). However, little or no change, or a decrease in creatine phosphokinase and myokinase have also been observed as a result of resistance training (116,186,189). Myosin ATPase has shown only minor changes in pooled muscle fibers (187). Resistance training programs that primarily stress the phosphagens (*i.e.*, readily available ATP and creatine phosphate [CP]) demonstrate reductions in glycolytic enzyme concentrations with pronounced hypertrophy, whereas intermittent high-intensity training, such as bodybuilding, may enhance glycolytic enzyme activity primarily in type II fibers. Phosphorylase activity has been shown to increase following resistance training (60,89). Phosphofructokinase (PFK) activity has been shown to increase or not change (or slightly decrease) (28,189). Lactate dehydrogenase (LDH) activity has been shown to increase, whereas no changes have been observed in hexokinase and malate dehydrogenase (28,60). Some increases in aerobic enzymes have been reported but are not typical because traditional resistance training poses little stress to aerobic metabolism (28). Aerobic enzyme activity has been shown to be lower in lifters compared with untrained individuals

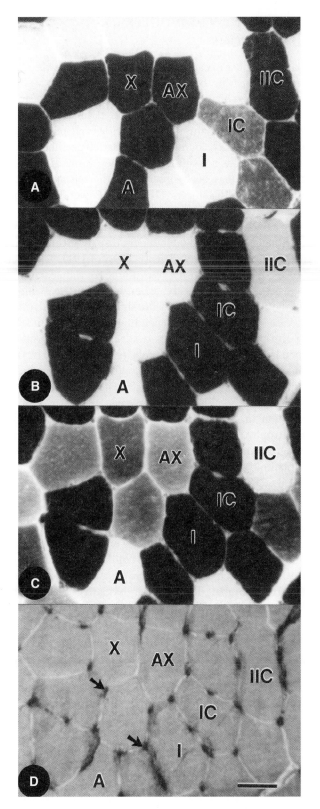

FIGURE 33-2. Muscle fiber types under different pH incubations. **A:** 10.4. **B:** 4.3. **C:** 4.6. **D:** The capillary stain with the black dots capillaries. X- and AX-marked fibers are type II. (Courtesy of Dr. Robert Staron, Ohio University, Athens, Ohio)

(190). Bodybuilders using high-volume programs, short rest periods between sets and exercises, and moderate-intensity training resistances have been shown to have higher citrate synthase activity in type II fibers than other types of lifters who train with heavier loads and longer rest periods between sets (187). However, it should be noted that bodybuilders typically perform aerobic exercise as well as resistance training, thus cross-sectional data should be viewed with caution. Therefore, most studies showing no change or a decrease in enzyme activity also reported significant muscle hypertrophy. Initially, enzyme activity may increase in response to resistance training but may not change or even decrease with subsequent training that produces significant muscle hypertrophy because of *protein dilution* (*i.e.,* a reduction in concentration per unit of muscle weight that is caused by increased muscle CSA). It appears that enzymatic changes associated with resistance training depend on the energy system demand, which is a composite of the interaction between intensity, volume, rest interval length, and muscle mass involvement. Traditional heavy resistance training will have minimal effects on enzyme activity, whereas a training program that minimizes hypertrophy and targets specific energy systems will most likely result in greater enzyme activities.

MUSCLE SUBSTRATE STORES

Anaerobic energy source substrates are enhanced with resistance training. Acute bouts of resistance exercise reduce ATP and CP concentrations and can increase storage of these compounds via a "supercompensation" effect. Five months of resistance training has been shown to increase resting intramuscular concentrations of CP and ATP by 28% and 18%, respectively; however, normal concentrations of CP and ATP have been reported in athletes having a significant amount of muscular hypertrophy (120,187). A 66% increase in intramuscular glycogen stores was shown after resistance training for 5 mo (120). Bodybuilders have been shown to have approximately a 50% greater concentration of glycogen than untrained individuals (187). However, muscle glycogen content has not always been shown to change with resistance training (187). Whether an increase in CP and ATP occurs with resistance training may depend on pretraining status, muscle group examined, and type of program performed. Lastly, a change in muscle triglyceride stores with resistance training remains equivocal, as lower and no difference from normal triglyceride content in the muscles of trained lifters have been reported (187). Although dietary practices and type of program may affect triglyceride concentrations, it can be hypothesized that intramuscular triglyceride concentrations are minimally affected by resistance training unless accompanied by significant weight loss.

CAPILLARY AND MYOGLOBIN ADAPTATIONS

A larger number of capillaries in muscle supports metabolism by increasing blood supply to the muscle. McCall et al. observed significant increases in numbers of capillaries (*capillarization*) per type I and II fibers following 12 wk of resistance training (131). However, no changes in *capillary density* (number of capillaries per fiber area) were observed as a result of fiber hypertrophy. Improved capillarization has been observed with resistance training in untrained subjects (183,187). Power lifters and weightlifters exhibit a similar capillary number and a lower capillary density when compared with nonathletic individuals; however, bodybuilders display greater capillarization and capillary density (79,174,191). Thus, it appears that high-intensity/low-volume resistance training decreases capillary density, whereas low-intensity/high-volume resistance training with short rest intervals may increase capillary density, depending on the magnitude of hypertrophy. These workouts result in large elevations in blood lactate; higher capillary density may facilitate lactate removal from the muscle to the blood (103). To conclude, capillarization can increase with resistance training, but this is typically, although not always, associated with a reduction in capillary density that is caused by muscle hypertrophy. Lastly, muscle myoglobin content following strength training may be decreased, yet the effect of this adaptation is not clear (69).

MITOCHONDRIAL DENSITY

In a manner similar to capillary density, mitochondrial density has been shown to decrease with resistance training because of the dilution effects of muscle hypertrophy (119). Decreased mitochondrial density is consistent with the minimal demands for oxidative metabolism placed on the musculature during most resistance training programs. Chilibeck et al. reported reduced mitochondrial density of regionally distributed mitochondria (*i.e.,* subsarcolemmal and intermyofibrillar mitochondrial density decreased similarly) following resistance training (23). Thus, mitochondrial density appears to decrease in response to resistance training because of the area measurement dilution, but absolute mitochondrial content has not been shown to decrease and appears to be similar in the transition from sedentary to strength or endurance trained individuals (150).

ENDOCRINE ADAPTATIONS

Hormones play a multitude of important regulatory roles in adaptation to resistance training. Neuroendocrine responses to resistance exercise take place in a unique physiologic environment and are a result of increased secretion, reduced hepatic clearance, plasma volume reductions, and/or reduced degradation rates (107). Acute elevations in circulating blood hormone concentrations observed during and immediately following a resistance exercise session increase the molar exposure of a hormone to its receptor on either the target tissue cell membrane (*e.g.*, peptides) or with nuclear/cytoplasmic receptors located within the target tissue (*e.g.*, steroid receptors) and increase receptor availability for binding and subsequent cellular changes. Receptor response from this interaction initiates events (through signaling cascades), ultimately leading to a specific cellular response, such as an increase in muscle protein synthesis or the use of a particular metabolic substrate. Endocrine release of hormones into the blood, paracrine release of hormones locally to affect other cells, and autocrine release of hormones to interact with the same cell are all involved with the hormonal control of cellular metabolism, repair, and remodeling.

The primary anabolic hormones are testosterone (T), growth hormone(s) (GH), insulin-like growth factors (IGF) and insulin, whereas cortisol is a catabolic hormone. *T* is a steroid hormone produced by the testes that increases protein synthesis, growth, strength and power, and controls secondary sex characteristics (198). It can also be produced in the adrenal gland via conversion from prohormones, which is the major way in which women produce T. The acidophilic cells of the anterior pituitary secrete the superfamily of *GH* polypeptides. The most commonly studied GH isoform, the 22-kD molecule, consists of 191 amino acids, yet the complexity of this GH superfamily is just starting to be understood (93). In addition, other monomeric, dimeric, protein-bound GH, and aggregates of GH have been identified that are included in this GH superfamily. GH is essential for promoting tissue anabolism. Some of the effects of GH are mediated by the anabolic protein hormone produced in the liver — *insulin-like growth factor-1* (IGF-1). *Insulin* has a potent upregulating effect on muscle protein synthesis when adequate amino acids are available. Insulin concentrations parallel changes in blood glucose, and its response is enhanced by protein/carbohydrates ingestion before, during, or immediately following the workout. Without such ingestion before exercise, serum insulin concentrations have been shown to decrease or show no change during an acute bout of resistance exercise (200). *Catecholamines* (epinephrine, norepinephrine, dopamine) reflect the acute demands of resistance exercise and are important for increasing force production, muscle contraction rate, energy availability, and augmenting other hormones, such as T. The adrenal cortex releases *cortisol*, which stimulates lipolysis in adipose cells, increases protein degradation (breakdown), and decreases protein synthesis in muscle cells. Cortisol may have a negative influence on mammalian target of rapamycin (mTOR) protein signaling cues and negatively affects protein synthesis. It is possible that the effects of cortisol may be greater in fast-twitch muscle fibers compared with slow-twitch muscle fibers, and the disinhibition of cortisol effects may occur with training in which the intensity of receptor interactions may decrease.

ACUTE HORMONAL RESPONSE

Hormonal adaptations are governed by their acute response to a workout, chronic changes in resting concentrations, and chronic changes in the acute response (*Table 33-2*) (71). Resistance exercise has been shown to

TABLE 33-2. Hormonal Adaptations to Resistance Training

Hormone	Acute Response to Resistance Training	Chronic Resting Adaptations	Chronic Changes to Acute Response
Testosterone	May ↑ or ↔; an ↑ is likely with high-intensity, high-volume programs with short rest intervals	Typically ↔ unless there are substantial changes in volume and intensity	May ↑ slightly if individual can train at higher levels
	Most critical for recovery and adaptation	May ↓ with overtraining	
Growth Hormone	↑ or ↔ with low-volume, low-intensity workouts is related to anaerobic nature of workout and to blood lactate when high- intensity, high-volume programs with short rest elicit large response	↔; however, overnight "bursts" may ↑ if workout is strenuous enough	Acute ↑ can be higher when individuals train harder over time
Insulin	↔, response related to diet or plasma volume ↓	↔	↔
IGF-1	Delayed response based on GH secretion patterns	Related to GH changes, ↔ or ↑ IGF-1 in muscle ↑	Related to GH
Cortisol	↑ or ↔ with low-volume, low-intensity workouts ↑ is related to anaerobic nature of workout when high-intensity, high-volume programs with short rest elicit large response	↔; ↓; may ↑ with overtraining	May not change
Catecholamines	↑ during workout and before in anticipation	↔	↔

↑, increase; ↓, decrease; ↔, no change; IGF-1, insulin-like growth factor-1; GH, growth hormone.

Modified from Hoffman J, Ratamess NA. *A Practical Guide to Developing Resistance-Training Programs.* Monterey (CA): Coaches Choice; 2006. 168 p.

result in elevated T (total and free) and GH and its molecular variants during and for up to 15–30 min postexercise in men (94–96). T elevations are most prominent in men, although some studies have shown slight T elevations in women, despite women having 10- to 30-fold lower T concentrations than men (145). The magnitude of T, cortisol, and GH elevation is greatest when large muscle mass exercises are performed during workouts of moderate to high in intensity and volume with short rest intervals (107). High correlations between blood lactate and GH concentrations have been reported, and it is thought that H^+ accumulation may be the primary factor influencing GH and cortisol release (64). When large muscle mass exercises are performed early in a workout, they have a positive effect (*i.e.*, greater strength and hypertrophy) on smaller muscle mass exercises performed later because, in part, of an enhanced T response (67). These data, in part, provide support for the ACSM's recommendation of performing large muscle mass exercises before small mass exercises for resistance exercise sequencing in addition to allowing for higher exercise intensity for the large muscle group exercise (*e.g.*, squat or leg press) (10). Resistance exercise increases concentrations of epinephrine, norepinephrine, and dopamine, and the catecholamine concentrations are elevated before resistance exercise (50,96,103). The magnitude may be dependent on the force of muscle contraction, amount of muscle stimulated, volume of resistance exercise, and rest interval length. In addition, the acute hormonal response to resistance exercise is attenuated when carbohydrates or protein are consumed before the workout (161). Yet, this may well be due to an increased amount of *upregulation* of receptors taking the hormones out of circulation (111).

CHRONIC CHANGES IN RESTING CONCENTRATIONS

Reported changes in resting T concentrations during resistance training have been inconsistent; with elevations, no differences and reductions reported, yet this is a function of the upregulation or downregulation of androgen receptors (ARs) (107,198). It appears that resting concentrations reflect the muscle tissue's current state relative to changes in training volume and intensity. Substantial changes in volume and intensity may elicit transient changes in resting T concentrations, and values may return to baseline when the individual returns to "normal" training. Chronic elevations in T may not be desirable in the sense that AR desensitization can occur; thus, the acute response may be most critical for tissue remodeling. Resistance training does not appear to affect resting concentrations of 22-kD GH in men and women (102). This contention is supported by data showing similar resting concentrations of GH in elite Olympic weightlifters/strength athletes compared

with lesser trained individuals (6). These findings are consistent with dynamic feedback mechanisms of GH and its roles in the homeostatic control of other variables (*e.g.*, glucose). This may be because of the lack of regulatory roles for the 22-kD monomer. One theory is that the larger molecular variants and binding proteins are more responsive to training adaptations. In a study by Kraemer et al., it was shown that different resistance training programs displayed different training effects based on the assay used to determine GH concentrations (102). Interestingly, the large aggregate GH isoforms were sensitive to training, and these affect muscle and connective tissue signaling and adaptations (93). Chronic exercise induces no consistent changes in immunoassayable GH variants, whereas bioassayable GH may increase across all fractions and training regimens.

Short-term resistance training does not appear to change resting levels of IGF-1, but long-term training may elicit some elevations. Resting IGF-1 concentrations have been shown to be higher in trained than untrained men and during high-volume multiple set training (127,169). Borst et al. reported significant elevations in resting serum IGF-1 following 13 wk of resistance training (16). However, these elevations were similar between single-set and multiple-set training groups, despite a significantly larger increase in strength for the multiple-set group. Thus, it appears that the intensity and volume of training significantly affects the chronic long-term IGF-1 adaptations. IGF-1 also appears to be related as a biomarker to aerobic fitness levels of men with higher values related to better aerobic fitness but not muscle strength or fat-free mass in men (146). Resting cortisol concentrations generally reflect long-term training stress. Resting cortisol concentrations do not appear to produce consistent patterns, as elevations, reductions and no change have been found (107). Thus, the acute cortisol response may reflect metabolic stress, whereas chronic changes (or lack of change) may be important to tissue homeostasis involving protein metabolism. Higher concentrations of cortisol may be indicative of an accumulated training stress that ultimately can cause problems with anabolic signaling and optimal muscle fiber adaptations (178).

CHRONIC CHANGES IN THE ACUTE HORMONAL RESPONSE

As a result of consistent resistance training, the acute hormonal response to a resistance exercise bout may improve as the individual exerts himself or herself to a greater extent. Thus, progressive overload is critical for potentially enhancing the acute hormonal response. It appears that a potentiated hormonal response takes several weeks to months of resistance training to occur. It has recently been shown that the short-term acute hormonal response to a standard resistance exercise protocol was not augmented, despite slightly higher resistance exercise volume in strength and power athletes (161). The associated metabolic and neural responses increased in stress typically result in higher hormonal response patterns. Yet, correlations of homeostatic hormonal signaling to accumulating variables such as muscle size and strength are inconsequential because of the temporal inequity of these two variables functions and movement over time (198).

AUTOCRINE/PARACRINE ACTIONS

IGF-1 has autocrine/paracrine functions within muscle cells. Two nonhepatic isoforms, IGF-1EA (similar to the circulating hepatic IGF-1) and *mechano-growth factor* (MGF), appear to increase protein synthesis, promote satellite cell activation, and are sensitive to the mechanical overload of resistance training. Bamman et al. found significant elevations in muscle IGF-1 mRNA following resistance exercise (13). However, a recent review indicates that data points toward the fact that IGF-1 splice variants may regulate myoblast differentiation through the actions of mature IGF-1 and not the E peptides, adding yet more complexity to the roles of the various peptides in the IGF superfamily (128). Nevertheless, it appears that overloaded muscle and subsequent mechanical damage associated with resistance training is a prominent stimulus for muscle IGF-1 isoform production and release.

ANDROGEN RECEPTOR ADAPTATIONS

ARs mediate the effects of androgens and are found in most tissues (198). Content depends on several factors, including muscle fiber type, contractile activity, and the concentrations of T. Resistance training has been shown to upregulate AR mRNA (13,78). The resistance exercise stimulus appears to mediate the magnitude of acute AR modifications. A typical profile sequence that one observes over a 1–24 h time frame after a resistance exercise protocol is a stabilization of the receptor followed by a catabolic *downregulation* of receptor content followed by the *upregulation* of the ARs if the stimulus is adequate (198). Higher volumes of exercise result in a shift from the static stabilization phase (162). It has been shown that women with lower molar concentrations of T go through this phasic pattern of AR binding more frequently than men (197). Workouts that stimulate T production also seem to enhance the AR upregulation (181). It has also been discovered that ingestion of a protein/carbohydrate supplement before and after the workout attenuates the AR downregulation, with higher volume resistance exercise observed 1-h postexercise (111). However, using a rat model, chronic alcohol consumption can downregulate AR content (196). Thus, nutritional intervention plays a critical role in AR modification postresistance exercise. In addition, significant correlations between baseline AR content in the vastus lateralis and 1-RM squat suggest that AR content, in part, assists in mediating strength changes during resistance training (162). Finally, although most human studies examine a mixed fiber-type muscle homogenate, it is interesting to note that using an animal model androgen content is downregulated in type I muscle fibers when anabolic exercise is used, indicating that type I muscle fibers have a potential upper limit for size to optimize oxygen kinetics (33).

CONNECTIVE TISSUE ADAPTATIONS

BONE

Bone is sensitive to intensity, compression, strain, and strain rate. Greater muscle strength increases the mechanical stress on bone, forcing bone to adapt by increasing mass and strength (an increase in *bone mineral density* [BMD]). Such forces are common in resistance training and relate to the type of exercise used, intensity of the resistance, number of sets, rate of loading, direction of forces, and frequency of training. It has been generally recommended that three to six sets of 1- to 10-RM loads for multiple-joint exercises be used, with 1–4 min of rest between sets for optimal bone loading (25). BMD increases during resistance training, provided that sufficient intensity and volume are used (85). Strength athletes — that is, weightlifters and power lifters — have been shown to have very high BMD values (hip, femur, lumbar spine, whole body) compared with untrained individuals (26,35,193). In a later investigation, Tsuzuku et al. reported significantly greater BMD in men resistance training with high intensity versus low intensity, thus showing that heavy loading is needed to see improvements in BMD (194). Recent research has indicated power training (light-to-moderate loads, high velocity) to be as, or more, effective than traditional resistance training for maintaining BMD in postmenopausal women (201).

Resistance training is effective for increasing BMD in men and women of all ages; however, the time course is rather long (*i.e.*, ~6 mo or longer) and depends on the structure of the program (22,86,142). Cussler et al. reported that the amount of weight lifted during 1 yr of resistance training was correlated to changes in BMD in postmenopausal women (30). In particular, weight lifted for the squat correlated highly to femur BMD, and the weighted march exercise (*i.e.*, hiking with a weighted backpack) correlated highly to total BMD. This study, as well as others, demonstrated the importance of intensity of resistance training for eliciting increases in BMD and osteoporosis risk reduction (194). Of significance have been recent studies demonstrating that many men and women resistance training in health clubs self-select intensities far below 60% of their respective 1-RM (45,58,158). Ratamess et al. have shown that women who trained on their own self-selected intensities of 38%–48% of their 1-RM, whereas women who were trained by a personal trainer self-selected intensities of 43%–57% of their 1-RM (158). Only 7% of the women tested self-selected at least 75% of 1-RM on at least one of the four exercises tested (158). These studies demonstrate that many individuals fail to adequately overload the skeletal system. Interestingly, in male athletes, estradiol levels, body mass index, and resistance training predicts BMD better than T (3). Therefore, it appears that only high-intensity resistance training may be effective for long-term progression in BMD enhancement.

Although increases in BMD accompanying resistance training take at least several months to be observed, the process of adaptation begins within the first few workouts as evidenced by blood elevations of two markers of bone anabolism: *bone alkaline phosphatase* and *osteocalcin* (81). Several studies have shown elevated serum osteocalcin (or bone alkaline phosphatase) concentrations during 1–18 mo of resistance training, and the magnitude of change has been shown to be affected by protein intake in some studies (12,54,133,160). Thus, the mechanisms of bone osteogenesis are engaged within the first few workouts, but it takes several months before measurable changes in BMD can be shown.

CARTILAGE, LIGAMENTS, TENDONS, AND FASCIA

Connective tissue is abundantly distributed throughout the body. As skeletal muscle strength increases, tendons, ligaments, cartilage, and fascia must also adapt to support greater loading. Extensive work is now being undertaken to better understand the morphological and intrinsic properties (90,185). In addition, data exited as to a differential response of exercise training and tendon responses with men being more responsive to training than women (124). The primary stimulus for growth of connective tissue is the mechanical forces created during resistance exercise. Signals from mechanical loading initiate a cascade of events ultimately leading from gene expression to greater protein synthesis incorporated into connective tissue. As with bone, the magnitude of connective tissue adaptation appears to be proportional to resistance exercise intensity. Changes in collagen size, number, and packing density within a tendon contribute to its size and strength. Exercise increases the size and strength of tendons and ligaments (184). Increased strength of the ligaments and tendons is a necessary adaptation to aid in preventing possible injury. It also appears that these structures hypertrophy somewhat slower than muscle because increases in *tendon stiffness* (force transmission per unit of strain), without changes in tendon CSA, have been reported despite increases in muscle strength and hypertrophy (112–114). Critical

is the intensity because heavy loads (80% of 1-RM) increase tendon stiffness, but light loads (20% of 1-RM) do not (113). Thus, structural changes (*e.g.*, mechanical quality of collagen) may precede tendon hypertrophy. Periodized heavy resistance training itself over 3 mo is capable of increasing the thickness of the patella tendon with or without protein supplementation (98). Connective tissue hypertrophy appears to occur in proportion to muscle size increases. This contention is supported by reports that bodybuilders do not differ from control subjects in the relative amount of connective tissue in the biceps brachii, and men and women bodybuilders possess similar relative amounts of connective tissue (9.7% vs. 10.7%, respectively) (9,117).

CARDIORESPIRATORY ADAPTATIONS

ACUTE RESPONSES TO RESISTANCE EXERCISE

Resistance exercise poses a high acute stress to the cardiovascular system. Heart rate, stroke volume, cardiac output, and blood pressure increase significantly to meet the demands of resistance exercise (41). The blood pressure response increases nonlinearly with the magnitude of active muscle mass (41). Although large elevations in blood pressure may occur, no negative effects on resting blood pressure have been reported. It has been known for some time that resistance training does reduce the pressor response to a weight training protocol demonstrating the health benefits of resistance training (42). During each set of resistance exercise, stroke volume and cardiac output increase, especially when a *Valsalva maneuver* is used (40). Interestingly, a recent study demonstrated that there was a significant inverse relationship between muscular strength and aortic stiffness independent of aerobic fitness, demonstrating that strength training had a positive effect on the heart from a peripheral perspective (39). In addition, ventilation is significantly elevated during each set, but this elevation quickly decreases to normal during the first minute of recovery (159). Ventilations in excess of 60 L · min^{-1} during resistance exercise have been observed with short rest intervals (159). Overall, the magnitude of the acute cardiovascular responses depends on the intensity and volume of exercise, muscle mass involvement, rest intervals used, and contraction velocity (106,108). However, resistance training does not significantly affect maximal aerobic capacity (see later in this chapter).

RESTING ADAPTATIONS

Decreased resting heart rate, or *bradycardia*, and blood pressure are positive cardiovascular adaptations that reduce cardiac workload and decrease the risk of myocardial infarction. Resistance training may reduce or not change resting heart rate, depending on one's level of fitness (as unfit individuals are most responsive). Highly resistance-trained athletes have an average or slightly below average resting heart rate (41). Resistance training has shown small, significant decreases in resting heart rate of 5%–12% (41). Decreases in resting heart rate are much more prominent during aerobic training. Resting systolic and diastolic blood pressure of strength-trained athletes is average or slightly below average (41). A meta-analysis of studies in which individuals performed weight training for 4 wk or more showed that resistance training decreases resting systolic and diastolic blood pressure approximately 2% and 4%, respectively (84). Stroke volume has been shown to increase in absolute magnitude but not relative to body surface area or lean body mass (41). Resistance training can be very important for patient populations and help improve their functional capabilities (74). In addition, resistance training may either not change or slightly decrease total cholesterol and low-density lipoprotein (LDL) cholesterol while increasing high-density lipo-protein (HDL) cholesterol (73). High-volume, short rest interval programs (*e.g.*, bodybuilding, circuit training) with high continuity appear most effective at eliciting cardiovascular adaptations at rest but still not as dramatic as aerobic training (56). Lastly, resistance training has been shown to increase left ventricular and intra-ventricular septal wall thicknesses, which are critical to tolerating greater cardiac pressure overload during resistance exercise (41). Increased wall thicknesses are also observed in several conditions that produce chronic elevations in afterload (systolic blood pressure), such as hypertension.

CHRONIC CHANGES TO THE ACUTE RESISTANCE EXERCISE RESPONSE

Resistance training has been shown to reduce the acute increases in heart rate and blood pressure during a workout of a similar absolute level of effort (173). In addition, resistance training leads to faster recovery of heart rate to resting values after a work bout (173). The decreases in heart rate and blood pressure during submaximal work are viewed as positive adaptations and reduce cardiovascular stress.

MAXIMAL OXYGEN CONSUMPTION

Resistance training does not significantly affect maximal oxygen consumption ($\dot{V}O_{2max}$) in fit individuals, although deconditioned individuals may see improvements. The lack of continuity during resistance exercise (*i.e.*, rest periods between sets) appears to pose limitations for potential improvements in $\dot{V}O_{2max}$. Large muscle mass workouts have been shown to elicit responses peaking at 60% of $\dot{V}O_{2max}$, which may not reach the critical threshold needed for improvement (187). Circuit training and high-volume, short rest period programs have been shown to improve $\dot{V}O_{2max}$, but the effects are considerably less than aerobic training (57).

It is important to note that some studies have shown that combining high-intensity resistance and aerobic training may interfere primarily with strength and power gains if the aerobic training is high in intensity, volume, and frequency (104). Yet improvement in $\dot{V}O_{2max}$ was not compromised with simultaneous training, but with strength training alone, no significant changes were observed (104). In contrast, most studies have shown no adverse effects on $\dot{V}O_{2max}$ from heavy resistance exercise despite the expected physiologic changes caused by resistance training, although a study has shown the addition of strength training can hinder $\dot{V}O_{2max}$ improvements (59). The physiologic mechanisms involved in the incompatibility may be related to alterations in neural recruitment patterns, attenuation of muscle hypertrophy, overtraining, inadequate recovery in between workouts, hormonal environment, and residual fatigue from aerobic workouts during resistance exercise. It is important to note that incompatibility may be seen at higher levels of training and may not be expected in a general health and fitness setting.

IMMUNE SYSTEM RESPONSES AND ADAPTATIONS

The overload associated with resistance exercise causes trauma and damage to skeletal muscle. The immune system responds with a series of reactions leading to an inflammatory response that contains and repairs the damage, removes debris from the injured area, and ultimately plays a key role in skeletal muscle hypertrophy. The immune system responds to infection, injury, and inflammation using many types of cells, including leukocytes (*e.g.*, neutrophils, monocytes, eosinophils, basophils, lymphocytes, and subsets), immunoglobulins, and cytokines (147). With exercise stress, the neuroendocrine and immune systems contributes to the mechanisms trying to accommodate the increase in physiological demands (47). The resulting adaptations alleviate the magnitude of subsequent stress or minimize the exercise challenge to fall within the normal homeostatic limits. This adaptive capacity of collaborating systems reflects the acquired, or adaptive, branch of the immune system.

Along with monocytes/macrophages, *neutrophils* are the first line of immune defense localized to the injury/inflammation site, especially with damaged skeletal muscle induced by exercise. *Monocytes* are involved in phagocytosis, antigen presentation, cytokine production, and cytotoxicity; differentiate into macrophages; and produce interleukin (IL)-1, IL-6, and tumor necrosis factor-alpha (TNF-α). Macrophages move to the injury site and secrete cytokines, growth factors, and other substances. *Lymphocytes* are involved with cytokine production, antigen recognition, antibody production, and cytotoxicity, which give rise to subpopulations of *T cells* (CD3+, CD8+, and CD4+), *B cells* (CD19+), and *natural killer* (NK) *cells* (CD16+ and CD56+). *Immunoglobulins* (*e.g.*, IgA, IgG, IgE, and IgM) are antibodies that react with antigens and are involved in phagocytosis. *Cytokines* are polypeptides involved in communication between lymphoid and other cells and perform virtually all immune functions. They are responsible for protein breakdown, removal of damaged muscle cells, and an increased production of prostaglandins (hormone-like substances that help to control the inflammation). Some major anti-inflammatory cytokines include IL-1 receptor antagonist, IL-4, IL-10, IL-11, IL-12, and IL-13. The cytokines IL-1, TNF-α, and IL-6 function as proinflammatory cytokines. Because of the mechanical stress to the neuromuscular system, it has been of interest to examine whether resistance training (*i.e.*, because of soreness, damage, etc.) could suppress immune function during the postworkout period. Interestingly, most studies have shown that resistance exercise does not lead to immunosuppression in young or elderly individuals unless overtraining is present (44,88,123,177).

The interactions of specific immune cells are also gaining a complexity of response indicative of the adaptive response to resistance exercise stress. In a recent study, it was found that glucocorticoid receptors on B lymphocytes were elevated in anticipation of the resistance exercise protocol (six sets of 5-RM loading) but were decreased during the exercise and then increased during the recovery (49). Thus, cortisol and its impact on immune function takes on a rapid temporal effect altering B lymphocyte functions over the course of a workout time frame. In addition, a potential difference between the sexes was observed with cortisol being higher in response to the exercise protocol in men, yet immune modulation by existing molar concentrations was similar.

LEUKOCYTES

Leukocyte concentrations increase during and after exercise for several hours, with the magnitude related to exercise intensity and volume (123). The increase is mostly attributed to neutrophils, although lymphocyte and monocyte counts also increase. During resistance exercise, total leukocytes significantly increase in a similar pattern to endurance exercise (44,92). However, the response is less pronounced in basophils and eosinophils (123). Following resistance exercise that causes muscle damage, the leukocyte response in skeletal muscle appears to be biphasic: There is an 8%–10% elevation

in the first 8 h after the workout, but a 14% elevation between the eighth and twenty-first hours postexercise, which corresponded to a period of halted recovery (157). The magnitude of increase appears to be similar between athletes and nonathletes. Resting leukocyte counts typically do not change unless the athlete is overtrained, then reductions may occur. A substantial portion of the exercise-induced changes in leukocyte number may be mediated by the endocrine system, in which hormones such as catecholamines, cortisol, GH, T, and estrogen have been shown to affect lymphocyte subpopulations and proliferation, NK cell activity, and the neutrophils response (149).

Lymphocytes and subsets increase in response to all types of exercise. Moderate and intense interval exercise results in 50%–200% increases, whereas long and prolonged exercise results in 25%–100% increases (122,123). Miles et al. have shown acute resistance exercise results in elevations in CD4+, CD8+, NK, and B cells by 42%–242%, with the response highest when blood lactates were high (135). Lymphocyte proliferation was studied during acute resistance exercise between women with high (~72 kg) and low (~40 kg) 1-RM squats. An increase was observed in the low-strength group, whereas a decrease was observed in the high-strength group, thereby demonstrating the potential factor of maximal strength and loading on the immune response (36). At rest, no differences have been observed between resistance-trained women and controls; however, male weightlifters have been shown to have higher values based on the training cycle (88,135,136). Resistance exercise may increase B cells and T-cell subsets (136,144). However, NK cell cytotoxic activity has been shown to be decreased by 40% at 2 h following intensive resistance exercise (144). Resting concentrations of lymphocytes do not differ between athletes (endurance and power) and nonathletes, and long-term training does not alter resting subset distribution (123). However, Miles et al. reported that after 3 mo of resistance training in previously untrained women, resting NK concentrations were higher but returned to baseline after 6 mo of training (135). Monocytes increase during resistance exercise by approximately 15%–50%, whereas prolonged endurance exercise results in a 50%–250% increase (123). Resting concentrations typically do not change. Interestingly, rest interval length may play a role. Mayhew et al. have recently shown that lymphocytosis and monocytosis are significantly greater by 1.5 h postexercise by 32%–67% when 1-min versus 3-min rest intervals were used for 10 sets of 10 repetitions of the leg press, thus showing the acute response depends on the program used (130).

In a recent study, the impact of the adrenergic response to resistance training was demonstrated as plasma epinephrine and norepinephrine increased during the exercise bout and returned to baseline during recovery in both men and women after six sets of 5-RM in the squat exercise (48). The β2-adrenergic receptor (β2-ADR) expression on circulating leukocyte were altered in a pattern reflective of the temporal changes in catecholamines. β2-ADR expression on monocytes were elevated in anticipation of the resistance exercise protocol. However, β2-ADR expression on monocytes and granulocytes decreased during the resistance exercise protocol. Interestingly, the β2-ADR expression on lymphocytes was elevated during the recovery time points. Thus, interactions of receptors on leukocytes present a differential pattern around a workout showing the dynamic nature of the immune system in response to resistance exercise stress.

IMMUNOGLOBULINS

Resting concentrations of IgA, IgG, IgE, and IgM are similar between athletes unless the athlete is overtrained (*i.e.*, reductions may be observed) (134). Acute exercise has been shown to produce small increases (8%–12%) of some immunoglobulins, but many studies show no effect (123). The combination of resistance and endurance training in the elderly has been shown to increase IgA at rest (7).

CYTOKINES

Cytokines are released in response to exercise (149). Proinflammatory cytokines increase significantly, as do anti-inflammatory cytokines during exercise, especially when there is a strong eccentric component. The role each of these cytokines play under different conditions can vary. With training, the hormonal and the cytokine responses to a resistance exercise workout will be altered to reflect the adaptation to a reduction in the stress response (76). It is thought that the rise in anti-inflammatory cytokines restrict the magnitude and duration of the inflammatory response (149). Acute resistance exercise has been shown to increase plasma concentrations of IL-6, IL-8, IL-10, and IL-1 receptor antagonist (143). In addition, muscle mRNA for IL-1β, IL-6, IL-8, and TNF-α increase following resistance exercise (143). IL-1 (α and β) may increase twofold to fivefold days after heavy eccentric exercise in skeletal muscle. IL-6 and TNF-α have been shown to increase significantly following resistance exercise (148). In the elderly, high levels of IL-6 and TNF-α were associated with low muscle size and strength (199). Greiwe et al. reported that 3 mo of resistance training in the elderly reduced skeletal muscle TNF-α mRNA and protein levels while protein synthesis rate was inversely related to levels of TNF-α (61). Thus, downregulation of proinflammatory cytokines may be another mechanism by which resistance training elicits muscle growth. It has been shown that IL-15 is found in high concentrations in muscle and has anabolic and angiogenic properties. Riechman et al. examined 10 wk of resistance training

and reported that plasma IL-15 concentrations were elevated following a workout and that the acute response was not enhanced over 10 wk (164). However, IL-15 protein was not associated with gains in muscle size. In addition, a polymorphism in the IL-15 receptor α gene was associated with greater amounts of muscle hypertrophy.

DELAYED ONSET MUSCLE SORENESS

Delayed onset muscle soreness (DOMS) is the pain or discomfort experienced 24–72 h after resistance exercising, which subsides within 2–3 d. DOMS is associated with localized pain in the exercised muscles, reduced range of motion, loss of muscle strength and power, greater muscle stiffness, and swelling. Resistance exercise with a strong eccentric component leads to the most substantial magnitude of muscle damage as measured directly via muscle biopsies or indirectly via blood markers, such as creatine kinase (CK), myoglobin, lactate dehydrogenase, troponin I, and MHC fragments (147). The extent of muscle damage depends on the intensity, volume, and type of muscle actions used, plus the training status of the individual. In fact, resistance-trained individuals have shown significantly less elevation in CK and myoglobin concentrations and less muscle damage 12–120 h following an acute resistance exercise protocol compared with untrained individuals (195). Repeated bouts of resistance exercise exert a protective effect on skeletal muscle, thereby making it less susceptible to damage and accelerating the rate of repair in young and elderly individuals (125,154). In addition, the extent of muscle damage has been attenuated, and recovery has been enhanced by amino acid and L-carnitine L-tartrate supplementation (110,180).

Several mechanisms have been proposed to explain DOMS. DOMS may result from mechanical stress via heavy resistance exercise or from metabolic stress characteristic of low-to-moderate intensity resistance exercise, coupled with high-volume or short rest intervals. Different (novel) muscle recruitment patterns (*e.g.*, performing an unfamiliar exercise) may lead to unaccustomed stress placed on muscles, ligaments, and tendons. Mechanical traumas to contractile proteins and cytoskeleton, acute inflammation, local ischemia, muscle spasm, connective tissue damage, and free radical proliferation have all been implicated in DOMS. It is likely that DOMS is multifactorial and a result of multiple conditions. Treatments for DOMS are limited. For example, stretching, nonsteroidal anti-inflammatory agents, hyperbaric oxygen therapy, cryotherapy, massage, ultrasound, and nutritional supplementation (vitamins C and E) have shown limited effectiveness (24). However, recent work showed that a pharmaceutical agent, Vicoprofen, was superior to ibuprofen or a placebo in helping the recovery and repair of skeletal muscle as determined via magnetic resonance imaging (99). Interestingly, this opioid medication seemed to augment the natural endogenous opioid proenkephalin peptides from the adrenal medulla known to have a potential immune modulatory positive effect (192). Thus, it appears that the cascade of events leading to muscle damage and DOMS (*i.e.*, swelling, inflammatory response, prostaglandin E_2 release, leukotriene synthesis, immune response) may be critical to the tissue remodeling process.

HEALTH AND FITNESS ADAPTATIONS

As mentioned previously, resistance training elicits positive cardiovascular adaptations related to pressure overload. $\dot{V}O_{2max}$ may improve only slightly, and this effect is greatest in unfit individuals. In addition, blood lipid profiles (decreased triglycerides, increased HDLs, decreased LDLs) may not change or improve (although aerobic exercise and diet have more substantial effects). However, resistance training may elicit other adaptations that benefit general health and fitness. Flexibility may improve as well as muscular strength, endurance, and power (109). Resistance training has been shown to reduce percent body fat; increase insulin sensitivity; decrease basal insulin levels and insulin response to a glucose challenge; increase basal metabolic rate; attenuate muscle sarcopenia; reduce the risk of osteoporosis, colon cancer, and low back pain; and maintain long-term independence and functional capacity (109,202). These benefits, as well as the performance-related benefits, have been shown to improve the quality of life in the elderly and clinical populations such as those with low back pain, osteoarthritis, cardiovascular disease, stroke, HIV (human immunodeficiency virus), neuromuscular disease (*e.g.*, myasthenia gravis, myotonic dystrophy), obesity, renal failure, chronic obstructive pulmonary disease, and Type 2 diabetes mellitus (109).

OVERTRAINING

Overtraining is long-term excessive frequency, volume, or intensity of training resulting in prolonged fatigue and decreased performance. Short-term excessive training is called *overreaching* (129). A popular training model is to overwork and then taper (reduce the training stimulus) to "rebound" in performance. Short-term overreaching followed by a tapering period has been shown to result in substantial strength and power gains, and this effect has been shown to be enhanced with creatine or amino acid supplementation (53,110,163). However, overreaching can become overtraining syndrome if it continues beyond a reasonable period of time. Overtraining syndrome may include a plateau or reduction in performance. The progression in the overtraining continuum follows: the *overload stimulus* to *acute fatigue* to *overreaching* to *overtraining*. Resistance or

anaerobic overtraining is not the same as aerobic overtraining, and the signs and symptoms may differ. Overtraining is associated with greater damage or negative physiologic alterations in the neuromuscular system. Overtraining classically was thought to be a function of either chronic use of high intensity, high volume, or a combination of both. Training periodization consists of careful planning to avoid overtraining. Overreaching has been shown to decrease resting concentrations of T and IGF-1 (65). If the source of overtraining is volume related, elevations in cortisol and reductions in resting luteinizing hormone (LH), total T, and free T concentrations have been reported (51,52). Intensity-related overtraining does not appear to alter resting concentrations of hormones (51,52). However, desensitization to the sympathetic response (*i.e.*, the ratio of epinephrine to the density of β2-ADRs) occurs, which can contribute to performance reductions (53). Other symptoms of overtraining include mood disturbances; decreased vigor, motivation, and confidence; higher levels of tension, depression, anger, fatigue, confusion, anxiety, and irritability; and impaired concentration.

DETRAINING

Detraining is the decrease in performance and loss of some physiologic adaptations that result from cessation of resistance training or a substantial reduction in its frequency, volume, or intensity. The magnitude of strength loss depends on the length of the detraining period and the training status of the individuals. Decrements may occur in as little as 2 wk and possibly sooner in highly strength-trained individuals, but little to no reductions may be seen in recreationally trained men within 6 wk of detraining (101). Strength loss appears related to neural mechanisms initially, with muscle atrophy predominating as the detraining period extends; however, the magnitude of strength lost rarely exceeds the strength gained through training (101). That is, residual resistance training effects are shown, as maximal strength after detraining is still higher than maximal strength assessed before beginning a weight training program. The high strength retainment suggests "muscle memory." In addition, the reason that previously trained muscle may be more responsive to retraining and more rapidly regain muscle size is related to the longer term retention of myonuclei produced with prior long-term training (18). Thus, muscle memory may be related to both neural and cellular mechanisms.

AGING INFLUENCES ON THE NEUROMUSCULAR SYSTEM

Physiologic limitations in endocrine and immune function, cell regeneration, cell water, neuronal death, and a host of other underlying changes are related to aging. Strength training has been one of the major modalities

BOX 33-1	**Neuromuscular Factors Associated with Age-Related Decreases in Strength and Power**

- Change in resting hormone levels
- Blunted acute hormonal response to exercise
- Decrease in muscular energy substrate content
- Decrease in anaerobic enzyme concentration and activity
- Decrease in mitochondrial mass
- Denervation or death of muscle cells
- Decreased muscle mass (atrophy of muscle fibers, particularly of type II)

- Decreased ability to develop force rapidly
- Antagonistic coactivation
- Changes in ability to maximally activate a muscle
- Changes at the neuromuscular junction
- Decreased firing rate of motor units
- Decreased insulin sensitivity and tolerance

used in the fight against the aging process (77). Ultimately, this leads to *sarcopenia*, a loss of muscle tissue (whether by reduced fiber size or number), which leads to reduced performance capacity (166). Strength is an important factor for functional abilities. Muscle weakness can advance to a stage at which an elderly individual cannot do common activities of daily living, such as getting out of a chair, sweeping the floor, or taking out the trash. Reduced functional ability may lead to a loss of independence. Thus, muscle strength is vital to our health, functional abilities, and independent living. Under normal conditions, strength performances appear to peak between the ages of 20 and 30 yr, after which changes in strength remain relatively stable or slightly decrease over the next 20 yr depending on an individual's activity level. Large dramatic decreases are observed in the sixth decade of life, and this decrease may be more dramatic in women. In fact, Bassey and Harries reported a loss of grip strength of 3% per year for men and nearly 5% for women over a 4-yr period (14). The muscle's ability to exert force rapidly (power) diminishes with age and may be more sensitive to reduction than maximal strength. Adequate muscle power may serve as a protective mechanism against falling in the elderly, which is one of the leading causes of injury and may lead to death. Thus, loss of power significantly reduces functional capacity. Participation in resistance training in older individuals has positive effects, but participation earlier in life can be more effective in combating the aging process and sarcopenia (151). *Box 33-1* overviews some basic changes with aging.

Resistance training can offset the magnitude of strength loss; however, some reductions may occur even in individuals who have strength trained most of their lives. The loss of strength in the lower extremities has been shown to be greater than that of the upper extremities. It appears that muscle strength losses are most dramatic after the age of 70 yr. Cross-sectional as well as longitudinal data indicate that muscle strength declines by approximately 15% per decade in the sixth and seventh decades of life and about 30% thereafter (68). Muscle power trainability

in seniors has received limited study but may be even more important for performance of activities of daily living (walking, climbing stairs, and lifting objects). Bassey et al. reported that leg extensor power was significantly correlated with chair-rising speed, stair-climbing speed and power, and walking speed in elderly men and women (14). Studies have investigated power training in the elderly and have revealed positive results. Integration of power exercises into resistance training has shown to be effective for improving performance (63,141). Henwood and Taaffe examined 8 wk of power training (three sets of eight repetitions with 35%–75% of 1-RM at maximal concentric velocity) and reported 21%–82% increases in muscle strength; 16%–33% increases in muscle power; and significant enhancement of stair-climbing ability, 6-m walk, and ability to rise from the chair and the floor (70). Bottaro et al. compared 10 wk of power training with traditional resistance training and reported similar increases in strength between groups; however, the power training group improved in up-and-go and 30-s chair stand performance by 15%–43%, whereas the traditional group did not improve in functional capacity (17). Similar findings were reported by Miszko et al. who reported power training to be more effective than traditional resistance training for improving functional performance (137). Other studies have shown similar findings (155). Thus, resistance training programs for the elderly also should address the need for power.

REFERENCES

1. Aagaard P, Andersen JL, Dyhre-Poulsen P, et al. A mechanism for increased contractile strength of human pennate muscle in response to strength training: changes in muscle architecture. *J Physiol.* 2001;534(Pt. 2):613–23.

2. Aagaard P, Simonsen EB, Andersen JL, Magnusson P, Dyhre-Poulsen P. Neural adaptation to resistance training: changes in evoked V-wave and H-reflex responses. *J Appl Physiol.* 2002;92(6): 2309–18.

3. Ackerman KE, Skrinar GS, Medvedova E, Misra M, Miller KK. Estradiol levels predict bone mineral density in male collegiate athletes: a pilot study. *Clin Endocrinol (Oxf).* 2012;76(3):339–45.

4. Adams GR, Harris RT, Woodard D, Dudley GA. Mapping of electrical muscle stimulation using MRI. *J Appl Physiol.* 1993;74(2):532–7.

5. Adams GR, Hather BM, Baldwin KM, Dudley GA. Skeletal muscle myosin heavy chain composition and resistance training. *J Appl Physiol.* 1993;74(2):911–5.

6. Ahtiainen JP, Pakarinen A, Kraemer WJ, Hakkinen K. Acute hormonal responses to heavy resistance exercise in strength athletes versus nonathletes. *Can J Appl Physiol.* 2004;29(5):527–43.

7. Akimoto T, Kumai Y, Akama T, et al. Effects of 12 months of exercise training on salivary secretory IgA levels in elderly subjects. *Br J Sports Med.* 2003;37(1):76–9.

8. Alegre LM, Jimenez F, Gonzalo-Orden JM, Martin-Acero R, Aguado X. Effects of dynamic resistance training on fascicle length and isometric strength. *J Sports Sci.* 2006;24(5):501–8.

9. Alway SE, Grumbt WH, Gonyea WJ, Stray-Gundersen J. Contrasts in muscle and myofibers of elite male and female bodybuilders. *J Appl Physiol.* 1989;67(1):24–31.

10. American College of Sports Medicine. American College of Sports Medicine position stand. Progression models in resistance training for healthy adults. *Med Sci Sports Exerc.* 2009;41(3):687–708.

11. Andrews TR, Mackey T, Inkrott TA, Murray SR, Clark IE, Pettitt RW. Effect of hang cleans or squats paired with countermovement vertical jumps on vertical displacement. *J Strength Cond Res.* 2011;25(9):2448–52.

12. Ballard TL, Clapper JA, Specker BL, Binkley TL, Vukovich MD. Effect of protein supplementation during a 6-mo strength and conditioning program on insulin-like growth factor I and markers of bone turnover in young adults. *Am J Clin Nutr.* 2005;81(6):1442–8.

13. Bamman MM, Shipp JR, Jiang J, et al. Mechanical load increases muscle IGF-I and androgen receptor mRNA concentrations in humans. *Am J Physiol Endocrinol Metab.* 2001;280(3):E383–90.

14. Bassey EJ, Fiatarone MA, O'Neill EF, Kelly M, Evans WJ, Lipsitz LA. Leg extensor power and functional performance in very old men and women. *Clin Sci (Lond).* 1992;82(3):321–7.

15. Bell GJ, Syrotuik D, Martin TP, Burnham R, Quinney HA. Effect of concurrent strength and endurance training on skeletal muscle properties and hormone concentrations in humans. *Eur J Appl Physiol.* 2000;81(5):418–27.

16. Borst SE, De Hoyos DV, Garzarella L, et al. Effects of resistance training on insulin-like growth factor-I and IGF binding proteins. *Med Sci Sports Exerc.* 2001;33(4):648–53.

17. Bottaro M, Machado SN, Nogueira W, Scales R, Veloso J. Effect of high versus low-velocity resistance training on muscular fitness and functional performance in older men. *Eur J Appl Physiol.* 2007;99(3):257–64.

18. Bruusgaard JC, Johansen IB, Egner IM, Rana ZA, Gundersen K. Myonuclei acquired by overload exercise precede hypertrophy and are not lost on detraining. *Proc Natl Acad Sci U S A.* 2010;107(34):15111–6.

19. Campos GE, Luecke TJ, Wendeln HK, et al. Muscular adaptations in response to three different resistance-training regimens: specificity of repetition maximum training zones. *Eur J Appl Physiol.* 2002;88(1–2):50–60.

20. Cannon RJ, Cafarelli E. Neuromuscular adaptations to training. *J Appl Physiol.* 1987;63(6):2396–402.

21. Carolan B, Cafarelli E. Adaptations in coactivation after isometric resistance training. *J Appl Physiol.* 1992;73(3):911–7.

22. Chilibeck PD, Calder A, Sale DG, Webber CE. Twenty weeks of weight training increases lean tissue mass but not bone mineral mass or density in healthy, active young women. *Can J Physiol Pharmacol.* 1996;74(10):1180–5.

23. Chilibeck PD, Syrotuik DG, Bell GJ. The effect of strength training on estimates of mitochondrial density and distribution throughout muscle fibres. *Eur J Appl Physiol Occup Physiol.* 1999;80(6):604–9.

24. Connolly DA, Sayers SP, McHugh MP. Treatment and prevention of delayed onset muscle soreness. *J Strength Cond Res.* 2003;17(1):197–208.

25. Conroy BP, Earle RW. Bone, muscle, and connective tissue adaptations to physical activity. In: Baechle TR, Earle RW, National Strength & Conditioning Association (U.S.), editors. *Essentials of Strength Training and Conditioning.* 2nd ed. Champaign: Human Kinetics; 2000. p. 57–72.

26. Conroy BP, Kraemer WJ, Maresh CM, et al. Bone mineral density in elite junior Olympic weightlifters. *Med Sci Sports Exerc.* 1993;25(10):1103–9.

27. Cormie P, McGuigan MR, Newton RU. Developing maximal neuromuscular power: part 2—training considerations for improving maximal power production. *Sports Med.* 2011;41(2):125–46.

28. Costill DL, Coyle EF, Fink WF, Lesmes GR, Witzmann FA. Adaptations in skeletal muscle following strength training. *J Appl Physiol.* 1979;46(1):96–9.

29. Crewther BT, Kilduff LP, Cook CJ, Middleton MK, Bunce PJ, Yang GZ. The acute potentiating effects of back squats on athlete performance. *J Strength Cond Res.* 2011;25(12):3319–25.

30. Cussler EC, Lohman TG, Going SB, et al. Weight lifted in strength training predicts bone change in postmenopausal women. *Med Sci Sports Exerc.* 2003;35(1):10–7.

31. De Luca CJ, Contessa P. Hierarchical control of motor units in voluntary contractions. *J Neurophysiol.* 2012;107(1):178–95.

32. Deschenes MR, Judelson DA, Kraemer WJ, et al. Effects of resistance training on neuromuscular junction morphology. *Muscle Nerve.* 2000;23(10):1576–81.

33. Deschenes MR, Maresh CM, Armstrong LE, Covault J, Kraemer WJ, Crivello JF. Endurance and resistance exercise induce muscle fiber type specific responses in androgen binding capacity. *J Steroid Biochem Mol Biol.* 1994;50(3–4):175–9.

34. Deschenes MR, Maresh CM, Crivello JF, Armstrong LE, Kraemer WJ, Covault J. The effects of exercise training of different intensities on neuromuscular junction morphology. *J Neurocytol.* 1993;22(8):603–15.

35. Dickerman RD, Pertusi R, Smith GH. The upper range of lumbar spine bone mineral density? An examination of the current world record holder in the squat lift. *Int J Sports Med.* 2000;21(7): 469–70.

36. Dohi K, Mastro AM, Miles MP, et al. Lymphocyte proliferation in response to acute heavy resistance exercise in women: influence of muscle strength and total work. *Eur J Appl Physiol.* 2001;85 (3–4):367–73.

37. Duchateau J, Enoka RM. Human motor unit recordings: origins and insight into the integrated motor system. *Brain Res.* 2011;1409:42–61.

38. Ebben WP. A brief review of concurrent activation potentiation: theoretical and practical constructs. *J Strength Cond Res.* 2006;20(4):985–91.

39. Fahs CA, Heffernan KS, Ranadive S, Jae SY, Fernhall B. Muscular strength is inversely associated with aortic stiffness in young men. *Med Sci Sports Exerc.* 2010;42(9):1619–24.

40. Falkel JE, Fleck SJ, Murray TF. Comparison of central hemodynamics between power lifters and bodybuilders during exercise. *J Strength Cond Res.* 1992;6(11):24–35.

41. Fleck SJ. Cardiovascular responses to strength training. In: *Strength and Power in Sport.* 2nd ed. Osney Mead, Oxford: Blackwell Science; 2003. p. 387–408.

42. Fleck SJ, Dean LS. Resistance-training experience and the pressor response during resistance exercise. *J Appl Physiol.* 1987;63(1):116–20.

43. Fleck SJ, Kraemer WJ. *Designing Resistance Training Programs.* 3rd ed. Champaign (IL): Human Kinetics; 2004. 377 p.

44. Flynn MG, Fahlman M, Braun WA, et al. Effects of resistance training on selected indexes of immune function in elderly women. *J Appl Physiol.* 1999;86(6):1905–13.

45. Focht BC. Perceived exertion and training load during selfselected and imposed-intensity resistance exercise in untrained women. *J Strength Cond Res.* 2007;21(1):183–7.

46. Folland JP, Williams AG. The adaptations to strength training: morphological and neurological contributions to increased strength. *Sports Med*. 2007;37(2):145–68.

47. Fragala MS, Kraemer WJ, Denegar CR, Maresh CM, Mastro AM, Volek JS. Neuroendocrine-immune interactions and responses to exercise. *Sports Med*. 2011;41(8):621–39.

48. Fragala MS, Kraemer WJ, Mastro AM, et al. Leukocyte beta2-adrenergic receptor expression in response to resistance exercise. *Med Sci Sports Exerc*. 2011;43(8):1422–32.

49. Fragala MS, Kraemer WJ, Mastro AM, et al. Glucocorticoid receptor expression on human B cells in response to acute heavy resistance exercise. *Neuroimmunomodulation*. 2011;18(3):156–64.

50. French DN, Kraemer WJ, Volek JS, et al. Anticipatory responses of catecholamines on muscle force production. *J Appl Physiol*. 2007;102(1):94–102.

51. Fry AC, Kraemer WJ. Resistance exercise overtraining and overreaching. Neuroendocrine responses. *Sports Med*. 1997;23(2):106–29.

52. Fry AC, Kraemer WJ, Ramsey LT. Pituitary-adrenal-gonadal responses to high-intensity resistance exercise overtraining. *J Appl Physiol*. 1998;85(6):2352–9.

53. Fry AC, Schilling BK, Weiss LW, Chiu LZ. Beta2-Adrenergic receptor downregulation and performance decrements during high-intensity resistance exercise overtraining. *J Appl Physiol*. 2006;101(6):1664–72.

54. Fujimura R, Ashizawa N, Watanabe M, et al. Effect of resistance exercise training on bone formation and resorption in young male subjects assessed by biomarkers of bone metabolism. *J Bone Miner Res*. 1997;12(4):656–62.

55. Gabriel DA, Kamen G, Frost G. Neural adaptations to resistive exercise: mechanisms and recommendations for training practices. *Sports Med*. 2006;36(2):133–49.

56. Garber CE, Blissmer B, Deschenes MR, et al. Quantity and quality of exercise for developing and maintaining cardiorespiratory, musculoskeletal, and neuromotor fitness in apparently healthy adults: guidance for prescribing exercise. *Med Sci Sports Exerc*. 2011;43(7):1334–59.

57. Gettman LR, Culter LA, Strathman TA. Physiologic changes after 20 weeks of isotonic vs isokinetic circuit training. *J Sports Med Phys Fitness*. 1980;20(3):265–74.

58. Glass SC, Stanton DR. Self-selected resistance training intensity in novice weightlifters. *J Strength Cond Res*. 2004;18(2):324–7.

59. Glowacki SP, Martin SE, Maurer A, Baek W, Green JS, Crouse SF. Effects of resistance, endurance, and concurrent exercise on training outcomes in men. *Med Sci Sports Exerc*. 2004;36(12):2119–27.

60. Green H, Dahly A, Shoemaker K, Goreham C, Bombardier E, Ball-Burnett M. Serial effects of high-resistance and prolonged endurance training on Na+-K+ pump concentration and enzymatic activities in human vastus lateralis. *Acta Physiol Scand*. 1999;165(2):177–84.

61. Greiwe JS, Cheng B, Rubin DC, Yarasheski KE, Semenkovich CF. Resistance exercise decreases skeletal muscle tumor necrosis factor alpha in frail elderly humans. *FASEB J*. 2001;15(2):475–82.

62. Hakkinen K, Alen M, Kraemer WJ, et al. Neuromuscular adaptations during concurrent strength and endurance training versus strength training. *Eur J Appl Physiol*. 2003;89(1):42–52.

63. Hakkinen K, Kraemer WJ, Pakarinen A, et al. Effects of heavy resistance/power training on maximal strength, muscle morphology, and hormonal response patterns in 60–75-year-old men and women. *Can J Appl Physiol*. 2002;27(3):213–31.

64. Hakkinen K, Pakarinen A. Acute hormonal responses to two different fatiguing heavy-resistance protocols in male athletes. *J Appl Physiol*. 1993;74(2):882–7.

65. Hakkinen K, Pakarinen A, Alen M, Kauhanen H, Komi PV. Daily hormonal and neuromuscular responses to intensive strength training in 1 week. *Int J Sports Med*. 1988;9(6):422–8.

66. Hakkinen K, Pakarinen A, Alen M, Kauhanen H, Komi PV. Neuromuscular and hormonal adaptations in athletes to strength training in two years. *J Appl Physiol*. 1988;65(6):2406–12.

67. Hansen S, Kvorning T, Kjaer M, Sjogaard G. The effect of short-term strength training on human skeletal muscle: the importance of physiologically elevated hormone levels. *Scand J Med Sci Sports*. 2001;11(6):347–54.

68. Harries UJ, Bassey EJ. Torque-velocity relationships for the knee extensors in women in their 3rd and 7th decades. *Eur J Appl Physiol Occup Physiol*. 1990;60(3):187–90.

69. Henneman E. Relation between size of neurons and their susceptibility to discharge. *Science*. 1957;126(3287):1345–7.

70. Henwood TR, Taaffe DR. Improved physical performance in older adults undertaking a short-term programme of high-velocity resistance training. *Gerontology*. 2005;51(2):108–15.

71. Hoffman J, Ratamess NA. *A Practical Guide to Developing Resistance-Training Programs*. Monterey (CA): Coaches Choice; 2006. 168 p.

72. Holtermann A, Roeleveld K, Engstrom M, Sand T. Enhanced H-reflex with resistance training is related to increased rate of force development. *Eur J Appl Physiol*. 2007;101(3):301–12.

73. Hurley BF. Effects of resistive training on lipoprotein-lipid profiles: a comparison to aerobic exercise training. *Med Sci Sports Exerc*. 1989;21(6):689–93.

74. Hwang CL, Chien CL, Wu YT. Resistance training increases 6-minute walk distance in people with chronic heart failure: a systematic review. *J Physiother*. 2010;56(2):87–96.

75. Ikegawa S, Funato K, Tsunoda N, Kanehisa H, Fukunaga T, Kawakami Y. Muscle force per cross-sectional area is inversely related with pennation angle in strength trained athletes. *J Strength Cond Res*. 2008;22(1):128–31.

76. Izquierdo M, Ibanez J, Calbet JA, et al. Cytokine and hormone responses to resistance training. *Eur J Appl Physiol*. 2009;107(4):397–409.

77. Jones TE, Stephenson KW, King JG, Knight KR, Marshall TL, Scott WB. Sarcopenia—mechanisms and treatments. *J Geriatr Phys Ther*. 2009;32(2):83–9.

78. Kadi F, Bonnerud P, Eriksson A, Thornell LE. The expression of androgen receptors in human neck and limb muscles: effects of training and self-administration of androgenic-anabolic steroids. *Histochem Cell Biol*. 2000;113(1):25–9.

79. Kadi F, Eriksson A, Holmner S, Butler-Browne GS, Thornell LE. Cellular adaptation of the trapezius muscle in strength-trained athletes. *Histochem Cell Biol*. 1999;111(3):189–95.

80. Kadi F, Schjerling P, Andersen LL, et al. The effects of heavy resistance training and detraining on satellite cells in human skeletal muscles. *J Physiol*. 2004;558(Pt 3):1005–12.

81. Karlsson MK, Vergnaud P, Delmas PD, Obrant KJ. Indicators of bone formation in weight lifters. *Calcif Tissue Int*. 1995;56(3):177–80.

82. Kawakami Y, Abe T, Kuno SY, Fukunaga T. Training-induced changes in muscle architecture and specific tension. *Eur J Appl Physiol Occup Physiol*. 1995;72(1–2):37–43.

83. Kearns CF, Abe T, Brechue WF. Muscle enlargement in sumo wrestlers includes increased muscle fascicle length. *Eur J Appl Physiol*. 2000;83(4–5):289–96.

84. Kelley GA, Kelley KS. Progressive resistance exercise and resting blood pressure: A meta-analysis of randomized controlled trials. *Hypertension*. 2000;35(3):838–43.

85. Kelley GA, Kelley KS, Tran ZV. Exercise and bone mineral density in men: a meta-analysis. *J Appl Physiol*. 2000;88(5):1730–6.

86. Kelley GA, Kelley KS, Tran ZV. Resistance training and bone mineral density in women: a meta-analysis of controlled trials. *Am J Phys Med Rehabil*. 2001;80(1):65–77.

87. Kemp TJ, Sadusky TJ, Saltisi F, et al. Identification of Ankrd2, a novel skeletal muscle gene coding for a stretch-responsive ankyrin-repeat protein. *Genomics*. 2000;66(3):229–41.

88. Kilgore JL, Pendlay GW, Reeves JS, Kilgore TG. Serum chemistry and hematological adaptations to 6 weeks of moderate to intense resistance training. *J Strength Cond Res*. 2002;16(4):509–15.

89. Komi PV, Suominen H, Heikkinen E, Karlsson J, Tesch P. Effects of heavy resistance and explosive-type strength training methods on mechanical, functional, and metabolic aspects of performance. In: Komi PV, editor. *Exercise and Sport Biology*. Champaign: Human Kinetics; 1982. p. 90–102.

90. Kongsgaard M, Nielsen CH, Hegnsvad S, Aagaard P, Magnusson SP. Mechanical properties of the human Achilles tendon, in vivo. *Clin Biomech (Bristol, Avon)*. 2011;26(7):772–7.

91. Kosek DJ, Kim JS, Petrella JK, Cross JM, Bamman MM. Efficacy of 3 days/wk resistance training on myofiber hypertrophy and myogenic mechanisms in young vs. older adults. *J Appl Physiol*. 2006;101(2):531–44.

92. Kraemer WJ, Clemson A, Triplett NT, Bush JA, Newton RU, Lynch JM. The effects of plasma cortisol elevation on total and differential leukocyte counts in response to heavy-resistance exercise. *Eur J Appl Physiol Occup Physiol*. 1996;73(1–2):93–7.

93. Kraemer WJ, Dunn-Lewis C, Comstock BA, Thomas GA, Clark JE, Nindl BC. Growth hormone, exercise, and athletic performance: a continued evolution of complexity. *Curr Sports Med Rep*. 2010;9(4):242–52.

94. Kraemer WJ, Fleck SJ, Callister R, et al. Training responses of plasma beta-endorphin, adrenocorticotropin, and cortisol. *Med Sci Sports Exerc*. 1989;21(2):146–53.

95. Kraemer WJ, Fleck SJ, Dziados JE, et al. Changes in hormonal concentrations after different heavy-resistance exercise protocols in women. *J Appl Physiol*. 1993;75(2):594–604.

96. Kraemer WJ, Fleck SJ, Maresh CM, et al. Acute hormonal responses to a single bout of heavy resistance exercise in trained power lifters and untrained men. *Can J Appl Physiol*. 1999;24(6):524–37.

97. Kraemer WJ, Fragala MS. Personalize it: Program design in resistance training. *ACSM's Health & Fitness Journal*. 2006;10(4):7–17.

98. Kraemer WJ, Hatfield DL, Volek JS, et al. Effects of amino acids supplement on physiological adaptations to resistance training. *Med Sci Sports Exerc*. 2009;41(5):1111–21.

99. Kraemer WJ, Joseph MF, Volek JS, et al. Endogenous opioid peptide responses to opioid and anti-inflammatory medications following eccentric exercise-induced muscle damage. *Peptides*. 2010;31(1):88–93.

100. Kraemer WJ, Koziris LP. Olympic weightlifting and power lifting. In: Lamb DR, Knuttgen HG, Murray R, editors. *Physiology and Nutrition for Competitive Sport*. Carmel: Cooper Pub Group; 1994. p. 1–54.

101. Kraemer WJ, Koziris LP, Ratamess NA, et al. Detraining produces minimal changes in physical performance and hormonal variables in recreationally strength-trained men. *J Strength Cond Res*. 2002;16(3):373–82.

102. Kraemer WJ, Nindl BC, Marx JO, et al. Chronic resistance training in women potentiates growth hormone in vivo bioactivity: characterization of molecular mass variants. *Am J Physiol Endocrinol Metab*. 2006;291(6):E1177–87.

103. Kraemer WJ, Noble BJ, Clark MJ, Culver BW. Physiologic responses to heavy-resistance exercise with very short rest periods. *Int J Sports Med*. 1987;8(4):247–52.

104. Kraemer WJ, Patton JF, Gordon SE, et al. Compatibility of high-intensity strength and endurance training on hormonal and skeletal muscle adaptations. *J Appl Physiol*. 1995;78(3):976–89.

105. Kraemer WJ, Ratamess NA. Endocrine responses and adaptations to strength and power training. In: Komi PV, IOC Medical Commission, International Federation of Sports Medicine, editors. *Strength and Power in Sport*. 2nd ed. Osney Mead, Oxford: Blackwell Science; 2003. p. 361–386.

106. Kraemer WJ, Ratamess NA. Fundamentals of resistance training: progression and exercise prescription. *Med Sci Sports Exerc*. 2004;36(4):674–88.

107. Kraemer WJ, Ratamess NA. Hormonal responses and adaptations to resistance exercise and training. *Sports Med*. 2005;35(4):339–61.

108. Kraemer WJ, Ratamess NA. Physiology of resistance training: current issues. In: Hughes C, editor. *Orthopaedic Physical Therapy Clinics of North America: Exercise Technologies*. Philadelphia: WB Saunders; 2000. p. 467–513.

109. Kraemer WJ, Ratamess NA, French DN. Resistance training for health and performance. *Curr Sports Med Rep*. 2002;1(3): 165–71.

110. Kraemer WJ, Ratamess NA, Volek JS, et al. The effects of amino acid supplementation on hormonal responses to resistance training overreaching. *Metabolism*. 2006;55(3):282–91.

111. Kraemer WJ, Spiering BA, Volek JS, et al. Androgenic responses to resistance exercise: effects of feeding and L-carnitine. *Med Sci Sports Exerc*. 2006;38(7):1288–96.

112. Kubo K, Kanehisa H, Fukunaga T. Effects of resistance and stretching training programmes on the viscoelastic properties of human tendon structures in vivo. *J Physiol*. 2002;538(Pt 1):219–26.

113. Kubo K, Komuro T, Ishiguro N, et al. Effects of low-load resistance training with vascular occlusion on the mechanical properties of muscle and tendon. *J Appl Biomech*. 2006;22(2):112–9.

114. Kubo K, Yata H, Kanehisa H, Fukunaga T. Effects of isometric squat training on the tendon stiffness and jump performance. *Eur J Appl Physiol*. 2006;96(3):305–14.

115. Lorenz D. Postactivation potentiation: an introduction. *Int J Sports Phys Ther*. 2011;6(3):234–40.

116. MacDougall JD. Adaptability of muscle to strength training: a cellular approach. In: Saltin B, editor. *Biochemistry of Exercise VI*. Champaign: Human Kinetics; 1986. p. 501–13.

117. MacDougall JD, Sale DG, Alway SE, Sutton JR. Muscle fiber number in biceps brachii in bodybuilders and control subjects. *J Appl Physiol*. 1984;57(5):1399–403.

118. MacDougall JD, Sale DG, Elder G, Sutton JR. Ultrastructural properties of human skeletal muscle following heavy resistance exercise and immobilization. *Med Sci Sports Exerc*. 1976;8:72–3.

119. MacDougall JD, Sale DG, Moroz JR, Elder GC, Sutton JR, Howald H. Mitochondrial volume density in human skeletal muscle following heavy resistance training. *Med Sci Sports*. 1979;11(2):164–6.

120. MacDougall JD, Ward GR, Sale DG, Sutton JR. Biochemical adaptation of human skeletal muscle to heavy resistance training and immobilization. *J Appl Physiol*. 1977;43(4):700–3.

121. Mackey AL, Esmarck B, Kadi F, et al. Enhanced satellite cell proliferation with resistance training in elderly men and women. *Scand J Med Sci Sports*. 2007;17(1):34–42.

122. Mackinnon LT. Chronic exercise training effects on immune function. *Med Sci Sports Exerc*. 2000;32(7 Suppl):S369–76.

123. MacKinnon L. Exercise and cytokines. In: Mackinnon LT, editor. *Advances in Exercise Immunology*. Champaign: Human Kinetics; 1999. p. 201–27.

124. Magnusson SP, Hansen M, Langberg H, et al. The adaptability of tendon to loading differs in men and women. *Int J Exp Pathol*. 2007;88(4):237–40.

125. Mair J, Mayr M, Muller E, et al. Rapid adaptation to eccentric exercise-induced muscle damage. *Int J Sports Med*. 1995;16(6): 352–6.

126. Martel GF, Roth SM, Ivey FM, et al. Age and sex affect human muscle fibre adaptations to heavy-resistance strength training. *Exp Physiol*. 2006;91(2):457–64.

127. Marx JO, Ratamess NA, Nindl BC, et al. Low-volume circuit versus high-volume periodized resistance training in women. *Med Sci Sports Exerc*. 2001;33(4):635–43.

128. Matheny RW,Jr, Nindl BC. Loss of IGF-IEa or IGF-IEb impairs myogenic differentiation. *Endocrinology*. 2011;152(5):1923–34.

129. Matos NF, Winsley RJ, Williams CA. Prevalence of nonfunctional overreaching/overtraining in young English athletes. *Med Sci Sports Exerc*. 2011;43(7):1287–94.

130. Mayhew DL, Thyfault JP, Koch AJ. Rest-interval length affects leukocyte levels during heavy resistance exercise. *J Strength Cond Res*. 2005;19(1):16–22.

131. McCall GE, Byrnes WC, Dickinson A, Pattany PM, Fleck SJ. Muscle fiber hypertrophy, hyperplasia, and capillary density in college men after resistance training. *J Appl Physiol*. 1996;81(5):2004–12.

132. McCann MR, Flanagan SP. The effects of exercise selection and rest interval on postactivation potentiation of vertical jump performance. *J Strength Cond Res*. 2010;24(5):1285–91.

133. Menkes A, Mazel S, Redmond RA, et al. Strength training increases regional bone mineral density and bone remodeling in middle-aged and older men. *J Appl Physiol*. 1993;74(5):2478–84.

134. Mero A, Miikkulainen H, Riski J, Pakkanen R, Aalto J, Takala T. Effects of bovine colostrum supplementation on serum IGF-I, IgG, hormone, and saliva IgA during training. *J Appl Physiol*. 1997;83(4):1144–51.

135. Miles MP, Kraemer WJ, Grove DS, et al. Effects of resistance training on resting immune parameters in women. *Eur J Appl Physiol*. 2002;87(6):506–8.

136. Miles MP, Kraemer WJ, Nindl BC, et al. Strength, workload, anaerobic intensity and the immune response to resistance exercise in women. *Acta Physiol Scand*. 2003;178(2):155–63.

137. Miszko TA, Cress ME, Slade JM, Covey CJ, Agrawal SK, Doerr CE. Effect of strength and power training on physical function in community-dwelling older adults. *J Gerontol A Biol Sci Med Sci*. 2003;58(2):171–5.

138. Mitchell CJ, Sale DG. Enhancement of jump performance after a 5-RM squat is associated with postactivation potentiation. *Eur J Appl Physiol*. 2011;111(8):1957–63.

139. Moritani T, deVries HA. Neural factors versus hypertrophy in the time course of muscle strength gain. *Am J Phys Med*. 1979;58(3):115–30.

140. Munn J, Herbert RD, Gandevia SC. Contralateral effects of unilateral resistance training: a meta-analysis. *J Appl Physiol*. 2004;96(5):1861–6.

141. Newton RU, Hakkinen K, Hakkinen A, McCormick M, Volek J, Kraemer WJ. Mixed-methods resistance training increases power and strength of young and older men. *Med Sci Sports Exerc*. 2002;34(8):1367–75.

142. Nichols DL, Sanborn CF, Love AM. Resistance training and bone mineral density in adolescent females. *J Pediatr*. 2001;139(4):494–500.

143. Nieman DC, Davis JM, Brown VA, et al. Influence of carbohydrate ingestion on immune changes after 2 h of intensive resistance training. *J Appl Physiol*. 2004;96(4):1292–8.

144. Nieman DC, Henson DA, Sampson CS, et al. The acute immune response to exhaustive resistance exercise. *Int J Sports Med*. 1995;16(5):322–8.

145. Nindl BC, Hymer WC, Deaver DR, Kraemer WJ. Growth hormone pulsatility profile characteristics following acute heavy resistance exercise. *J Appl Physiol*. 2001;91(1):163–72.

146. Nindl BC, Santtila M, Vaara J, Hakkinen K, Kyrolainen H. Circulating IGF-I is associated with fitness and health outcomes in a population of 846 young healthy men. *Growth Horm IGF Res*. 2011;21(3):124–8.

147. Paul GL, DeLany JP, Snook JT, Seifert JG, Kirby TE. Serum and urinary markers of skeletal muscle tissue damage after weight lifting exercise. *Eur J Appl Physiol Occup Physiol*. 1989;58(7):786–90.

148. Peake JM, Nosaka K, Muthalib M, Suzuki K. Systemic inflammatory responses to maximal versus submaximal lengthening contractions of the elbow flexors. *Exerc Immunol Rev*. 2006;12:72–85.

149. Pedersen BK, Hoffman-Goetz L. Exercise and the immune system: regulation, integration, and adaptation. *Physiol Rev*. 2000;80(3):1055–81.

150. Pesta D, Hoppel F, Macek C, et al. Similar qualitative and quantitative changes of mitochondrial respiration following strength and endurance training in normoxia and hypoxia in sedentary humans. *Am J Physiol Regul Integr Comp Physiol*. 2011;301(4):R1078–87.

151. Peterson MD, Sen A, Gordon PM. Influence of resistance exercise on lean body mass in aging adults: a meta-analysis. *Med Sci Sports Exerc*. 2011;43(2):249–58.

152. Pette D, Staron RS. Mammalian skeletal muscle fiber type transitions. *Int Rev Cytol*. 1997;170:143–223.

153. Ploutz LL, Tesch PA, Biro RL, Dudley GA. Effect of resistance training on muscle use during exercise. *J Appl Physiol*. 1994;76(4):1675–81.

154. Ploutz-Snyder LL, Giamis EL, Formikell M, Rosenbaum AE. Resistance training reduces susceptibility to eccentric exercise-induced muscle dysfunction in older women. *J Gerontol A Biol Sci Med Sci*. 2001;56(9):B384–90.

155. Porter MM. Power training for older adults. *Appl Physiol Nutr Metab*. 2006;31(2):87–94.

156. Putman CT, Xu X, Gillies E, MacLean IM, Bell GJ. Effects of strength, endurance and combined training on myosin heavy chain content and fibre-type distribution in humans. *Eur J Appl Physiol*. 2004;92(4–5):376–84.

157. Raastad T, Risoy BA, Benestad HB, Fjeld JG, Hallen J. Temporal relation between leukocyte accumulation in muscles and halted recovery 10–20 h after strength exercise. *J Appl Physiol*. 2003;95(6):2503–9.

158. Ratamess NA, Faigenbaum AD, Hoffman JR, Kang J. Self-selected resistance training intensity in healthy women: the influence of a personal trainer. *J Strength Cond Res*. 2008;22(1):103–11.

159. Ratamess NA, Falvo MJ, Mangine GT, Hoffman JR, Faigenbaum AD, Kang J. The effect of rest interval length on metabolic responses to the bench press exercise. *Eur J Appl Physiol*. 2007;100(1):1–17.

160. Ratamess NA, Hoffman JR, Faigenbaum AD, Mangine GT, Falvo MJ, Kang J. The combined effects of protein intake and resistance training on serum osteocalcin concentrations in strength and power athletes. *J Strength Cond Res*. 2007;21(4):1197–203.

161. Ratamess NA, Hoffman JR, Ross R, Shanklin M, Faigenbaum AD, Kang J. Effects of an amino acid/creatine energy supplement on the acute hormonal response to resistance exercise. *Int J Sport Nutr Exerc Metab*. 2007;17(6):608–23.

162. Ratamess NA, Kraemer WJ, Volek JS, et al. Androgen receptor content following heavy resistance exercise in men. *J Steroid Biochem Mol Biol*. 2005;93(1):35–42.

163. Ratamess NA, Kraemer WJ, Volek JS, et al. The effects of amino acid supplementation on muscular performance during resistance training overreaching. *J Strength Cond Res*. 2003;17(2):250–8.

164. Riechman SE, Balasekaran G, Roth SM, Ferrell RE. Association of interleukin-15 protein and interleukin-15 receptor genetic variation with resistance exercise training responses. *J Appl Physiol*. 2004;97(6):2214–9.

165. Roberts MD, Dalbo VJ, Kerksick CM. Postexercise myogenic gene expression: are human findings lost during translation? *Exerc Sport Sci Rev*. 2011;39(4):206–11.

166. Rosenberg IH. Sarcopenia: origins and clinical relevance. *Clin Geriatr Med*. 2011;27(3):337–9.

167. Roth SM, Ferrell RE, Peters DG, Metter EJ, Hurley BF, Rogers MA. Influence of age, sex, and strength training on human muscle gene expression determined by microarray. *Physiol Genomics*. 2002;10(3):181–90.

168. Roth SM, Martel GF, Ferrell RE, Metter EJ, Hurley BF, Rogers MA. Myostatin gene expression is reduced in humans with heavy-resistance strength training: a brief communication. *Exp Biol Med (Maywood)*. 2003;228(6):706–9.

169. Rubin MR, Kraemer WJ, Maresh CM, et al. High-affinity growth hormone binding protein and acute heavy resistance exercise. *Med Sci Sports Exerc*. 2005;37(3):395–403.

170. Sale DG. Neural adaptations to strength training. In: Komi PV, IOC Medical Commission, International Federation of Sports Medicine, editors. *Strength and Power in Sport*. 2nd ed. Osney Mead, Oxford: Blackwell Science; 2003. p. 281–314.

171. Sale DG. Postactivation potentiation: role in human performance. *Exerc Sport Sci Rev*. 2002;30(3):138–43.

172. Sale DG, MacDougall JD, Upton AR, McComas AJ. Effect of strength training upon motoneuron excitability in man. *Med Sci Sports Exerc*. 1983;15(1):57–62.

173. Sale DG, Moroz DE, McKelvie RS, MacDougall JD, McCartney N. Effect of training on the blood pressure response to weight lifting. *Can J Appl Physiol.* 1994;19(1):60–74.

174. Schantz P. Capillary supply in hypertrophied human skeletal muscle. *Acta Physiol Scand.* 1982;114(4):635–7.

175. Schoenfeld BJ. The mechanisms of muscle hypertrophy and their application to resistance training. *J Strength Cond Res.* 2010; 24(10):2857–72.

176. Seynnes OR, de Boer M, Narici MV. Early skeletal muscle hypertrophy and architectural changes in response to high-intensity resistance training. *J Appl Physiol.* 2007;102(1):368–73.

177. Simonson SR, Jackson CG. Leukocytosis occurs in response to resistance exercise in men. *J Strength Cond Res.* 2004;18(2):266–71.

178. Spiering BA, Kraemer WJ, Anderson JM, et al. Effects of elevated circulating hormones on resistance exercise-induced Akt signaling. *Med Sci Sports Exerc.* 2008;40(6):1039–48.

179. Spiering BA, Kraemer WJ, Anderson JM, et al. Resistance exercise biology: manipulation of resistance exercise programme variables determines the responses of cellular and molecular signalling pathways. *Sports Med.* 2008;38(7):527–40.

180. Spiering BA, Kraemer WJ, Vingren JL, et al. Responses of criterion variables to different supplemental doses of L-carnitine L-tartrate. *J Strength Cond Res.* 2007;21(1):259–64.

181. Spiering BA, Kraemer WJ, Vingren JL, et al. Elevated endogenous testosterone concentrations potentiate muscle androgen receptor responses to resistance exercise. *J Steroid Biochem Mol Biol.* 2009;114(3–5):195–9.

182. Staron RS, Karapondo DL, Kraemer WJ, et al. Skeletal muscle adaptations during early phase of heavy-resistance training in men and women. *J Appl Physiol.* 1994;76(3):1247–55.

183. Staron RS, Malicky ES, Leonardi MJ, Falkel JE, Hagerman FC, Dudley GA. Muscle hypertrophy and fast fiber type conversions in heavy resistance-trained women. *Eur J Appl Physiol Occup Physiol.* 1990;60(1):71–9.

184. Stone MH, Karatzaferi C. Connective tissue and bone response to strength training. In: Komi PV, IOC Medical Commission, International Federation of Sports Medicine, editors. *Strength and Power in Sport.* 2nd ed. Osney Mead, Oxford; Malden: Blackwell Science; 2003. p. 343–60.

185. Svensson RB, Hansen P, Hassenkam T, et al. Mechanical properties of human patellar tendon at the hierarchical levels of tendon and fibril. *J Appl Physiol.* 2012;112(3):419–26.

186. Tesch PA. Skeletal muscle adaptations consequent to long-term heavy resistance exercise. *Med Sci Sports Exerc.* 1988;20(5 Suppl): S132–4.

187. Tesch PA, Alkner BA. Acute and chronic muscle metabolic adaptations to strength training. In: Komi PV, IOC Medical Commission, International Federation of Sports Medicine, editors. *Strength and Power in Sport.* 2nd ed. Osney Mead, Oxford: Blackwell Science; 2003. p. 265–80.

188. Tesch PA, Karlsson J. Muscle fiber types and size in trained and untrained muscles of elite athletes. *J Appl Physiol.* 1985;59(6): 1716–20.

189. Tesch PA, Komi PV, Hakkinen K. Enzymatic adaptations consequent to long-term strength training. *Int J Sports Med.* 1987;8 Suppl 1:66–9.

190. Tesch PA, Thorsson A, Essen-Gustavsson B. Enzyme activities of FT and ST muscle fibers in heavy-resistance trained athletes. *J Appl Physiol.* 1989;67(1):83–7.

191. Tesch PA, Thorsson A, Kaiser P. Muscle capillary supply and fiber type characteristics in weight and power lifters. *J Appl Physiol.* 1984;56(1):35–8.

192. Triplett-McBride NT, Mastro AM, McBride JM, et al. Plasma proenkephalin peptide F and human B cell responses to exercise stress in fit and unfit women. *Peptides.* 1998;19(4):731–8.

193. Tsuzuku S, Ikegami Y, Yabe K. Effects of high-intensity resistance training on bone mineral density in young male powerlifters. *Calcif Tissue Int.* 1998;63(4):283–6.

194. Tsuzuku S, Shimokata H, Ikegami Y, Yabe K, Wasnich RD. Effects of high versus low-intensity resistance training on bone mineral density in young males. *Calcif Tissue Int.* 2001;68(6):342–7.

195. Vincent HK, Vincent KR. The effect of training status on the serum creatine kinase response, soreness and muscle function following resistance exercise. *Int J Sports Med.* 1997;18(6):431–7.

196. Vingren JL, Koziris LP, Gordon SE, Kraemer WJ, Turner RT, Westerlind KC. Chronic alcohol intake, resistance training, and muscle androgen receptor content. *Med Sci Sports Exerc.* 2005;37(11):1842–8.

197. Vingren JL, Kraemer WJ, Hatfield DL, et al. Effect of resistance exercise on muscle steroid receptor protein content in strength-trained men and women. *Steroids.* 2009;74(13–14):1033–9.

198. Vingren JL, Kraemer WJ, Ratamess NA, Anderson JM, Volek JS, Maresh CM. Testosterone physiology in resistance exercise and training: the up-stream regulatory elements. *Sports Med.* 2010;40(12):1037–53.

199. Visser M, Pahor M, Taaffe DR, et al. Relationship of interleukin-6 and tumor necrosis factor-alpha with muscle mass and muscle strength in elderly men and women: the Health ABC Study. *J Gerontol A Biol Sci Med Sci.* 2002;57(5):M326–32.

200. Volek JS. Influence of nutrition on responses to resistance training. *Med Sci Sports Exerc.* 2004;36(4):689–96.

201. Von Stengel S, Kemmler W, Kalender WA, Engelke K, Lauber D. Differential effects of strength versus power training on bone mineral density in postmenopausal women: a 2-year longitudinal study. *Br J Sports Med.* 2007;41(10):649–55; discussion 655.

202. Williams MA, Haskell WL, Ades PA, et al. Resistance exercise in individuals with and without cardiovascular disease: 2007 update: a scientific statement from the American Heart Association Council on Clinical Cardiology and Council on Nutrition, Physical Activity, and Metabolism. *Circulation.* 2007;116(5):572–84.

SELECTED REFERENCES FOR FURTHER READING

Baechle TR, Earle RW. *Essentials of Strength Training and Conditioning.* 3rd ed. Champaign (IL): Human Kinetics; 2008. 656 p.

Dochateau J, Enoka RM. Human motor unit recordings: origins and insight into the integrated motor system. *Brain Res.* 2011;1409: 42–61.

Hoffman J. *Physiological Aspects of Sport Training and Performance.* Champaign (IL): Human Kinetics; 2002. 352 p.

Kraemer WJ, Adams K, Cafarelli E, et al. American College of Sports Medicine position stand. Progression models in resistance training for healthy adults. *Med Sci Sports Exerc.* 2002;34(2):364–80.

Kraemer WJ, Ratamess NA. Fundamentals of resistance training: progression and exercise prescription. *Med Sci Sport Exerc.* 2004;36:674–8.

Ratamess NA. *ACSM's Foundations of Strength Training and Conditioning.* Baltimore (MD): Lippincott Williams & Wilkins; 2011. 560 p.

Schoenfeld BJ. The mechanisms of muscle hypertrophy and their application to resistance training. *J Strength Cond Res.* 2010;24(10): 2857–72.

Zatsiorsky VM, Kraemer WJ. *Science and Practice of Strength Training.* 2nd ed. Champaign (IL): Human Kinetics; 2006. 264 p.

INTERNET RESOURCES

- American College of Sports Medicine: http://www.acsm.org
- National Strength and Conditioning Association: http://www.nsca-lift.org

Group Exercise Programming

As with any form of exercise, the overall purpose of **group exercise** programming is to help participants enhance their quality of life through beneficial movement experiences and social interaction. One of the underlying goals is to help participants improve their health-related components of fitness, which include cardiorespiratory capacity and endurance, muscular strength and endurance, flexibility, and body composition, and thus enjoy their lives more fully. Research demonstrates that exercising in a group can enhance overall adherence to exercise (10). Group exercise has been shown to increase balance and postural stability in older adults (12) as well as to improve functional and psychological well-being of women who are overweight (23). It is important that group exercise program design revolve around the health-related components of fitness and social aspects of wellness.

Group exercise has grown from traditional high- and low-impact classes (high/low) in the late 1970s to now include indoor cycling; boot camp; sports conditioning; water exercise; dance options such as Zumba; use of strength and conditioning equipment such as dumbbells, barbells, stability balls, and suspension training devices; Pilates; mind/body classes such as yoga (*Fig. 34-1*), **fusion** classes that combine two or more formats; stretching-only classes; and much more.

TRENDS IN GROUP EXERCISE

According to Tharrett and Peterson, future programs for group exercise include branded group classes (such as BodyPump), fusion fitness (blend styles such as indoor cycling/yoga or cardio/strength), extreme fitness (boot camp, SWAT fitness), and core and functional fitness classes (53). The IDEA 2011 fitness trends survey (1) lists **core conditioning** classes, Pilates, yoga, and group strength training among the top 10 most frequently offered programs. In addition, fitness professionals surveyed in the 2011 report stated that small group personal training, indoor and outdoor boot camp training, and branded choreography group classes have grown the most. Highly choreographed workouts have declined, for example, step programming in facilities has decreased from 65% to 58% in the past year, yet branded choreographed programs have increased from 22% to 47% in the last 2 yr. Zumba, which is a branded, choreographed program, appears to be popular because the moves tend to be simpler with large amounts of repetition, and participants generally feel it is less important to be "in sync" with everyone than it is to simply have fun. The American College of Sports Medicine (ACSM) 2011 trends survey (54) points to educated fitness professionals, fitness programs for older adults, and strength training as the top three trends in the industry. The IDEA 2010 Fitness Trends Survey (45) reported that class duration length varies with 60-min and 45-min classes being offered most frequently. What is found in surveys from fitness facility staff may not always be what is best for the general public. As obesity continues to increase and fewer people participate in movement experiences in general, one may question why duration is increasing in health clubs when fewer people are participating in regular exercise (27). Principles of exercise progression

KEY TERMS

Core conditioning: A group exercise format focusing on muscles of the trunk. This format typically uses muscle strength and endurance exercises and may incorporate posture, balance, and flexibility exercises as well, with the overall goal of developing core stability.

Fusion: Group exercise programs that use more than one format in the same class, such as indoor cycling plus resistance training or yoga plus stability balls.

Group exercise: A class format in which several people participate in a given exercise mode in unison, led by an instructor, and, although patterns of movement may be uniform among participants, intensity level varies individually and the instructor gives modifications for various fitness abilities.

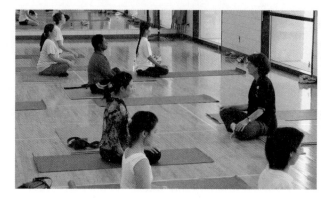

FIGURE 34-1. Group exercise has grown from a purely cardio-respiratory activity to include yoga and relaxation formats also.

would warrant the need to have class sessions start at 30 min and progress in duration. It is important that fitness professionals remain in touch with the general public and tailor programming to improve the overall health and wellness of the population at large rather than cater to a population that is already moving and would continue to move even if there were not any fitness facilities available. Reaching out to all participants is an important goal of the group exercise programmer.

GROUP EXERCISE INSTRUCTOR RESPONSIBILITIES

Balancing being a motivator and an educator with being effective as a mentor of healthy movement experiences is the main charge of a group exercise instructor. The motivational/inspirational aspect of instructing includes having new moves, new music, and state-of-the-art equipment. The educational part of instructing includes knowing why certain moves are more appropriate than others and why some moves are controversial, making sure current research and knowledge are incorporated into the group exercise session, and making educated choices and decisions about the information given to participants. Both parts help establish a professional and caring attitude. Learning to take responsibility for the health and well-being of participants starts with understanding the importance of establishing a positive attitude and atmosphere.

CREATING A HEALTHY MOVEMENT EXPERIENCE

Creating a comfortable and safe movement experience involves establishing a healthy emotional outlook for participants. Education and motivation alone may not suffice to keep participants coming back to group exercise. It is necessary to tap into the feelings and emotions of participants to affect adherence. Ornish believes that interpersonal interaction might be the single most

important concept that breeds an accepting environment in a group exercise experience (36). One study concerning overweight women's perceptions of an exercise class revealed that the most powerful influences affecting their exercise behavior were concerns about embarrassment and judgment by others (3). Another author found that independent of body image concerns, women participating in rooms with mirrors felt worse after exercising than women in an environment without mirrors (22). Finally, it is noted that enjoyment during physical activity is optimized when a positive and supportive leadership style is coupled with an enriched and supportive group environment (16).

Instructors should realize that what they do and say has a major impact on the class atmosphere. Group exercise instructors affect exercise adherence and may be an important predictor of exercise behavior (6). Having social intelligence in any group setting dictates the success of the group experience. A specific example of poor social intelligence within a group exercise setting would be for an instructor to be located in the front of the class and talking only to those in the front row. The participants in the middle and back rows may not feel their presence is acknowledged. The instructor who knows everyone's name, greets them when they come into class, and moves around the class throughout the workout will be creating a healthier emotional/social atmosphere for the participants; this is a positive example of social intelligence.

It is important for all group exercise instructors to get out among the participants and observe and assist during the entire workout. Staying in one place gives only one frame of reference to participants. When the instructor is nearby and observing, the participants may improve their attention and their practicing of skills, so it is ideal to move around the room and affect as many participants as possible. The instructor as coach applies to all segments of the class format and needs to be evaluated throughout the class. It is important to allow participants to see that the group exercise instructor has empathy and is there to instruct participants rather than perform his or her own workout. Instructors with exceptional social intelligence skills make it clear they are there for the participants.

ROLE MODELING

Group exercise instructors should take care of themselves in order to be good role models for their students. Leg and foot pain as well as laryngeal discomfort are common overuse problems experienced by group exercise instructors (30). Role modeling healthy behavior includes taking time off to rest the injured area when necessary, modifying troublesome moves, using a microphone, performing an appropriate warm-up, and providing flexibility exercises in the cool-down. It's important that instructors model a reasonable level of fitness within the domains of cardiorespiratory and muscular fitness as well as appropriate body composition. Yet, instructors should also model a healthy body image and not fall prey to unrealistic and frequently changing societal views (15). This includes the avoidance of pejorative words such as "fat" or "flabby," which may keep participants focused on appearance and lead to them feeling negatively about their own bodies rather than enjoying the movement experience.

OVERALL CLASS FORMAT

Group exercise classes may include segments such as preclass preparation, warm-up, cardiorespiratory training, resistance training, neuromuscular or balance exercises, and flexibility/cool-down (28). Preclass preparation insures physiological readiness for a safe and effective class. The warm-up incorporates dynamic movements, performed at a low-to-moderate intensity and using full range of motion to increase the temperature and blood flow within the specific muscles to be targeted in the remainder of the class. The cardiorespiratory segment is aimed at improving cardiorespiratory capacity and endurance, as well as body composition, by keeping the body working in a desired target range for 10–30 min typically or even longer. Following the cardiorespiratory workout, a gradual cool-down reduces the heart rate (HR) toward resting levels and prevents pooling of blood in the lower extremities. A resistance training segment, aimed at improving muscular strength and endurance, can be included either before, after, or in place of the cardiorespiratory segment. If both are to be performed, the cardiorespiratory segment is usually performed before the resistance training segment so that the former serves as a thorough warm-up for the latter. Core conditioning exercises as well as neuromotor exercises, especially those promoting balance, are ideally included also. The class ends with a flexibility/cool-down component that includes stretching and relaxation exercises designed to further lower HR and enhance overall flexibility. In "fusion" classes, the segments might include, for example, 30 min of indoor cycling followed by 30 min of strength work (*Fig. 34-2*). The most important concept is to employ safe and effective programming to improve the health-related components of fitness regardless of the class format.

Individual segments of a group exercise class are described in detail later in this chapter and are summarized in *Box 34-1*.

PRECLASS PREPARATION

There are a few common principles in the preclass preparation for any group exercise class, which will be reviewed in this section.

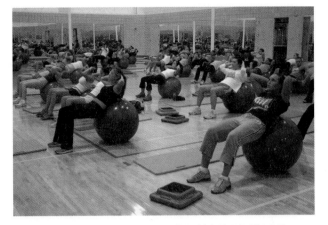

FIGURE 34-2. This group strength class was followed by a 30-min cardio segment. This combination is an example of a "fusion class."

Know the Participants

Chapter 11 provides a review of acquiring health information. The information gathered from these sources needs to be transferred into making a safe and effective class. For example, if two participants say they have occasional lower back pain, incorporating abdominal and low back strengthening as well as hamstring stretching into the class format on a regular basis would help their conditions. Make sure participants are aware that the time they took to fill out the health information is useful by asking participants questions and also by letting them know about any pertinent modifications specific to their information. Of course, some modifications will need to be explained directly to an individual participant if it is not appropriate to address the issue to the entire class.

Orient New Participants

A professional group exercise instructor takes the time to meet and orient new participants and also makes himself or herself available if any participants have questions or concerns. This can be a time when instructors give the most amount of feedback about the class in general, which helps establish a positive and comfortable class environment and may also enhance adherence of the participants. Orientation does not always have to be performed one-on-one but can also be accomplished through brochures and information posted when participants enter the class.

Choose Appropriate Attire

Appropriate attire for a specific group exercise format is an important consideration. For certain class formats, such as indoor cycling, special attire is needed and should be modeled by the instructor. However, when teaching a senior class, it would not be appropriate to

BOX 34-1   Class Format Summary

PRECLASS PREPARATION

- Know the participants' health histories and survey new participants.
- Be available before class; orient new participants.
- Discuss and model appropriate attire and footwear.
- Have music cued up and equipment ready before class begins.
- Acknowledge class and introduce self.
- Preview class format and participant responsibilities.
- Encourage participants to bring water to classes and provide breaks to drink.

WARM-UP SEGMENT

- Beginning segment includes an appropriate amount of dynamic movement.
- Focus on rehearsal moves as a large part of the movement selection.
- If stretching is used after the dynamic warm-up, hold only briefly (5–10 s) and keep upper or lower body moving.
- Verbal directions are clear, and volume and tempo of music are appropriate.

CARDIORESPIRATORY SEGMENT

- Promote independence and self-responsibility among participants.
- Gradually increase intensity.
- Provide options for varying impact and/or intensity.
- Build sequences logically and progressively.
- Use various muscle groups.

- Use music to create a motivational atmosphere.
- Monitor intensity through heart rate and/or rating of perceived exertion checks.
- Incorporate a postcardio cool-down segment.

RESISTANCE TRAINING SEGMENT

- Muscle balance and functional fitness are encouraged.
- Instructor's form is appropriate, and instructor observes and corrects participants' form.
- Provide verbal, visual, and physical cues on posture and body mechanics.
- Describe adaptations for participants with injuries or special needs.
- Use the functional exercise continuum (which organizes various exercises from easiest to hardest) to help choose the most appropriate exercise or variation for all participants.
- Use equipment safely and effectively.
- Create a motivational/instructional atmosphere.

NEUROMOTOR SEGMENT

- Provide exercises for both static and dynamic balance.
- Provide modifications and progressions as necessary.

FLEXIBILITY SEGMENT

- Stretching of major muscle groups is performed in a safe and effective manner.
- Relaxation/visualization concludes the flexibility segment.

Adapted with permission from Kennedy CA, MM Yoke. *Methods of group exercise instruction.* Champaign (IL): Human Kinetics; 2005. 254 p.

---

wear a midriff outfit because it might be intimidating. In many group exercise classes, correct spinal alignment and form should be visible with each movement the instructor demonstrates, requiring the use of form-fitting clothing. The instructor must balance the comfort level of the class with functional wear for effective teaching.

Equipment Preparation

With the large variety of equipment available for group exercise (stability balls, handheld weights, resistance bands, balance devices, kettlebells, yoga blocks, etc.), it is important to be prepared ahead of time and inform participants about what will be used. If participants are expected to obtain individual items (such as from an equipment closet), posting an explanation of which exercise tubing device is harder/easier would be helpful. Instructors may have a white board at the class entrance that has a welcome to the class and a list of equipment needed for the class. Personal equipment used by the

instructor (exercise equipment, microphone, etc.) ought to be ready before the class start time.

Use of Music

Many group exercise classes use music as a way to motivate participants and create more overall enjoyment in the movement experience. Research has validated the idea that music is beneficial from a motivational standpoint (5,22). In terms of using music to create a beat to follow, research has found that external auditory cues, such as rhythmic music and percussion pulses, favorably affect coordinated walking and proprioceptive control (48). However, moving to the beat of music is not always necessary in a group exercise setting. Some yoga, Pilates, and outdoor group exercise sessions do not use music. Although using the beat is important in most choreographed classes, such as Zumba, kickboxing, and step, music is also used in cycling, boot camp, and water exercise as background sound to help motivate or set a mood. It is important to balance music volume and verbal cueing. If the music is so loud that the verbal cueing is not heard, that can be a problem for the participants. Seniors, especially, need to be asked about the volume of the music. IDEA published an opinion statement on the volume of music based on standards established by the United States Occupational Safety and Health Administration. IDEA stated that music volume during group exercise classes should measure no more than 90 decibels (dB), and because the instructor's voice needs to be about 10 dB louder than the music to be heard, the instructor's voice should measure no more than 100 dB (38). A study on voice problems with group exercise instructors found that 44% of instructors surveyed experienced partial or complete voice loss during and after instructing (32). Instructors also had increased episodes of voice loss, hoarseness, and sore throat unrelated to illness since they began instructing. To protect the voice of instructors, it is important to use a microphone system.

Always ask participants about their preference in music. Just as many personal fitness trainers make the mistake of giving their own workout to potential clients, group fitness instructors often choose music that is personally motivating. Although it is important that music motivates the instructor, it is imperative that it motivates the participants (*Fig. 34-3*).

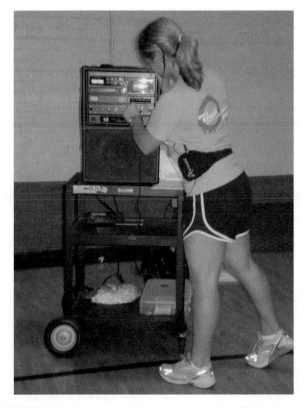

FIGURE 34-3. A group exercise instructor needs sufficient time to prepare the stereo system and microphone during the preclass preparation.

Acknowledge Class Participants

Creating a positive attitude and atmosphere begins with the instructor welcoming people before class begins and introducing himself or herself, especially when teaching in a facility where different people come to class every week and there is no set class roster. If participants are aware of the instructor's name, they will be more likely to come up and ask questions afterward. New people coming to a group exercise class are often afraid of asking questions or may feel out of place. Understanding this and asking for feedback will create a more open, safe environment for all participants and not just the regular participants. Also, try to approach all new participants individually at the end of each of their first few classes; ask if they have any questions and make certain to invite them back.

Preview Class Format

An overview of what the specific class format will be should accompany the instructor's introduction. Make sure to introduce the class format before each class begins. After previewing the class format, it is also important that participants understand their individual responsibilities. Intensity is the responsibility of the participant, not the instructor. The instructor provides modifications for various intensities to allow participants to make a choice. Encourage, demonstrate, and promote various exercise choices so participants are comfortable working at their own pace.

WARM-UP

There are a few common principles in the warm-up that apply to any group exercise class; these will be reviewed in the following section.

Appropriate Dynamic Movement

The purpose of the warm-up is to prepare the body for the more rigorous demands of the cardiorespiratory and/or resistance training segments by raising the body temperature. A higher core temperature increases the metabolism of the muscles as well as the blood flow and release of oxygen. Appropriate dynamic movement involves the use of large muscle groups exercising at a low to moderate intensity, for example, low kicks and half-time punches as preparation for a kickboxing or a walking/jogging segment prior to sprints and running in a boot camp class.

Rehearsal Moves

Rehearsal moves are a less intense version of the movement patterns that participants will perform during the cardiorespiratory portion of class. Rehearsal moves should make up most warm-up, thus preparing participants mentally and physically for the challenges of the workout ahead. Examples of these would be using the bench to warm up during a step class, or teaching participants how to hill climb briefly in an indoor cycling class.

The concept of rehearsal moves relates to the principle of specificity of training. This principle states that the body adapts specifically to whatever demands are placed on it. Specificity applies not only to energy systems and muscle groups but also to movement patterns. In a group exercise session, participants may become frustrated if they are not able to perform the movements effectively. Introducing these movement patterns in the warm-up will assist with learning the proper technique. For example, a fast salsa step may be used in the cardiorespiratory segment of a Zumba class, so it would be appropriate to include it at half speed in the warm-up. This helps participants not only physiologically and psychologically but also specifically helps the neuromuscular system by practicing the pathways that will be needed later on during the workout (*Fig. 34-4*).

Stretches, If Appropriate

Whether to stretch during the warm-up is a debated issue. A literature review found that insufficient evidence existed to conclude that preexercise stretching prevents injuries (52). However, the authors stated that "the evidence is not of sufficient strength, quality, and generalizability to recommend altering or eliminating preexercise stretching" (52). With this in mind, the warm-up should contain mostly dynamic warm-up activities. If static stretches are included, they should be held only briefly during the warm-up (*e.g.*, 5–10 s) to lengthen the muscles in preparation for activity. For sport activities where muscular strength, power, and endurance are needed for performance, it is recommended that stretching be performed after the activity rather than before (52). The decision on how to go about warming up and stretching, therefore, is an individual one. Flexibility is an important health-related component of fitness and should be included in the workout. However, the optimum use of flexibility exercises may be at the end of the workout (*Fig. 34-5*).

CARDIORESPIRATORY SEGMENT

There are a few common principles in the cardiorespiratory segment of most group exercise classes, which will be reviewed in this section.

Promote Self-Responsibility

Whether teaching classes such as yoga, Zumba, or a boot camp class, it is impossible to be everywhere or help everyone simultaneously. Each participant is working at a different fitness level and has different goals. If participants try to exercise at the instructor's level or at another participant's level, they may work too hard and sustain an injury, or they may not work hard enough to meet their goals. A few ways to help promote independence and self-responsibility are to encourage participants to work at their own pace, use rating of perceived exertion (RPE) checks, and inform them about how they should feel through common examples. Demonstrate high-, medium-, and low-intensity options for individual movements or activities within a class. Group exercise instructors should educate participants about achieving the level of effort they need to reach and continually

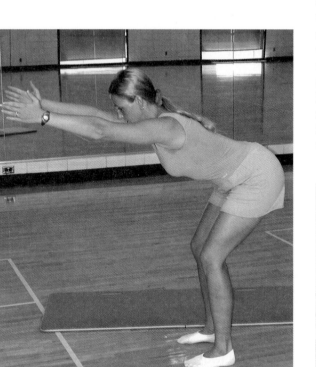

FIGURE 34-4. Long-lever spinal flexion with hips flexed is a good rehearsal move for performing standing upper-body free-weight exercises.

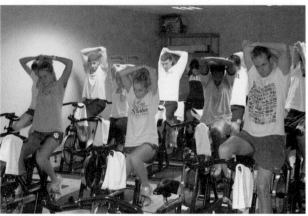

FIGURE 34-5. Enhancing flexibility in an indoor cycling group exercise class at the end of the workout.

remind them that intensity is their responsibility, not the instructor's. It is recommended that the group exercise instructor not only personally maintain an intermediate level of intensity most of the time but also present other options and intensities as the need arises. Mastering this concept is the true "art" of group exercise and one reason why group exercise is more difficult than one-on-one instruction.

Impact and/or Intensity Options

In most group exercise classes, movement selection can affect impact and/or intensity. For example, marching in place entails moderate impact, as some of the person's weight strikes the floor while some of the weight is supported by the other foot. Jumping activities are high impact in that the entire body weight strikes the ground when landing. Impact is not an issue in an indoor cycling class, yet intensity options are still important. For example, a hill climb out of the saddle at a high resistance is considered a higher intensity option, whereas seated at a lower resistance (while maintaining a moderate cycling cadence) would be a lower intensity option. All group exercise sessions have movements that can vary impact and intensity.

More recently, high-intensity training (HIT) and high-intensity interval training (HIIT) have become popular. Some boot camp-style classes now feature HIT. This type of training generally involves short bursts (<60 s) of all-out effort; each high-intensity interval is followed by a short recovery (21). Because this type of training is, by design, very intense and requires maximal or near-maximal effort, it is appropriate only for low-risk populations. Even in HIT/HIIT classes, lower intensity and low-impact options should always be made available.

Building Sequences

In most group exercise classes, sequence building is important in order for participants to feel successful. In other words, moves should progress logically from one to the other. In a high/low class, an example of building sequences logically would be teaching a group a grapevine move for the first time by breaking down the movement. Perform two-step touches to the right followed by two-step touches to the left. Then perform the same step touches, only this time, step behind to make a grapevine move. Progressing properly in a water exercise class would mean marking a specific move by performing it, then increasing the speed of movement, traveling with the move, and then resisting the movement. If sequences are logical and progressive, there is a certain "flow" to the class. Without such continuity, participants may end up standing and watching, feel confused while doing the movement, execute it improperly, or not enjoy the experience because they are uncomfortable.

Methods of Monitoring Cardiorespiratory Intensity

Monitoring exercise intensity within the cardiorespiratory segment is important. HR is a common choice but has several limitations. During high/low impact, for example, a given HR value is associated with a lower amount of oxygen consumption than the same HR during treadmill exercise (37). This may be because of the various intermittent movements using small amounts of muscle mass during high/low as compared with continuous movement with a large amount of muscle mass (hips and thighs) during treadmill exercise. The higher HR that results from the continuous use of elevated arms is a pressor response. This HR discrepancy may be true for other similar forms of group exercise such as kickboxing. During water exercise, HR values are lower than those observed in land exercise likely because of a shift in blood volume caused by the water pressure (18). Although differences in HR between certain modes of exercise may make it difficult to accurately predict energy expenditure, HR can still be used as a relative indicator of changes in intensity within each mode. Indoor cycling classes use a mode of exercise involving an upright posture and continuous use of a large amount of muscle mass. Therefore, HR can be an excellent means of monitoring intensity. The power readout in watts available on some cycling machines also provides an excellent means of monitoring intensity and provides nearly instantaneous feedback, whereas HR responds more slowly to changes in effort. When measuring HR, wearing a chest strap monitor greatly improves the ease of use. If participants are to measure HR by palpation, they must be taught to do so accurately.

Other disadvantages of the HR method include the effect of certain medications on HR and the problem inherent in maximal HR (HR_{max}) formulas. Certain medications, most notably some antihypertensive drugs, can alter the HR response to exercise; consequently, RPE may be preferred for monitoring intensity of participants on these medications. Traditional HR_{max} formulas have been shown to have a high degree of variability and a newer, more accurate formula [$HR_{max} = 207 - (0.7 \times age)$] should be considered (20). Even so, it's important to realize that if the maximum HR is estimated by any formula, rather than a known value derived from testing, then the subsequent calculations for target HR will also be an estimate, either underestimating or overestimating the appropriate training zone (this is true even if one is wearing an HR monitor).

RPE and the talk test are subjective means of monitoring exercise intensity. RPE is a practical way to help participants listen to their bodies and work at levels that feel appropriate for them. See *Chapter 30* for more detail.

Application of Intensity Monitoring to the Group Exercise Setting

Whether using target HR, RPE, or the talk test to monitor exercise intensity, there are a few points of practical application within a group exercise setting:

- If using music, turn off the music during manual measurement of HR, so the beats do not influence the counting.
- Palpation of the radial artery is preferred over the carotid pulse; if using the carotid pulse, press lightly to avoid slowing the HR through stimulation of the carotid baroreceptors.
- Check intensity several times during a workout so it can be modified if needed.
- Keep participants moving to prevent blood from pooling in the lower extremities when checking HR or asking about perceived exertion.
- Use a brief counting period, such as 10 s, to facilitate ease and accuracy of HR measurement.

Postcardio Cool-Down

If the cardiorespiratory segment is to be followed by a different segment, such as resistance training, a brief cool-down (*e.g.*, 5 min) should be performed in between. Cooling down prevents blood from pooling in the lower extremities and allows the cardiopulmonary system to transition to less intense workloads. Encourage participants to relax, slow down, keep arms below the level of the heart, and put less effort into the movements. Using less intense music, changing one's tone of voice, and verbalizing the transition to the participants can create this atmosphere. If the cardiorespiratory segment is the last training segment of the workout, then a longer cool-down (5–10 min) should be performed, along with stretching. See the following text for more information in the section describing the flexibility segment of the group exercise class.

Resistance Training/Muscle Conditioning Segment

Various group exercise formats involve resistance training for the development of muscular strength/ endurance. Resistance can be provided by body weight, resistance bands and tubing, and handheld weights. Detailed information regarding the prescription of resistance training is provided in *Chapter 31*.

Progression in Programming

A method of exercise selection and progression that has been developed by Yoke and Kennedy can be tailored to the group exercise setting (59). This system involves progressing along a continuum from simple to complex, from easy to hard, and from beginner to advanced exercise in six steps, as described in *Box 34-2* and illustrated in *Figures 34-6* through *34-11*. Organizing exercises in this way can make it easier for an instructor to think on his or her feet and adjust an exercise to suit individual needs. For example, if a participant complains of shoulder pain when doing a triceps dip off a bench, a skilled instructor could suggest a safer, easier, more stable alternative that doesn't

---

BOX 34-2 | **Six-Step Exercise Progression Model for Resistance Training Segment of Group Exercise Classes**

Level #1: Isolate and educate.

The participant is learning how to focus on the muscle and movement. Exercises in this level are often performed in the supine or prone position.

Level #2: Isolate and educate and add resistance.

Resistance is added to the exercise in Level #1.

Level #3: Add functional training position.

To better challenge the stabilizing muscles, an exercise in a seated or standing position (for the targeted muscles) is performed.

Level #4: Combine increasing function with resistance.

Some type of overload (e.g., weights, tubing, bands) is added to challenge the body's stabilizers in the functional position.

Level #5: Challenge multiple muscle groups with increasing resistance and core challenge.

More complex exercises (e.g., squats and lunge variations) are added that combine muscular fitness, balance, coordination, and stability.

Level #6: Add balance, increased functional challenge, speed, or rotational movements.

The use of stability balls, Bosu balls (half stability balls), wobble boards, or spinal rotation to exercise movements is added. Some individuals may never reach this level because of their fitness level, health history, or past or current musculoskeletal injury.

Reprinted with permission from Yoke M, Kennedy C. *Functional Exercise Progressions.* Monterey (CA): Healthy Learning Publisher; 2004. 126 p.

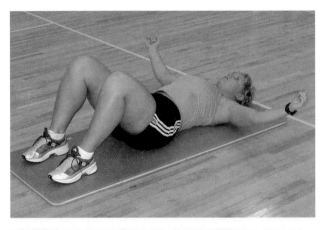

FIGURE 34-6. Level 1 short-lever pectoral fly exercise that focuses on isolation and education in a supine position.

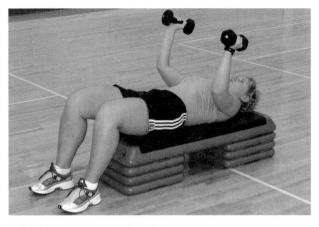

FIGURE 34-7. Level 2 short-lever pectoral fly exercise that adds resistance to the Level 1 position using weights.

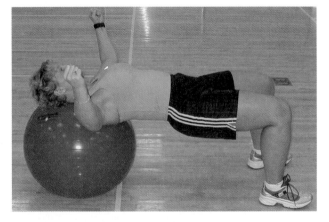

FIGURE 34-8. Level 3 pectoral fly performed in a supine position on a stability ball to destabilize the movement.

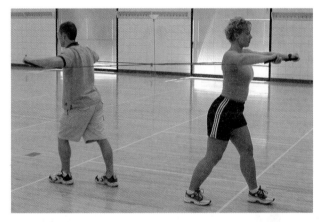

FIGURE 34-9. Level 4 pectoral press with a partner using resistance tubing.

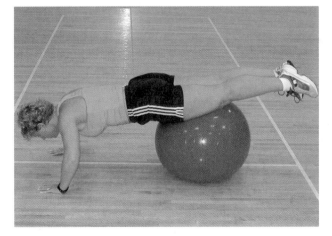

FIGURE 34-10. Level 5 pectoral push-up using a stability ball challenges neuromotor capacities.

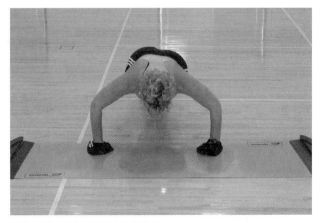

FIGURE 34-11. Level 6 pectoral exercise performing a push-up using a slide board to destabilize the upper body for increased functional challenge.

require as much shoulder joint range of motion or weight bearing; the participant could instead perform a seated or standing unilateral triceps press-down with an elastic tube or band. In this position, the shoulder joint is in neutral and the upper arm is much easier to stabilize. A seated or standing triceps press down with a tube is an excellent level 1 choice — safe, effective, and easy for most participants to perform correctly with an appropriate resistance. Understanding what makes an exercise safer and easier to perform versus what makes an exercise controversial is a critical skill for all group exercise instructors. Imagine a scenario where an instructor gives a challenging exercise, such as a dead lift, to a group of participants. If most participants continue to perform the exercise with poor form and alignment, even after diligent, clear cues have been given, safety is still an issue. If participants have inflexible hamstring muscles and poor core stability, they will most likely perform the dead lifts with a rounded, flexed spine, which can be a mechanism of back injury. Clearly, the exercise (in this case, a dead lift) is inappropriate for this particular group of participants. A competent instructor will immediately discontinue the dead lift and introduce an exercise that most participants can perform safely and effectively. If the goal is to strengthen the gluteus maximus and hamstrings, a safer alternative would be hip extension in the all-fours position or, even safer, in the prone position. On the exercise continuum proposed by Yoke and Kennedy, a dead lift is on the far right end (advanced — level 6), the all-fours position is near the middle (intermediate — level 3), and the prone position is on the far left (beginner — level 1). It is very helpful if group exercise instructors understand and can apply this concept, thus enhancing safety and effectiveness for all participants.

Utilize Equipment Safely and Effectively

Portable resistance training equipment, such as exercise bands, stability balls, BOSU balance trainers, kettlebells, handheld weights, and weighted bars are often used in a group exercise class. Research has shown that stability ball training (*Fig. 34-12*) helps improve spinal stability (11). One study concluded that the unstable nature of the ball elicits a greater neuromuscular response when compared with training on a stable surface (4). Another new trend in group exercise is body weight leverage training (*e.g.*, the TRX Suspension Trainer). Special equipment is required that is an investment for a facility, but according to the IDEA 2010 Fitness Trends Survey, this type of program has top growth potential. With so many "toys" and tools at their disposal, group exercise instructors must ensure proper participant usage and form and must always keep safety as a priority.

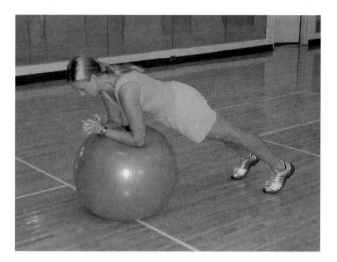

FIGURE 34-12. Stability balls can be used to enhance trunk stabilizer muscles.

Core Training

Eighty percent of facilities offer core-conditioning classes, according to the IDEA 2010 Fitness Trends Survey (45). Traditionally, core conditioning refers to training the abdominal and lower back muscles, so as to develop spinal stability and help prevent or manage low back pain. However, some disciplines (such as Pilates) consider core training to include all the major muscles of the pelvis, spine, scapulae, and neck. The Pilates technique also focuses on mobility of these areas as well as stability, stamina, and endurance of core musculature. Approximately 90% of facilities now offer Pilates training, generally in the form of mat Pilates. Pilates, a discipline named after its originator, Joseph Pilates, has been shown to help in the management of lower back pain (24), particularly when Pilates apparatus, such as the reformer, Cadillac, barrel, or chair, is used (42). Whether using Pilates techniques or not, group exercise instructors will want to make certain that the benefit of any core-conditioning exercise used in class outweighs the potential risk of injury. All core exercises can be organized along the functional exercise continuum, and appropriate exercises need to be chosen for any given group of participants.

It is important to separate resistance training from cardiorespiratory training. A study evaluated the effects of step-class training with and without the use of light handheld weights (31). Both group's improved aerobic fitness and strength, but the group using weights did not experience any greater improvement in aerobic fitness or strength compared with the group that did not use weights. Therefore, if the goal is to improve aerobic fitness, greater progression of aerobic activity within the cardiorespiratory segment of a class is needed. And similarly, if the goal is to improve strength or muscular endurance, greater progression within the resistance training segment is needed. Attempting to accomplish both goals simultaneously is not an effective technique, particularly for beginners, and may compromise form, leading to injury.

NEUROMOTOR EXERCISE

Neuromotor exercise includes training for balance, agility, and improved proprioception or coordination. Balance exercises, especially, are important for older adults who are at risk for falling and have declining abilities in activities of daily living (40). Static balance exercises may be provided, which can involve standing on one leg while moving other extremities, standing on an unstable surface (e.g., foam cushion or BOSU balance trainer), or maintaining a narrow base of support (e.g., a tandem stance). According to 2011 ACSM Guidelines for exercise prescription (19), studies that have resulted in improvements in neuromotor exercise have mostly used training frequencies of >2–3 d · wk^{-1} with exercise sessions of >20–30 min in duration for a total of >60 min of neuromotor exercise per week; however, more research is needed before any definitive recommendations can be made. There is no available evidence concerning the number of repetitions of exercises needed, the intensity of the exercise, or optimal methods for progression. Dynamic balance exercises may also be helpful; these may include pretending to walk along a "tightrope" (a piece of masking tape placed along the floor), stepping from "stone to stone" while balancing, or maneuvering around obstacles such as a cone, chair, or book. Tai chi is yet another form of group exercise that promotes balance and coordination (26).

Functional Exercise

More recently, the concepts of functional fitness and functional exercise have been promoted as a way to enhance neuromotor abilities. A functional exercise is one that helps improve an individual's activities of daily living, whatever those activities may be. However, some experts and promotional materials mix the terms functional training with core training. Others have labeled a functional exercise as one that involves multiple muscles and multiple joints, often with the weight, or resistance, being held farther away from the body and is an exercise that requires many muscles to work together to perform a smooth, coordinated movement. A classic example of a multiple muscle and joint exercise is the woodchopper, in which a weight (kettlebell or medicine ball) is swung from a position high above one shoulder down across the front of the body to finish near the floor on the outside of the opposite foot. Although all of these concepts and exercises can be valid, group exercise instructors will want to use them appropriately, making certain to give the right exercise to the right person at the right time. In general, an exercise such as a woodchopper is at the advanced end of the functional exercise continuum because it requires multimuscle strength, endurance, flexibility, balance, coordination, and core stability all at once, and is relatively difficult to perform correctly.

FLEXIBILITY SEGMENT

There are a few common principles in the flexibility segment of most group exercise classes that will be reviewed in this section.

Stretching

It is important to stretch the muscle groups that have been used in the group exercise activity as well as muscles that are commonly tight. For instance, after an indoor cycling class, not only stretching the quadriceps, calves, and gluteus is appropriate because they are major muscles used for cycling but also the hamstrings as they remain in a shortened position during cycling. In a kickboxing session, it is important to stretch the muscles that surround the hip as well as the muscles of the anterior chest. However, other muscle groups should not be ignored, as a balanced approach incorporates stretching all the major muscle groups (*Fig 34-13*). Props, such as stretching straps, yoga blocks, cushions, foam rollers, and stability balls, may all be used to enhance flexibility during the stretch segment. Flexibility exercises, similar to resistance training exercises, can exist along a continuum from easiest to hardest. For example, a hamstring stretch that is safe and relatively easy for almost everyone to perform correctly is the supine hamstring stretch. A more difficult hamstring stretch is the seated, one-leg forward bend; here, sufficient hamstring flexibility is required before a participant can even get into proper spinal alignment. An advanced example of a hamstring stretch could be forward bending while in a full split on the floor. All these stretches involve hip flexion and knee extension, ensuring that hamstrings will be elongated, but not all of these examples are appropriate for all participants. Group exercise instructors need to

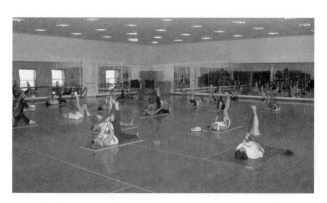

FIGURE 34-13. Flexibility can be enhanced in a group exercise setting using stretching bands.

know various exercises in order to best serve the general public. *Chapter 31* provides additional information regarding exercise prescription for flexibility.

Relaxation and Visualization

A popular activity to complete a group exercise class is relaxation. This may be structured or free flowing. Guided imagery or creative visualization might help deepen the relaxation as, for example, the instructor describes quiet forests, gentle breezes, peaceful ocean waves, or a warm fire. Tightening and releasing muscle groups in a progression through the body is another effective relaxation technique. One of the simplest techniques for both relaxation and meditation is for the participants to mindfully focus on their breathing, feeling the rising and falling of the abdomen (if supine), and slowing and lengthening each breath. Positive affirmations or intentions for the day may also be suggested. Complete silence, or the use of quiet music, may be used to set the appropriate mood for this aspect of the class session.

POPULAR GROUP EXERCISE PROGRAMS

A diverse number of group exercise programs have emerged in an effort to meet the needs of regular exercisers and to attract new fitness participants. Some of the popular group programs briefly highlighted in this section include high/low or cardio, step training, kickboxing, boot camp, water fitness, indoor cycling, yoga, stability ball workouts, and Pilates.

HIGH/LOW OR MIXED IMPACT GROUP EXERCISE CLASSES

Mixed-impact (or high/low) classes combine high-impact cardiorespiratory movements that are associated with greater stresses on the lower extremities (*e.g.*, running, jumping, and hopping) with low-impact movements that provide minimal stress on the lower extremities (*e.g.*, side lunges and march in place). Combinations and routines are choreographed to music and incorporate various arm movements, leg movements, traveling patterns, and directional turns. An advantage of mixed-impact classes is the ability to modify the intensity and/or the impact of the exercise. One study found a large difference in energy cost between low-impact (4–5 kcal · min^{-1}) and high-impact (10–11 kcal · min^{-1}) movement styles (57). Typically, the most common ways to modify any group-led exercise are to alter the speed of movement, modify the range of motion of the movement, vary the amount of traveling completed with a movement, and change the vertical component of the movement. A few safety considerations specific to mixed-impact classes are to not

hop repeatedly on one foot (*e.g.*, more than eight times in a row) to avoid excessive impact-related stress, avoid twisting hop variations that may lead to spinal stress, and use a music tempo of 135–155 beats per minute (bpm). Jazzercise is an example of a mixed-impact group exercise branded classes.

STEP TRAINING

Step training is a mainstay cardiorespiratory class format (*Fig. 34-14*). Step training has been described as a safe, low-impact exercise that may potentially provide high-intensity cardiorespiratory conditioning (42). Steps are also often used in sports conditioning/boot camp circuit classes as a way to increase intensity in a small space. The workouts can be as challenging as a rigorous jogging workout and yet produce impact forces as safe as walking. However, use of fast stepping cadences appear to result in greater vertical ground reaction forces on the body in less experienced step enthusiasts (43). It is recommended that the cadence of step classes generally range from 118 to 128 bpm (35,47). Research demonstrates that changing bench height is the most consequential variable to alter step exercise intensity (17,39,42,55,58). The most widely used step platforms have adjustable heights from 4 to 12 in (10–30 cm), with a stepping surface 14-in wide by 42-in long (36 cm × 107 cm). Instructors may instruct participants to use increasing step heights to accomplish progression of intensity, although some impact and power variations significantly increase intensity as well. The typical riser increase allows for a 2 in (5 cm) change in step height. *Box 34-3* provides safety tips to follow when implementing a step training program.

KICKBOXING AND BOOT CAMP

Kickboxing and cardioboxing are two of the many martial arts–based exercise class formats that have become a staple component of the group fitness industry. Movements

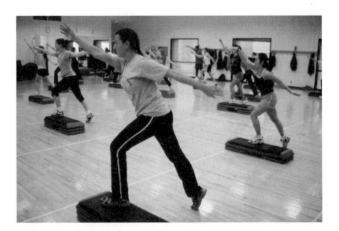

FIGURE 34-14. A group exercise step class.

BOX 34-3   Safety Considerations for Step Training Classes

- Step entirely on the top part of the platform with each step, not allowing any part of the foot to hang over an edge.
- Discourage flexing the knees more than 90 degrees; vary step height as needed. Avoid flexing the knees more than 60 degrees for participants predisposed to patellofemoral pain.
- Adding handheld weights to step training is not recommended because of a lack of additional gains in fitness (31).
- To lower the exercise intensity quickly, stop stepping and switch to marching in place on the ground.
- Use cross-training shoes or indoor fitness shoes for step workouts. Most running shoes do not provide suitable support for step movements.
- Avoid step combinations that travel forward and down off the bench, which increase eccentric stress.

- Maintain an upright posture and bend at the knees for ascending and descending movements. Too much hip flexion while stepping may place unwanted stress on the spine.
- Frequently change the leading foot when doing the step patterns to avoid overstressing one leg (e.g., at least once per minute).
- Avoid excessive repetition of movement patterns on one leg to avoid orthopedic stress.
- Include movement choices for a variety of muscle groups to include those that may not receive much use in activities of daily living (e.g., hamstrings, adductors, abductors).

Reprinted with permission from Smith J. Injury prevention in step classes. *IDEA Health & Fitness Source.* 2000;18:36–45; Aerobics and Fitness Association of America. *AFAA Step Training: A Manual for Instructors.* Sherman Oaks (CA): Aerobics and Fitness Association of America; 2010. 88 p.

include kicks, punches, elbow strikes, jabs, knee strikes, and combinations thereof, which are similar to those used in boxing and martial arts. The combative drills in these classes are mixed with recovery bouts of basic aerobic movements such as boxer-style rope skipping (with or without a rope), walking, and light jogging in place. Some kickboxing group exercise classes involve boxing gloves, punching bags, and martial arts equipment, although other programs incorporate "shadow boxing," with no equipment. Most of these classes are driven by moderately paced music (approximately 120–135 bpm),

although the music may be used only for motivation rather than to control the choreography.

A key concern with martial arts-based exercise classes is the preparation of instructors to properly teach the programs (56). Instructors need to have proper knowledge of correct punching techniques as well as the progressive teaching skills to minimize joint-related injuries among class participants. *Box 34-4* provides some safety guidelines to consider with martial arts-based exercise classes.

Boot camp classes are currently very popular, with many instructors taking to the outdoors with their

BOX 34-4   Safety Considerations for Kickboxing Classes

- Perform a satisfactory warm-up to properly prepare the muscles and joints for the ensuing challenge of the workout.
- With all upper-body strikes and jabs, make sure the elbow is not taken past its normal range of motion (ROM).
- To protect the supporting leg, execute no more than 10 kicks consecutively.
- Do not kick beyond the normal ROM. Control for any "snapping" movements during leg extension.
- Kicking and pivoting together may be contraindicated for many learners. Beginners should master the basic moves before progressing to advanced kickboxing movements.

- Use a music tempo of 120 to 135 bpm to discourage movements being performed incorrectly and hastily.
- Be aware that the novelty of martial arts movements may lead to delayed-onset muscle soreness in those just starting classes.
- To protect ligaments, turn out the toes slightly and flex the knee of the supporting leg when kicking.
- Deliver punches from the body as opposed to from the shoulders.

bpm, beats per minute.

Reprinted with permission from Williams A. Injury prevention in kickboxing classes. *IDEA Health & Fitness Source.* 2000;18:58–67; Aerobics and Fitness Association of America. *AFAA Kickboxing: A Manual for Instructors.* Sherman Oaks (CA): Aerobic and Fitness Association of America; 2010. 72 p.

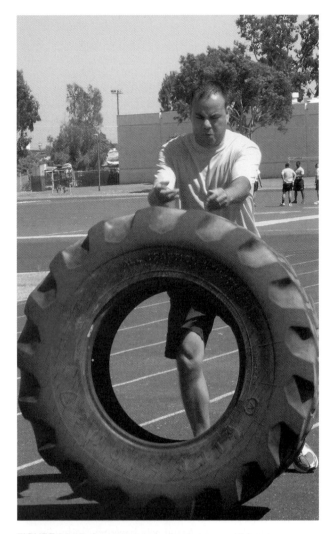

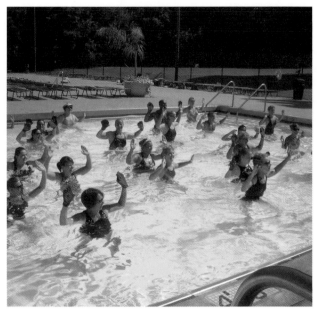

FIGURE 34-16. A group water exercise class.

FIGURE 34-15. A group exercise boot camp participant performing a tire flip.

participants. A boot camp workout is inspired by military training regimens and typically incorporates short sprints, shuttle runs, burpees, reaction drills, push-ups, sit-ups, lunges, medicine ball throws, pull-ups, and tug-of-war. Some programs use tire flips and sled pulls with weights to simulate more functional activities (*Fig. 34-15*). Although many participants find this type of program to be fun, high energy, and motivating, instructors must take care to accommodate all fitness levels and offer modifications and options.

WATER FITNESS CLASSES

Water fitness classes are staple, with older adults especially (*Fig. 34-16*). However, there is a general lack of awareness about the benefits and special techniques associated with water fitness classes. Water exercise training programs have been shown to reduce percent body fat in women who are overweight (34), improve

activities of daily living on land (51), and provide various fitness- and health-related benefits (8,13,50). A practical consideration is to progressively increase intensity by increasing speed of movement and by using equipment overload (surface area or buoyancy-resisted devices) to increase resistance to movement of the limbs through the water (33).

INDOOR CYCLING

A stationary indoor group cycling class is a unique group-led exercise format that has attracted many devoted supporters. IDEA 2011 Fitness Trends (54) show that this activity is continuing to increase in popularity with a 20% increase in the past year. Because of its non–weight-bearing nature, the indoor cycling class offers some orthopedic advantages for special populations who are not able to perform traditional weight-bearing exercise. Also, for seasoned cyclists, indoor cycling offers a viable option to the hazards of wintertime weather cycling.

Instructors lead exercise enthusiasts through a "virtual" outdoor road ride, complete with valleys, hills, straightaways, and finish lines (7). Music for indoor cycling classes is selected for motivation and geared toward enhancing the mood during various portions of the class. No beats-per-minute guidelines have been established with indoor cycling classes; however, faster and slower tempos are used in support of changes in exercise intensity (46). The success of an indoor cycling class depends heavily on the instructors' exercise program design knowledge as well as their ability to motivate the participants (29). *Box 34-5* provides safety guidelines for indoor cycling.

BOX 34-5	Safety Considerations for Indoor Cycling Classes

- Seat height should be adjusted so that the knee is flexed 25–30 degrees as the pedal travels through the bottom of the stroke. (If the participant stops at the bottom of the stroke and lowers his or her heel so that the foot is parallel to the floor, knee flexion should be 5–10 degrees.)
- The front-to-back seat position should be set so that the front of the knee is directly above the center of the pedal halfway through the down stroke.
- Handlebar height is based on the comfort of the participant. Low handlebars that create a flat back position should only be used by those who are accustomed to such posture, such as competitive road cyclists.
- Review the operation of the emergency brake with participants; suddenly stopping the pedaling action without using the brake can cause injury.
- Have participants wear correct cycling apparel. Cycling shorts with padded inserts help to lessen the discomfort of prolonged cycling. Hard-soled cycling shoes are preferred to minimize the pressure on the feet when pedaling. Many cycling shoes have a cleat that can snap into the pedal,

improving cycling mechanics and power transfer from the body.
- Because of the multiple fitness levels in a class, provide resistance or cadence options during the various class segments. In general, maintaining a relatively high cadence (such as 80–100 revolutions per minute [rpm]) with a low resistance produces less stress on the knees than does a low-cadence/high-resistance combination.
- Encourage participants to bring water bottles to stay hydrated.
- Vary the riding position during the class to minimize lower back discomfort.
- To minimize wrist and upper body tension, instruct participants not to place too much weight on the handlebars while in a standing position.

Source: Bryant CX, Wenson J, Peterson JA. Safe and enjoyable group cycling for your members: reviewing these group cycling basics can help you guide your members through a fun and effective exercise experience. *Fitness Management*. 2001;17(6):38–40;42; Kolovou T. Launching and indoor cycling program: these marketing tactics and tips for indoor cycling instruction will help with the launch and profitable continuation of your program. *Fitness Management*. 2000;16(6):40–2; Sherman RM. The indoor cycling revolution: designing classes that chart the course to success. *IDEA Today*. 1997;15(3):30–3;35–6;39; and Vogel AE. Injury prevention in indoor cycling classes. *IDEA Health & Fitness Source*. 2000;18:48–57.

YOGA

With origins in India, yoga has existed for at least 5,000 yr. **Yoga** means *union*, and it refers to one of the symbolic systems of Hindu philosophy that strive to bring together and develop the body, mind, and spirit. Hatha yoga is the form with which Westerners are most familiar and is defined by a series of physical postures (*asanas*) and breathing patterns. There are several different forms of Hatha yoga that are popularly practiced. Some of the most popular forms of yoga are briefly described here. Iyengar yoga incorporates traditional Hatha techniques into fluid, dance-like sequences. It uses props such as chairs, pillows, blankets, and belts to accommodate persons with special needs (9). Ashtanga yoga is a fast-paced, athletic style that is the foundation for power yoga classes (9,25). These classes provide more vigorous workouts than other forms of yoga. Hot yoga, popularized as Bikram yoga, is done in a sauna-style room that is heated to approximately 100° F (38° C), so the muscles are warm for stretching (25). Kripalu yoga focuses on personal growth and self-improvement through the practice of meditation during poses (9,25). Kundalini yoga merges stretching, breathing, and meditation.

Some considerations for teaching yoga classes include the following (9,25):

- Consider the ability of the participants in a given class when selecting postures because some postures require significant levels of strength or flexibility. Yoga postures and variations of postures may be ranked along a continuum from easiest to hardest.
- Provide modifications of postures for participants who have muscle or joint problems or whose strength and flexibility are below the class average.
- Avoid poses that place significant stress on the low back or the neck (*e.g.*, the plow) unless working with advanced students.
- Participants with high blood pressure or glaucoma should not perform postures in which the head is positioned below the level of the heart, such as headstands.
- Always teach proper body alignment specific to each posture.

Many certifications exist in yoga; the Yoga Alliance encourages instructors to become registered yoga teachers (RYTs).

STABILITY BALL WORKOUTS

Originating in Europe, stability ball training has spread throughout North America. Although originally used in rehabilitation, stability ball training is frequently used in group exercise classes. The unstable nature of the ball disturbs the position of one's body if the center of mass is not well controlled. Thus, the body's neuromuscular balance-regulating mechanisms are challenged when performing stability ball exercises, as opposed to performing the same movements on a solid base of support, such as a bench. Stability balls can be a useful part of an instructor's equipment repertoire and can be used to help fulfill the ACSM neuromotor exercise guidelines (19). Balls come in various sizes. Proper ball size is observed when the individual is seated on the apex of the ball with the feet flat on the floor, and the hips and knees are bent at 90 degrees. The "peanut" shape is less challenging to one's balance and may be more appropriate for beginners. Many stability ball exercises are designed to work muscles of the trunk, but upper- and lower-body exercises are performed as well.

Some considerations for teaching stability ball classes include the following (14,44):

- Initially, have the participants sit on the ball and become aware of their center of gravity on this unstable base of support. Progress with exercises once participants have mastered the sitting position.
- Less skilled participants should place the ball close to a wall, with their back toward the wall or, preferably, be spotted.
- Individuals with advanced osteoporosis or with vestibular dysfunction (i.e., vertigo) should not use stability balls.
- Smooth floor surfaces (e.g., wood as opposed to carpet) are more difficult because of the reduced friction and should not be used with less skilled participants (such as older adults).

BOSU Balance Trainers are also popular. These half-dome-shaped devices may be used with either the rubber dome side up or the rigid plastic side up. Various exercises can be performed on the BOSU; most are used to add additional core and balance challenges.

PILATES

The historic roots of Pilates are from World War I, when Joseph Pilates (1880–1967) invented rehabilitation equipment and created a series of strength and flexibility exercises for prisoners of war. Pilates eventually opened a training studio in New York City, helping professional dancers with their conditioning. He wrote two books describing his training methods, *Return to Life Through Contrology* and *Your Health*. Pilates-based programs today are popular in the United States. Pilates uses many different types of equipment, such as the reformer, trapeze table, combo chair, and Barrel, although these are most often done in one-on-one training and require specialty certifications. Mat Pilates is very popular in group exercise and focuses on posture, alignment, and core conditioning. It is not considered a cardiorespiratory form of exercise (2). A great variety of Pilates instructor certification courses are available (49), with the Pilates Method Alliance being the major unifying association for Pilates instructors.

SUMMARY

Teaching group exercise is challenging because of the various modalities available and the wide range of fitness and skill levels evident in any group of participants. Effective group exercise instructors understand that modifications, variations, and individualized intensity monitoring are essential to ensure safe and enjoyable participation by all. Many group exercise classes involve some form of cardiovascular conditioning, along with strengthening exercises, flexibility exercises, neuromotor activities, and proper warm-up and cool-down activities. For specialized group-led classes, it is recommended that instructors obtain additional training specific to the instructional method (*Fig. 34-17*).

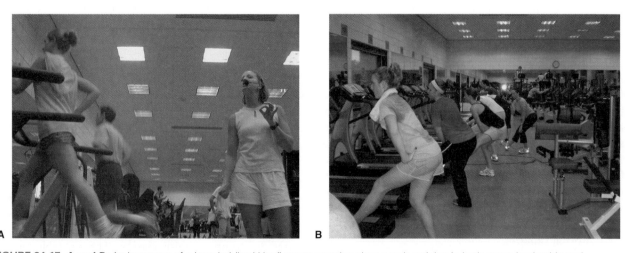

FIGURE 34-17. A and B: An instructor of a branded "trekking" group exercise class needs training in both group leadership and treadmill skills.

REFERENCES

1. 2011 IDEA Fitness Programs and Equipment Trends. *IDEA Fitness Manager.* 2011;July/Aug:1–7.

2. American Council on Exercise. Can Pilates Do It All? *ACE FitnessMatters.* 2005;November/December:10–1.

3. Bain LL, Wilson T, Chaikind E. Participant perceptions of exercise programs for overweight women. *Res Q Exerc Sport.* 1989; 60(2):134–43.

4. Behm DG, Anderson KG. The role of instability with resistance training. *J Strength Cond Res.* 2006;20(3):716–22.

5. Boutcher SH, Trenske M. The effects of sensory deprivation and music on perceived exertion and affect during exercise. *J Sport Exercise Psychol.* 1990;12(2):167–76.

6. Bray SR, Gyurcsik NC, Culos-Reed SN, Dawson KA, Martin KA. An exploratory investigation of the relationship between proxy efficacy, self-efficacy and exercise attendance. *Journal of Health Psychology.* 2001;6(4):425–34.

7. Bryant CX, Wenson J, Peterson JA. Safe and enjoyable group cycling for your members: reviewing these group cycling basics can help you guide your members through a fun and effective exercise experience. *Fitness Management.* 2001;17(6): 38–40;42.

8. Bushman BA, Flynn MG, Andres FF, Lambert CP, Taylor MS, Braun WA. Effect of 4 wk of deep water run training on running performance. *Med Sci Sports Exerc.* 1997;29(5):694–9.

9. Carrico M. Contraindications of yoga. *IDEA Health & Fitness Source.* 1998;16(10):34–40.

10. Carron AV, Hausenblas HA, Mack D. Social influence and exercise: a meta-analysis. *J Sport Exercise Psychol.* 1996;18(1):1–16.

11. Carter JM, Beam WC, McMahan SG, Barr ML, Brown LE. The effects of stability ball training on spinal stability in sedentary individuals. *J Strength Cond Res.* 2006;20(2):429–35.

12. Clary S, Barnes C, Bemben D, Knehans A, Bemben M. Effects of ballates, step aerobics, and walking on balance in women aged 50–75 years. *Journal of Sports Science and Medicine.* 2006;5(3):390–9.

13. Davidson K, McNaughton L. Deep water running training and road running training improve VO2max in untrained women. / L'entrainement de course en eau profonde et de course sur route ameliorent la capacite aerobie maximale chez les femmes non entrainees. *Journal of Strength & Conditioning Research.* 2000;14(2):191–5.

14. Eckmann TF. Older adults get on the ball: the stability ball is an effective training tool that can add a fun twist to your work with mature clients. *IDEA Health & Fitness Source.* 1998;16(1):81–5.

15. Evans E, Kennedy C. The body image problem in the fitness industry. *IDEA Today.* 1993;May:50–6.

16. Fox LD, Rejeski WJ, Gauvin L. Effects of leadership style and group dynamics on enjoyment of physical activity. *Am J Health Promot.* 2000;14(5):277–83.

17. Francis PR, Poliner J, Buono MJ, Francis LL. Effects of choreography, step height, fatigue and gender on metabolic cost of step training. *Med Sci Sports Exerc.* 1992;24(5):S12.

18. Frangolias DD, Rhodes EC. Maximal and ventilatory threshold responses to treadmill and water immersion running. *Med Sci Sports Exerc.* 1995;27(7):1007–13.

19. Garber CE, Blissmer B, Deschenes MR, et al. Quantity and quality of exercise for developing and maintaining cardiorespiratory, musculoskeletal, and neuromotor fitness in apparently healthy adults: guidance for prescribing exercise. *Med Sci Sports Exerc.* 2011;43(7):1334–59.

20. Gellish RL, Goslin BR, Olson RE, McDonald A, Russi GD, Moudgil VK. Longitudinal modeling of the relationship between age and maximal heart rate. *Med Sci Sports Exerc.* 2007;39(5):822–9.

21. Gibala MJ, Little JP. Just HIT it! A time-efficient exercise strategy to improve muscle insulin sensitivity. *J Physiol.* 2010;588(Pt 18): 3341–2.

22. Ginis KAM, Jung ME, Gauvin L. To see or not to see: Effects of exercising in mirrored environments on sedentary women's feeling states and self-efficacy. *Health Psychology.* 2003;22(4):354–61.

23. Grant SK, Todd T, Atchison P, Kelly P, Stoddart D. The effects of a 12 week group exercise program on physiological and psychological variables and function in overweight women. *Public Health.* 2004;118(1):31–4.

24. Graves BS, Quinn JV, O'Kroy JA, Torok DJ. Influence of Pilates-based mat exercise on chronic lower back pain. *Med Sci Sports Exerc.* 2005;37(5):S27.

25. Hollingshead S. Yoga: for sports performance. *IDEA Health & Fitness Source.* 2002;20(4):30–9.

26. Jahnke R, Larkey L, Rogers C, Etnier J, Lin F. A comprehensive review of health benefits of qigong and tai chi. *Am J Health Promot.* 2010;24(6):e1–25.

27. Jakicic JM, Otto AD. Physical activity considerations for the treatment and prevention of obesity. *Am J Clin Nutr.* 2005;82(1 Suppl): 226S–9S.

28. Kennedy CA, MM Yoke. *Methods of group exercise instruction.* Champaign (IL): Human Kinetics; 2005. 254 p.

29. Kolovou T. Launching and indoor cycling program: these marketing tactics and tips for indoor cycling instruction will help with the launch and profitable continuation of your program. *Fitness Management.* 2000;16(6):40–2.

30. Komura Y, Inaba R, Fujita S, et al. Health condition of female aerobic dance instructors. Subjective symptoms and related factors. *Sangyo Igaku.* 1992;34(4):326–34.

31. Kravitz L, Heyward VH, Stolarczyk LM, Wilmerding V. Does step exercise with handweights enhance training effects? *Journal of Strength & Conditioning Research.* 1997;11(3):194–9.

32. Long J, Williford HN, Olson MS, Wolfe V. Voice problems and risk factors among aerobics instructors. *J Voice.* 1998;12(2): 197–207.

33. Mayo JJ. Practical guidelines for the use of deep-water running. *Strength Cond J.* 2000;22(1):26–9.

34. Nagle EF, Robertson RJ, Jakicic JJ, Otto AD, Ranalli JR, Chiapetta LB. Effects of aquatic exercise and walking in sedentary obese women undergoing a behavioral weight-loss intervention. *International Journal of Aquatic Research & Education.* 2007;1(1): 43–56.

35. Olson MS, Williford HN, Blessing DL, Greathouse R. The cardiovascular and metabolic effects of bench stepping exercise in females. *Med Sci Sports Exerc.* 1991;23(11):1311–7.

36. Ornish D. *Love & Survival: The Scientific Basis for the Healing Power of Intimacy.* 1st ed. New York (NY): HarperCollins; 1998. 284 p.

37. Parker SB, Hurley BF, Hanlon DP, Vaccaro P. Failure of target heart rate to accurately monitor intensity during aerobic dance. *Med Sci Sports Exerc.* 1989;21(2):230–4.

38. Recommendations for music volume in fitness classes. *IDEA Today.* 1997;15(6):50.

49. Riker HA, Zabik RM, Dawson ML, Frye PA. The effect of step height and upper body involvement on oxygen consumption and energy expenditure during step aerobics. *Med Sci Sports Exerc.* 1998;30(5):S945.

40. Rubenstein LZ. Falls in older people: epidemiology, risk factors and strategies for prevention. *Age Ageing.* 2006;35 Suppl 2:ii37–41.

41. Rydeard R, Leger A, Smith D. Pilates-based therapeutic exercise: effects on subjects with nonspecific chronic low back pain and functional disability. *J Orthop Sports Phys Ther.* 2011;36(7):472–84.

42. Scharff-Olson M, Williford HN, Blessing DL, Brown JA. The physiological effects of bench/step exercise. *Sports Med.* 1996;21(3): 164–75.

43. Scharff-Olson M, Williford HN, Blessing DL, Moses R, Wang T. Vertical impact forces during bench-step aerobics: exercise rate and experience. *Percept Mot Skills.* 1997;84(1):267–74.

44. Schlicht J. Stability balls: an injury risk for older adults? *ACSM's Health & Fitness Journal.* 2002;6(4):14–7.

45. Schroeder J, Dotan S. 2010 Idea Fitness Programs & Equipment Trends. *IDEA Fitness Journal.* 2010;7(7):22–31.

46. Sherman RM. The indoor cycling revolution: designing classes that chart the course to success. *IDEA Today.* 1997;15(3):30–3;35–6;39.

47. Smith J. Injury prevention in step classes. *IDEA Health & Fitness Source.* 2000;18(6):36–42;45.

48. Staum MJ. Music and rhythmic stimuli in the rehabilitation of gait disorders. *J Music Ther.* 1983;20(2):69–87.

49. Stott M. How to start a Pilates-based program. *Fitness Management.* 2000;16:44–8.

50. Takeshima N, Rogers ME, Watanabe E, et al. Water-based exercise improves health-related aspects of fitness in older women. *Med Sci Sports Exerc.* 2002;34(3):544–51.

51. Templeton MS, Booth DL, O'Kelly WD. Effects of aquatic therapy on joint flexibility and functional ability in subjects with rheumatic disease. *J Orthop Sports Phys Ther.* 1996;23(6):376–81.

52. Thacker SB, Gilchrist J, Stroup DF, Kimsey CD Jr. The impact of stretching on sports injury risk: a systematic review of the literature. *Med Sci Sports Exerc.* 2004;36(3):371–8.

53. Tharrett S, Peterson JA. The health/fitness club industry: challenge and change. In: *Fitness Management: A Comprehensive Resource for Developing, Leading, Managing, and Operating a Successful Health/Fitness Club.* Monterey (CA): Healthy Learning; 2006. p. 34.

54. Thompson WR. Worldwide survey of fitness for 2011. *ACSM's Health & Fitness Journal.* 2010;14(6):8–17.

55. Wang N, Scharff-Olson M, Williford HN. Energy cost and fuel utilization during step aerobics exercise. *Med Sci Sports Exerc.* 1993;25(5):S630.

56. Williams A. Injury prevention in Kickboxing classes. *IDEA Health & Fitness Source.* 2000;18(6):58–64;67.

57. Williford HN, Scharff-Olson M, Blessing DL. The physiological effects of aerobic dance. A review. *Sports Med.* 1989;8(6):335–45.

58. Woodby-Brown S, Berg K, Latin RW. Oxygen cost of aerobic dance bench stepping at three heights. *Journal of Strength & Conditioning Research.* 1993;7(3):163–7.

59. Yoke MM, Kennedy C. *Functional Exercise Progressions.* Monterey (CA): Healthy Learning; 2004. 126 p.

SELECTED REFERENCES FOR FURTHER READING

Kennedy C, Yoke M. *Methods of Group Exercise Instruction.* Champaign (IL): Human Kinetics; 2009. 348 p.

Yoke M, Kennedy C. *Functional Exercise Progressions.* Monterey (CA): Healthy Learning; 2004. 126 p.

INTERNET RESOURCES

- Aerobics and Fitness Association of America: http://www.afaa.com
- American College of Sports Medicine: http://www.acsm.org
- American Council on Exercise: http://www.acefitness.org
- IDEA Health and Fitness Association: http://www.ideafit.com

Obesity (body mass index [BMI] $\geq$30 kg $\cdot$ m^{-2}) and overweight (BMI $=$ 25$-$29.9 kg $\cdot$ m^{-2}) are serious health issues in the United States. Based on the 2009–2010 National Health and Nutrition Examination Survey (NHANES), approximately 36% of U.S. adults were considered obese, with 35.8% of women and 35.5% of men obese (26), as illustrated in *Figure 35-1*. The mean age-adjusted BMI was 28.7 kg $\cdot$ m^{-2} for men and women. Obesity, which is considered a multifactorial condition, is related to many chronic diseases, such as coronary heart disease, hypertension, stroke, Type 2 diabetes mellitus, dyslipidemia, gallbladder disease, and some cancers (4,34,54). Taken together, several of these conditions—obesity, hypertension, dyslipidemia and insulin resistance (leading to Type 2 diabetes mellitus)—are known as the metabolic syndrome. Weight loss by those persons who are overweight or obese, and prevention of weight gain in others, would likely decrease chronic disease, improve quality of life, and decrease health care costs in the United States.

Although there are many factors that play a role in the rise in obesity in the United States and throughout the world, the main reason for the significant rise in obesity is caused by lifestyle factors. Individuals are eating more and exercising less. This is obvious in the larger portion sizes at restaurants (24) as well as people watching more television and driving their cars more than in the past (39). The primary goal of this chapter is to discuss the impact nutrition, exercise, behavioral interventions, and bariatric surgery have on weight management.

KEY TERMS

Adipocyte: Fat cell.

Anorexia nervosa: A severe form of eating disorder, whereby the individual consumes little to no food energy each day and typically exercises excessively; this may or may not be coupled with use of other methods for decreasing intake (*e.g.*, vomiting, diuretic use, laxative use); the individual is typically severely underweight.

Bariatrics: A branch of medicine that addresses the causes, prevention, and treatment of obesity.

Body fat distribution: An assessment of how body fat is distributed; android obesity ("apple shape"), in which more fat is stored in the abdominal area, is more strongly related to an increased risk of cardiovascular disease and Type 2 diabetes mellitus than gynoid obesity ("pear shape"), in which more fat is stored in the hip area. A separate consideration of body fat distribution is visceral (fat surrounding the internal organs) versus subcutaneous (fat directly beneath the skin); as with android obesity, visceral fat carries greater risk than subcutaneous fat.

Body mass index (BMI): A measure of a person's stockiness (body mass in kilograms divided by height in meters squared, kg $\cdot$ m^{-2}) used to assess if a person is underweight, of healthy weight, overweight, or obese.

Bulimia nervosa: A severe form of eating disorder, whereby the individual consumes normal or, more typically, much higher than needed amounts of food energy each day, followed by purging (*e.g.*, vomiting, diuretic use, laxative use, overexercising); the individual is often of normal body weight.

Fat-free mass (FFM): Body mass minus the mass of all body fat, that is, both essential fat (found within bone marrow, nervous tissue, and internal organs) and storage fat (visceral and subcutaneous adipose stores). Most body composition techniques estimate fat mass and FFM.

Lean body mass (LBM): Body mass minus the mass of storage fat. LBM and FFM are often erroneously used interchangeably, as FFM exceeds LBM.

Metabolic syndrome: A condition conferring elevated risk for Type 2 diabetes mellitus and cardiovascular disease and is defined (by the National Cholesterol Education Program — Adult Treatment Panel III [25]) but modified for impaired fasting glucose as defined by the American Diabetes Association (31) as having at least three of the following signs:

- Fasting plasma glucose $\geq$100 mg $\cdot$ dL^{-1} or on medication for hyperglycemia
- Blood pressure $\geq$130/85 mm Hg or on medication for hypertension
- Fasting triglycerides $\geq$150 mg $\cdot$ dL^{-1}
- High-density lipoprotein cholesterol (HDL-C) <40 mg $\cdot$ dL^{-1} for men and <50 mg $\cdot$ dL^{-1} for women
- Abdominal obesity, waist circumference >102 cm (40 in) for men and >88 cm (35 in) for women

Obesity: Having a marked excess of body fat, generally categorized as a BMI $\geq$30 kg $\cdot$ m^{-2}.

Overweight: Having an excess of body fat less pronounced than obesity, generally categorized as a BMI of 25.0–29.9 kg $\cdot$ m^{-2}.

Percent body fat: The percentage of an individual's mass that is fat. This can be estimated by dual-energy X-ray absorptiometry (DEXA), plethysmography (e.g., BOD POD®), hydrostatic weighing, skinfold assessment, or other methods (the first three methods listed are considered the most accurate).

Resting metabolic rate (RMR): The amount of energy needed to sustain life at rest, typically measured as kilocalorie per day. RMR is usually measured after a person has fasted for at least 12 h.

Thermogenesis: The production of heat, especially the increased heat production associated with digestion of a meal.

ESTABLISHING A HEALTHY BODY WEIGHT GOAL

Several methods can be used to determine a person's "ideal body weight"; however, in many cases, especially for athletes, ideal body weight may be unrealistic. Thus, it is better to focus on a "healthy body weight" rather than an "ideal body weight." A healthy body weight is different for each individual, athlete, or nonathlete and is one that is relative to a person's overall health profile (e.g., serum lipid levels, glucose levels, blood pressure). The simplest method to determine a healthy body weight is by using the BMI. BMI

is defined as a person's mass (in kilograms) divided by his or her height in meters squared (m^2). BMI is not perfect because it does not take into account percent body fat; thus, a muscular athlete may have a BMI that is considered "obese," whereas an individual with a narrow frame could have too much body fat and yet be considered of normal weight. Nor does BMI account for body fat distribution, the location of body fat within a given person, such as android versus gynoid and visceral versus subcutaneous. BMI is a better indicator for determining the prevalence of overweight and obesity in a large population rather than for determining body composition in an individual. Nonetheless, for the average sedentary person, BMI typically works well. For an overview of body composition measurement, refer to *Chapter 18*. *Table 4-1* in *GETP9* lists the different BMI levels and how they match to overweight and obesity.

Note that a BMI between 18.5 kg $\cdot$ m^{-2} and 24.9 kg $\cdot$ m^{-2} is considered healthy because individuals within this range are at the lowest risk for developing chronic disease. Although obesity increases the risk of major chronic diseases (such as Type 2 diabetes mellitus and cardiovascular disease), a BMI of <18.5 kg $\cdot$ m^{-2} can place a person at risk for osteoporosis, gastrointestinal diseases, immune impairment, and diseases of the heart that are related to electrolyte imbalances. In addition, a low BMI may also be an indication of an eating disorder, such as anorexia nervosa or bulimia nervosa, which can also lead to the aforementioned risks. Aside from being overweight or obese, other risk factors to consider are hypertension, high levels of low-density lipoprotein cholesterol (LDL-C), low levels of high-density lipoprotein cholesterol (HDL-C), high serum triglyceride levels, high blood glucose levels, family history of heart disease,

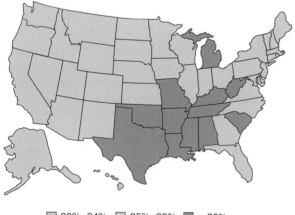

20%–24%   25%–29% $\geq$30%

FIGURE 35-1. Percentage of adults who are obese in the United States for 2010 (body mass index $\geq$30 kg $\cdot$ m^{-2}). The data from this map show even more "new" colors from previous years, denoting a greater percentage of obesity in more states. (Adapted from Centers for Disease Control and Prevention, 2010; http://www.cdc.gov/obesity/data/trends.html.)

sedentary lifestyle and cigarette smoking (see *Table 2-3* in *GETP9*).

VARIOUS WEIGHT LOSS METHODS

Although many individuals know that they should increase their physical activity levels, only 50.6% of adults in the United States are moderately active for $30 \text{ min} \cdot \text{d}^{-1}$ for $5 \text{ d} \cdot \text{wk}^{-1}$, or are vigorously active for $20 \text{ min} \cdot \text{d}^{-1}$ for $>3 \text{ d} \cdot \text{wk}^{-1}$ (58). By encouraging accumulated activity, this may allow for greater adherence to daily physical activity. In addition, accumulated activity is well documented to result in equal amounts of weight loss and improvement in cardiovascular fitness when compared with exercising for a single continuous bout (35,37,38,64). From 60% to 74% of U.S. adults are inactive or underactive (15,51). This lack of physical activity contributes to the increasing prevalence of obesity and, in turn, escalating health care costs. If this issue is not properly addressed, it is predicted that the majority of the U.S. population will be obese by the 23rd century (28). Lifestyle interventions (diet and exercise programs) reduce body weight and lead to significant reductions in comorbidities (*e.g.*, diabetes mellitus, coronary heart disease) (33). For example, Hamman et al. (33) reported that for every kilogram of weight lost, there was a 16% reduction in diabetes risk, emphasizing that small changes in body weight can lead to significant reductions in chronic disease risk.

In conjunction with increasing physical activity levels, individuals need to decrease energy intake and consume healthier diets that will not only help with weight reduction/maintenance but also provide positive effects to help stave off diseases such as cancer, diabetes mellitus, and coronary heart disease. In some cases, drastic dietary (*i.e.*, very-low-calorie diets [VLCDs]) and surgical approaches (*i.e.*, bariatric surgery) may be used. In all cases, behavioral changes need to be made to ensure long-term success.

Jakicic et al. (36) studied the "dose response" of physical activity in women who were overweight and obese (BMI = $27–40 \text{ kg} \cdot \text{m}^{-2}$; 21–45 yr of age). Participants were randomly assigned to one of four weight loss intervention groups based on energy expenditure (1,000 vs. 2,000 kcals expended during physical activity per week) or intensity (moderate vs. vigorous). In addition, the women were asked to decrease their energy intake to $1,200–1,500 \text{ kcal} \cdot \text{d}^{-1}$. The researchers reported that participants who maintained a weight loss of 10% or more of initial body weight at 24 mo engaged in significantly more physical activity ($1,835 \text{ kcal} \cdot \text{wk}^{-1}$ or $275 \text{ min} \cdot \text{wk}^{-1}$) than those who maintained a weight loss of less than 10% of initial body weight ($p < .001$). Jakicic et al. (36) emphasized the need for interventions with greater energy expenditure per week, combined with a decrease in energy intake, for sustained weight loss in individuals who are obese.

DIET, EXERCISE, AND A COMBINATION OF DIET PLUS EXERCISE

Researchers have assessed the effects of diet alone, exercise alone, and a combination of diet plus exercise on weight loss, maintenance of weight loss, and the prevention of weight gain. When considering the role of exercise, researchers have also evaluated the impact of exercise intensity and the number of exercise sessions. The effects of various weight loss methods on muscle mass have also been studied.

Brinkworth et al. (11) reported that a 12-wk exercise program led to reductions in body weight, cardiovascular risk factors, and risk factors for diabetes mellitus. In an attempt to evaluate the effects of a combined exercise and dietary weight loss strategy on serum LDL-C concentrations, Varady et al. (68) evaluated a low-fat diet combined with moderate endurance training on LDL particle size and distribution in 20 women who were obese and hypercholesterolemic. They reported a significant mean weight loss of 14.8% with the combined low-fat diet (<30% fat, 50%–60% carbohydrate, 20% protein) and endurance training program (>40 min moderate training, three times per week). In addition, serum total cholesterol, LDL-C, and triglyceride concentrations significantly decreased by 8.9%, 7.5%, and 27.1%, respectively, with a concomitant 9.9% increase (significant) in HDL-C concentrations.

In an effort to establish if individuals will continue their exercise and diet program after they have been in a supervised program, Volpe and colleagues (69) examined the effects of diet alone, exercise alone, and a combination of diet and exercise on body weight, body composition, and other physiological variables in 90 sedentary women and men with mild obesity. The three interventions were compared in a randomized longitudinal study design with data collected across 12 mo. The exercise programs were supervised for 6 mo, after which participants in the exercise only and exercise plus diet groups were provided with exercise equipment (skiing machines) to take home. At 6 and 9 mo in women and 9 mo in men, the diet plus exercise group significantly lost body weight compared to the diet only and exercise only groups. However, by 1 yr, recidivism was high, and thus, no significant differences existed among groups in any of the measures.

LaFortuna et al. (42) examined intensity of exercise in men and women with a BMI of about $41 \text{ kg} \cdot \text{m}^{-2}$. Although body weight loss was equal between the low- and high-intensity exercise groups, the authors concluded that the higher intensity exercise program achieved greater generalized improvement in muscle performance and physical fitness as well as a stronger motivation for spontaneous physical activity compared with the low-intensity group (42).

In addition to exercise intensity, some researchers demonstrate that exercising in multiple bouts throughout the day is as effective for weight loss and cardiovascular benefits as exercising in for a single, continuous bout (37,38). Exercising in multiple short bouts throughout the day may provide greater adherence for some individuals who have erratic schedules. Jakicic et al. (38) also reported that weight loss is greatest if energy expended is >150 min $\cdot$ wk^{-1}.

The National Weight Control Registry (NWCR) was established in 1993 to assess the characteristics of individuals who can consistently maintain body weight. Individuals on the registry consistently report high levels of physical activity. Catenacci et al. (14) examined the physical activity levels in NWCR participants compared to physical activity in normal-weight and overweight controls. Physical activity was documented using a triaxial accelerometer for 1 wk. These researchers reported that individuals in NWCR spent significantly ($p = .004$) more time per day in sustained bouts of moderate-to-vigorous physical activity (MVPA) compared to overweight controls (41.5 $\pm$ 35.1 min $\cdot$ d^{-1} vs. 19.2 $\pm$ 18.6 min $\cdot$ d^{-1}) and nearly significantly ($p = .080$) more than normal-weight controls (25.8 $\pm$ 23.4 min $\cdot$ d^{-1}). These results demonstrate the important role that physical activity plays in the long-term maintenance of weight loss. Furthermore, researchers concluded that continued activity, which is ≥ 10 min in duration, could play a major role in weight loss maintenance.

In addition to weight maintenance, exercise appears to preserve muscle mass compared with diet alone. Weiss et al. (74) evaluated whether energy restriction decreases muscle mass and whether exercise preserves or improves muscle mass. Healthy men and women, 50–60 yr of age, with an average BMI of 23.5–29.9 kg $\cdot$ m^{-2}, were evaluated before and after a 1-yr energy restriction via weight loss ($n = 18$) or exercise ($n = 16$). They reported that muscle mass was decreased in response to energy restriction but not in response to a similar weight loss induced by exercise.

Exercise not only preserves muscle mass but may also affect regional fat loss. Murphy et al. (53) examined if exercise-induced weight loss would elicit greater decreases in intermuscular and visceral adipose tissue compared with energy-restricted weight loss. They also examined whether changes in the respective adipose tissues would result in improved glucose regulation. Thirty-nine sedentary men and women, 50–60 yr of age, with a BMI between 23.5 and 29.9 kg $\cdot$ m^{-2}, were randomly assigned to either 1 yr of calorie restriction, 1 yr of exercise, or a control group. Researchers found that weight loss was similar ($p = .25$) in the energy restriction ($-10.8 \pm 1.4\%$) and exercise groups ($-8.3 \pm 1.5\%$) but significantly greater than the control group ($-2.0 \pm 2.4\%$; $P < .05$). Intermuscular and visceral fat

were significantly decreased in the energy restriction and exercise groups compared to the control group ($p \leq .05$). Both the energy restriction and exercise groups showed significant improvements in insulin sensitivity.

The 2009 American College of Sports Medicine (ACSM) position stand summarizes the role of exercise and diet as strategies for weight loss and weight loss maintenance (21). Although exercise alone may not provide the greatest weight loss over time, exercise results in modest levels of weight loss and is important in preventing weight regain. For even greater weight loss, exercise combined with lower energy intake is most effective. If weight loss or prevention of weight gain is the key, then the intensity of physical activity is not as important. However, if greater spontaneous exercise and, hence, greater energy expenditure will occur with higher intensity exercise (and perhaps with multiple bouts of exercise), then these may be other motivational tools used with some individuals.

Perceived Barriers to Physical Activity and Healthier Eating

Although studies on combined diet and exercise have shown positive effects on weight loss and/or in the reduction of chronic disease risk (33,68), often they have not been able to maintain long-term weight loss, even with successful weight loss during the intervention trial (32).

Aaltonen et al. (3) evaluated the motives and perceived barriers to long-term engagement in physical activity in 16 same-sex twin pairs (mean age of 60 yr) who had either been physically active or who had been sedentary for more than 30 yr. More than half of the participants reported no reasons for being sedentary other than various health problems. Overall, however, Aaltonen et al. (3) reported no differences in perceived barriers between active and inactive cotwins. From their results, they concluded that consistent physical activity was maintained because of (a) the participants' wishes to improve or maintain physical skills or techniques, (b) a feeling that exercise would improve mental and physical health, and (c) the activity was enjoyable. These researchers emphasized the importance of motivation and suggested that perceived barriers play a smaller role with respect to exercise or sedentary behavior.

The loss of social support from research personnel after the completion of diet and exercise interventions could be a reason for high recidivism. Providing opportunities for increased physical activity and healthier eating are not the only issues that need to be addressed. Although facilities or time may be available, individuals will often not begin an exercise program and/or diet program because of their perceived barriers and lack of knowledge to initiate a program. Once an exercise and/ or diet program is initiated, however, perceived benefits and barriers disappear (40). Kao et al. (40) found that providing an exercise program that assisted participants to develop individualized approaches significantly improved perceived exercise benefits and self-efficacy and decreased perceived barriers. Motivation and social support play primary roles in whether a person will begin an exercise program and/or diet. Counseling may be one avenue through which this goal can be achieved.

DIETARY COUNSELING AND WEIGHT LOSS

In an attempt to evaluate counseling people to exercise and eat within energy needs, Welty et al. (75) evaluated the effects of on-site dietitian counseling on weight loss and serum lipid concentrations in an outpatient physician's office. They assessed the effects of counseling 80 patients who are overweight or obese (average age = 55 ± 12 yr; average BMI = 30.1 ± 6.4 kg · m^{-2}) to exercise 30 min · d^{-1} and eat an adapted dietary approaches to stop hypertension (DASH) diet. They reported a mean weight loss of 4.9 kg at 1.75 yr follow-up. More importantly, 64 of the patients were able to maintain a significant weight loss of 5.3% at 2.6 yr of follow-up. They also reported significantly improved serum lipid levels. Welty et al. (75) reported that a dietitian who is counseling patients to exercise and eat nutritiously in a physician outpatient setting is successful for weight loss as well as for weight loss maintenance and improving coronary heart disease risk.

Dansinger et al. (19) conducted a meta-analysis of studies from 1980 to 2006 on the impact of dietary counseling on long-term weight loss. They reported that, compared with usual care, dietary counseling interventions resulted in modest weight loss that seemed to lessen over time. They added, however, that more studies are required that will focus on decreasing loss of participants to follow-up as well as emphasizing factors that are most effective in weight loss.

More recently, Low et al. (48) evaluated the efficacy of motivational interviewing compared to nutritional counseling for weight loss in 56 male and female patients who were obese and with heart disease. Participants were assigned to either motivational interviewing or nutrition counseling and followed-up over 3 mo. They used trained undergraduate students to provide the motivational interviewing. They reported significant weight loss in women, but not in men, with the motivational interviewing. Note that, although effective, the authors pointed out that some limitations of their study included a small sample size and nonrandomization of participants to their respective groups.

DIFFERENT TYPES OF DIETS AND WEIGHT LOSS

It is clear that energy balance is the key to weight maintenance and that altering energy balance through changes in intake and expenditure can result in weight loss (or weight gain). Although individual dietary needs differ, research on the effects of different types of diets continues. In addition, work on genetic predisposition to types of weight loss treatments is also under way and in the near future may provide important information regarding the treatment most likely to be successful in a given individual based on genetic makeup.

The most popularly studied diets are the low-carbohydrate versus high-fat diets, or high-carbohydrate versus low-fat diets. Rankin and Turpyn (60) studied 29 women who are overweight or obese (BMI = 32 ± 5 kg · m^{-2}) who were randomly assigned to a self-selected low-carbohydrate/high-fat diet or a high-carbohydrate/low-fat diet for 4 wk. The two diets were similar in energy intake (about 1,360 kcal · d^{-1}). A significantly greater weight loss was reported in the low-carbohydrate diet group; however, there was a significant increase in C-reactive protein (a marker of inflammation) in the low-carbohydrate group compared with the high-carbohydrate group.

Although the aforementioned results are interesting, they are short term. A 12-yr study on the long-term effects of a low-carbohydrate diet in Sweden (the Women's Lifestyle and Health cohort study that was initiated in 1991–1992) included 42,237 women, 30–49 yr of age (43). Researchers reported that a low-carbohydrate/high-protein intake was related to increased total mortality, with a greater increase in cardiovascular disease in this cohort of women. This is the first long-term study evaluating low-carbohydrate diets on disease risk.

Krebs et al. (41) studied individuals with Type 2 diabetes mellitus, 30–75 yr of age. Participants were randomized either to a low-fat, high-protein group (30% of energy from protein, 40% from carbohydrate, 30% from fat) or a low-fat, high-carbohydrate group (15% protein, 55% carbohydrate, 30% fat). Of the 419 participants enrolled in the study, 294 completed the study. There were no differences seen between groups in body weight or waist circumference during the 1-yr trial or the 12-mo follow-up. Both groups significantly lost body weight and decreased their waist circumference. No significant differences between groups were found in the following: body fat, glycosylated hemoglobin (HbA1C), blood lipid levels, blood pressure, and renal function.

Four popular diets (Atkins, Zone, LEARN, and Ornish) were compared in a study over a 1-yr period in 311 premenopausal women who were overweight or obese (BMI ranged from 27 to 40 kg · m^{-2}) (30). The women were randomly assigned to one of the four diets. At 1 yr, weight loss was greater for the Atkins group compared to the other diet groups (average weight loss: Atkins = 4.7 kg; Zone = 1.6 kg; LEARN = 2.6 kg; Ornish = 2.2 kg). In contrast, Sacks et al. placed more than 800 adults who were overweight on one of four diet plans, with the composition ranging from 20% fat/65% carbohydrates to 40% fat/35% carbohydrates (61). All groups lost statistically similar amounts in the first 6 mo

(~6 kg on average), and all groups regained about half that in the following 18 mo.

Aside from a low-carbohydrate or high-carbohydrate diet, the glycemic index may affect weight loss. Ebbeling et al. (23) examined whether a low-glycemic load diet (40% carbohydrate, 35% fat) fared better with weight loss and insulin secretion compared with a low-fat diet (55% carbohydrate, 20% fat). Their participants were 18–35 yr of age and followed the respective diets for 6 mo, with a 12-mo follow-up. They found that plasma HDL-C and triglyceride concentrations improved more on the low-glycemic load diet; however, LDL-C concentration improved more on the low-fat diet. They concluded that decreasing glycemic load may be particularly important to achieve weight loss amid individuals with high insulin secretion.

The Mediterranean diet has been found to be beneficial for heart disease and cancer prevention; however, it is not well studied with respect to weight loss. Recently, Andreoli et al. (7) studied the effects of a moderately hypoenergetic Mediterranean diet and exercise program on body composition and cardiovascular disease risk factors in women who were obese. Of the 60 participants who began the study, 47 completed the entire study, resulting in a 22% attrition rate. Mean age of the subjects was 39.7 ± 13.2 yr. Body weight, BMI, and fat mass were significantly decreased ($P < .001$) at 2 and 4 mo. Body weight decreased from 80.5 ± 15.8 to 75.2 ± 14.7 kg and BMI from 30.7 ± 6.0 to 28.7 ± 5.6 kg $\cdot$ m^{-2}. In addition, cardiovascular risk factors were significantly improved (7).

VLCDs are often used for weight loss for individuals who are morbidly obese (BMI ≥ 40 kg $\cdot$ m^{-2}) or have grade II obesity (BMI = 35–39.9 kg $\cdot$ m^{-2}) with comorbid conditions (7). These diets routinely consist of highly engineered powdered supplements that are rich in protein and average in the range of 500–800 kcal $\cdot$ d^{-1}. They are typically associated with hospitals or specialized clinics, and individuals undergoing these diets are monitored by physicians as well as a team of other medical personnel, including registered dietitians, exercise physiologists, and registered nurses.

A potential value of the VLCD is the rapid weight loss that occurs, typically at the rate of 3–5 lb $\cdot$ wk^{-1}. This rate of loss can be motivating to the individual and often allows him or her to lose very large amounts of weight. Individual programs report many who lose 50–100 lb — occasionally those who lose more than 200 lb — using a VLCD and often a 20% group average weight loss for those engaged for at least 6 mo. The length of a typical VLCD is 12–26 wk; however, select individuals with careful monitoring have maintained a VLCD plan for more than a year to achieve very large amounts of weight loss. An individual who correctly implements a VLCD is typically not hungry despite taking in only 500–800 kcal $\cdot$ d^{-1}. This is a result of the makeup of the food (high-quality protein, carbohydrates, and little fat) and the limited calories that produce a mild ketotic state

(undetectable via urine dipstick assessment), which in turn curbs hunger. The allied health professional who counsels these patients often must request that they eat more supplements per day because they tend to eat fewer supplements because of not being hungry. This principle of VLCD (*i.e.*, ketosis) is similar to the Atkins diet, which aims to deplete the liver and skeletal muscles of carbohydrate stores, which in turn requires the body to metabolize fat stores for energy production. The difference with the VLCD is its heart-healthy low-fat makeup.

The VLCD is often criticized as potentially dangerous. It is true that in the 1970s, there were several cardiac arrhythmic deaths linked to the VLCD, but increases in protein and micronutrients and careful medical monitoring have essentially eliminated this risk, and contemporary VLCD studies do not report significant dangers or side effects. Typical risks include dehydration and gallstones. Dehydration risk is minimized by requiring adequate water each day (more than 64 oz), removing patients from diuretics as indicated, and adding a small amount of salt to the low-sodium VLCD. Gallstone risk can be minimized by eating a bolus of fat each day (~5–10 g) or by using the medication ursodiol.

The VLCD is also criticized for not being able to maintain the losses often achieved in the initial months of the diet. However, much of the research points to potential shortcomings in long-term maintenance planning. Leser et al. (46) reported that 3 yr after weight loss using a VLCD, the women who were most successful were those who maintained physical activity and low-fat diets. Wadden et al. (72) reported that women who were first placed on a VLCD (420 kcal $\cdot$ d^{-1} for 16 wk) and then placed on a balanced deficit diet of 1,200 kcal $\cdot$ d^{-1} lost the same amount of body weight (~11 kg) after 1 yr compared with those individuals who were placed on the balanced deficit diet for the entire year.

Some are also concerned that using a VLCD will result in difficulty losing weight during subsequent diet attempts. Li et al. (47) assessed 480 patients who restarted a VLCD at least once, and some up to four times, to assess the ability to lose weight on subsequent attempts. During the initial attempt, the mean weight loss was 21.3 kg for women and 28.8 kg for men. In all subsequent weight loss attempts using VLCD, the rate of weight loss was not different from the initial attempt. Interestingly, the restart initial weight was lower than the first attempt weight, but the final weight was higher than the first attempt weight, on average. Patients also did not stay on the VLCD as long during subsequent attempts, potentially leading to not being able to achieve a lower final weight. An important part of a VLCD is various supplements used. Patients will get bored quickly simply drinking a vanilla or chocolate shake as some programs offer. A goal is to offer the patient variety. Recently, commercial supplement companies have developed a wide array of food types (shakes, puddings, soups, hot or cold drinks, bars, snacks, etc.) and flavors that reduces the boredom of previous iterations of the VLCD.

These high-protein supplements may also be used in a partial meal replacement diet strategy (often termed *low-calorie diet* or LCD). These diets often are in the range of 1,000–1,200 kcal · d^{-1} and are used for portion control along with some "regular" food. This type of plan is excellent for patients with diabetes. A report of the Look AHEAD study, which is assessing patients with Type 2 diabetes for the long-term (11 yr) health effects of lifestyle intervention — including exercise and a low-calorie, low-fat diet with prescribed use of meal replacement products — found that attendance at meetings and the regular use of meal replacement supplements were associated with the best weight loss success in the 5,000 patients enrolled in this study (73). On the average, patients in the intervention group achieved an 8.6% ± 6.9% weight loss at 1 yr into the treatment protocol. Tsai and Wadden (67), using a meta-analysis approach, reported a similar long-term weight loss for a partial meal replacement (LCD) versus VLCD, thus suggesting the effectiveness of the partial meal replacement approach. This reference also provides an excellent overview of the history of the VLCD.

Malandrucco et al. (50) used a VLCD (400 kcal · d^{-1}) to evaluate if there would be improvements in insulin sensitivity, insulin secretion, or both after 1 wk of energy restriction in 14 patients who were severely obese (BMI ≥40 kg · m^{-2}) with Type 2 diabetes mellitus. Participants were placed on this VLCD for 7 d. The researchers reported a 3.22 ± 0.56% reduction in body weight ($P < .001$), with 42% of the weight loss from fat. They also reported significant decreases in fasting plasma glucose and triacylglycerol concentrations. The researchers suggested that the improvement in the participants' metabolic profile was "primarily due to the amelioration of β cell function, whereas no contribution of insulin sensitivity was shown."

Although most individuals who are trying to lose weight would prefer to do so rapidly, it has been well documented that a slower weight loss, through diet and exercise, is the best way to maintain body weight once the weight is lost. Lutes et al. (49) assessed the impact of a weight loss program that emphasized small changes over a 3-mo intervention followed by a 6-mo follow-up. Twenty-five adult women who were obese (BMI = 31.8 kg · m^{-2}) were asked to choose and implement small changes in their diet and exercise during weekly group-based meetings over a 3-mo period. Participants then received phone calls every other week over a 6-mo follow-up period. The participants lost, on average, 3.2 ± 0.47 kg ($P < .001$) during the 3-mo period and continued to lose weight during the 6-mo phone-based follow-up program, leading to a >5% weight loss over the 9-mo program. This research demonstrates the need to emphasize slower changes in body weight, which

leads to more permanent weight loss. Weight loss can be achieved using small changes to dietary intake and physical activity that can lead to long-term weight loss and maintenance. Indeed, Senechal et al. (63) compared rapid and slow weight loss on the body composition and metabolic risk factors following energy restriction in postmenopausal women who are obese. Although both the slow and rapid weight loss groups significantly lost weight, the rapid weight loss group also lost lean body mass (LBM). However, only the slow weight loss group had significant decreases in fasting triacylglycerol concentrations and diastolic blood pressure. Senechal et al. concluded, "A slower [weight loss] seems to be more beneficial to improve body composition as well as metabolic risk factors in postmenopausal women."

BEHAVIORAL APPROACHES TO WEIGHT LOSS

Behavioral change is the key to weight loss and maintenance. Certainly, behavior/lifestyle counseling should be incorporated into any weight management program, including both the least and most aggressive methods. There have been several studies evaluating the effects of a combined behavioral, diet, exercise, and/or diet-plus-exercise approach to weight loss. Many have found positive results; however, recidivism usually occurs when the intervention is completed. In an interesting approach to using a behavioral treatment with weight loss, Ledikwe et al. (44) evaluated if energy density and energy intake changed with behavioral approaches to weight loss. They reported energy density and energy intake decreased, along with body weight with various behavioral interventions. In some cases, even if energy density was increased, energy intake was decreased.

Burke et al. (13) compared a standard (omnivorous) diet with a lacto-ovo vegetarian diet in 176 sedentary adults who were overweight (average BMI = 34 kg · m^{-2}). The participants were either randomly assigned to one of the two diets or assigned to the diet of their preference, and the intervention included both exercise goals and 12 mo of behavioral counseling. Seventy-five percent of the participants completed the study. The researchers reported that all groups significantly lost weight, ranging from 4% to 8%, with no difference between the two types of diets.

Nakade et al. (55), in a 1-yr randomized controlled trial with 235 adults in Japan who were overweight and obese, examined a behavioral approach that emphasized tailored behavior counseling, diet, weight loss, and weight maintenance. The 119 participants in the intervention group received an individual-based counseling using a behavioral approach; alterations made to dietary intake and physical activity were individualized for each participant compared to a control group. One year later, the intervention group lost significantly more weight than the control group (-5.0 kg vs. 0.1 kg for men and -3.9 kg vs. -0.2 kg for women). After 1-yr follow-up, the intervention group maintained significantly lower body weight, lower energy intake, and improvements in overall nutritional intake compared to the control group. This individualized behavioral approach led to significant changes in dietary intake, physical activity, and weight loss and maintenance. The researchers did report specific differences between men and women and suggested that sex-specific approaches should be implemented.

INTERNET-BASED APPROACHES TO WEIGHT LOSS

In the 21st century, it is rare to find people who have not or do not use a computer. Therefore, a tool for weight loss that cannot be ignored is the Internet. Because a complete review of this tool is beyond the scope of this chapter, a brief update on Internet-based weight loss programs will be presented. Saperstein et al. (62) published a review article on the impact of the Internet for weight loss. They reported that the general public is definitely using the Internet for diet and fitness information. More importantly, they found that the Internet had affected behavior.

Collinson et al. (18) evaluated the efficacy of an Internet-based weight loss program that included foods with a low glycemic index in 103 individuals with a BMI ≥ 28 kg $\cdot$ m^{-2}. A dietitian counseled the participants during weekly chat rooms and monthly e-mail messages. A significant reduction in body weight, BMI, and waist circumference from baseline to 6 mo in the 70 participants who completed the program was reported. Although this program was effective, there was no control group with which to compare the results.

Morgan et al. (52) reported the 12-mo follow-up results of the SHED-IT (self-help, exercise, and diet using information technology) trial, an Internet-based weight loss program designed for men. Sixty-five men who were overweight or obese (35.9 ± 11.1 yr of age; BMI $= 30.6 \pm 2.8$ kg $\cdot$ m^{-2}) were randomly assigned to either the Internet group ($n = 34$) or an information-only control group ($n = 31$). Both groups of men received one face-to-face information session and a program booklet. The Internet group was asked to use the study Web site for 3 mo. All participants were evaluated at baseline 3, 6, and 12 mo for body weight, waist circumference, BMI, blood pressure, and resting heart rate. The Internet group who self-monitored as instructed ("compliers") maintained greater weight loss at 12 mo (-8.8 kg) compared to the Internet group "non-compliers" (-1.9 kg) and controls (-3.0 kg). Although successful, this intervention demonstrates the need for individuals who use an Internet-based weight loss program to self-monitor for greater success in weight loss maintenance. Successful Internet programs included the use of self-monitoring, altering energy balance, use of behavioral strategies, and providing feedback and support. It is important, therefore, to realize that patients may be obtaining other information (which may or may not be sound) from Internet-based weight loss sites. Also, the studies performed using Internet-based interventions typically used these in lieu of clinic visits with an allied health professional, such as a registered dietitian or exercise physiologist. Future investigations will likely focus on integrated models combining Internet technology and clinic visits.

SURGICAL METHODS OF WEIGHT LOSS

Individuals who are morbidly obese (BMI ≥ 40.0 kg $\cdot$ m^{-2}) or have class II obesity (BMI 35.0–39.9 kg $\cdot$ m^{-2}) with comorbidities may be candidates for bariatric surgical techniques to induce weight loss. Such individuals should initially exhaust all attempts to lose weight through dietary and exercise interventions. However, for those who find it too difficult to lose weight successfully through standard methods, bariatric surgery is becoming increasingly popular. The number of bariatric surgeries in the United States peaked at approximately 136,000 in 2004 and had leveled off at approximately 125,000 in 2008 (56). Bariatric surgery is highly effective at inducing significant weight loss and has beneficial effects on Type 2 diabetes mellitus, dyslipidemia, hypertension, and sleep apnea (12). Proczko-Markuszewska et al. (59) examined the effects of Roux-en-Y gastric bypass on Type 2 diabetes mellitus in 73 patients who were morbidly obese (41 females and 32 males). Type 2 diabetes mellitus was regressed in 61 (70%) patients while they were still in the hospital postsurgery, whereas 14 patients showed improvement in HbA1C 12 wk postsurgery. Additionally, two important studies (5,65) reported significant long-term weight loss coupled with reductions in long-term mortality in patients who underwent bariatric surgery. These studies suggest not only that bariatric surgery is an effective treatment option in the morbidly obese but also that long-term intentional weight loss definitively improves lifespan (10). And this positive effect is not thought to just be limited to bariatric surgery as the method for weight loss but true for any method of intentional weight loss.

There are several bariatric surgical techniques. The two most common are Roux-en-Y gastric bypass and gastric banding (45). The Roux-en-Y procedure involves attaching the jejunum of the small intestine to a small portion of the proximal stomach. The lower portion of the stomach, the duodenum, and a short length of the jejunum are bypassed but are reattached to the intact jejunum distal to the stomach pouch (forming one limb of the "Y" and allowing digestive enzymes from the duodenum to enter the distal jejunum). Weight loss is induced primarily by restricting the amount of food that can be eaten at one time because of the very small size of the stomach pouch and secondarily because of malabsorption caused by the stomach contents not passing through the duodenum. Gastric banding is a simpler procedure in which a band is placed around the proximal stomach and cinched to create a small pouch. As with gastric bypass, the small size of the stomach pouch restricts the amount of food that can be eaten. Unlike gastric bypass, gastric banding allows the contents of the pouch to enter the lower portion of the stomach and then proceed through the duodenum. Gastric banding is performed laparoscopically (through a small abdominal incision, guided with an endoscope) and, thus, has fewer surgical complications. Another advantage is that a greater percentage of weight loss is fat weight as opposed to fat-free weight following gastric banding as compared with gastric bypass and another bariatric technique, biliopancreatic diversion (16).

Both gastric bypass and gastric banding currently have relatively low surgical mortality, approximately 0.5% and 0.1%, respectively (45). However, there are several common postoperative complications, including vomiting (very prevalent and lasting up to 6 mo), "dumping syndrome" (sweating, dizziness, and fatigue occurring after ingestion of sugar; very prevalent after gastric bypass), vitamin B_{12} and iron deficiencies, and gallstone formation (29). Weight regain can also be an issue. Patients can adopt a habit of consuming multiple small meals and, thus, overcome the restrictive effect of the small stomach pouch. Bariatric surgery patients must be counseled regarding proper nutrition and caloric intake. It is important that behavior changes are adopted and continued after surgery. It has been reported that individuals with binge-eating disorder before bariatric surgery are likely to continue binge eating postsurgery (57).

Another common complication of bariatric surgery and subsequent weight loss is redundant skin that does not regress. The excessive skin is susceptible to rashes and infections and may cause the patient significant psychological distress (66). The excess skin may be removed in circumferential abdominoplasty or other types of "body contouring" plastic surgery. The incidence of such procedures in postbariatric surgery patients peaked at approximately 68,000 in 2005 (8) and has since fallen to 59,000 in 2008 (1) and 50,000 in 2011 (2), paralleling changes in bariatric surgery incidence as mentioned previously.

Bariatric surgery is a highly effective weight loss method for the morbidly obese with the potential to reduce mortality. However, patients must be encouraged to use diet and exercise as the first approach and, if choosing surgical intervention, be counseled regarding the lengthy period required to manage the postoperative complications.

IMPORTANCE OF AN ADEQUATE DAILY ENERGY INTAKE FOR HEALTHY WEIGHT MANAGEMENT

The basic premise of weight maintenance is that energy intake equals energy expenditure. If weight loss is to be achieved, then energy intake must be less than energy expenditure (or energy expenditure must be greater than energy intake). It is important to maintain adequate energy intake because micronutrients (vitamins and minerals) are required for physiologic processes in the body. If micronutrients are not adequately consumed, other problems, such as impairment of the immune system, may occur.

Typically, a weight loss of no more than 2 lb $\cdot$ wk^{-1} (~1 kg) is often a goal for several reasons: (a) this smaller amount of weight loss may help to preserve LBM when a large amount of weight is lost; (b) although slower, this lower amount of weight loss may result in better adherence and better ability of the person to maintain that weight loss because, typically, the person has made lifestyle changes rather than drastic changes to his or her dietary intake; and (c) slower weight loss typically means less water loss and, thus, that a "false weight loss" has not occurred. However, in select individuals using properly designed aggressive weight loss methods (e.g., VLCD or surgery) that result in a greater per week rate of weight loss, these issues can be overcome.

To lose 1 lb $\cdot$ wk^{-1} of body fat, a person should be in a 500-kcal deficit $\cdot$ d^{-1} because 1 lb of fat stores 3,500 kcal. It is important to note that not everyone loses 1 lb of fat with a 3,500-kcal deficit, but this is an average. Some individual variation occurs. Nonetheless, in general, a person can achieve this deficit by, for example, exercising enough to burn 250 kcal and decrease intake by 250 kcal daily. These values would need to be doubled if a 2-lb $\cdot$ wk^{-1} weight loss is desired. This level of deficit is moderate and reduces the risk of inadequate levels of energy and nutrient intake; it also increases compliance while also decreasing a person's likelihood of regaining the body weight lost. Although a combination of a moderate energy intake deficit and moderately increased energy expenditure may provide the best method to achieve weight loss, weight loss can be achieved by exercise alone. Donnelly et al. (22) reported that after 16 mo, exercise alone prevented weight gain in women and resulted in a significant weight loss for men (~5.2 kg weight loss on average) compared with a sedentary control group.

DETERMINING ENERGY NEEDS

Energy needs can be determined in several ways. Two important equations are the Harris-Benedict equation and the Mifflin-St. Jeor equation. These equations take into account a person's age, sex, weight, and height; however, the Harris-Benedict equation may overpredict a person's energy needs (9). Simply multiplying a person's body weight in pounds by 11 (providing a crude estimate of a person's **resting** metabolic rate [RMR]), then adding appropriate factors based on energy expenditure is another way. ACSM defines resting metabolism as 1 metabolic equivalent (MET) or an oxygen consumption of 3.5 mL $\cdot$ min^{-1} $\cdot$ kg^{-1}, which equals to 1 kcal $\cdot$ hr^{-1} $\cdot$ kg^{-1}. This yields a daily value for RMR of 24 × body mass (kg) (or 10.9 × body weight in pounds).

Determining a person's intake over time and assessing body weight is a more tedious method of assessing energy needs; however, this provides a more accurate estimate. Another more tedious but more accurate method is to assess an individual's RMR (kcal $\cdot$ d^{-1} used at rest), dietary-induced thermogenesis (energy expended after a meal; this must be conducted for up to 4 h after a meal), and energy expended during exercise all through indirect calorimetry (either using a metabolic cart or a whole-room calorimeter). These methods measure oxygen consumption and expiration of carbon dioxide, and then energy expenditure is calculated. Doubly labeled water provides the best estimate of a person's energy expenditure each day; however, it is expensive and does not partition how much energy is used for each activity.

Because many of these methods may not be practical, a useful tool for determining energy needs is to refer to the Food and Nutrition Board of the Institute of Medicine, National Academy of Sciences' (27) recommendations for energy intake based on energy expenditure.

ESTIMATING THE THERMIC EFFECT OF ACTIVITY

The thermic effect of activity varies based on an individual's activity patterns. The greater the duration and intensity of the exercise, the greater the energy expenditure. The Compendium of Physical Activities is a resource to estimate energy expenditure (6). The compendium provides gross MET values (*i.e.*, resting metabolism is included); therefore, RMR (*i.e.*, 1 MET) must be subtracted to avoid counting it twice. Also, the compendium does not take into account factors such as the individual's body mass or the individual's personal choice of intensity for a given activity. For specific activities that have highly predictable energy expenditures, such as walking, running, and stationary cycling, the ACSM has developed metabolic equations that provide relatively accurate values (see *Chapter 30*).

THE MACRONUTRIENTS: CARBOHYDRATES, FAT, AND PROTEIN

Equally as important as consuming the proper amount of energy is the consumption of a proper balance of energy sources, macronutrients, and micronutrients (vitamins and minerals) (see *Chapter 4*). Although proper nutrition should be individualized, it is generally recommended that individuals consume about 45%–65% of their total energy intake from carbohydrates (which provide 4 kcal $\cdot$ g^{-1}) (27). These carbohydrates should consist mostly of whole grains (*e.g.*,

whole wheat products; brown rather than white rice). The consumption of whole grains provides more micronutrients as well as greater amounts of fiber, all of which can help to stave off cardiovascular disease and cancer. Protein is another macronutrient that is often perceived as the "building block" of muscle in the body. Although it is true that protein (which provides 4 kcal $\cdot$ g^{-1}) is required for muscle growth, if protein intake is above what the body requires, much of it is stored as fat in adipocytes. In general, adults need about 0.8 g of protein $\cdot$ kg^{-1} of body weight (sedentary healthy person), which is equal to about 0.4 g of protein $\cdot$ lb^{-1} of body weight (27). For example, a 70-kg (154-lb) person requires, on average, about 56 g of protein $\cdot$ d^{-1}. Each ounce of a protein food provides about 7 g of protein. A person who exercises strenuously may require slightly more protein per day (*e.g.*, about 1.1–1.6 g $\cdot$ kg^{-1} of body mass or 0.5–0.7 g $\cdot$ lb^{-1} of body weight), especially if he or she is novice to the specific exercise program.

Fat is required for proper bodily function. Fat provides 9 kcal $\cdot$ g^{-1} of energy. It is recommended that individuals consume about 20%–35% of their total energy intake from fat (27); however, the type of fat consumed is most important. Monounsaturated fats (prevalent in olive oil, nuts, avocados) and polyunsaturated fats (*e.g.*, safflower oil, sunflower oil) should be consumed in higher amounts than saturated fats (*e.g.*, butter, lard, fat from meat) and hydrogenated fats. Hydrogenated fats are unsaturated fats that have been chemically altered to make them more stable. The hydrogenation process creates "trans" fats (referring to the molecular structure of double bonds within the fatty acid). Saturated and hydrogenated fats lead to increased risk of heart disease because they increase blood levels of LDL-C. Although alcohol provides energy (7 kcal $\cdot$ g^{-1}), it should be consumed in moderation because high consumption of alcohol can lead to malnutrition and other disorders.

THE MICRONUTRIENTS

Vitamins and minerals are required for life, but they are required in much lower quantities than the macronutrients. Their functions are many, but they do *not* provide energy as do the macronutrients. However, many vitamins and minerals are required for energy metabolism and can affect exercise performance and overall health if they are not consumed in the right balance. It is beyond the scope of this chapter to review all the vitamins and minerals; therefore, the reader is referred to *Chapter 4* and to an article in *ACSM's Health & Fitness Journal* (70).

INAPPROPRIATE WEIGHT LOSS METHODS

Fad diets are promoted by television, newspaper, and magazine articles on a daily basis. The weight loss industry is a billion-dollar industry, and dieting books are among the top sellers. However, many times, these fad diets are promoted by individuals who are not qualified or trained in any way to provide this information. Furthermore, because the weight loss may be unhealthy, these fad diets may be dangerous.

When assessing diet books, those that restrict certain food groups, especially fruits and vegetables, and state that their diets will cure everything are not appropriate. Furthermore, exercise books that state that a person only needs to exercise 5 min $\cdot$ d^{-1} to lose weight are greatly overstating the truth.

Other inappropriate weight loss methods that can be dangerous are use of saunas or steam rooms, exercising in the heat wearing heavy clothing to "sweat off the pounds," starvation diets, liquid diets that are not supervised by physicians and other health care professionals, diets that require megadosing of vitamin and mineral supplements (megadosing can be dangerous because many minerals compete for one another within the body if they share the same carrier), and diets that are only several weeks long, promising rapid weight loss. Often, these rapid weight loss diets can be dangerous and can lead to loss of large amounts of muscle mass and water. If the claims seem too good to be true, they probably are, and that weight loss regimen should be avoided.

Furthermore, rapid weight loss that is not under medical supervision is not recommended because negative consequences can ensue. These consequences can be as serious as electrolyte imbalances leading to cardiac dysrhythmias. Individuals who lose weight rapidly also tend to lose more lean muscle mass, which can lead to an overall decline in RMR. This decline in RMR may make it more difficult for weight loss to occur in the future. In addition, if those who lose weight rapidly do not change the behavior that led to their obesity, their weight loss may not be maintained over time.

GENERAL GUIDELINES FOR PROPER WEIGHT LOSS

ACSM published a position stand on weight loss in 2009 (21). In brief, a combination of decreased energy intake and increased energy expenditure was emphasized with a recommended energy deficit of 500–1,000 kcal $\cdot$ d^{-1}. Furthermore, it was reported that although health benefits can be attained with a minimum of 150 min $\cdot$ wk^{-1} (2.5 h) of moderate-intensity exercise, individuals who are overweight or obese may better maintain weight loss if they gradually increase exercise to 200–300 min $\cdot$ wk^{-1} (3.3–5.0 h) of exercise. The incorporation of resistance training was also encouraged to increase strength and function, but it may not prevent the loss of fat-free mass (FFM) more than aerobic training when incorporated with a weight loss program.

In 2011, the United States Department of Agriculture (USDA) replaced MyPyramid.gov with ChooseMyPlate.gov (17). ChooseMyPlate.gov food tracker is an excellent way for individuals to participate in interactive learning about their energy intake, energy expenditure, and quality of the foods they consume.

The Dietary Guidelines for Americans 2010 (20) is also a helpful guide for eating more healthily. If people simply increase their fruit and vegetable intake, their overall energy intake usually decreases, and they are consuming products that provide a good deal of fiber and antioxidants, both of which help stave off some chronic diseases. In 2010, the seventh edition of the Dietary Guidelines for Americans (20) was published and stressed the importance of eating well and exercising. *Box 35-1* lists the key points for achieving and maintaining weight loss.

| **BOX 35-1** | **Guidelines for Achieving and Maintaining Weight Loss** |

ACHIEVING WEIGHT LOSS

Negative Caloric Balance

- Increase exercise and decrease caloric intake to create a negative energy balance of 500–1,000 kcal $\cdot$ d^{-1}.

Exercise Recommendations

- Exercise 5–7 d $\cdot$ wk^{-1} for 30–60 min $\cdot$ d^{-1}, beginning with moderate intensity (40%–59% $\dot{V}O_2R$ or HRR); consider progressing to vigorous intensity (>60% $\dot{V}O_2R$ or HRR); see *Chapter 30* for details on prescribing exercise.
- Total duration of moderate-intensity exercise should be ≥150 min $\cdot$ wk^{-1} and progress to ≥300 min $\cdot$ wk^{-1} (if exercise intensity is vigorous, duration may be proportionally less).
- Include resistance training as part of an overall exercise plan.

Dietary Recommendations

- Reduce caloric intake to accomplish negative caloric balance in combination with exercise.
- Maintain a well-balanced diet composed of fruits, vegetables, whole grains, and lean protein sources.
- Keep dietary fat <30% of total calories, with reduction in saturated and hydrogenated sources for health benefits.

MAINTAINING WEIGHT LOSS

- Continue appropriate dietary and exercise patterns as permanent behavior change.
- Duration of moderate-intensity exercise should be >250 min $\cdot$ wk^{-1}.

$\dot{V}O_2R$, oxygen consumption reserve; HRR, heart rate reserve.

SUMMARY

Proper weight loss takes time. People do not gain excess weight in a short period of time; therefore, they need to be reminded that weight loss will not occur in a short period of time. A small deficit in food consumption (e.g., 250 kcal $\cdot$ d^{-1}), coupled with an increase in energy expenditure (e.g., 250 kcal $\cdot$ d^{-1}), can lead to a weight loss of about 1 lb $\cdot$ wk^{-1}. Properly designed aggressive weight loss methods, such as surgery or VLCD, can be successful in select individuals. Individuals who are successful at maintaining weight loss consume a moderately lower energy intake, exercise on a daily basis, and have implemented behavioral change to improve their overall lifestyle. Wadden et al. (71) reported that long-term weight control included "continued patient-practitioner contact (whether on-site or by e-mail), high levels of physical activity, and the long-term use of pharmacotherapy [if warranted] combined with lifestyle modification." A lifestyle change is the key to successful weight loss. Individuals should be cautioned regarding inappropriate weight loss methods to prevent potentially serious side effects from occurring.

REFERENCES

1. *2008 Plastic Surgery Statistics Report: 2008 Body Contouring After Massive Weight Loss* [Internet]. Arlington Heights (IL): American Society of Plastic Surgeons; [cited 2011 May 10]. Available from: http://www.plasticsurgery.org/Documents/news-resources/statistics/2008-statistics/2008-plastic-surgery-after-weight-loss-statistics.pdf

2. *2011 Plastic Surgery statistics Report: 2011 Body Contouring After Massive Weight Loss* [Internet]. Arlington Heights, IL: American Society of Plastic Surgeons; [cited 2011 May 10]. Available from: http://www.plasticsurgery.org/Documents/news-resources/statistics/2011-statistics/2011_Stats_BodyCont_Procedures.pdf

3. Aaltonen S, Leskinen T, Morris T, et al. Motives for and barriers to physical activity in twin pairs discordant for leisure time physical activity for 30 years. *Int J Sports Med.* 2012;33(2):157–63.

4. Adamo KB, Tesson F. Genotype-specific weight loss treatment advice: how close are we? *Appl Physiol Nutr Metab.* 2007;32(3):351–66.

5. Adams TD, Gress RE, Smith SC, et al. Long-term mortality after gastric bypass surgery. *N Engl J Med.* 2007;357(8):753–61.

6. Ainsworth BE, Haskell WL, Whitt MC, et al. Compendium of physical activities: an update of activity codes and MET intensities. *Med Sci Sports Exerc.* 2000;32(9 Suppl):S498–504.

7. Andreoli A, Lauro S, Di Daniele N, Sorge R, Celi M, Volpe SL. Effect of a moderately hypoenergetic Mediterranean diet and exercise program on body cell mass and cardiovascular risk factors in obese women. *Eur J Clin Nutr.* 2008;62(7):892–7.

8. *Body Contouring After Major Weight Loss* [Internet]. Arlington Heights (IL): American Society of Plastic Surgeons; [cited 2011 Mar 22]. Available from: http://www1.plasticsurgery.org/ebusiness4/ProductCatalog/pdf/brochures/Body_Contouring.pdf

9. Boullata J, Williams J, Cottrell F, Hudson L, Compher C. Accurate determination of energy needs in hospitalized patients. *J Am Diet Assoc.* 2007;107(3):393–401.

10. Bray GA. The missing link — lose weight, live longer. *N Engl J Med.* 2007;357(8):818–20.

11. Brinkworth GD, Noakes M, Buckley JD, Clifton PM. Weight loss improves heart rate recovery in overweight and obese men with features of the metabolic syndrome. *Am Heart J.* 2006;152(4):693.e1–6.

12. Buchwald H, Avidor Y, Braunwald E, et al. Bariatric surgery: a systematic review and meta-analysis. *JAMA.* 2004;292(14):1724–37.

13. Burke LE, Warziski M, Styn MA, Music E, Hudson AG, Sereika SM. A randomized clinical trial of a standard versus vegetarian diet for weight loss: the impact of treatment preference. *Int J Obes (Lond).* 2008;32(1):166–76.

14. Catenacci VA, Grunwald GK, Ingebrigtsen JP, et al. Physical activity patterns using accelerometry in the National Weight Control Registry. *Obesity (Silver Spring).* 2011;19(6):1163–70.

15. Centers for Disease Control and Prevention. Physical activity trends — United States, 1990–1998. *MMWR Morb Mortal Wkly Rep.* 2001;50(9):166–9.

16. Chaston TB, Dixon JB, O'Brien PE. Changes in fat-free mass during significant weight loss: a systematic review. *Int J Obes (Lond).* 2007;31(5):743–50.

17. ChooseMyPlate.gov [Internet]. Alexandria (VA): U.S. Department of Agriculture; [cited 2011 Sep 1]. Available from: http://www.choosemyplate.gov

18. Collinson A, Lindley R, Campbell A, Waters I, Lindley T, Wallace A. An evaluation of an Internet-based approach to weight loss with low glycaemic load principles. *J Hum Nutr Diet.* 2011;24(2):192–5.

19. Dansinger ML, Tatsioni A, Wong JB, Chung M, Balk EM. Meta-analysis: the effect of dietary counseling for weight loss. *Ann Intern Med.* 2007;147(1):41–50.

20. *Dietary Guidelines for Americans* [Internet]. Washington (DC): U.S. Department of Health and Human Services and U.S. Department of Agriculture; [cited 2011 Mar 31]. Available from: http://www.cnpp.usda.gov/DGAs2010-PolicyDocument.htm

21. Donnelly JE, Blair SN, Jakicic JM, et al. American College of Sports Medicine Position Stand. Appropriate physical activity intervention strategies for weight loss and prevention of weight regain for adults. *Med Sci Sports Exerc.* 2009;41(2):459–71.

22. Donnelly JE, Hill JO, Jacobsen DJ, et al. Effects of a 16-month randomized controlled exercise trial on body weight and composition in young, overweight men and women: the Midwest Exercise Trial. *Arch Intern Med.* 2003;163(11):1343–50.

23. Ebbeling CB, Leidig MM, Feldman HA, Lovesky MM, Ludwig DS. Effects of a low-glycemic load vs low-fat diet in obese young adults: a randomized trial. *JAMA.* 2007;297(19):2092–102.

24. Ello-Martin JA, Ledikwe JH, Rolls BJ. The influence of food portion size and energy density on energy intake: implications for weight management. *Am J Clin Nutr.* 2005;82(1 Suppl):236S–41S.

25. Executive Summary of the Third Report of the National Cholesterol Education Program (NCEP) Expert Panel on Detection, Evaluation, and Treatment of High Blood Cholesterol in Adults (Adult Treatment Panel III). *JAMA.* 2001;285:2486–97.

26. Flegal KM, Carroll MD, Kit BK, Ogden CL. Prevalence of obesity and trends in the distribution of body mass index among US adults, 1999–2010. *JAMA.* 2012;307(5):491–7.

27. Food and Nutrition Board, Institute of Medicine, National Academy of Sciences. *Dietary Reference Intakes for Energy, Carbohydrate, Fiber, Fat, Fatty Acids, Cholesterol, Protein, and Amino Acids.* Washington (DC): The National Academies Press. 2005. 1357 p.

28. Foreyt J, Goodrick K. The ultimate triumph of obesity. *Lancet.* 1995;346(8968):134–5.

29. Fujioka K. Follow-up of nutritional and metabolic problems after bariatric surgery. *Diabetes Care.* 2005;28(2):481–4.

30. Gardner CD, Kiazand A, Alhassan S, et al. Comparison of the Atkins, Zone, Ornish, and LEARN diets for change in weight and related risk factors among overweight premenopausal women: the A TO Z Weight Loss Study: a randomized trial. *JAMA.* 2007;297(9):969–77.

31. Genuth S, Alberti KG, Bennett P, et al. Follow-up report on the diagnosis of diabetes mellitus. *Diabetes Care.* 2003;26(11):3160–7.

32. Gilden Tsai A, Wadden TA. The evolution of very-low-calorie diets: an update and meta-analysis. *Obesity (Silver Spring).* 2006;14(8):1283–93.

33. Hamman RF, Wing RR, Edelstein SL, et al. Effect of weight loss with lifestyle intervention on risk of diabetes. *Diabetes Care*. 2006; 29(9):2102–7.

34. Healthy People 2010 [Internet]. Washington (DC): U.S. Dept. of Health and Human Services; [cited 2011 Mar 22]. Available from: http://www.healthypeople.gov/2010

35. Jakicic JM, Clark K, Coleman E, et al. American College of Sports Medicine position stand. Appropriate intervention strategies for weight loss and prevention of weight regain for adults. *Med Sci Sports Exerc*. 2001;33(12):2145–56.

36. Jakicic JM, Marcus BH, Lang W, Janney C. Effect of exercise on 24-month weight loss maintenance in overweight women. *Arch Intern Med*. 2008;168(14):1550–59, discussion 1559–60.

37. Jakicic JM, Wing RR, Butler BA, Robertson RJ. Prescribing exercise in multiple short bouts versus one continuous bout: effects on adherence, cardiorespiratory fitness, and weight loss in overweight women. *Int J Obes Relat Metab Disord*. 1995;19(12):893–901.

38. Jakicic JM, Winters C, Lang W, Wing RR. Effects of intermittent exercise and use of home exercise equipment on adherence, weight loss, and fitness in overweight women: a randomized trial. *JAMA*. 1999;282(16):1554–60.

39. Jeffery RW, Utter J. The changing environment and population obesity in the United States. *Obes Res*. 2003;11 Suppl:12S–22S.

40. Kao YH, Lu CM, Huang YC. Impact of a transtheoretical model on the psychosocial factors affecting exercise among workers. *J Nurs Res*. 2002;10(4):303–10.

41. Krebs JD, Elley CR, Parry-Strong A, et al. The Diabetes Excess Weight Loss (DEWL) Trial: a randomised controlled trial of high-protein versus high-carbohydrate diets over 2 years in type 2 diabetes. *Diabetologia*. 2012;55(4):905–14.

42. Lafortuna CL, Resnik M, Galvani C, Sartorio A. Effects of non-specific vs individualized exercise training protocols on aerobic, anaerobic and strength performance in severely obese subjects during a short-term body mass reduction program. *J Endocrinol Invest*. 2003;26(3):197–205.

43. Lagiou P, Sandin S, Weiderpass E, et al. Low carbohydrate-high protein diet and mortality in a cohort of Swedish women. *J Intern Med*. 2007;261(4):366–74.

44. Ledikwe JH, Rolls BJ, Smiciklas-Wright H, et al. Reductions in dietary energy density are associated with weight loss in overweight and obese participants in the PREMIER trial. *Am J Clin Nutr*. 2007;85(5): 1212–21.

45. Lee CW, Kelly JJ, Wassef WY. Complications of bariatric surgery. *Curr Opin Gastroenterol*. 2007;23(6):636–43.

46. Leser MS, Yanovski SZ, Yanovski JA. A low-fat intake and greater activity level are associated with lower weight regain 3 years after completing a very-low-calorie diet. *J Am Diet Assoc*. 2002;102(9): 1252–6.

47. Li Z, Hong K, Wong E, Maxwell M, Heber D. Weight cycling in a very low-calorie diet programme has no effect on weight loss velocity, blood pressure and serum lipid profile. *Diabetes Obes Metab*. 2007; 9(3):379–85.

48. Low KG, Giasson H, Connors S, Freeman D, Weiss R. Testing the effectiveness of motivational interviewing as a weight reduction strategy for obese cardiac patients: a pilot study [published online ahead of print February 12, 2012]. *Int J Behave Med*.

49. Lutes LD, Daiss SR, Barger SD, Read M, Steinbaugh E, Winett RA. Small changes approach promotes initial and continued weight loss with a phone-based follow-up: nine-month outcomes from ASPIRES II. *Am J Health Promot*. 2012;26(4):235–38.

50. Malandrucco I, Pasqualetti P, Giordani I, et al. Very-low-calorie diet: a quick therapeutic tool to improve β cell function in morbidly obese patients with type 2 diabetes. *Am J Clin Nutr*. 2012;95(3):609–13.

51. Marcus BH, Forsyth LH. How are we doing with physical activity? *Am J Health Promot*. 1999;14(2):118–24.

52. Morgan PJ, Lubans DR, Collins CE, Warren JM, Callister R. 12-month outcomes and process evaluation of the SHED-IT RCT: an internet-based weight loss program targeting men. *Obesity (Silver Spring)*. 2011;19(1):142–51.

53. Murphy JC, McDaniel JL, Mora K, Villareal DT, Fontana L, Weiss EP. Preferential reductions in intermuscular and visceral adipose tissue with exercise-induced weight loss compared with calorie restriction. *J Appl Physiol*. 2012;112(1):79–85.

54. Must A, Anderson SE. Effects of obesity on morbidity in children and adolescents. *Nutr Clin Care*. 2003;6(1):4–12.

55. Nakade M, Aiba N, Suda N, et al. Behavioral change during weight loss program and one-year follow-up: Saku Control Obesity Program (SCOP) in Japan. *Asia Pac J Clin Nutr*. 2012;21(1):22–34.

56. Nguyen NT, Masoomi H, Magno CP, Nguyen XM, Laugenour K, Lane J. Trends in use of bariatric surgery, 2003–2008. *J Am Coll Surg*. 2011;213(2):261–6.

57. Niego SH, Kofman MD, Weiss JJ, Geliebter A. Binge eating in the bariatric surgery population: a review of the literature. *Int J Eat Disord*. 2007;40(4):349–59.

58. *Prevalence and Trends Data: Nationwide 2009 Physical Activity* [Internet]. Atlanta (GA): Centers for Disease Control and Prevention; [cited 2012 Mar 26]. Available from: http://apps.nccd.cdc.gov/brfss/display.asp?cat=PA&yr=2009&qkey=4418&state=US

59. Proczko-Markuszewska M, Stefaniak T, Kaska L, Kobiela J, Sledziński Z. Impact of Roux-en-Y gastric bypass on regulation of diabetes type 2 in morbidly obese patients [published online ahead of print February 21, 2012]. *Surg Endosc*.

60. Rankin JW, Turpyn AD. Low carbohydrate, high fat diet increases C-reactive protein during weight loss. *J Am Coll Nutr*. 2007;26(2):163–9.

61. Sacks FM, Bray GA, Carey VJ, et al. Comparison of weight-loss diets with different compositions of fat, protein, and carbohydrates. *N Engl J Med*. 2009;360(9):859–73.

62. Saperstein SL, Atkinson NL, Gold RS. The impact of Internet use for weight loss. *Obes Rev*. 2007;8(5):459–65.

63. Sénéchal M, Arguin H, Bouchard DR, et al. Effects of rapid or slow weight loss on body composition and metabolic risk factors in obese postmenopausal women. A pilot study. *Appetite*. 2012; 58(3):831–4.

64. Serwe KM, Swartz AM, Hart TL, Strath SJ. Effectiveness of long and short bout walking on increasing physical activity in women. *J Womens Health*. 2011;20(2):247–53.

65. Sjostrom L, Narbro K, Sjostrom CD, et al. Effects of bariatric surgery on mortality in Swedish obese subjects. *N Engl J Med*. 2007;357(8):741–52.

66. Song AY, Rubin JP, Thomas V, Dudas JR, Marra KG, Fernstrom MH. Body image and quality of life in post massive weight loss body contouring patients. *Obesity (Silver Spring)*. 2006;14(9):1626–36.

67. Tsai AG, Wadden TA. The evolution of very-low-calorie diets: an update and meta-analysis. *Obesity (Silver Spring)*. 2006;14(8): 1283–93.

68. Varady KA, Lamarche B, Santosa S, Demonty I, Charest A, Jones PJ. Effect of weight loss resulting from a combined low-fat diet/exercise regimen on low-density lipoprotein particle size and distribution in obese women. *Metabolism*. 2006;55(10):1302–7.

69. Volpe SL, Kobusingye H, Bailur S, Stanek E. Effect of diet and exercise on body composition, energy intake and leptin levels in overweight women and men. *J Am Coll Nutr*. 2008;27(2):195–208.

70. Volpe SL, Soolman J. Minerals for weight-loss fact or fiction? *ACSM Health Fitness J*. 2007;11(3):20–6.

71. Wadden TA, Butryn ML, Wilson C. Lifestyle modification for the management of obesity. *Gastroenterology*. 2007;132(6):2226–38.

72. Wadden TA, Foster GD, Letizia KA. One-year behavioral treatment of obesity: comparison of moderate and severe caloric restriction and the effects of weight maintenance therapy. *J Consult Clin Psychol*. 1994;62(1):165–71.

73. Wadden TA, West DS, Neiberg RH, et al. One-year weight losses in the Look AHEAD study: Factors associated with success. *Obesity (Silver Spring)*. 2009;17(4)713–22.

74. Weiss EP, Racette SB, Villareal DT, et al. Lower extremity muscle size and strength and aerobic capacity decrease with caloric restriction but not with exercise-induced weight loss. *J Appl Physiol.* 2007;102(2):634–40.

75. Welty FK, Nasca MM, Lew NS, Gregoire S, Ruan Y. Effect of onsite dietitian counseling on weight loss and lipid levels in an outpatient physician office. *Am J Cardiol.* 2007;100(1):73–5.

SELECTED REFERENCES FOR FURTHER READING

Donnelly JE, Blair SN, Jakicic JM, et al. American college of Sports Medicine Position Stand. Appropriate physical activity intervention strategies for weight loss and prevention of weight regain for adults. *Med Sci Sports Exerc.* 2009;41(2):459–71.

Gardner CD, Kiazand A, Alhassan S, et al. Comparison of the Atkins, Zone, Ornish, and LEARN diets for change in weight and related risk factors among overweight premenopausal women: the A to Z Weight Loss Study: a randomized trial. *JAMA.* 2007;297(9):969–77.

Gilden Tsai A, Wadden TA. The evolution of very-low-calorie diets: an update and meta-analysis. *Obesity (Silver Spring).* 2006;14(8):1283–93.

Kennedy MS. Making progress against childhood obesity. *Am J Nurs.* 2007;107(9):22.

Volpe SL, Soolman J. Minerals for weight loss: fact or fiction? *ACSM's Health & Fitness Journal.* 2007;11(3):1–7.

INTERNET RESOURCES

- American Dietetic Association: http://www.eatright.org/Public
- American Society for Metabolic and Bariatric Surgery: http://www.asbs.org
- Centers for Disease Control and Prevention. Obesity and Overweight: http://www.cdc.gov/nccdphp/dnpa/obesity/resources.htm
- Medline Plus. Obesity: http://www.nlm.nih.gov/medlineplus/obesity.html
- National Heart, Lung, and Blood Institute. Clinical Guidelines on the Identification, Evaluation, and Treatment of Overweight and Obesity in Adults: http://www.nhlbi.nih.gov/guidelines/obesity/ob_home.htm
- North American Association for the Study of Obesity: http://www.naaso.org
- U.S. Department of Agriculture. Dietary Guidelines for Americans, 2010: http://www.cnpp.usda.gov/dgas2010-policydocument.htm
- U.S. Department of Agriculture. Healthy School Meals Resource System: http://schoolmeals.nal.usda.gov
- U.S. Department of Agriculture. MyPlate: http://www.choosemyplate.gov
- U.S. Department of Agriculture, Food and Nutrition Information Center. Childhood Obesity: A Food and Nutrition Resource List for Educators and Researchers: http://www.nal.usda.gov/fnic/pubs/bibs/topics/weight/childhoodobesity.html

Exercise Prescription in Special Populations: Women, Pregnancy, Children, and Older Adults

This chapter describes exercise testing and exercise prescription for several special populations, specifically women, especially during pregnancy; children and adolescents; and older adults.

WOMEN

Women have become increasingly more interested in physical activity and sport as a result of the passing of Title IX legislation. The recent obesity epidemic has also provided an impetus for many women to begin taking part in physically active lifestyles. This interest in improving activity and fitness levels has led to more focus on women and exercise. Physiologic differences between men and women may necessitate special considerations when developing exercise prescriptions.

EXERCISE RESPONSE

Compared with men, women have lower absolute and relative maximal volume of oxygen consumed per unit time $\dot{V}O_{2max}$ values. This difference in $\dot{V}O_{2max}$ is because men have a greater amount of muscle mass as well as increased hemoglobin levels. Women also have a lower blood volume compared with men and, consequently, lower stroke volumes, which lead to increased heart rates (HRs) to maintain cardiac output (124). In terms of strength, women are able to generate nearly the same force as men when the weight lifted is compared with lean body mass (123).

EXERCISE TESTING

Generally, the adult guidelines for standard exercise testing apply to both men and women (see *Chapters 21 and 22*).

EXERCISE PRESCRIPTION

Generally, the adult guidelines for standard exercise prescription apply to both men and women (see *Chapters 30 and 31*).

SPECIAL CONSIDERATIONS

Women have an increased level of body fat, which is necessary to maintain a healthy menstrual cycle and support pregnancy. Lean body mass is lower compared with men because of the higher levels of body fat. Lower lean body mass is related to lower $\dot{V}O_{2max}$ and decreased overall strength in women compared with men (40). Because of monthly hormonal flux, women experience regular menstrual cycles. The menstrual cycle typically does not affect the ability to continue regular exercise. Estrogen has a protective effect against heart disease in women, hence the later development of cardiovascular disease (CVD) in women (87). Female athletes may experience amenorrhea, a cessation of the menstrual cycle, as a result of reduced energy availability or energy deficiency. Energy deficiency is defined in the literature as an energy imbalance that may emerge if excessive expenditure demands are not compensated with an increase in dietary intake (78–80).

KEY TERMS

Adolescent: A person between the onset of puberty and maturation, approximately 13–18 yr old.

Child: A person between birth and puberty, defined as younger than approximately 13 yr old.

Growth: Increase in size of a body part or body as a whole.

Maturation: The process and progress toward reaching the adult state.

Oftentimes in athletes, amenorrhea is accompanied by eating disorders and osteoporosis, contributing to the female athlete triad. Middle-aged women experience menopause, which is the cessation of the menstrual cycle, because of age-related lower levels of estrogen and progesterone. Symptoms of menopause may be attenuated by regular exercise in these women (34). As a result of menopause, women lose the protective effect of estrogen against heart disease (87). CVD risk then approaches that of men; therefore, regular exercise should be continued.

PREGNANCY

Pregnancy is a time when a woman's body undergoes significant anatomic and physiologic changes. These changes are caused by the release of gestational hormones that allow for appropriate changes to occur in the body to create an optimal environment for the fetus. Healthy pregnant women without exercise contraindications (see *Box 8-1* in *ACSM's Guidelines for Exercise Testing and Prescription*, 9th edition) are encouraged to exercise throughout the pregnancy. Regular exercise during pregnancy provides benefits to the mother and the child (37,39). Benefits include reduced risk of excessive weight gain and a decreased risk of development of conditions associated with pregnancy, such as gestational diabetes mellitus and pregnancy-induced hypertension (101).

The American College of Sports Medicine (ACSM) endorses guidelines (88) regarding exercise in pregnancy and the postpartum period set forth by the American College of Obstetricians and Gynecologists (4,30) and the Joint Committee of the Society of Obstetricians and Gynecologists of Canada and the Canadian Society for Exercise Physiology (CSEP) (37). These guidelines outline the importance of exercise during pregnancy and provide guidance on exercise prescription and contraindications for beginning and continuing exercise during pregnancy.

EXERCISE RESPONSE

Pregnancy has a major effect on the physiologic responses women have to exercise. *Table 8-1* in *ACSM's Guidelines for Exercise Testing and Prescription*, 9th edition provides an overview of these responses that are detailed in this chapter.

Metabolic Response

Changes in the anatomy and physiology of pregnant women lead to differing exercise responses compared with a nonpregnant woman. Oxygen uptake during weight-dependent exercise is increased, whereas oxygen uptake during weight-independent exercise is unchanged during pregnancy (28).

Cardiovascular Response

During exercise, pregnant women have increased HRs primarily caused by increased levels of gestational hormones in the first trimester (27). During subsequent trimesters, HR is elevated to maintain blood pressure. Blood volume increases by approximately 50% during pregnancy to accommodate the needs of both mother and fetus (41). This increase in blood volume increases stroke volume and cardiac output. Systolic and diastolic blood pressures remain unchanged during pregnancy. A decrease in total peripheral resistance attenuates the increase in blood volume that typically would cause blood pressure to increase (125).

Ventilatory Response

Minute ventilation ($\dot{V}_E$) increases during pregnancy because of increased ventilatory sensitivity. A lower ventilatory threshold and an increase in the sensitivity to CO_2 cause tidal volume and breathing frequency to increase (125). Because of the increased $\dot{V}_E$, both ventilatory equivalent for oxygen ($\dot{V}_E/\dot{V}O_2$) and ventilatory equivalent for carbon dioxide ($\dot{V}_E/\dot{V}CO_2$) increase.

Fetal Response

Factors that can elicit a fetal response to exercise include blood flow and oxygen delivery, heat dissipation, and glucose availability. A decrease in any of these factors can adversely affect the fetus. The degree of the effect depends on the intensity of the exercise. High-intensity exercise will cause a greater decrease in any of the factors compared with moderate-intensity exercise. Women who exercise regularly before and during pregnancy have increased blood flow, oxygen, and nutrient delivery to the uterus, which reduces the risk of adversely affecting the fetus during exercise. Also, women who exercise tend to divert more blood flow to the skin and begin to sweat sooner, allowing heat to dissipate more quickly without causing a dangerous increase in fetal temperature (26). These adaptations allow women to comfortably exercise during pregnancy without risk to fetal health. Additionally, exercise during pregnancy may impact fetal birth weight and mode of delivery. Women who exercise during pregnancy are less likely to give birth to overweight or low-birth-weight babies and may be at lower risk for cesarean delivery (19,52,62,96).

EXERCISE TESTING

Maximal exercise testing should not be performed in pregnant women unless medically necessary. If a maximal exercise test is warranted, the test should be performed with physician supervision. An equation for predicting peak oxygen uptake ($\dot{V}O_{2peak}$) from peak HR and peak speed and grade achieved during incremental, submaximal treadmill exercise has been validated for women during pregnancy (88). Women who have been sedentary before pregnancy or who have a medical condition (see *Box 8-1* in the *ACSM's Guidelines for Exercise Testing and Prescription*, 9th edition) should receive clearance from their physician before beginning an exercise program.

EXERCISE PRESCRIPTION

The CSEP Physical Activity Readiness Medical Examination for Pregnancy (PARmed-X for Pregnancy) is used for screening pregnant women before participating in exercise programs (see *Fig. 8-1* in the *ACSM's Guidelines for Exercise Testing and Prescription*, 9th edition) (98). The recommended exercise prescription for pregnant women is generally consistent with recommendations for the general adult population. However, it is important to monitor and adjust exercise prescriptions according to the woman's symptoms, discomforts, and abilities.

Physical activity should be performed on at least 3 d, preferably every day of the week. Physical activity should be moderate intensity (40%–60% oxygen uptake reserve [$\dot{V}O_2R$]). If $\dot{V}O_{2peak}$ is known, workloads associated with 40%–60% of $\dot{V}O_2R$ may be calculated. In nonpregnant women, $\dot{V}O_2R$ is typically translated into a target HR using equivalent percentages of heart rate reserve (HRR). However, because pregnancy raises resting HR and lowers maximal HR (HR_{max}), the HRR method is ineffective unless true resting and HR_{max} are known. Given the rarity of maximal testing during pregnancy, neither the $\dot{V}O_2R$ nor HRR method of prescribing exercise intensity is commonly used. Alternatives include using rating of perceived exertion (RPE) (12–14 on a 6–20 scale) or the "talk test" (being able to maintain a conversation during activity) to monitor exercise intensity. General guidelines for physical activity during pregnancy are summarized in *Table 36-1*. If HR is used to establish intensity, ranges that correspond to moderate-intensity exercise have been developed for pregnant women based on age (*Table 36-2*) (37).

The duration of physical activity should be at least 15 min $\cdot$ d^{-1}, gradually increasing to at least 30 min $\cdot$ d^{-1} of accumulated physical activity. The type of physical activity should be dynamic and rhythmic in nature and use large muscle groups. Aerobic activities include walking, cycling, and swimming. Pregnant women should avoid contact sports and sports/activities that may cause loss of balance or trauma to the mother or fetus. Examples of sports/activities to avoid include soccer, basketball, ice hockey, horseback riding, and vigorous-intensity racquet sports.

SPECIAL CONSIDERATIONS

Pregnant women who have been sedentary or who have a condition that inhibits them from engaging in recommended levels of physical activity should gradually increase activity with the goal of meeting the guidelines previously mentioned. Women who are morbidly obese and women with medical conditions related to pregnancy, gestational diabetes mellitus, or pregnancy-induced hypertension should receive clearance from their physician before beginning an exercise program. Exercise prescriptions should be adjusted according to each woman's medical condition, symptoms, and functional capacity.

Exercise should be terminated should any of the following occur: vaginal bleeding, dyspnea before exertion, dizziness, headache, chest pain, muscle weakness, calf pain or swelling, preterm labor, decreased fetal movement, and amniotic fluid leakage. In the case of calf pain and swelling, thrombophlebitis should be ruled out (30).

Pregnant women should avoid exercising in the supine position after the first trimester to ensure that venous obstruction to the fetus does not occur. They should also avoid the Valsalva maneuver during exercise. For the safety of the woman and fetus, exercise should take place in a thermoneutral environment, and the woman should be adequately hydrated to avoid heat stress.

During pregnancy, the metabolic demand increases by approximately 300 kcal $\cdot$ d^{-1}. Exercise also increases the metabolic demand, which depends on the intensity and duration of the workout. Women should increase caloric intake to meet the caloric costs of both pregnancy and

TABLE 36-2. Modified Heart Rate Target Zones for Moderate-Intensity Aerobic Exercise in Pregnancy Based on Maternal Age and Weight Status (Body Mass Index) (36,37,88)

BMI (kg $\cdot$ m^{-2})	Age (yr)	Fitness Level	HR Range (bpm)
<25	<20	Any	140–155
	20–29	Low	129–144
		Active	135–150
		Fit	145–160
	30–39	Low	128–144
		Active	130–145
		Fit	140–156
≥25	20–29	Any	102–124
	30–39	Any	101–120

bpm, beats per minute.

TABLE 36-1. Physical Activity Recommendations for Pregnant Women

Frequency	3 d $\cdot$ wk^{-1}, preferably daily
Intensity	Moderate (40%–60% $\dot{V}O_2R$) RPE 12–14 (on 6–20 scale) Talk test
Duration	15–30 min
Mode	Aerobic activity

RPE, rating of perceived exertion; $\dot{V}O_2R$, oxygen consumption reserve.

exercise. This will ensure that the mother and fetus are receiving proper nutrients to sustain the pregnancy.

Pregnant women may participate in a strength-training program. The program should incorporate low-resistance lifts (40%–60% of estimated one repetition maximum [1-RM]) and high-repetition sets (12–15 repetitions). During strength training, women should avoid the supine position and the Valsalva maneuver.

Generally, exercise in the postpartum period may begin approximately 4–6 wk after delivery and with permission from a physician. Women who deliver via cesarean section may require more than 6 wk after delivery to begin exercise. Deconditioning typically occurs during the initial postpartum period, so women should gradually increase exercise until prepregnancy physical fitness levels are achieved.

CHILDREN AND ADOLESCENTS

In 2007–2008, 31.7% of U.S. children and adolescents were classified as overweight or obese (92). Current trends indicate that this number will increase over the next few years. Most children participate in adequate amounts of physical activity (22). However, physical activity levels decrease through adolescence such that most adolescents are not participating in sufficient amounts of physical activity to meet recommended guidelines (42). Decreased levels of physical activity during childhood and adolescence tend to track as lower levels of physical activity in adulthood (82). These findings provide evidence that children who adopt a physically active lifestyle may have a better chance of continuing this behavior later in life.

CVD risk factors that are present in youth also have a tendency to track into adulthood. Youth who are overweight are more likely to have a higher prevalence of CVD risk factors than their normal-weight peers. In children and adolescents, the presence of CVD risk factors may indicate the future development of disease, which manifests much later in life. Risk factors that track into adulthood include dyslipidemia, hypertension, obesity, impaired glucose tolerance, and sedentary behavior (117). Each of these risk factors can be modified positively through physical activity. Therefore, it is important that children become physically active during childhood and continue this behavior through adolescence into adulthood to reduce their risk of CVD and all-cause mortality.

In addition to benefits on health and fitness, physical activity also has a positive influence on academic performance (29) and self-esteem. Because of the protective and health benefits of habitual physical activity, it is important that children maintain an active lifestyle and that they continue this behavior through adolescence into adulthood (117).

EXERCISE RESPONSE

As a result of growth and maturation processes, children's physiologic responses to exercise differ from those of adults (see *Table 8-2* in the *ACSM's Guidelines for Exercise Testing and Prescription*, 9th edition). Children's smaller stature and body weight, in addition to the immaturity of their physiologic regulatory systems, requires special consideration when exercising.

Children have lower absolute oxygen uptake ($\dot{V}O_2$ [$L \cdot min^{-1}$]) values compared with adults. However, because of the immaturity of their metabolic system and scaling, children's relative oxygen uptake ($\dot{V}O_2$ [$mL \cdot kg^{-1} \cdot min^{-1}$]) is higher than in adults. Children are also less economical than adults, resulting in a greater relative oxygen consumption, especially during locomotor activities. According to the geometric principles of scaling, smaller organisms are expected to have higher metabolic rates (relative to body mass) than larger organisms.

Cardiovascular Response

Children's stroke volumes at submaximal and maximal exercise are lower than the adults'. Children's submaximal HRs and HR_{max} are generally higher than adult HRs at corresponding workloads. Cardiac output is slightly lower in children. Because of lower cardiac outputs, the systolic and diastolic blood pressures are lower in children (60,105).

Ventilatory Response

$\dot{V}_E$ is lower in children than in adults. Children have a higher breathing frequency than adults; however, children tend not to breathe as deeply. Children use less oxygen per breath, which may be caused by a shorter ventilatory cycle, a result of higher breathing frequency. The oxygen cost of ventilation is also higher in children because of their more frequent, shallow breaths (60,105).

Thermoregulatory Response

Children have immature thermoregulatory systems. They have a higher threshold for sweating and have a lower perspiration rate than adults. These thermoregulatory responses require that youth exercise in thermoneutral environments and be properly hydrated so as not to overheat. Special care must be taken to avoid ambient temperatures that are greater than body temperature because children will gain heat more quickly than the adults because of their greater surface area to body mass ratio (60,105).

EXERCISE TESTING

Generally, adult guidelines for standard exercise testing apply to children and adolescents (see *Chapters 21* and *22*). The exercise testing protocol and mode of testing (treadmill vs. cycle) should be based on the reason the test is being performed and the functional capacity of the child or adolescent. Typically, treadmills elicit a higher $\dot{V}O_{2peak}$ and HR_{max}. Cycle ergometers provide less risk for injury but need to be adjustable to the size of the child or adolescent. Before testing, children and adolescents should be familiarized with the test protocol and procedure. This familiarization serves to minimize stress and maximize the potential for a successful test. Compared with adults, children and adolescents are mentally and psychologically immature and may require extra motivation and support during the exercise test (97).

In addition to traditional clinical fitness testing, health/fitness testing may be performed outside of the clinical setting. Fitness testing may occur in places such as schools or community centers. In these types of settings, the FITNESSGRAM test battery may be used to assess the components of health-related fitness in youth (32), including cardiorespiratory capacity, muscular strength, muscular endurance, flexibility, and body composition. Criterion-referenced standards are available for this test.

EXERCISE PRESCRIPTION

Aerobic Activity

Exercise prescription guidelines outlined later in this chapter for children and adolescents establish the minimal amount of physical activity needed to achieve the various components of health-related fitness. These recommendations are included in the 2008 Physical Activity Guidelines for Americans and are based on a combination of evidence-based guidelines developed by an expert panel and the National Association for Sport and Physical Education (NASPE), the governing body for physical education (1,33,114).

Physical activity should be performed at least 3–4 d · wk^{-1}, preferably daily. It should be of moderate (physical activity that noticeably increases breathing, sweating, and HR) to vigorous (physical activity that substantially increases breathing, sweating, and HR) intensity. These intensities are intended to approximate 40%–59% and 60%–85% of $\dot{V}O_2R$, respectively. RPE scales, such as the OMNI Scale, may also be used to set the intensity of activity (see *Fig. 28-2*). Youth should participate in 30 min · d^{-1} of moderate and 30 min · d^{-1} of vigorous intensity to total 60 min · d^{-1} of accumulated physical activity. To achieve these recommended levels of physical activity, youth should participate in various activities that are enjoyable and developmentally appropriate, which may include locomotor activities, active games, dance, sports, as well as bone and muscle strengthening activities. *Table 36-3* presents a summary of physical activity guidelines for children and adolescents.

TABLE 36-3. Physical Activity Recommendations for Children and Adolescents

Frequency	3–4 d · wk^{-1}, preferably daily
Intensity	Moderate to vigorous
Duration	60 min (accumulated)
Mode	Activities that are enjoyable and developmentally appropriate

Strength Training

Research indicates that children and adolescents may safely participate in strength-training activities (9,46). Strength gains achieved by prepubescent youth typically occur as a result of neuromuscular adaptations; postpubescent youth can achieve hypertrophic adaptations because of the presence of anabolic hormones. Recommendations for resistance training include moderate intensity (60%–80% of estimated 1-RM), 8–15 repetitions for one to three sets, and no more than 2 d · wk^{-1}. It is of primary importance that youth receive proper instruction and supervision (9,46). Also, youth should be able to properly fit the equipment being used for training. Equipment that is too large for children and adolescents impedes them from using proper form while training, which may increase their risk of injury.

Flexibility

Youth should regularly participate in activities that promote increased levels of flexibility and range of motion for at least 3 d · wk^{-1}, preferably every day. Intensity of the stretch should be to the point of mild discomfort and should be held for 10–30 s. Static stretching should be emphasized, with each major muscle group targeted during stretching sessions.

Special Considerations

Because of the increasing prevalence of childhood obesity and decreasing levels of daily physical activity in youth, children and adolescents may not be able to achieve 60 min · d^{-1} of physical activity. It is important to gradually increase the duration and frequency of physical activity to achieve this goal. Gradual progression will lower the risks of program dropout and injury. In this population, every effort should be made to decrease sedentary activities, such as watching television, surfing the Internet, and playing stationary video games. It is also important that youth are exposed to various activities that promote lifelong activity and fitness (*i.e.*, walking and cycling).

Children and adolescents with diseases or disabilities such as asthma, diabetes mellitus, obesity, cystic fibrosis, and cerebral palsy should have their exercise prescriptions tailored to their condition, symptoms, and functional capacity. With most of these disease states, youth have a lower level of cardiorespiratory fitness compared with their healthy counterparts. This low level of fitness may be the result of the children being sedentary, either because of the inability to exercise or the physicians and/or parents encourage inactivity (6). In most cases, youth with these diseases are able to exercise, usually resulting in improved fitness and decreased symptoms of the disease.

OLDER ADULTS

Currently, disparities exist among population groups in levels of physical activity that exaggerate the negative health consequences of a sedentary lifestyle. According to the 2008 Physical Activity Guidelines Advisory Committee report, demographic groups at highest risk for inactivity are older adults, women, minorities, those with low income or educational background, and those with disabilities, obesity, or chronic health conditions (1). These are the same demographic groups that bear a large burden of the diseases amenable to prevention and treatment with exercise (110) and yet have the least access and opportunity for health-promotion efforts related to physical activity. Therefore, exercise and fitness specialists should identify and understand the barriers to physical activity faced by particular population groups and be prepared to develop programs and tools that address these barriers.

Previous goals for older adults focused on physical activities designed to improve cardiorespiratory fitness and prolong life. However, it is now recognized that older adults can benefit from various physical activities that promote functional independence throughout life (3). An exercise program should include muscle strength, cardiovascular and muscular endurance, balance, and flexibility. The problems of mobility impairment, falls, arthritis, osteoporotic fractures, and functional status are related in part to muscle strength and mass (38,68,108,112,119), and thus strengthening activities, although important for all age groups, are particularly important for older adults. Age-related loss of muscle strength and mass (sarcopenia) and bone density, which are most dramatic in women, may be attenuated by strengthening exercises. With appropriate resistance training, losses in strength can be regained even after decades of muscle disuse (2,10,58,108,115). Unfortunately, national survey data indicate that women report lower than average participation in strength training (11% vs. 16%) (23). Additionally, despite the evidence on safety and efficacy, the prevalence of resistive exercise is even lower among the old (6%, ages 65–74 yr) and the very old (4%, older than the age of 75 yr) (23). Individuals in this latter age group, particularly older than the age of 85 yr, are primarily women, making an understanding of the risks and benefits of exercise in this most vulnerable cohort a priority.

RATIONALE FOR EXERCISE IN OLDER ADULTS

The rationale for the integration of a physical activity prescription into health care for older adults is based on four essential concepts (99,100). First, physiologic changes attributable to disuse are similar to those that have been observed in aging populations, leading to the speculation that the way in which we age may in fact be greatly modulated with attention to activity levels. Second, chronic diseases increase with age, and exercise has been shown to be an independent risk factor and/or potential treatment for most of the major causes of morbidity and mortality in western societies, a potential which is currently vastly underused (15,49,65,100). Third, traditional medical interventions do not typically address disuse syndromes accompanying chronic disease, which may be responsible for much of the disability associated with the disease. Exercise is particularly good at targeting syndromes of disuse (118). Finally, many pathophysiologic aberrations that are central to a disease or its treatment are addressed only by exercise, which therefore deserves a place in the mainstream of medical care and not as an optional adjunct.

It is clear that the optimum approach to "successful aging" or to health care in the older population cannot ignore the overlap of these areas. In some cases, exercise can be used to avert "age-related" decrements in physiologic function and thereby maximize function and quality of life in older adults. On the other hand, the combination of exercise and sound nutrition, particularly in relation to favorable alterations in body composition, will have numerous important effects on risk factors for chronic disease as well as the disability that accompanies such conditions. Therefore, understanding the effects of aging on exercise capacity and how habitual physical activity can modify this relationship in the older adult, including its specific utility in treating medical diseases, is critical for health care practitioners of all disciplines.

ASSESSMENT OF ACTIVITIES OF DAILY LIVING

Exercising frail older adults requires higher levels of supervision, attention to setting and safety, and prioritization of physical activities so that those most directly applicable to mobility and independence are emphasized first. Identification of functional deficits can be done using a variety of tools that assess independence in both basic activities of daily living (ADLs), such as feeding and clothing oneself (69), as well as instrumental, or higher level activities (instrumental activities of daily

TABLE 36-4. Activities of Daily Living Assessment

BATHING

Either sponge bath, rub bath, or shower	☐ Receives no assistance (gets in/out of tub by self if tub is the usual means of bathing)	0
	☐ Receives assistance in bathing only one part of the body (such as back or leg)	1
	☐ Receives assistance in bathing more than one part of the body (or not bathed)	2

DRESSING

Gets clothes from closet and drawers, including underclothes, outer garments, and uses of fasteners (including braces, if worn)	☐ Gets clothes and gets completely dressed without assistance	0
	☐ Gets clothes and gets dressed without assistance except for assistance in tying shoes	1
	☐ Receives assistance in getting clothes or in getting dressed or stays partly or completely undressed	2

TOILETING

Going to the "toilet room" for bowel and urine elimination, cleaning self after elimination, and arranging clothes	☐ Goes to the toilet room, cleans self, and arranges clothes without any assistance (may use object for support such as a cane, walker, wheelchair and may manage night bedpan or commode, emptying same in the morning)	0
	☐ Receives assistance in going to the toilet room, in cleansing self, or in arranging clothes after elimination or in the use of night bedpan or commode	1
	☐ Doesn't go the room termed as "toilet for the elimination process"	2

TRANSFERS

	☐ Moves in and out of bed as well as in and out of a chair without assistance (may use an object for support such as a walker or cane)	0
	☐ Moves in or out of bed or a chair with assistance	1
	☐ Doesn't get out of bed	2

CONTINENCE

	☐ Controls urination and bowel movement completely by self	0
	☐ Has occasional accidents	1
	☐ Supervision helps keep urine or bowel control; catheter is used; or is incontinent	2

FEEDING

	☐ Feeds self without assistance	0
	☐ Feed self except for getting assistance in cutting meat or buttering bread	1
	☐ Receives assistance in feeding, is partially fed, or is completely fed using tubes or intravenous fluids	2

Assistance means supervision, direction, or physical assistance. Higher scores indicate greater degrees of disability.

Modified with permission from Katz S, Akpom CA. A measure of primary sociobiological functions. *Int J Health Serv*. 1976;6:493–508.

living [IADLs]) required for independent living, such as shopping, cooking, cleaning, paying bills, using transportation services, etc. (77). *Table 36-4* provides a commonly used form for assessing basic ADLs. If deficits are identified in basic ADLs, therapeutic exercise prescription may ameliorate these by relieving the contribution of physiological impairments such as low muscle power, aerobic capacity, or balance. Exercise will be unlikely to compensate for severe deficits because of cognitive impairment. However, improved mobility and safety because of better balance and strength are still a worthwhile goal in the frail older adult with dementia, for example, even if ADL independence itself is not achieved.

EXERCISE TESTING

When exercise is prescribed for health care goals, its use by the individual should be systematically reviewed and adjusted over time with exercise testing. Such assessments and tracking should be built into any exercise prescription for older adults, as outlined in *Chapters 4* and 7 of *GETP9*.

Periodically performing exercise-capacity assessments and reviewing activity logs will form the primary means of assessing compliance and adaptation over time, and it is recommended that such discussions be included in counseling sessions/group meetings at regular intervals (see *Chapter 11, GETP9* for more details on theoretical models and effective techniques). Often, suboptimal training habits (particularly lack of sufficient volume or regularity, progression, and appropriate intensity) will be discovered. The primary goal of the exercise prescription is to change the exercise behavior itself and, thereby, physical fitness. Additionally, secondary goals may be improvements in specific symptoms or conditions, such as obesity, arthritis pain, depression, sleep disturbance, angina, time to claudication, or *metabolic fitness*, (*e.g.*, glucose control, blood pressure, or systemic inflammation), and appropriate measurements may be made to gauge progress in these areas as well. However, as some things are slow to change — that is, the effects are not dramatic in the short term — it is best not to overly emphasize the goals such as weight loss or the need for antihypertensive medicines as the participant may be discouraged rather than be encouraged by the pace or consistency of the results.

Many health outcomes appear to be related to the accumulated volume and/or intensity of exercise, and therefore, monitoring compliance will theoretically provide evidence that the benefits are occurring (16,17,25, 93,99,100,108,112). However, it is also beneficial to monitor improvements in cardiovascular fitness because aerobic capacity itself has a stronger relationship to mortality than level of physical activity (50).

Documenting improvements in fitness may reinforce long-term behavioral adaptations. Improved fitness may be shown by the following:

- Improved measurements of maximal aerobic capacity
- Decreased HR and blood pressure response to a submaximal workload
- Decreased RPE for a submaximal workload
- Improved strength
- Ability to lift a submaximal load more times
- Ability to withstand postural stress or negotiate obstacles
- Improved joint range of motion

EXERCISE TESTING FOR THE OLDEST SEGMENT OF THE POPULATION

Aerobic Capacity Testing

Because treadmill testing and indirect calorimetry are not always available or feasible, particularly in frail older adults, field estimates of aerobic capacity are usually substituted. The 6-min walk test is a simple way to do this in a clinical setting and requires minimal equipment (56). This test has been used as an index of rehabilitation in patients with heart and pulmonary disease, and results are known to improve with effective interventions. With exercise training, pulse and blood pressure at 6 min should decrease, and distance covered should increase. Alternatives to the 6-min walk test are walking a fixed distance (*e.g.*, 400 m), climbing multiple flights of stairs as rapidly as possible, or stepping up and down a single step for several minutes, followed by the measurement of HR and blood pressure. However, the potential for musculoskeletal injury because of balance, hip and knee arthritis, or vision problems make rapid-stepping tests less desirable in the older adults. Fixed distance tests are excluded in those who cannot walk the minimum distance because of comorbidities or frailty, and thus fixed time tests such as the 6-min walk are more widely applicable across a spectrum of older adults and can even be used in those with walkers, canes, or wheelchairs.

In evaluating the responses to aerobic exercise, reduced fatigue and/or breathlessness during submaximal exercise will be more significant to individuals than the increase in maximal aerobic capacity. Because most ADLs take place at submaximal workloads, this benefit should be readily appreciable to the older adult. Large improvements

in maximal aerobic capacity are not seen in "lifestyle" approaches to aerobic exercise and are likely to occur only after structured, high-intensity progressive or interval aerobic training (25). Therefore, it is best to concentrate on the improved tolerance for submaximal workloads to avoid discouraging a compliant exerciser who is doing an appropriate *volume* of exercise to achieve health benefits, but perhaps not at an *intensity* required for improvements in maximal aerobic capacity. Also, ask older adults to report their current RPE for tasks performed at home. Providing this as written or visual "proof of progress" over the course of several months will reinforce the positive change in behavior that has occurred and emphasize the relevance of the exercise prescription to daily life.

Strength Testing

As an alternative to 1-RM testing, a perceived exertion scale, such as the Borg Scale, may be considered to rate effort during a lift (13). On this 6–20 scale, a rating of 15–18 (hard to very hard) is equivalent to 80% of maximum lifting capacity in studies conducted in young and older adults and is therefore an appropriate peak training goal (53,76). The technique is as follows: A person lifts an initial weight and is asked to rate its difficulty. If the rating is less than 15, increase weight gradually on succeeding lifts until a rating of 15–18 is reached. Older adults rarely choose weights that are too heavy. On the other hand, there is a tendency to choose weights that are too light to be optimally therapeutic. The negative effects of exercising at a subtherapeutic intensity are numerous: discouragement at lack of progress; delayed recovery from atrophy and illness; and limited improvements in arthritis, mobility, balance, and other outcomes. There is little evidence that the often presumed positive benefits of using very light weights (*e.g.*, prevention of injury, minimizing dropout, addressing fears of lifting heavy objects, avoiding cardiovascular events) outweigh the negative consequences of minimal anabolic efficacy.

PREEXERCISE ASSESSMENT IN OLDER ADULTS

Most older adults, despite the presence of chronic diseases and disabilities, are able to undertake and benefit from an exercise prescription that is tailored to their physiologic capacities, comorbidities, and neuropsychological and behavioral needs. The permanent exclusions to any structured exercise are generally severe irreversible conditions where exercise would impose a risk on the health status of the individual (59,122) (see *Chapter 4, GETP9*). For some older adults, such as those with critical aortic stenosis, cardiac or peripheral vascular ischemia at rest, a large or unstable aortic aneurysm, or known cerebral aneurysm (when surgery is not an option because of advanced age or other medical considerations), any exercise that significantly elevates cardiac workload or blood pressure is considered high risk and therefore not recommended. Relatively few older adults, even those in long-term care, would be excluded from all exercise programs based on items in this category (*Table 36-5*) outside of those with severe forms of dementia or end-stage cardiac or other terminal disease.

Most questions about exercise prescription eligibility are items in the "temporary exclusion" category. Judgments must be made based on the severity of the diagnosis, timing of the event in question, and reevaluation after a diagnostic workup or medication adjustments. Most older adults in this category will be able to

TABLE 36-5. Evaluation of Appropriateness of Exercise Prescription in Older Adults

I. Stop! Permanent Exclusion	II. Wait! Temporary Exclusion	III. Go! Exercise Recommended
If any boxes in this column are checked, individual is ineligible for any exercise prescription at this time.	If any boxes in this column are checked, follow protocols for further evaluation of these concerns with medical personnel before reevaluating for appropriateness/modification of exercise prescription.	If only boxes in this column are checked, individual is suitable for exercise rescription without additional evaluation by medical personnel at this time.
End-stage congestive heart failure	Acute change in mental status or delirium, psychosis	Arthritis, stable
Permanent bedbound status	Cerebral hemorrhage within the past 3 mo	Chronic obstructive pulmonary disease, asthma
Severe cognitive impairment or behavioral disturbance	Exacerbation of chronic inflammatory joint disease or osteoarthritis	Stable joint disease, or osteoarthritis
Unstable abdominal, thoracic, or cerebral aneurysm	Eye surgery within the past 2 wk	Coronary artery disease, stable
Untreated severe aortic stenosis	Fracture in healing stage	Chronic renal failure
Other _____	Hernia, symptomatic (abdominal or inguinal) or bleeding hemorrhoids	Cancer (history or current)
	Myocardial infarction or cardiac surgery within 3 mo	Chronic liver disease surgery within past 3 mo
		Chronic venous stasis symptoms
	Proliferative diabetic retinopathy or severe nonproliferative retinopathy	Dementia, cognitive impairment
	Pulmonary embolism or deep venous thrombosis within 3 mo	Depression, anxiety, low morale thrombosis within 3 mo
	Soft tissue injury, healing	Diabetes
	Active suicidality or suicidal ideation	Drugs causing muscle wasting (steroids)
	Systemic infection	Frailty
	Uncontrolled blood pressure (>160/100 mm Hg)	Falls, history of hip fracture
	Uncontrolled diabetes mellitus (FBG >200 mg · dL^{-1})	Gait and balance disorders, mobility impairment
	Uncontrolled malignant cardiac arrhythmia (ventricular tachycardia, complete heart block, atrial flutter, symptomatic bradycardia)	Hypertension
	Unstable angina (at rest or crescendo pattern, ECG changes)	HIV infection
	Other _____	Hyperlipidemia
		Malnutrition, poor appetite
		Neuromuscular disease
		Obesity
		Osteoporosis
		Parkinson disease
		Peripheral vascular disease
		Stroke, stable

FBG, fasting blood glucose; ECG, electrocardiogram; HIV, human immunodeficiency virus.

be reclassified as appropriate for exercise once their condition has been treated or stabilized. Each of the items listed in *Table 36-5* are discussed briefly later in this chapter, with a rationale for the approach to management that maximizes safety of the exercise prescription and is consistent with the current ACSM guidelines for healthy (50) or older adults (3). For older adults with no exclusion items, a clinical exercise specialist or other health care professional may initiate an exercise program without further review. However, should a significant change in health status occur after exercise has begun (such as one of the items from the temporary exclusion category), physician review may be required.

Acute Change in Mental Status or Delirium

Because these symptoms may be indicative of an emerging disease process, such as metabolic disorder, fluid imbalance, drug toxicity, systemic infection, or transient ischemic attack, exercise must be delayed until appropriate diagnostic tests have determined the cause of the altered mental status. It is sometimes difficult to recognize delirium when it is superimposed on a chronic dementia, but the characteristic features of fluctuation throughout the day and decreased attention span should differentiate it from stable cognitive impairment. Once delirium has cleared, or the cause of the cognitive impairment or psychosis is identified and stable, exercise participation is no longer restricted. Residual underlying mental impairment will require lower exercise leader-to-older adult ratios than can be used with cognitively intact older adults. Some individuals with dementia may have an exacerbation of symptoms of disorientation, paranoia, or behavioral disturbance toward the late afternoon or evening hours ("sundowning"). If this syndrome is present, it is important to plan exercise sessions for such older adults at a more favorable time of the day to facilitate optimal participation.

Cerebral Hemorrhage within the Past 3 Months

Hemorrhagic stroke from intracerebral or subarachnoid bleeding is far less common than ischemic stroke from thrombosis or embolism, accounting for about 30% of all strokes. In its acute phase, activities are contraindicated that have the potential to significantly raise intracerebral or systemic arterial pressure for fear of extending the area of bleeding. There is no clear evidence to indicate when progressive resistance or aerobic exercise may begin, but general physical therapy is initiated as soon as the patient is able. Many neurologists suggest waiting for 3 mo after hemorrhagic stroke before initiating progressive resistance training or other kinds of strenuous exercise. In the absence of more definitive data, waiting until the subacute stage of recovery, approximately 8–12 wk after intracerebral bleeding, is recommended. If other features of cardiovascular status and blood pressure are stable at that time, the program can be initiated without modification.

By contrast, thrombotic or embolic stroke is not a contraindication to exercise training. If hemodynamic status is stable, progressive resistance and aerobic and balance training may be added to other elements of physical therapy during the recovery from ischemic stroke. Alternatively, exercise training may be initiated once formal physical therapy has ended as a means to continue and extend the benefits of acute rehabilitation to the subacute and chronic phases of recovery.

In all forms of stroke, proper breathing technique should be emphasized to avoid excessive rises in mean arterial pressure that may occur during the Valsalva maneuver (straining against a closed glottis). Although the cerebral and ocular circulations are protected to some extent against acute rises in blood pressure via autoregulatory pathways governing the vasoconstriction of the cerebral vessels, this pathway can be overridden by extreme rises in pressure. Such rises are associated with very heavy loads, sustained contractions, breath holding, and the Valsalva maneuver, which is why such techniques are not indicated whether or not stroke is present. More data are needed on the use of resistance or aerobic training during the early recovery period from ischemic stroke.

Exacerbation of Chronic Inflammatory Joint Disease or Osteoarthritis

Although both resistance and aerobic exercise have been shown to be beneficial for function and pain in chronic arthritis, there are times during a flare-up of the disease that such exercise needs to be avoided or modified. Usually, this is a temporary condition affecting one or more joints that will resolve with appropriate diagnosis, treatment, and time, thus allowing exercise prescription to be initiated in standard or modified form. Appropriate steps may include the following:

- Evaluation of other possible causes of joint pain, including fracture, dislocation, rotator cuff, cartilage or ligament tear, septic or gout-related inflammation in the joint, referred neurologic pain, spinal stenosis, and carpal tunnel syndrome, which require specific therapeutic interventions
- Modification of pain or anti-inflammatory medications to provide better coverage of symptoms
- Prescription of isometric strength training of the muscles around the affected joint(s), with a transition to dynamic strength training as soon as symptoms have stabilized
- Modification of positions or ranges of motion of the standard exercises to accommodate particular musculoskeletal restrictions.

Individuals whose independence and mobility are threatened by progressive joint disease in hips or knees and surrounding muscle atrophy from disuse are in *great need* of strengthening exercises for their upper body. They will increasingly rely on shoulder and triceps strength to assist with transfers when lower extremity pain and reduced range of motion are present and progressive. Such prophylactic use of progressive resistance training to offset impending disability is preferable to using assistive devices such as higher chair seats or "adaptive maneuvers" such as rocking back and forth to rise from a chair. Assistive devices or alternative strategies such as rocking do not improve the underlying physiologic capacity of the individual and should therefore be used as adjuncts when needed but not considered appropriate as an isolated approach to such impairments.

Eye Surgery within the Past 2 Weeks

Recent ophthalmologic procedures, such as cataract extraction, laser treatments, or other surgery, require a period of healing during which elevations of intraocular pressure are contraindicated. The exact duration of this recovery period is not known with precision, and ophthalmologists may impose restrictions for periods ranging from a few days to 2 wk. Therefore, it is recommended that any older adult who has had such procedures should have a clearance by his or her ophthalmologist before engaging in exercise. Activities that should be avoided in older adults who are healing from an eye surgery include the following:

- Lowering the head below the heart
- Direct impact to eye or surrounding tissues
- High-impact, jolting activities (jumping, jogging)
- Any activity or situation that causes very high elevations in blood pressure

Thus, walking, stepping, or cycling at low-to-moderate intensities, or typical resistance training as outlined in these guidelines can be resumed as soon as clearance is obtained.

Fracture in Healing Stage

Specific timing of resistance training after a fracture will depend on the type and stability of fracture, surgical treatment, casting or immobilization, and pain control. Therefore, clearance should be sought from the orthopedic surgeon, physiatrist, or physical therapist directing the care during acute rehabilitation. For fractures involving a cast, isometric resistance exercises should be initiated immediately after fixation in most cases and will prevent the rapid muscle atrophy associated with periods of immobilization. Once immobilization is no longer needed, isometric training can be replaced with dynamic training to regain the maximum range of motion and strength across the affected joints.

Hip fractures will be followed by a period of partial weight bearing and restrictions in hip motion and will depend on the type of surgical fixation used, stability of the fracture site, and underlying degree of osteopenia

around the prosthesis. Hip adduction, flexion, and internal rotation are often prohibited for a period after prosthetic joint implantation, for example. Communication with the therapist or surgeon will be required to establish the nature and the time course of such restrictions. In general, by 6 wk postoperation, most patients with fractured hips who have regained ambulatory status will be full weight bearing and will no longer require hip movement restrictions. At this time, or whenever the surgeon approves, standard exercises may be initiated to complement and extend other aspects of rehabilitation. Lower extremity resistance exercises (hip abduction, extension, flexion, knee extension and flexion, and plantar flexion) and balance training are particularly important to the recovery of gait, balance, and function in this cohort and do not place the person at risk for prosthetic dislocation once surgically stable. For those patients who do not regain ambulatory status, arm strengthening will be critical for optimizing independence in transfer activities, and leg exercises in seated or modified standing postures should be included as tolerated. The combination of high-intensity strength and balance training in the year after hip fracture has been shown to reduce both rate of institutionalization and mortality compared to usual physical therapy and medical treatment (111) and is, thus, recommended for such patients whenever feasible.

Symptomatic Hernia (Abdominal or Inguinal) or Bleeding Hemorrhoids

The elevation in intra-abdominal pressure during weight-lifting exercise may increase symptoms in an unrepaired hernia or bleeding hemorrhoid. In some cases, avoiding breath holding, straining, and the Valsalva maneuver will be sufficient to prevent symptoms, and training can be initiated. In other cases, any elevation in pressure is intolerable, and it may be necessary to treat the hernia surgically or with mechanical supports. In general, umbilical hernias that are small and reducible are not associated with pain, bowel obstruction, or strangulation, and do not preclude training with moderate loads, although they may enlarge with higher loads. More worrisome are large or painful inguinal hernias, which may require surgical evaluation and delay exercise initiation. Previously repaired hernias are not a contraindication to resistance training; however, careful instruction on breathing techniques and monitoring for hernia pain or protrusion during exercise should be carried out because these individuals are at risk for recurrence.

Myocardial Infarction or Cardiac Surgery within Past 3 Months

Exercise has been shown to be an effective strategy after myocardial infarction or cardiac surgery to improve mortality, reduce secondary events, and improve quality of life. Cardiac rehabilitation programs include both aerobic and resistive training after medical stabilization and, therefore, are appropriate for such patients as part of their overall recovery. However, older adults with a recent cardiac event should be cleared by a physician and monitored for physical signs or symptoms of heart disease because they are at risk for recurrent events. Precautions that apply to the patient with heart disease include the following:

- Avoiding the Valsalva maneuver at all times
- Avoiding sustained, isometric contractions
- Observing rest periods between repetitions and sets
- Exercising in supervised setting with emergency plan in place for facility
- Stopping exercise immediately if there is any suspicion of angina, arrhythmias, or ischemia during exercise
- Warming up and cooling down with slow walking or biking before and after more vigorous exercise

Proliferative Diabetic Retinopathy or Severe Nonproliferative Retinopathy

There are case reports of retinal bleeding or detachment occurring in response to extreme elevations in blood pressure associated with very heavy power lifting or sustained isometric contractions with Valsalva maneuver. Individuals with severe retinopathy are at high risk for retinal detachment and bleeding under normal conditions, and therefore, significant elevations in arterial and intraocular pressure, such as those associated with strenuous exercise or head-down positioning, should be avoided. Milder degrees of retinopathy and nonproliferative retinopathy seen with hypertensive disease or Type 2 diabetes do not preclude resistive or aerobic exercises as normally prescribed. It is recommended that older adults with retinopathy of moderate-to-severe degree be evaluated by an ophthalmologist before beginning an exercise regimen. Because retinal hemorrhage or detachment are, in many cases, preventable with prophylactic laser treatment, annual eye examinations are indicated in all adults with hypertension and diabetes, regardless of exercise participation. Most adults with mild or moderate retinopathy are appropriate for moderate-to-high intensity aerobic and resistive exercises. Avoiding sustained and isometric contractions, breath holding, Valsalva maneuver, and holding the head below the level of the heart minimize risk.

Pulmonary Embolism or Deep Venous Thrombosis within 3 Months

In the acute phase, it is possible that mechanical and hemodynamic factors associated with exercise of any kind could cause a clot to break off or move in the circulation, causing further symptoms or pulmonary infarction. It is not known precisely what the risk of exercise is in this situation. Therefore, it is prudent to avoid strenuous activity until full anticoagulation has been achieved and the clot has organized and is unlikely to expand or embolize further. Although the precise timing of such a period of waiting is unknown, a conservative approach is to wait until 3 mo before initiating exercise in older adults with a pulmonary or deep venous thrombosis. However, it is likely that most such individuals may begin exercise earlier than 3 mo after the event, as long as anticoagulant status is stable and hemodynamic or respiratory status is not compromised. Falling while on anticoagulants will increase the risk of soft tissue bleeding and bruising, so particular care should be taken during transfer activities before and after exercises, when postural blood pressure changes may be prevalent, as well as in the handling of weights that could be dropped onto legs or feet. Padding the front of the shin with a woolen leg warmer or thick sock may be necessary to prevent bruising from the use of ankle weights.

Soft Tissue Injury (Healing)

Depending on the nature of the injury, various periods of rest may be needed in the face of acute soft tissue trauma or surgery. Once sutures are removed and skin closure has occurred, exercise may usually be resumed. Sprains, strains, bruises, skin lacerations, dislocations, and other injuries should be evaluated on a case-by-case basis for the timing of exercise. In general, it is best to continue exercising the unaffected body parts to avoid disuse and behavioral disruption. In addition, isometric exercises of the affected body part may be continued to prevent muscle atrophy without causing additional injury to joints, tendons, ligaments, or other affected tissues.

Suicidal Ideation

Although depression may be treated with moderate-to-high intensity exercise, an older adult who currently expresses passive ("I wish I was dead") or active ("I have a plan to take my life") suicidal ideation must be immediately referred to a qualified psychiatric/medical professional. Older men who live alone are the cohort at the highest risk of suicide, and such sentiments should never be dismissed. Once antidepressant treatment has been initiated, exercise may be a strong adjunctive or alternative form of therapy prescribed for clinical depression.

Systemic Infection

During acute systemic infections, there is an increased risk of dehydration, arrhythmias, pericarditis, myocarditis, ischemia, delirium, and fatigue, all of which affect both the safety and feasibility of exercise training. Therefore, it is recommended that while a febrile condition or systemic infection exists, exercise be temporarily put on hold. For nonsystemic minor infections, such as a small skin infection or minor upper respiratory symptoms, clinical judgment should be used to direct the nature and intensity of physical activities.

Uncontrolled Blood Pressure (>160/100 mm Hg)

Although most exercises elevate blood pressure acutely during muscle contraction, the chronic effect of training in nonhypertensives and hypertensives is to lower blood pressure slightly. Weightlifting exercises cause moderate elevations in systolic and diastolic blood pressure for several beats while the muscle is contracted, followed by a rapid return to baseline values or below baseline values in the recovery period between lifts. Therefore, if blood pressure is currently uncontrolled, exercise should not be initiated until better levels are achieved (*e.g.*, approximately 150/95 mm Hg or lower on most readings). There are no definitive data on exactly what cutoff should be used, but hypertension needs to be controlled whether exercise is planned or not, so general recommendations for monitoring and treating hypertension in older adults should be followed. This is particularly true for patients with Type 2 diabetes who are at higher risk for vascular complications if hypertension is uncontrolled. For individuals with mild-to-moderate elevations in pressure (140–170/90–100 mm Hg), review by a physician with a plan for dietary, pharmacologic, and physical activity management of the hypertension is recommended. Resistive and aerobic exercises are appropriate for these patients. Until blood pressure is better controlled, it may be prudent to monitor blood pressure and pulse responses to exercise. In addition, individuals with hypertension should avoid very strenuous aerobic exercise, very heavy loads, sustained contractions, isometric handgrip, and Valsalva maneuver during lifting to minimize blood pressure excursions.

Uncontrolled Diabetes Mellitus (Fasting Blood Glucose >200 mg · dL^{-1})

As with hypertension, diabetes is generally an indication *for* exercise; however, in the acute stage when metabolic control is poor, exercise may cause blood glucose levels to deteriorate further. In the insulin-resistant patient with Type 2 diabetes, severe ketosis or acidosis are unlikely, but the rise in blood glucose may produce symptoms of fatigue or altered mental state as well as infections, diuresis, and dehydration. Therefore, it is recommended that glucose control be improved before initiating an exercise regimen. Fasting glucose values between 140 and 200 mg · dL^{-1} are not a contraindication to exercise prescription but require physician review of the overall management plan. Both aerobic and resistance training exert marked beneficial effects on insulin resistance and glucose tolerance, even in the absence of weight loss or dietary change and should therefore be

a central part of the management of Type 2 diabetes. Decreasing overall sedentary time by inserting episodes of low-intensity physical activity, such as standing up and moving around during commercial breaks, is preferable to uninterrupted long bouts of sedentary behavior. Sedentary behavior has been shown to be a significant risk factor for metabolic impairment (48).

Optimally, exercise sessions should coincide with peak elevations in blood glucose 1–2 h after meals (particularly after breakfast) and, thus, minimize swings in glucose levels throughout the day. Those who require insulin injections should not exercise directly after taking insulin unless they have had a meal in between injections. In some cases, doses of medications may need to be lowered if sustained, regular exercise regimens are incorporated into the lifestyle of the patient. Monitoring glycosylated hemoglobin (Hb$_{A1c}$) levels every 3 mo during exercise training will help define the effects of exercise and any needed adjustments in dietary or pharmacologic management.

Uncontrolled Malignant Cardiac Arrhythmia (Ventricular Tachycardia, Complete Heart Block, Atrial Flutter, Symptomatic Bradycardia)

These arrhythmias require attention by the physician regardless of the intent to prescribe exercise. In some cases, control cannot be achieved with drugs or pacemakers, and the patient may be unsuitable for exercise because of the potential danger of inducing sustained ventricular tachycardia, hypotension, complete heart block, or ischemia. Nonmalignant arrhythmias — such as isolated premature atrial or ventricular contractions, couplets, atrial fibrillation at a controlled rate, or totally paced rhythms — do not preclude aerobic or resistive training. The underlying etiologies should be ruled out, such as dehydration, thyroid disease, electrolyte disturbance, ischemia, or pulmonary disease, and such conditions should be evaluated and treated before the introduction of significant changes in physical activity levels.

Unstable Angina (at Rest or Crescendo Pattern, Electrocardiogram Changes)

Although chronic stable angina and ischemic heart disease are indications for exercise, unstable angina and undiagnosed chest pains must be evaluated fully before commencing exercise. The evaluation will depend on the clinical presentation and the level of medical intervention agreed on by the patient and caregivers. Once the cardiac diagnosis is made and symptoms are controlled surgically or pharmacologically, exercise may begin as in other kinds of cardiac rehabilitation situations. Both resistance training and aerobic exercise are safe and effective in such patients. Resistance training is sometimes more tolerable than aerobic training in patients with a low threshold for ischemia because of the more modest HR response and nonsustained blood pressure response to resistive exercise, resulting in a lower average double product (heart rate–pressure product). The double product is a noninvasive index of myocardial oxygen demand and therefore can be used as a marker of the ischemic threshold. In addition, diastolic pressure and therefore coronary perfusion tends to rise rather than fall, minimizing ischemic potential. The same precautions listed previously that reduce the risk of blood pressure and intraocular pressure elevations are relevant here to minimize the likelihood of ischemia in this setting. A small proportion of patients will have uncontrolled ischemia at rest despite treatment, and exercise is contraindicated in such individuals.

Management of Older Adults with No Exclusions to Exercise

All the listed conditions (*Table 36-5*) are indications to exercise, rather than reasons to limit exercise participation (57). This assumes that the condition is currently medically managed and no recent changes in symptoms or level of disease have occurred. Reintroduction of exercise after prolonged periods of injury or convalescence is crucial to prevent functional decline.

EXERCISE PRESCRIPTION IN OLDER ADULTS

Exercise Prescription Implementation: Prioritize Physical Activity Needs in Relation to Risks

After initial screening, many problems and needs will be identified in the typically sedentary older individual. It is therefore important to know how to deliver the prescription in logical stages that are palatable and feasible. In most cases, it is recommended to start with one component of exercise (balance, strength, endurance, flexibility) and allow the older adult a time to get comfortable with the new routine of exercise before adding other components. This approach requires attention to risk factors, medical history, physical examination findings, and personal preferences and will be different for each individual.

If significant deficits in muscle strength or balance are identified, these should be addressed before the initiation of aerobic training. Prescribing progressive aerobic training in the absence of sufficient balance or strength is likely to result in knee pain, fear of falling, falls, and limited ability to progress aerobically. Attempting to ambulate those who cannot lift themselves out of a chair or maintain standing balance is a suboptimal approach. Paying attention to the physiologic determinants of transfer ability and ambulation,

and targeting these specifically with the appropriate exercise prescription when reversible deficits are uncovered, is recommended.

In some cases, the older adults may benefit equally from resistance and aerobic training (*e.g.*, for the treatment of depression), but exercise prescription decisions are made based on their ability to tolerate one form of exercise over another (11,112). Severe osteoarthritis of the knee, recurrent falls, and a low threshold for ischemia may make resistance training safer or more tolerable than aerobic training as an antidepressant treatment. Prioritization requires careful consideration of the risks and benefits of each mode of activity as well as current health status and physical fitness level.

Aerobic Activity

Cardiovascular endurance training refers to the exercise in which large muscle groups contract repeatedly against little or no resistance other than that imposed by gravity. The purpose of this type of training is to increase the maximal amount of aerobic work that can be carried out as well as to decrease the physiologic response and perceived difficulty of submaximal aerobic workloads. Extensive adaptations in the cardiopulmonary system, peripheral skeletal muscle, circulation, and metabolism are responsible for these changes in exercise capacity and tolerance. Many types of exercise fall into this category, including walking, hiking, running, dancing, stair climbing, biking, swimming, rowing, and cross-country skiing. The key distinguishing feature between activities that are primarily aerobic versus anabolic in nature is the larger degree of overload to the muscle in resistance training. Resistance training causes the kinds of adaptations in the nervous system and muscle that lead to marked strength gain and hypertrophy.

Modes of Aerobic Exercise

The decision about how to train aerobically depends on factors such as preference, access, likelihood of injury, health-related restrictions, and desired benefits. Although there are differences in oxygen consumption among various kinds of aerobic exercise, personal preference has the strongest link to long-term compliance. Most activities, when performed regularly, can contribute to improvements in cardiovascular efficiency, reduction of metabolic risk factors, and reduced risk of many chronic diseases.

Two other factors assume importance regarding aerobic exercise modality in older adults and in women in particular. The first is the differential effects of various aerobic activities on bone mineral density (BMD). It is clear from recent meta-analyses (63,84,85) that the beneficial effect of exercise on bone in older adults is both modality and intensity dependent. Clinical trials of low-impact, low-intensity exercises such as stretching/calisthenics or low-intensity weightlifting in postmenopausal women have not been shown to significantly improve BMD compared to controls at any site (63,85). Walking alone has not been shown to significantly improve BMD at the spine or hip or reduce fractures in randomized clinical trials (RCTs) (63,85), although earlier epidemiological studies suggested this. Thus, older recommendations (12) suggesting that basic weight-bearing exercise, such as simple walking, is sufficient for optimization of bone health, are not consistent with the most robust evidence from RCTs to date (85). High-impact activities, such as jogging, jumping, and running, although beneficial for bone formation in children and premenopausal women (61,67), have been associated with high rates of knee and ankle injuries, even in healthy older adults, and have not yet been shown to increase BMD by themselves in older women (7). A recent meta-analysis of seven controlled trials in postmenopausal women found that high or novel impact-only protocols were ineffective in increasing BMD at any site (84). However, the combination of such high-impact exercise and high-intensity resistance training was effective for BMD improvements (63,81). In older adults with preexisting arthritis, such high-impact activities are neither feasible nor recommended because they are more likely to result in injuries and exacerbations of arthritis in this cohort. Balancing the skeletal need for weight-bearing or high-impact loading and the safety requirements of the joints and connective tissues for low-impact loading favors exercises such as walking, dancing, hiking, or stair climbing over running, step aerobics, or jumping rope. Men and women without underlying arthritis may perform high-impact activities safely as long as muscle and ligament strength and joint structure are normal, or if the activities are combined with or preceded by resistance training. Concurrent resistance training may prevent much of the joint problems and injuries incurred during typical high-impact aerobic pursuits, but this remains to be shown experimentally.

Overall, walking and its derivations are the most widely studied, feasible, safe, accessible, and economical mode of aerobic training for men and women of most ages and states of health. These activities do not require special equipment or locations and do not need to be taught or supervised (except in the individuals who are cognitively impaired, very frail, or medically unstable). Walking bears a natural relationship to ordinary ADLs, making it easier to integrate into lifestyle and functional tasks than any other mode of exercise. Therefore, it is theoretically more likely to translate into improved functional independence and mobility than other types of aerobic exercise.

Intensity of Aerobic Exercise

The intensity of aerobic exercise refers to the amount of oxygen consumed ($\dot{V}O_2$) or energy expended per minute while performing the activity, which will vary from about 5 kcal $\cdot$ min^{-1} for light activities, to 7.5 kcal $\cdot$ min^{-1} for moderate activities, and to 10–12 kcal $\cdot$ min^{-1} for very heavy activities. Energy expenditure increases with increasing body weight for weight-bearing aerobic activities as well as with inclusion of larger muscle mass and increased work (force × distance) and power output (work/time) demands of the activity. The most intensive activities are those that involve the muscles of the arms, legs, and trunk simultaneously; necessitate moving the full body weight through space; and are done at a rapid pace (e.g., cross-country skiing). Adding extra loads to the body weight (backpack, weight belt, wrist weights) increases the force needed to move the body parts through space and therefore increases the aerobic intensity of the work performed.

The intensity of aerobic work can be calculated by measuring the actual consumption of oxygen using measurements of inspired and expired gases, which are analyzed for their oxygen and carbon dioxide content. Because this method is normally only available in research facilities or clinical laboratories, estimations are usually made by assessing cardiovascular responses or subjective rating of effort by the participant. In normal individuals in sinus rhythm, the rise in HR is directly proportional to the increasing oxygen consumption or aerobic workload. Thus, monitoring HR has traditionally been a primary means of both prescribing appropriate intensity levels as well as following training adaptations when direct measurements of oxygen consumption are not available. The HRR method is the most useful estimate of intensity, and training is normally recommended at a moderate (40%–59%) to vigorous (60%–89%) level (50). Calculation of target HRs using HRR is described in *Chapter 30*.

Difficulties with an intensity prescription based on HR in older adults include the presence of arrhythmias, pacemakers, or β-blockers (systemic or ophthalmologic) that may alter the HR response to exercise. An easier and more obtainable estimate of aerobic intensity is to prescribe a moderate level as 12–14 ("somewhat hard") or a vigorous level as 15–17 ("hard") on the 6–20 RPE Scale (13). (Similar intensities on the 0–10 scale are 5–6 for moderate and 7–8 for vigorous.) At a moderate level, the exerciser should note increased pulse and respiratory rate but still be able to talk. This scale has been validated for use in men and women, young and old, those with coronary disease, and healthy adults and is therefore of widespread applicability (70). This scale is easy to teach and is a means to "supervise" training intensity from afar by means of written diaries or telephone calls, making it cost-effective in community programs and health care settings. Usually, a visual representation of the RPE Scale is used to increase accuracy, but assessment can be done without this prop in patients who are blind or cannot read.

As is the case with all forms of exercise, to maintain the same relative training intensity over time, the absolute

TABLE 36-6. Increasing the Intensity of Aerobic Exercise for Older Adults

Mode of Exercise	Ways to Increase Intensity
Walking	Add small weights around wrists Swing arms Use "race walking" style Add inclines, hills, stairs Carry weighted backpack or waist belt[a] Push a wheelchair or stroller (with someone in it)
Cycling	Increase pedaling speed Increase resistance to pedals Add hills Add backpack[a] Add child carrier to back of bike
Water activities	Use arms and legs in strokes Add resistive equipment for water Increase pace
Tennis	Convert from doubles to singles game
Golf	Carry golf clubs[a] Eliminate golf cart
Dance	Increase pace of movements Add more arm and leg movements

[a]Avoid flexing the spine when doing this to prevent excessive compressive forces on the thoracic spine.

training load must be increased as fitness improves. In younger individuals, walking may be changed to jogging and then running to increase intensity as needed. More appropriate in older or frail adults are progressive alterations in workload that increase energy expenditure without converting to a high-impact form of activity. Examples of how to prescribe such progression for various modes of aerobic exercise are given in *Table 36-6*. Workloads should be progressed based on the ratings of effort at each training session. Once the perceived exertion slips below 11–12 ("fairly light") on the RPE Scale, the workload should be increased to maintain the physiologic stimulus for continued cardiovascular adaptation. As with resistance training, the most common error in aerobic training is failure to progress, which results in an early suboptimal plateau in cardiovascular and metabolic improvement.

Volume of Aerobic Exercise

In most very old, frail adults, aerobic exercise is not used for the *prevention* of premature mortality, CVD, diabetes, or hypertension, or for the treatment of obesity. It is therefore likely that 60–120 min of exercise each week will be sufficient to provide benefits in maximal and submaximal cardiovascular efficiency, psychological well-being, and control of chronic diseases such as arthritis, diabetes, peripheral vascular disease, chronic lung disease, coronary artery disease, and congestive heart failure, for example (99). It should be noted, however, that little research on aerobic training in very

old or frail adults has been conducted, and most recommendations are simply extrapolated from studies in younger individuals. For older adults in general, the standard adult guidelines of 150–300 min · wk^{-1} of moderate intensity, or 75–150 min · wk^{-1} of vigorous intensity, are recommended (1).

It has been shown that aerobic exercise does not need to be carried out at a single session to provide training effects and may be broken up into 10 min bouts to reach the desired volume of training (99). Shorter sessions have not been evaluated for efficacy, although public health recommendations for integrating short bouts of 5 min into the daily routine have been recently made. Very frail adults may initially only tolerate 2–5 min of walking or other aerobic activities, and a reasonable goal is to increase tolerance for longer workloads until 10–20 min of exercise can be sustained without resting. This would provide substantial functional benefits in the nursing home because walking for 20 min would likely enable the older adults to get to almost any location in the home without having to stop and rest.

Overall, a session or sessions of aerobic exercise carried out at least once every 3 d adding up to 60 min · wk^{-1} appears to be the minimal prescription based on currently available literature. Higher volumes of exercise such as 30 min · d^{-1}, 5 d · wk^{-1} are frequently recommended (1). It is not recommended to exercise long bouts once or twice a week as an alternative to several shorter sessions because this is likely to result in overuse muscle soreness and injuries. The risk of sudden death during physical activity appears to be limited to those who do not exercise on a regular basis (at least 1 h · wk^{-1}), which is another reason for advocating regular, moderate doses of exercise rather than periodic high-volume training.

Supervision and Setting

Most people will be familiar with the basic principles of common forms of aerobic exercise (*e.g.*, walking, biking, swimming), so this is frequently carried out in unsupervised settings. Exceptions to this general rule may be made in special circumstances, such as in cardiac rehabilitation settings or with frail adults, when safety may be a concern. In addition, when new techniques are introduced (*e.g.*, aerobic dance, aqua aerobics) or when compliance needs to be more intensively monitored for efficacy (as in the treatment of obesity or diabetes), supervision may be required. It is often possible to graduate to a partially monitored program after a new routine has been established to increase flexibility and yet maintain reinforcing contact and supervision. A group setting or supervised program does not automatically ensure higher exercise compliance in older adults. King et al. have shown that *choice* is the most important determinant of compliance, and if barriers to supervised participation away from home (such as dislike of group exercise, need to care for a family member, lack of transportation, financial costs, inclement weather, inconvenient scheduling, or work commitments) outweigh the benefits (perceived safety, access to trainers, support of group members, socialization), there is no advantage to prescribing center-based, supervised exercise (72). Assessing an older adult's preferences is the most important factor in the early prescription process to avoid failure and behavioral relapse.

Monitoring Progress

The best way to monitor progress in an aerobic training program is to review a participant's activity log, including frequency, duration, and HR or RPE of exercise sessions. This can be simply recorded on an ordinary calendar posted on the refrigerator in the spaces for each day of the month, as follows:

Walking, 20 min, RPE 14

If such monthly calendars are reviewed periodically by a member of the health care team, advice can be given on a timely basis about patterns, volume, and intensity of exercise to enhance compliance and optimize efficacy. For example, if an individual with diabetes is noted to be exercising long bouts at 5 d intervals, advice may be given to change to shorter bouts every 3 d. Events that typically trigger long bouts of noncompliance (*e.g.*, illness, injury, depression, work commitments, vacation, babysitting responsibilities) can be identified, and relapse prevention strategies are put into place to avert such patterns.

Benefits of Aerobic Exercise

The benefits of aerobic exercise have been extensively studied over the past 40 yr, and the most important of these for older adults are listed in *Table 36-7*. They include a broad range of physiologic adaptations that are opposite to the effects of aging on most body systems as well as major health-related clinical outcomes. The health conditions responsive to aerobic exercise include most of those of concern to older adults: osteoporosis, heart disease, stroke, breast cancer, diabetes, obesity, hypertension, arthritis, depression, and insomnia (100). These physiologic and clinical benefits form the basis for the inclusion of aerobic exercise as an essential component of the overall physical activity prescription for healthy aging.

Risks of Aerobic Exercise

The major potential risks associated with aerobic exercise are listed in *Table 36-8*. Most of these adverse events are preventable with attention to the underlying medical conditions present, appropriate choice of exercise modality, avoiding exercise during extreme environmental conditions, wearing proper footwear and clothing, and minimizing or avoiding exercise during acute illness or in the presence of new, undefined symptoms. All older adults should have yearly ophthalmologic examinations

for glaucoma and retinal changes, and therefore, exercise programming should be delayed until this routine health screen has been completed to avoid complications. If someone has had recent ophthalmologic surgery, exercise is contraindicated for several weeks to avoid

TABLE 36-7. Benefits of Aerobic Exercise in Older Adults

Physiologic Adaptation	Prevention or Treatment of Disease
Increased bone density	Arthritis
Decreased total body and visceral adipose tissue	Breast cancer
Decreased fibrinogen levels	Chronic insomnia
Decreased sympathetic and hormonal response to exercise	Colon cancer
Decreased LDL, increased HDL levels	Coronary artery disease
Decreased postural blood pressure response to stressors	Depression
Increased heart rate variability	Hyperlipidemia
Increased neural reaction time	Hypertension
Increased blood volume and hematocrit	Impotence
Increased energy expenditure	Obesity
Increased glycogen storage in skeletal muscle	Osteoporosis
Increased oxidative enzyme capacity in skeletal muscle	Overall and cardiovascular mortality
Increased glucose disposal rate	Peripheral vascular disease
Increased mitochondrial volume density in skeletal muscle	Prostate cancer
Decreased resting heart rate and blood pressure	Stroke
Increased GLUT4 receptors in skeletal muscle	Type 2 diabetes mellitus
Decreased arterial stiffness	
Increased maximal aerobic capacity	
Increased stroke volume during exercise[a]	
Increased capillary density in skeletal muscle	
Increased insulin sensitivity	
Improved glucose tolerance	
Increased cardiac contractility during exercise[a]	
Decreased heart rate/BP response to submaximal exercise	
Increased oxygen extraction by skeletal muscle	

LDL, low-density lipoprotein; HDL, high-density lipoprotein; GLUT4, glucose transporter; BP, blood pressure.

[a]Observed only in older endurance-trained men thus far.

TABLE 36-8. The Risks of Aerobic Exercise in Older Adults

Musculoskeletal	Cardiovascular	Metabolic
Falls	Arrhythmia	Dehydration
Foot ulceration or laceration	Cardiac failure	Electrolyte imbalance
Fracture, osteoporotic or traumatic	Hypertension	Energy imbalance
Hemorrhoids[a]	Hypotension	Heat stroke
Hernia[a]	Ischemia	Hyperglycemia
Joint or bursa inflammation, exacerbation of arthritis	Pulmonary embolism	Hypoglycemia
Ligament or tendon strain or rupture	Retinal hemorrhage or detachment, lens detachment	Hypothermia
Muscle soreness or tear	Ruptured cerebral or other aneurysm	Seizures
Stress incontinence	Syncope or postural symptoms	

[a]Primarily associated with increased intra-abdominal pressure during resistive exercise but may occur if Valsalva maneuver occurs during aerobic activities.

raising intraocular pressure, and specific recommendations should be obtained from the ophthalmologist. Metabolic complications are rare unless diabetes is out of control at the time exercise is initiated or dehydration or acute illness is present. Most fluid balance problems can be handled by only exercising in reasonable temperature and humidity and drinking extra fluid on exercise days.

Cardiovascular complications are most likely if ischemic heart disease is not well controlled medically or surgically before exercise initiation, if warning signs are ignored, or if sudden vigorous exercise is attempted by a previously sedentary individual. When exercising appropriately, both aerobic and resistance training have been shown to reduce the incidence of angina and medication use in cardiac rehabilitation settings and are indicated as part of standard medical management of coronary artery disease. Although claudication is mentioned as a possible adverse side effect of exercise in those with peripheral vascular disease, aerobic exercise has been shown to significantly increase exercise tolerance in these patients (*i.e.*, increased time to claudication) (51). However, some studies have suggested that it is most effective if exercise is continued for 30–90 s after the onset of claudication and then a rest period taken. This is different from angina or any of the other symptoms listed in *Table 36-8*, where exercise should be stopped immediately if they occur. Insisting on continuing exercise after the onset of claudication pain may result in aversion to physical activity and thus is not required. Many studies not prescribing exercise in this way have also been shown to significantly improve peripheral arterial disease symptoms.

Musculoskeletal problems are more common than any other risk of aerobic exercise, particularly in the novice or very frail older adult. Often, if significant weakness or balance impairment is present, it is best to avoid aerobic exercise altogether until strength and balance have been improved sufficiently to allow safe weight-bearing exercises such as walking. If this is not done, falls, arthritis pain, fear of falling, and muscle fatigue will be limiting, and effective aerobic training will be precluded. Gently warming up

muscles with slow movements before aerobic exercise is important to avoid soft tissue injury. Avoid high-impact activities such as jumping, step aerobics, and jogging in those with arthritis or weak muscles and ligaments because this is a principle cause of sports-related injury.

Muscle-Strengthening Activity

Progressive resistance training (PRT) is one of the four basic modalities of exercise that is recommended for older adults as part of a balanced physical activity program, whether this is formalized as an exercise prescription or integrated into lifestyle changes. PRT is the process of challenging the skeletal muscle with an unaccustomed stimulus, or load, such that neural and muscle tissue adaptations take place, leading ultimately to increased muscle force producing capacity (strength) and muscle mass. In this kind of exercise, the muscle is contracted slowly a few times in each session against a relatively heavy load. Any muscle may be trained in this way, although usually, 8–10 major muscle groups with clinical relevance are trained for a balanced and functional outcome (116,122).

Equipment

Equipment to carry out PRT (121) ranges from only body weight to technologically sophisticated pneumatic or hydraulic resistance training machines. In general, in the older adult, machine-based training allows the most robust adaptations to be achieved, offers maximum safety, and requires less technique. Free weights, on the other hand, offer significant advantages in terms of cost and flexibility in programming, may provide a better stimulus for motor coordination and balance, and are the only option in most home and limited-space settings.

Intensity

Many consensus panels have recommended that elderly or frail adults should initially use a lower intensity (approximately 60% of 1-RM, or a weight that can be lifted 10–15 times before fatiguing). However, most of the RCTs of resistance training in older adults that have resulted in large gains in strength have used an intensity of approximately 80% of 1-RM after a short period of adaptation. There is little evidence that this intensity is unsafe or poorly tolerated in men or women, healthy or frail, up to 100 yr of age (47,110), or those in early outpatient cardiac rehabilitation (116). By contrast, low-intensity training results in negligible or modest gains in strength and associated clinical benefits (38,108) and is therefore not recommended as the optimal mode of training if the primary intent is to increase muscle size and strength.

Volume

The volume of resistance training refers to the frequency of sessions and the number of sets and repetitions (lifts) performed during each session for each muscle group. This subject has generated a great deal of debate among scientists, trainers, and athletes, but a review of the existing scientific data does allow useful conclusions to be drawn.

Frequency

Depending on the access to training, motivation of the individual, and other circumstances, training frequency should be tailored to maximize adherence without compromising physiologic and clinical benefits. It is most effective to recommend training frequencies of $3 \text{ d} \cdot \text{wk}^{-1}$ in the older adult. Because long-term compliance generally does not exceed 60%–70% of recommendations, two sessions per week on average will be performed. Thus, a reasonable physiologic response is achievable. If only one session per week is planned, and it is missed due to illness, vacation, or other activities, then 2 full weeks elapse between training, which may result in lost strength, disruption of progress, soreness, or loss of commitment to the new behavior. In addition, with only one session per week (with the possible exception of trunk muscle training) (102), it will take longer for a level of competence and clinical benefit to be reached that will lead to sustained adherence.

Some individuals like to train every day, particularly if they notice psychological benefits from participation. This can be accomplished by exercising different muscle groups on different days, for example, arm exercises on Monday, Wednesday, and Friday and leg exercises on Tuesday, Thursday, and Saturday. This allows individual muscle groups to recover between training sessions but provides an activity $6 \text{ d} \cdot \text{wk}^{-1}$. Such shorter sessions (15–20 min) may fit better into some schedules than a few long sessions each week and may, thus, enhance overall compliance. A similar approach has been advocated with cardiovascular training because intermittent short bouts of exercise appear to be as beneficial as longer sessions. In all cases, a balance must be achieved between preferences, convenience, barriers such as time

or transportation, access to trainers or equipment, and known physiologic requirements before a rational prescription can be formulated that maximizes compliance and adaptation.

Setting and Supervision

Resistance training is a novel activity for most older men and women, and supervision is recommended initially to ensure proper technique, provide confidence, and ensure progression to appropriate levels of intensity. This supervision may take the form of hands-on training or a combination of visits, videos, telephone calls, mail, or feedback on activity logs. Most unsupervised weight-lifting programs in older adults suffer more from low intensity than from low compliance. This will markedly limit adaptations that accrue and therefore needs to be addressed in any program implementation or exercise prescription. Success in getting older adults to progress to higher weights requires continuous supervision, although this may gradually shift from direct supervision to more remote means of providing feedback. Given adherence to the principles of intensity, form, and volume, the setting is flexible and will primarily depend on issues such as cost, transportation, availability of trainers, spouse, or other dependent needs at home, living situation, health status, cognition, and functional or mobility impairments. Cognitive impairment does not preclude training, but it does mandate long-term supervision. It has been demonstrated that compliance is highest when older adults are allowed to choose the setting in which they exercise. It is incorrectly assumed that all older adults want to exercise in a group (72). A major factor that predicts lack of involvement in a nursing home exercise program is the patient's characteristic of not participating in groups of any kind as assessed by the nursing staff. So determination of such barriers to adoption and preferences for setting is crucial to successful behavior change in relation to all modes of exercise.

Benefits

Increases in muscle size and strength following appropriate PRT are not seen with other forms of exercise and are also not obtainable with low-intensity PRT. Therefore, if a primary goal of exercise is to prevent or treat sarcopenia, there is no effective substitute for this modality of exercise. The hypertrophic response to training does appear to be affected by health status, anabolic hormonal milieu, nutritional substrate availability, changes in protein synthesis with age, and other factors yet to be identified (20,74,83,90,120,121). Suggestions that women do not undergo hypertrophy as effectively as men appear to be partially related to differences in training intensity and age of the trial subjects as well as a probable sex difference in training adaptation because of hormonal milieu. It is clear that exogenous anabolic steroids can augment the hypertrophic response to resistive exercise in young men (73); they appear to have the same effect in older men as well (14). However, trials with growth hormone or its secretagogues, or estrogen, have thus far largely failed to show significant benefit in terms of muscle mass or strength in older adults when given alone or in combination with resistance training.

Risks

PRT has been considered a relatively risky form of exercise in the past and has therefore been sometimes avoided by health care professionals in their counseling of older adults. However, a wealth of literature over the past 20 yr indicates that this modality of exercise is in fact quite safe and is more feasible in many groups of patients and frail elders than is cardiovascular exercise, as illustrated in *Box 36-1*. There are few medical contraindications to PRT, as outlined in *Box 36-2*. Apart from these specific circumstances, resistance training is a realistic option even in very frail elderly individuals. Frailty is not a contraindication to strength training but conversely one of the most important reasons to prescribe it.

The potential risks of resistance training are primarily musculoskeletal injury and cardiovascular events. Musculoskeletal injury is preventable with attention to the following points:

- Adherence to proper form
- Isolation of the targeted muscle group
- Slow velocity of lifting
- Limitation of range of motion to the pain-free arc of movement
- Avoidance of momentum and ballistic movements to complete a lift
- Use of machines or chairs with good back support
- Use of rest periods between sets and rest days between sessions

---

BOX 36-1 | **Indications for Choosing Resistance Training over Aerobic Training**

- Severe arthritis preventing weight-bearing activity
- Lower extremity fracture with casting
- Inability to support body weight
- Foot ulceration or ankle injury
- Severe balance disorder or recurrent falls precluding safe standing or walking
- Amputation of lower extremities without prostheses
- Chronic lung disease and hypoxia with aerobic exercise
- Low threshold for ischemia with aerobic exercise

BOX 36-2 | **Medical Contraindications to Resistance Training**

- Unstable angina, untreated severe left main coronary artery disease
- Angina, hypotension, or arrhythmias provoked by resistance training
- Significant exacerbation of musculoskeletal pain with resistance training
- End-stage congestive heart failure
- Failure to thrive, terminal illness
- Severe valvular heart disease

A distinction should be made between delayed onset muscle soreness (DOMS), a normal response to the initiation or increase in intensity of PRT, and an acute musculoskeletal injury such as a ligament tear, sprain, hernia, or muscle rupture. DOMS presents as a dull, diffuse aching sensation over the trained muscle group that starts the day following exercise and peaks about 48 h after the session and may take several days to completely resolve. This symptom complex gradually diminishes and disappears in the first few weeks of continuous training but will resurface after interruptions to the training schedule. Delayed onset muscle soreness is related to the damage caused to the muscle by mechanical stretch and loading, which in turn stimulates a reactive inflammatory response, characterized by damage to muscle cell membranes, cytokine elevations, intracellular edema, and leukocyte infiltrates (31). Ultimately, this process is not harmful and does not need to be suppressed or treated because the repair to this damage results in a desirable adaptation of increased protein synthesis and fiber hypertrophy. Eccentric (lowering, lengthening) contraction produces most of the damage. However, because the damage ultimately leads to hypertrophy, eccentric contractions should not be avoided but in fact be emphasized in training programs for older adults with low muscle mass.

An acute injury, by contrast, will be felt during or just after the exercise session itself and is more likely to be perceived as sudden in onset, sharp, easily localizable, often allowing identification of the exact site of injury. Such events should always provoke a response known as RICE:

- Rest
- Ice
- Compression
- Elevation

Ice can be applied via use of a cold pack for 15–20 min every hour in the acute phase. Compression with an elastic bandage so as to limit fluid accumulation will minimize pain, as does elevating the injured site. Such a protocol serves to immobilize the affected joint and lessen the edema and inflammatory infiltrate that will otherwise occur. If there is a dislocation, fracture, or other serious injury, stabilization of the bones and ligaments is crucial before definitive diagnosis and treatment. Weight bearing and all other activity should be restricted until appropriate medical care is available.

In patients with preexisting arthritis, there may be intermittent exacerbation of joint symptoms or inflammation with the initiation of PRT. However, the overall effect of training is to decrease chronic arthritis pain over time (45,64,103,107). During periods of disease flare-up, it may be necessary to switch to isometric contractions, lower the weight lifted, limit the range of motion through which the load is lifted, or insert additional days of rest between training sessions. It is advisable to continue isometric contractions because this will prevent loss of strength during periods of flare-up. Once the symptoms have lessened, normal exercise sessions may resume.

The circulatory response to PRT has been a matter of controversy, and there is much misperception about the actual changes that occur. Blood pressure changes are difficult to measure during PRT because of the transient nature of the rises and the fact that blood pressure falls almost immediately after a repetition is completed. This makes monitoring of intra-arterial pressure the only accurate way to gather such information. A study of these factors has been completed in older men by Benn et al. (8) and additional reviews of the literature provided by McCartney (86). The HR response to PRT is generally lower than the response to aerobic exercise such as walking up an incline or stair climbing. The increase in systolic blood pressure tends to be similar between walking and stair climbing. Diastolic pressure elevations are greater with PRT than aerobic exercise, thus increasing mean arterial pressure to a greater degree. The rate–pressure product (the product of systolic blood pressure and HR), which is representative of myocardial oxygen demand, is greatest for stair climbing, followed by weightlifting and walking. The authors concluded from these studies that older adults engaged in high-intensity weightlifting exercise are exposed to no greater peak circulatory stress than that created by a few minutes of inclined walking and much less than that elicited by climbing three to four flights of stairs. In addition, the double product during weightlifting and some forms of aerobic work are similar; the contribution of HR is much higher in aerobic work, whereas the mean pressure is higher in weightlifting. The slower HR and increased diastolic pressure during PRT compared with aerobic work would facilitate diastolic filling and coronary artery perfusion, both desirable outcomes in an older individual, particularly one with diastolic dysfunction (impaired relaxation and filling) or coronary artery disease (15). Consistent

with these observations are the reports of patients who exhibit ischemia or angina during treadmill work but not during weightlifting exercises at a similar elevation of the double product. In the largest series of maximum strength tests, in 26,000 individuals undergoing testing, no cardiovascular event occurred (54). Additionally, the literature suggests a reduction in ischemic signs and symptoms after PRT in patients with heart disease, attesting to the safety of this form of exercise.

In contrast to typical weightlifting regimens, the response to a sustained isometric contraction of a small muscle mass is a more substantial increase in arterial pressure; therefore, this mode of training is not recommended. Circulatory responses increase with the intensity of the relative load and the number of repetitions in a set. Intrathoracic pressure during a Valsalva maneuver, which is transmitted directly to the arterial vasculature, also causes a rise in blood pressure. The Valsalva maneuver is difficult to avoid when lifting loads is >85% of 1-RM and is invoked with lower loads when muscles are fatigued. Thus, keeping lifting intensity at 80% of 1-RM and limiting sets to eight repetitions (rather than "to fatigue" as has sometimes been suggested) should minimize the contribution to circulatory stress during the Valsalva. The circulatory response is lowest during the eccentric (lengthening) phase of the contraction and highest during the static and early part of the concentric phase. Emphasizing the duration of the eccentric contraction will both moderate cardiovascular stress and maximize hypertrophic adaptations and is thus highly recommended for older adults in particular. A summary of the major factors related to circulatory responses in weightlifting exercise is presented in Box 36-3.

Patients with unstable cardiovascular signs and symptoms, as noted in Box 36-2, should not begin any exercise regimen, including weightlifting, without medical evaluation.

BOX 36-3	**Factors Related to Increased Circulatory Stress during Resistance Training**

- Higher relative intensity of load lifted
- Static contractions
- Early phase of concentric contraction
- Greater muscle mass used
- Performance of a Valsalva maneuver
- Increasing number of repetitions
- Fatigue of muscles

Circulatory stress, increase of heart rate and blood pressure in response to resistive exercise.

Special Considerations in Older Men and Women

Older men and women will lift lower absolute loads than younger adults because of their generally smaller muscle mass, but the relative load recommended is the same after initial introduction and learning of proper technique. The adaptations observed in older men and women should be similar to those seen in their younger counterparts.

Special consideration should be given to erector spinae and upper back muscles, which contribute to back extension (104). Stimulation of these muscle groups will strengthen the bones of the thoracic and lumbar spine and counteract the forces promoting osteopenic vertebral compression fractures in high-risk men and women. In addition, isometric and dynamic exercises including scapular retraction and depression will attenuate the upward migration of the humeral head, which otherwise promotes the common problems of subacromial bursitis, impingement syndromes, and rotator cuff degeneration and tears.

Falls and disorders of gait and balance are prevalent in older men and women, and therefore, training programs should include the ankle dorsiflexors and plantar flexors, hip abductors, hip extensors, and knee extensors and flexors if possible. Those who are wheelchair restricted will benefit from triceps and shoulder exercises to increase wheelchair mobility and independence in transfers.

Abdominal muscle strengthening is important to many older men and women for perceived aesthetic reasons (even in 90-yr-old patients in nursing homes) and to therapists for its contribution to good posture, balance, and control of low back pain symptoms because of degenerative changes in the spine and surrounding tissues.

Monitoring Progress

It is imperative to monitor progress in PRT because adaptation depends on maintenance of the training stimulus, which requires continuous increases in absolute load. Techniques suitable for enhancing compliance are discussed in *Chapters 45* and *46* of this *Resource Manual* and *Chapter 11* of *GETP9*, but regarding this modality of training, the need for documentation of the training load, by the individual or the trainer, is paramount (127). Providing this feedback in graphic form is particularly useful for reinforcing the presence or absence of appropriate progression because training loads should increase steadily and continuously if appropriate technique is being followed. For some individuals, it may be important to monitor target symptoms or functions that may change during the course of training, such as angina, shortness of breath, falls, insomnia, depressive symptoms, ability to climb stairs, use of assistive devices, fear of falling, blood glucose levels, waist, and arm or calf circumference. Deciding what goals are important

and realistic at the beginning of an exercise program and monitoring progress in domains that are meaningful to the older adult will provide the most effective motivation. Because strength increases are usually the most dramatic outcome, periodic testing of maximum strength may be helpful for reevaluating goals. Another option is a simple test of recording the amount of time it takes to stand up and sit down for 5 or 10 times in a row. Results will provide a proxy index of lower extremity muscle power. In addition, the perceived exertion in response to lifting the weights that were used in the first week of training can be remeasured over time to demonstrate how much easier tasks that once seemed difficult are after training. Any adverse events attributable to the exercise should also be tracked so that appropriate investigation and/or adjustments in training regimens can be made.

Enhancing Balance with Resistance Training

Standard high-intensity PRT has been shown to improve mobility and balance (94). The feasibility and efficacy of a specific balance-enhancing technique incorporated directly into the PRT routine in a group of older adults (average age 84 yr) with a history of falls or gait and balance problems have been recently tested. As outlined in *Box 36-4*, participants were instructed to gradually reduce the hand support during their standing weight-lifting exercises but otherwise follow the general principles outlined previously. They exercised 3 d · wk^{-1} over a 12-wk period. The balance-enhancing postural exercises targeted hip extensors, hip flexors, hip abductors, knee flexors, and plantar flexors. This training regimen resulted in large improvements in static and dynamic balance as follows:

Usual gait speed:	6% increase
Maximal gait speed:	10% increase
Tandem stand time:	162% increase
One-legged stand time:	126% increase
Tandem walk time:	6% increase
Errors made during tandem walk:	55% decrease

BOX 36-4 | **Adding Balance Training to Resistive Exercises**

Step 1: Hold onto chair or table with two hands during standing resistive exercises (hip flexion, hip abduction, hip extension, knee flexion, and plantar flexion).

Step 2: Hold on with one hand only.

Step 3: Hold on with one fingertip only.

Step 4: Keep both hands 2 in above chair or table.

Even if an adult does not have balance impairments at the time of initial prescription, it is prudent to include standard balancing exercises in his or her prescription to prevent decrements from occurring in the future. Studies are continuing on the long-term adaptations to this enhanced form of resistance training.

Integration of Strength Training into Daily Activities

Although PRT is usually conceptualized as a discreet "exercise" activity, there are ways of incorporating elements of PRT into daily life in the same way that aerobic activities are incorporated. The guiding principles underlying such incorporation are listed in *Table 36-9*.

Balance Exercises for Frequent Fallers or Individuals with Mobility Problems

Balance training is probably the least well defined of the various exercise modalities. Despite the use of balance-enhancing modalities for decades by physical therapists and others working with adults and children with developmental or degenerative neurologic diseases affecting balance, only recently have there been well-controlled formalized studies of techniques and outcomes (21,75,99). The recognition that balance impairment is a risk factor for falls and hip fracture even in adults without identifiable neurologic disease has expanded the potential target population for balance training to the general aging cohort. The pressing need for definitive outcome data on feasibility and efficacy of various intervention techniques has stimulated quantitative research that will assist in the development of clinical protocols. In the meantime, the balance prescription must be formulated from various evidence collected in epidemiologic studies, experimental trials, and clinical practice. It should be noted that in many cases, it is difficult to compare the results across trials because investigators have used unique training interventions and different outcome measures (21,24,66,106,109).

Any activity that increases one's ability to maintain balance in the face of a threat to stability may be considered a balance-enhancing activity. Common stressors include the following:

- Narrowing the base of support
- Perturbation of the ground support
- Decrease in proprioceptive sensation
- Diminished or misleading visual inputs
- Disturbed vestibular system input
- Increased compliance of the support surface
- Movement of the center of mass of the body away from the vertical

On a day-to-day basis, stressors may also include things such as environmental hazards, postural hypotension, and drugs that affect central nervous system function. The plethora of conditions that contribute to gait and balance abnormalities in older adults requires a multifactorial approach to balance enhancement and falls prevention. Presented later in this chapter is a summary of exercise techniques that have favorable effects on this physiologic capacity and therefore forms an important part of the exercise prescription for older adults.

Balance-enhancing activities affect the central nervous system control of balance and coordination of movement and augment the peripheral neuromuscular system response to signals that balance is threatened. Resistance training improves balance by enhancing the strength of postural control muscles of the trunk and lower

TABLE 36-9. Incorporating Strengthening into Daily Activities	
Principle	**Examples**
Use smallest possible muscle mass to accomplish task.	Rise from a chair without using arms to assist. Lift heavy objects with one arm instead of two. Stand on one leg. Climb stairs using hands only lightly for balance on rails.
Resist gravity.	Sit down slowly. Lower body weight slowly up and down stairs. Lower packages slowly. Lift slowly rather than swinging objects into position.
Do not use momentum to assist with tasks.	Don't rock body to rise from a low chair or sofa.
Perform isometric contractions when resting.	Push down on floor with toes when sitting. Hook toes under sofa and pull up while sitting. Stand on one leg whenever waiting in line. Push out against armchairs with forearms and upper arm while sitting. Extend spine and retract and depress scapulae against back of chair while sitting. Press legs together when sitting or lying. Do abdominal crunches while riding in cars or buses. Place hands palms up under desk and pull up while sitting. Push head back against high-backed seat. Perform Kegel (pelvic floor) exercises anytime.

extremities, particularly the ankles, hips, and knees, so a person is able to mount a more robust response to a given stressor (94). It is not known whether resistance training also changes the neural recruitment of these muscles in response to perturbations in balance so that they are activated more quickly or in better sequence, but this may be an additional beneficial adaptation. Even when seated resistance training only is performed, improvements in static and dynamic balance can be demonstrated in older adults. Inclusion of standing postures, particularly if hand support is gradually withdrawn, has an even greater effect on balance.

General Technique

The general approach to improving balance should rely on theoretical principles designed to elicit adaptations in the central neurologic control of posture and equilibrium. The basic idea is to progressively challenge the system with stressors of increasing difficulty in three different domains:

1. Narrowing the base of support for the body
2. Displacing the center of mass to the limits of tolerance
3. Removing or minimizing contributions of visual, vestibular, and proprioceptive pathways to balance

Each of these will be considered in turn.

Narrowing the Base of Support. This is one of the most commonly used techniques and is quite effective. The person is instructed to stand in postures of increasing difficulty as follows:

- Feet apart with assistive device
- Feet apart without assistive device
- Feet together (tandem; touching along entire length)
- Semitandem stand (feet touching but the toe of one foot is at the instep of the other foot)
- Heel-to-toe stand (toe of one foot is touching the heel of the foot in front)
- One-legged stand (one foot only is on the ground)
- Toe stand (standing on tiptoe with both or only one foot)
- Heel stand (standing on both heels)

These postures have been presented in order of increasing difficulty, with the possible exception of the final two postures (toe stand and heel stand), which may present variable challenges to an individual depending not only on balance capacity but also on muscle strength, presence of arthritis, peripheral edema, range of motion in the ankle, and other podiatric issues. Each of the aforementioned listed postures should be tried under direct supervision to see where in this hierarchy that he or she begins to have difficulties maintaining balance. A useful technique is to ask the person to hold the desired posture for 15 s. If done successfully (without moving feet, grabbing for support, or falling), the next more difficult posture is tried. It is essential that the examiner be close

to the person at all times to prevent a fall. Wherever difficulty is first noted (defined as inability to hold the stance for the full 15 s), this is the level prescribed as the initial "training" posture. Training involves practicing this posture (see the following text for volume) until it is mastered, then progressing to the next higher level of difficulty. Community-dwelling men and women of average age of 80 yr begin to have difficulty at the level of the heel-to-toe stand (44,55,94,95). By contrast, frailer individuals in a nursing home may find the feet-together position initially difficult or impossible.

In addition to the static postures noted earlier, the principle of narrowing the base of support can be applied to dynamic movements as well, such as during heel-to-toe walking. This can be taken to a higher level of difficulty by tandem walking backward or with the eyes closed, or on a flat board 3–4 in wide that serves as a balance beam.

As long as the basic principle is followed, it does not matter whether the stances are done by themselves as a discreet training session; are incorporated into strength-training sessions; are practiced while carrying out daily activities, such as standing in line, cooking, doing housework, or talking on the phone; or form part of a more extensive routine of yoga, tai chi, or dance. The essential feature is progression, driven by challenging the person with difficult tasks to induce favorable adaptations.

Displacing the Center of Mass. The goal of this mode of training is to move the body weight through space toward the limits of sway, just short of where the balance is lost. All movement involves some displacement of the center of mass, including walking, but as a person's resources improve, more difficult and challenging displacement tasks can be mastered. In its simplest form, the person can be asked to stand still with his or her feet slightly apart and keeping the body rigid, lean forward, backward, and to each side as far as possible without having to move one's feet to maintain balance. Other ways of displacing the center of mass include the following:

- Turning in a circle
- Shifting weight from side to side
- Stepping over obstacles, such as a step or a book
- Turning or leaning while holding a heavy object, such as a book or a dumbbell, out in front of the chest
- Crossover walking, sideways walking, heel walking
- Moving weighted arms or legs out to the front or side (as in standing resistive exercises with free weights)
- Balancing on a large ball or rocker platform (available in many physical therapy settings)

Tai chi and yoga involve many postures that similarly perturb the center of the mass as well as diminish the base of support within simple or more complex movements; thus, these exercises fall into the theoretical constructs mentioned previously (75,128). If complicated forms of these exercises cannot be mastered, simpler versions have been tested and found to be feasible and effective in older adults, resulting in reduced fall rates as well as decreased fear of falling. By contrast, training using sophisticated balance platforms has not been shown to improve these clinical outcomes, although improvements in balance capacity tested on the same machine may be seen (126). Exercise classes including tai chi are now available in many senior centers and local gyms and are thus economical and highly accessible to many older adults. Compared with the high cost and lack of access to computerized balance training systems, as well as greater efficacy in falls prevention (129), tai chi or other kinds of functional balance-stressing movements are preferred to balance platform training for most older adults. However, there are many groups of clinical patients, such as those with Parkinson disease, stroke, brain injury, or other neurologic conditions, who may benefit from balance platform training in an acute rehabilitation setting. There is a need for research into appropriate transition protocols for such clinical populations, which may involve use of the low-tech methods outlined earlier for more chronic rehabilitation or home settings.

Minimizing Contributions of Visual and Proprioceptive Pathways. The ability to tolerate a narrowed base of support or shift in the center of mass will be markedly impaired if sensory inputs to balance control are reduced. This is most simply accomplished by closing the eyes during any of the movements mentioned in the preceding two sections. This should only be done after the posture in question has been completely mastered with eyes open. It is also recommended to try this under direct supervision of a trainer or other professional, particularly in high-risk adults. In addition, positioning in between a wall and a chair or other object is recommended for maximal safety.

Decreased proprioceptive input can be accomplished by practicing standing postures on a highly compliant surface, such as a pillow, piece of foam, mattress, or quilt. Using a mattress has the added advantage of providing a "safety net" should balance be lost during the attempt. This should allow safer progression to higher levels of difficulty without fear of injury. It is a good idea to teach adults strategies on how to get up from a fall before undertaking any balance training, so the fear of this outcome is reduced. No progression to reduced proprioceptive input should be made until the standard movements on a hard surface can be completed competently (without loss of balance). The combination of decreased vision and proprioception will be even more difficult than either adaptation alone. Proprioceptive input can be lessened in stages by inserting foam or mattresses of increasing thickness under the feet during training. A simple log sheet can be made to track the postures and these additional modifications on a weekly basis to monitor progress.

All balance movements should be done slowly and with deliberation because this stresses the control systems more and produces better physiologic adaptation. As with resistance training, increased speed uses momentum for the appropriate physiologic domain (strength, balance) and therefore undercuts desired stress on the system. For example, heel walking is actually easier when done rapidly rather than slowly, so the challenge and adaptation will be greater when done slowly. One of the outcomes of the tai chi intervention was that the older participants walked and moved more slowly after training, and their deliberation in movement was felt to be related to their reduced fear of falling and subsequent fall rates (126).

Intensity

Intensity in balance training refers to the degree of difficulty of the postures, movements, or routines practiced. The appropriate level of difficulty or "intensity" for any balance-enhancing exercise is the highest level that can be tolerated without inducing a fall or near-fall. In a supervised session, the individual can be pushed to the limits of such tolerance because safety is assured by the presence of the trainer. In an unsupervised setting, the person should be told to try movements only up to the level that they fail to master completely. For example, if the goal is to hold the heel-to-toe stand for 15 s and the person can only hold the posture for 10 s before grabbing the wall for support, this is the appropriate initial training intensity. Progression in intensity is the key to improvement as in other exercise domains, but this concept of mastery of the previous level before progression must be adhered to for safety. This is particularly important in frail elders who are at highest risk for falls, osteoporotic fractures, and other injuries.

Volume and Frequency

No definite statement can be made at this time about the minimum effective dose of balance training techniques described previously. Regimens have ranged from 1–7 d · wk^{-1} and from once a day to several times per day (5,109). A reasonable recommendation would appear to be 2–3 d · wk^{-1}, but this is more a matter of convention rather than an evidence-based recommendation. It is likely that as with other forms of training, a dose-response relationship exists, although thresholds have not been defined. There is no evidence that any negative effects are seen with high-volume training. Therefore, for adults with significant balance impairments, training 3–7 d · wk^{-1} may be advantageous. On the other hand, healthy adults may require only preventive practice 1 d · wk^{-1} for maintenance of mobility and function. Many more studies are needed in this area to define the recommendation further.

Choose several basic types of exercises (narrowed base of support, displacement of center of mass) and repeat each exercise two to three times at the most difficult level that falls short of being "mastered." It is unlikely that increasing the number of repetitions of a task that can be easily accomplished (*e.g.*, the semitandem stand) will lead to improvements in balance, but a few repetitions of a difficult task (such as standing on one leg) will lead to favorable adaptations. As with PRT, the emphasis should be on progressing to higher degrees of difficulty rather than high volumes of training. Tai chi and similar forms of exercise have been successfully prescribed from 45 min to 1 h for 2–3 d $\cdot$ wk^{-1}, but minimum effective doses are unknown.

Supervision and Setting

Balance training can be accomplished without the need for specialized equipment, which means that it can be done anywhere. The only supervision requirement relates to safety considerations and the level of fall risk. In the case of tai chi or yoga, an instructor may be needed to teach the discipline and assure correct form. Practicing balance on a carpeted or other soft surface (such as a lawn) is desirable. If balance is impaired, supervision is highly recommended until capacity improves. Progression to each higher level of intensity should only be attempted after mastery has been achieved. A group setting is convenient because exercisers can learn from each other's form, provide supervision and encouragement, and thereby challenge each other to progress with more confidence. Many trainers have used such group settings not only to teach balance exercises but also to deliver psychological interventions designed to reduce fear of falling and increase self-efficacy, talk about the safety enhancements of the home environment, practice techniques for getting up from a fall, discuss ways to get help in an emergency, and uncover other fall and fracture risks (*e.g.*, postural hypotension, impaired vision, nutritional habits). Thus, the multifactorial nature of falls makes the use of a group setting for balance exercise delivery perhaps more important than it is in other modalities of exercise.

Benefits

Balance training has been shown to result in improved balance performance, decreased fear of falling, decreased incidence of falls, and increased ability to participate in other activities that have been limited by gait and balance difficulties (99,109). It is expected, although not proven, that such changes would ultimately lead to improvements in functional independence, reduced hip fractures and other serious injuries, and improved overall quality of life. Such long-term outcomes will require larger studies of longer duration than those that have been reported to date. In particular, there is a need for data on the feasibility and efficacy of balance training in the very old and frail, in whom deficits are larger, fall risk is usually multifactorial, and cognitive impairments or degenerative neurologic diseases exist. All of these factors may alter the robustness of the physiologic adaptation achieved with training.

Balance training does not result in increased strength or aerobic capacity by itself. However, there may be some maintenance of muscle strength from the isometric contractions that occur during many of the balance-enhancing and one-legged postures and the bent-knee stance during tai chi.

Risks

The primary risk of balance training is loss of balance, resulting in a fall, injury, or increased fear of falling. This is preventable with attention to the factors governing progression, intensity, setting, and supervision. There is little or no elevation in pulse or blood pressure during these kinds of exercises, so cardiovascular events are not an expected or reported consequence. Musculoskeletal injury, other than that resulting from a fall, would also be unlikely.

It should be noted that there might be exacerbation of preexisting arthritic pain or inflammation of the knee during prolonged one-legged standing or tai chi postures requiring a semicrouched stance. These positions need to be adapted or avoided in those with significant weight-bearing pain in the joint. However, once quadriceps muscle strength improves with appropriate resistive exercises (see previous discussion), balance movements may be tolerable. Impaired flexibility may also limit some tai chi or yoga postures and may lead to injury if range of motion is forced. Gradual progression over time in the complexity of postures should prevent most injuries to soft tissues.

Integrating the Balance Prescription into Daily Life

Many activities in daily life can be turned into a balance-enhancing movement or position with a little creativity, making balance training one of the easiest modalities of exercise to integrate. Some examples of how this can be accomplished are listed as follows:

- While standing in line, cooking, combing your hair, or doing dishes, move your feet closer together or stand on one leg if possible during the task; alternate legs every 15–30 s.
- When crossing a room or other short distance, tandem, heel, toe, crossover, or sideways walk for 10–20 ft instead of normal walking.
- Carry small items (books, cartons of milk) by holding them out at arm's length while you walk (without bending the spine).
- Close your eyes or stand on one leg while riding a moving bus or train (lightly hold onto a bar for support if needed).

- Attempt to rise from a chair without use of the arms. Next, advance to rising using only one leg for support. The same may be practiced when sitting back down.

As with balance training sessions, none of these "integrated exercises" should be tried if they are beyond the current capacity of the individual. With time, these habits will become reinforced, and more opportunities to improve balance will appear throughout the normal daily routine. Challenge groups to think of creative ways to modify tasks and activities that are relevant to them in this way. Such group participation in exercise recommendations will serve as a motivational tool to increase overall training volume and optimally enhance the functional benefits of this modality of exercise. By turning "waiting in line" into an opportunity to exercise, one will never look at standing in line the same way again.

SPECIAL CONSIDERATIONS

Special Considerations in the Older Woman

Women respond as well as men to the same level of aerobic training. Less robust responses of aerobic capacity or weight loss appear to be related to reduced volume and/or intensity of training in many studies involving women. However, there does appear to be a difference in the way in which men and women adapt to cardiovascular training. Endurance-trained older men have been shown to increase exercise-related cardiac contractility and stroke volume during aerobic work (43), whereas this central adaptation has not yet been observed in older women (89,91,113). Older women adapt to aerobic training with peripheral changes, such as increased oxidative enzyme capacity, mitochondrial volume density, and capillary density in skeletal muscle. These peripheral changes are responsible for the overall increase in maximal oxygen consumption achieved.

Another consideration in older women is exercise-induced or exacerbated urinary incontinence (35). This symptom may be so limiting that it precludes exercise participation entirely in some women and should be considered when compliance is low despite delivery of appropriate training and behavioral methods. Incontinence in this case is usually stress incontinence related to weak pelvic floor muscles and collagen from low estrogenic state of postmenopausal women who are not on hormone replacement therapy as well as aging muscle and connective tissue and birth trauma. Although a complete discussion of urinary incontinence is beyond the scope of this chapter, a few points are worth emphasizing. Losses of urine when standing, coughing, sneezing, or initiating exercise are often from stress incontinence secondary to the rise in intra-abdominal pressure caused by these activities. The presence of such symptoms should be part of the preexercise assessment of older women. If any other urinary symptoms are present such as dysuria, frequency, urge incontinence, or hematuria, referral for medical

BOX 36-5	**Steps to Minimize Urinary Incontinence related to Exercise**

- Void before activity.
- Drink extra fluid after exercise rather than before or during sessions.
- Avoid all caffeine- and alcohol-containing foods and beverages for at least 3 h before exercise.
- Minimize breath holding and use of Valsalva maneuver during exercise.
- Practice pelvic muscle-strengthening exercises (Kegel exercises).
- Minimize high-impact activities.
- Use intravaginal support or external pad during exercise.
- Review medications and dosing schedule with physician.

evaluation is necessary. If not, the measures outlined in *Box 36-5* can be instituted to minimize the occurrence of incontinent episodes. Pelvic floor muscle exercises are isometric resistance training for the levator ani muscles, which prevent the urethra from descending in response to increases in intra-abdominal pressure as noted previously (18,71). An effective regimen is as follows:

- Hold a maximal contraction of levator ani muscles (without Valsalva) for 5 s; these muscles can be identified during a pelvic examination and are the muscles used to voluntarily stop the stream of urine (also called Kegel exercises).
- Rest for 10 s.
- Repeat preceding steps for a total of 10 min.
- Complete this 10-min session four times per day everyday.

Success rates for pelvic muscle exercises vary widely (30%–60%), most likely because compliance is low, and contractions are submaximal. Biofeedback has been used to show women when they are effectively producing contractile force with these muscles (18). An approach to compliance that may be behaviorally attractive is to have women with stress incontinence perform the pelvic muscle contractions whenever they are sitting at rest or riding in a car or during rest periods between sets of a weightlifting regimen. In this way, pelvic training does not take "extra" time during the day and will become automatic once the habit is established. If the problem is not resolved with these simple measures, referral to a specialist is indicated for more specific treatment or medication management.

Finally, the lower muscle mass and tendency for gait disorders and falls seen in older women compared with men means that aerobic training is rarely indicated as an isolated exercise prescription in this population. It is reasonable, therefore, to start with strength and balance training and to add aerobic training only when there has been some improvement in these other areas. It should be noted that there is little evidence that aerobic training significantly improves strength, muscle mass, or balance, although such statements are often made in general exercise guidelines for the older adult.

Integration of Exercise into Daily Activities

Among all the modalities of exercise, cardiovascular exercise is the easiest to integrate into daily activities. It requires a few behavioral decisions that can be adhered to with reasonable success. For example, decisions could be made to the following:

- Never use an escalator or elevator when stairs are available.
- Never take the car for errands that can be accomplished with a 10-min walk.
- Do not use remote control devices.
- Substitute manual devices (lawn mowers, egg beaters, brooms) for mechanical devices whenever possible.
- Park in the most remote corner of the parking lot whenever shopping.

If these suggestions appear too difficult initially (such as climbing five flights of stairs while carrying groceries), add them gradually. For example, a person might start by taking the elevator four flights, walking the final flight, and advance to walking the entire way. This approach is very effective because it adheres to both the behavioral principle of "shaping" — taking small steps at a time — as well as the physiologic principle of incremental progression of volume and intensity of training. Immediate feedback on fitness is available as well, as the person notices the ability to climb all five flights of stairs with minimal effort after a few weeks. Although it may seem that these alterations in routine are time consuming, the advantage is that no additional time is required for a discrete endurance training session of 20–30 min during the course of a day. Often, waiting for a busy elevator actually takes longer than climbing the stairs, and the time taken circling the parking lot looking for a close space could have been better spent walking the extra distance.

Older adults of long-term care facilities present a special problem in terms of "lifestyle" exercise prescription. In a nursing home, it is difficult to find stairs to climb or lawns to mow, so walking groups initiated around regularly scheduled activities when staff is available may have the best chance of success. As older adults improve in fitness, extra laps around the ward can be added to extend the walk to at least 10 min. Three such walks a day will complete a 30-min aerobic regimen for 7 d · wk^{-1}. The most fit older adults should be encouraged to push older adults who are wheelchair-bound on these walks because

this will free staff to help less able older adults ambulate and will also increase the aerobic intensity of the walk for the fitter older adults. Additionally, the psychological benefits of increased self-esteem and morale can be substantial when older adults are encouraged to do this because they are given back an essential caregiving role that may have been lost on entry to the long-term care facility.

REFERENCES

1. *2008 Physical Activity Guidelines for Americans* [Internet]. Washington (DC): U.S. Department of Health and Human Services; [cited 2011 Sep 2]. Available from: http://www.health.gov/paguidelines/pdf/paguide.pdf
2. Ades PA, Savage PD, Cress ME, Brochu M, Lee NM, Poehlman ET. Resistance training on physical performance in disabled older female cardiac patients. *Med Sci Sports Exerc.* 2003;35(8):1265–70.
3. American College of Sports Medicine, Chodzko-Zajko WJ, Proctor DN, et al. American College of Sports Medicine position stand. Exercise and physical activity for older adults. *Med Sci Sports Exerc.* 2009;41(7):1510–30.
4. Artal R, O'Toole M. Guidelines of the American College of Obstetricians and Gynecologists for exercise during pregnancy and the postpartum period. *Br J Sports Med.* 2003;37(1):6–12; discussion 12.
5. Baker MK, Atlantis E, Fiatarone Singh MA. Multi-modal exercise programs for older adults. *Age Ageing.* 2007;36(4):375–81.
6. Bar-Or O. Pathophysiological factors which limit the exercise capacity of the sick child. *Med Sci Sports Exerc.* 1986;18(3):276–82.
7. Bassey EJ, Rothwell MC, Littlewood JJ, Pye DW. Pre- and postmenopausal women have different bone mineral density responses to the same high-impact exercise. *J Bone Miner Res.* 1998;13(12):1805–13.
8. Benn SJ, McCartney N, McKelvie RS. Circulatory responses to weight lifting, walking, and stair climbing in older males. *J Am Geriatr Soc.* 1996;44(2):121–5.
9. Bernhardt DT, Gomez J, Johnson MD, et al. Strength training by children and adolescents. *Pediatrics.* 2001;107(6):1470–2.
10. Binder EF, Yarasheski KE, Steger-May K, et al. Effects of progressive resistance training on body composition in frail older adults: results of a randomized, controlled trial. *J Gerontol A Biol Sci Med Sci.* 2005;60(11):1425–31.
11. Blumenthal JA, Babyak MA, Moore KA, et al. Effects of exercise training on older patients with major depression. *Arch Intern Med.* 1999;159(19):2349–56.
12. Bonaiuti D, Shea B, Iovine R, et al. Exercise for preventing and treating osteoporosis in postmenopausal women. *Cochrane Database Syst Rev.* 2002;(3):CD000333.
13. Borg G, Linderholm H. Perceived exertion and pulse rate during graded exercise in various age group. *Acta Med Scand.* 1970;472(Suppl):194–206.
14. Borst SE. Interventions for sarcopenia and muscle weakness in older people. *Age Ageing.* 2004;33(6):548–55.
15. Braith RW, Stewart KJ. Resistance exercise training: its role in the prevention of cardiovascular disease. *Circulation.* 2006;113(22):2642–50.
16. Brown DW, Brown DR, Heath GW, et al. Associations between physical activity dose and health-related quality of life. *Med Sci Sports Exerc.* 2004;36(5):890–6.
17. Bucksch J. Physical activity of moderate intensity in leisure time and the risk of all cause mortality. *Br J Sports Med.* 2005;39(9):632–8.
18. Burns PA, Pranikoff K, Nochajski TH, Hadley EC, Levy KJ, Ory MG. A comparison of effectiveness of biofeedback and pelvic muscle exercise treatment of stress incontinence in older community-dwelling women. *J Gerontol.* 1993;48(4):M167–74.

19. Campbell MK, Mottola MF. Recreational exercise and occupational activity during pregnancy and birth weight: a case-control study. *Am J Obstet Gynecol.* 2001;184(3):403–8.

20. Campbell WW, Leidy HJ. Dietary protein and resistance training effects on muscle and body composition in older persons. *J Am Coll Nutr.* 2007;26(6):696S–703S.

21. Carter ND, Kannus P, Khan KM. Exercise in the prevention of falls in older people: a systematic literature review examining the rationale and the evidence. *Sports Med.* 2001;31(6):427–38.

22. Centers for Disease Control and Prevention. Physical activity levels among children aged 9–13 years—United States, 2002. *MMWR Morb Mortal Wkly Rep.* 2003;52(33):785–8.

23. Centers for Disease Control and Prevention. Strength training among adults aged >/=65 years—United States, 2001. *MMWR Morb Mortal Wkly Rep.* 2004;53(2):25–8.

24. Chang JT, Morton SC, Rubenstein LZ, et al. Interventions for the prevention of falls in older adults: systematic review and meta-analysis of randomised clinical trials. *BMJ.* 2004;328(7441):680.

25. Church TS, Earnest CP, Skinner JS, Blair SN. Effects of different doses of physical activity on cardiorespiratory fitness among sedentary, overweight or obese postmenopausal women with elevated blood pressure: a randomized controlled trial. *JAMA.* 2007;297(19):2081–91.

26. Clapp JF. *Exercising through Your Pregnancy.* Omaha (NE): Addicus Books; 2002. 245 p.

27. Clapp JF,3rd. Maternal heart rate in pregnancy. *Am J Obstet Gynecol.* 1985;152(6 Pt 1):659–60.

28. Clapp JF,3rd. Oxygen consumption during treadmill exercise before, during, and after pregnancy. *Am J Obstet Gynecol.* 1989;161(6 Pt 1):1458–64.

29. Coe DP, Pivarnik JM, Womack CJ, Reeves MJ, Malina RM. Effect of physical education and activity levels on academic achievement in children. *Med Sci Sports Exerc.* 2006;38(8):1515–9.

30. Committee on Obstetric Practice. ACOG committee opinion. Exercise during pregnancy and the postpartum period. Number 267, January 2002. American College of Obstetricians and Gynecologists. *Int J Gynaecol Obstet.* 2002;77(1):79–81.

31. Connolly DA, Sayers SP, McHugh MP. Treatment and prevention of delayed onset muscle soreness. *J Strength Cond Res.* 2003;17(1):197–208.

32. Cooper Institute for Aerobic Research. *Fitnessgram & Activitygram Test Administration Manual.* 4th ed. Champaign (IL): Human Kinetics; 2010. 152 p.

33. Corbin CB, Pangrazi RP, National Association for Sport and Physical Education, Council on Physical Education for Children, National Association for Sport and Physical Education. *Physical Activity for Children: A Statement of Guidelines for Children Ages 5–12.* 2nd ed. Reston (VA): National Association for Sport and Physical Education; 2004. 28 p.

34. Daley A, Macarthur C, Stokes-Lampard H, McManus R, Wilson S, Mutrie N. Exercise participation, body mass index, and health-related quality of life in women of menopausal age. *Br J Gen Pract.* 2007;57(535):130–5.

35. Danforth KN, Shah AD, Townsend MK, et al. Physical activity and urinary incontinence among healthy, older women. *Obstet Gynecol.* 2007;109(3):721–7.

36. Davenport MH, Charlesworth S, Vanderspank D, Sopper MM, Mottola MF. Development and validation of exercise target heart rate zones for overweight and obese pregnant women. *Appl Physiol Nutr Metab.* 2008;33(5):984–9.

37. Davies GA, Wolfe LA, Mottola MF, MacKinnon C, Society of Obstetricians and gynecologists of Canada, SOGC Clinical Practice Obstetrics Committee. Joint SOGC/CSEP clinical practice guideline: exercise in pregnancy and the postpartum period. *Can J Appl Physiol.* 2003;28(3):330–41.

38. De Vos NJ, Singh NA, Ross DA, Stavrinos TM, Orr R, Fiatarone Singh MA. Optimal load for increasing muscle power during explosive resistance training in older adults. *J Gerontol A Biol Sci Med Sci.* 2005;60(5):638–47.

39. Dempsey JC, Butler CL, Williams MA. No need for a pregnant pause: Physical activity may reduce the occurrence of gestational diabetes mellitus and preeclampsia. *Exerc Sport Sci Rev.* 2005;33(3):141–9.

40. Drinkwater BL. Women and exercise: physiological aspects. *Exerc Sport Sci Rev.* 1984;12:21–51.

41. Duvekot JJ, Cheriex EC, Pieters FA, Menheere PP, Peeters LH. Early pregnancy changes in hemodynamics and volume homeostasis are consecutive adjustments triggered by a primary fall in systemic vascular tone. *Am J Obstet Gynecol.* 1993;169(6):1382–92.

42. Eaton DK, Kann L, Kinchen S, et al. Youth risk behavior surveillance—United States, 2009. *MMWR Surveill Summ.* 2010;59(5):1–142.

43. Ehsani AA, Ogawa T, Miller TR, Spina RJ, Jilka SM. Exercise training improves left ventricular systolic function in older men. *Circulation.* 1991;83(1):96–103.

44. Era P, Sainio P, Koskinen S, Haavisto P, Vaara M, Aromaa A. Postural balance in a random sample of 7,979 subjects aged 30 years and over. *Gerontology.* 2006;52(4):204–13.

45. Ettinger WH,Jr, Burns R, Messier SP, et al. A randomized trial comparing aerobic exercise and resistance exercise with a health education program in older adults with knee osteoarthritis. The Fitness Arthritis and Seniors Trial (FAST). *JAMA.* 1997;277(1):25–31.

46. Faigenbaum AD, Kraemer WJ, Blimkie CJ, et al. Youth resistance training: updated position statement paper from the national strength and conditioning association. *J Strength Cond Res.* 2009;23(5 Suppl):S60–79.

47. Fiatarone MA, O'Neill EF, Ryan ND, et al. Exercise training and nutritional supplementation for physical frailty in very elderly people. *N Engl J Med.* 1994;330(25):1769–75.

48. Ford ES, Kohl HW,3rd, Mokdad AH, Ajani UA. Sedentary behavior, physical activity, and the metabolic syndrome among U.S. adults. *Obes Res.* 2005;13(3):608–14.

49. Galper DI, Trivedi MH, Barlow CE, Dunn AL, Kampert JB. Inverse association between physical inactivity and mental health in men and women. *Med Sci Sports Exerc.* 2006;38(1):173–8.

50. Garber CE, Blissmer B, Deschenes MR, et al. Quantity and quality of exercise for developing and maintaining cardiorespiratory, musculoskeletal, and neuromotor fitness in apparently healthy adults: guidance for prescribing exercise. *Med Sci Sports Exerc.* 2011;43(7):1334–59.

51. Gardner AW, Katzel LI, Sorkin JD, et al. Exercise rehabilitation improves functional outcomes and peripheral circulation in patients with intermittent claudication: a randomized controlled trial. *J Am Geriatr Soc.* 2001;49(6):755–62.

52. Gavard JA, Artal R. Effect of exercise on pregnancy outcome. *Clin Obstet Gynecol.* 2008;51(2):467–89.

53. Gearhart RE, Goss FL, Lagally KM, Jakicic JM, Gallagher J, Robertson RJ. Standardized scaling procedures for rating perceived exertion during resistance exercise. *J Strength Cond Res.* 2001;15(3):320–5.

54. Gordon NF, Kohl HW,3rd, Pollock ML, Vaandrager H, Gibbons LW, Blair SN. Cardiovascular safety of maximal strength testing in healthy adults. *Am J Cardiol.* 1995;76(11):851–3.

55. Guralnik JM, Simonsick EM, Ferrucci L, et al. A short physical performance battery assessing lower extremity function: association with self-reported disability and prediction of mortality and nursing home admission. *J Gerontol.* 1994;49(2):M85–94.

56. Guyatt GH, Sullivan MJ, Thompson PJ, et al. The 6-minute walk: a new measure of exercise capacity in patients with chronic heart failure. *Can Med Assoc J.* 1985;132(8):919–23.

57. Haskell WL, Lee IM, Pate RR, et al. Physical activity and public health: updated recommendation for adults from the American College of Sports Medicine and the American Heart Association. *Med Sci Sports Exerc.* 2007;39(8):1423–34.

58. Hauer K, Specht N, Schuler M, Bartsch P, Oster P. Intensive physical training in geriatric patients after severe falls and hip surgery. *Age Ageing*. 2002;31(1):49–57.

59. Heath JM, Stuart MR. Prescribing exercise for frail elders. *J Am Board Fam Pract*. 2002;15(3):218–28.

60. Hebestreit HU, Bar-Or O. Differences between children and adults for exercise testing and exercise prescription. In: Skinner JS, editor. *Exercise Testing and Exercise Prescription for Special Cases: Theoretical Basis and Clinical Application*. 3rd ed. Philadelphia: Lippincott Williams & Wilkins; 2005. p. 68–84.

61. Heinonen A, Kannus P, Sievanen H, et al. Randomised controlled trial of effect of high-impact exercise on selected risk factors for osteoporotic fractures. *Lancet*. 1996;348(9038):1343–7.

62. Hopkins SA, Baldi JC, Cutfield WS, McCowan L, Hofman PL. Exercise training in pregnancy reduces offspring size without changes in maternal insulin sensitivity. *J Clin Endocrinol Metab*. 2010;95(5):2080–8.

63. Howe TE, Shea B, Dawson LJ, et al. Exercise for preventing and treating osteoporosis in postmenopausal women. *Cochrane Database Syst Rev*. 2011;7(7):CD000333.

64. Hughes SL, Seymour RB, Campbell RT, et al. Long-term impact of Fit and Strong! On older adults with osteoarthritis. *Gerontologist*. 2006;46(6):801–14.

65. Janssen I, Jolliffe CJ. Influence of physical activity on mortality in elderly with coronary artery disease. *Med Sci Sports Exerc*. 2006;38(3):418–7.

66. Kannus P, Sievanen H, Palvanen M, Jarvinen T, Parkkari J. Prevention of falls and consequent injuries in elderly people. *Lancet*. 2005;366(9500):1885–93.

67. Kato T, Terashima T, Yamashita T, Hatanaka Y, Honda A, Umemura Y. Effect of low-repetition jump training on bone mineral density in young women. *J Appl Physiol*. 2006;100(3):839–43.

68. Katsiaras A, Newman AB, Kriska A, et al. Skeletal muscle fatigue, strength, and quality in the elderly: the Health ABC Study. *J Appl Physiol*. 2005;99(1):210–6.

69. Katz S, Ford AB, Moskowitz RW, Jackson BA, Jaffe MW. Studies of illness in the aged. The index of ADL: a standardized measure of biological and psychosocial function. *JAMA*. 1963;185:914–9.

70. Kaufman C, Berg K, Noble J, Thomas J. Ratings of perceived exertion of ACSM exercise guidelines in individuals varying in aerobic fitness. *Res Q Exerc Sport*. 2006;77(1):122–30.

71. Kim H, Suzuki T, Yoshida Y, Yoshida H. Effectiveness of multidimensional exercises for the treatment of stress urinary incontinence in elderly community-dwelling Japanese women: a randomized, controlled, crossover trial. *J Am Geriatr Soc*. 2007;55 (12):1932–9.

72. King AC, Taylor CB, Haskell WL. Effects of differing intensities and formats of 12 months of exercise training on psychological outcomes in older adults. *Health Psychol*. 1993;12(4):292–300.

73. King DS, Sharp RL, Vukovich MD, et al. Effect of oral androstenedione on serum testosterone and adaptations to resistance training in young men: a randomized controlled trial. *JAMA*. 1999;281(21):2020–8.

74. Kryger AI, Andersen JL. Resistance training in the oldest old: consequences for muscle strength, fiber types, fiber size, and MHC isoforms. *Scand J Med Sci Sports*. 2007;17(4):422–30.

75. Kuramoto AM. Therapeutic benefits of Tai Chi exercise: research review. *WMJ*. 2006;105(7):42–6.

76. Lagally KM, Amorose AJ. The validity of using prior ratings of perceive exertion to regulate resistance exercise intensity. *Percept Mot Skills*. 2007;104(2):534–42.

77. Lawton MP, Brody EM. Assessment of older people: self-maintaining and instrumental activities of daily living. *Gerontologist*. 1969;9(3):179–86.

78. Loucks AB, Callister R. Induction and prevention of low-T3 syndrome in exercising women. *Am J Physiol*. 1993;264(5 Pt 2): R924–30.

79. Loucks AB, Heath EM. Induction of low-T3 syndrome in exercising women occurs at a threshold of energy availability. *Am J Physiol*. 1994;266(3 Pt 2):R817–23.

80. Loucks AB, Laughlin GA, Mortola JF, Girton L, Nelson JC, Yen SS. Hypothalamic-pituitary-thyroidal function in eumenorrheic and amenorrheic athletes. *J Clin Endocrinol Metab*. 1992;75(2): 514–8.

81. Maddalozzo GF, Snow CM. High intensity resistance training: effects on bone in older men and women. *Calcif Tissue Int*. 2000; 66(6):399–404.

82. Malina RM. Tracking of physical activity and physical fitness across the lifespan. *Res Q Exerc Sport*. 1996;67(3 Suppl):S48–57.

83. Martel GF, Roth SM, Ivey FM, et al. Age and sex affect human muscle fibre adaptations to heavy-resistance strength training. *Exp Physiol*. 2006;91(2):457–64.

84. Martyn-St James M, Carroll S. A meta-analysis of impact exercise on postmenopausal bone loss: the case for mixed loading exercise programmes. *Br J Sports Med*. 2009;43(12):898–908.

85. Martyn-St James M, Carroll S. Meta-analysis of walking for preservation of bone mineral density in postmenopausal women. *Bone*. 2008;43(3):521–31.

86. McCartney N. Acute responses to resistance training and safety. *Med Sci Sports Exerc*. 1999;31(1):31–7.

87. Mendelsohn ME, Karas RH. The protective effects of estrogen on the cardiovascular system. *N Engl J Med*. 1999;340(23): 1801–11.

88. Mottola MF, Davenport MH, Brun CR, Inglis SD, Charlesworth S, Sopper MM. VO_{2peak} prediction and exercise prescription for pregnant women. *Med Sci Sports Exerc*. 2006;38(8):1389–95.

89. Neilan TG, Ton-Nu TT, Jassal DS, et al. Myocardial adaptation to short-term high-intensity exercise in highly trained athletes. *J Am Soc Echocardiogr*. 2006;19(10):1280–5.

90. Norrbrand L, Fluckey JD, Pozzo M, Tesch PA. Resistance training using eccentric overload induces early adaptations in skeletal muscle size. *Eur J Appl Physiol*. 2008;102(3):271–81.

91. Ogawa T, Spina RJ, Martin WH,3rd, et al. Effects of aging, sex, and physical training on cardiovascular responses to exercise. *Circulation*. 1992;86(2):494–503.

92. Ogden CL, Carroll MD, Curtin LR, Lamb MM, Flegal KM. Prevalence of high body mass index in US children and adolescents, 2007–2008. *JAMA*. 2010;303(3):242–9.

93. Okazaki K, Iwasaki K, Prasad A, et al. Dose-response relationship of endurance training for autonomic circulatory control in healthy seniors. *J Appl Physiol*. 2005;99(3):1041–9.

94. Orr R, Raymond J, Fiatarone Singh M. Efficacy of progressive resistance training on balance performance in older adults: a systematic review of randomized controlled trials. *Sports Med*. 2008;38(4):317–43.

95. Ostchega Y, Harris TB, Hirsch R, Parsons VL, Kington R, Katzoff M. Reliability and prevalence of physical performance examination assessing mobility and balance in older persons in the US: data from the Third National Health and Nutrition Examination Survey. *J Am Geriatr Soc*. 2000;48(9):1136–41.

96. Owe KM, Nystad W, Bø K. Association between regular exercise and excessive newborn birth weight. *Obstet Gynecol*. 2009;114(4): 770–6.

97. Paridon SM, Alpert BS, Boas SR, et al. Clinical stress testing in the pediatric age group: a statement from the American Heart Association Council on Cardiovascular Disease in the Young, Committee on Atherosclerosis, Hypertension, and Obesity in Youth. *Circulation*. 2006;113(15):1905–20.

98. PARmed-X for Pregnancy [Internet]. Gloucester (Ontario): Canadian Society for Exercise Physiology; [cited 2011 Feb 24]. Available from: http://www.csep.ca/english/view.asp?x=698

99. Paterson DH, Jones GR, Rice CL. Ageing and physical activity: evidence to develop exercise recommendations for older adults. *Can J Public Health*. 2007;98 Suppl 2:S69–108.

100. Pedersen BK, Saltin B. Evidence for prescribing exercise as therapy in chronic disease. *Scand J Med Sci Sports*. 2006;16 Suppl 1:3–63.

101. Pivarnik JM, Chambliss HO, Clapp JF, et al. Impact of physical activity during pregnancy an d postpartum on chronic disease risk. *Med Sci Sports Exerc*. 2006;38(5):989–1006.

102. Pollock ML, Graves JE, Bamman MM, et al. Frequency and volume of resistance training: effect on cervical extension strength. *Arch Phys Med Rehabil*. 1993;74(10):1080–6.

103. Rejeski WJ, Ettinger WH,Jr, Martin K, Morgan T. Treating disability in knee osteoarthritis with exercise therapy: a central role for self-efficacy and pain. *Arthritis Care Res*. 1998;11(2):94–101.

104. Risch SV, Norvell NK, Pollock ML, et al. Lumbar strengthening in chronic low back pain patients. Physiologic and psychological benefits. *Spine (Phila Pa 1976)*. 1993;18(2):232–8.

105. Rowland TW. *Children's Exercise Physiology*. 2nd ed. Champaign (IL): Human Kinetics; 2004. 312 p.

106. Rubenstein LZ. Falls in older people: epidemiology, risk factors and strategies for prevention. *Age Ageing*. 2006;35 Suppl 2:ii37–41.

107. Sevick MA, Bradham DD, Muender M, et al Cost-effectiveness of aerobic and resistance exercise in seniors with knee osteoarthritis. *Med Sci Sports Exerc*. 2000;32(9):1534–40.

108. Seynnes O, Fiatarone Singh MA, Hue O, Pras P, Legros P, Bernard PL. Physiological and functional responses to low-moderate versus high-intensity progressive resistance training in frail elders. *J Gerontol A Biol Sci Med Sci*. 2004;59(5):503–9.

109. Sherrington C, Lord SR, Finch CF. Physical activity interventions to prevent falls among older people: update of the evidence. *J Sci Med Sport*. 2004;7(1 Suppl):43–51.

110. Singh MA. Exercise comes of age: rationale and recommendations for a geriatric exercise prescription. *J Gerontol A Biol Sci Med Sci*. 2002;57(5):M262–82.

111. Singh NA, Quine S, Clemson LM, et al. Effects of high-intensity progressive resistance training and targeted multidisciplinary treatment of frailty on mortality and nursing home admissions after hip fracture: a randomized controlled trial. *J Am Med Dir Assoc*. 2012;13(1):24–30.

112. Singh NA, Stavrinos TM, Scarbek Y, Galambos G, Liber C, Fiatarone Singh MA. A randomized controlled trial of high versus low intensity weight training versus general practitioner care for clinical depression in older adults. *J Gerontol A Biol Sci Med Sci*. 2005;60(6):768–76.

113. Spina RJ, Miller TR, Bogenhagen WH, Schechtman KB, Ehsani AA. Gender-related differences in left ventricular filling dynamics in older subjects after endurance exercise training. *J Gerontol A Biol Sci Med Sci*. 1996;51(3):B232–7.

114. Strong WB, Malina RM, Blimkie CJ, et al. Evidence based physical activity for school-age youth. *J Pediatr*. 2005;146(6):732–7.

115. Suetta C, Magnusson SP, Rosted A, et al. Resistance training in the early postoperative phase reduces hospitalization and leads to muscle hypertrophy in elderly hip surgery patients—a controlled, randomized study. *J Am Geriatr Soc*. 2004;52(12):2016–22.

116. Taaffe DR. Sarcopenia—exercise as a treatment strategy. *Aust Fam Physician*. 2006;35(3):130–4.

117. U.S. Department of Health and Human Services, Centers for Disease Control and Prevention, National Center for Chronic Disease Prevention and Health Promotion, The President's Council on Physical Fitness and Sports. *Physical Activity and Health: A Report of the Surgeon General*. Atlanta (GA): President's Council on Physical Fitness and Sports; 1996. 278 p.

118. Verhaeghe J, Thomsen JS, van Bree R, van Herck E, Bouillon R, Mosekilde L. Effects of exercise and disuse on bone remodeling, bone mass, and biomechanical competence in spontaneously diabetic female rats. *Bone*. 2000;27(2):249–56.

119. Visser M, Simonsick EM, Colbert LH, et al. Type and intensity of activity and risk of mobility limitation: the mediating role of muscle parameters. *J Am Geriatr Soc*. 2005;53(5):762–70.

120. Welle S, Totterman S, Thornton C. Effect of age on muscle hypertrophy induced by resistance training. *J Gerontol A Biol Sci Med Sci*. 1996;51(6):M270–5.

121. Wernbom M, Augustsson J, Thomee R. The influence of frequency, intensity, volume and mode of strength training on whole muscle cross-sectional area in humans. *Sports Med*. 2007; 37(3):225–64.

122. Williams MA, Haskell WL, Ades PA, et al. Resistance exercise in individuals with and without cardiovascular disease: 2007 update: a scientific statement from the American Heart Association Council on Clinical Cardiology and Council on Nutrition, Physical Activity, and Metabolism. *Circulation*. 2007; 116(5):572–84.

123. Wilmore JH. Alterations in strength, body composition and anthropometric measurements consequent to a 10-week weight training program. *Med Sci Sports*. 1974;6(2):133–8.

124. Wilmore JH, Stanforth PR, Gagnon J, et al. Cardiac output and stroke volume changes with endurance training: the HERITAGE Family Study. *Med Sci Sports Exerc*. 2001;33(1):99–106.

125. Wolfe LA. Pregnancy. In: Skinner JS, editor. *Exercise Testing and Exercise Prescription for Special Cases: Theoretical Basis and Clinical Application*. 3rd ed. Philadelphia: Lippincott Williams & Wilkins; 2005. p. 377–91.

126. Wolf SL, Barnhart HX, Kutner NG, McNeely E, Coogler C, Xu T. Reducing frailty and falls in older persons: an investigation of Tai Chi and computerized balance training. Atlanta FICSIT Group. Frailty and Injuries: Cooperative Studies of Intervention Techniques. *J Am Geriatr Soc*. 1996;44(5):489–97.

127. Woodard CM, Berry MJ. Enhancing adherence to prescribed exercise: structured behavioral interventions in clinical exercise programs. *J Cardiopulm Rehabil*. 2001;21(4):201–9.

128. Wu G. Evaluation of the effectiveness of Tai Chi for improving balance and preventing falls in the older population—a review. *J Am Geriatr Soc*. 2002;50(4):746–54.

129. Zijlstra GA, van Haastregt JC, van Rossum E, van Eijk JT, Yardley L, Kempen GI. Interventions to reduce fear of falling in community-living older people: a systematic review. *J Am Geriatr Soc*. 2007;55(4):603–15.

SELECTED REFERENCES FOR FURTHER READING

American College of Obstetricians and Gynecologists. ACOG committee opinion (No. 267, January 2002). Exercise during pregnancy and the postpartum period. *Int J Gynaecol Obstet*. 2002;77: 79–81.

Artal R, O'Toole M. Guidelines of the American College of Obstetricians and Gynecologists for exercise during pregnancy and the postpartum period. *Br J Sports Med*. 2003;37:6–12; discussion 12.

Fiatarone Singh M. Exercise comes of age: rationale and recommendations for a geriatric exercise prescription. *J Gerontol Med Sci*. 2002; 57(A):M262–82.

Haskell WL, Lee IM, Pate RR, et al. Physical activity and public health: updated recommendation for adults from the American College of Sports Medicine and the American Heart Association. *Med Sci Sports Exerc*. 2007;39(8):1423–34.

Hebestreit HU, Bar-Or O. Differences between children and adults for exercise testing and prescription. In: Skinner JS, editor. *Exercise Testing and Exercise Prescription for Special Cases*. Philadelphia: Lippincott Williams & Wilkins; 2005. p. 68–84.

INTERNET RESOURCES

- American College of Obstetricians and Gynecologists: http://www.acog.org
- American College of Sports Medicine: http://www.acsm.org

IV

Exercise Prescription for Clinical Populations

CLINTON A. BRAWNER, MS, FACSM, ACSM-CES, ACSM-RCEP, *Section Editor*

Exercise Prescription and Medical Considerations

Regular exercise training is associated with health benefits that include prolonged life, reduced chronic illness, and improved quality of life. However, undiagnosed cardiovascular, pulmonary, and metabolic abnormalities are sometimes unmasked during exercise testing and training. They may occasionally result in illness and death. In addition, musculoskeletal injuries are not uncommon in the physically active population. These challenges and threats to personal health and safety must be balanced against the health benefits of an active lifestyle. This chapter reviews the medical considerations of exercise testing and training. Pertinent information is presented concerning the causes, recognition, care, and prevention of injuries and illnesses unique to exercise training. In addition, environmental influences during exercise and their associated health risks are discussed.

PREPARTICIPATION SCREENING

The beneficial impact of exercise on many diseases is well known. Several observational studies as well as large-scale trials demonstrate an inverse relationship between physical activity and chronic medical conditions such as cardiovascular disease, hypertension, stroke, osteoporosis, Type 2 diabetes mellitus (DM), obesity, colon cancer, breast cancer, anxiety, and depression (31,41,44,45,49, 56,61,70,74,76,77,81). It is important to remember that compared with sedentary adults, physically fit individuals have one-quarter to one-half of the risk of developing cardiac disease (57,79). Another goal of exercise is to preserve or improve fitness and quality of life.

Expanded exercise participation by a larger and older population increases the likelihood of injury as the number of participants and volume of training increases. Participants should be screened for medical conditions that could lead to injury or disease when starting a new exercise program or increasing the intensity of their current training. Additionally, it is well documented that during an acute bout of exercise, a sedentary individual is at an increased risk for sudden cardiac death (SCD); however, this risk is balanced by the reduced long-term risk of heart disease and SCD as a result of regular physical activity (75). Exercise professionals are encouraged to perform health and fitness screenings before participants begin exercise programs (see *Chapter 11*). These screenings should be used to detect not only cardiopulmonary and metabolic abnormalities but also musculoskeletal problems that are a contraindication to exercise. The American Heart Association (AHA)/American College of Sports Medicine (ACSM) Health/Fitness Screening Questionnaire is a useful first step in a multistage assessment process (*Box 37-1*)(12).

When a medical evaluation is indicated (see *Chapter 2* in *GETP9*), it should include a focused history and physical exam. A focused history should identify any history of cardiac, pulmonary, metabolic disease, and/or musculoskeletal injury before the implementation of an exercise program. A focused physical exam is intended to identify signs necessitating further evaluation. This would include listening to heart and lung sounds, checking pulses, evaluating for edema, and a musculoskeletal exam. Examples of findings that would require further evaluation are a history of syncope, angina pectoris, unusual

KEY TERMS

Air quality index: An index for reporting daily air quality that indicates how clean or polluted the air is and what associated health effects might be a concern.

Angina pectoris: Transient pain or discomfort in the chest (or adjacent areas) caused by myocardial ischemia.

Chondromalacia: Softening of any cartilage.

Musculotendinous degeneration: Deterioration of the muscle-tendon area.

Myocardial ischemia: Insufficient blood supply to the heart muscle.

| **BOX 37-1** | **AHA/ACSM Health/Fitness Facility Preparticipation Screening Questionnaire** |

Assess your health status by marking all *true* statements.

History

You have had:

___ A heart attack
___ Heart surgery
___ Cardiac catheterization
___ Coronary angioplasty (PTCA)
___ Pacemaker/implantable cardiac defibrillator/
rhythm disturbance
___ Heart valve disease
___ Heart failure
___ Heart transplantation
___ Congenital heart disease

Symptoms

___ You experience chest discomfort with exertion.
___ You experience unreasonable breathlessness.
___ You experience dizziness, fainting, or blackouts.
___ You experience ankle swelling.
___ You experience unpleasant awareness of a forceful
or rapid heart rate.
___ You take heart medications.

*If you marked any of these statements in this section, consult your physician or other appropriate health care provider before engaging in exercise. You may need to use a facility with a **medically qualified staff**.*

Other health issues

___ You have diabetes.
___ You have asthma or other lung disease.
___ You have burning or cramping sensation in your
lower legs when walking short distance.
___ You have musculoskeletal problems that limit your
physical activity.
___ You have concerns about the safety of exercise.
___ You take prescription medications.
___ You are pregnant.

Cardiovascular risk factors

___ You are a man ≥45 yr.
___ You are a woman ≥55 yr.
___ You smoke or quit smoking within the previous
6 mo.
___ Your BP is ≥140/90 mm Hg.
___ You don't know your BP.
___ You take BP medication.
___ Your blood cholesterol level is ≥200 mg · dL^{-1}.
___ You don't know your cholesterol level.
___ You have a close blood relative who had a heart
attack or heart surgery before age 55 yr (father or
brother) or age 65 yr (mother or sister).
___ You are physically inactive (*i.e.*, you get <30 min
of physical activity on at least 3 d · wk^{-1}).
___ You have a body mass index ≥30 kg · m^{-2}.
___ You have prediabetes.
___ You don't know if you have prediabetes.

*If you marked two or more of the statements in this section, you should consult your physician or other appropriate health care provider as part of good medical care and progress gradually with your exercise program. You might benefit from using a facility with a **professionally qualified exercise staff**[a] to guide your exercise program.*

___ None of the above.

You should be able to exercise safely without consulting your physician or other appropriate health care provider in a self-guide program or almost any facility that meets your exercise program needs.

....

[a]Professionally qualified exercise staff refers to appropriately trained individuals who possess academic training, practical and clinical knowledge, skills, and abilities commensurate with the credentials defined in *Appendix A*.

Note: Individuals with multiple CVD risk factors should be encouraged to consult with their physician prior to initiating a vigorous intensity exercise program as part of good medical care and should progress gradually with their exercise program of any exercise intensity.

AHA, American Heart Association; ACSM, American College of Sports Medicine; PTCA, percutaneous transluminal coronary angioplasty; BP, blood pressure.

Reprinted with permission from *ACSM's Guidelines for Exercise Testing and Prescription*. 9th ed. Baltimore (MD): Lippincott Williams and Wilkins; 2014; adapted from Balady GJ, Chaitman B, Driscoll D, et al. American Heart Association/American College of Sports Medicine Joint Scientific Statement: Recommendations for cardiovascular screening, staffing, and emergency policies at health/fitness facilities. *Med Sci Sports Exerc.* 1998;30:1009–18.

shortness of breath; a new or previously unknown heart murmur, unequal or absent pulses; or wheezing, rales, or crackles heard in the lung fields, which may be a sign of bronchospasm or fluid accumulated in the airways, irregular heartbeats, and uncontrolled hypertension. Peripheral edema can also indicate an acute process, such as a deep venous thrombosis, in the setting of asymmetric lower-extremity edema, or a chronic disease that leads to fluid retention. A more complete list of the major signs and symptoms of cardiopulmonary and metabolic disease can be found in *Box 37-2*.

If indicated, a musculoskeletal exam assesses the range of motion of major joints of the upper and lower extremities and the cervical and lumbar spines. It is important to determine previous orthopedic surgery history, particularly knee and hip replacements. In addition, muscle strength, motor control, and balance may be assessed using functional activities for the purpose of determining the individual's ability to participate or perform a specific activity (72).

In addition to assessing risk factors for cardiovascular disease, a complete list of current medications, both prescription and over the counter, including dose and frequency, should be obtained for any individual wishing to undergo exercise testing. Many common medications directly alter the physiologic response to exercise. For example, β-blockers, which are commonly used for heart failure, hypertension, or coronary artery disease, will attenuate the heart rate (HR) and blood pressure (BP) response to exercise. Some antidepressants can increase HR and lower BP during rest or exercise. A more complete list of common medications and their effects on HR, BP, electrocardiogram (ECG), and exercise capacity can be found in *Table A-1* of the *GETP9*.

CONTRAINDICATIONS TO EXERCISE TESTING AND TRAINING

Through preparticipation screening, individuals may be found with contraindications to exercise such that the risks outweigh the benefits. The absolute and relative contraindications to exercise testing are listed in *Box 3.5* in *GETP9* (1). Those with absolute contraindications should refrain from exercise until further medical evaluation can be performed and their disease process treated and stabilized. Individuals with relative contraindications may only need further evaluation of the risk–benefit ratio before starting an exercise program. See *Chapter 3* of *GETP9* for further information.

HEALTH CONSIDERATIONS

MUSCULOSKELETAL CONDITIONS

Most types of physical activities are beneficial because moderate exercise is an important element for general well-being (76). The risk of musculoskeletal injury increases for all levels of participation with increasing physical activity, intensity, and duration of training (59). Understanding the associated risks, preventive measures, and procedures of immediate care can reduce the incidence and severity of exercise-related musculoskeletal injuries.

INJURY RISK FACTORS

Musculoskeletal injuries are among the most common adverse effects of regular exercise and physical activity for individuals of all ages (8,9). Musculoskeletal injuries can be attributed to the complex interaction of intrinsic and extrinsic risk factors (*Box 37-3*) that predispose physically active individuals to specific types of injuries (64,65,73). Poor baseline physical fitness, excessive training, improper biomechanics, and improper training techniques also affect the incidence of injury. Helping exercise participants identify modifiable short- and long-term injury risks could assist in developing strategies to decrease injuries.

The annual injury rate for recreational adult fitness participants is between two and three injuries per participant per year (66). Most of these injuries (76%) result in time lost from physical activity. The risk of musculoskeletal injury associated with various physical activities and cardiorespiratory fitness levels among recreationally active adults has also been reported (36). The findings indicate that moderate types and duration of physical activity promoted by the ACSM and other national health organizations have lower injury risk than more vigorous types and longer durations of physical activity (32,76). The risk of physical activity–related injury among adults increases for runners, sports participants, persons engaging in more than 1.25 h · wk^{-1} of physical activity, and individuals with moderate-to-high cardiorespiratory fitness levels. However, walking for exercise does not appear to be associated with a significant increased risk of activity-related injuries, even among walkers with the highest duration of activity per week. This low risk of musculoskeletal injury suggests that participation in walking can be safely recommended as a way to improve health and fitness for virtually any individual (21,36).

Comparisons of injury rates of athletes and exercise participants provide a perspective for understanding the magnitude of the problem of fitness-related injuries. The annual overall incidence of injury among distance runners is reported to range from 24% to 65% for heterogeneous populations of recreational and competitive runners (39). The cause of musculoskeletal running injuries is related to the runner, the running activity itself, and the environment (60). Training errors are reported in 60%–80% of injuries to runners and are commonly caused by exceeding limits of duration and intensity, high rates of progression, and excessive hill running (42).

BOX 37-2	**Major Signs or Symptoms Suggestive of Cardiovascular, Pulmonary, or Metabolic Disease**[a]

SIGN OR SYMPTOM	CLARIFICATION/SIGNIFICANCE
Pain or discomfort (or other anginal equivalent) in the chest, neck, jaw, arms, or other areas that may result from myocardial ischemia	One of the cardinal manifestations of cardiac disease, in particular, coronary artery disease Key features *favoring an ischemic origin* include the following: • *Character*: Constricting, squeezing, burning, "heaviness" or "heavy feeling" • *Location*: Substernal, across midthorax, anteriorly; in both arms, shoulders; in neck, cheeks, teeth; in forearms, fingers; in interscapular region • *Provoking factors*: Exercise or exertion, excitement, other forms of stress, cold weather, occurrence after meals Key features *against an ischemic origin* include the following: • *Character*: Dull ache; "knifelike," sharp, stabbing; "jabs" aggravated by respiration • *Location*: In left submammary area; in left hemithorax • *Provoking factors*: After completion of exercise, provoked by a specific body motion
Shortness of breath at rest or with mild exertion	*Dyspnea* (defined as an abnormally uncomfortable awareness of breathing) is one of the principal symptoms of cardiac and pulmonary disease. It commonly occurs during strenuous exertion in healthy, well-trained persons and during moderate exertion in healthy, untrained persons. However, it should be regarded as abnormal when it occurs at a level of exertion that is not expected to evoke this symptom in a given individual. Abnormal exertional dyspnea suggests the presence of cardiopulmonary disorders, in particular, left ventricular dysfunction or chronic obstructive pulmonary disease.
Dizziness or syncope	*Syncope* (defined as a loss of consciousness) is most commonly caused by a reduced perfusion of the brain. Dizziness and, in particular, syncope *during* exercise may result from cardiac disorders that prevent the normal rise (or an actual fall) in cardiac output. Such cardiac disorders are potentially life threatening and include severe coronary artery disease, hypertrophic cardiomyopathy, aortic stenosis, and malignant ventricular dysrhythmias. Although dizziness or syncope shortly *after* cessation of exercise should not be ignored, these symptoms may occur even in healthy persons as a result of a reduction in venous return to the heart.
Orthopnea or paroxysmal nocturnal dyspnea	*Orthopnea* refers to dyspnea occurring at rest in the recumbent position that is relieved promptly by sitting upright or standing. *Paroxysmal nocturnal dyspnea* refers to dyspnea, beginning usually 2–5 h after the onset of sleep, which may be relieved by sitting on the side of the bed or getting out of bed. Both are symptoms of left ventricular dysfunction. Although nocturnal dyspnea may occur in persons with chronic obstructive pulmonary disease, it differs in that it is usually relieved after the person relieves himself or herself of secretions rather than specifically by sitting up.
Ankle edema	Bilateral ankle edema that is most evident at night is a characteristic sign of heart failure or bilateral chronic venous insufficiency. Unilateral edema of a limb often results from venous thrombosis or lymphatic blockage in the limb. Generalized edema (known as anasarca) occurs in persons with the nephrotic syndrome, severe heart failure, or hepatic cirrhosis.
Palpitations or tachycardia	*Palpitations* (defined as an unpleasant awareness of the forceful or rapid beating of the heart) may be induced by various disorders of cardiac rhythm. These include tachycardia, bradycardia of sudden onset, ectopic beats, compensatory pauses, and accentuated stroke volume resulting from valvular regurgitation. Palpitations also often result from anxiety states and high cardiac output (or hyperkinetic) states, such as anemia, fever, thyrotoxicosis, arteriovenous fistula, and the so-called idiopathic hyperkinetic heart syndrome.

BOX 37-2	Major Signs or Symptoms Suggestive of Cardiovascular, Pulmonary, or Metabolic Disease[a] (*Continued*)

SIGN OR SYMPTOM	CLARIFICATION/SIGNIFICANCE
Intermittent claudication	*Intermittent claudication* refers to the pain that occurs in a muscle with an inadequate blood supply (usually as a result of atherosclerosis) that is stressed by exercise. The pain does not occur with standing or sitting, is reproducible from day to day, is more severe when walking upstairs or up a hill, and is often described as a cramp, which disappears within 1–2 min after stopping exercise. Coronary artery disease is more prevalent in persons with intermittent claudication. Patients with diabetes are at increased risk for this condition.
Known heart murmur	Although some may be innocent, heart murmurs may indicate valvular or other cardiovascular disease. From an exercise safety standpoint, it is especially important to exclude hypertrophic cardiomyopathy and aortic stenosis as underlying causes because these are among the more common causes of exertion-related sudden cardiac death.
Unusual fatigue or shortness of breath with usual activities	Although there may be benign origins for these symptoms, they also may signal the onset or change in the status of cardiovascular, pulmonary, or metabolic disease.

[a]These signs or symptoms must be interpreted within the clinical context in which they appear because they are not all specific for cardiovascular, pulmonary, or metabolic disease.

High-impact aerobic dance is also associated with a substantial incidence of injury (33). The incidence of injury in aerobic dance is reported to be approximately 45% of students and 75% of instructors (53). Eighty percent of these injuries affect the lower legs and are related to frequency of exercise; improper footwear; or exercise on hard, nonresilient surfaces (67). Low-impact aerobics participation is now common and is used as an alternative to high-impact aerobics, which was primarily performed in earlier years. The injury rates for low- and high-impact aerobic dance has been reported as 24% and 38%, respectively (37). Injury rates of more recent derivations of aerobic dance, such as kickboxing, boot camp, P90X, Tae Bo, and other intensive "floor routine"–based training programs have not been published.

BOX 37-3	Injury Risk Factors

INTRINSIC RISK FACTORS

History of previous injury
Inadequate fitness or conditioning
Body composition
Bony alignment abnormalities
Strength or flexibility imbalances
Joint or ligamentous laxity
Predisposing musculoskeletal disease

EXTRINSIC RISK FACTORS

Excessive load on the body
Type of movement
Speed of movement
Number of repetitions
Footwear
Surface
Training errors

Excessive distances
Fast progression
High intensity
Running on hills
Poor technique
Fatigue
Adverse environmental conditions
Air quality
Darkness
Heat or cold
High humidity
Altitude
Wind
Worn or faulty equipment

Modified with permission from Renstrom P, Kannus P. Prevention of sports injuries. In: Strauss RH, editor. *Sports Medicine*. 2nd ed. Philadelphia: Saunders; 1991. p. 307–29.

It is estimated that more than 970,000 emergency department (ED) visits occurred from 1990 through 2007 in the United States as a direct result of weight-training injuries (40). This comprehensive survey of ED data revealed that younger (average age 28 yr) men (82%) sustained most of the injuries; the most common injury was a strain/sprain (46%) most frequently caused by weights dropping on the person (66%); approximately 90% of injuries occurred with free weights. Previous estimates of the risk of acute injury from weight training and weight equipment ranged from 2.4% to 7.6% of participants per year. A previous study showed a 35% increase in the number of ED injuries related to weight-training activities from 1978 to 1998 (38). From 1990 to 2007, the number of ED injuries related to weight training increased to 48%; however, it is not clear if the rising incidence is caused by higher injury rates or increased overall participation. Injuries reported included soft tissue injury, lacerations, concussions, and fractures and dislocations. Most weight-training injuries occur from excessive training, improper techniques, and the misuse of weight-training equipment, with the most important precipitating factor being inadequate recovery (17,63).

Disorders of the musculoskeletal system may directly increase the risk of acute or chronic injury by interrupting normal structure and function of bone, joint, and soft tissue. The most common musculoskeletal risk factors include osteoarthritis, osteoporosis, chondromalacia, age-related musculotendinous degeneration, and malalignments of the lower extremities (55). Excessive body weight predisposes individuals to acute and overuse injuries, including osteoarthritic changes of the hip and knee with weight-bearing recreational activities (28,30). Weight loss reduces the risk of developing knee osteoarthritis, but its effect on the progression of the disease is unknown (29). In addition, vigorous physical activity may predispose participants to osteoarthritis by means of mechanical trauma to the joint (30). For example, there is an increased risk of osteoarthritis for competitive sports and running but not for recreational running (43).

Concerns for Exercise Testing and Programming

Musculoskeletal injuries are a health burden because they may lead to permanent reductions in activity, thereby resulting in deconditioning. To reduce the incidence and severity of injury, it is important to identify predisposing risk factors through education and clinical intervention. Behavior modification regarding early detection of symptoms of overuse is important for preventing injury. Participants should be encouraged to report injuries and symptoms to their health care provider and exercise professional (if they have one) because untreated musculoskeletal injuries are likely to worsen the problem or predispose to future

exercise-related injury (2). Strenuous exercise is contraindicated in the presence of acute joint injury, chronic joint inflammation (osteoarthritis), or uncontrolled systemic joint disease (rheumatoid arthritis). Under medical management, submaximal and symptom-limited fitness testing along with exercise program participation is not contraindicated. The progression and level of physical activity must be pain free, individualized, and otherwise limited by precautions and contraindications associated with specific medical conditions. The goal of exercise programs for individuals after musculoskeletal injury or those with orthopedic disease and disability should be to prevent debilitation caused by inactivity and to improve endurance, exercise tolerance, strength, and flexibility (26). The goal is, of course, primary prevention of musculoskeletal injury. As such, proper warm-up, stretching, and cool-down should be performed as part of an exercise program, and particularly with strenuous exercise.

Treatment Considerations

Most activity-related injuries result from either *macrotrauma* (tension, shear, or compression) or *microtrauma* (overuse or repetitive motion). Damage to tissue caused by trauma is defined as the *primary injury*. With the exception of controlling hemorrhage, initial treatment has little effect on the extent or severity of primary injury. Improper care or delay in treatment may cause additional pain, swelling, and tissue damage of healthy tissues. Secondary hypoxic/inflammatory injury (the death of healthy cells caused by lack of oxygen or inflammation) is caused by the body's natural response to hemorrhage with a decrease in blood flow to the injured body segment. Secondary injury may continue even after bleeding is controlled, which necessitates that the initial treatment protocol consists of rest, ice, compression, elevation, and stabilization during the 24–72 h after injury.

Exercise professionals are often asked for advice regarding the management of musculoskeletal problems or injuries. This may entail making recommendations about training and modifications in exercise programs, rendering immediate first aid, or referring participants to physicians. To help in decision making, knowledge of common exercise injuries (*Table 37-1*) and their causative mechanisms (*Table 37-2*) is important.

Basic first-aid procedures for common exercise-related musculoskeletal injuries are outlined in *Table 37-3*. The combination of *Rest, Ice, Compression, Elevation*, and *Stabilization* (RICES) is the appropriate treatment for immediate care of patients with acute injuries (62). When used properly, the RICES treatment regimen reduces the total amount of tissue damage; decreases swelling and pain; and aids in controlling the inflammatory response, which results in quicker rehabilitation and recovery. Rest allows time to control the effects of trauma and to avoid additional tissue damage. Rest is a continuum ranging from complete rest or immobilization to restricted activity

TABLE 37-1. Descriptions of General Exercise Injuries

Condition	Description	Characteristics
Sprain	A stretch or tear to the ligaments and stabilizing connective tissues of a joint	Swelling, pain, joint instability, loss of function
Strain	A stretch or tear in the muscle or adjacent tissue, such as the fascia or muscle tendon	Movement pain, local tenderness, loss of strength and ROM
Contusion	A bruise that occurs from a sudden traumatic blow to soft or bony tissue	Soft tissue hemorrhage, hematoma, ecchymosis, movement restriction
Acute fracture	A sudden break of a bone	Deformity, bone point tenderness, swelling, ecchymosis
Stress fracture	Microscopic damage to the bone caused by repetitive stress	Insidious onset of pain that persists when attempting activity; tenderness
Bursitis	Inflammation of a bursa between bony prominences and muscle or tendon	Swelling, pain, some loss of function
Tendonitis	Inflammation of a tendon	Gradual onset, diffuse or local pain, tenderness, loss of strength
Plantar fasciitis	Inflammatory condition to the plantar surface of the foot	Inferior heel pain, pain increased with weight bearing
Shin splints	An overuse injury that indicates pain in the anteromedial shin	Pain occurring before, during, or after activity; bone tenderness
Patellofemoral pain syndrome	Knee pain caused by lateral deviation of the patella as it tracks in the femoral groove	Tenderness of the lateral patella, pain, swelling
Low back pain	Condition resulting from trauma or multiple episodes of microtrauma resulting in muscular or joint pain	Pain accentuated by sudden flexion, extension, or rotation; muscle weakness
Rotator cuff tendonitis	Inflammation of the rotator cuff muscles or tendons	Diffuse pain, increased with overhead activities; muscle weakness in external rotation
Tennis elbow	Inflammation of the lateral epicondyle of the humerus	Pain in lateral elbow during and after activity; weakness of the wrist in extension

ROM, range of motion.

(relative rest) of the involved body part. The application of ice or some form of cold application helps lower tissue temperature, thus slowing cell metabolism. Cold applications also are beneficial for reducing pain and muscle spasms that accompany musculoskeletal injuries. Both compression and elevation contribute to swelling control. Stabilization allows musculature around the injury to relax, which, along with the ice, aids in limiting the pain–spasm cycle (62). Therapeutic treatments, such as heat modalities and exercise rehabilitation (*e.g.*, physical therapy), are often prescribed after the initial treatment and are designed to promote healing and allow return to regular physical activity.

Concussion injuries are unique from musculoskeletal injuries and occur as a result of linear or rotational accelerations to the brain induced by impact or trauma. Incidence rates are greatest in contact sports such as football, soccer, ice hockey, lacrosse, and combative arts (*e.g.*, boxing, martial arts). Common acute and delayed signs and symptoms may include loss of consciousness, amnesia, confusion or slurred speech, blurred or double vision, headache, dizziness, emotional lability, and sleep disturbances among others. The most important acute treatment consideration is to delay return to play if concussion is either diagnosed or suspected to prevent further trauma to the brain. Exercise should be withheld

until cleared by a physician to begin training and, specifically, competition. This is important because symptoms can linger for extended durations (*i.e.*, months) and be worsened with premature return to play with long-term adverse health impacts (34).

CARDIOVASCULAR CONDITIONS

In addition to the many musculoskeletal injuries that have been discussed, various additional health-related conditions can potentially affect exercise participants. The stress of physical exertion during exercise, accompanied by risk factors or environmental conditions, can increase the risk for cardiopulmonary or metabolic complications that can affect the individual's health.

The AHA/ACSM Health/Fitness Facility Preparticipation Screening Questionnaire uses history, symptoms, and risk-factor information to help direct people to either begin an exercise program or contact a physician before starting exercise (see *Box 37-1*)(11). The AHA and ACSM have jointly published guidelines for classifying exercise participants according to disease risk (11). The recommendation states that participants should be classified into one of three risk strata: apparently healthy persons, persons at increased risk, and persons with known cardiovascular disease. These risk strata are based on traditional risk

TABLE 37-2. Common Acute and Chronic Exercise Injuries and Causes

Body Region	Injury	Mechanism of Injury
Upper Extremities		
Shoulders	Rotator cuff strain	Throwing; swimming
	Rotator cuff tendonitis	Use of arm above horizontal; repetitive overhead activities
	Anterior glenohumeral dislocation	Forced horizontal abduction, external rotation
Upper arms	Bicipital tenosynovitis	Repeated forceful external rotation of the arm
Elbows	Lateral epicondylitis	Repeated forceful extension of the elbow (tennis elbow)
	Medial epicondylitis	Repeated forceful flexion of the elbow
Wrists and hands	Carpal tunnel syndrome	Activities that require repeated wrist flexion
	Strains and sprains	Falling on the wrist or outstretched hand
	Fractures	Falling on the outstretched hand
Lower Extremities		
Feet	Heel bruise	Contusion; sudden stop-and-go movements in running
	Plantar fasciitis	Unequal leg length; inflexible longitudinal arch; tight gastrocnemius–soleus muscle
	Metatarsalgia	Excessive pressure under the forefoot; fallen metatarsal arch
	Metatarsal stress fracture	Training overload; unequal leg length; hyperpronation of foot
Ankle, lower legs	Inversion ankle sprain	Foot forced into inversion-plantarflexion
	Achilles tendon strain	Sudden excessive dorsiflexion of foot
	Achilles tendonitis	Training errors; tight gastrocnemius–soleus muscle
	Anterior, posterior tibial tendonitis	Faulty posture alignment; falling arches; overuse stress
	Stress fracture of the tibia, fibula	Overuse stress; biomechanical foot problems
	Shin splints	Overtraining; running on hard surface; malaligned lower leg
Knees	Patellofemoral pain syndrome	Overuse (*e.g.*, hill running); patellar compression
	Joint sprain	Direct straight-line or rotary forces
	Meniscal lesion	Excessive pressure (squatting); shear forces
	Patellar subluxation, dislocation	Alignment abnormalities; quadriceps weakness
	Chondromalacia patella	Abnormal patellar tracking; anatomic variation
	Degenerative arthritis	Overuse stress; obesity
	Patellar or quadriceps tendonitis	Sudden or repetitive forceful extension of knee
	Iliotibial band friction syndrome	Overuse stress associated with running, cycling
Upper legs	Quadriceps muscle strain	Weak muscles; sudden contraction, as during jumping
	Hamstring muscle strain	Strength imbalance; tightness; explosive movements
Hips	Trochanteric bursitis	Increased Q-angle; unequal leg length; faulty running form
Trunk		
Abdomen	Muscle strain	Sudden twisting of the trunk; reaching overhead
Spine	Lumbar strain and sprain	Poor posture; lumbar lordosis; sudden abrupt extension or contraction, sometimes with trunk rotation
	Low back pain	Acute traumatic event; overuse; poor sitting posture; static or repeated flexion activities

factor, medical history and diagnoses, and, in some cases, maximal exercise testing results. After an individual has been stratified, decisions can be made regarding the need for and the types of medical examination and exercise testing. People at higher risk for coronary heart disease are directed to seek exercise facilities providing appropriate levels of staff supervision (*Table 37-4*) (3).

Attempting to identify the individual at risk for SCD is the major purpose of the athletic preparticipation screening process. The risk of SCD in the young athlete is 0.01% or less (1/200,000) (71). When discussing the risk of SCD, athletes are divided into two groups based on age (<35 yr and >35 yr). The athlete <35 yr is more likely to have a congenital heart lesion as the cause of SCD, whereas

TABLE 37-3. Basic First-Aid Guidelines for Exercise-Related Musculoskeletal and Skin Injuries

Condition	First-Aid Procedures
Acute musculoskeletal injuries: contusion, sprain, strain	If no fracture, follow the RICES guidelines: set the area at rest (immobilize), apply an ice bag or cold pack with an elastic wrap for 20–30 min, and elevate the extremity above the heart. Reevaluate after initial first aid, support the injured area, and apply an elastic wrap to maintain compression, keeping the extremity elevated, if possible. Reapply ice or cold packs every 2 h for 30 min and then continue to maintain compression and elevation during periods when cold is not being applied. Repeat these procedures for the first 24–72 h depending on the severity of injury and symptoms.
Fracture	Keep the individual still with the extremity in the position found, without moving the extremity or individual, if possible. Activate EMS or the facility's emergency response system to transport the individual to an ER. Do not apply a commercial or homemade splint unless the individual must be moved. Apply a cold pack. Calm and reassure the individual. Monitor the individual for signs and symptoms of shock, internal bleeding, and other life-threatening conditions. If splinting is warranted, proper splinting technique includes the following: (a) check distal pulse, skin temperature, color, and sensation for damage to nerves and blood vessels; (b) keep the individual still and immobilize the joints above and below the suspected fracture site along with the broken bone ends with splinting materials, the ground, or other body part; and (c) recheck for circulation and sensation distal to the injury site.
Open skin wounds	With all open wounds, be sure to place a barrier (*e.g.*, disposable latex gloves) between yourself and the individual's blood or body fluids and follow universal precautions to prevent the transfer of blood-borne pathogens. Be sure to wash your hands immediately after providing care. Minor wounds without significant bleeding (*e.g.*, blisters, abrasions, lacerations, and incisions) should be cleaned with soap and water and treated with a germicide cream or solution, followed by the application of a sterile dressing (such as an adhesive plastic strip, gauze pad, or other commercial wound cover). The individual should be reminded to watch for signs of infection, keep the area clean and dry, and change the dressing as needed. Significant wounds that are bleeding severely should be treated by one or more of the following procedures: (a) apply direct pressure by applying a sterile dressing directly to the wound and applying pressure with the flat of the hand and fingers (if the dressing becomes saturated, apply additional dressings on top of the previous without removing the saturated dressing); (b) elevate the limb (if no fracture is suspected) while maintaining direct pressure elevate the wound above the individual's heart; (c) apply a bandage snugly over the dressing; or (d) if the preceding methods fail to stop the wound from bleeding, apply pressure to the brachial artery in the arm for upper-extremity wounds or femoral artery in the groin for lower-extremity wounds. Activate EMS or the facility's emergency response system.

RICES, rest, ice, compression, elevation, and stabilization; EMS, emergency medical services; ER, emergency room.

TABLE 37-4. Emergency Plans and Equipment for Health Fitness Facilities

	Level 1	Level 2	Level 3	Level 4	Level 5
Type of Facility	Unsupervised exercise room (*e.g.*, hotel, commercial building)	Single exercise leader	Fitness center for general membership	Fitness center offering special programs for clinical populations	Medically supervised clinical exercise program (*e.g.*, cardiac rehabilitation)
Personnel	None	Exercise leader; recommended: medical liaison	General manager; H/F instructor; exercise leader; recommended: medical liaison	General manager; exercise specialist; H/F instructor; medical liaison	General manager; exercise specialist; H/F instructor; exercise leader; medical liaison
Emergency Plan	Present	Present	Present	Present	Present
Emergency Equipment	Telephone in room Signs; encouraged: PAD plan with AED as part of the composite PAD plan in the host facility (hotel, commercial building)	Telephone; signs Encouraged: BP kit, stethoscope, PAD plan with AED	Telephone; signs Encouraged: BP kit, stethoscope, PAD plan with AED (the latter are strongly encouraged in facilities with membership >2,500 and those in which EMS response time is expected to be <5 min from recognition of arrest)	Telephone; signs BP kit, stethoscope; strongly encouraged: PAD plan with AED	Telephone; signs BP kit, stethoscope, oxygen, crash cart defibrillator[a]

H/F, health and fitness; PAD, public access to defibrillation; AED, automated external defibrillator; BP, blood pressure; EMS, emergency medical services .

[a]Standard equipment in Level 5 facilities includes a defibrillator (1,14).

Reprinted with permission from Balady GJ, Chaitman B, Driscoll D, et al. Recommendations for cardiovascular screening, staffing, and emergency policies at health/fitness facilities. *Circulation.* 1998;97(22):2283–93..

the athlete >35 yr is more likely to have coronary artery disease as the cause of SCD (51). In the United States, the incidence of congenital heart disease in the young athlete has been estimated to be 0.2%–0.7% or about 30,000 young competitive athletes (50,71). The most common causes of SCD in the young athletes are hypertrophic cardiomyopathy, arrhythmogenic right ventricular cardiomyopathy, and anomalous coronary arteries.

In those older than 35 yr who die during exercise, coronary artery disease is the most common cause. **Myocardial ischemia** may manifest as a continuum of diastolic dysfunction, a decrease in left ventricular ejection fraction, abnormal BP responses, ECG abnormalities, arrhythmias, or angina. Atrial and ventricular tachycardias are serious arrhythmias that can lead to ventricular fibrillation and sudden death (24). Unstable tachycardia exists when the heart beats too fast, resulting in reduced diastolic filling time and reduced stroke volume. This tachycardia may lead to hemodynamic instability and signs and symptoms such as pain, myocardial infarction, hypotension, congestive heart failure, or SCD (*Table 37-5*).

A natural consequence of endurance training is a decreased resting HR. The actual mechanisms responsible for this decrease are not entirely clear, but training appears to alter the intrinsic HR, probably as a function of structural remodeling of the sinus node, increased left ventricular dimension and stroke volume, and by increases in parasympathetic activity while sympathetic activity is reduced (46). However, in untrained individuals, pronounced *bradycardia* (resting HR <40 beats per minute [bpm]) may be the result of conduction abnormalities, such as complete heart

block and sinus node disease. In particular, acute myocardial infarction can lead to ischemic damage to the conducting system of the heart, producing bradycardias that range from sinus bradycardia to complete heart block (see *Table 37-5*) (24). Both autonomic influences and the intrinsic pathology of the conduction system can lead to bradycardia. Therefore, it is necessary to distinguish between training-induced bradycardia and pathologic bradycardia, which can be a serious cause for concern. Typically, if a person is asymptomatic and is physically active or performing regular intentional exercise training, it is likely that the bradycardia is not pathologic. Also a treadmill stress test with normal HR response supports the opinion that the bradycardia is secondary to exercise training.

Concerns for Exercise Testing and Programming

In patients with multiple coronary risk factors, exercise testing may provide important insight into exercise capacity as well as diagnostic and prognostic information. Some of the indicators of poor prognosis that can be assessed during a symptom-limited maximal exercise test are ST-segment depression at a low workload, peak capacity <5 metabolic equivalents (METs), a hypotensive response to exercise, chronotropic incompetence (*e.g.*, failure to achieve 85% of age-predicted maximal HR), and a low HR recovery (*e.g.*, failure of HR to decrease from peak exercise by at least 12 bpm within the first minute post exercise) (1,22).

Although the general principles of exercise prescription hold for patients with cardiovascular disease, as

TABLE 37-5. Cardiopulmonary and Metabolic Conditions

Condition or Abnormality	Definition	Signs and Symptoms
Hypertrophic cardiomyopathy	Hypertrophy of the myocardium	Cardiac palpitations, angina, syncope, vertigo; asymptomatic
Tachycardia	HR ≥100 bpm in adults at rest	Chest palpitations; difficulty breathing, severe chest pressure, chest pain, shortness of breath while exercising
Bradycardia	HR <60 bpm in adults at rest	Chest pain, shortness of breath, fatigue, exercise intolerance, hypotension, decrease in BP when standing
Tachypnea	Abnormal rapidity of respiration	Hyperventilation syndrome (also known as behavioral breathlessness *or* psychogenic dyspnea)
Hypertension	Systolic BP ≥140 mm Hg Diastolic BP ≥90 mm Hg	Headache; most people are symptom free until complications arise
Hypotension	Decreased systolic and diastolic BP	Syncope and fatigue; occurs in shock, hemorrhage, and dehydration
Fainting	Feeling weak as though about to lose consciousness	Paleness; weakness; dizziness; weak, rapid, irregular pulse
Syncope	Transient loss of consciousness caused by inadequate blood flow to the brain	Peripheral circulatory failure; cardiac arrhythmia; hyperventilation
Hypoglycemia	Abnormal decreased blood glucose level	Headache; shakiness, confusion, faintness, blurred or double vision, tachycardia, pallor, convulsions, unconsciousness
Hyperglycemia	Abnormal increased blood glucose level	Nausea, dizziness when rising, polyuria, blurred vision, weight loss

HR, heart rate; bpm, beats per minute; BP, blood pressure.

outlined in *Chapters 7* and *8* of *GETP9*, particular attention should be paid to the warm-up and cool-down phases. An adequate warm-up may aid in preventing ST-segment depression, arrhythmias, and transient left ventricular dysfunction (13,14). An adequate cool-down allows for HR and BP to return to baseline values, reducing post-exercise hypotension, dizziness, and catecholamine surges (25). Other potential adverse health effects from exercise include cardiac dysfunction, ischemic arrhythmias, and an excessive hypertensive response (see *Table 37-5*).

Although sufficiently powered studies evaluating the safety of resistance training in patients with moderate- to high-risk cardiovascular disease do not yet exist, there are data that show benefit in low-risk individuals. A low-risk individual is defined as no evidence of myocardial ischemia with exercise, no severe left ventricular dysfunction, and without complex ventricular arrhythmias. It is generally recommended that low- to moderate-risk individuals with heart disease complete at least 2–4 wk of an aerobic exercise training program before initiating resistance training. Resistance training should be at a low-to-moderate intensity, and the Valsalva maneuver should be avoided. Resistance training in patients with moderate- to high-risk disease should be closely monitored. ACSM endorses guidelines regarding resistance exercise in individuals with cardiovascular disease, including heart failure, set forth by the AHA (78).

Individuals with hypertension can benefit from exercise. Exercise programs that primarily include endurance activity, resistance training, or both are beneficial in preventing the development and management of hypertension. An exercise training program can decrease systolic or diastolic BP by 5–7 mm Hg in patients with hypertension (58). This is important because a decrease of 2 mm Hg of systolic and diastolic pressures reduces the risk of stroke by 14% and 17% and the risk of coronary artery disease by 9% and 6%, respectively (58).

There is emerging evidence that high-intensity exercise training at levels up to 95% of the age-predicted peak HR may be beneficial for patients with heart disease (80). A pilot study found that exercise intensity was an important factor for reversing left ventricular remodeling and improving aerobic capacity, endothelial function, and quality of life in patients with chronic heart failure. Currently, however, there is no sufficient data to recommend high-intensity training for patients with heart disease.

PULMONARY CONDITIONS

Obstructive lung disease and restrictive pulmonary disease are two conditions that require special consideration for exercise prescription. *Obstructive lung disease* is characterized by air trapping and lung hyperinflation and is often diagnosed as emphysema, chronic bronchitis, or small airway disease. Asthma is included in this category, but it is characterized by reversible airflow obstruction and may be induced by exercise. In obstructive lung disease, hypoxia can develop as a result of ventilation/perfusion mismatch caused by hyperventilation of emphysematous areas in the lung, leading to an increase in dead-space ventilation (20). However, dyspnea that is caused by mechanical constraints and hyperinflation may occur without hypoxemia and may respond well to supplemental oxygen. During exercise, the goal is to optimize airflow by controlling inflammation, bronchospasm, airway mucus, and predisposing conditions (including tobacco use or triggers such as allergens and cold air).

Restrictive lung disease encompasses multiple disease processes that involve the lung parenchyma, pleura, or chest wall and result in reduced filling of the lung. The incidence of restrictive lung disease is low compared with obstructive lung disease. Diagnosis is made by pulmonary function testing with a reduced total lung capacity. During exercise, the reduction in ventilatory volume may lead to hypoxemia secondary to an increase in dead-space ventilation from a higher respiratory rate (rapid shallow breathing).

In general, exercise testing and training may be safely performed by patients with chronic lung disease, given that the subject's specific lung disease is accounted for and guidelines for pulmonary rehabilitation are followed. Pulmonary rehabilitation is a program used to progressively increase exercise capacity in patients with lung disease, but its role has not been well established in restrictive disease. Pulse oximetry and supplemental oxygen may be needed during testing or training, depending on the severity of the patient's lung disease. See *Chapter 39* for a more detailed description of pulmonary considerations in exercise and pulmonary rehabilitation.

METABOLIC CONDITIONS

DM is a chronic metabolic disorder marked by hyperglycemia. DM results either from failure of the pancreas to produce insulin (Type 1 DM) or from insulin resistance with inadequate insulin secretion to sustain normal metabolism (Type 2 DM). Type 1 DM usually presents as an acute illness with dehydration and often diabetic ketoacidosis. Individuals with Type 2 DM can be asymptomatic during the initial years with the disease (4). Diagnosis is based on a fasting plasma glucose level, an oral glucose tolerance test, and/or glycated hemoglobin (HbA1C) (4).

Complications of DM include heart disease, renal dysfunction, retinopathies, peripheral arterial disease, slowly healing lower limb/foot ulcers, and an inability to control blood glucose with a propensity for hyperglycemia or hypoglycemia. If any of these are present, consultation with a physician is warranted. Guidelines to avoid exercise-induced hypoglycemia in individuals with DM are shown in *Box 37-4* (5). In patients with poorly controlled diabetes (*i.e.*, a blood sugar >300 mg · dL^{-1}), exercise may actually increase glucose levels because of counterregulatory hormones. Exercise should be avoided if urinary or blood

<table>
<tr><td>

BOX 37-4

</td><td>

Guidelines for Avoiding Exercise-Induced Hypoglycemia

</td></tr>
</table>

- Check blood glucose before exercise.
- If blood glucose <100 mg · dL^{-1}, consume 15–20 g carbohydrate 15–30 min before training.
- Recheck blood glucose after 30 min of training or sooner if symptoms are present.
- Exercise 1–2 h after eating.
- Avoid exercise during insulin peak time.
- Avoid insulin injection into exercising limbs; suggest injection into abdominal tissue.
- Have fast-acting glucose available at all times (*e.g.*, glucose tablets).
- Check blood glucose immediately after exercise; if blood glucose <60 mg · dL^{-1}, then consume 15–20 g carbohydrate (glucose preferred).

ketones are present (47). *Chapter 40* provides specifics for exercise training for persons with diabetes.

NEUROMUSCULAR CONDITIONS

Often, patients presenting to clinical exercise programs for treatment of cardiac, pulmonary, or metabolic disease have concomitant neuromuscular conditions. These conditions may result in physical disability. Therefore, physical accessibility of the exercise facility is an important consideration for this population, consistent with the Americans with Disabilities Act of 2002 (7). Adequate and safe access to exercise facilities including entrances, equipment, bathrooms, pools, locker rooms, and elevators should be maintained as much as is reasonably possible (68). The following paragraphs and *Table 37-6* briefly review some of these conditions.

Multiple sclerosis (MS) is a neuromuscular process that leads to dysfunction of the central nervous system. Current recommendations are for baseline fitness evaluation using a cycle ergometer. Common issues that affect patients with MS and should be considered in exercise prescription include lower-extremity muscle weakness, including foot

TABLE 37-6. Neuromuscular Conditions, Signs or Symptoms, and Training Considerations

Neuromuscular Condition	Major Signs or Symptoms	Aerobic Training Considerations	Strength Training Considerations
Stroke	• Hemiplegia • Ataxia (wide variability in severity)	• Arm/leg ergometry or seated stepping if unsteady gait • Treadmill walking as tolerated • Monitor exercise BP to prevent hypertension (>220/110 mm Hg)	• Gravity only, bands, or weights as able • Adaptive gloves or assistive aids to safely hold weight • Focus on weakest side to increase ability to use • Monitor exercise BP to prevent hypertension (>220/110 mm Hg)
Multiple sclerosis	• Profound diurnal pattern fatigue and specifically motor fatigue • Heat intolerance • Incoordination • Spasticity • Blurred vision • Facial and/or tongue numbness • Urinary frequency and urgency • Abnormal or loss of skin sensations	• Precooling and/or early morning exercise to minimize heat intolerances	• Perform on nonaerobic training days, consider seated or supine posture, avoid free weights if upper extremity sensory deficits
Parkinson disease	• Tremor • Bradykinesia • Rigidity • Impaired postural reflexes	• Adjust aerobic mode to reduce fall risk • Slow static stretching • ROM exercises	• Consider machine instead of free weights to minimize injury risk
Peripheral neuropathy and neuropathic pain	• Chronic and persistent pain sometimes worse at night and discordant with stimulus (*i.e.*, blanket on affected limb) • Lack of normal pain perception (*i.e.*, diabetic neuropathy)	• May be deconditioned due to avoidance of exercise • Choose mode to avoid pain • Monitor for other signs and symptoms of angina because it may not be felt or recognized by patient	• May have weakness and limited ROM of affected muscles • Active and passive ROM exercises • Strength training as tolerated to minimize acute and post exercise pain

BP, blood pressure; ROM, range of motion.

Adapted from Myers J, Nieman DC, American College of Sports Medicine. *ACSM's Resources for Clinical Exercise Physiology: Musculoskeletal, Neuromuscular, Neoplastic, Immunologic, and Hematologic Conditions.* 2nd ed. Philadelphia (PA): Wolters Kluwer Health/Lippincott Williams & Wilkins Health; 2010. 323 p.

drop; loss of sensation, balance, and muscle coordination; muscle spasticity; and visual disturbances. As such, low-impact exercises such as walking, cycling, and water aerobics may be necessary for safe training. Patients with MS are also known to have a greater sensitivity to heat with exacerbation of neural deficits and may benefit from precooling with water immersion as well as early morning exercise training to control the rise in core body temperature. Regular stretching may enhance the effects of medications in the management of spasticity in patients with MS (16). See *Chapter 3* in *ACSM's Resources for Clinical Exercise Physiology, Second Edition* for a more detailed description of MS and exercise considerations (54).

Parkinson disease is a progressive neuromuscular disease that affects the central nervous system, leading to resting tremors, bradykinesia, rigidity, and postural instability. In ambulatory patients, walking is the preferred method of exercise testing or endurance training, whereas a stationary, recumbent, or upper-extremity ergometer is more appropriate for those patients with postural instability. If a treadmill is used, a safety harness system may be necessary. See *Chapter 4* in *ACSM's Resources for Clinical*

Exercise Physiology, Second Edition for more information on Parkinson disease and exercise testing and training (54).

Patients with Parkinson disease or MS benefit from adequate warm-up and flexibility activities because they are often quite inflexible from their conditions and associated sedentary living. It would be wise to assess flexibility and begin a program to enhance range of motion as an adjunct to a cardiorespiratory and/or resistance exercise training program. This will likely assist to improve functional status and potentially allow some additional exercise modalities to be used that require a minimal amount of flexibility to use.

ENVIRONMENTAL CONSIDERATIONS

The human body experiences unique challenges and occasionally adverse health effects when performing physical activity in extreme environmental conditions (*e.g.*, high or low temperature, high humidity, high altitude, underwater submersion, and pollution). Special precautions and modifications of exercise programming are sometimes needed to reduce health risks related to the exercise environment (*Table 37-7*). It is vitally

TABLE 37-7. Basic First-Aid Guidelines for Environmental and Exercise Intolerance Conditions

Condition	Guidelines
Environmental and exercise intolerance	Stop activity; calm and reassure the individual; monitor vital signs; activate EMS, if warranted.
Dizziness	Stop activity; position patient supine with legs elevated; monitor vital signs and seek medical attention if symptoms persist.
Fainting	Position patient in supine with the legs elevated, provided no injury is suspected; monitor vital signs and seek medical attention if symptoms persist. If individual has fallen, check for additional injuries before moving.
Syncope	Position patient in supine with the legs elevated, provided no injury is suspected; monitor vital signs; assess for heat stress or other conditions that may predispose syncope; maintain normal body temperature; seek medical attention if symptoms persist or worsen. If individual has fallen, check for additional injuries before moving.
Heat cramps	Stop activity; attempt to reduce muscular cramp by stretching, relaxation, and massage; replace lost salt and fluids with salty snacks and sodium-containing fluids; continue to monitor the individual's hydration status for the next few days.
Heat exhaustion	Stop activity and move the individual to a shaded or air-conditioned area; remove excess clothing and cool individual if body temperature is elevated; place the individual in a reclining position with the legs above the heart; if not nauseated, vomiting, or experiencing any CNS dysfunction, rehydrate with chilled water or sports drink; monitor vital signs, core temperature, and CNS status; activate EMS system if rapid improvement is absent.
Heat stroke	Aggressive and immediate whole-body cooling via cold-water immersion (35° to 58° F or 1.67° to 14.5° C) if constant monitoring of core temperature is possible; alternative cooling strategies include spraying body with cold water, using fans, placing ice or cold towels over as much of the body possible, or moving to shaded or air-conditioned facility; activate EMS and monitor ABCs, core temperature, and CNS; cease cooling when core temperature reaches approximately 101° F (38.3° C).
Hyponatremia	Distinguish between hyponatremia, heat exhaustion, dehydration, and heat stroke; activate EMS and transfer to medical facility; individuals with suspected hyponatremia should not be administered fluids unless directed by a physician. Weight gain during exercise resulting in hyponatremia is because of overdrinking fluids.
Systemic hypothermia	Carefully move individual to a warm place; activate EMS; arrange rapid transport to emergency facility; monitor vital signs and provide care for shock; remove wet clothing and cover with blankets to retain body heat; provide external heat; encourage drinking hot liquids.
Local injury (frostbite, chilblain, frostnip)	Remove wet clothing; soak area in warm water (100° to 105° F or 37.8° to 40.5° C); cover the affected area with dry, sterile dressings; check ABCs, monitor vital signs, and care for shock; do not rewarm a frostbitten area if there is danger of refreezing; activate EMS or transport individual to an emergency medical facility.

EMS, emergency medical services; CNS, central nervous system; ABC, airway, breathing, circulation.

important that exercise professionals have knowledge about environmental factors in order to establish safe exercise prescriptions and programs. These environmental conditions are more important for some individuals than for others, depending on their baseline status and specific disease(s) or condition(s). *Chapter 3* provides detailed information on the physiologic effects of exercise in different environmental conditions.

Heat

The stress of physical exertion is often complicated by environmental thermal conditions that result in elevated body temperature above the normal range (*i.e.*, hyperthermia). Heat stress is not always accurately reflected by air temperature alone. Humidity, air velocity (or wind), and thermal radiation also contribute to the total heat stress when exercising (*Box 37-5*). The human body regulates temperature by increasing skin blood flow up to 12–15 L · min^{-1}, which leads to increased sweat production as well as better cooling through convection and conduction mechanisms. During exercise, sweat evaporation becomes the most important avenue of heat loss. Because sweat must evaporate to provide cooling, high humidity limits sweat evaporation and the subsequent transfer of heat from the body. Patients with diabetes, particularly those with peripheral neuropathy,

and those with neuromuscular conditions, particularly MS, do not sweat normally and may be prone to hyperthermia (48). Care must be taken to assist them in maintaining a safe body temperature, such as exposing skin and using a fan to facilitate convective heat loss. Patients who have had gastric bypass surgery are also at risk for hyperthermia during exercise because of a reduced ability to drink large boluses of water. They must learn and practice continual sipping of water throughout the day, even when they are not exercising, to remain adequately hydrated and maintain their ability to sweat properly during exercise. Another particular concern is that body temperature regulation may be compromised in patients with heart failure who cannot generate an adequate cardiac output to transfer excess body heat to the environment (23). Consequently, body temperature can increase to critical levels, seriously jeopardizing health (10,15).

Heat illnesses are more likely in hot, humid weather but can also occur in the absence of hot and humid conditions (*Box 37-6*). When the exercise session is conducted in hot, humid conditions or if the individual is not acclimated to exercise in the heat, special precautions and modifications of exercise programming for exertional heat illnesses must be undertaken. The most important factors in reducing heat illness are to limit the intensity and duration of activity, choose clothing designed to allow heat dissipation from the body, increase the

BOX 37-5	Heat Index

TEMPERATURE (° F)

RH	80	82	84	86	88	90	92	94	96	98	100	102	104	106	108	110
40	80	81	83	85	88	91	94	97	101	105	109	114	119	124	130	136
45	80	82	84	87	89	93	96	100	104	109	114	119	124	130	137	
50	81	83	85	88	91	95	99	103	108	113	118	124	131	137		
55	81	84	86	89	93	97	101	106	112	117	124	130	137			
60	82	84	88	91	95	100	105	110	116	123	129	137				
65	82	85	89	93	98	103	108	114	121	128	136					
70	83	86	90	95	100	105	112	119	126	134						
75	84	88	92	97	103	109	116	124	132							
80	84	89	94	100	106	113	121	129								
85	85	90	96	102	110	117	126	135								
90	86	91	98	105	113	122	131									
95	86	93	100	108	117	127										
100	87	95	103	112	121	132										

RH, relative humidity.

130 or above, heat stroke highly likely with continued exposure; 105–130, heat stroke likely with prolonged exposure; 90–105, heat stroke possible with prolonged exposure.

Adapted from the National Oceanic and Atmospheric Administration, Office of Climate, Water, and Weather Services. *Heat: A Major Killer* [Internet]. [cited 2012 May 21]. Available from: http://www.nws.noaa.gov/om/heat/index.shtml#heatindex

BOX 37-6 Common Exertional Heat Illnesses

EXERCISE-ASSOCIATED MUSCLE (HEAT) CRAMPS

- Acute, painful, involuntary muscle contraction
- Present during or after intense exercise sessions
- Caused by fluid deficiencies (dehydration), electrolyte imbalances, neuromuscular fatigue

HEAT SYNCOPE (ORTHOSTATIC DIZZINESS)

- Occurs when exposed to high environmental temperatures or dehydration
- Individuals may be vulnerable during initial exercise sessions in the heat (unacclimated state)
- Caution for individuals with heart disease and those taking diuretics
- Can occur immediately after cessation of activity or after rapid assumption of upright posture after lying or sitting

EXERCISE (HEAT) EXHAUSTION

- The inability to continue exercise associated with any combination of heavy sweating, dehydration, sodium loss, and energy depletion
- Body core temperature generally ranges between 36° C (97° F) and 40° C (104° F); pallor, weakness, headache, dizziness, diarrhea

- Difficult to distinguish from exertional heat stroke without measuring rectal temperature

EXERTIONAL HEAT STROKE

- Elevated core temperature (usually >40° C [104° F]) associated with signs of organ system failure caused by hyperthermia
- Tachycardia, hypotension, sweating (skin may be wet or dry at time of collapse), altered mental status, and vomiting
- Can result in death

EXERTIONAL HYPONATREMIA

- Relatively rare condition defined as a blood sodium level <130 mmol · L^{-1}, producing intracellular swelling that causes potentially fatal neurologic and physiologic dysfunction
- Disorientation, altered mental status, headache, vomiting, lethargy, swelling of hands and feet, pulmonary and cerebral edema
- Can result in death

---

number and length of rest breaks, and encourage proper hydration. Several other factors important to preventing heat illnesses are listed in *Box 37-7* (15,18).

Cold

Increasing year-round participation in such sporting activities as the triathlon, hiking, running, and cycling has created new concerns about exercise in the cold. The two major cold stressors, ambient temperature (air) and water, cause a loss of body heat that threatens homeostasis. *Hypothermia* occurs when body temperature falls below 36° C (97° F) and is a risk when a person is exposed to cold conditions (air or water) or after trauma (10). Ambient temperature and wind influence the effective temperature of an environment. The wind chill index determines the wind's cooling effect on exposed tissue and can be used as a guide to determine suitable outdoor exercise conditions (*Box 37-8*). When exposed to cold, the body attempts to increase internal heat production by increasing muscular activity, such as shivering, and by increasing the individual's basal metabolic rate. After the body temperature falls below 34.5° C (94° F), the hypothalamus begins to lose its ability to regulate body temperature. This ability is completely lost when

the internal temperature falls to about 29.5° C (85° F). Predisposing factors to cold injury include inadequate insulation from wind and cold, restricted circulation because of arterial disease or tight clothing (including footwear), fatigue, and the body's shunting of blood away from the skin when exposed to the cold. *Box 37-9* provides a list of characteristics increasing the risk of cold injury (19).

The hazards of excessive cold exposure include potential injury to both peripheral tissues and the life-supporting cardiovascular and respiratory systems. Considerable water loss from the respiratory passages can lead to dehydration during exercise in the cold because of the very low humidity of cold air (52). Inspired ambient air temperature generally does not pose a danger to the respiratory tract tissues. However, in some cases, cold air inhalation may exacerbate asthma symptoms or result in chest pain in those with coronary artery disease. The use of a scarf or mask to allow heating and humidifying of inspired cold air may help in these situations. But for some, avoidance of cold air during exercise may be the best choice.

The early warning signs of peripheral cold injury include tingling and numbness in the fingers and toes or a burning sensation in the nose and ears (6). Effects

BOX 37-7   Recommendations for Preventing Heat Illness

- Modify activity under high-risk conditions (wet bulb globe temperature >28° C [82° F]); consider rescheduling or delaying the session until safer conditions prevail.
- Schedule exercise sessions to avoid the hottest time of the day (10 a.m. to 5 p.m.).
- Avoid radiant heating from direct sunlight.
- Progressively increase the intensity and duration of work in the heat over days or weeks to allow time for acclimatization.
- Instruct individuals to drink water and sodium-containing fluids to keep their urine clear to light yellow to improve hydration.
- Individual should weigh themselves before and after exercise to estimate the amount of body water lost during exercise and to ensure a return to preexercise weight before the next exercise session.
- Consume approximately 1.00–1.25 L (16–20 oz) of fluid for each kilogram of body water lost during exercise.
- Wear loose-fitting, absorbent, light-colored clothing, mesh clothing, or new-generation cloth blends specially designed to allow effective cooling.
- Conduct warm-up and stretching sessions in the shade (for outdoor activities).
- Individuals who have lost 2% of body weight should be excluded from participation (as should those who exhibit heat illness symptoms).

BOX 37-8   Windchill Chart

WIND (MPH)

Calm	5	10	15	20	25	30	35	40	45	50	55	60
40	36	34	32	30	29	28	28	27	26	26	25	25
35	31	27	25	24	23	22	21	20	19	19	18	17
30	25	21	19	17	16	15	14	13	12	12	11	10
25	19	15	13	11	9	8	7	6	5	4	4	3
20	13	9	6	4	3	1	0	−1	−2	−3	−3	−4
15	7	3	0	−2	−4	−5	−7	−8	−9	−10	−11	−11
10	1	−4	−7	−9	−11	−12	−14	−15	−16	−17	−18	−19
5	−5	−10	−13	−15	−17	−19	−21	−22	−23	−24	−25	−26
0	−11	−16	−19	−22	−24	−26	−27	−29	−30	−31	−32	−33
−5	−16	−22	−26	−29	−31	−33	−34	−36	−37	−38	−39	−40
−10	−22	−28	−32	−35	−37	−39	−41	−43	−44	−45	−46	−48
−15	−28	−35	−39	−42	−44	−46	−48	−50	−51	−52	−54	−55
−20	−34	−41	−45	−48	−51	−53	−55	−57	−58	−60	−61	−62
−25	−40	−47	−51	−55	−58	−60	−62	−64	−65	−67	−68	−69
−30	−46	−53	−58	−61	−64	−67	−69	−71	−72	−74	−75	−76
−35	−52	−59	−64	−68	−71	−73	−76	−78	−79	−81	−82	−84
−40	−57	−66	−71	−74	−78	−80	−82	−84	−86	−88	−89	−91
−45	−63	−72	−77	−81	−84	−87	−89	−91	−93	−95	−97	−98

TEMPERATURE (° F)

Frostbite occurs in 15 min or less.

Windchill (° F) = 35.74 + 0.6215T − 35.75 (V$^{0.16}$) + 0.4275T (V$^{0.16}$)

where

T = air temperature (° F)

V = wind speed (mph)

Adapted from National Oceanic and Atmospheric Administration. Meteorological tables. *National Weather Service, Easter Region Headquarters* [Internet]. [cited 2012 Oct 1]. Available from: http://www.nws.noaa.gov/om/windchill/index.shtml

| BOX 37-9 | Risk Factors for Cold Injury and Hypothermia |

- Exercising in water or rain significantly increases the risk for developing hypothermia.
- Individuals with lower combined values of subcutaneous fat thickness, fat percentage, and muscle mass may not maintain core temperature appropriately.
- Older individuals (>60 yr) are at an increased risk of hypothermia because of blunted physiologic and behavioral responses to cold.
- Children are at a greater risk of hypothermia than adults because of differences in body composition and anthropometry.
- Hypoglycemia impairs shivering and increases the risk for hypothermia.
- Winter athletes have a higher incidence of exercise-induced bronchospasm than the general population.
- Individuals with coronary artery disease may be at increased risk because of hemodynamic changes from cold stress.

of cold on body function and local injury include the following:

1. Systemic hypothermia (both core and shell temperatures decrease)
   - Slowing of body functions
   - Cardiac arrhythmias
   - Cardiac arrest and possible death at very low core body temperatures
2. Local injury (core temperature is maintained, but shell [skin] temperature is decreased)
   - Frostnip: mild cold injury resulting in reversible blanching of the skin
   - Chilblain: mild cold injury marked by localized redness, burning, and swelling on exposed body parts
   - Frostbite: severe tissue and cell damage caused by freezing of a body part

The principles of care for cold injuries are to prevent further heat loss, rewarming, and watch for complications. Specific prevention strategies include the following:
- Practice prevention through preparation and anticipate length of exposure and potential for weather changes.
- Layer clothing properly.
- Have dry clothing available, if possible.
- Avoid overdressing; excessive sweating and poor evaporation of sweat can promote heat loss in the cold.
- Recognize individuals susceptible to cold injury.
- Be able to recognize the signs and symptoms of hypothermia, frostbite, and cold injury.

Altitude

Acute exercise or sports competition at high altitude is associated with performance impairment of about 1% for every 100 m above 1,200 m (~4,000 ft) for nonathletic individuals. The lower barometric pressure of high altitude results in lower partial pressures of oxygen, which limits pulmonary diffusion and oxygen transport to tissues (52). Hyperventilation and increased submaximal cardiac output via elevated HR are the primary immediate responses to altitude exposure.

Clinical problems associated with exercise at high altitude can include increased susceptibility to cold-related disorders and dehydration caused by colder and dryer air temperature as altitude increases. In addition, because the atmosphere is thinner and drier, solar radiation is more intense. Individuals with cardiac or pulmonary disease that limits oxygen exchange at the lungs and/or transport to tissues may have a difficult time at altitudes above 1,500 m (5,000 ft) (35). Patients with coronary artery disease may experience myocardial ischemia at lower activity intensities while at altitude compared to sea level. If a person has obstructive pulmonary disease, he or she may experience hypoxemia as a result of the low oxygen partial pressures. Both of these patient groups should be advised to allow several days for acclimatization after traveling to higher altitudes, they should be aware of symptoms that may be associated with inadequate perfusion and to adjust their level of exertion as needed, and they should consult their physician before travel. A symptom-limited maximal exercise test may be indicated (35). Individuals with pulmonary limitations may require supplemental oxygen if their hemoglobin saturation falls below 88%. Travel to very high altitudes (above 2,500 m or 8,000 ft) may not be prudent, especially for those with moderate-to-severe cardiac or pulmonary disease (35).

Three medical problems resulting from exercising at moderate-to-high altitudes (above 3,658 m or 12,000 ft) include the following (52):

1. Acute mountain sickness (headache, dyspnea on exertion, light-headedness, fatigue, nausea, difficulty sleeping)
2. High-altitude pulmonary edema (severe fatigue and weakness, dyspnea, and cough)
3. High-altitude cerebral edema (severe headaches, nausea, vomiting, impaired mental processing, ataxia, and ashen skin color)

Exercise considerations when exercising at altitude include the following:

- The length of time required for altitude acclimatization increases as altitude increases.
- Observable improvements in exercise tolerance occur within 5–7 d of initial altitude exposure. Full adaptations require about 2 wk, although acclimatization to relatively high altitudes may require 4–6 wk. Individuals with cardiac or pulmonary disease may

require additional acclimation time, and those with severe disease may never fully acclimate.

- Aerobic and endurance-related exercise capacity is reduced because acclimatization does not fully compensate for reduced partial pressure of oxygen at altitude for any individual.

Pollution

The U.S. Environmental Protection Agency (EPA) is responsible for informing and alerting the general population about air quality (27). The EPA uses the air quality index (AQI) for five major pollutants: ground-level ozone, particulate matter, carbon monoxide, sulfur dioxide, and nitrogen dioxide. For each of these pollutants, the EPA has established national air quality standards to protect against harmful health effects. AQI levels can vary, depending on the time of day or from one season to the next. *Table 37-8* provides a health advisory statement for the major pollutants and guidelines to

follow that protect health and prevent unsafe exercise participation (27). As for altitude, patients with cardiac and pulmonary disease may be more adversely affected by pollutants than healthy individuals. Avoiding outdoor exercise on ozone action/alert days is prudent in these instances.

Hyperbaric Environment

Hyperbaria can be defined as exposure of the body to increased pressure, such as occurs during underwater diving. For every 10 m of increasing depth in sea water, the pressure increases by 1 atmosphere (ATM) or 760 mm Hg. Increasing pressures can cause nitrogen to accumulate in body fluids and tissues and lead to decompression illness. Decompression illness is the major safety concern when diving at greater depths and lengths of time; for example, when diving with self-contained underwater breathing apparatus (SCUBA) gear, if the ascent is not slow enough, nitrogen dissolved

TABLE 37-8. Air Quality Index[a]

Index Values	Levels of Health Concern	Health Advisory: Ozone	Health Advisory: PM$_{2.5}$	Health Advisory: CO	Health Advisory: SO$_2$	Health Advisory: NO$_2$
0–50	Good	None	None	None	None	None
51–100	Moderate	Unusually sensitive people should limit prolonged outdoor exertion	None	None	None	None
101–150	Unhealthy for sensitive groups	Active children and adults and people with respiratory disease such as asthma	None	People with CVD (*e.g.,* such as angina) should limit heavy exertion and avoid sources of CO (*e.g.,* heavy traffic).	People with asthma should consider limiting outdoor exertion.	None
151–200	Unhealthy	Active children and adults and people with respiratory disease (*e.g.,* asthma); everyone else, especially children, should avoid prolonged outdoor exertion.	People with respiratory or heart disease, the elderly, and children should avoid prolonged exertion; everyone else should limit prolonged exertion.	People with CVD (*e.g.,* angina) should limit moderate exertion and sources of CO, such as heavy traffic.	Children, asthmatics, and people with heart or lung disease should limit outdoor exertion.	None
201–300	Very unhealthy	Active children and adults and people with respiratory disease (*e.g.,* asthma) should avoid all outdoor exertion; everyone else should limit outdoor exertion.	People with respiratory or heart disease, the elderly, and children should avoid any outdoor activity; everyone else should avoid prolonged exertion.	People with CVD (*e.g.,* angina) should avoid exertion and sources of CO (*e.g.,* heavy traffic).	Children, asthmatics, and people with heart or lung disease should avoid outdoor exertion; everyone else should limit outdoor exertion.	Children and people with respiratory disease (*e.g.,* asthma) should limit heavy outdoor exertion.
301–500	Hazardous	Everyone should avoid all outdoor exertion.	Everyone should avoid any outdoor exertion; people with respiratory or heart disease, the elderly, and children should remain indoors.	People with CVD (*e.g.,* angina) should avoid exertion and sources of CO (*e.g.,* heavy traffic); everyone else should limit heavy exertion.	Children, asthmatics, and people with heart or lung disease should remain indoors; everyone else should avoid outdoor exertion.	Children and people with respiratory disease (*e.g.,* asthma) should limit moderate and heavy outdoor exertion.

CVD, cardiovascular disease.

[a]Pollutants: ground-level ozone, particulate matter (PM$_{2.5}$), carbon monoxide (CO), sulfur dioxide (SO$_2$), and nitrogen dioxide (NO$_2$).

Adapted from U.S. Environmental Protection Agency. Air quality index—a guide to air quality and your health. *AirNow* [Internet]. [cited 2012 May 19]. Available from: http://airnow.gov/index.cfm?action=aqibasics.aqi

in body fluids and tissues is forced to escape as bubbles of gas rather than as dissolved gas. Each dive should be preplanned to account for the amount of time at given pressures (depths), particularly during ascent, to allow nitrogen to be exhaled as gas and prevent decompression illness (69).

Other physiologic consequences of submersion include decreased cutaneous blood flow, increased central blood volume, increased venous return, and lower HR. Increased heat transfer of water and decreased cutaneous blood flow place divers at risk for hypothermia.

SUMMARY

Musculoskeletal injuries, chronic diseases, and environmental factors may complicate exercise participation. Adequate screening and evaluation are important to identify and counsel individuals about special considerations that may be relevant to their situation before beginning an exercise. Health and fitness facility personnel involved in the management or delivery of exercise programs must possess the knowledge to recognize at-risk individuals and take steps to prevent and respond to exercise-related injuries and illnesses.

REFERENCES

1. *ACC/AHA 2002 Guideline Update for Exercise Testing. A report of the American College of Cardiology/American Heart Association Task Force on Practice Guidelines (Committee on Exercise Testing)* [Internet]. Dallas (TX): American College of Cardiology/American Heart Association; [cited 2011 Mar 14]. Available from: http://www.americanheart.org/downloadable/heart/1032279013658 exercise.pdf

2. Almeida SA, Trone DW, Leone DM, Shaffer RA, Patheal SL, Long K. Gender differences in musculoskeletal injury rates: a function of symptom reporting? *Med Sci Sports Exerc.* 1999;31(12):1807–12.

3. American Association of Cardiovascular & Pulmonary Rehabilitation. *Guidelines for Cardiac Rehabilitation and Secondary Prevention Programs.* 4th ed. Champaign (IL): Human Kinetics; 2004. 280 p.

4. American Diabetes Association. Diagnosis and classification of diabetes mellitus. *Diabetes Care.* 2011; 34 Suppl 1:S62–9.

5. American Diabetes Association. Physical activity/exercise and diabetes mellitus: position statement. *Diabetes Care.* 2003;26(Suppl 1):S73–7.

6. American Red Cross. *Community First Aid and Safety.* San Bruno (CA): StayWell; 2002. 240 p.

7. *Americans with Disabilities Act Accessibility Guidelines for Buildings and Facilities; Recreation Facilities* [Internet]. Washington (DC): U.S. Access Board, U.S. Department of Justice; [cited 2012 Jan 31]. Available from: http://www.access-board.gov/recreation/final.htm

8. Andrews JR. Overuse syndromes of the lower extremity. *Clin Sports Med.* 1983;2(1):137–48.

9. Arendt EA. Common musculoskeletal injuries in women. *Phys Sportsmed.* 1996;24(7):39–48.

10. Armstrong LE, Epstein Y, Greenleaf JE, et al. American College of Sports Medicine position stand. Heat and cold illnesses during distance running. *Med Sci Sports Exerc.* 1996;28(12):i–x.

11. Artal R, O'Toole M. Guidelines of the American College of Obstetricians and Gynecologists for exercise during pregnancy and the postpartum period. *Br J Sports Med.* 2003;37(1):6–12; discussion 12.

12. Balady GJ, Chaitman B, Driscoll D, et al. Recommendations for cardiovascular screening, staffing, and emergency policies at health/fitness facilities. *Circulation.* 1998;97(22):2283–93.

13. Barnard RJ, Gardner GW, Diaco NV, MacAlpin RN, Kattus AA. Cardiovascular responses to sudden strenuous exercise—heart rate, blood pressure, and ECG. *J Appl Physiol.* 1973;34(6):833–7.

14. Barnard RJ, MacAlpin R, Kattus AA, Buckberg GD. Ischemic response to sudden strenuous exercise in healthy men. *Circulation.* 1973;48(5):936–42.

15. Binkley HM, Beckett J, Casa DJ, Kleiner DM, Plummer PE. National Athletic Trainers' Association position statement: Exertional heat illnesses. *J Athl Train.* 2002;37(3):329–43.

16. Brar SP, Smith MB, Nelson LM, Franklin GM, Cobble ND. Evaluation of treatment protocols on minimal to moderate spasticity in multiple sclerosis. *Arch Phys Med Rehabil.* 1991;72(3):186–9.

17. Bruin G, Kuipers H, Keizer HA, Vander Vusse GJ. Adaptation and overtraining in horses subjected to increasing training loads. *J Appl Physiol.* 1994;76(5):1908–13.

18. Casa DJ, Armstrong LE, Hillman SK, et al. National athletic trainers' association position statement: fluid replacement for athletes. *J Athl Train.* 2000;35(2):212–24.

19. Castellani JW, Young AJ, Ducharme MB, et al. American College of Sports Medicine position stand: prevention of cold injuries during exercise. *Med Sci Sports Exerc.* 2006;38(11):2012–29.

20. Celli BR. Pathophysiology of chronic obstructive pulmonary disease. In: Hodgkin JE, Celli BR, Connors GL, editors. *Pulmonary Rehabilitation: Guidelines to Success.* 3rd ed. Philadelphia: Lippincott Williams & Wilkins; 2000. p. 41–55.

21. Colbert LH, Hootman JM, Macera CA. Physical activity-related injuries in walkers and runners in the aerobics center longitudinal study. *Clin J Sport Med.* 2000;10(4):259–63.

22. Cole CR, Blackstone EH, Pashkow FJ, Snader CE, Lauer MS. Heart-rate recovery immediately after exercise as a predictor of mortality. *N Engl J Med.* 1999;341(18):1351–7.

23. Cui J, Arbab-Zadeh A, Prasad A, Durand S, Levine BD, Crandall CG. Effects of heat stress on thermoregulatory responses in congestive heart failure patients. *Circulation.* 2005;112(15):2286–92.

24. Cummins RO, Field JM, Hazinski MF, Babbs CF, American Heart Association. *ACLS Provider Manual.* Dallas (TX): American Heart Association; 2001. 252 p.

25. Dimsdale JE, Hartley LH, Guiney T, Ruskin JN, Greenblatt D. Postexercise peril. Plasma catecholamines and exercise. *JAMA.* 1984;251(5):630–2.

26. Durstine JL, Moore GE, American College of Sports Medicine. *ACSM's Exercise Management for Persons with Chronic Diseases and Disabilities.* 2nd ed. Champaign (IL): Human Kinetics; 2003. 374 p.

27. *EPA-454/K-03-002* [Internet]. Research Triangle Park (NC): U.S. Environmental Protection Agency; [cited 2011 Mar 14]. Available from: http://www.airnow.gov/

28. Ettinger WH Jr, Burns R, Messier SP, et al. A randomized trial comparing aerobic exercise and resistance exercise with a health education program in older adults with knee osteoarthritis. The Fitness Arthritis and Seniors Trial (FAST). *JAMA.* 1997;277(1):25–31.

29. Felson DT, Zhang Y, Anthony JM, Naimark A, Anderson JJ. Weight loss reduces the risk for symptomatic knee osteoarthritis in women. The Framingham Study. *Ann Intern Med.* 1992;116(7):535–9.

30. Felson DT, Zhang Y, Hannan MT, et al. Risk factors for incident radiographic knee osteoarthritis in the elderly: the Framingham Study. *Arthritis Rheum.* 1997;40(4):728–33.

31. Feskanich D, Willett W, Colditz G. Walking and leisure-time activity and risk of hip fracture in postmenopausal women. *JAMA.* 2002;288(18):2300–6.

32. Garber CE, Blissmer B, Deschenes MR, et al. Quantity and quality of exercise for developing and maintaining cardiorespiratory, musculoskeletal, and neuromotor fitness in apparently healthy adults: guidance for prescribing exercise. *Med Sci Sports Exerc.* 2011;43(7):1334–59.

33. Garrick JG, Gillien DM, Whiteside P. The epidemiology of aerobic dance injuries. *Am J Sports Med.* 1986;14(1):67–72.

34. Herring SA, Cantu RC, Guskiewicz KM, et al. Concussion (mild traumatic brain injury) and the team physician: a consensus statement—2011 update. *Med Sci Sports Exerc.* 2011;43(12): 2412–22.

35. Higgins JP, Tuttle T, Higgins JA. Altitude and the heart: is going high safe for your cardiac patient? *Am Heart J.* 2010;159(1):25–32.

36. Hootman JM, Macera CA, Ainsworth BE, Martin M, Addy CL, Blair SN. Association among physical activity level, cardiorespiratory fitness, and risk of musculoskeletal injury. *Am J Epidemiol.* 2001;154(3):251–8.

37. Janis LR. Aerobic dance survey. A study of high-impact versus low-impact injuries. *J Am Podiatr Med Assoc.* 1990;80(8):419–23.

38. Jones CS, Christensen C, Young M. Weight training injury trends: a 20-year survey. *Phys Sportsmed.* 2000;28(7):61–72.

39. Kaufman KR, Brodine S, Shaffer R. Military training-related injuries: surveillance, research, and prevention. *Am J Prev Med.* 2000;18(3 Suppl):54–63.

40. Kerr ZY, Collins CL, Comstock RD. Epidemiology of weight training-related injuries presenting to United States emergency departments, 1990 to 2007. *Am J Sports Med.* 2010;38(4):765–71.

41. Kesaniemi YK, Danforth E,Jr, Jensen MD, Kopelman PG, Lefebvre P, Reeder BA. Dose-response issues concerning physical activity and health: an evidence-based symposium. *Med Sci Sports Exerc.* 2001;33(6 Suppl):S351–8.

42. Koplan JP, Rothenberg RB, Jones EL. The natural history of exercise: a 10-yr follow-up of a cohort of runners. *Med Sci Sports Exerc.* 1995;27(8):1180–4.

43. Lane NE. Physical activity at leisure and risk of osteoarthritis. *Ann Rheum Dis.* 1996;55(9):682–4.

44. Lee IM, Rexrode KM, Cook NR, Manson JE, Buring JE. Physical activity and coronary heart disease in women: is "no pain, no gain" passe? *JAMA.* 2001;285(11):1447–54.

45. Leitzmann MF, Rimm EB, Willett WC, et al. Recreational physical activity and the risk of cholecystectomy in women. *N Engl J Med.* 1999;341(11):777–84.

46. Lewis SF, Nylander E, Gad P, Areskog NH. Non-autonomic component in bradycardia of endurance trained men at rest and during exercise. *Acta Physiol Scand.* 1980;109(3):297–305.

47. Lopez-Jimenez F, Kramer VC, Masters B, et al. Recommendations for managing patients with diabetes mellitus in cardiopulmonary rehabilitation: an American Association of Cardiovascular and Pulmonary Rehabilitation statement. *J Cardiopulm Rehabil Prev.* 2012;32(2):101–12.

48. Luo KR, Chao CC, Chen YT, et al. Quantitation of sudomotor innervation in skin biopsies of patients with diabetic neuropathy. *J Neuropathol Exp Neurol.* 2011;70(10):930–8.

49. Manson JE, Greenland P, LaCroix AZ, et al. Walking compared with vigorous exercise for the prevention of cardiovascular events in women. *N Engl J Med.* 2002;347(10):716–25.

50. Maron BJ, Thompson PD, Ackerman MJ, et al. Recommendations and considerations related to preparticipation screening for cardiovascular abnormalities in competitive athletes: 2007 update: a scientific statement from the American Heart Association Council on Nutrition, Physical Activity, and Metabolism: endorsed by the American College of Cardiology Foundation. *Circulation.* 2007;115(12):1643–55.

51. Maron BJ, Zipes DP. Introduction: eligibility recommendations for competitive athletes with cardiovascular abnormalities-general considerations. *J Am Coll Cardiol.* 2005;45(8):1318–21.

52. McArdle WD, Katch FI, Katch VL. *Exercise Physiology: Energy, Nutrition, and Human Performance.* 5th ed. Baltimore (MD): Lippincott Williams & Wilkins; 2001. 1158 p.

53. Mutoh Y, Sawai S, Takanashi Y, Skurko L. Aerobic dance injuries among instructors and students. *Physician Sportsmed.* 1988; 16(12):80–8.

54. Myers J, Nieman DC, American College of Sports Medicine. *ACSM's Resources for Clinical Exercise Physiology: Musculoskeletal, Neuromuscular, Neoplastic, Immunologic, and Hematologic Conditions.* 2nd ed. Philadelphia (PA): Wolters Kluwer Health/Lippincott Williams & Wilkins Health; 2010. 323 p.

55. Nieman DC. *Exercise Testing and Prescription: A Health Related Approach.* 5th ed. Boston (MA): McGraw-Hill; 2003. 774 p.

56. Paffenbarger RS,Jr, Hyde RT, Wing AL, Lee IM, Jung DL, Kampert JB. The association of changes in physical-activity level and other lifestyle characteristics with mortality among men. *N Engl J Med.* 1993;328(8):538–45.

57. Pescatello LS, Arena R, Riebe D, American College of Sports Medicine. *ACSM's Guidelines for Exercise Testing and Prescription.* 9th ed. Philadelphia (PA): Lippincott Williams & Wilkins; 2012. 380 p.

58. Pescatello LS, Franklin BA, Fagard R, et al. American College of Sports Medicine position stand. Exercise and hypertension. *Med Sci Sports Exerc.* 2004;36(3):533–53.

59. Powell KE, Heath GW, Kresnow MJ, Sacks JJ, Branche CM. Injury rates from walking, gardening, weightlifting, outdoor bicycling, and aerobics. *Med Sci Sports Exerc.* 1998;30(8):1246–9.

60. Powell KE, Kohl HW, Caspersen CJ, Blair SN. An epidemiological perspective on the causes of running injuries. *Physician Sportsmed.* 1986;14(6):100–14.

61. Powell KE, Thompson PD, Caspersen CJ, Kendrick JS. Physical activity and the incidence of coronary heart disease. *Annu Rev Public Health.* 1987;8:253–87.

62. Prentice WE, Arnheim DD. *Arnheim's Principles of Athletic Training: A Competency-Based Approach.* 14th ed. New York (NY): McGraw-Hill Higher Education; 2011. 940 p.

63. Reeves RK, Laskowski ER, Smith J. Weight training injuries: part 2: diagnosing and managing chronic conditions. *Phys Sportsmed.* 1998;26(3):54–73.

64. Renström P, International Olympic Committee, Medical Commission, International Federation of Sports Medicine. *The Encyclopaedia of Sports Medicine. Vol. 4. Sports Injuries: Basic Principles of Prevention and Care.* Oxford, United Kingdom: Blackwell Scientific Publications; 1993. 482 p.

65. Renstrom P, Kannus P. Prevention of sports injuries. In: Strauss RH, editor. *Sports Medicine.* 2nd ed. Philadelphia: Saunders; 1991. p. 307–29.

66. Requa RK, DeAvilla LN, Garrick JG. Injuries in recreational adult fitness activities. *Am J Sports Med.* 1993;21(3):461–7.

67. Richie DH,Jr, Kelso SF, Bellucci PA. Aerobic dance injuries: a retrospective study of instructors and participants. *Physician Sportsmed.* 1985;13(2):130–40.

68. Riley BB, Rimmer JH, Wang E, Schiller WJ. A conceptual framework for improving the accessibility of fitness and recreation facilities for people with disabilities. *J Phys Act Health.* 2008;5(1):158–68.

69. Robergs RA, Roberts SO. *Exercise Physiology: Exercise, Performance, and Clinical Applications.* St. Louis (MO): Mosby; 1997. 840 p.

70. Rockhill B, Willett WC, Manson JE, et al. Physical activity and mortality: a prospective study among women. *Am J Public Health.* 2001;91(4):578–83.

71. Schairer JR. Cardiovascular assessment for risk of sudden cardiac death in athletes. *J Clin Exerc Physiol.* 2012;1:9–14.

72. Schenck RC, American Academy of Orthopaedic Surgeons. *Athletic Training and Sports Medicine.* 3rd ed. Rosemont (IL): American Academy of Orthopaedic Surgeons; 1999. 925 p.

73. Shephard RJ, Åstrand P-. *Endurance in Sport: The Encyclopaedia of Sports Medicine.* Oxford, United Kingdom: Blackwell Scientific Publications; 1992. 1008 p.

74. Tanasescu M, Leitzmann MF, Rimm EB, Willett WC, Stampfer MJ, Hu FB. Exercise type and intensity in relation to coronary heart disease in men. *JAMA.* 2002;288(16):1994–2000.

75. Thompson PD, Franklin BA, Balady GJ, et al. Exercise and acute cardiovascular events placing the risks into perspective: a scientific statement from the American Heart Association Council on Nutrition, Physical Activity, and Metabolism and the Council on Clinical Cardiology. *Circulation.* 2007;115(17):2358–68.

76. U.S. Department of Health and Human Services, Centers for Disease Control and Prevention, National Center for Chronic Disease Prevention and Health Promotion, The President's Council on Physical Fitness and Sports. *Physical Activity and Health: A Report of the Surgeon General.* Atlanta (GA): President's Council on Physical Fitness and Sports; 1996. 278 p.

77. Wenger NK, Froelicher ES, Smith LK, et al. Cardiac rehabilitation as secondary prevention. Agency for Health Care Policy and Research and National Heart, Lung, and Blood Institute. *Clin Pract Guidel Quick Ref Guide Clin.* 1995;17:1–23.

78. Williams MA, Haskell WL, Ades PA, et al. Resistance exercise in individuals with and without cardiovascular disease: 2007 update: a scientific statement from the American Heart Association Council on Clinical Cardiology and Council on Nutrition, Physical Activity, and Metabolism. *Circulation.* 2007;116(5):572–84.

79. Williams PT. Physical fitness and activity as separate heart disease risk factors: a meta-analysis. *Med Sci Sports Exerc.* 2001;33(5):754–61.

80. Wisloff U, Stoylen A, Loennechen JP, et al. Superior cardiovascular effect of aerobic interval training versus moderate continuous training in heart failure patients: a randomized study. *Circulation.* 2007;115(24):3086–94.

81. Yu S, Yarnell JW, Sweetnam PM, Murray L, Caerphilly study. What level of physical activity protects against premature cardiovascular death? The Caerphilly study. *Heart.* 2003;89(5):502–6.

SELECTED REFERENCES FOR FURTHER READING

Armstrong LE, Casa DJ, Millard-Stafford M, Moran DS, Pyne SW, Roberts WO. American College of Sports Medicine position stand. Exertional heat illness during training and competition. *Med Sci Sports Exerc.* 2007;39(3):556–72.

Castellani JW, Young AJ, Ducharme MB, Giesbrecht GG, Glickman E, Sallis RE. American College of Sports Medicine position stand: prevention of cold injuries during exercise. *Med Sci Sports Exerc.* 2006;38(11):2012–29.

Fletcher GF, Balady GJ, Amsterdam EA, et al. Exercise standards for testing and training. American Heart Association scientific statement. *Circulation.* 2001;104:1644–740.

Garber CE, Blissmer B, Deschenes MR, et al. American College of Sports Medicine position stand. Quantity and quality of exercise for developing and maintaining cardiorespiratory, musculoskeletal, and neuromotor fitness in apparently healthy adults: guidance for prescribing exercise. *Med Sci Sports Exerc.* 2011;43(7):1334–59.

Higgins JP, Tuttle T, Higgins JA. Altitude and the heart: is going high safe for your cardiac patient? *Am Heart J.* 2010;159(1):25–32.

Sawka MN, Burke LM, Eichner ER, Maughan RJ, Montain SJ, Stachenfeld NS. American College of Sports Medicine position stand. Exercise and fluid replacement. *Med Sci Sports Exerc.* 2007;39(2):377–90.

INTERNET RESOURCES

- AirNow: http://www.airnow.gov
- American Academy of Orthopaedic Surgeons: http://www.aaos.org
- American Heart Association: http://www.americanheart.org
- American Lung Association: http://www.lung.org
- American Medical Society for Sports Medicine: http://www.amssm.org

38

Exercise Prescription for Patients with Cardiovascular Disease

Exercise is recommended for virtually all adults, including individuals who have (94,119) cardiovascular disease (CVD). For individuals with CVD, physical activity is therapeutic and should be prioritized to prevent further development of disease and disability. However, prior to commencing with an exercise training regimen, it is recommended that individuals with CVD consult with an appropriate health care provider (47,103). Prescribing exercise in individuals with CVD can be both complex and challenging, and this chapter reviews the important disease-specific issues that warrant consideration.

DISEASE-SPECIFIC EFFECTS ON PHYSIOLOGIC RESPONSES AND FITNESS

Patients with CVD may demonstrate a normal or abnormal cardiovascular response to an acute bout of exercise depending on the severity of disease and other factors (*Table 38-1*) (70,71). Potential cardiovascular responses are discussed in the following section.

HEART RATE

A normal response to maximal exercise testing involves the patient achieving a heart rate (HR) that is within two standard deviations of an age-predicted maximum value (24,42). Failure to achieve ≥85% (10,25) of the age-predicted maximum HR in the absence of β-adrenergic blocking agents or other medications that affect the chronotropic response is termed chronotropic incompetence. In patients on a β-adrenergic blocking agent, chronotropic incompetence is defined as failure to achieve ≥62% of age-predicted maximum (73). The finding of chronotropic incompetence during exercise, even as an isolated anomaly, can be predictive of the presence of coronary artery disease (CAD) and is associated with increased risk of morbidity and mortality (24,80). After a bout of exercise, a normal increase in parasympathetic tone causes the HR to decrease fairly quickly. Comparison of the HR at 1 or 2 min into recovery with peak HR is termed *HR recovery*. Abnormal HR recovery, defined as a decrease in HR of <12 bpm at 1 min while walking in recovery and <22 bpm at

KEY TERMS

Angina: Chest pain, pressure, discomfort, or fullness that typically occurs as a result of coronary artery stenosis, which prevents adequate blood flow and oxygen delivery to the myocardium, creating a temporary mismatch between the delivery and the demand for oxygen. Typically, angina is brought on by exertion or psychological stress and resolves with rest or nitroglycerin.

Chronotropic incompetence: An attenuated heart rate response to exercise; failure to achieve a heart rate that is ≥85% or within two standard deviations of the age-predicted maximum. In patients on a β-adrenergic blocking agent, chronotropic incompetence is defined as failure to achieve ≥62% of age-predicted maximum.

Heart failure: Condition created by disease or injury to cardiac myocytes, in which myocardial contraction/relaxation function is abnormal to the extent that the heart is no longer able to pump blood at a rate commensurate with the requirement of metabolizing tissues.

Ischemic cascade: The temporal sequence of cellular, hemodynamic, electrocardiographic, and symptomatic expressions occurring during myocardial ischemia.

Rate–pressure product: Surrogate of myocardial oxygen consumption, computed as the product of heart rate and systolic blood pressure.

TABLE 38-1. Comparison of Peak Arm and Leg Responses in Healthy Subjects and Those with Heart Failure and Cardiac Transplant

	Peak HR (beats · min^{-1})	Oxygen Consumption (L · min^{-1})	Rate–Pressure Product × 10^2 (beats · mm Hg · min^{-1})
Healthy			
Arm	140 ± 13	1.50 ± 0.38	285 ± 39
Leg	162 ± 45	2.28 ± 0.150	325 ± 45
Heart Failure			
Arm	128 ± 17	1.08 ± 0.22	205 ± 52
Leg	144 ± 14	1.48 ± 0.30	241 ± 40
Cardiac Transplant			
Arm	135 ± 4	1.15 ± 0.07	248 ± 20
Leg	145 ± 4	1.60 ± 0.09	278 ± 19

HR, heart rate.

Rate–pressure product = peak HR × peak systolic blood pressure.

Source: Keteyian SJ, Marks CR, Brawner CA, Levine AB, Kataoka T, Levine TB. Responses to arm exercise in patients with compensated heart failure. *J Cardiopulm Rehabil.* 1996;16(6):366–71; Keteyian S, Marks CR, Levine AB, et al. Cardiovascular responses of cardiac transplant patients to arm and leg exercise. *Eur J Appl Physiol Occup Physiol.* 1994;68(5):441–4.

2 min if supine, also predicts future cardiac mortality (25,33,65).

BLOOD PRESSURE

Because of a reduction in systemic vascular resistance in the metabolically more active muscles during exercise, the normal diastolic blood pressure (BP) response is to remain constant or decrease slightly during exercise. Conversely, the normal response of systolic BP during incremental exercise is to increase progressively with a plateau at peak exercise. In patients with CAD, systolic BP during exercise may respond normally or may disproportionately increase or inappropriately decrease. Although there are test termination criteria based on an excessive BP response (*i.e.*, systolic BP >250 mm Hg or diastolic BP >115 mm Hg), there is no clear definition for exertional hypertension during an exercise test. *Exertional hypotension* is defined as a drop in systolic BP >10 mm Hg despite an increase in workload (103). In the absence of BP-lowering or afterload-reducing medications such as β-adrenergic blocking agents and angiotensin-converting enzyme inhibitors, a failure of systolic BP to increase with increasing exercise intensity is also considered an abnormal systolic BP response to exercise (47,103). Exertional systolic hypotension and hypertension are both associated with an increased risk of cardiac events (34,63). An increase in diastolic BP of 10 mm Hg or more may be associated with CAD, but it is more often a marker for future hypertension (41,116,133).

CARDIAC OUTPUT AND OXYGEN UPTAKE

Maximum oxygen uptake ($\dot{V}O_2$) in healthy, active adults is typically between 30 and 45 mL · kg^{-1} · min^{-1}. In patients with CAD, however, maximum $\dot{V}O_2$ is likely reduced and may not be attained during exercise because of limitation by symptoms. In such cases, the highest $\dot{V}O_2$ attained is termed peak $\dot{V}O_2$. In a two-site study involving more than 2,800 patients, Ades et al. showed that peak $\dot{V}O_2$ was 19.3 ± 6.1 mL · kg^{-1} · min^{-1} and 14.5 ± 3.9 mL · kg^{-1} · min^{-1} for men and women with CAD, respectively (2). In general, the reduction in peak $\dot{V}O_2$ in patients with CVD often exceeds 50% when compared with age-matched, healthy persons.

A patient's reduced ability to transport and use oxygen is typically caused by several factors, including a diminished cardiac output, a reduced peak blood flow within the peripheral musculature, and peripheral skeletal muscle cellular abnormalities that affect oxygen use and energy production. Cardiac output (HR × stroke volume) during exercise may be reduced because of chronotropic incompetence or left ventricular dysfunction secondary to prior myocardial infarction (MI), transient coronary ischemia, or a nonischemic cardiomyopathy that results in a reduced ejection fraction and stroke volume (29). With regular exercise training, peak $\dot{V}O_2$ can be increased by approximately 15%–30% in previously sedentary patients with CAD (53,57,126).

SCIENTIFIC AND PHYSIOLOGIC RATIONALE FOR EXERCISE THERAPY IN PATIENTS WITH HEART DISEASE

Typical symptoms associated with heart disease are angina, dyspnea at rest or at low levels of exertion, orthopnea, peripheral edema, palpitations, dizziness, and syncope. Symptoms can occur in isolation or in combination. Other than chest pain or pressure, symptoms that occur with physical activity may be considered as an anginal equivalent. Management of symptoms is of paramount importance in the treatment of patients with heart disease and an important reason for referral to a cardiac rehabilitation program.

The development of angina represents the cumulative impact of a sequence of pathophysiologic events referred to as the ischemic cascade (60,95). The ischemic cascade has been studied during percutaneous transluminal coronary angioplasty, atrial pacing, and exercise testing. It begins with the imbalance between myocardial oxygen supply and demand and produces an ischemic event that first causes cellular abnormalities leading to abnormalities in diastolic function (reduced ventricular compliance and impaired filling), with subsequent abnormalities in systolic function. Next, electrocardiographic (ECG) changes, such as ST-segment depression, occur, and, finally, the patient may experience angina. After the myocardial oxygen supply and demand imbalance is corrected at the cellular level, the process is reversed: angina resolves first, then the ECG changes, followed by improvement in systolic function, and, finally, normalization of diastolic dysfunction.

Berger et al. (17) found that although hemodynamic abnormalities were seen in nearly all patients with CAD studied during ischemia, radionuclide evidence of global or regional wall motion abnormalities were only noted in 80% of patients and ECG and symptomatic evidence of ischemia occurred in only 50% and 30% of patients, respectively. Thus, it is of fundamental importance to understand that although ischemia results in abnormalities of diastolic and systolic function in most patients, ECG changes and angina are seen less frequently. Finally, some patients — such as those with diabetes mellitus or those who have undergone cardiac transplant — experience ST-segment depression without angina (i.e., silent ischemia), whereas others may experience angina without ST-segment depression.

MYOCARDIAL OXYGEN DEMAND

Physiologic variables that determine myocardial oxygen demand are HR, left ventricular preload, and myocardial contractility. At rest and during exercise, myocardial oxygen consumption can be reliably estimated by the product of HR and systolic BP. This is called the rate–pressure product (RPP) (i.e., double product). The normal maximal exercise response results in an RPP of 25,000 mm Hg $\cdot$ beats $\cdot$ min^{-1} or higher (129).

For patients with CAD and angina symptoms, the RPP is generally a reproducible indicator of the myocardial oxygen demand at which angina initially occurs (i.e., the angina threshold). For example, consider the patient who undertakes a graded exercise test walks for 6 min and stops because of angina at an RPP of 19,300 (HR of 140 bpm times a systolic BP of 138 mm Hg). After the test, this patient's physician prescribes a β-adrenergic

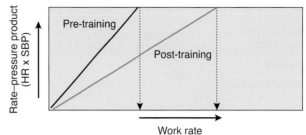

FIGURE 38-1. Regular exercise training attenuates myocardial O$_2$ demand during exercise, as estimated by the rate–pressure product. HR, heart rate; SBP, systolic blood pressure.

blocking agent (i.e., β-blocker) as a means to attenuate the increases in both HR and systolic BP during exercise. After 1 mo of taking this medication, a repeat test is conducted and reveals a longer total exercise time of 7.2 min, a lower peak RPP of 15,600 (HR of 120 bpm times a systolic BP of 130 mmHg), an increased peak metabolic equivalent (MET) level, and a test that is now stopped because of fatigue rather than angina. This means that this patient can now exercise longer and do so in a symptom-free manner. Regular exercise training also lowers HR and BP responses during submaximal exercise and also creates a rightward shift in the RPP–work rate relationship (Fig. 38-1). This shift in the RPP curve demonstrates how regular exercise can lead to patients experiencing fewer symptoms during routine and leisure-time activities.

MYOCARDIAL OXYGEN SUPPLY

As mentioned previously, myocardial ischemia occurs as a result of an imbalance between oxygen supply and demand. To better appreciate the pathophysiology leading to angina in patients with stable CAD, one must understand the four basic pathogenic factors that affect myocardial oxygen (O$_2$) supply: coronary artery stenosis with endothelial dysfunction, microvascular dysfunction, abnormalities of the autonomic nervous system, and abnormalities of coagulation and fibrinolytic systems. This section focuses on how a chronic exercise program might contribute to ameliorating several of these components (Table 38-2).

Coronary artery stenosis can be further divided into the components of plaque formation, collateral artery formation, and endothelial dysfunction. Several trials demonstrated that a combined intervention of aggressive risk factor modification and exercise training is associated with a slowing of progression, and sometimes regression, of CAD (58,100). The Stanford Coronary Risk Intervention Project revealed that the mean rate of plaque progression in the combined risk factor modification and exercise training group was half that of patients in the usual care group (58).

TABLE 38-2. Pathophysiologic Effects of Exercise and Exercise Training

Pathophysiologic Variable	Acute Exercise	Chronic Exercise Training
Vascular		
Vascular stenosis	—	Partial regression ($>2,200$ kcal $\cdot$ wk^{-1})
Coronary collaterals	—	—
Endothelial dysfunction	—	↓
Capillary flow	—	↑
Autonomic Nervous System		
Parasympathetic	↓	↑
Sympathetic	↑	↓
Hemostatic		
Fibrinogen	↑	↓
Factor VII	—	—
Platelet aggregation	↑	↓
Fibrinolysis	↓	↑
Viscosity	↑	↓

↑, increase; ↓, decrease; —, no effect.

Schuler et al. (115) randomized patients with heart disease to either a combined risk factor modification plus exercise ($n = 56$) group or a usual care ($n = 55$) group. At 1 yr, the intervention group demonstrated no change in the luminal diameter, whereas the usual care group experienced a significant decrease in diameter (i.e., plaque progression). Repeat angiography at 6 yr demonstrated significantly less atherosclerotic progression in the intervention group. Interestingly, a secondary analysis of subjects in the exercise intervention group revealed that those expending $<1,000$ kcal $\cdot$ wk^{-1} experienced the greatest amount of disease progression, whereas subjects expending $>1,500$ kcal $\cdot$ wk^{-1} demonstrated the slowest rate of disease progression. Regression of CAD was observed in patients training at an average energy expenditure of $2,200$ kcal $\cdot$ wk^{-1} (54).

Currently, the evidence that exercise causes collateral coronary blood vessel formation in humans is equivocal and involves a limited number of trials with small sample sizes. Belardinelli et al. (15) randomized 46 patients with chronic CAD and impaired left ventricular function into a group that exercised versus a sedentary control group. The group that exercise trained had significant improvement in contractile response to dobutamine. In a subgroup of the trained patients, improvements in contractile response correlated with an increase in coronary collateral score, suggesting additional coronary collateral formation. However, Hambrecht et al. (54) and Niebauer et al. (96) assessed the combined effects of <3 h of exercise per week and a low-fat diet on collateral formation in patients with CAD compared with patients receiving usual care.

After 1 yr, there was no significant difference between the groups with respect to coronary collateral formation.

Abnormal endothelial function in patients with CAD was first described in 1986 by Ludmer et al. (82). Whereas normal coronary arteries dilate in response to intracoronary acetylcholine, a paradoxical vasoconstriction is observed in patients with CAD or chronic heart failure. Endothelial dysfunction is thought to result from a decreased production of nitric oxide within vascular smooth muscle cells. Using invasive techniques, Hambrecht et al. (55) showed that exercise training partially normalizes coronary endothelial dysfunction and improves myocardial blood flow.

ADDITIONAL PHYSIOLOGIC VARIABLES

The autonomic nervous system, through a complex interplay of the parasympathetic and sympathetic components, mediates changes in HR, BP, and vascular tone (i.e., systemic resistance). Patients with a previous MI (19,46) and those with chronic heart failure (97,98) often have abnormalities of autonomic function at rest and during exercise because of a decrease in parasympathetic and an increase in sympathetic activity. This dysfunction often manifests itself as an elevated resting HR and an attenuated peak exercise HR response.

Another measure of autonomic function, the beat-to-beat (measured in milliseconds) variation in R-R intervals known as HR variability (HRV), serves as a surrogate assessment for parasympathetic activity. After an MI, mean values of HRV are attenuated by up to one-third when compared with age- and sex-matched healthy control subjects and improve with time but never return to normal. The magnitude of the attenuation in HRV reflects the amount of the myocardial damage. Even after making adjustments for abnormal left ventricular function and ventricular ectopy, patients with attenuated parasympathetic activity, as measured by a reduced HRV, have a fivefold increase in mortality (75). Although much less precise, plasma norepinephrine represents another marker for sympathetic activity. Patients with heart failure often have elevated plasma norepinephrine levels at rest, with such elevations associated with worsening heart failure and representing a strong and independent predictor of future mortality (32).

Chronic exercise training partially reverses autonomic dysfunction in patients with CVD. Among patients with chronic heart failure, Roveda et al. (107) showed a 33% decrease in muscle sympathetic nervous system activity after 4 mo of exercise training to levels similar to that in normal controls. Additionally, exercise trials involving patients recovering from an MI demonstrate significant improvement in HRV (83,127). Finally, exercise training results in decreased resting and exercise plasma norepinephrine levels in both patients with MI and patients with heart failure (14,31,68,84).

Koenig (62,77) and Imhof and Koenig (62) describe the relationship between hemostatic components, CVD risk, and exercise. Abnormalities in the concentrations of hemostatic elements, such as fibrinogen, factor VII, and platelet hyperactivity, as well as fibrinolytic elements, such as tissue plasminogen activator, have been identified as cardiovascular risk factors (63,77,89,125). The viscosity of the blood is also important to coronary blood flow. The major determinants of blood viscosity are hematocrit and fibrinogen levels. Increased fibrinogen levels are associated with a twofold increase in the risk for cardiovascular events. Increased factor VII levels, platelet hyperactivity, and decreased tissue plasminogen activator levels have also been shown to be predictors of coronary events but to a lesser degree (27,59,135). Much, but not all, of the literature describes an inverse relationship for moderate- to vigorous-intensity exercise training and fibrinogen levels. Although there is no evidence that factor VII levels are affected by acute exercise, endurance exercise increases activity in the fibrinolytic system. Long-term exercise training trials in patients with a history of an MI report reductions in erythrocyte rigidity, platelet aggregation, and adherence. Carroll et al. (27) and others (43,78) demonstrate an inverse relationship between hematologic parameters, such as plasma viscosity and hematocrit, and physical activity parameters, such as leisure-time physical activity and peak $\dot{V}O_2$ in patients with a history of MI. Importantly, most of the studies addressing the relationship between exercise and the level of hemostatic components involved individuals without known CAD.

CARDIAC REHABILITATION AND EXERCISE TRAINING: GENERAL OVERVIEW, MORBIDITY, MORTALITY, AND SAFETY

Cardiac rehabilitation is a program that addresses the continuum of care including inpatient, early outpatient, and long-term follow-up (11). To prevent deconditioning while in the hospital following a cardiac-related event, patients can start with slow ambulation as soon as they are medically stable. In fact, much of the deterioration in exercise tolerance during an inpatient stay can be countered through simple exposure to orthostatic or gravitational stress (by intermittent sitting or standing) and range-of-motion exercises (35). While a patient is hospitalized, education about CVD and how it is treated is initiated and activity level is increased from sitting to standing to ambulation. If there are no adverse responses noted, the patient may progress with ambulation as tolerated. Monitoring may include HR, BP, and cardiac ECG telemetry before and during activity (5).

Prior to discharge from the hospital, patients with CVD should also be referred to outpatient cardiac rehabilitation. Early outpatient and long-term follow-up cardiac rehabilitation both strive to further a patient's education but differ based on extent of supervision and monitoring during exercise, a patient's level of independence and functional capacity, and time from the index event (5).

Participation in outpatient cardiac rehabilitation represents guideline-based care to reduce the risk for experiencing a second event, improve exercise tolerance, manage symptoms, and facilitate healthier lifestyle changes (5,8,119). However, at present, cardiac rehabilitation is significantly underused. For example, among Medicare beneficiaries, in 1997, only 14% of patients experiencing an MI and 31% of those who had undergone coronary artery bypass graft surgery (CABG[S]) participated in cardiac rehabilitation (9,122).

A 2004 meta-analysis of exercise training trials involving patients with heart disease indicated that exercise-based cardiac rehabilitation was associated with a 25% reduction in subsequent risk for all-cause mortality but no significant effect on reducing nonfatal MI (124). Among patients with a recent MI enrolled in the multicenter and multifactorial lifestyle, the Global Secondary Prevention Strategies to Limit Event Recurrence After Myocardial Infarction (GOSPEL) trial, there was a nonsignificant ($P = 0.12$) 12% reduction in the primary combined endpoint of cardiovascular mortality; nonfatal MI; nonfatal stroke; or hospitalization for angina, heart failure, or urgent revascularization. However, there were significant exercise training–related reductions in risk for other important clinical endpoints, including the combined outcome of cardiac mortality, MI or stroke (33% reduction), or nonfatal MI alone (48% reduction) (50). Suaya et al. (123) observed that among older patients with CAD, after controlling for potential confounding factors, the relative risk for mortality was reduced almost 20% in those who attended 25 or more sessions of cardiac rehabilitation over 5 yr versus patients who attended 24 or fewer sessions.

For patients with stable chronic heart failure due to a reduced ejection fraction (HFREF), the multicenter Heart Failure and a Controlled Trial Investigating Outcomes of Exercise Training (HF-ACTION) trial compared the effects of exercise training plus usual care versus usual care alone and showed an 11% reduction in the adjusted risk for all-cause mortality or hospitalization and 15% reduction in the adjusted risk for cardiovascular mortality or heart failure hospitalization (99). A meta-analysis from Davies et al. (37) showed no effect on mortality alone because of exercise in patients with HFREF and a 28% decrease in heart failure–related hospitalization. Finally, Hammill et al. (56) reported that among elderly Medicare beneficiaries with a diagnosis of heart failure, mortality and MI were reduced by approximately 19% and 18%, respectively, over 4 yr in patients who attended 36 cardiac rehabilitation sessions versus those patients who attended 12 sessions. Considering the totality of the clinical outcome data, it is reasonable to conclude that cardiac rehabilitation and exercise training favorably affect several important clinical endpoints in patients with CVD.

With a goal of increasing program participation and optimizing patient outcomes, multiple models for the delivery of outpatient services have been employed. These models differ regarding the program frequency and duration, on-site versus remote monitoring and supervision, the focus of the interventions provided, use of kiosk or computer-based coordinated programs, and patient care coordinated through nurse case management (18,26,39,51,64,81). Monitoring patients remotely appears to be safe (1), and use of activity monitors, accelerometers, and global positioning system devices are related to improved patient outcomes (38,136). In the future, cellular and Web-based technologies may provide opportunities to expand the reach of programs to offer services to patients who heretofore were unable to access cardiac rehabilitation services (136).

The incidence of fatal and nonfatal cardiac events occurring during or shortly after a traditional cardiac rehabilitation exercise session is low. Fatal events occur at a rate of 1 in ~900,000 patient hours of participation in supervised exercise training, with most events occurring in patients considered to be at high risk for cardiac events. The rate of nonfatal MI during cardiac rehabilitation is approximately 1 in 250,000 patient hours

(124,131). Among patients with HFREF enrolled in HF-ACTION, 3% of patients randomized to the exercise group were hospitalized for an event that occurred during or within 3 h of exercise; an event rate that was quite similar to the 2% of patients in the usual care arm that reported experiencing an event requiring hospitalization during or within 3 h of exercise (99).

EXERCISE PRESCRIPTION AND PROGRAMMING

Table 38-3 provides a brief overview of some of the unique challenges and specific considerations associated with developing an exercise training regimen for individuals with CVD. Individuals with chronic illnesses have rates of sedentary behavior of 30%–40%, exceeding the general population rate of 24% (28,36). Instituting a regular exercise regimen in these patients may help modify several of the risk factors associated with CVD (*Table 38-4*).

Activity levels assessed by pedometers of participants at the start of cardiac rehabilitation reveals that nearly 80% would be classified as "sedentary" or "low active." In fact, on noncardiac rehabilitation exercise training days, average daily step counts were only about 5,300 steps, well below the 10,000 steps per day that has been incorporated into physical activity recommendations (109).

TABLE 38-3. Summary of Unique Exercise Prescription Issues among Patients with Cardiovascular Disease

Illness	Intensity	Comments
Coronary artery disease	40%–80% HRR	To affect mortality, frequency, duration, and intensity of training should result in a weekly energy expenditure of 1,500–2,000 kcal.[a,b]
Angina or equivalent	40%–80% HRR with necessary adjustment to keep upper HR more than 10 beats below ischemic threshold	Consider a prophylactic nitroglycerin 15 min before anticipated exertion if symptoms limit routine ADL or ability to exercise.
Myocardial infarction	40%–80% HRR	Achieve 1,500–2,000 kcal of energy expenditure through physical activity each week.[a,b]
Percutaneous coronary angioplasty	40%–80% HRR	Achieve 1,500–2,000 kcal of energy expenditure through physical activity each week.[a,b]
CABG or valve surgery	40%–80% HRR	Restrict upper-body movement until sternum is healed (8–12 wk).
Chronic heart failure	40%–80% HRR	If needed, initially guide exercise intensity at 40%–60% HRR and adjust duration to three bouts of 10 min each, progressing to 30–40 min.
Cardiac transplant	RPE 11–14	Restrict upper-body resistance exercises until sternum is healed (8–12 wk).
Pacemaker, ICD, biventricular, CRT	40–80% HRR with necessary adjustment to keep HR at least 10 bpm below defibrillation threshold	Avoid activities that stretch the arms for 3–4 wk and strength training for 4–6 wk.

HRR, heart rate reserve; ADL, activities of daily living; CABG, coronary artery bypass graft; RPE, rating of perceived exertion; ICD, implantable cardiac defibrillator; CRT, cardiac resynchronization therapy.

[a]American Association of Cardiovascular and Pulmonary Rehabilitation. *Guidelines for Cardiac Rehabilitation and Secondary Prevention.* 4th ed. Champaign (IL): Human Kinetics; 2004. p. 65–66, 118–120.

[b]Schuler G, Hambrecht R, Schlierf G, et al. Regular exercise and low fat diet—effects on progression of coronary artery disease. *Circulation.* 1992;86:1–11.

TABLE 38-4. Summary of Effects of Cardiorespiratory Exercise Training on Selected Cardiovascular Risk Factors

Risk Factor	Effect
Smoking	By itself: little or no effect
	Exercise should be part of a comprehensive smoking cessation program.
Lipid abnormalities	
Cholesterol	Little or no effect
LDL cholesterol	Little or no effect
HDL cholesterol	Mild-to-moderate increase
Hypertension	Reduces incidence (especially among white men)
Systolic blood pressure	Reduced: average, 6 mm Hg
Diastolic blood pressure	Reduced: average, 5 mm Hg
Obesity	Exercise alone: mild effect
	Exercise should be part of a comprehensive weight management program

LDL, low-density lipoprotein; HDL, high-density lipoprotein.

In addition, the average weekly exercise energy expenditure that typically occurs during monitored cardiac rehabilitation is quite low at approximately 800 kcal · wk^{-1} (110,113), remarkably similar to the weekly caloric exercise energy expenditure among patients participating in a long-term maintenance cardiac rehabilitation program (~830 kcal · wk^{-1}) (112). Patients in that maintenance program expended another 675 kcal · wk^{-1} participating in activities removed from cardiac rehabilitation. Combining rehabilitation-based and home-based activity, 72% of patients exceeded 1,000 kcal · wk^{-1} and 43% exceeded 1,500 kcal · wk^{-1} in weekly energy expenditure (112). This level of caloric expenditure is less than the >1,500 kcal suggested by Hambrecht and colleagues (54). Consequently, alternatives to the traditional cardiac rehabilitation exercise prescription may need to be considered to optimize CAD risk factors and favorably impact future clinical events in patients with CAD.

For example, high-calorie-expenditure exercise (i.e., targeting 3,000–3,500 kcal · wk^{-1} exercise-related energy expenditure) combined with a comprehensive behavioral weight loss intervention is associated with marked improvements in abdominal obesity, insulin resistance, lipid profiles, BP (3), endothelial function (111), platelet aggregation (66), and self-reported quality of life (105). Further study is needed, however, to determine whether higher volumes of exercise and consequent improvements in cardiovascular risk factors result in further reductions in mortality and morbidity.

After any index cardiac event and prior to commencing with an exercise training program, it is optimal for a patient to perform a symptom-limited exercise tolerance test (e.g., exercise stress test). Information obtained from an exercise test is necessary for developing an appropriate exercise prescription and is useful for guiding a patient's return to work or home/leisure activities. Unfortunately, patients are frequently referred to or participate in exercise training or cardiac rehabilitation without having an exercise test. For these patients, the exercise prescription should be implemented conservatively with close surveillance. Exercise intensity should be guided by rating of perceived exertion (RPE) of 11–14 (85,103) and titrated to provide the most efficacious program while maintaining the patients within their physical limitations and below their symptomatic threshold.

Regardless of whether an exercise tolerance test is performed, it is generally recommended that patients who have experienced a cardiovascular event start at the lower end of their training intensity (40%–60% HR reserve [HRR] or 11–13 on the RPE scale) (5). Typically, a cardiac rehabilitation session consists of a 5–10-min warm-up and cool-down period in addition to the aerobic training phase (5). These warm-up and cool-down phases should include stretching, range of motion, and low-intensity aerobic activities.

Following warm-up and prior to cool-down phases of cardiac rehabilitation or exercise training, an aerobic phase is completed and should involve exercising large muscle groups through rhythmic activities such as walking, cycling, or stationary rowing. Because training benefits are specific to the activity performed, both the legs and the arms need to be trained (30).

The duration of the aerobic phase should be progressively increased to at least 30 min and then time permitting, preferably titrated up to 60 min per session. Ideally, this amount of exercise per session should be performed most days per week. Exercise intensity is also progressively increased, as tolerated, up to 80% HRR. The actual number of sessions attended by patients in the formal cardiac rehabilitation setting is usually individualized, dictated by a multitude of factors including medical necessity, insurance coverage, program availability, and the patient's work and family obligations. Encouraging maximum program participation is recommended because observational studies have shown that long-term outcomes are positively correlated with the number of cardiac rehabilitation sessions attended (56,123).

Over the past 5 yr, there has been expanding interest to employ higher intensity aerobic interval training in patients with MI or heart failure or those with risk factors for CAD. Current research suggests that this type of training results in significantly greater improvement in fitness and endothelial function compared to moderately intense exercise (91,92,134). Aerobic interval training employs an exercise training intensity of approximately 90%–95% of peak HR (80%–90% HRR) for a brief interval of approximately 4 min, interspersed with a 3-min period of lower-intensity exercise (60%–70% of peak HR, 40%–50% HRR) for recovery purposes. It should be emphasized, however, that the studies using the regimen of aerobic interval training have included a small number of subjects and, as such, have not been adequately powered to resolve questions regarding patient safety or whether such training results in greater reductions in clinical events than the moderate, continuous training that is routinely employed today.

In addition to cardiovascular exercise, it is important for patients with CAD to include a resistance training program. A 2007 scientific statement of the American Heart Association (132) endorsed by the American College of Sports Medicine recommended mild-to-moderate resistance training for improving muscular strength and endurance, preventing and managing various chronic medical conditions, and modifying risk factors. Although dynamic resistance exercise for the upper and lower body is now recommended as part of a structured cardiac rehabilitation program (104), there are still limited data on the effects of resistance training on clinical endpoints among moderate- to high-risk patients with CVD. Also, it remains unclear to what extent, if any; cardiovascular risk factors such as hyperlipidemia and hypertension are favorably modified by resistance training in patients with CVD (104,132).

Isometric exercises are not recommended among patients with CAD because of a potential significant rise in systolic and diastolic BP. Moderate-intensity dynamic resistance exercise (defined as 50%–60 % of one repetition maximum [1-RM]) results in improved muscle strength and endurance, both of which are important for the safe return to activities of daily living, vocational and avocational activities, and maintaining independence. Higher intensity (80% of 1-RM) resistance training has also been shown to be well tolerated and effective in increasing strength and physical function in elderly individuals with CAD.

A commonly recommended resistance training program involves performing one set of 8–10 regional exercises performed 2–3 d · wk^{-1} (22,49,79,132). Typically, these programs involve starting at a low weight and progressing to 10–15 repetitions. While resistance training is at 50%–80% of 1-RM, the RPP should not exceed that prescribed for endurance exercise, and perceived exertion should remain between 11 and 14 on the Borg scale (79,132). Patients undergoing a catheterization with or without percutaneous coronary intervention and those recovering from an uncomplicated MI may begin a resistance training program as early as 3 and 5 wk after the event, respectively (5). Patients undergoing CABG or valve surgery involving a sternotomy should avoid upper-limb resistance training until sternal healing has occurred, which is generally 8–12 wk after surgery. Patients may benefit by first training the upper limbs with elastic bands and hand weights before progressing to resistance-type exercise machines (5).

Concerning the use and efficacy of ECG monitoring in cardiac rehabilitation programs in the United States, presently, it is left to the clinicians in the program to decide whether to incorporate ECG telemetry monitoring when exercising patients with CVD, usually based on a patient's risk for exercise-related events (5). Although ECG telemetry monitoring during cardiac rehabilitation is common in the United States, it is important to point out that such an approach is not used in either Canada or Europe. Albeit limited, analysis of safety data from several clinical studies suggest that ECG monitoring may not be necessary when exercising patients with chronic heart failure (44,72,87).

CORONARY ARTERY DISEASE

Among patients with CAD, a lower intensity and longer warm-up might help them avoid the occurrence of angina, ST-segment depression, threatening arrhythmias, and transient left ventricular dysfunction (12,13). Similar to recovery from a maximal exercise stress test, the cool-down phase after exercise training facilitates the gradual return of HR and BP to resting values and therefore reduces the likelihood of hypotension/dizziness after exercise. Training parameters may need to be modified based on an individual patient's symptoms and medication use.

ANGINA AND MYOCARDIAL INFARCTION

Exercise, lifestyle behavior changes, and medical compliance are key for people with stable angina or after an MI to help reduce overall cardiac risk and prevent or retard progression of atherosclerotic plaques (100). It was initially thought that the threshold at which the myocardium becomes ischemic and angina occurs is reproducible and, as mentioned earlier, can be estimated by the RPP. Subsequent work by Garber et al. (49) and others (16,88,106) demonstrated that the angina threshold varies with the type of exercise performed. They found that the RPP at the ischemic threshold varied depending on whether one was performing a maximal stress test or a longer submaximal exercise session. The ischemic threshold occurred at a lower HR during sustained submaximal exercise and daily activities at home than during a maximal stress test. Circadian rhythm also plays a role (106), in that the ischemic threshold was found to be lower at 1 p.m. than 8 a.m. and 9 p.m. Forearm vascular resistance was increased at 8 a.m. and 9 p.m. compared with 1 p.m., suggesting that increased vascular resistance may be one of the causes for the variability in angina threshold. However, for a given patient performing a specific activity at the same time of the day, there did appear to be reproducibility in the RPP at which angina occurs (106). Therefore, one goal for patients with angina is to perform routine daily activities at an RPP that is below their ischemic threshold, thus reducing the amount of angina and fatigue they experience. Another goal is to increase the amount of work, home activity, or exercise they can perform at a given RPP (5,47) or below their ischemic threshold (*Fig. 38-1*).

Exercise programming for patients with angina or those having suffered an MI requires that they first identify and understand their symptoms. Specifically, individuals need to be able to identify the nature of their angina (*e.g.*, location, precipitating factors, associated symptoms, and radiation pattern) and understand that there are no clinical benefits derived from exercising with such discomfort or pain. In cardiac rehabilitation, there are angina rating scales (*e.g.*, 1–4) to help assess the severity of symptoms. Patients also need to identify which activities precipitate their angina and modify the situation accordingly. For example, if walking in the cold causes chest discomfort, then they should exercise indoors or consider wearing a scarf or other protective wear over their mouth to warm inhaled air. Similarly, if a routine daily activity or mild exercise regularly causes chest pain, they should talk with their physician about possibly taking sublingual nitroglycerin beforehand. In the cardiac rehabilitation setting, it is not uncommon for patients who regularly experience angina at relatively low workloads (*e.g.*, 2 METs) to take one sublingual nitroglycerin about 15 min before starting their warm-up. This practice usually allows these patients to exercise in a pain-free manner and at slightly higher workloads. Also, it may be beneficial to include a longer warm-up (≥10 min) to help minimize or avoid ischemia.

Regardless of having suffered a previous MI or not, for patients with evidence of exercise-induced ischemia (*i.e.*, angina, ECG changes), the upper limit for HR during exercise training should be 10 or more beats below the HR or RPP at which ischemia was first identified during a graded exercise test (5,48). If a patient does not experience symptoms and the ECG is uninterpretable, it is difficult to determine the ischemic threshold during an exercise test with echocardiographic or radionuclide imaging. Myocardial ischemia may manifest itself as angina, ST-segment depression, ventricular arrhythmias, or an abnormal BP response (61). A stress imaging study may be positive for ischemia but does not determine the intensity at which the ischemia began. In situations like this, it may be prudent to be conservative and avoid vigorous intensity exercise by prescribing exercise at 40%–60% HRR.

Medications such as β-blockers, nitrates, and calcium channel blockers may influence the ischemic threshold. As a result, patients should take their medications between 3 and 10 h before undergoing an exercise test administered for the purpose of establishing an exercise training HR range. The exercise test should be rescheduled if a patient fails to take the medication, because the HR response will not be representative of what the patient will experience during exercise training. Optimally, another exercise test should be completed if a patient's medication or dose is changed, although this is not always possible because of insurance reimbursement issues. Ideally, a symptom-limited exercise tolerance test is performed prior to or very soon after initiation of exercise training in cardiac rehabilitation.

REVASCULARIZATION (CORONARY ARTERY BYPASS GRAFT AND PERCUTANEOUS CORONARY ANGIOPLASTY)

The three medical/surgical treatment modalities for CAD — medications, percutaneous coronary angioplasty, and CABG — are discussed in *Chapter 6*. In general, the benefits and limitations of exercise are quite similar for patients after revascularization as they are for patients after an MI. Signs of ischemia during exercise, such as angina, ST-segment depression, and hemodynamic abnormalities (*i.e.*, chronotropic incompetence, blunted BP response) are often eliminated or occur at higher intensity activities after revascularization.

The recommendations for starting cardiac rehabilitation and exercise programming for patients after angioplasty are generally the same as for other patients with CAD. However, because patients undergoing angioplasty frequently do not experience myocardial damage or extensive surgery, they can return to physical activities sooner. This may include beginning cardiac rehabilitation within 72 h after the procedure (114). Patients undergoing CABG begin rehabilitation as early as 2 wk after surgery, with the initial focus on aerobic-type exercises. All upper-body exercise should be limited to range-of-motion and light-resistance activities such as arm ergometry until 4–8 wk after surgery (5). Following the initial wound healing of revascularization, patients should be able to exercise up to 80% HRR, 3–4 d · wk^{-1}, and for 20–60 min. After approximately 10–12 wk, adequate healing of the sternum has occurred, and patients can safely initiate a resistance training program similar to other patients with CVD (5).

VALVE DYSFUNCTION/REPAIR/REPLACEMENT

Heart valve abnormalities, such as stenosis and regurgitation, reduce cardiac output and thus increase the work that the heart must perform to meet the body's physiologic demands (21). As a result, myocardial hypertrophy can develop. Over time, this may lead to a decrease in ventricular distensibility and diastolic dysfunction. Exercise will not improve or change the function of the valves, but it will help to improve the efficiency of oxygen extraction by the skeletal muscles and improve the work capacity of the individual (21). In general, asymptomatic patients with mild valvular disease and normal left ventricular function and normal pulmonary artery pressures are not restricted from exercise training or participating in competitive sports (21,101). Patients with aortic or mitral regurgitation with a more than mildly dilated left ventricle or abnormal systolic function should avoid competitive sports (21). Because of the risk of sudden death, it is recommended that patients with moderate-to-severe aortic stenosis not participate in vigorous or competitive exercise (21).

Patients with bioprosthetic or mechanical valves should limit themselves to moderate-intensity exercise training. Patients on anticoagulation therapy (warfarin) for mechanical valves or atrial fibrillation should avoid contact sports (21). Most of the changes in the myocardium that develop because of faulty valve function are partially reversible after surgery, provided that cardiac function has not been compromised long enough for permanent remodeling to occur. This length of time varies among individuals (21).

Most valve abnormalities can be corrected with surgical procedures. Following surgery, patients are encouraged to begin an exercise program to improve exercise tolerance and prevent other heart problems (101). It is advised that patients follow the same post surgery guidelines as those for patients who are post-CABG.

HEART FAILURE

Current evidence indicates that moderately intense aerobic exercise safely improves exercise tolerance in patients with heart failure, partially reverses much of the abnormal pathophysiology that accompanies the disease, and improves health-related quality of life and several important clinical outcomes (67). When prescribing exercise for patients with heart failure, one must also consider the etiology. Specifically, the cause of the heart failure may be either ischemic or nonischemic, and if it is the former, then the guidelines for prescribing exercise in patients with angina may also need to be followed. Initially, the duration of activity may need to be adjusted to allow these patients more opportunity for rest and to progress at their own pace. In fact, some patients may better tolerate discontinuous training involving short bouts of exercise interspersed with bouts of rest (90,134).

An exercise intensity between 55% and 75% HRR is able to increase exercise tolerance and yield generally similar relative gains in cardiorespiratory fitness (67). Based on these data, for the first few exercise sessions, it is appropriate to limit the upper end of exercise intensity to 60% HRR, titrated based on a patient's subjective feelings of fatigue using the RPE scale (e.g., 11–14 on Borg 6–20 scale). For patients with atrial fibrillation or those with frequent ectopic beats that interfere with the accurate measurement of HR during exercise, training intensity can be guided by RPE alone.

Because disorders of skeletal muscle function (i.e., strength and endurance) also contribute to the reduction in exercise tolerance observed in patients with heart failure, consideration should be given to incorporating resistance or strength training into the overall exercise plan for selected patients. Similar to what was described earlier for aerobic or cardiorespiratory training, patient effort during resistance training also needs to be increased in a progressive manner. For example, the intensity should be progressively increased over several weeks from ~30%–40% of 1-RM to 70% of 1-RM. Higher intensity (80% of 1-RM) resistance training has also been shown to be well tolerated and effective in increasing strength and physical function in individuals with heart failure (108).

Increasingly common is the use of left ventricular assist devices (LVAD) for patients with end-stage heart failure. In brief, the LVAD pump is implanted intra-abdominally or in a preperitoneal pocket external to the abdominal viscera. The left ventricle is cannulated at the apex of the heart for inflow to the pump, which then sends blood into the ascending aorta distal to the aortic valve. Current-generation LVADs have smaller internal components because of the use of continuous versus pulsatile flow pumps and have resulted in less mechanical device failures and a longer lifespan for the device (52).

An obvious benefit of cardiac rehabilitation with this patient population is reversal of the skeletal muscle atrophy and exercise intolerance that occurs with prolonged sedentary behavior. Although patients receiving an LVAD may be more functional than those with severe heart failure without an LVAD, those with a recently (i.e., <3 mo) implanted device are still likely to be extremely deconditioned and have unique medical concerns requiring attention by the cardiac rehabilitation staff. To date, there are no large, multicenter prospective trials investigating the effects of exercise training in patients with LVADs; hence, the optimal training prescriptions have not yet been established. That said, similar to cardiac transplant recipients, maintaining a moderate level of perceived exertion (Borg scale 11–13) while gradually increasing exercise intensity likely represents an appropriate method. It is not uncommon for initial exercise workload to begin at or below 2 METs in most patients with an LVAD with future increases in intensity guided by perceived exertion. Factors that can influence the overall functional capacity of a patient and initial workloads chosen for rehabilitation include time from LVAD implantation, current activity habits, comorbidities, and age. Response to training can be safely evaluated with the 6-min walk test.

Cardiac rehabilitation staff should also be familiar with the LVAD and work with the patient and the LVAD coordinator at their institution regarding emergency procedures and complications common to the device (e.g., device failure, hypovolemia). Also, because of the nonpulsatile flow of blood in the newer, continuous LVAD models, auscultatory BP assessment may not be reliable at rest. In these patients, it may be helpful to measure mean arterial BP via Doppler ultrasound.

Contraindications to exercise will be similar to other cardiac rehabilitation participants; additionally, exercise should be withheld if mean arterial pressure is less than 65 mm Hg or if the low flow device alarm is activated (117). Should an LVAD patient lose consciousness, chest compressions should not be performed because this may damage the LVAD and dislodge the lines attached to the heart.

It is important to acknowledge that most literature to date concerning the physiologic and clinical responses of patients with heart failure to exercise training pertains to patients with HFREF. However, patients with heart failure and preserved ejection fraction represent up to 50% of patients with heart failure; unfortunately, very little exercise research has been conducted on these patients. Two trials involving patients with heart failure and preserved ejection fraction showed that regular exercise improves exercise intolerance to a magnitude that is similar to patients with HFREF (74,118).

CARDIAC TRANSPLANT

Despite receiving a donor heart with normal systolic function and subsequent improvement in functional capacity, cardiac transplant recipients continue to experience exercise intolerance after surgery that is about 40%–50% below that of age-matched normal individuals (6). This exercise intolerance is believed to be primarily attributable to the absence of efferent sympathetic innervation of the myocardium, affecting HR and contractility responses, residual skeletal muscle abnormalities developed before transplantation because of heart failure, and decreased skeletal muscle strength (6).

After surgery, medical management focuses on preventing rejection of the donor heart by suppressing immune system function while avoiding complicating side effects such as infections, hyperlipidemia, hypertension, osteoporosis, diabetes, certain cancers, and accelerated graft atherosclerosis of the epicardial and intramural coronary arteries. Because of the denervated myocardium, at least during the first year after transplantation, many differences in the cardiorespiratory and neuroendocrine responses are evident at rest, during exercise, and in recovery in cardiac transplant recipients (120,121). These abnormalities include an elevated resting HR (often >90 bpm); elevated systolic and diastolic BP at rest, partly attributable to increased plasma norepinephrine and the immunosuppressive medications (*i.e.*, cyclosporine and prednisone); an attenuated increase in HR during submaximal work; a lower peak HR and peak stroke volume; a greater increase in plasma norepinephrine during exercise; and a delayed slowing of HR in recovery (6). Failure of HR to recover in a normal time course is thought to be attributable to increased levels of plasma norepinephrine, exerting a positive chronotropic effect in the absence of vagal efferent innervation (4).

To prescribe exercise and guide exercise intensity in cardiac transplant recipients in the first year after surgery, it is best to disregard all HR-based methods because of the abnormal control of HR in these patients (69,120). For example, it is common to find persons with cardiac transplant within the past year achieving an exercise HR during training that not only exceeds 85% of peak HR but is also often equal to or greater than the peak HR attained during their last symptom-limited exercise test. RPE between 11 and 14 should be used to guide exercise training intensity (7,69).

Among patients with cardiac transplant who undergo exercise training, exercise capacity increases by about 15%–40%, resting HR is unchanged or decreases slightly, peak HR increases, there is little change in peak stroke volume or cardiac dimensions, and quality of life is favorably altered (7). In a comprehensive prospective, randomized trial, Kobashigawa et al. (76) showed a 49% increase in peak $\dot{V}O_2$ and a 23 bpm increase in peak HR.

In addition, patients with cardiac transplant can benefit from a systematic program of resistance training because leg strength deficit contributes to the reduced exercise capacity after surgery. Braith, Beck, and Edwards (22,23) showed that resistance training improves muscular endurance and also partially restores bone mineral density and addresses the skeletal muscle abnormalities (*i.e.*, strength development, lipid content, fiber size) that commonly occur because of long-term corticosteroid therapy. A progressive resistance training program of 7–10 exercises that focus on the legs, back, arms, and shoulders, started 6–12 wk after transplant surgery and performed two times per week, is recommended (23).

PACEMAKERS, RESYNCHRONIZATION THERAPY, IMPLANTABLE CARDIAC DEFIBRILLATORS, AND ARRHYTHMIAS

Pacemakers and implantable cardiac defibrillators (ICD) are devices typically implanted in the upper chest to monitor and regulate the electrical activity of the heart. Functional capacity may be improved with pacemakers because of an improved HR response to exercise. Rate-responsive pacemakers respond to exercise by sensing movement or ventilation and gradually increase HR until the upper rate of the pacemaker is reached. The type of ramp-up programmed into the pacemaker determines how quickly the HR is increased in response to exercise. Both the ramp and the upper rate limit of the pacemaker are adjustable to maximize a patient's exercise performance. The pacemaker upper rate limit is usually set so it is 10 or more beats below ischemic threshold (102,104). Biventricular pacemakers (*i.e.*, cardiac resynchronization therapy) are used for the treatment of heart failure. Indications for a biventricular pacemaker include left ventricular dysfunction with left bundle-branch block, poor functional capacity, and evidence of asynchronous ventricular contraction. Unlike traditional pacemakers, these pace both the right and left ventricles. Biventricular pacemakers are designed to act just like other pacemakers and may or may not have ICD capacity (40). Data demonstrate that functional capacity (*i.e.*, peak $\dot{V}O_2$) and quality of life are improved with the use of a biventricular pacemaker (45,86,130).

ICDs are devices that detect abnormal heart rhythms and deliver an electrical shock if a dangerous rhythm is detected (102). Exercise intensity in patients with an ICD should be set at least 10 beats below the programmed firing threshold. For many patients, this is not a big concern because they are taking a medication (*i.e.*, β-adrenergic blocking agents) that prevents their HR from increasing to the ICD firing threshold, which is often between 150 and 180 bpm. Exercise tests performed to evaluate ischemia in patients with pacemakers require imaging studies during the test because of the abnormal resting ECG.

Unfortunately, return to activity guidelines after device implantation are poorly defined. For example, Naffe et al. (93), surveyed 48 hospitals in the United States regarding instructions provided to patients after implant surgery and reported discharge instructions as diverse as no activity restrictions to directing patients to use a sling to prohibit arm movement for up to 4 wk. In fact, the authors reported receiving so many different responses that it was impossible to categorize them. In general, to maintain device and incision integrity, vigorous upper-extremity activities such as swimming, bowling, lifting weights, elliptical machines, and golfing should be avoided for 3–4 wk after implant. Lower-extremity activities can resume as tolerated immediately after implantation. Although evidence suggests that current activity guidelines may be overly restrictive (93), participation in cardiac rehabilitation has been shown to improve functional capacity in patients with an implanted device.

Often, patients with CVD will also have atrial and/or ventricular arrhythmias during exercise. Regular exercise training favorably alters cardiac autonomic regulation, which provides a possible means of preventing dangerous arrhythmias (20). Patients with atrial fibrillation have irregular HRs that prevent the use of standard exercise HR prescriptions. These patients should guide their exercise intensity using the Borg RPE scale. Patients presenting with frequent premature ventricular contractions should also be monitored closely and for longer periods. If there is a set HR at which they become more frequent, the exercise prescription may be set 10 beats below this HR, especially if they become symptomatic.

Most of these patients will also require further testing to determine the impact of these arrhythmias and to help the physician better control them.

SUMMARY

Exercise programming as reviewed in this chapter allows patients with various CVDs to exercise safely (5,128,132). The inclusion of exercise in the treatment of these patients is beneficial because of its favorable effects on risk factors, symptoms, functional capacity, physiology, and quality of life. Finally, and possibly most important, all patients with CVD should be encouraged to participate in exercise because of its real or likely positive impact on mortality and morbidity.

REFERENCES

1. Ades PA, Pashkow FJ, Fletcher G, Pina IL, Zohman LR, Nestor JR. A controlled trial of cardiac rehabilitation in the home setting using electrocardiographic and voice transtelephonic monitoring. *Am Heart J.* 2000;139(3):543–8.
2. Ades PA, Savage PD, Brawner CA, et al. Aerobic capacity in patients entering cardiac rehabilitation. *Circulation.* 2006;113(23):2706–12.
3. Ades PA, Savage PD, Toth MJ, et al. High-calorie-expenditure exercise: a new approach to cardiac rehabilitation for overweight coronary patients. *Circulation.* 2009;119(20):2671–8.
4. Albrecht AE, Lillis D, Pease MO, et al. Heart rate and catecholamine responses during exercise and recovery in cardiac transplant recipients. *J Cardiopulm Rehabil.* 1993;13(3):182–7.
5. American Association of Cardiovascular & Pulmonary Rehabilitation. *Guidelines for Cardiac Rehabilitation and Secondary Prevention Programs.* 4th ed. Champaign (IL): Human Kinetics; 2004. 280 p.
6. Arena R, Humphrey R. Cardiac transplant. In: Durstine JL, Moore GE, Painter PL, Roberts SO, editors. *ACSM's Exercise Management for Persons with Chronic Disease and Disabilities.* Champaign: Human Kinetics; 2009. p. 99–106.
7. Arena R, Myers J, Williams MA, et al. Assessment of functional capacity in clinical and research settings: a scientific statement from the American Heart Association Committee on Exercise, Rehabilitation, and Prevention of the Council on Clinical Cardiology and the Council on Cardiovascular Nursing. *Circulation.* 2007;116(3):329–43.
8. Arnold JM, Liu P, Demers C, et al. Canadian Cardiovascular Society consensus conference recommendations on heart failure 2006: diagnosis and management. *Can J Cardiol.* 2006;22(1):23–45.
9. Balady GJ, Ades PA, Bittner VA, et al. Referral, enrollment, and delivery of cardiac rehabilitation/secondary prevention programs at clinical centers and beyond: a presidential advisory from the American Heart Association. *Circulation.* 2011;124(25):2951–60.
10. Balady GJ, Arena R, Sietsema K, et al. Clinician's guide to cardiopulmonary exercise testing in adults: a scientific statement from the American Heart Association. *Circulation.* 2010;122(2):191–225.
11. Balady GJ, Williams MA, Ades PA, et al. Core components of cardiac rehabilitation/secondary prevention programs: 2007 update: a scientific statement from the American Heart Association Exercise, Cardiac Rehabilitation, and Prevention Committee, the Council on Clinical Cardiology; the Councils on Cardiovascular Nursing, Epidemiology and Prevention, and Nutrition, Physical Activity, and Metabolism; and the American Association of Cardiovascular and Pulmonary Rehabilitation. *Circulation.* 2007;115(20):2675–82.
12. Barnard RJ, Gardner GW, Diaco NV, MacAlpin RN, Kattus AA. Cardiovascular responses to sudden strenuous exercise—heart rate, blood pressure, and ECG. *J Appl Physiol.* 1973;34(6):833–7.

13. Barnard RJ, MacAlpin R, Kattus AA, Buckberg GD. Ischemic response to sudden strenuous exercise in healthy men. *Circulation.* 1973;48(5):936–42.

14. Belardinelli R, Georgiou D, Cianci G, Purcaro A. Randomized, controlled trial of long-term moderate exercise training in chronic heart failure: effects on functional capacity, quality of life, and clinical outcome. *Circulation.* 1999;99(9):1173–82.

15. Belardinelli R, Georgiou D, Ginzton L, Cianci G, Purcaro A. Effects of moderate exercise training on thallium uptake and contractile response to low-dose dobutamine of dysfunctional myocardium in patients with ischemic cardiomyopathy. *Circulation.* 1998;97(6):553–61.

16. Benhorin J, Pinsker G, Moriel M, Gavish A, Tzivoni D, Stern S. Ischemic threshold during two exercise testing protocols and during ambulatory electrocardiographic monitoring. *J Am Coll Cardiol.* 1993;22(3):671–7.

17. Berger HJ, Reduto LA, Johnstone DE, et al. Global and regional left ventricular response to bicycle exercise in coronary artery disease. Assessment by quantitative radionuclide angiocardiography. *Am J Med.* 1979;66(1):13–21.

18. Berra K. Does nurse case management improve implementation of guidelines for cardiovascular disease risk reduction? *J Cardiovasc Nurs.* 2011;26(2):145–67.

19. Bigger JT,Jr, Fleiss JL, Steinman RC, Rolnitzky LM, Kleiger RE, Rottman JN. Frequency domain measures of heart period variability and mortality after myocardial infarction. *Circulation.* 1992;85(1):164–71.

20. Billman GE. Aerobic exercise conditioning: a nonpharmacological antiarrhythmic intervention. *J Appl Physiol.* 2002;92(2):446–54.

21. Bonow RO, Cheitlin MD, Crawford MH, Douglas PS. Task force 3: valvular heart disease. *J Am Coll Cardiol.* 2005;45(8):1334–40.

22. Braith RW, Beck DT. Resistance exercise: training adaptations and developing a safe exercise prescription. *Heart Fail Rev.* 2008;13(1):69–79.

23. Braith RW, Edwards DG. Exercise following heart transplantation. *Sports Med.* 2000;30(3):171–92.

24. Brener SJ, Pashkow FJ, Harvey SA, Marwick TH, Thomas JD, Lauer MS. Chronotropic response to exercise predicts angiographic severity in patients with suspected or stable coronary artery disease. *Am J Cardiol.* 1995;76(17):1228–32.

25. Brubaker PH, Kitzman DW. Chronotropic incompetence: causes, consequences, and management. *Circulation.* 2011;123(9):1010–20.

26. Carlson JJ, Johnson JA, Franklin BA, VanderLaan RL. Program participation, exercise adherence, cardiovascular outcomes, and program cost of traditional versus modified cardiac rehabilitation. *Am J Cardiol.* 2000;86(1):17–23.

27. Carroll S, Cooke CB, Butterly RJ. Physical activity, cardiorespiratory fitness, and the primary components of blood viscosity. *Med Sci Sports Exerc.* 2000;32(2):353–8.

28. Chobanian AV, Bakris GL, Black HR, et al. The seventh report of the Joint National Committee on Prevention, Detection, Evaluation, and Treatment of High Blood Pressure: the JNC 7 report. *JAMA.* 2003;289(19):2560–72.

29. Clausen JP. Circulatory adjustments to dynamic exercise and effects of physical training in normal subjects and in patients with coronary artery disease. In: Sonnenblick EH, Lesch M, editors. *Exercise and Heart Disease.* New York: Grune & Stratton; 1977. p. 39–75.

30. Clausen JP, Trap-Jensen J, Lassen NA. The effects of training on the heart rate during arm and leg exercise. *Scand J Clin Lab Invest.* 1970;26(3):295–301.

31. Coats AJS, Adamopoulos S, Radaelli A, et al. Controlled trial of physical training in chronic heart failure: Exercise performance, hemodynamics, ventilation, and autonomic function. *Circulation.* 1992;85(6):2119–31.

32. Cohn JN, Levine TB, Olivari MT, et al. Plasma norepinephrine as a guide to prognosis in patients with chronic congestive heart failure. *N Engl J Med.* 1984;311(13):819–23.

33. Cole CR, Blackstone EH, Pashkow FJ, Snader CE, Lauer MS. Heart-rate recovery immediately after exercise as a predictor of mortality. *N Engl J Med.* 1999;341(18):1351-7.

34. Comess KA, Fenster PE. Clinical implications of the blood pressure response to exercise. *Cardiology.* 1981;68(4):233–44.

35. Convertino VA. Effect of orthostatic stress on exercise performance after bed rest: Relation to inhospital rehabilitation. *J Cardiac Rehabil.* 1983;3(9):660–3.

36. Crespo CJ, Keteyian SJ, Heath GW, Sempos CT. Leisure-time physical activity among US adults. Results from the Third National Health and Nutrition Examination Survey. *Arch Intern Med.* 1996; 156(1):93–8.

37. Davies EJ, Moxham T, Rees K, et al. Exercise training for systolic heart failure: Cochrane systematic review and meta-analysis. *Eur J Heart Fail.* 2010;12(7):706–15.

38. de Blok BM, de Greef MH, ten Hacken NH, Sprenger SR, Postema K, Wempe JB. The effects of a lifestyle physical activity counseling program with feedback of a pedometer during pulmonary rehabilitation in patients with COPD: a pilot study. *Patient Educ Couns.* 2006;61(1):48–55.

39. DeBusk RF, Haskell WL, Miller NH, et al. Medically directed at-home rehabilitation soon after clinically uncomplicated acute myocardial infarction: a new model for patient care. *Am J Cardiol.* 1985;55(4):251–7.

40. Delnoy PP, Ottervanger JP, Luttikhuis HO, et al. Sustained benefit of cardiac resynchronization therapy. *J Cardiovasc Electrophysiol.* 2007;18(3):298–302.

41. Dlin RA, Hanne N, Silverberg DS, Bar-Or O. Follow-up of normotensive men with exaggerated blood pressure response to exercise. *Am Heart J.* 1983;106(2):316–20.

42. Ellestad MH, Wan MK. Predictive implications of stress testing. Follow-up of 2700 subjects after maximum treadmill stress testing. *Circulation.* 1975;51(2):363–9.

43. Elwood PC, Yarnell JW, Pickering J, Fehily AM, O'Brien JR. Exercise, fibrinogen, and other risk factors for ischaemic heart disease. Caerphilly Prospective Heart Disease Study. *Br Heart J.* 1993;69(2):183–7.

44. Experience from controlled trials of physical training in chronic heart failure. Protocol and patient factors in effectiveness in the improvement in exercise tolerance. European Heart Failure Training Group. *Eur Heart J.* 1998;19(3):466–75.

45. Fan S, Lyon CE, Savage PD, Ozonoff A, Ades PA, Balady GJ. Outcomes and adverse events among patients with implantable cardiac defibrillators in cardiac rehabilitation: a case-controlled study. *J Cardiopulm Rehabil Prev.* 2009;29(1):40–3.

46. Farrell TG, Paul V, Cripps TR, et al. Baroreflex sensitivity and electrophysiological correlates in patients after acute myocardial infarction. *Circulation.* 1991;83(3):945–52.

47. Fletcher GF, Balady GJ, Amsterdam EA, et al. Exercise standards for testing and training: a statement for healthcare professionals from the American Heart Association. *Circulation.* 2001;104(14):1694–740.

48. Friedman D, Roberts SD. Angina and silent ischemia. In: Durstine JL, Moore GE, Painter PL, Roberts SO, editors. *ACSM's Exercise Management for Persons with Chronic Disease and Disabilities.* Champaign: Human Kinetics; 2009. p. 66–72.

49. Garber CE, Carleton RA, Camaione DN, Heller GV. The threshold for myocardial ischemia varies in patients with coronary artery disease depending on the exercise protocol. *J Am Coll Cardiol.* 1991;17(6):1256–62.

50. Giannuzzi P, Temporelli PL, Marchioli R, et al. Global secondary prevention strategies to limit event recurrence after myocardial infarction: results of the GOSPEL study, a multicenter, randomized controlled trial from the Italian Cardiac Rehabilitation Network. *Arch Intern Med.* 2008;168(20):2194–204.

51. Gordon NF, English CD, Contractor AS, et al. Effectiveness of three models for comprehensive cardiovascular disease risk reduction. *Am J Cardiol.* 2002;89(11):1263–8.

52. Griffith BP, Kormos RL, Borovetz HS, et al. HeartMate II left ventricular assist system: from concept to first clinical use. *Ann Thorac Surg.* 2001;71(3 Suppl):S116–20; discussion S114–6.

53. Hambrecht R, Niebauer J, Fiehn E, et al. Physical training in patients with stable chronic heart failure: effects on cardiorespiratory fitness and ultrastructural abnormalities of leg muscles. *J Am Coll Cardiol.* 1995;25(6):1239–49.

54. Hambrecht R, Niebauer J, Marburger C, et al. Various intensities of leisure time physical activity in patients with coronary artery disease: effects on cardiorespiratory fitness and progression of coronary atherosclerotic lesions. *J Am Coll Cardiol.* 1993;22(2): 468–77.

55. Hambrecht R, Wolf A, Gielen S, et al. Effect of exercise on coronary endothelial function in patients with coronary artery disease. *N Engl J Med.* 2000;342(7):454–60.

56. Hammill BG, Curtis LH, Schulman KA, Whellan DJ. Relationship between cardiac rehabilitation and long-term risks of death and myocardial infarction among elderly Medicare beneficiaries. *Circulation.* 2010;121(1):63–70.

57. Hartung GH, Rangel R. Exercise training in post-myocardial infarction patients: comparison of results with high risk coronary and post-bypass patients. *Arch Phys Med Rehabil.* 1981;62(4): 147–50.

58. Haskell WL, Alderman EL, Fair JM, et al. Effects of intensive multiple risk factor reduction on coronary atherosclerosis and clinical cardiac events in men and women with coronary artery disease. The Stanford Coronary Risk Intervention Project (SCRIP). *Circulation.* 1994;89(3):975–90.

59. Heinrich J, Balleisen L, Schulte H, Assmann G, van de Loo J. Fibrinogen and factor VII in the prediction of coronary risk. Results from the PROCAM study in healthy men. *Arterioscler Thromb.* 1994;14(1):54–9.

60. Heller GV, Ahmed I, Tilkemeier PL, Barbour MM, Garber CE. Comparison of chest pain, electrocardiographic changes and thallium-201 scintigraphy during varying exercise intensities in men with stable angina pectoris. *Am J Cardiol.* 1991;68(6):569–74.

61. Hoberg E, Schuler G, Kunze B, et al. Silent myocardial ischemia as a potential link between lack of premonitoring symptoms and increased risk of cardiac arrest during physical stress. *Am J Cardiol.* 1990;65(9):583–9.

62. Imhof A, Koenig W. Exercise and thrombosis. *Cardiol Clin.* 2001; 19(3):389–400.

63. Irving JB, Bruce RA, DeRouen TA. Variations in and significance of systolic pressure during maximal exercise (treadmill) testing. *Am J Cardiol.* 1977;39(6):841–8.

64. Jolly K, Lip GY, Sandercock J, et al. Home-based versus hospital-based cardiac rehabilitation after myocardial infarction or revascularisation: design and rationale of the Birmingham Rehabilitation Uptake Maximisation Study (BRUM): a randomised controlled trial [ISRCTN72884263]. *BMC Cardiovasc Disord.* 2003;3:10.

65. Jolly MA, Brennan DM, Cho L. Impact of exercise on heart rate recovery. *Circulation.* 2011;124(14):1520–6.

66. Keating FK, Schneider DJ, Savage PD, Bunn JY, Toth MJ, Ades PA. Platelet reactivity decreases after exercise training and weight loss in overweight patients with coronary artery disease. *Circulation.* 2009;120:S512.

67. Keteyian SJ. Exercise training in congestive heart failure: risks and benefits. *Prog Cardiovasc Dis.* 2011;53(6):419–28.

68. Keteyian SJ, Brawner CA, Schairer JR, et al. Effects of exercise training on chronotropic incompetence in patients with heart failure. *Am Heart J.* 1999;138(2 Pt 1):233–40.

69. Keteyian S, Ehrman J, Fedel F, Rhoads K. Heart rate-perceived exertion relationship during exercise in orthotopic heart transplant patients. *J Cardiopulm Rehabil.* 1990;10(8):287–93.

70. Keteyian SJ, Marks CR, Brawner CA, Levine AB, Kataoka T, Levine TB. Responses to arm exercise in patients with compensated heart failure. *J Cardiopulm Rehabil.* 1996;16(6):366–71.

71. Keteyian S, Marks CR, Levine AB, et al. Cardiovascular responses of cardiac transplant patients to arm and leg exercise. *Eur J Appl Physiol Occup Physiol.* 1994;68(5):441–4.

72. Keteyian SJ, Mellett PA, Fedel FJ, McGowan CM, Stein PD. Electrocardiographic monitoring during cardiac rehabilitation. *Chest.* 1995;107(5):1242–6.

73. Khan MN, Pothier CE, Lauer MS. Chronotropic incompetence as a predictor of death among patients with normal electrograms taking beta blockers (metoprolol or atenolol). *Am J Cardiol.* 2005;96(9):1328–33.

74. Kitzman DW, Brubaker PH, Morgan TM, Stewart KP, Little WC. Exercise training in older patients with heart failure and preserved ejection fraction: a randomized, controlled, single-blind trial. *Circ Heart Fail.* 2010;3(6):659–67.

75. Kleiger RE, Miller JP, Bigger JT,Jr, Moss AJ. Decreased heart rate variability and its association with increased mortality after acute myocardial infarction. *Am J Cardiol.* 1987;59(4):256–62.

76. Kobashigawa JA, Leaf DA, Lee N, et al. A controlled trial of exercise rehabilitation after heart transplantation. *N Engl J Med.* 1999;340(4):272–7.

77. Koenig W. Haemostatic risk factors for cardiovascular diseases. *Eur Heart J.* 1998;19 Suppl C:C39–43.

78. Koenig W, Sund M, Doring A, Ernst E. Leisure-time physical activity but not work-related physical activity is associated with decreased plasma viscosity. Results from a large population sample. *Circulation.* 1997;95(2):335–41.

79. Kraemer WJ, Adams K, Cafarelli E, et al. American College of Sports Medicine position stand. Progression models in resistance training for healthy adults. *Med Sci Sports Exerc.* 2002;34(2): 364–80.

80. Lauer MS, Okin PM, Larson MG, Evans JC, Levy D. Impaired heart rate response to graded exercise. Prognostic implications of chronotropic incompetence in the Framingham Heart Study. *Circulation.* 1996;93(8):1520–6.

81. Lee AJ, Shepard DS. Costs of cardiac rehabilitation and enhanced lifestyle modification programs. *J Cardiopulm Rehabil Prev.* 2009; 29(6):348–57.

82. Ludmer PL, Selwyn AP, Shook TL, et al. Paradoxical vasoconstriction induced by acetylcholine in atherosclerotic coronary arteries. *N Engl J Med.* 1986;315(17):1046–51.

83. Malfatto G, Facchini M, Bragato R, Branzi G, Sala L, Leonetti G. Short and long term effects of exercise training on the tonic autonomic modulation of heart rate variability after myocardial infarction. *Eur Heart J.* 1996;17(4):532–8.

84. Malfatto G, Facchini M, Sala L, Branzi G, Bragato R, Leonetti G. Effects of cardiac rehabilitation and beta-blocker therapy on heart rate variability after first acute myocardial infarction. *Am J Cardiol.* 1998;81(7):834–40.

85. McConnell TR. Exercise prescription when the guidelines do not work. *J Cardiopulm Rehabil.* 1996;16(1):34–7.

86. McCullough PA, Abraham WT. Does quality of life evidence assist in the selection of patients for resynchronization therapy? *Card Electrophysiol Rev.* 2003;7(1):71–6.

87. McKelvie RS, Teo KK, Roberts R, et al. Effects of exercise training in patients with heart failure: the Exercise Rehabilitation Trial (EXERT). *Am Heart J.* 2002;144(1):23–30.

88. McLenachan JM, Weidinger FF, Barry J, et al. Relations between heart rate, ischemia, and drug therapy during daily life in patients with coronary artery disease. *Circulation.* 1991;83(4):1263–70.

89. Meade TW, Ruddock V, Stirling Y, Chakrabarti R, Miller GJ. Fibrinolytic activity, clotting factors, and long-term incidence of ischaemic heart disease in the Northwick Park Heart Study. *Lancet.* 1993;342(8879):1076–9.

90. Meyer K, Schwaibold M, Westbrook S, et al. Effects of short-term exercise training and activity restriction on functional capacity in patients with severe chronic congestive heart failure. *Am J Cardiol.* 1996;78(9):1017–22.

91. Moholdt T, Aamot IL, Granøien I, et al. Aerobic interval training increases peak oxygen uptake more than usual care exercise training in myocardial infarction patients: a randomized controlled study. *Clin Rehabil*. 2012;26(1):33–44.

92. Munk PS, Staal EM, Butt N, Isaksen K, Larsen AI. High-intensity interval training may reduce in-stent restenosis following percutaneous coronary intervention with stent implantation: A randomized controlled trial evaluating the relationship to endothelial function and inflammation. *Am Heart J*. 2009;158(5):734–41.

93. Naffe A, Iype M, Easo M, et al. Appropriateness of sling immobilization to prevent lead displacement after pacemaker/implantable cardioverter-defibrillator implantation. *Proc (Bayl Univ Med Cent)*. 2009;22(1):3–6.

94. Nelson ME, Rejeski WJ, Blair SN, et al. Physical activity and public health in older adults: recommendation from the American College of Sports Medicine and the American Heart Association. *Circulation*. 2007;116(9):1094–105.

95. Nesto RW, Kowalchuk GJ. The ischemic cascade: temporal sequence of hemodynamic, electrocardiographic, and symptomatic expressions of ischemia. *Am J Cardiol*. 1987;59(7):23C–30C.

96. Niebauer J, Hambrecht R, Marburger C, et al. Impact of intensive physical exercise and low-fat diet on collateral vessel formation in stable angina pectoris and angiographically confirmed coronary artery disease. *Am J Cardiol*. 1995;76(11):771–5.

97. Nolan J, Batin PD, Andrews R, et al. Prospective study of heart rate variability and mortality in chronic heart failure: results of the United Kingdom heart failure evaluation and assessment of risk trial (UK-heart). *Circulation*. 1998;98(15):1510–6.

98. Nolan J, Flapan AD, Capewell S, MacDonald TM, Neilson JM, Ewing DJ. Decreased cardiac parasympathetic activity in chronic heart failure and its relation to left ventricular function. *Br Heart J*. 1992;67(6):482–5.

99. O'Connor CM, Whellan DJ, Lee KL, et al. Efficacy and safety of exercise training in patients with chronic heart failure: HF-ACTION randomized controlled trial. *JAMA*. 2009;301(14):1439–50.

100. Ornish D, Brown SE, Scherwitz LW, et al. Can lifestyle changes reverse coronary heart disease? The Lifestyle Heart Trial. *Lancet*. 1990;336(8708):129–33.

101. Parker MW, Thompson PD. Exercise in valvular heart disease: risks and benefits. *Prog Cardiovasc Dis*. 2011;53(6):437–46.

102. Pashkow FJ. Patients with implanted pacemakers or implanted cardioverter defibrillators. In: Wenger NK, Hellerstein HK, editors. *Rehabilitation of the Coronary Patient*. 3rd ed. New York: Churchill Livingstone; 1992. p. 431–438.

103. Pescatello LS, Arena R, Riebe D, American College of Sports Medicine. *ACSM's Guidelines for Exercise Testing and Prescription*. 9th ed. Philadelphia, PA: Lippincott Williams & Wilkins; 2012. 380 p.

104. Pollock ML, Franklin BA, Balady GJ, et al. AHA Science Advisory. Resistance exercise in individuals with and without cardiovascular disease: benefits, rationale, safety, and prescription: an advisory from the Committee on Exercise, Rehabilitation, and Prevention, Council on Clinical Cardiology, American Heart Association; position paper endorsed by the American College of Sports Medicine. *Circulation*. 2000;101(7):828–33.

105. Pope L, Harvey-Berino J, Savage P, et al. The impact of high-calorie-expenditure exercise on quality of life in older adults with coronary heart disease. *J Aging Phys Act*. 2011;19(2):99–116.

106. Quyyumi AA, Panza JA, Diodati JG, Lakatos E, Epstein SE. Circadian variation in ischemic threshold. A mechanism underlying the circadian variation in ischemic events. *Circulation*. 1992;86(1):22–8.

107. Roveda F, Middlekauff HR, Rondon MU, et al. The effects of exercise training on sympathetic neural activation in advanced heart failure: a randomized controlled trial. *J Am Coll Cardiol*. 2003;42(5):854–60.

108. Savage PA, Shaw AO, Miller MS, et al. Effect of resistance training on physical disability in chronic heart failure. *Med Sci Sports Exerc*. 2011;43(8):1379–86.

109. Savage PD, Ades PA. Pedometer step counts predict cardiac risk factors at entry to cardiac rehabilitation. *J Cardiopulm Rehabil Prev*. 2008;28(6):370–7; quiz 378–9.

110. Savage PD, Brochu M, Scott P, Ades PA. Low caloric expenditure in cardiac rehabilitation. *Am Heart J*. 2000;140(3):527–33.

111. Savage PD, Ludlow M, Toth MJ. Exercise and weight loss improves endothelial dependant vasodilatory capacity in overweight individuals with coronary heart disease [abstract]. *J Cardiopulm Rehabil Prev*. 2009;29(4):264.

112. Schairer JR, Keteyian SJ, Ehrman JK, Brawner CA, Berkebile ND. Leisure time physical activity of patients in maintenance cardiac rehabilitation. *J Cardiopulm Rehabil*. 2003;23(4):260–5.

113. Schairer JR, Kostelnik T, Proffitt SM, et al. Caloric expenditure during cardiac rehabilitation. *J Cardiopulm Rehabil*. 1998; 18(4):290–4.

114. Schelkum PH. Exercise after angioplasty: How much? How soon? *Phys Sportsmed*. 1992;20:199–212.

115. Schuler G, Hambrecht R, Schlierf G, et al. Regular physical exercise and low-fat diet. Effects on progression of coronary artery disease. *Circulation*. 1992;86(1):1–11.

116. Sheps DS, Ernst JC, Briese FW, Myerburg RJ. Exercise-induced increase in diastolic pressure: indicator of severe coronary artery disease. *Am J Cardiol*. 1979;43(4):708–12.

117. Slaughter MS, Pagani FD, Rogers JG, et al. Clinical management of continuous-flow left ventricular assist devices in advanced heart failure. *J Heart Lung Transplant*. 2010;29(4 Suppl):S1–39.

118. Smart N, Haluska B, Jeffriess L, Marwick TH. Exercise training in systolic and diastolic dysfunction: effects on cardiac function, functional capacity, and quality of life. *Am Heart J*. 2007;153(4):530–6.

119. Smith SC,Jr, Benjamin EJ, Bonow RO, et al. AHA/ACCF Secondary Prevention and Risk Reduction Therapy for Patients With Coronary and Other Atherosclerotic Vascular Disease: 2011 Update: a guideline from the American Heart Association and American College of Cardiology Foundation. *Circulation*. 2011;124(22):2458–73.

120. Squires RW. Exercise therapy for cardiac transplant recipients. *Prog Cardiovasc Dis*. 2011;53(6):429–36.

121. Squires RW, Leung TC, Cyr NS, et al. Partial normalization of the heart rate response to exercise after cardiac transplantation: frequency and relationship to exercise capacity. *Mayo Clin Proc*. 2002;77(12):1295–300.

122. Suaya JA, Shepard DS, Normand SL, Ades PA, Prottas J, Stason WB. Use of cardiac rehabilitation by Medicare beneficiaries after myocardial infarction or coronary bypass surgery. *Circulation*. 2007;116(15):1653–62.

123. Suaya JA, Stason WB, Ades PA, Normand SL, Shepard DS. Cardiac rehabilitation and survival in older coronary patients. *J Am Coll Cardiol*. 2009;54(1):25–33.

124. Taylor RS, Brown A, Ebrahim S, et al. Exercise-based rehabilitation for patients with coronary heart disease: systematic review and meta-analysis of randomized controlled trials. *Am J Med*. 2004;116(10):682–92.

125. Thaulow E, Erikssen J, Sandvik L, Stormorken H, Cohn PF. Blood platelet count and function are related to total and cardiovascular death in apparently healthy men. *Circulation*. 1991;84(2):613–7.

126. Thompson PD. The benefits and risks of exercise training in patients with chronic coronary artery disease. *JAMA*. 1988;259(10):1537–40.

127. Tiukinhoy S, Beohar N, Hsie M. Improvement in heart rate recovery after cardiac rehabilitation. *J Cardiopulm Rehabil*. 2003;23(2):84–7.

128. U.S. Department of Health and Human Services, Centers for Disease Control and Prevention, National Center for Chronic Disease Prevention and Health Promotion, The President's Council on Physical Fitness and Sports. *Physical Activity and Health: A Report of the Surgeon General*. Atlanta (GA): President's Council on Physical Fitness and Sports; 1996. 278 p.

129. Wasserman K. *Principles of Exercise Testing & Interpretation: Including Pathophysiology and Clinical Applications*. 3rd ed. Philadelphia (PA): Lippincott Williams & Wilkins; 1999. 556 p.

130. Wasserman K, Sun XG, Hansen JE. Effect of biventricular pacing on the exercise pathophysiology of heart failure. *Chest*. 2007;132(1):250–61.

131. Wenger NK, United States. Cardiac Rehabilitation Guideline Panel, United States, Agency for Health Care Policy and Research. *Cardiac Rehabilitation Clinical Practice Guideline: AHCPR Publication no. 96-0672*. Rockville, MD: U.S. Department of Health and Human Services, Public Health Service, Agency for Health Care Policy and Research; 1995. 202 p.

132. Williams MA, Haskell WL, Ades PA, et al. Resistance exercise in individuals with and without cardiovascular disease: 2007 update: a scientific statement from the American Heart Association Council on Clinical Cardiology and Council on Nutrition, Physical Activity, and Metabolism. *Circulation*. 2007;116(5):572–84.

133. Wilson NV, Meyer BM. Early prediction of hypertension using exercise blood pressure. *Prev Med*. 1981;10(1):62–8.

134. Wisloff U, Stoylen A, Loennechen JP, et al. Superior cardiovascular effect of aerobic interval training versus moderate continuous training in heart failure patients: a randomized study. *Circulation*. 2007;115(24):3086–94.

135. Womack CJ, Nagelkirk PR, Coughlin AM. Exercise-induced changes in coagulation and fibrinolysis in healthy populations and patients with cardiovascular disease. *Sports Med*. 2003;33(11):795–807.

136. Worringham C, Rojek A, Stewart I. Development and feasibility of a smartphone, ECG, and GPS based system for remotely monitoring exercise in cardiac rehabilitation. *PLoS One*. 2011;6(2):e14669.

SELECTED REFERENCES FOR FURTHER READING

American Association of Cardiovascular and Pulmonary Rehabilitation. *Guidelines for Cardiac Rehabilitation and Secondary Prevention Programs*. 4th ed. Champaign (IL): Human Kinetics; 2004. 280 p.

American College of Sports Medicine. *ACSM's Exercise Management for Persons with Chronic Diseases and Disabilities*. 3rd ed. Champaign (IL): Human Kinetics; 2009. 456 p.

Brubaker P, Kaminsky LA, Whaley, MH. *Coronary Artery Disease: Essentials of Prevention and Rehabilitation Programs*. Champaign (IL): Human Kinetics; 2002. 376 p.

Ehrman J, Gordon PM, Visich PS, Keteyian SJ. *Clinical Exercise Physiology*. 2nd ed. Champaign (IL): Human Kinetics; 2009.

Graves JE, Franklin BA. *Resistance Training for Health and Rehabilitation*. Champaign (IL): Human Kinetics; 2001.

INTERNET RESOURCES

- AACVPR: American Association of Cardiovascular and Pulmonary Rehabilitation: http://www.aacvpr.org
- American College of Sports Medicine (position stands): http://www.acsm.org/publications/positionStands.htm
- American Heart Association (scientific statements and practice guidelines list): http://www.americanheart.org/presenter.jhtml?identifier ≥2158
- National Clinical Guideline Clearinghouse: http://www.guideline.gov
- National Heart Lung and Blood Institute Clinical Guidelines: http://www.nhlbi.nih.gov/guidelines

Exercise Prescription for Patients with Pulmonary Disease

EPIDEMIOLOGY

Acute and chronic diseases of the upper and lower pulmonary pathways are responsible for significant morbidity and mortality. By definition, pulmonary diseases affect the lungs, including the airways, blood vessels, and parenchyma. The common symptoms of pulmonary disease are shortness of breath, wheezing, cough, expectoration of sputum, and chest pain or discomfort. Given the prevalence of pulmonary diseases, it can be appreciated how frequently these symptoms manifest themselves in the population and how they are highly likely to impact the ability to participate in physical activities. The most common pulmonary diseases in order of importance are chronic obstructive pulmonary disease (COPD; encompassing emphysema and chronic bronchitis), asthma, sleep apnea, and pulmonary vascular disease. Sleep apnea will not be discussed further in this chapter, but one of its symptoms, daytime

hypersomnolence (excessive sleepiness), can affect physical activity with predictable limitations. Other conditions, such as bronchiectasis, cystic fibrosis, pleural effusion, ventilatory muscle weakness, and disorders of ventilatory control, will be discussed briefly where they have distinguishing features that differ from the common diseases.

CHRONIC OBSTRUCTIVE PULMONARY DISEASE

COPD is a major cause of mortality, morbidity, and disability worldwide and within the United States (108). The National Health and Nutritional Examination Survey III (NHANES III) estimated the prevalence of COPD to be 24 million adults (76). COPD is ranked as the fourth leading cause of death worldwide and is projected to rise to the third leading cause by 2015, just behind cardiovascular disease and cancer. The socioeconomic

KEY TERMS

Asthma: A disease of the lung characterized by airflow obstruction that is usually completely reversible and is usually associated with airway hyperreactivity.

Atelectasis: Collapse of part or all of a lung caused by a blockage of an airway (bronchus) or by external pressure on the lung.

Bronchiectasis: A relatively uncommon destructive lung disease characterized by irreversible dilatation of the distal bronchi, impaired clearance of sputum, and chronic infection.

Chronic bronchitis: Chronic inflammation of the conducting airways associated with the inhalation of noxious particles or gases (usually tobacco smoke).

Chronic obstructive pulmonary disease (COPD): Chronic bronchitis and emphysema.

Emphysema: Considered an element of COPD that primarily destroys the connective tissue structure of the lung, resulting in enlargement of distal air spaces.

Interstitial lung disease (ILD): A group of restrictive pulmonary diseases involving pathology primarily confined to the lung parenchyma.

Obstructive pulmonary disease: A category of diseases of the pulmonary system characterized by increased airway resistance, which is a major physiologic limitation.

Pulmonary arterial hypertension (PAH): Elevation of pulmonary arterial pressure usually associated with pulmonary vascular disease.

Pulmonary vascular disease: A category of lung diseases that affect the pulmonary vasculature by destruction or remodeling.

Restrictive pulmonary disease: A category of lung diseases in which the underlying pathologic process involved with each disease interferes with ability for normal lung expansion.

Ventilatory control: Mechanism that adjusts pulmonary ventilation to match metabolic requirements or to control acid-base state.

implications are enormous. According to the Centers for Disease Control and Prevention, COPD is responsible for 8 million outpatient medical visits and 1.5 million emergency department visits per year. It is estimated that COPD is responsible for 1.9% or 726,000 of all hospitalizations and is a major contributing illness for 25 million additional hospitalizations (76). An estimated $50 billion was spent on this disorder in 2010, with $30 billion linked to direct costs such as medication, hospitalizations, and oxygen therapy. In addition, approximately $10 billion has been linked to indirect medical costs, such as lost work productivity and disability (58). COPD accounts for approximately 120,000 deaths per year in the United States, and consistently since 2000, more women than men have died from this disease (56).

ASTHMA

Asthma is a common disease and is estimated to affect approximately 16 million Americans, one-third of whom are children, making it the most common chronic childhood disease (51). Asthma has attracted public attention because it affects children and young adults. This disease claims more than 4,000 lives per year in the United States. Many of the deaths because of acute severe asthma occur in the young and may have been preventable (35). Asthma is characterized by chronic airway inflammation and reversible airflow obstruction, at least in its earlier stages (44). Asthma is linked to 100 million days missed from work or school and 470,000 hospitalizations annually in the United States (35). The monetary costs are substantial (146) and reflect both direct medical costs (hospital admissions and cost of medications) and indirect nonmedical costs (time lost from work, premature death) (130).

INTERSTITIAL LUNG DISEASE

Interstitial lung disease (ILD) encompasses several distinct disease entities, each of which tends to result in pulmonary fibrosis or scarring of the lung parenchyma. The most significant of these diseases is called *idiopathic* (unknown etiology) *pulmonary fibrosis* (IPF). Conditions that are associated with pulmonary fibrosis include connective tissue disease, such as rheumatoid arthritis and systemic lupus erythematosus; pneumoconioses, such as coal workers lung and asbestosis; and extrinsic allergic alveolitis in response to inhaled organic materials like fungi. Although much less common than the obstructive diseases (COPD and asthma), pulmonary fibrosis can result in markedly deranged physiology and severely reduced exercise performance.

PULMONARY VASCULAR DISEASE

In recent years, pulmonary vascular diseases have been gaining attention. Although less common, like ILDs, they might affect exercise performance and require special precautions in exercise testing and prescription. As pulmonary vascular disease progresses, vascular remodeling tends to increase pulmonary vascular resistance, resulting in pulmonary hypertension. The World Health Organization categorizes pulmonary hypertension into (a) pulmonary arterial hypertension (PAH), (b) pulmonary venous hypertension, (c) pulmonary hypertension associated with pulmonary diseases including chronic hypoxemia, (d) pulmonary hypertension as a result of thromboembolic disease, and (e) miscellaneous disorders directly affecting the pulmonary vasculature (121). There are several causes associated with PAH; the most devastating of which is called *primary pulmonary hypertension* (PPH). Secondary causes include connective tissue diseases, such as progressive systemic sclerosis (scleroderma), human immunodeficiency virus (HIV), and exposure to anorexigenic (appetite suppressant) drugs. The estimated incidence of PPH is one to two cases per million persons in the general population, and it is more common in women than men (1.7 women per man) (112). Secondary causes of pulmonary hypertension may be relatively common but underdiagnosed. Reliable estimates of the prevalence of this condition are difficult to obtain because of the diversity of identifiable causes.

PATHOPHYSIOLOGY

A basic understanding of the pathophysiology of the different pulmonary diseases, particularly in the context of exercise performance, improves the efficacy and success of exercise programs for these patients. The design of the exercise program can be enhanced by recognizing disease features that can be used to individualize the program and optimize the individual exercise response. Acquiring this knowledge base can be a complicated task, particularly if the diseases are approached in an individual manner. This task can be simplified by grouping diseases based on physiologic similarities. Four groups of diseases can be defined and named for their primary limitation: obstructive pulmonary disease, restrictive pulmonary disease, pulmonary vascular disease, and disturbances in ventilatory control. The physiologic pattern associated with each category can be generally applied to all the diseases within the respective category.

CHRONIC OBSTRUCTIVE PULMONARY DISEASE

COPD is a preventable and treatable disease in which the characteristic abnormality is chronic airway inflammation in response to exposure to noxious particles and gases (11,108). The most common etiology by far is tobacco smoking, which includes exposure to environmental tobacco smoke (passive smoking). Occupational or environmental exposures are now thought to be responsible for about 20% of the cases of COPD. The term COPD

TABLE 39-1. Global Initiative for Chronic Obstructive Lung Disease: Guidelines for Chronic Obstructive Pulmonary Disease Staging

Severity	Stage	$FEV_{1.0}{}^{a}$	Symptoms[b]
Mild	I	>80%	Intermittent symptoms
Moderate	II	50%–80%	Persistent symptoms
Severe	III	30%–50%	Exacerbations
Very severe	IV	<30% or <50% with chronic respiratory failure	Respiratory failure

[a]$FEV_{1.0}$ values are based on postbronchodilator measurements.

[b]Symptom categories are useful in clinical management but might not correlate with $FEV_{1.0}$.

$FEV_{1.0}$, forced expiratory volume in 1 s.

Adapted from Cooper CB, Tashkin DP. Recent developments in inhaled therapy in stable chronic obstructive pulmonary disease. *BMJ.* 2005;330(7492):640–4; (50) Global Initiative for Chronic Obstructive Lung Disease Web site [Internet]. Global Initiative for Chronic Obstructive Lung Disease; [cited 2011 Mar 15]. Available from: http://www.goldcopd.com/.

encompasses chronic bronchitis and emphysema. Disease severity is staged according to guidelines set by the Global Initiative for Chronic Obstructive Lung Disease (GOLD) (108) (*Table 39-1*). Chronic bronchitis is defined by its histopathology, which is predominantly neutrophilic airway inflammation, but the clinical syndrome is still defined by symptoms such as sputum production on most days of the week for more than 3 mo for at least two consecutive years (37). By contrast, the primary abnormality in emphysema involves destruction of alveolar septae and enlargement of the air spaces distal to the terminal bronchioles (60). COPD is recognized as an inflammatory disease of the airways with increased numbers of alveolar macrophages, neutrophils, and cytotoxic T lymphocytes, accompanied by release of multiple inflammatory mediators (*e.g.*, oxygen free radicals, chemokines, cytokines, and growth factors) (11). An imbalance between neutrophil-derived proteases (*e.g.*, neutrophil elastase and matrix metalloproteinases) and antiprotease defense mechanisms are characteristic of emphysema (11). One example of the genetic predisposition to developing emphysema is α-1 protease inhibitor deficiency, an inherited condition that accounts for 1%–2% of cases of emphysema (55). From a practical standpoint, it is usually difficult to separate chronic bronchitis from emphysema, and most individuals manifest a combination of both conditions.

The chronic inflammation common to COPD leads to progressive narrowing of small airways in the lung, thus increasing airway resistance. The destruction of lung connective tissue and loss of alveolar attachments in emphysema reduces lung elastic recoil. Both mechanisms hinder exhalation and tend to cause air trapping in regions of the lung with increased time constants for lung emptying. This process results in static hyperinflation that can be measured at rest. However, of particular importance during exercise as a result of increased ventilation rate and increased ventilation ($\dot{V}_E$) is dynamic hyperinflation. With dynamic hyperinflation, lung volumes increase even further.

Hyperinflation is central to understanding the pathophysiology of lung mechanics in COPD (*Fig. 39-1*) (29). Of all the spirometric measures in obstructive pulmonary disease, inspiratory capacity, a measure of hyperinflation, correlates best with patient-reported outcomes such as dyspnea, exercise capacity, and quality of life (QOL) (95,96). At higher operational lung volumes, the increased elastic and threshold work of breathing

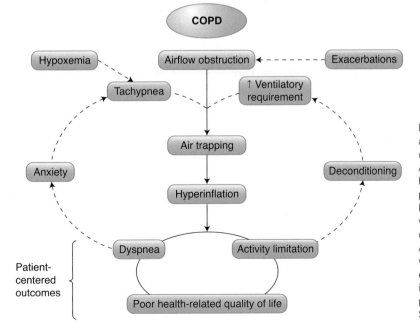

FIGURE 39-1. Central role of air trapping and hyperinflation in the pathophysiology of chronic obstructive pulmonary disease (COPD). Although related to increased airway resistance, hyperinflation correlates more directly with patient-centered outcomes. Activity limitation leads to deconditioning, which in turn, increases ventilatory requirements establishing a cycle of decline leading to worsening hyperinflation. Anxiety and hypoxemia cause tachypnea, which worsens hyperinflation by allowing less time for exhalation. (Adapted from Cooper CB. Exercise in chronic pulmonary disease: aerobic exercise prescription. *Med Sci Sports Exerc.* 2001;33[7 Suppl]:S671–9.)

contributes to dyspnea. Also, the configuration of the diaphragm tends to be low and flat, which diminishes its mechanical efficiency during inhalation. Factors that increase ventilatory work also affect energy expenditure and oxygen requirement. When ventilatory muscle work exceeds oxygen supply, ventilatory muscle fatigue and exercise termination can result (29). The negative effects of dynamic hyperinflation during exercise include increased elasticity; increased threshold work of breathing, which contributes to dyspnea and early exercise termination; and the potential for reduced venous return and cardiac output as a result of the increased intrathoracic pressure (96).

Celli et al. (25) proposed the use of a multidimensional index, the BODE index, to more accurately rate the severity of COPD and predict the risk of death attributable to pulmonary and nonpulmonary causes. The BODE index is a 10-point scale that assigns points based on the results of four measures: body mass index (B), airflow obstruction (O), dyspnea (D), and exercise capacity (E). Airflow obstruction is measured by the forced expiratory volume in 1 s ($FEV_{1.0}$) (85,103); dyspnea with the Medical Research Council (MRC) dyspnea scale (16); and exercise capacity, measured by the best of two trials on the 6-min walking test (7) (*Table 39-2*).

Optimizing pulmonary system mechanics before implementing an exercise program is essential for patients with COPD. Many patients with COPD demonstrate a degree of reversibility with bronchodilator therapy, particularly when assessed in terms of inspiratory capacity and hyperinflation. The GOLD guidelines have outlined the list of pharmacologic interventions advocated for COPD but do not provide a clear selection sequence for these agents. A review of inhaled therapies in COPD proposed a simple three-step approach for mild, moderate, and severe disease (46,101). A combination of an inhaled short-acting anticholinergic agent (*e.g.*, ipratropium) plus a short-acting β-agonist agent (SABA) (*e.g.*, albuterol) is beneficial before exercise and useful to relieve dyspnea (65). Long-acting bronchodilator

therapies are recommended for maintenance therapy of COPD in patients with persistent symptoms. These include the long-acting muscarinic antagonist (LAMA) (*e.g.*, tiotropium) and the long-acting β-adrenoreceptor agonists (LABA) (*e.g.*, salmeterol, formoterol, and indacaterol). These long-acting drugs are recommended because of their sustained bronchodilator efficacy and convenience (*e.g.*, tiotropium is a once-daily medication). Evidence suggests that inhaled corticosteroids should be prescribed for patients with severe COPD ($FEV_{1.0}$ <50% of predicted) to reduce the frequency of acute exacerbations. They are most efficacious in those patients who have frequent exacerbations (*e.g.*, two or more per year) (31,122). Prophylactic use of oral medications, such as the antibiotic azithromycin and the selective phosphodiesterase inhibitor roflumilast, has also been shown to reduced exacerbations in patients with severe COPD.

After lung mechanics are optimized by bronchodilator therapy, the need for oxygen supplementation should be assessed. The underlying mechanism for hypoxia in COPD involves regional mismatching between ventilation and perfusion (23). Within regions of the lung where emphysema is the dominant pathology, the capillary bed is destroyed. Ventilation to these areas, dead-space ventilation, is wasted and does not contribute to gas exchange. Regions of the lungs where chronic bronchitis is dominant have impaired ventilation because of airway narrowing while perfusion is relatively preserved. This results in lung units with low ventilation/perfusion (V/Q) ratios and poor oxygenation of pulmonary capillary blood. Venous admixture of deoxygenated blood with oxygenated blood from other regions of the lung results in a net reduction in the oxygen content of systemic arterial blood. Thus, dead-space ventilation and venous admixture can be viewed as opposite ends of the spectrum of gas exchange abnormality or V/Q mismatching, with low V/Q ratios resulting in hypoxemia.

Increased dead-space ventilation affects exercise performance by increasing the ventilatory requirement at a given metabolic rate. In circumstances in which ventilatory capacity is limited, dead-space ventilation can result in ventilatory limitation and directly contribute to exercise limitations. Venous admixture lowers arterial oxyhemoglobin saturation and can result in desaturation during exercise, particularly when blood flows through V/Q mismatch areas increases with increased cardiac output. Desaturation, or failure of adequate gas exchange, is a serious cause of exercise limitation but can be overcome to some extent by providing supplemental oxygen.

ASTHMA

The relationship between COPD and asthma has undergone much debate throughout the years (11,38,117). The classic definition for asthma is airflow obstruction

TABLE 39-2. BODE Index

Points on BODE Index

Variable	0	1	2	3
$FEV_{1.0}$ (% predicted)	≥56	50–64	36–49	≤35
Distance walked in 6 min (m)	≥350	250–349	150–249	≤149
MMRC dyspnea scale	0–1	2	3	4
BMI	>21	≤21		

BODE, body mass index (B), airflow obstruction (O), dyspnea (D), and exercise capacity (E); $FEV_{1.0}$, forced expiratory volume in 1 s; MMRC, Modified Medical Research Council; BMI, body mass index.

Adapted from Celli BR, Cote CG, Marin JM, et al. The body-mass index, airflow obstruction, dyspnea, and exercise capacity index in chronic obstructive pulmonary disease. *N Engl J Med.* 2004;350(10):1005–12.

that is completely reversible and usually associated with airway hyperreactivity (38). One perspective considers chronic bronchitis, emphysema, and asthma as distinct diseases, sometimes with overlapping features (1). An alternative perspective, the so-called Dutch hypothesis (38,106,117), claims that asthma, chronic bronchitis, and emphysema are components of a single disease. The reality of varying degrees of disease overlap adds to the difficulty in differentiating these diseases clinically. The general consensus is that COPD refers to chronic bronchitis and emphysema alone. It is erroneous, however, to differentiate asthma as being reversible or responsive to bronchodilator therapy and COPD as being irreversible. The reality is that COPD is, by definition, partially reversible, and often the bronchodilator response is impressive, particularly after combined classes of bronchodilators (65). Asthma, on the other hand, becomes less responsive to bronchodilator therapy with poor control and over time (66,131).

The pathology of asthma consists of chronic airway inflammation, smooth muscle hyperplasia and hypertrophy, mucous hypersecretion, distal airway mucus plugging, and atelectasis. The disruption of V/Q matching in the lungs also causes hypoxemia (128).

Triggers that induce the inflammatory cascade are important to recognize and avoid if possible (44,128). Triggers can include inhaled allergens and irritants, even cold air. Common aeroallergen triggers are dust mites, animal dander, pollen, and mold spores. Inhaled irritants include smoke, fumes, and airborne particulates. Occupational or nonallergenic triggers include invisible particulate matter (*e.g.*, particulate matter <10 μm [PM-10], fumes, diesel exhaust) and gases (oxides of nitrogen, oxides of sulphur, and ozone). Some individuals exhibit aspirin sensitivity, often in association with nasal polyps. The effect of these triggers is dose dependent and often immediate. However, symptoms that occur after allergen exposure can sometimes manifest a delayed onset that occurs 6–8 h after exposure. Seasonal variations are not uncommon. In sensitive individuals, cool air and humidity can also serve as triggers because of the effect on airway tone. Some patients have exercise-induced asthma (EIA) in which the stimulus to bronchoconstriction is thought to be pulmonary heat exchange at higher levels of ventilation. Trigger avoidance, suppression of inflammation, and prophylaxis (*i.e.*, before exercise) are essential elements in asthma management (44).

Asthma is a clinical diagnosis, although bronchial provocation studies are used by some to confirm or refute the diagnosis (44,128). The traditional test for EIA recommends an exercise stimulus of >80% of maximum heart rate for 6 min. A maximal cardiopulmonary exercise test can be also used as a provocation study to identify EIA in some cases (30,32). A 10% fall in $FEV_{1.0}$ after the exercise test is considered abnormal; a fall of 15% appears to be more diagnostic of exercise-induced bronchoconstriction (EIB) (32). This usually occurs about 10 min after exercise, with recovery by 30 min after the exercise stimulus.

Asthma severity can be divided into four levels: mild intermittent, mild persistent, moderate persistent, and severe persistent (45,51). See *Box 39-1* for classifications

---

BOX 39-1   Classification of Asthma Severity by Clinical Features before Treatment

INTERMITTENT

Symptoms less than once a week
Brief exacerbations
Nocturnal symptoms not more than twice a month
- FEV_1 or PEF ≥80% predicted
- PEF variability <20%

MILD PERSISTENT

Symptoms more than once a week but less than once a day
Exacerbations may affect activity and sleep
Nocturnal symptoms more than twice a month
- FEV_1 or PEF ≥80% predicted
- PEF variability 20–30%

MODERATE PERSISTENT

Symptoms daily
Exacerbations may affect activity and sleep

Nocturnal symptoms more than once a week
Daily use of inhaled short-acting β_2-agonist
- FEV_1 or PEF 60%–80% predicted
- PEF variability >30%

SEVERE PERSISTENT

Symptoms daily
Frequent exacerbations
Frequent nocturnal asthma symptoms
Limitation of physical activities
- FEV_1 or PEF ≤60% predicted
- PEF variability >30%

....

FEV_1, forced expiratory volume in 1 second; PEF, peak expiratory flow.

From the *Global Strategy for Asthma Management and Prevention, 2011*, used with permission from the Global Initiative for Asthma (GINA), www.ginasthma.org

TABLE 39-3. Levels of Asthma Control

Characteristic	Controlled (all of the following)	Partly Controlled (any measure present in any week)	Uncontrolled
Daytime symptoms	None ($\leq$2 times/wk)	>2 times/wk	Three or more features of partly controlled asthma present in any week
Limitations of activities	None	Any	
Nocturnal symptoms/awakening	None	Any	
Need for reliever/rescue treatment	None (twice or less/week)	>2 times/wk	
Lung function (PEF or $FEV_{1.0}$)[a]	Normal	<80% predicted or personal best (if known)	
Exacerbations	None	$\geq$1 time/yr[b]	One in any week[c]

PEF, peak expiratory flow; $FEV_{1.0}$, forced expiratory volume in 1 s.

[a]Lung function is not a reliable test for children 5 yr and younger.

[b]Any exacerbation should prompt review of maintenance treatment to ensure that it is adequate.

[c]By definition, an exacerbation in any week makes that an uncontrolled asthma week.

Adapted from Global Initiative for Chronic Obstructive Lung Disease Web site [Internet]. Global Initiative for Chronic Obstructive Lung Disease; [cited 2011 Mar 15]. Available from: http://www.goldcopd.com/.

of asthma severity (51). The frequency and severity of both basal symptoms and exacerbations determine the level of severity. The most recent guidelines, however, emphasize the importance of including the level of asthma control in the evaluation of disease severity (*Table 39-3*). Each severity level corresponds to a specific step approach, which defines general treatment options.

SABA bronchodilators, such as albuterol, have an effectiveness lasting 4–6 h. They are the drugs of choice for rapid relief of symptoms related to acute bronchoconstriction (10,44,91). LABA bronchodilators, such as salmeterol and formoterol, result in improvement of airflow for up to 12 h (10,44,91). Because of their delayed onset of action, LABA inhalers are not recommended for "rescue" relief of bronchoconstriction. Side effects of β-agonists — such as tachycardia, palpitations, dysrhythmias, and tremor — require consideration in the context of exercise and could potentially compromise the exercise response (10,44,91).

In summary, successful asthma management requires trigger awareness, environmental controls, peak flow monitoring, and pharmacotherapy based on illness severity. Important considerations in the management of EIA include recognition of symptoms and pretreatment with bronchodilator therapy. Management of EIA is much more easily accomplished when chronic bronchial inflammation is kept under control.

BRONCHIECTASIS

Bronchiectasis is an inflammatory condition characterized by irreversible damage and dilatation of the bronchi (113,120). Regions of bronchiectasis in the lung commonly become chronically infected. Acute exacerbations of this disease influence the amount, color, and consistency of mucus produced. Mucociliary clearance is impaired in bronchiectasis, with retained secretions imposing a significant clinical problem.

Cystic fibrosis (CF) is an important cause of bronchiectasis in the United States and Europe, and this disorder has a genetic basis. The age at onset for CF is characteristically childhood, but genetic testing has enabled the identification of adult onset. Recurrent and chronic lung infection with resistant bacterial pathogens, particularly gram-negative organisms such as Pseudomonas species and nontuberculous Mycobacteria, is common in CF.

Airflow obstruction occurs in up to 50% of individuals with bronchiectasis (86). In some patients, the airflow obstruction is associated with bronchial hyperresponsiveness, as demonstrated by bronchial provocation with methacholine. This observation may represent coexisting asthma (9). Administration of an inhaled bronchodilator should be considered but should be determined on an individual basis. One study (86) demonstrated improved airflow after inhalation of the short-acting muscarinic antagonist (SAMA) ipratropium bromide, suggesting that bronchoconstriction in bronchiectasis is mediated by reflex vagal mechanism related to airway irritation (66,131).

Bronchopulmonary hygiene is fundamental to the management of bronchiectasis (113,120). The treatment involves a combination of adequate hydration to reduce mucous tenacity and chest physiotherapy implemented either manually or with the aid of mechanical devices (18,113,120). Theoretically, exercise performance could be improved in patients with bronchiectasis by implementing bronchopulmonary hygiene and clearing mucous plugging, thereby improving gas exchange.

INTERSTITIAL LUNG DISEASE

ILD implies that the primary site of pathophysiologic abnormality is the lung parenchyma (86). Multiple classifications are proposed for ILDs. The classification scheme used in this chapter includes infiltrating (edema, amyloid, or tumor), inflammatory (idiopathic interstitial pneumonias and acute respiratory distress syndrome), and infectious processes. As a result of inflammation of fibrosis of the interstitial space, the lungs become stiff and noncompliant, causing restrictive physiology and diffusion impairment. Reduced compliance limits the increase in tidal volume during exercise and results in a disproportionate rise in the breathing frequency. Ventilation rates will often exceed 50 breaths per minute at maximum exercise, and the breathing pattern is rapid and shallow. As with obstructive disease, when the ventilatory requirement of exercise reaches the limited ventilatory capacity, there will be exercise impairment. Some ILDs are classically characterized by a combination of both restriction and obstruction (86). The diseases typically associated with both processes include sarcoidosis, hypersensitivity pneumonitis, pulmonary (Langerhans) histiocytosis, and lymphangiomyomatosis (86). Different natural histories are encountered for each ILD, and fluctuations in disease severity are likely to influence the exercise potential.

Compared with COPD, there has been relatively little investigation of the exercise physiology of ILDs (57,78–80). Some experts have argued for the usefulness of exercise testing in the evaluation of select restrictive pulmonary diseases (82). Abnormalities of gas exchange are particularly evident with ILDs. Loss of pulmonary capillary bed and V/Q mismatching cause increased dead-space ventilation and exercise-induced hypoxemia (57,78–80,82). The diffusing capacity is usually low, with restrictive disease reflecting impaired gas diffusion through the alveolar-capillary membrane (86). This abnormality might not translate into clinically significant hypoxemia at rest because there is adequate pulmonary capillary transit time to allow complete diffusion equilibrium of the oxygen molecules. However, during exercise, the reduced pulmonary capillary transit time in conjunction with slowed diffusion can result in significant hypoxemia (57,78,79,81,83).

OTHER RESTRICTIVE PULMONARY DISEASES

Whereas ILDs can be viewed as causing restriction by reducing lung compliance, there are other extrapulmonary diseases that cause restriction (86). The most important to consider are pleural effusion, chest wall deformity, and ventilatory muscle weakness. There are many causes of pleural effusions, including pneumonia, heart failure, renal disease, liver disease, and malignancy. Chest wall deformities can be related to kyphoscoliosis

or they may accompany chronic neuromuscular diseases, such as muscular dystrophy, myopathy, or postpolio syndrome. The same neuromuscular diseases, plus others such as acute postinfectious polyneuropathy (Guillain-Barre syndrome) and myasthenia gravis, can cause ventilatory muscle weakness.

The extrapulmonary causes of restriction have common pathophysiologic features that pertain to exercise. Both reduced chest wall compliance and ventilatory muscle weakness compromise ventilatory capacity by limiting the ability to increase in tidal volume. As a result, increases in ($\dot{V}_E$) tend to rely more on increased breathing frequency. During maximal incremental exercise, it is not unusual to see a breathing frequency >50 breaths per minute in this type of patient. In those circumstances in which the ventilatory requirement for exercise approaches or equals the reduced ventilatory capacity, ventilatory limitation will be the cause of exercise limitation.

PULMONARY VASCULAR DISEASES

Under normal conditions, the pulmonary vascular system is a low-pressure circuit with a low vascular resistance (86). Vascular resistance can be altered by disease. The mechanism depends on whether the vessel is a primary disease target. *Box 39-2* shows the World Health Organization disease classifications based on the cause of pulmonary hypertension. The distinction of etiology has both prognostic and therapeutic value. PPH exemplifies the vessel wall as the primary disease target (86). This disease is rare and mostly sporadic in occurrence, with only 10% of the cases demonstrating genetic linkage (86). Risk factors predisposing to PPH include connective tissue diseases, chronic liver disease, HIV infection, cocaine or amphetamine use, and

---

BOX 39-2 | **World Health Organization Disease Classification of the Cause of Pulmonary Hypertension**

1. Pulmonary arterial hypertension
2. Pulmonary venous hypertension
3. Pulmonary hypertension associated with pulmonary disease or chronic hypoxemia
4. Pulmonary hypertension because of chronic thromboembolic disease
5. Pulmonary hypertension because of disorders directly affecting pulmonary vasculature

Adapted from Simonneau G, Galie N, Rubin LJ, et al. Clinical classification of pulmonary hypertension. *J Am Coll Cardiol.* 2004;43(12 Suppl S):5S–12S.

World Health Organization Classification of the Severity of Illness for Pulmonary Hypertension

Class I   Asymptomatic, no physical limitations

Class II   Mild limitation of physical activity; comfortable at rest; breathless on exertion

Class III   Marked limitation of physical activity; comfortable at rest; unduly breathless on exertion

Class IV   Unable to perform any physical activity; symptomatic at rest; right heart failure

Adapted from Simonneau G, Galie N, Rubin LJ, et al. Clinical classification of pulmonary hypertension. *J Am Coll Cardiol.* 2004;43(12 Suppl S):5S–12S.

anorexigenic agents, such as fenfluramine and tryptophan. Diagnosis of PPH is complex, and readers are referred to McGoon et al. (83) for a detailed overview. The determination of disease severity of pulmonary hypertension follows the criteria used by the American Heart Association outlined for congestive heart failure (*i.e.*, New York Heart Association classification) (*Box 39-3*) (64).

Secondary pulmonary hypertension demonstrates an indirect effect of disease on pulmonary vascular resistance. Diseases that can lead to the development of secondary pulmonary hypertension include pulmonary fibrosis, COPD, and left-sided heart disease (86). Prognostic and therapeutic implications underscore the importance of making the distinction between primary and secondary pulmonary hypertension (64,86).

EXERCISE RESPONSES IN PULMONARY DISEASE

Exercise intolerance is the hallmark of chronic lung disease. Foremost among the symptoms that limit exercise is dyspnea and/or fatigue because of some combination of the pathologic changes in lung function noted earlier. These may be exacerbated by physical deconditioning, anxiety secondary to exertional shortness of breath, and declining motivation. As shown in *Figure 39-2* (28), there is a vicious cycle whereby dyspnea leads to further exercise intolerance, deconditioning, and increased ventilatory requirements at a given workload. Exercise capacity is reduced in patients with chronic lung diseases because of ventilatory and gas exchange limitations, cardiac and respiratory muscle dysfunction, and skeletal muscle disuse and/or dysfunction. Specific limitations to exercise in chronic pulmonary disease and their influence on exercise prescription are shown in *Table 39-4*.

ACUTE RESPONSES TO EXERCISE

The acute responses to exercise resulting from those factors that limit exercise tolerance because of the specific limitations imposed by chronic lung diseases are listed in *Box 39-4*. The goals surrounding the exercise component of pulmonary rehabilitation are to alleviate these functional limitations (*Box 39-5*).

CHRONIC EXERCISE RESPONSES: EVIDENCE-BASED OUTCOMES

The chronic responses to exercise training in patients with lung disease are dependent on several factors, including disease severity, initial level of fitness, supplemental oxygen, and optimal management of bronchodilator therapy in patients with airflow limitation

FIGURE 39-2. Diagram to illustrate the vicious cycle (on left) of disabling breathlessness, physical inactivity, and deconditioning in chronic pulmonary disease. Pulmonary rehabilitation that includes exercise training offers a favorable cycle (on right) of reconditioning, restoration of functional capacity, and improved quality of life. (Adapted from Cooper CB. The connection between chronic obstructive pulmonary disease symptoms and hyperinflation and its impact on exercise and function. *Am J Med.* 2006;119[10 Suppl 1]:21–31.)

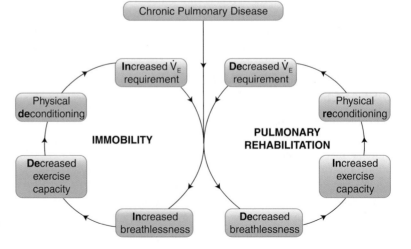

TABLE 39-4. Specific Limitations to Exercise in Chronic Pulmonary Disease and How They Influence Exercise Prescription

Specific Exercise Limitation	Thresholds Influencing Intensity Prescription	Goals and Targets for Exercise Prescription
Physical deconditioning (*i.e.*, premature lactic acidosis)	Metabolic (lactate) threshold	Reconditioning exercise Exercise intensity should be above metabolic threshold
Ventilatory limitation (*e.g.*, $\dot{V}E_{max}$, MVV)	Dyspnea Metabolic (lactate) threshold Hypoventilation Hypoxemia (desaturation)	Increase ventilatory capacity Improve ventilatory system mechanics Mitigate lactic acidosis through reconditioning Reduce ventilatory requirement Increase respiratory muscle strength Offer ventilatory assistance Improve breathing efficiency (reduce VD/VT) Prevent desaturation with supplemental oxygen
Ventilatory inefficiency (*e.g.*, dynamic hyperinflation in COPD or high VD/VT)	Bronchoconstriction or airway collapse Tachypnea Hypoventilation	Relieve expiratory airflow obstruction Optimize bronchodilator therapy Reduce respiratory rate Teach breathing techniques Teach panic control
Gas exchange failure (*i.e.*, hypoxemia or hypercapnia)	Desaturation Respiratory acidosis	Prevent hypoxemia and hypoventilation Use supplemental oxygen Offer assisted ventilation
Cardiovascular limitations (*e.g.*, myocardial ischemia, hypertension, pulmonary vascular disease)	Angina Hypertension Dysrhythmia	Symptom monitoring and management Monitor BP during exercise, as indicated Monitor ECG during exercise, as indicated Adjust intensity, as indicated
Symptomatic limitations	Dyspnea Anxiety Fear	Psychotherapy Desensitization Mastery Panic control

$\dot{V}E_{max}$, maximum ventilation per unit of time; MVV, maximum voluntary ventilation; VD/VT, dead-space to tidal volume ratio; COPD, chronic obstructive pulmonary disease; ECG, electrocardiogram; BP, blood pressure.

Adapted from Cooper CB. Exercise in chronic pulmonary disease: aerobic exercise prescription. *Med Sci Sports Exerc.* 2001;33(7 Suppl):S671–9.

(110). A patient's ability to tolerate endurance exercise at intensities above the lactate threshold may also influence the extent to which endurance performance is improved (21). Typical adaptations to exercise training are shown in *Box 39-6*. Supporting evidence for these adaptations will be noted throughout this chapter. Evidence is based on the American College of Chest Physicians (ACCP)/American Association of Cardiovascular and Pulmonary Rehabilitation (AACVPR) report on evidence-based clinical practice guidelines for pulmonary rehabilitation, which includes a grading of the strength of evidence and balance of benefits to risks/burdens (110). *Table 39-5* contains a key for the ACCP grading of these benefits. Also included are recently published, evidenced-based clinical practice guidelines for physiotherapists (69) and systematic reviews of progressive resistance exercise training for improving strength and activities of daily living in patients with COPD (99); effects of resistance training for improving pulmonary function in patients with COPD (127); and of great recent interest, a systematic review of interval versus continuous endurance exercise training in patients with COPD (13).

THE EXERCISE PRESCRIPTION

The joint ACCP/AACVPR evidence-based clinical practice guidelines for pulmonary rehabilitation (110) provide strong recommendations for exercise training as a mandatory component of pulmonary rehabilitation. In addition, the 2006 American Thoracic Society (ATS)/European Respiratory Society (ERS) statement on pulmonary rehabilitation (93) has provided the scientific evidence for the physiologic effects of chronic lung disease and the role of pulmonary rehabilitation in affecting change in the ensuing functional limitations.

Exercise training improves exercise tolerance and may also improve motivation to exercise as well as psychological and cognitive outcomes (54,102,136). The exercise training component of pulmonary rehabilitation programs should be comprehensive, providing cardiorespiratory exercise, muscle strengthening, and joint range-of-motion exercise. The addition of inspiratory

BOX 39-4	Acute Responses to Exercise in Chronic Lung Diseases

OBSTRUCTIVE DISEASES

Reduced $\dot{V}O_{2max}$

Early-onset lactic acidosis and reduced metabolic (lactate) threshold

Reduced muscular strength

Reduced ventilatory reserve

Increased VD/VT

Increased ventilatory equivalents for O_2 ($\dot{V}E/\dot{V}O_2$) and CO_2 ($\dot{V}E/\dot{V}CO_2$)

Increased difference between arterial and end-tidal partial pressures for CO_2 ($PaCO_2 - P_{ET}CO_2$)

Increased difference between alveolar and end-tidal partial pressures for O_2 ($PAO_2 - PaO_2$)

No increase in ventilatory equivalent for CO_2 at maximum exercise

Respiratory acidosis

Hypoxemia depending on the presence of low V_A/Q lung units

Low peak heart rate and low percent of predicted maximum heart rate achieved

Low O_2 pulse

RESTRICTIVE DISEASES

Reduced $\dot{V}O_{2max}$

Reduced metabolic (lactate) threshold

Reduced $\Delta \dot{V}O_2/\Delta WR$ slope

Increased VD/VT

Increased ventilatory equivalents for O_2 ($\dot{V}E/\dot{V}O_2$) and CO_2 ($\dot{V}E/\dot{V}CO_2$)

Increased difference between arterial and end-tidal partial pressures for CO_2 ($PaCO_2 - P_{ET}CO_2$)

No increase in ventilatory equivalent for CO_2 at maximum exercise

Respiratory acidosis

Hypoxemia that is usually progressive

Ratio of tidal volume to inspiratory capacity (VT/IC) that ≈ 1 at low levels of work

Muscular weakness

VO_{2max}, maximal volume of oxygen consumed per unit of time; VD/VT, dead space to tidal volume ratio; O_2, oxygen; VE, volume of expired air per unit time; VO_2, volume of oxygen consumed per unit time; CO_2, carbon dioxide; VCO_2, volume of carbon dioxide produced per unit time ; $PaCO_2$ partial pressure of arterial CO_2; $P_{ET}CO_2$, partial pressure of end tidal CO_2; V_A/Q, alveolar ventilation to perfusion ratio; $\Delta VO_2/\Delta WR$, ratio of change in oxygen uptake to change in work rate.

Adapted from (141) Wasserman K. Exercise tolerance in the pulmonary patient. In: Casaburi R, Petty TL, editors. *Principles and Practice of Pulmonary Rehabilitation*. Philadelphia: Saunders; 1993. p. 119–121.

BOX 39-5	**Goals of Pulmonary Rehabilitation**

Improve exercise performance and activities of daily living

Alleviate dyspnea

Restore a positive outlook

Reduce the work of breathing

Normalize arterial blood gases

Increase mechanical efficiency

Improve nutrition

Improve emotional state

Decrease health-related costs

Lengthen survival

Adapted from (24) Celli BR. Pulmonary rehabilitation for COPD. A practical approach for improving ventilatory conditioning. *Postgrad Med.* 1998;103(4): 159–60, 167–8, 173–6.

muscle training may be of value for some patients, particularly those with low inspiratory muscle strength (107,110).

Most research studying the effects of exercise training in chronic lung diseases has been undertaken in patients with COPD. To date, there are no evidence-based guidelines for exercise training in other forms of lung disease. It is reasonable to believe, however, that the general principles of training recommended by expert groups and evidence-based practice guidelines for the COPD population can also be applied to other forms of chronic lung disease when appropriate, as long as disease-specific modifications are employed. The following sections summarize recommendations for endurance training, resistance training, flexibility exercise, and inspiratory muscle training in patients with COPD. Subsequent sections will describe concerns and modifications that should be considered in disease-specific applications for exercise training in patients with chronic lung diseases other than COPD.

After medical evaluation and optimization of bronchodilator and oxygen therapy, a maximal cardiopulmonary exercise test can be valuable in defining the specific

BOX 39-6	**Chronic Adaptations to Exercise in Individuals with Chronic Lung Disease**

1. Maximal endurance exercise
   Increased aerobic capacity ($\dot{V}O_{2max}$)
   Increased maximal work rate
   Increased 6-min walking distance
2. Submaximal endurance exercise
   Higher metabolic (lactate) threshold
   Increased endurance (longer duration at same work rate)
   Reduced heart rate[a]
   Reduced $\dot{V}O_2$[a]
   Reduced perception of effort[a]
   Reduced blood lactate[a]
   Reduced $\dot{V}CO_2$[a]
   Reduced minute ventilation[a]

3. Peripheral muscle performance
   Increased upper- and lower-body peripheral muscle strength and endurance
   Increased rate of force development
   Improved mechanical efficiency
4. Symptoms
   Decreased dyspnea
   Less fear and anxiety because of sensations of breathlessness
   Improved quality of life

....

$\dot{V}O_{2max}$, maximal volume of oxygen consumed per unit of time; $\dot{V}O_2$, volume of oxygen consumed per unit time; $\dot{V}CO_2$, volume of carbon dioxide produced per unit time.

[a]Compared with the same absolute pretraining work rates.

physiologic limitations to exercise, assessing the safety of exercise, helping formulate the exercise prescription, and provide a baseline for monitoring progress and program efficacy. When this is not possible or is inappropriate, functional exercise assessments, such the 6-min walk test (7) or the shuttle walk test (123), can provide helpful information for setting the exercise prescription and for progress monitoring. See *Chapter 25* for information on exercise assessments for patients with pulmonary disease.

Exercise assessments may also be used to identify relationships between exercise intensity and symptoms such as hypoxemia, exercise-induced bronchospasm, cardiac abnormalities, or musculoskeletal limitations. Constant work rates tests are particularly appealing because of their ability to precisely identify work rate and therefore provide good reproducibility and for their clinical applicability especially for monitoring of therapeutic interventions (2). Unlike incremental exercise testing that investigates the limits of tolerance, constant work rate testing assesses the type of work more likely to be encountered in everyday life (22). For resistance training, the one repetition maximum (1-RM) procedure (8) may be useful and can be safely applied in patients with chronic pulmonary diseases (67).

Cardiorespiratory Exercise Training

Individualized exercise prescriptions for people with chronic lung disease include application of the familiar

TABLE 39-5. American College of Chest Physicians Relationship of Strength of the Supporting Evidence to the Balance of Benefits to Risks and Burdens

Strength of Evidence	Balance of Benefits to Risks and Burdens[a]			
	Benefits Outweigh Risks/Burdens	**Risks/Burdens Outweigh Benefits**	**Evenly Balanced**	**Uncertain**
High	1A	1A	2A	
Moderate	1B	1B	2B	
Low or very low	1C	1C	2C	2C

DESCRIPTION OF BALANCE OF BENEFITS TO RISKS/BURDENS SCALE

Benefits clearly outweigh the risks and burdens	Certainty of imbalance
Risks and burdens clearly outweigh the benefits	Certainty of imbalance
The risks/burdens and benefits are closely balanced	Less certainty
The balance of benefits to risks and burdens is uncertain	Uncertainty

[a]1A, 1B, 1C, strong recommendation; 2A, 2B, weak recommendation; 2C, weak recommendation.

Adapted from Ries AL, Bauldoff GS, Carlin BW, et al. Pulmonary Rehabilitation: Joint ACCP/AACVPR Evidence-Based Clinical Practice Guidelines. *Chest.* 2007;131(5 Suppl):4S–42S.

FITT (Frequency, Intensity, Time, and Type) principle adjusted to the patient's capabilities, disease-specific limitations, therapeutic objectives, and goals. Intensity and duration guidelines should be considered together because they dictate the total energy expenditure of an exercise session. For example, interval training has been shown to elicit effects similar to continuous endurance training when equivalent amounts of total work performed are the same (69). Warm-up and cool-down periods should be integrated into the training session as described in the following section. A summary of current evidence-based guidelines for endurance exercise training in patients with COPD and, for comparison, in older healthy adults is presented in *Table 39-6*.

Warm-up

A 5–10-min warm-up, including whole-body, low- to moderate-intensity cardiorespiratory and local muscle endurance exercise, provides a gradual transition to higher intensity exercise performed during the conditioning phase. The warm-up period is valuable for increasing muscle temperature, improving oxygen exchange, and speeding nerve impulse transmission (6). Warm-up activities should be similar to those to be performed in the subsequent training period and not induce shortness of breath. Joint readiness, the gradually increasing movement of the joints to be used during the conditioning period, should be included. Stretching exercise is often incorporated into the warm-up period but should be considered as a distinct segment and performed after warm-up exercise or cool-down. See "Flexibility" section as follows.

Cool-down

The purpose of the cool-down period is to return the body to preexercise conditions by gradually decreasing the exercise intensity. Avoiding an abrupt stop in the activity maintains blood pressure through the action of the peripheral muscle pump and thus helps prevent blood pooling that can precipitate hypotension, dizziness, syncope, and cardiac arrhythmias. Cool-down also reduces the risk of postexercise bronchospasm (1). The duration of the cool-down is dependent on the intensity of the previous exercise and is typically 3–10 min. Stretching can be added at the end of the cool-down but should not be considered as the primary cool-down activity.

TABLE 39-6. Summary of Evidence-Based Guidelines for Cardiorespiratory Exercise Training

Reference	Group	Frequency	Intensity	Time	Type	Strength of Evidence
(5)	Patients with COPD	≥3 d · wk^{-1}	Low intensity High intensity High and low	>30 min	Walking Cycling Swimming Upper-body ergometer	IB[a] IA[a]
(69)	COPD: Able to tolerate moderate-intensity, continuous exercise	3 d · wk^{-1}	≥50%–60% WR$_{peak}$		Cycle ergometer treadmill	2B[b] vs. no training
(69)	COPD: Those with severe dyspnea unable to sustain continuous exercise and/or others if treatment goals are consistent with interval training	3 d · wk^{-1}	≥70%–90% WR$_{peak}$ (No guideline for recovery intensity)	30–180 s high intensity (No guideline for high:low intensity ratio)	Cycle ergometer treadmill	2A[c] 2B[b] vs. continuous endurance exercise
(3)	Older, healthy adults	5 d · wk^{-1} 3 d · wk^{-1}	Moderate[d] Vigorous[d] Combinations	≥30 min ≥20 min	Walking Other aerobic activity	I (A)[e] IIa (B)[e]

COPD, chronic obstructive pulmonary disease; WR$_{peak}$, peak work rate.

[a]See *Table 39-5*.

[b]Supported by at least one randomized controlled trial of good quality (PEDro [Physiotherapy Evidence Database] score >6/10) with sufficient power OR two randomized controlled trial OR controlled studies including case-control of cohort study).

[c]Supported by at least one randomized controlled trial with sufficient power and PEDro score >6/10.

[d]Rating exercise at 5–6 on a 10-point scale for "moderate" exercise (5 d · wk^{-1}) and 7–8 on the 10-point scale for vigorous exercise (3 d · wk^{-1}) or a combination of these.

[e]Based on the American College of Cardiology/American Heart Association approach to assigning the classification of recommendations and level of evidence.

Classification of Recommendations

I: Conditions for which there is evidence and/or general agreement that a given procedure or treatment is useful and effective (should; is recommended; is indicated; is useful/effective, beneficial)

IIa: Weight of evidence/opinion is in favor of usefulness/efficacy (is reasonable; can be useful, effective, or beneficial; is probably recommended or indicated)

Levels of Evidence

A: Data derived from multiple randomized clinical trials

B: Data derived from a single randomized trial or from nonrandomized studies

Frequency

Three to 5 d · wk^{-1} of endurance exercise training is recommended to achieve optimal health-related and physiologic benefits (1,69,93,110) and should be supervised by at least one clinical exercise professional. This guideline is consistent with recommendations for frequency of endurance exercise training in healthy older adults (89). Two supervised sessions plus one or more home sessions may be an acceptable alternative to three supervised sessions. However, the efficacy of home exercise alone in patients with pulmonary disease is not clear.

Intensity

Defining appropriate or optimal intensity targets for patients with chronic lung disease is difficult. In some cases, general exercise intensity recommendations for healthy individuals may be used (104). However, ventilatory limitations, dyspnea, skeletal muscle dysfunction, exercise tolerance, motivation, oxygen transport, cardiac function, and patient safety may limit the tolerable levels of exertion in these patients (see *Table 39-4*). In response to this, alternative approaches such as high-intensity interval training (13,69,139) or one-legged cycling (40) have been proposed.

According to the American College of Sports Medicine (ACSM), individuals with asthma should perform cardiorespiratory exercise at an intensity near the ventilatory threshold or 80% of maximal walking speed as determined during a 6-min walk test. For patients with COPD, the ACSM recommends an intensity of 60%–80% of peak work rate and titrated based on dyspnea. See *Chapter 10* in *GETP9*.

Intensity targets based on percentage of estimated maximal heart rate or heart rate reserve may be difficult in patients with chronic lung disease (27). Resting heart rate is often elevated in individuals with chronic lung disease, particularly if their severity is advanced (118). The exercise limitations seen in these patients, as well as the effects of some medication, prohibit attainment of the predicted value of maximal heart rate and thus its use in intensity calculations. Maximal cardiopulmonary exercise testing obviates this problem because a symptom-limited maximum heart rate can be measured along with maximum work rate. The volume of oxygen consumed per unit of time ($\dot{V}O_2$) and work rate at the metabolic or gas exchange threshold may also be determined. These data may then be used with symptom scores (*e.g.*, rating of perceived exertion [RPE], dyspnea scales) collected during the maximal cardiopulmonary exercise test to generate appropriate training intensities (17,26,62,134).

When maximal exercise test data are not available, submaximal testing may prove useful. Although there are no specific intensity guidelines that use heart rate indices, heart rates that are correlated with symptom scores, such as the Borg RPE (17) or dyspnea scales (62,75), determined during submaximal exercise, such as a 6-min walk test, can provide an objective measure of training intensity and progress monitoring. In clinical practice, RPE and dyspnea scores provide self-adjusting anchors for intensity prescriptions. That is, as fitness improves, work rates will increase at the same symptom score. Periodic assessment of this relationship provides a mechanism for progress monitoring. Intensity targets of 12–14 on the traditional Borg RPE scale or 4–6 on the Borg 0–10 category/ratio scale (17) are reasonable (93). Regardless of the intensity used, monitoring oxygen saturation in patients with more severe disease should be part of the exercise regimen, at least during the initial few weeks of training. Oxygen saturation during exercise should be maintained at ≥88% by the use of supplemental oxygen if necessary (1). This therapeutic strategy enables a higher intensity of exercise to be sustained for longer, thus enhancing any physiological training effect.

Research into the optimal exercise intensity for individuals with pulmonary disease continues to evolve. Examples include the use of high intensities, interval training, and one-legged exercise training. Higher training intensities have been shown to produce greater benefits in patients with COPD than lower intensities (21) and should be considered when appropriate (94). Alternatively, lower intensity prescriptions may be more appropriate at the onset of rehabilitation for those with poor exercise tolerance and may promote long-term adherence and "metabolic fitness" (39) that may lead to health benefits other than improved physical function. For patients with mild-to-moderate COPD or controlled asthma, use of intensity guidelines set for older adults (89) may be used (see *Table 39-6*). Current evidence-based clinical practice guidelines grade the recommendation of higher versus lower training intensity as moderately strong or 1B (see *Table 39-5*), whereas both high- and low-intensity exercise training are given a grade of strong or 1A for their ability to produce clinical benefits in patients with COPD (110).

In one study, high-intensity but not moderate-intensity exercise resulted in reduced dyspnea at rest and submaximal exercise and increased 12-min walk distance (49). *High intensity* and *moderate intensity* are relative terms and do not indicate high absolute workloads because peak workload is significantly reduced in patients with COPD (110). However, there may be reluctance to use high-intensity exercise in individuals with moderate-to-severe lung disease. Estimating the maximum sustainable exercise intensity may be determined by (a) recognizing the difference between "perceived level of exertion" and "dyspnea"; (b) avoiding sustained ventilatory loads close to ventilatory capacity, which would correlate to a "moderate" dyspnea index; and (c) aiming for constant work rate exercise intensity that is

60%–80% of peak work rate or >70%–90% peak work rate used in an interval training format. Sustained exercise intensity levels higher than these recommendations predispose to muscle fatigue and exhaustion. If ventilatory muscle fatigue occurs, ventilatory failure can ensue. Although skeletal muscle fatigue is better tolerated, it still influences the frequency at which exercise can be performed (28,75,115). Distinguishing between perceived exertion and dyspnea is essential but difficult because they are not mutually exclusive (75). The former represents the degree of peripheral muscle fatigue and weakness, and the latter represents the degree of breathlessness.

Application of interval exercise training in patients with COPD that allows higher intensity exercise (>70%–90% of peak work rate) for short durations (30–180 s) interspersed with rest intervals in work-to-rest ratios of 1:1 or 1:2 has undergone significant scientific inquiry over the last several years (13,68,69,74,140). The rationale for interval training centers on avoidance of symptoms and perceptions of dyspnea that lead to ventilatory limitation and decreased duration of higher intensity exercise. Patients with COPD experience early lactic acidosis because of impaired oxygen delivery to peripheral muscle. Together with the skeletal muscle dysfunction often seen in patients with COPD (73), ventilation can be severely taxed. Blood lactate concentrations have been shown to be lower during interval training relative to continuous exercise (68), thereby reducing some of the stimulus to breathe. In patients with severe COPD, Vogiatzis (139) have shown threefold increases in exercise time with high-intensity interval training (30 s at 100% peak work rate interspersed with 30 s unloaded cycling) compared with constant work rate exercise (80% peak work rate). Ratings of dyspnea and leg fatigue and arterial lactate concentrations measured at the same time point (i.e., "iso-time") of interval and continuous exercise (the end of constant work rate exercise, 10.3 min) were significantly lower in interval training. Additionally, $\dot{V}O_2$ and $\dot{V}_E$ were stable across the 32 min of interval training and were 16% and 12% lower, respectively, compared at end exercise with continuous training.

Systematic reviews (13) and clinical practice guidelines for physiotherapists (69) support the use of interval training, especially when disease severity or symptoms preclude continuous higher intensity exercise. Most studies contained within these reviews held total work completed equal in interval and continuous training with both methods yielding significant improvements in aerobic capacity, lactate threshold, peak work rate, 6-min walk distance, and several measures of health-related QOL with no differences in degree of improvement between methods (13). It should be noted, however, that given the possibility of threefold differences in high-intensity training duration as shown by Vogiatzis (139), interval training in the appropriate setting might prove more beneficial than continuous, constant work rate exercise (68).

According to a review by Zainuldin et al. (148), conflicting data have been reported among studies investigating whether higher versus lower intensity or interval versus continuous training elicited significantly different results. They assessed randomized controlled trials that compared either higher versus lower intensity leg exercise or interval versus continuous training. Three studies (119 patients) were evaluated for differences between higher and lower intensity leg exercise (1 treadmill) on change in constant work rate endurance time, and two studies were examined for differences in 6-min walk performance. Neither constant work rate time nor 6-min walk was shown to be significantly different between groups. It should be noted that two of these studies held the volume of work equal between groups but varied the duration, whereas the third used the same session duration resulting in different volumes of work. Analysis of mean differences in peak work rate (eight studies), peak $\dot{V}O_2$ (five studies), peak $\dot{V}_E$ (three studies), and lactate threshold (three studies) also showed no significant differences between subjects performing continuous or interval training.

One-legged cycling has been investigated as a strategy for endurance training in patients with COPD (40). The conceptual framework suggests that by using a smaller muscle mass but with the same load as with two-legged cycling, the ventilatory requirement may be lower, whereas the metabolic demands are the same. Many patients with COPD are limited by shortness of breath during exercise even at moderate levels of ventilation and thus relegated to lower training intensities to avoid dyspnea. Available evidence suggests that patients with COPD can generate a greater percentage of their peak power from a two-legged incremental exercise test during a one-legged cycling incremental exercise test than healthy controls, 80% peak power versus 50% peak power (41). During constant work rate exercise, healthy individuals could exercise twice as long compared with single-leg exercise, but the subjects with COPD exercised four times longer with lower ventilatory requirements (41). Training studies comparing one- and two-legged cycling in patients with COPD have reported between group differences revealing large effect sizes (Cohen's $d \geq 0.8$) for peak work rate, peak $\dot{V}O_2$, and peak rate of elimination of carbon dioxide ($\dot{V}CO_{2peak}$) favoring one-legged training, all $P < .05$. Moderate effect sizes ($d = 0.5–0.6$) were shown for peak $\dot{V}_E$ and dyspnea scores favoring one-legged training for peak $\dot{V}_E$ ($P < .05$) and two-legged training for dyspnea score. Larger studies are needed to confirm these results. Especially for the most severely limited patients, one-legged cycling may provide a viable alternative with the possibility of yielding greater training effects (40).

Time (Duration)

The ACSM recommends at least 20–30 min per exercise session for individuals with asthma. No specific guidelines for exercise duration have been set for patients with other chronic lung diseases. However, an initial goal of 30 (range 20–60) min has been suggested, with a goal of progressing to 60–90 min as tolerated (1,27). Individuals with moderate or severe COPD may only be able to tolerate a few minutes at the start of a training program. Because training intensity in part dictates achievable training duration, attempting to achieve an intensity target that is set too high may preclude attainment of target duration. Patients with chronic lung disease often do not achieve 30 min of continuous endurance training until several weeks into their rehabilitation program, even at lower intensities. In the initial phases of endurance exercise training, one approach to achieving target duration is to decrease the exercise intensity. Although this might be a desirable solution until the individual has adapted to regular exercise, another option is to apply the aerobic exercise prescription in intervals for several weeks with the goal of achieving 30 min or more of cumulative aerobic exercise with each session.

The ACSM recommends training frequencies of 3–5 d $\cdot$ wk^{-1} for patients with asthma and COPD. The same frequency is recommended for healthy older adults depending on the intensity with which the exercise is performed (89) (see *Table 39-6*). These general guidelines for healthy individuals may be successfully adapted to patients with other chronic lung diseases as well.

Type (Mode)

Patients with chronic lung disease typically use lower-extremity modalities, such as treadmills and cycle ergometers. This has practical value in improving performance of the muscles of ambulation. Treadmill exercise is usually preferred by patients and exercise professionals because of its similarity to everyday walking and greater relevance to many activities of daily living. Cycle ergometry can be used as a means of varying the exercise mode and may be preferred in patients with arthritis, joint deformities, or morbid obesity because of its low impact on the musculoskeletal system.

Other modes of endurance exercise training may be used successfully, including indoor or outdoor walking, rowing, arm ergometry, stepping, swimming, water aerobics, modified aerobic dance, and seated aerobics (1). According to the ACSM, for patients with asthma, swimming (preferably in a nonchlorinated pool) is less asthmogenic and therefore a better tolerated form of exercise. Patient participation in selecting one or more appropriate (*e.g.*, large muscle group, rhythmic exercise) exercise training modes will likely add enjoyment and contribute to long-term compliance and is recommended. Previous ACCP/AACVPR evidence-based guidelines for pulmonary rehabilitation emphasized the scientific evidence in favor of aerobic exercise training using the large muscle groups of the legs (107). Current evidence-based (94) and practice guidelines (110) provide new support for the use of upper-extremity exercise specifically for developing upper-limb exercise capacity and reduced ventilation and oxygen cost during unsupported arm activity. In addition, a recent systematic review (69) recommended arm exercise as adjunctive therapy in selected patients with upper-extremity weakness who desire improvements in performing upper-extremity activities of daily living. Although conclusive evidence was absent, both free-weight exercises and arm ergometry were recommended with greater emphasis on resistance exercise for improving activities of daily living. No studies have been done that identify an optimal training regimen for improvement in upper extremity function (69).

Supplemental Oxygen during Exercise

Oxyhemoglobin saturation (SaO_2) should be $\geq$88% during exercise (1). Incremental exercise testing will aid in identifying the intensity at which patients become hypoxemic. Periodic monitoring of SaO_2 by pulse oximetry will help guide administration of supplemental oxygen therapy. Supplemental oxygen administered during exercise training is recommended (grade 1C, see *Table 39-5*) for patients with severe resting or exercise-induced hypoxemia (69,110). Although inconclusive, supplemental oxygen administered to patients who do not experience significant exercise-induced desaturation has been shown to allow higher training intensities and improved constant work rate performance (grade 2C, see *Table 39-5*) (110); however, because of the low strength of the evidence, it's routine use is not currently recommended in these cases.

Resistance Exercise Training

Deconditioning and muscle atrophy is common in patients with COPD because of the vicious cycle of increasing ventilatory limitations, shortness of breath, and consequent decreases in physical activity. This contributes to skeletal muscle atrophy and loss of muscle strength, power, and endurance. In addition, myopathies in skeletal muscle attributable to systemic inflammation, oxidative stress, blood gas abnormalities, and use of corticosteroids have also been proposed as mechanisms contributing to skeletal muscle dysfunction (124). Evidence suggests that loss of muscle strength is proportional to the loss of muscle mass in patients with COPD and that there is preferential loss of muscle size and strength in the lower limbs (15). Peripheral muscle dysfunction that contributes to the exercise intolerance seen in chronic lung diseases has received considerable attention (99,100,124) and is

TABLE 39-7. Summary of Recommendations and Suggestions for Resistance Exercise Training in Patients with COPD and Older Adults

Reference	Group	Frequency	Intensity	Sets	Repetitions	Rest	Exercises
(126)	COPD	2–3 d · wk^{-1}	50%–60% 1-RM initially Progress to 85% 1-RM	1–3	10–12 initially Progress to 6–10	1–3 min	8–10
(98)	COPD	2–3 d · wk^{-1}	50%–85% 1-RM	2–4	6–12		3–9
(89)	Healthy, older adults	≥2 d · wk^{-1}	Moderate to high[a]	1 or more	10–15		8–10

COPD, chronic obstructive pulmonary disease; 1-RM, one repetition maximum.

[a]Moderate intensity is defined as 5–6 on a 0–10 scale; high intensity is 7–8 on a 0–10 scale.

shown to be significantly and independently related to increased use of health care resources (36), poorer prognosis (36), and mortality (129). Recent evidence-based and scientific guidelines for pulmonary rehabilitation (69,93,110) and systematic reviews of resistance training in COPD (99) clearly emphasize the value of resistance exercise training for increasing muscle strength and muscle mass for both upper and lower extremities. Strength of evidence for these outcomes is graded at 1A (i.e., highest recommendation). A summary of resistance training recommendations is shown in *Table 39-7*. The Canadian Thoracic Society recommends the addition of resistance training to aerobic training because the combination has been shown to be more effective than cardiorespiratory training alone in improving endurance and functional ability (grade 2B; see *Table 39-5*) (77).

Data examining the effectiveness of progressive resistance exercise training on measures of physical function tend to favor resistance training over comparison groups (e.g., endurance training or no intervention). A recent systematic review of progressive resistance exercise training in patients with COPD focused not only on muscle performance outcomes but also on changes in physical function and showed large effect sizes for changes in stair-climbing speed and repeated chair stands, with greater benefit seen in patients who participated in resistance training (99). Resistance training had no effect on $\dot{V}O_2$ walking distance or submaximal cycling endurance when compared to cardiorespiratory training or concurrent aerobic and resistance training (99).

Resistance training has also been explored for its potential in improving measures of pulmonary function such as forced vital capacity (FVC), $FEV_{1.0}$, or peak $\dot{V}_E$. Strasser et al. (127) have recently provided insight into this important question through their systematic review and meta-analysis. The pooled effect of resistance training (expiratory muscle training was not included) demonstrated a significant increase in FVC of 0.37 L, (95% confidence interval [CI], 0.26–0.49; $P < .001$), a strong trend for an increase in peak $\dot{V}_E$ (effect size = 3.77 L · min^{-1}; 95% CI, −0.51–8.04, $P = .08$), but no change in $FEV_{1.0}$ whether expressed

as percent predicted (effect size 2.7% predicted, 95% CI, −1.86–7.27, $P = .25$) or in absolute liters (0.08 L, 95% CI, −0.03–0.09; $P = .14$). Additionally, this review examined whether a dose-response relationship was evident for resistance training volume and pulmonary function. The meta-analysis was unable to detect such a relationship but reported a tendency toward a low negative effect of resistance exercise frequency on $FEV_{1.0}$ and FVC; three or more resistance training sessions per week negatively impacted $FEV_{1.0}$ and FVC relative to two sessions per week. Intensity of training was inconsistently related to improved lung function; however, intensities using 60%–70% 1-RM had more beneficial effects on $FEV_{1.0}$ and peak $\dot{V}_E$ than intensities of 80%–90% 1-RM. A notable exception is a study in which 12 patients with COPD ($FEV_{1.0}$ <60% of predicted) were randomized to perform high-intensity leg press exercise training three times weekly for 8 wk or to a nonexercising control group (59). Compared with controls, the exercising subjects showed significant improvements in $FEV_{1.0}$ (+21%) and mechanical efficiency of leg cycling (+31%). Summarizing, their meta-analysis and in view of the limited number of study groups and heterogeneity of outcome results for trials comprising it, Strasser et al. (127) concluded that resistance training does not alter $FEV_{1.0}$ but does increase FVC and peak $\dot{V}_E$, which may result in significant reductions in breathlessness and improved ventilatory capacity. Finally, the authors recommended 2 d · wk^{-1} of resistance training at 70% 1-RM with two or more sets per muscle group per week. Monitoring pulmonary function might be of value in downwardly adjusting the training intensity if $FEV_{1.0}$ falls.

There is no consensus regarding the characteristics of an optimal resistance training program for patients with pulmonary disease, and from the earlier discussion, training for changes in muscle size, strength, and physical function might require different approaches than training to improve lung function. Templates for program design have emerged from reviews of research in resistance training for individuals with COPD that have resulted in successful outcomes (98,126) and guidelines for resistance training in healthy older adults are available and applicable (89) (see *Table 39-7*). The ACSM encourages resistance training for individuals with COPD based on guidelines outlined for healthy persons (see *Chapter 10* of *GETP9*).

The same FITT framework used with endurance training is applicable for resistance training as well. If resistance training is not preceded by several minutes of cardiorespiratory exercise training, then a warm-up period is likely indicated. This can be accomplished using very light resistance and gradually increasing the range of motion.

Frequency

Two to 3 nonconsecutive days per week of resistance training is recommended for patients with COPD (1,98,110,126) and is consistent with recommendations for strength training in older adults (90). On each of these days, participants perform sets of resistance training for at least the large muscle groups of the upper and lower extremity.

Intensity

The current recommendation for resistance training intensity in older individuals is 60%–70% 1-RM or a workload that allows the individual to perform 10–15 repetitions. When testing is conducted by experienced personnel, the 1-RM procedure has been shown to be safe in patients with COPD (67). However, because the 1-RM is a highly effort-dependent measure requiring maximal force production and some exercise professionals may be hesitant in performing this in older individuals, Nelson et al. (89) proposed an alternative approach to guiding resistance training intensity that makes use of perceptual ratings in which moderate exercise is rated at 5–6 and high intensity at 7–8 on a 0–10-point scale (89).

Time

Strength training should be a component of a comprehensive exercise rehabilitation program for patients with COPD that includes endurance training and flexibility exercise as well as resistance training. Total training session time for endurance and strength exercise, when reported, has ranged between 40 and 90 min. Using reasonable assumptions for time per repetition, the strength-training portion of a comprehensive pulmonary rehabilitation program could be completed within 20–40 min, assuming one set of 8–12 repetitions performed for 8–10 exercises interspersed with 2–3 min rest between sets (126). This estimate may be modified based on disease severity and program design. The number and choice of exercises may be dictated by patient goals and needs assessment (*e.g.*, improving ability to climb stairs in the patient's domicile) or by contraindications such as arthritic joints or osteoporosis (a potential problem in

patients undergoing long-term corticosteroid therapy). A free-weight squat, for example, would typically not be appropriate in the COPD population. However, a seated leg press exercise or repetitions of standing up from a bench or chair while holding progressively heavier weights may be acceptable alternatives. If patients cannot stand up from the chair or bench with their body weight alone, the seat height may be elevated or direct supervision may be necessary.

The rest interval between sets should also be considered. An ideal rest period between sets is difficult to establish for the patient with COPD primarily because of varying degrees of dyspnea and/or oxyhemoglobin desaturation. Although a 1-min rest interval between sets might be attempted in selected patients who are performing a higher intensity training bout, in practice, most patients will require a 2- to 3-min period of rest.

Type

Many types of resistance training are available, including machine weights, free weights, elastic resistance, weighted balls, and body weight. Choice of equipment is often dictated by what is available. However, almost any form of resistance will suffice as long as it can be graded in its application, is safe to use, and has some motivational appeal to the participant. Consideration should be given to the minimal weight that can be set for any given exercise. Some types of weight machines have minimal resistances that are too high or weights that are in increments that are too large for some patients who exhibit significant atrophy and weakness. For some, the use of free weights may be contraindicated because of balance/safety issues. Elastic resistance can provide low force requirements and may be ideal for some very debilitated patients.

Sustainability of Resistance Training in COPD

Without continuing in a maintenance program, the benefits related to exercise tolerance and QOL derived from comprehensive pulmonary rehabilitation programs decline after program completion. However, some benefits are sustained to the extent that they do not return to baseline for 6–12 mo (5). Whether patients with COPD who complete an initial resistance training program sustain the benefits accrued from these short-term programs is not well known. Houchen et al. (63) examined this question through an extensive literature review of studies in which participants had COPD and completed an intervention that included resistance training, a follow-up period of at least 12 wk, and a measure of muscle strength. Only three studies met inclusion criteria with an aggregate of 198 patients with COPD. These three studies yielded conflicting results — two showed muscle strength decrease 12 mo and 12 wk after cessation of training, but strength was statistically higher than baseline, whereas the third study reported that none of the benefits gained from 12 wk of resistance training were maintained 12 wk later. Several ideas may be gleaned from the Houchen et al. review (63). First, there is a need for high-quality trials investigating the extent to which changes in muscle strength, endurance, and power are maintained after the initial training program. When available, these data will inform the design and execution of continued resistance exercise training required to maintain, or better, improve upon initial gains. Second, studies investigating sustainability of improvements in muscle performance should include different modes of delivering the maintenance program including home exercise and community-based resources (3,42,43,135) and use technology to remotely monitor compliance with training.

Flexibility

Flexibility is recognized as a component of a comprehensive exercise training regimen and should be performed with the objective of "maintaining the flexibility necessary for regular physical activity and daily life" (89). The health-related benefits of good flexibility are not well established, and no specific guidelines for patients with chronic respiratory diseases are available. However, recent recommendations for flexibility exercise training in healthy older adults (89) are relevant as are general guidelines for healthy individuals (104). These include performing flexibility exercises at least 2 d · wk^{-1} for at least 10 min each day (89). *Table 39-7* summarizes the recommendations for healthy older adults and general ACSM guidelines for prescriptions to improve flexibility. Additional research is needed to demonstrate the extent to which flexibility is lost with aging, whether regular stretching reduces or reverses this loss, and whether improved flexibility confers health benefits not obtained from other forms of exercise.

Ventilatory (Inspiratory) Muscle Training

Many patients with COPD experience inspiratory muscle weakness that leads to increased breathlessness and decreased exercise tolerance. As reported in the 2007 Joint ACCP/AACVPR Practice Guidelines, several recent randomized controlled trials (70,72,114,144,145) have demonstrated positive physiologic and patient-centered effects from inspiratory muscle training. However, the results of these studies, as well as their single-center design with relatively few patients, have not convinced the ACCP/AACVPR to change their previous evidence-based practice guidelines (107), which now state that (a) inspiratory muscle training should be considered in selected patients who have decreased inspiratory muscle strength and breathlessness despite receiving optimal medical therapy, and (b) overall, the scientific

evidence does not support the routine use of inspiratory muscle training as an essential component of pulmonary rehabilitation (grade 1B) (110). The ATS/ERS practice guidelines (93) provide similar recommendations that "although the data are inconclusive, inspiratory muscle training could be considered as adjunctive therapy in pulmonary rehabilitation, primarily in patients with suspected or proven ventilatory muscle weakness."

Guidelines for inspiratory muscle training have been provided by the AACVPR (1) and include the following:

- Frequency of 4–5 d · wk^{-1}
- Intensity of 30% maximal inspiratory pressure measured at the mouth (Pimax)
- Time of two 15-min sessions per day or one 30-min session per day
- Type — Three types of inspiratory muscle training are used: inspiratory resistance training (14), threshold loading (52), and normocapnic hyperventilation (116). There is no demonstrated superiority of one method over another to suggest its preferred use (93).

Neuromuscular Electrical Stimulation

Neuromuscular electrical stimulation (NMES) might be considered as a means to elicit passive peripheral muscular contractions in patients with advanced COPD, ILD, or PAH who are severely deconditioned and unable to perform recommended aerobic or resistance training. The low metabolic and ventilatory demands of NMES make it a particularly attractive modality in these patient groups. Handheld NMES devices deliver biphasic impulse currents with stimulation frequencies and intensities of 10–50 Hz and 20–100 mA, respectively (137). In their systematic review, Sillen et al. (119) report that intensity of stimulation should lead to a visible, strong muscle contraction or to patients' tolerance. Training protocols for NMES vary considerably from 3–7 d · wk^{-1}, with session durations of 20–120 min once or twice daily for 24–70 total sessions (119,137). Training can be used safely at home during acute exacerbations (88). Although only a limited number of studies are available in patients with COPD, NMES training has resulted in significant improvements in muscle function, exercise tolerance, and dyspnea during activities of daily living (88,138). One study, however, found no significant differences in peak quadriceps torque, leg muscle mass, or 6-min walk distance between patients with COPD receiving 6 wk of NMES compared to a sham treatment group (34). In their review, Sillen et al. (119) concluded that NEMS is safe, with patient complaints limited to mild muscle cramps or soreness. The benefits of NMES for patients with COPD remain to be confirmed in large randomized controlled trials.

DISEASE-SPECIFIC CONSIDERATIONS

General Safety Concerns for Exercise Training in People with Chronic Lung Disease

Exercise training in patients with chronic lung disease is generally considered safe, even with high relative intensities, when training guidelines are correctly applied with due consideration of individual patients' exercise tolerance and thresholds limiting exercise intensity (see *Table 39-4*).

Cardiopulmonary exercise testing is valuable in assessing overall safety of exercise training. The availability of supplemental oxygen during training helps maintain appropriate levels of oxygen saturation, thus reducing hypoxemia and dyspnea. Periodic monitoring by pulse oximetry and visual analog scales for dyspnea are helpful in this regard (16,26). Optimal bronchodilator therapy improves lung function by reducing airflow obstruction and thereby reduces breathlessness and wheeze. Pursed-lip breathing should be taught, practiced, and performed as needed to lower end-expiratory lung volume and improve the inspiratory capacity (94,132,133). During resistance training, proper biomechanics for lifting technique reduces the risk of musculoskeletal injury; avoidance of the Valsalva maneuver during lifting reduces the risk of developing high intrathoracic pressures, thereby decreasing venous return and cardiac output (147). Periodic blood pressure measurements may be necessary in select patients with hypertension.

Asthma

Ram et al. (109) reviewed the effects of exercise training in patients with asthma, noting several limitations in the studies. Bearing this in mind, the authors concluded from their review that exercise training generally resulted in statistically significant improvements in maximum work rate, peak $\dot{V}O_2$, maximum heart rate, and maximum exercise ventilation. However, the absolute changes were small. There was no evidence of improved lung function or evidence that the improved measures of cardiopulmonary performance translate into improved physical function.

The airflow obstruction in asthma is generally considered reversible. Recommendations for exercise training include avoidance of triggers resulting in bronchoconstriction, adequate warm-up, and use of bronchodilators before exercise (1). Exercise can induce bronchoconstriction (*i.e.*, EIB), especially when the asthma is inadequately controlled (71). However, EIB is less problematic when asthma is well controlled with optimal therapy (20,105). EIB may also occur in those who do not otherwise have asthma (143). Tests to determine the presence of EIB are described in detail elsewhere (30,32). Briefly, the test requires a two-step process. First, an exercise stimulus of >80% of maximum heart rate is applied for 6–8 min

of exercise on a treadmill or cycle ergometer to increase the $\dot{V}_E$ to 40%–60% of the expected value. Second, serial $FEV_{1.0}$ measurements are obtained by spirometry at 5, 10, 15, 20, and 30 min postexercise; in some protocols, measurements at 1 and 3 min are also obtained. An abnormal response is defined as a fall of >10% below the baseline $FEV_{1.0}$ at each interval, although a fall of >15% has also been recommended, particularly if challenge tests are performed in the field (32). Blood pressure and oxygen saturation should be measured throughout the test and recovery periods. Although unusual, upper-airway abnormalities other than asthma may also exhibit positive challenge tests and may be distinguished from EIB through examination of the flow-volume loop (32). A diagnostic cardiopulmonary exercise test may also be used as a provocation study to identify EIA (2,30). Severe bronchoconstriction is a potential hazard following challenge testing. Immediate administration of nebulized bronchodilator therapy and oxygen usually provide successful treatment (32). Tests should be appropriately supervised by trained technicians and, in the case of higher risk individuals, by a physician.

The comprehensive exercise training program described for patients with COPD is directly applicable to individuals with asthma when airway obstruction is adequately managed with bronchodilator therapy and triggers to bronchoconstriction (such as cold, dry, dusty air, and inhaled pollutants) are removed. Warm-up and bronchodilator therapy before exercise will often reduce the occurrence of EIB (1).

Interstitial Lung Disease

Currently, no evidence-based guidelines for exercise training in pulmonary rehabilitation are available for patients with ILD, although these so-called "non-COPD" patients are reported to benefit from such training (107). Relatively few studies of exercise training have been conducted in patients with ILD, and most follow guidelines appropriate for use in patients with COPD. Functional improvements from pulmonary rehabilitation seen in patients with ILD are similar (33,87) or slightly less (48) than those observed in patients with COPD. In their review, Markovitz and Cooper (81) noted that compared with controls, studies of exercise training in patients with ILD showed significant improvements in submaximal endurance (47,61,87), reductions in dyspnea and fatigue (47,61,87), improved QOL, and reduced hospitalizations (87). One study that performed follow-up analysis at 6 mo observed that improvements in 6-min walk distance, dyspnea, and fatigue achieved after 8 wk of twice weekly supervised exercise training were not maintained (61). As in patients with COPD (110), the loss of functional and QOL improvements achieved after initial exercise training in patients with ILD, maintenance programs are required to sustain benefits (53,111).

In general, the exercise training recommendations used in patients with COPD apply to those with the ILDs when modifications are adapted to the individual's exercise tolerance. During exercise training, careful application of intensity and duration guidelines is recommended in these patients. Despite the benefits of high-intensity training in patients with COPD, it may not be indicated in patients with ILD because it may result in deranged gas exchange, desaturation, and incapacitating dyspnea.

Bronchiectasis

Very few studies have investigated the role of rehabilitative exercise in patients with bronchiectasis. Smidt et al. (125) identified only one study that qualified for inclusion in their best evidence summary of exercise training in chronic diseases (18). Based on this single study, it was concluded that there is insufficient evidence to support or refute the effectiveness of exercise therapy for patients with bronchiectasis. Published contemporaneously with the Smidt et al. report, Newall et al. (90) found that a small number of patients with bronchiectasis who were randomized to 8 wk of three-times-weekly sessions of 45 min of high-intensity exercise training improved exercise tolerance, but the addition of inspiratory muscle training provided no added benefit. Neither exercise training nor inspiratory muscle training affected 24-h sputum clearance.

A retrospective analysis of a pulmonary rehabilitation program in 95 patients with bronchiectasis provides additional insight into responsiveness to exercise training in this subgroup of COPD (97). Program efficacy was evaluated from baseline to 12 mo with comparisons to patients with COPD who were matched for sex, age, and 6-min walk distance. All patients completed 6–8 wk of twice weekly supervised exercise training consisting of 15 min each of progressive walking and cycling plus resistance training. Two to three sessions of walking at home were recommended. After training, patients with bronchiectasis increased 6-min walk distance by 53 m and Chronic Respiratory Disease Questionnaire (CRQ) total score by 14 units. Thirty-five patients in both groups were assessed at 12 mo. At 12 mo, the 6-min walk distance remained significantly higher than baseline (+21 m), although this was below the minimum clinically important difference (35 m). The CRQ score was 12 units above baseline at 12 mo, which was considered clinically important. There were no significant differences between patients with bronchiectasis and COPD for outcome measures after rehabilitation or at 3-mo intervals up to 12 mo. These data suggest that patients with bronchiectasis respond well to pulmonary rehabilitation with changes similar to those with COPD. Future prospective randomized trials are needed to confirm this observation. Although data are limited at this time, application of exercise training guidelines suggested for patients with COPD appear to be appropriate for patients with bronchiectasis.

Pulmonary Arterial Hypertension

Exercise training in PAH is a serious undertaking with the necessity for precautions that exceed those employed in other chronic lung diseases. In patients with PAH, pulmonary arterial pressures can increase suddenly and dramatically during exercise, predisposing them to right ventricular decompensation and cardiovascular collapse (12). Sudden death has been reported during exercise in individuals with PAH. The underlying mechanism is postulated as acute right ventricular pressure overload or cardiac dysrhythmia. This suggests that some patients with PAH may require electrocardiographic monitoring. Hypoxemia reflects the severity of PAH, and when significant during exercise, it often requires supplemental oxygen (86). Fatigue and weakness are important manifestations of PAH and reflect the inability to meet metabolic demands of exercise. This is accentuated by early-onset lactic acidosis. Other symptoms include resting tachycardia, substernal chest pain, presyncope, and syncope. These, along with oxygen saturation, should be carefully monitored (1).

Before exercise training, patients' medical treatment should be optimized and exercise training sessions closely supervised by experienced personnel (1). Recommendations for exercise training in patients with PAH include lower intensity exercise training, avoidance of arm ergometry or resistance exercise training that may result in a Valsalva maneuver, and avoidance of floor exercise (1). One recent recommendation has suggested that patients with stable PAH first undergo moderate-intensity aerobic exercise training until established and well tolerated. Afterward, resistance exercise may be initiated and added to the training routine. In those individuals who are severely deconditioned and/or with advanced PAH, NMES should be considered (4). In contrast, Mereles et al. (84) demonstrated that stable, medically optimized patients with severe chronic PAH could undergo vigorous exercise training. In this 15-wk randomized controlled trial with crossover design, patients completed a closely supervised inpatient training phase (7 d · wk^{-1} for 3 wk) that was immediately followed by 12 wk of home training. The inpatient training consisted of 10–25 min of progressive interval training (up to 60%–80% peak heart rate) and 5 d · wk^{-1} of walking for 60 min. Additionally, patients performed light (0.5–1.0 kg) dumbbell resistance training for 30 min, 5 d · wk^{-1}. Home training consisted of 5 d · wk^{-1} of leg cycling for 15–30 min at target heart rate, 3 d · wk^{-1} dumbbell training, and 2 d · wk^{-1} of walking. Home training was monitored by twice weekly telephone calls. Significant improvements in 6-min walk distance of 85 m and 75 m were seen after 3 wk of training in the primary training group and in the control group that crossed over to training, respectively. Further, slight improvement or maintenance of change was noted at 15 wk. In addition, significant improvements were observed in QOL (Short Form 36 [SF-36]), maximum work rate, maximum heart rate, peak $\dot{V}O_2$, as well as $\dot{V}O_2$ and work rate at the ventilatory threshold. The training was well tolerated, with no adverse events reported. The authors cautioned, however, that exercise training in patients with PAH can have serious adverse effects. It is important to note that the Mereles et al. (84) study began in the hospital and was carefully supervised and monitored by personnel experienced with these patients. As noted in an accompanying editorial, carefully designed exercise is safe and beneficial, at least in the short term, for patients with PAH (92). These data are encouraging but remain to be confirmed in larger groups of patients with PAH in which there is more random selection and perhaps greater diversity in patient characteristics. Although the results are impressive, considerable training time was invested, which begs the question whether other patients with PAH can tolerate and/or complete such a program and whether a less rigorous regimen would produce similar results.

IMPLEMENTATION OF PULMONARY REHABILITATION PROGRAMS

Pulmonary rehabilitation is a structured, "evidence-based, multidisciplinary, and comprehensive intervention for patients with chronic lung diseases who are symptomatic and often have decreased daily life activities" (93).

The comprehensive nature of pulmonary rehabilitation addresses both physical and psychological needs and facilitates a holistic approach to lung disease management with well-defined objectives (see *Box 39-5*) and evidence-based practice guidelines and outcomes (93,110). The components of a comprehensive pulmonary rehabilitation program are outlined in *Box 39-7*. Recommended guidelines for implementing the exercise training component are summarized in *Tables 39-6* and *39-7*. The building blocks for these guidelines are discussed throughout this chapter, along with the observed responses to the exercise.

The optimal length of time over which to implement the initial pulmonary rehabilitation program is not clear (110). In general, although the evidence is weak, programs that are of longer duration (*e.g.*, >12 wk) result in greater sustained benefits than shorter programs (ACCP/AACVRP grade 2C; see *Table 39-5*). Recent Canadian Thoracic Society evidence-based clinical practice guidelines also recommend longer duration pulmonary rehabilitation programs with durations beyond 6–8 wk (77). The available research suggests that many variables, including the variations in types of programs, program participants, and program content, affect benefits that may be derived. Somewhat surprising, even 6–12 wk of pulmonary rehabilitation have yielded durable benefits that have persisted for 12–18 mo following completion of the program. However, despite the apparent sustainability of benefit from relatively short-term rehabilitation, these benefits eventually disappear when exercise training ceases (53,111). This, as well as the unquestioned value of exercise training in patients

---

BOX 39-7	**Components of Pulmonary Rehabilitation Program**

Patient education

Pulmonary anatomy, physiology, and disease pathophysiology

Diagnostic testing

Treatment (including oxygen, medications, surgery)

Bronchial hygiene techniques

Breathing retraining

Exercise training, including endurance, strength, and flexibility training of the upper and lower extremities

Ventilatory muscle training

Education on energy conservation techniques, self-management, self-assessment, symptom management, sleep, sexuality, nutrition, stress management, and indications for seeking medical advice and resources

Infection control (avoidance, early intervention, and immunization)

Environmental control

Smoking cessation

Psychosocial intervention and support

Community services including patient and family support groups

Advance care planning

Counseling on recreation and leisure activities and travel

Adapted from Haynes JM. AARC clinical practice guideline: pulmonary rehabilitation. *Respir Care.* 2002;47:617–25.

with chronic lung disease, clearly suggests the need for long-term maintenance strategies. Possible approaches include repeat courses, participation in maintenance programs, guided and monitored home exercise, self-management, participation in exercise programs available in community settings, or combinations of these. Community-based maintenance programs are appealing because of their potential for increased accessibility, cost savings, resources, expertise for individualized training, and opportunity to mix with members of the local community (43). Several studies conducted in the United States (3), United Kingdom (43,142), and the Netherlands (19,42,135) have revealed successful application of community-based exercise training resulting in significant improvements favoring those assigned to community-based exercise versus controls. Improvements included measures of aerobic endurance, muscle strength and power, dyspnea scores, and cost savings. Heterogeneity of program and study design, severity of COPD among subjects, inclusion of asthmatics, and delivery of the program make it difficult to arrive at a single set of recommendations. However, in their recently published clinical practice guidelines, the Canadian Thoracic Society has provided the highest level of evidence, grade 1A (see *Table 39-5*), for the effectiveness of nonhospital based compared with hospital-based pulmonary rehabilitation (77). The Canadian Thoracic Society strongly recommends that all patients with COPD have access to pulmonary rehabilitation regardless of site (77).

Research is needed to identify successful options for long-term maintenance programs that address problems such as sustainable motivation, adherence, cost, and accessibility. Additionally, randomized controlled trials are needed to improve understanding of the more unique needs of patients with nonobstructive lung diseases such as ILD and PAH.

SUMMARY

By adapting basic exercise training guidelines to patient capabilities and disease-specific concerns, individuals with chronic lung disease can successfully perform exercise training regardless of the illness severity level. Disease-specific concerns can be easily identified with a basic understanding of lung pathophysiology because it relates to pattern recognition for each of the disease categories. These principles also facilitate identification of the proper therapeutic interventions. Incorporating modifications based on the individual's response to exercise can further augment individualization of the exercise program. The response to exercise is best judged by understanding basic pathophysiology and recognizing the meaning and measurement of certain signs and symptoms.

REFERENCES

1. American Association of Cardiovascular and Pulmonary Rehabilitation. *Guidelines for Pulmonary Rehabilitation Programs.* 3rd ed. Champaign (IL): Human Kinetics; 2004. 188 p.
2. American Thoracic Society, American College of Chest Physicians. ATS/ACCP Statement on cardiopulmonary exercise testing. *Am J Respir Crit Care Med.* 2003;167(2):211–77.
3. Amin S, Abrazado M, Quinn M, Storer TW, Tseng CH, Cooper CB. Feasibility of community-based exercise training in patients with moderate COPD: a controlled pilot study. *Eur Respr J.* In press.
4. Arena R. Exercise testing and training in chronic lung disease and pulmonary arterial hypertension. *Prog Cardiovasc Dis.* 2011;53(6):454–63.
5. Arnardottir RH, Boman G, Larsson K, Hedenstrom H, Emtner M. Interval training compared with continuous training in patients with COPD. *Respir Med.* 2007;101(6):1196–204.
6. Åstrand P, Rodahl K. *Textbook of Work Physiology: Physiological Bases of Exercise.* 3rd ed. New York (NY): McGraw Hill; 1986. 756 p.
7. ATS Committee on Proficiency Standards for Clinical Pulmonary Function Laboratories. ATS statement: guidelines for the six-minute walk test. *Am J Respir Crit Care Med.* 2002;166(1):111–7.
8. Baechle TR, Earle RW, Wathen D. Resistance training. In: Baechle TR, Earle RW, National Strength & Conditioning Association (U.S.), editors. *Essentials of Strength Training and Conditioning.* 2nd ed. Champaign: Human Kinetics; 2000. p. 406–417.
9. Barnes PJ. *Asthma and COPD: Basic Mechanisms and Clinical Management.* London (United Kingdom): Academic Press; 2002. 780 p.
10. Barnes PJ. Asthma management: can we further improve compliance and outcomes? *Respir Med.* 2004;98 Suppl A:S8–9.
11. Barnes PJ, Shapiro SD, Pauwels RA. Chronic obstructive pulmonary disease: molecular and cellular mechanisms. *Eur Respir J.* 2003;22(4):672–88.
12. Barst RJ, McGoon M, Torbicki A, et al. Diagnosis and differential assessment of pulmonary arterial hypertension. *J Am Coll Cardiol.* 2004;43(12 Suppl S):40S–7S.
13. Beauchamp MK, Nonoyama M, Goldstein RS, et al. Interval versus continuous training in individuals with chronic obstructive pulmonary disease—a systematic review. *Thorax.* 2010;65(2):157–64.
14. Belman MJ, Shadmehr R. Targeted resistive ventilatory muscle training in chronic obstructive pulmonary disease. *J Appl Physiol.* 1988;65(6):2726–35.
15. Bernard S, LeBlanc P, Whittom F, et al. Peripheral muscle weakness in patients with chronic obstructive pulmonary disease. *Am J Respir Crit Care Med.* 1998;158(2):629–34.
16. Bestall JC, Paul EA, Garrod R, Garnham R, Jones PW, Wedzicha JA. Usefulness of the Medical Research Council (MRC) dyspnoea scale as a measure of disability in patients with chronic obstructive pulmonary disease. *Thorax.* 1999;54(7):581–6.
17. Borg G. *Borg's Perceived Exertion and Pain Scales.* Champaign (IL): Human Kinetics; 1998. 104 p.
18. Bradley J, Moran F, Greenstone M. Physical training for bronchiectasis. *Cochrane Database Syst Rev.* 2002(3):CD002166.
19. Cambach W, Chadwick-Straver RV, Wagenaar RC, van Keimpema AR, Kemper HC. The effects of a community-based pulmonary rehabilitation programme on exercise tolerance and quality of life: a randomized controlled trial. *Eur Respir J.* 1997;10(1):104–13.
20. Carlsen KH, Carlsen KC. Exercise-induced asthma. *Paediatr Respir Rev.* 2002;3(2):154–60.
21. Casaburi R, Patessio A, Ioli F, Zanaboni S, Donner CF, Wasserman K. Reductions in exercise lactic acidosis and ventilation as a result of exercise training in patients with obstructive lung disease. *Am Rev Respir Dis.* 1991;143(1):9–18.
22. Casaburi R, Porszasz J. Constant work rate exercise testing: a tricky measure of exercise tolerance. *COPD.* 2009;6(5):317–9.
23. Celli BR. Pathophysiology of chronic obstructive pulmonary disease. In: Hodgkin JE, Celli BR, Connors GL, editors. *Pulmonary*

Rehabilitation: Guidelines to Success. 3rd ed. Philadelphia: Lippincott Williams & Wilkins; 2000. p. 41–55.

24. Celli BR. Pulmonary rehabilitation for COPD. A practical approach for improving ventilatory conditioning. *Postgrad Med.* 1998;103(4):159–60, 167–8, 173–6.

25. Celli BR, Cote CG, Marin JM, et al. The body-mass index, airflow obstruction, dyspnea, and exercise capacity index in chronic obstructive pulmonary disease. *N Engl J Med.* 2004;350(10): 1005–12.

26. Chida M, Inase N, Ichioka M, Miyazato I, Marumo F. Ratings of perceived exertion in chronic obstructive pulmonary disease— a possible indicator for exercise training in patients with this disease. *Eur J Appl Physiol Occup Physiol.* 1991;62(6):390–3.

27. Cooper CB. Exercise in chronic pulmonary disease: aerobic exercise prescription. *Med Sci Sports Exerc.* 2001;33(7 Suppl):S671–9.

28. Cooper CB. Exercise in chronic pulmonary disease: limitations and rehabilitation. *Med Sci Sports Exerc.* 2001;33(7 Suppl):S643–6.

29. Cooper CB. The connection between chronic obstructive pulmonary disease symptoms and hyperinflation and its impact on exercise and function. *Am J Med.* 2006;119(10 Suppl 1):21–31.

30. Cooper CB, Storer TW. *Exercise Testing and Interpretation: A Practical Approach*. New York (NY): Cambridge University Press; 2001. 278 p.

31. Cooper CB, Tashkin DP. Recent developments in inhaled therapy in stable chronic obstructive pulmonary disease. *BMJ.* 2005; 330(7492):640–4.

32. Crapo RO, Casaburi R, Coates AL, et al. Guidelines for methacholine and exercise challenge testing—1999. This official statement of the American Thoracic Society was adopted by the ATS Board of Directors, July 1999. *Am J Respir Crit Care Med.* 2000;161(1): 309–29.

33. Crouch R, MacIntyre NR. Pulmonary rehabilitation of the patient with nonobstructive lung disease. *Respir Care Clin N Am.* 1998;4(1):59–70.

34. Dal Corso S, Napolis L, Malaguti C, et al. Skeletal muscle structure and function in response to electrical stimulation in moderately impaired COPD patients. *Respir Med.* 2007;101(6):1236–43.

35. *Data Fact Sheet: Asthma Statistics* [Internet]. Bethesda (MD): National Institutes of Health, National Heart, Lung, and Blood Institute; 1999 [cited 2011 Mar 15]. 4p. Available from: http:// www.nhlbi.nih.gov/health/prof/lung/asthma/asthstat.pdf

36. Decramer M, Gosselink R, Troosters T, Verschueren M, Evers G. Muscle weakness is related to utilization of health care resources in COPD patients. *Eur Respir J.* 1997;10(2):417–23.

37. Definition and classification of chronic bronchitis for clinical and epidemiological purposes. A report to the Medical Research Council by their Committee on the Aetiology of Chronic Bronchitis. *Lancet.* 1965;1(7389):775–9.

38. Desai TJ, Karlinsky JB. OPD: clinical manifestations, diagnosis, and treatment. In: Baum GL, Crapo JD, editors. *Baum's Textbook of Pulmonary Diseases*. 7th ed. Philadelphia: Lippincott Williams & Wilkins; 2004. p. 204–246.

39. Despres JP, Lamarche B. Low-intensity endurance exercise training, plasma lipoproteins and the risk of coronary heart disease. *J Intern Med.* 1994;236(1):7–22.

40. Dolmage TE, Goldstein RS. Effects of one-legged exercise training of patients with COPD. *Chest.* 2008;133(2):370–6.

41. Dolmage TE, Goldstein RS. Response to one-legged cycling in patients with COPD. *Chest.* 2006;129(2):325–32.

42. Effing T, Zielhuis G, Kerstjens H, van der Valk P, van der Palen J. Community based physiotherapeutic exercise in COPD self-management: a randomised controlled trial. *Respir Med.* 2011;105(3):418–26.

43. Elliott M, Watson C, Wilkinson E, Musk AW, Lake FR. Short- and long-term hospital and community exercise programmes for patients with chronic obstructive pulmonary disease. *Respirology.* 2004;9(3):345–51.

44. *Expert Panel Report 2: Guidelines for the Diagnosis and Management of Asthma* [Internet]. Bethesda (MD): National Asthma Education and Prevention Program, Second Expert Panel on the Management of Asthma; 1997 [cited 2011 Mar 15]. 146 p. Available from: http://www.ncbi.nlm.nih.gov/books/NBK2358/

45. *Expert Panel Report 3: Guidelines for the Diagnosis and Management of Asthma* [Internet]. Bethesda (MD): National Heart, Lung, and Blood Institute National Asthma Education and Prevention Program; 2007 [cited 2011 Mar 15]. 417 p. Available from: http://www.nhlbi.nih.gov/guidelines/asthma/asthgdln.pdf

46. Ferguson GT, Cherniack RM. Management of chronic obstructive pulmonary disease. *N Engl J Med.* 1993;328(14):1017–22.

47. Ferreira A, Garvey C, Connors GL, et al. Pulmonary rehabilitation in interstitial lung disease: benefits and predictors of response. *Chest.* 2009;135(2):442–7.

48. Foster S, Thomas HM 3rd. Pulmonary rehabilitation in lung disease other than chronic obstructive pulmonary disease. *Am Rev Respir Dis.* 1990;141(3):601–4.

49. Gimenez M, Servera E, Vergara P, Bach JR, Polu JM. Endurance training in patients with chronic obstructive pulmonary disease: a comparison of high versus moderate intensity. *Arch Phys Med Rehabil.* 2000;81(1):102–9.

50. Global Initiative for Chronic Obstructive Lung Disease Web site [Internet]. Global Initiative for Chronic Obstructive Lung Disease; [cited 2011 Mar 15]. Available from: http://www.goldcopd.com/

51. *Global Strategy for Asthma Management and Prevention* [Internet]. GINA: Global Initiative for Asthma; 2009 [cited 2008 Oct 8]. 456 p. Available from: http://www.ginasthma.org/Guidelineitem .asp??l1=2&l2=1&intId=1561

52. Gosselink R, Wagenaar RC, Decramer M. Reliability of a commercially available threshold loading device in healthy subjects and in patients with chronic obstructive pulmonary disease. *Thorax.* 1996;51(6):601–5.

53. Griffiths TL, Burr ML, Campbell IA, et al. Results at 1 year of outpatient multidisciplinary pulmonary rehabilitation: a randomised controlled trial. *Lancet.* 2000;355(9201):362–8.

54. Guell R, Resqueti V, Sangenis M, et al. Impact of pulmonary rehabilitation on psychosocial morbidity in patients with severe COPD. *Chest.* 2006;129(4):899–904.

55. Guidelines for the approach to the patient with severe hereditary alpha-1-antitrypsin deficiency. American Thoracic Society. *Am Rev Respir Dis.* 1989;140(5):1494–7.

56. Han MK, Postma D, Mannino DM, et al. Gender and chronic obstructive pulmonary disease: why it matters. *Am J Respir Crit Care Med.* 2007;176(12):1179–84.

57. Harris-Eze AO, Sridhar G, Clemens RE, Zintel TA, Gallagher CG, Marciniuk DD. Role of hypoxemia and pulmonary mechanics in exercise limitation in interstitial lung disease. *Am J Respir Crit Care Med.* 1996;154(4 Pt 1):994–1001.

58. Hilleman DE, Dewan N, Malesker M, Friedman M. Pharmacoeconomic evaluation of COPD. *Chest.* 2000;118(5):1278–85.

59. Hoff J, Tjonna AE, Steinshamn S, Hoydal M, Richardson RS, Helgerud J. Maximal strength training of the legs in COPD: a therapy for mechanical inefficiency. *Med Sci Sports Exerc.* 2007;39(2): 220–6.

60. Hogg JC, Senior RM. Chronic obstructive pulmonary disease—part 2: pathology and biochemistry of emphysema. *Thorax.* 2002;57(9): 830–4.

61. Holland AE, Hill CJ, Conron M, Munro P, McDonald CF. Short term improvement in exercise capacity and symptoms following exercise training in interstitial lung disease. *Thorax.* 2008;63(6):549–54.

62. Horowitz MB, Littenberg B, Mahler DA. Dyspnea ratings for prescribing exercise intensity in patients with COPD. *Chest.* 1996;109(5):1169–75.

63. Houchen L, Steiner MC, Singh SJ. How sustainable is strength training in chronic obstructive pulmonary disease? *Physiotherapy.* 2009;95(1):1–7.

64. Hunt SA, Baker DW, Chin MH, et al. ACC/AHA Guidelines for the Evaluation and Management of Chronic Heart Failure in the Adult: Executive Summary A Report of the American College of Cardiology/American Heart Association Task Force on Practice Guidelines (Committee to Revise the 1995 Guidelines for the Evaluation and Management of Heart Failure): developed in collaboration with the International Society for Heart and Lung Transplantation; Endorsed by the Heart Failure Society of America. *Circulation.* 2001;104(24):2996–3007.

65. In chronic obstructive pulmonary disease, a combination of ipratropium and albuterol is more effective than either agent alone. An 85-day multicenter trial. COMBIVENT Inhalation Aerosol Study Group. *Chest.* 1994;105(5):1411–9.

66. Jeffery PK, Godfrey RW, Adelroth E, Nelson F, Rogers A, Johansson SA. Effects of treatment on airway inflammation and thickening of basement membrane reticular collagen in asthma. A quantitative light and electron microscopic study. *Am Rev Respir Dis.* 1992;145(4 Pt 1):890–9.

67. Kaelin ME, Swank AM, Adams KJ, Barnard KL, Berning JM, Green A. Cardiopulmonary responses, muscle soreness, and injury during the one repetition maximum assessment in pulmonary rehabilitation patients. *J Cardiopulm Rehabil.* 1999;19(6):366–72.

68. Kortianou EA, Nasis IG, Spetsioti ST, Daskalakis AM, Vogiatzis I. Effectiveness of interval exercise training in patients with COPD. *Cardiopulm Phys Ther J.* 2010;21(3):12–9.

69. Langer D, Hendriks E, Burtin C, et al. A clinical practice guideline for physiotherapists treating patients with chronic obstructive pulmonary disease based on a systematic review of available evidence. *Clin Rehabil.* 2009;23(5):445–62.

70. Larson JL, Covey MK, Wirtz SE, et al. Cycle ergometer and inspiratory muscle training in chronic obstructive pulmonary disease. *Am J Respir Crit Care Med.* 1999;160(2):500–7.

71. Lee TH, Anderson SD. Heterogeneity of mechanisms in exercise induced asthma. *Thorax.* 1985;40(7):481–7.

72. Lisboa C, Villafranca C, Leiva A, Cruz E, Pertuze J, Borzone G. Inspiratory muscle training in chronic airflow limitation: effect on exercise performance. *Eur Respir J.* 1997;10(3):537–42.

73. Mador MJ, Bozkanat E. Skeletal muscle dysfunction in chronic obstructive pulmonary disease. *Respir Res.* 2001;2(4):216–24.

74. Mador MJ, Krawza M, Alhajhusian A, Khan AI, Shaffer M, Kufel TJ. Interval training versus continuous training in patients with chronic obstructive pulmonary disease. *J Cardiopulm Rehabil Prev.* 2009;29(2):126–32.

75. Mahler DA, Horowitz MB. Perception of breathlessness during exercise in patients with respiratory disease. *Med Sci Sports Exerc.* 1994;26(9):1078–81.

76. Mannino DM, Buist AS. Global burden of COPD: risk factors, prevalence, and future trends. *Lancet.* 2007;370(9589):765–73.

77. Marciniuk DD, Brooks D, Butcher S, et al. Optimizing pulmonary rehabilitation in chronic obstructive pulmonary disease—practical issues: a Canadian Thoracic Society Clinical Practice Guideline. *Can Respir J.* 2010;17(4):159–68.

78. Marciniuk DD, Sridhar G, Clemens RE, Zintel TA, Gallagher CG. Lung volumes and expiratory flow limitation during exercise in interstitial lung disease. *J Appl Physiol.* 1994;77(2):963–73.

79. Marciniuk DD, Watts RE, Gallagher CG. Dead space loading and exercise limitation in patients with interstitial lung disease. *Chest.* 1994;105(1):183–9.

80. Markovitz GH, Cooper CB. Exercise and interstitial lung disease. *Curr Opin Pulm Med.* 1998;4(5):272–80.

81. Markovitz GH, Cooper CB. Rehabilitation in non-COPD: mechanisms of exercise limitation and pulmonary rehabilitation for patients with pulmonary fibrosis/restrictive lung disease. *Chron Respir Dis.* 2010;7(1):47–60.

82. Mascolo MC, Truwit JD. Role of exercise evaluation in restrictive lung disease: new insights between March 2001 and February 2003. *Curr Opin Pulm Med.* 2003;9(5):408–10.

83. McGoon M, Gutterman D, Steen V, et al. Screening, early detection, and diagnosis of pulmonary arterial hypertension: ACCP evidence-based clinical practice guidelines. *Chest.* 2004;126 (1 Suppl):14S–34S.

84. Mereles D, Ehlken N, Kreuscher S, et al. Exercise and respiratory training improve exercise capacity and quality of life in patients with severe chronic pulmonary hypertension. *Circulation.* 2006; 114(14):1482–9.

85. Miller MR, Hankinson J, Brusasco V, et al. Standardisation of spirometry. *Eur Respir J.* 2005;26(2):319–38.

86. Murray JF, Nadel JA. Part 2: Manifestations and diagnosis of respiratory disease. In: Murray JF, Nadel JA, editors. *Textbook of Respiratory Medicine.* 3rd ed. Philadelphia: Saunders; 2000. p. 539–912.

87. Naji NA, Connor MC, Donnelly SC, McDonnell TJ. Effectiveness of pulmonary rehabilitation in restrictive lung disease. *J Cardiopulm Rehabil.* 2006;26(4):237–43.

88. Neder JA, Sword D, Ward SA, Mackay E, Cochrane LM, Clark CJ. Home based neuromuscular electrical stimulation as a new rehabilitative strategy for severely disabled patients with chronic obstructive pulmonary disease (COPD). *Thorax.* 2002;57(4):333–7.

89. Nelson ME, Rejeski WJ, Blair SN, et al. Physical activity and public health in older adults: recommendation from the American College of Sports Medicine and the American Heart Association. *Med Sci Sports Exerc.* 2007;39(8):1435–45.

90. Newall C, Stockley RA, Hill SL. Exercise training and inspiratory muscle training in patients with bronchiectasis. *Thorax.* 2005;60(11):943–8.

91. Newman KB, Mason UG 3rd, Schmaling KB. Clinical features of vocal cord dysfunction. *Am J Respir Crit Care Med.* 1995;152(4 Pt 1):1382–6.

92. Newman JH, Robbins IM. Exercise training in pulmonary hypertension: implications for the evaluation of drug trials. *Circulation.* 2006;114(14):1448–9.

93. Nici L, Donner C, Wouters E, et al. American Thoracic Society/ European Respiratory Society statement on pulmonary rehabilitation. *Am J Respir Crit Care Med.* 2006;173(12):1390–413.

94. Nield MA, Soo Hoo GW, Roper JM, Santiago S. Efficacy of pursedlips breathing: a breathing pattern retraining strategy for dyspnea reduction. *J Cardiopulm Rehabil Prev.* 2007;27(4):237–44.

95. O'Donnell DE, Fluge T, Gerken F, et al. Effects of tiotropium on lung hyperinflation, dyspnoea and exercise tolerance in COPD. *Eur Respir J.* 2004;23(6):832–40.

96. O'Donnell DE, Revill SM, Webb KA. Dynamic hyperinflation and exercise intolerance in chronic obstructive pulmonary disease. *Am J Respir Crit Care Med.* 2001;164(5):770–7.

97. Ong HK, Lee AL, Hill CJ, Holland AE, Denehy L. Effects of pulmonary rehabilitation in bronchiectasis: a retrospective study. *Chron Respir Dis.* 2011;8(1):21–30.

98. O'Shea SD, Taylor NF, Paratz J. Peripheral muscle strength training in COPD: a systematic review. *Chest.* 2004;126(3):903–14.

99. O'Shea SD, Taylor NF, Paratz JD. Progressive resistance exercise improves muscle strength and may improve elements of performance of daily activities for people with COPD: a systematic review. *Chest.* 2009;136(5):1269–83.

100. Palange P, Wagner PD. "The skeletal muscle in chronic respiratory diseases", summary of the ERS research seminar in Rome, Italy, February 11–12 1999. *Eur Respir J.* 2000;15(4):807–15.

101. Pauwels RA, Buist AS, Ma P, Jenkins CR, Hurd SS, GOLD Scientific Committee. Global strategy for the diagnosis, management, and prevention of chronic obstructive pulmonary disease: National Heart, Lung, and Blood Institute and World Health Organization Global Initiative for Chronic Obstructive Lung Disease (GOLD): executive summary. *Respir Care.* 2001;46(8):798–825.

102. Paz-Diaz H, Montes de Oca M, Lopez JM, Celli BR. Pulmonary rehabilitation improves depression, anxiety, dyspnea and health

status in patients with COPD. *Am J Phys Med Rehabil.* 2007; 86(1):30–6.

103. Pellegrino R, Viegi G, Brusasco V, et al. Interpretative strategies for lung function tests. *Eur Respir J.* 2005;26(5):948–68.

104. Pescatello LS, Arena R, Riebe D, American College of Sports Medicine. *ACSM's Guidelines for Exercise Testing and Prescription.* 9th ed. Philadelphia (PA): Lippincott Williams & Wilkins; 2012. 380 p.

105. Pierson WE, Voy RO. Exercise-induced bronchospasm in the XXIII summer Olympic games. *N Engl Reg Allergy Proc.* 1988;9(3): 209–13.

106. Postma DS, Boezen HM. Rationale for the Dutch hypothesis. Allergy and airway hyperresponsiveness as genetic factors and their interaction with environment in the development of asthma and COPD. *Chest.* 2004;126(2 Suppl):96S–104S; discussion 159S–61S.

107. Pulmonary rehabilitation: joint ACCP/AACVPR evidence-based guidelines. ACCP/AACVPR Pulmonary Rehabilitation Guidelines Panel. American College of Chest Physicians. American Association of Cardiovascular and Pulmonary Rehabilitation. *Chest.* 1997;112(5):1363–96.

108. Rabe KF, Hurd S, Anzueto A, et al. Global strategy for the diagnosis, management, and prevention of chronic obstructive pulmonary disease: GOLD executive summary. *Am J Respir Crit Care Med.* 2007;176(6):532–55.

109. Ram FS, Robinson SM, Black PN, Picot J. Physical training for asthma. *Cochrane Database Syst Rev.* 2005;(4):CD001116.

110. Ries AL, Bauldoff GS, Carlin BW, et al. Pulmonary Rehabilitation: Joint ACCP/AACVPR Evidence-Based Clinical Practice Guidelines. *Chest.* 2007;131(5 Suppl):4S–42S.

111. Ries AL, Kaplan RM, Limberg TM, Prewitt LM. Effects of pulmonary rehabilitation on physiologic and psychosocial outcomes in patients with chronic obstructive pulmonary disease. *Ann Intern Med.* 1995;122(11):823–32.

112. Rubin LJ. Primary pulmonary hypertension. *N Engl J Med.* 1997;336(2):111–7.

113. Ryu JH, Myers JL, Swensen SJ. Bronchiolar disorders. *Am J Respir Crit Care Med.* 2003;168(11):1277–92.

114. Sanchez RH, Montemayor RT, Ortega RF, et al. Inspiratory muscle training in patients with COPD: effect on dyspnea, exercise performance, and quality of life. *Chest.* 2001;120(3):748–56.

115. Sassi-Dambron DE, Eakin EG, Ries AL, Kaplan RM. Treatment of dyspnea in COPD. A controlled clinical trial of dyspnea management strategies. *Chest.* 1995;107(3):724–9.

116. Scherer TA, Spengler CM, Owassapian D, Imhof E, Boutellier U. Respiratory muscle endurance training in chronic obstructive pulmonary disease: impact on exercise capacity, dyspnea, and quality of life. *Am J Respir Crit Care Med.* 2000;162(5): 1709–14.

117. Sciurba FC. Physiologic similarities and differences between COPD and asthma. *Chest.* 2004;126(2 Suppl):117S–24S; discussion 159S–61S.

118. Sietsema K. Cardiovascular limitations in chronic pulmonary disease. *Med Sci Sports Exerc.* 2001;33(7 Suppl):S656–61.

119. Sillen MJ, Speksnijder CM, Eterman RM, et al. Effects of neuromuscular electrical stimulation of muscles of ambulation in patients with chronic heart failure or COPD: a systematic review of the English-language literature. *Chest.* 2009;136(1):44–61.

120. Silverman E, Ebright L, Kwiatkowski M, Cullina J. Current management of bronchiectasis: review and 3 case studies. *Heart Lung.* 2003;32(1):59–64.

121. Simonneau G, Galie N, Rubin LJ, et al. Clinical classification of pulmonary hypertension. *J Am Coll Cardiol.* 2004;43(12 Suppl S): 5S–12S.

122. Sin DD, McAlister FA, Man SF, Anthonisen NR. Contemporary management of chronic obstructive pulmonary disease: scientific review. *JAMA.* 2003;290(17):2301–12.

123. Singh SJ, Morgan MD, Scott S, Walters D, Hardman AE. Development of a shuttle walking test of disability in patients with chronic airways obstruction. *Thorax.* 1992;47(12):1019–24.

124. Skeletal muscle dysfunction in chronic obstructive pulmonary disease. A statement of the American Thoracic Society and European Respiratory Society. *Am J Respir Crit Care Med.* 1999;159(4 Pt 2):S1–40.

125. Smidt N, de Vet HC, Bouter LM, et al. Effectiveness of exercise therapy: a best-evidence summary of systematic reviews. *Aust J Physiother.* 2005;51(2):71–85.

126. Storer TW. Exercise in chronic pulmonary disease: resistance exercise prescription. *Med Sci Sports Exerc.* 2001;33(7 Suppl): S680–92.

127. Strasser B, Siebert U, Schobersberger W. Effects of resistance training on respiratory function in patients with chronic obstructive pulmonary disease: a systematic review and meta-analysis. *Sleep Breath.* 2012.

128. Sutherland ER, Kraft M, Crapo JD. Diagnosis and treatment of asthma. In: Baum GL, Crapo JD, editors. *Baum's Textbook of Pulmonary Diseases.* 7th ed. Philadelphia: Lippincott Williams & Wilkins; 2004. p. 179–198.

129. Swallow EB, Reyes D, Hopkinson NS, et al. Quadriceps strength predicts mortality in patients with moderate to severe chronic obstructive pulmonary disease. *Thorax.* 2007;62(2):115–20.

130. Thompson S. On the social cost of asthma. *Eur J Respir Dis Suppl.* 1984;136:185–91.

131. Tiddens H, Silverman M, Bush A. The role of inflammation in airway disease: remodeling. *Am J Respir Crit Care Med.* 2000;162 (2 Pt 2):S7–S10.

132. Tiep BL. Pursed lips breathing-easing does it. *J Cardiopulm Rehabil Prev.* 2007;27(4):245–6.

133. Tiep BL, Burns M, Kao D, Madison R, Herrera J. Pursed lips breathing training using ear oximetry. *Chest.* 1986;90(2):218–21.

134. Vallet G, Ahmaidi S, Serres I, et al. Comparison of two training programmes in chronic airway limitation patients: standardized versus individualized protocols. *Eur Respir J.* 1997;10(1):114–22.

135. van Wetering CR, Hoogendoorn M, Mol SJ, Rutten-van Molken MP, Schols AM. Short- and long-term efficacy of a community-based COPD management programme in less advanced COPD: a randomised controlled trial. *Thorax.* 2010;65(1):7–13.

136. Verrill D, Barton C, Beasley W, Lippard WM. The effects of short-term and long-term pulmonary rehabilitation on functional capacity, perceived dyspnea, and quality of life. *Chest.* 2005;128(2):673–83.

137. Vivodtzev I, Lacasse Y, Maltais F. Neuromuscular electrical stimulation of the lower limbs in patients with chronic obstructive pulmonary disease. *J Cardiopulm Rehabil Prev.* 2008;28(2): 79–91.

138. Vivodtzev I, Pepin JL, Vottero G, et al. Improvement in quadriceps strength and dyspnea in daily tasks after 1 month of electrical stimulation in severely deconditioned and malnourished COPD. *Chest.* 2006;129(6):1540–8.

139. Vogiatzis I. Strategies of muscle training in very severe COPD patients. *Eur Respir J.* 2011;38(4):971–5.

140. Vogiatzis I, Nanas S, Roussos C. Interval training as an alternative modality to continuous exercise in patients with COPD. *Eur Respir J.* 2002;20(1):12–9.

141. Wasserman K. Exercise tolerance in the pulmonary patient. In: Casaburi R, Petty TL, editors. *Principles and Practice of Pulmonary Rehabilitation.* Philadelphia: Saunders; 1993. p. 119–121.

142. Waterhouse JC, Walters SJ, Oluboyede Y, Lawson RA. A randomised 2 × 2 trial of community versus hospital pulmonary rehabilitation, followed by telephone or conventional follow-up. *Health Technol Assess.* 2010;14(6):i–v, vii–xi, 1–140.

143. Weiler JM. Exercise-induced asthma: a practical guide to definitions, diagnosis, prevalence, and treatment. *Allergy Asthma Proc.* 1996;17(6):315–25.

144. Weiner P, Magadle R, Beckerman M, Weiner M, Berar-Yanay N. Comparison of specific expiratory, inspiratory, and combined muscle training programs in COPD. *Chest.* 2003;124(4):1357–64.

145. Weiner P, Magadle R, Beckerman M, Weiner M, Berar-Yanay N. Maintenance of inspiratory muscle training in COPD patients: one year follow-up. *Eur Respir J.* 2004;23(1):61–5.

146. Weiss KB, Sullivan SD. The economic costs of asthma: a review and conceptual model. *Pharmacoeconomics.* 1993;4(1):14–30.

147. Williams MA, Haskell WL, Ades PA, et al. Resistance exercise in individuals with and without cardiovascular disease: 2007 update: a scientific statement from the American Heart Association Council on Clinical Cardiology and Council on Nutrition, Physical Activity, and Metabolism. *Circulation.* 2007;116(5):572–84.

148. Zainuldin R, Mackey MG, Alison JA. Optimal intensity and type of leg exercise training for people with chronic obstructive pulmonary disease. *Cochrane Database Syst Rev.* 2011(11):CD008008.

SELECTED REFERENCES FOR FURTHER READING

American Association of Cardiovascular and Pulmonary Rehabilitation. *AACVPR Guidelines for Pulmonary Rehabilitation Programs.* 4th ed. Champaign (IL): Human Kinetics; 2010. 184 p.

Durstine JL, Moore GE, Painter PL, Roberts SO, editors. *ACSM's Exercise Management for Persons with Chronic Diseases and Disabilities.* 3rd ed. Champaign (IL): Human Kinetics; 2009. 456 p.

Leung RW, Alison JA, McKeough ZJ, Peters MJ. Ground walk training improves functional exercise capacity more than cycle training in people with chronic obstructive pulmonary disease (COPD): a randomised trial. *J Physiother.* 2010;56(2):105–12.

Song B, Wolf KH, Gietzelt M, et al. Decision support for teletraining of COPD patients. *Methods Inf Med.* 2010;49(1):96–102.

INTERNET RESOURCES

- American Thoracic Society (statements): http://www.thoracic.org/statements
- Global Initiative for Asthma (GINA) Workshop Reports: http://www.ginasthma.com/
- Global Initiative for Chronic Lung Disease: http://www.goldcopd.com
- National Asthma Education and Prevention Program (Expert Panel report 2: Guidelines for the diagnosis and management of asthma): http://www.nhlbi.nih.gov/guidelines/asthma/asthgdln.htm
- National Clinical Guideline Clearinghouse (Pulmonary Rehabilitation): http://guidelines.gov/content.aspx?id=10856

Exercise Prescription for Patients with Diabetes

Diabetes mellitus is characterized by abnormal glucose metabolism resulting from defects in insulin release, action, or both (7). This complex metabolic disease requires rigorous self-management combined with an appropriate balance of nutritional intake, medication(s), and regular physical activity (PA)/exercise for blood glucose control.

This chapter focuses on the most common forms of diabetes, including Type 1 diabetes mellitus (T1DM), Type 2 diabetes mellitus (T2DM), and gestational diabetes mellitus (GDM). Each type of diabetes is distinct in etiology (7) and, subsequently, in exercise programming. Safe and effective exercise recommendations are presented to assist in diabetes management and accompanying diabetes-related health complications.

EPIDEMIOLOGY AND CHARACTERIZATION OF DIABETES MELLITUS

According to the latest estimates, nearly 26 million Americans have diabetes, with one-quarter of cases still undiagnosed, and another 79 million adults have prediabetes (127). Four types of diabetes are recognized based on etiologic origin: Type 1, Type 2, gestational

KEY TERMS

Autonomic neuropathy: Disease affecting the nerves innervating the heart, gastrointestinal, and genitourinary tract; cardiovascular autonomic neuropathy (CAN) is the most common and clinically important type of this neuropathy.

Continuous glucose monitoring: Newer technologies that allow for subcutaneous monitoring of glucose levels with frequent readings (usually every 5 min) for a week or more per probe insertion.

Diabetic ketoacidosis (DKA): High level of blood ketones (*e.g.*, β-hydroxybutyrate, acetoacetate, acetone), accompanied by hyperglycemia, that can result in coma or death if not treated.

Estimated average glucose: Alternate method to report glycated hemoglobin (HbA1C) levels, in $mg \cdot dL^{-1}$ of plasma glucose, in which estimated average glucose = $(28.7 \times HbA1C) - 46.7$ (*e.g.*, HbA1C value of 6.0% equates to an estimated average glucose of $126 \, mg \cdot dL^{-1}$).

Gestational diabetes mellitus (GDM): A hyperglycemic condition developing most often during the third trimester of pregnancy (when placental hormones decrease insulin action); although it usually resolves postpartum, it is associated with a greater risk for the mother of developing Type 2 diabetes later in life (102).

Glycated hemoglobin (HbA1C): Test to assess glycemic control over the previous 2–3 mo based on the percentage of hemoglobin that is glycated (bound with glucose); a normal value is ~4.0%–6.0%.

Hyperglycemia: High plasma glucose level (*e.g.*, $\geq 126 \, mg \cdot dL^{-1}$).

Hypoglycemia: Low plasma glucose level (*e.g.*, $< 70 \, mg \cdot dL^{-1}$).

Insulin resistance: A condition in which there is a relative lack of insulin action in insulin-sensitive tissues (primarily skeletal muscle) needed to maintain normal glucose levels.

Latent autoimmune diabetes of the adult (LADA): A form of Type 1 diabetes that is often slower in onset and diagnosed in adults; also known as Type 1.5 diabetes.

Metabolic syndrome: A syndrome characterized by a constellation of disorders, including insulin resistance/glucose intolerance/diabetes, obesity, central adiposity, dyslipidemia, and hypertension.

Nephropathy: A disease affecting the kidneys resulting in excessive urinary protein (microalbuminuria) as a marker of end-stage renal disease.

Peripheral neuropathy: Disease affecting the nerves in the extremities, especially the lower legs and feet, resulting in pain and/or loss of sensation and increased risk of amputation.

Retinopathy: A disease caused by long-term damage to blood vessels of the retina caused by elevated blood glucose levels; the stages include nonproliferative (less severe) and proliferative (more advanced and severe form), which is the leading cause of new blindness in adults.

Self-monitoring of blood glucose: The practice of using blood glucose monitoring devices outside of clinical settings to monitor changes in blood glucose levels.

Type 1 diabetes mellitus (T1DM): Immune-mediated disease that selectively destroys the pancreatic β-cells, leading to a central defect in insulin release upon stimulation; although associated more with youth, this type of diabetes is often diagnosed in adults as LADA.

Type 2 diabetes mellitus (T2DM): Disease formerly afflicting persons older than 40 yr, is directly related to insulin resistance, and is increasing in prevalence among younger children and adolescents; accounts for 90%–95% of all diabetes.

(*i.e.*, diagnosed during pregnancy), and other specific origins (*i.e.*, genetic defects, drug induced); however, most cases are of Type 2 (90% of all cases), followed by Type 1 (5%–10% of all cases) (37,38). Diagnostic and classification criteria of diabetes focus on cause and pathogenesis (7) (see *Chapter 8*).

Although T1DM is one of the most common chronic diseases diagnosed in children, about half of all cases occur in adults of varying ages — known as latent autoimmune diabetes of the adult (LADA) (7). Likewise, although T2DM was formerly seen mostly among older adults, its diagnosis in youth has risen dramatically over the past two decades (175). GDM is associated with a 40%–60% chance of developing T2DM in the next 5–10 yr (127). The burden of diabetes disproportionately affects minorities. The prevalence rates are about twofold greater in Hispanic/Latino, non-Hispanic Black, Native American, Asian, and Pacific Islander populations compared with non-Hispanic Whites (127). It is now estimated that one in three Americans born in 2000 or later will develop diabetes during their lifetimes, with rates closer to 50% in high-risk, ethnic populations (125,126).

Diabetes increases the onset of diabetes-related complications, which exacerbate morbidity and increase the likelihood of physical limitation or disability (11,92). Hyperglycemia for an extended period is linked with chronic diabetes-related complications that worsen macrovascular, microvascular, and neural processes. Because of daily fluctuations in blood glucose occurring in diabetes, therapeutic interventions are aimed at blood glucose control, management of heart disease risk factors, and prevention of diabetes-related complications (11,65,69,163).

CLINICAL MANAGEMENT OF DIABETES MELLITUS

The diagnosis of diabetes mellitus is based on established criteria (7) (see *Chapter 8*). *Table 40-1* provides the major characteristics of T1DM and T2DM. Effective management involves use of self-monitoring of blood glucose, use of appropriate medications to regulate blood glucose levels,

regular participation in PA/exercise, and body weight management, as well as good dietary habits (7,11,167). Exercise interventions for individuals with diabetes should ideally involve a multidisciplinary team of specialists that includes a physician (*e.g.*, endocrinologist/diabetologist, internist), certified diabetes educator, registered dietician, and exercise professional to facilitate individual education and lifestyle changes to manage this disease (11). Self-management skills are essential to success, and diabetes education is an important tool to improve glycemic control (11).

BLOOD GLUCOSE MANAGEMENT

Precise hormonal and metabolic events that normally regulate glucose homeostasis are frequently disrupted in diabetes because of defects in insulin release, action, or both (7,47). Glucose control requires near-normal balance between hepatic glucose production and peripheral glucose uptake, combined with effective insulin responses (184). With diabetes, a reduced ability to precisely match glucose production and utilization results in daily glucose fluctuations and requires adjustments in dosages of exogenous insulin and/or antihyperglycemic medications. These adjustments should be combined with adequate changes in dietary intake, particularly when anticipating PA/exercise (143). Information about the use of insulin and oral agents to treat diabetes is provided in *Chapter 8*.

After diagnosis, clinical emphasis is placed on self-monitoring of blood glucose, which benefits glycemic control regardless of the type of diabetes (167). It usually involves at least three to six glucose checks per day by individuals with T1DM but much less frequent blood glucose monitoring by non-insulin users with T2DM (63). Continuous glucose monitoring can be very useful in detecting patterns in blood glucose across multiple days and evaluating both acute and delayed effects of exercise (3). Adjustments to insulin dose, oral medications, and/or carbohydrate intake can be fine-tuned using the detailed information provided by continuous glucose monitoring.

TABLE 40-1. Major Characteristics of Type 1 and Type 2 Diabetes

Factor	Type 1	Type 2
Age at onset	More often early in life but may occur at any age	Usually older than age 30 yr but may occur at any age
Type of onset	Rapid, with short duration of symptoms in children; slower progression with LADA later in life	Slow progression (*e.g.*, years)
Genetic susceptibility	HLA-related DR3 and DR4, ICAs, IAAs; limited family history	Frequent genetic background; not HLA related
Environmental factors	Virus, toxins, autoimmune stimulation	Obesity, poor nutrition, physical inactivity, POP exposure
Islet cell antibody	Present at onset	Usually not observed
Endogenous insulin	Minimal or absent	Stimulated response either adequate with delayed secretion or reduced but not absent; insulin resistance present
Nutritional status	Thin or overweight; catabolic state (recent weight loss)	Obese, overweight, or normal; little or no recent weight loss
Symptoms	Thirst, polyuria, polyphagia, fatigue	Mild or frequently none; acanthosis nigricans; PCOS in females
Ketosis	Common at onset or during insulin deficiency	Unusual (resistant to ketosis except during infection or stress)
Control of diabetes	Often difficult, with wide glucose fluctuation	Variable; helped by dietary adherence, weight loss, exercise
Dietary management	Essential but must be balanced with insulin dosage	Essential; may suffice for glycemic control
Insulin	Required for all	Required for ~40%
Oral hypoglycemics	Usually not effective (unless insulin resistant as well)	Effective

LADA, latent autoimmune diabetes of the adult; HLA, human leukocyte antigen; DR, D-related antigen; ICA, islet cell antibodies; IAA, insulin autoantibodies; POP, persistent organic pollutants; PCOS, polycystic ovary syndrome.

Concomitant lifestyle improvements (*i.e.*, dietary changes and PA/exercise) assist in the control of blood glucose levels and reduce the risk of acute and long-term diabetes-related complications (8,11). Overall glycemic control is assessed by measuring glycated hemoglobin (HbA1C or A1C), which reflects a time-averaged blood glucose concentration over the previous 2–3 mo. The recommended HbA1C goal is <7.0% (12). Using the estimated average glucose conversion, this goal equates to <154 mg · dL^{-1} (or 8.6 mmol · L^{-1}). HbA1C levels should ideally be assessed every 3–4 mo (7,11).

Insulin Injections or Continuous Subcutaneous Insulin Infusion

Treatment of T1DM requires multiple daily insulin injections or continuous subcutaneous insulin infusion (via a pump) to facilitate glucose uptake and control glucose levels (11). Insulin dosages (via pump or injection) may be reduced before, during, and/or following exercise to avoid hypoglycemia depending on the intensity, duration, and timing of the activity (1,52,55). Insulin adjustments involve a trial-and-error process that requires understanding of insulin action and the impact of exercise, food intake, and medication on glucose variability, combined with frequent self-monitoring of blood glucose

(1,24,52,55,171,172). Self-monitoring of blood glucose and appropriate regimen changes are the cornerstones of safe and effective blood glucose control during and following PA in insulin users (63,167).

Many individuals with T2DM are also prescribed insulin to assist in blood glucose management (179). In such cases, insulin may only be basal in nature (such as a once-daily injection of long-acting insulin like glargine or detemir) or may involve premeal injections of faster acting insulin. However, fear of weight gain, more frequent hypoglycemia, and other barriers to insulin use in T2DM may limit its effectiveness in this population (152). All insulin users, regardless of the type of diabetes, have a higher risk of exercise-induced hypoglycemia and should use self-monitoring of blood glucose, along with appropriate use of increased carbohydrate intake and decreased insulin dosages, to prevent hypoglycemia (77,89,173).

Some insulin users take injections of a synthetic analog (*i.e.*, pramlintide) to replace the hormone amylin that is usually cosecreted with insulin by the β-cells of the pancreas. The use of such an analog can complicate the treatment of exercise-induced hypoglycemia given that it slows the absorption of ingested carbohydrate from the gut and should likely not be taken before engaging in an acute bout of exercise (185).

Oral and Other Antihyperglycemic Medications

Oral agents are widely prescribed for T2DM when onset is recent and little (*e.g.*, <20 units) or no insulin is taken (11). Oral agents are prescribed individually or in combination to optimize glucose control. At present, oral and other injectable agents (besides insulin) that target different areas of the body are prescribed, including the pancreas (insulin release), liver (glucose production), and muscles (insulin action). Their general mechanisms of action are discussed briefly in the following section. Their relative risk of causing exercise-associated hypoglycemia is additionally listed in *Table 40-2*.

β-Cell Stimulants to Enhance Insulin Release

Medications that stimulate insulin release (primarily sulfonylureas and meglitinides) are taken at mealtime to better manage postprandial glycemia. Because of their effect on insulin release, these oral agents may lead to hypoglycemia with or without exercise (101). The prolonged length of action of some of these agents (*i.e.*, early generation sulfonylureas) increases the risk for low blood glucose and requires more frequent self-monitoring of blood glucose when individuals are regularly exercising.

Medications to Improve Insulin Sensitivity

Some diabetes medications improve insulin sensitivity in muscle tissue, adipose tissue, and the liver, whereas others promote muscle glucose uptake and inhibit hepatic glucose output. The most widely prescribed diabetes medication, metformin, targets both hepatic glucose output and peripheral insulin action (148). In general,

these medications mainly improve the action of insulin or lower hepatic glucose production at rest, not during exercise, so their risk of causing exercise-associated hypoglycemia is low (98).

Medications to Slow Intestinal Absorption of Carbohydrates

Medications that decrease carbohydrate absorption rate and slow the increase in postprandial blood glucose levels have no direct effect on exercise responses. However, they can delay effective treatment of hypoglycemia during activities by slowing the absorption of carbohydrates ingested to treat this condition (98). Some newer peptide analogs that are injectable (*e.g.*, exenatide and liraglutide) delay gastric emptying and also suppress the release of glucagon (145).

Medications to Mimic the Effects of Peptides

Some newer medications mimic the body's natural peptides (*i.e.*, incretin mimetics) or increase concentrations of peptides that prevent degradation of natural insulin-stimulating enzymes. One such medication, sitagliptin, blocks an enzyme (dipeptidyl peptidase-4 or DPP-4) that normally deactivates a protein (glucagon-like peptide-1 or GLP-1) that keeps insulin circulating in the blood longer. The injectable medications that mimic the action of incretin hormones (GLP-1 receptor agonists: exenatide and liraglutide) also help the body make more insulin while slowing the rate of digestion so that glucose enters the blood more slowly (145).

ROLE OF PHYSICAL ACTIVITY/EXERCISE

In individuals with any type of diabetes, regular PA/exercise has many benefits, including improvement of cardiovascular, metabolic, and psychological health; primary and secondary prevention of cardiovascular disease; and prevention of diabetes-related complications (34). Engaging in regular PA/exercise is an important therapeutic intervention to assist in managing diabetes and its complications, and, when combined with other lifestyle measures, it reduces cardiovascular disease risk factors (15,29,34,156). Regular PA/exercise facilitates improved blood glucose control in T2DM and may offer a similar benefit in GDM (8,37,38). Although regular exercise does not uniformly provide glycemic management in those with T1DM unless appropriate regimen changes are made, exercise is still considered a safe and effective adjunct therapy for the management of T1DM (11).

Improved blood glucose control attenuates the progression of cardiovascular disease (168). Exercise, in combination with dietary improvements and weight loss, has been demonstrated to favorably modify lipids and lipoproteins, thereby lowering cardiovascular disease risk in diabetes (15). Also, reductions in blood pressure (BP) have been demonstrated through exercise and

TABLE 40-2. Risk of Hypoglycemia with Use of Diabetic Medications	
No or Minimal Risk	**Higher Risk**
Acarbose: Precose	Glimepiride: Amaryl
Metformin and combinations with metformin:	Glipizide and combinations with glipizide:
Glucophage	Glucotrol, Glucotrol XL
Avandamet	Metaglip (glipizide/metformin)
(metformin/rosiglitazone)	Glyburide and combinations
Miglitol: Glyset	with glyburide:
Pioglitazone: Actos	DiaBeta
Rosiglitazone: Avandia	Glynase
Exenatide:	Pres Tab
Byetta (daily)	Micronase
Bydureon (weekly)	Glucovance
Liraglutide: Victoza	(glyburide/metformin)
Sitagliptin: Januvia	Nateglinide: Starlix
Saxagliptin: Onglyza	Repaglinide: Prandin
Pramlintide: Symlin	Insulin: All types and delivery methods

Well-known brand names are listed following the generic names.

Reprinted with permission from Colberg-Ochs S. Physical activity. In: Mensing C, editor. *The Art and Science of Diabetes Self-Management Education Desk Reference.* 2nd ed. Chicago: American Association of Diabetes Educators. 2011. pp. 385–416.

weight loss and may be partially explained by improved insulin sensitivity and loss of visceral fat (168). Glucose control is improved through exercise in individuals with T2DM and in some women with GDM. A lower HbA1C generally reduces the risk for diabetes-related complications, including cardiovascular disease (29,148,165).

BODY WEIGHT MANAGEMENT

Whereas body weight is more frequently normal or near normal at onset of T1DM (28), obesity and overweight are highly prevalent in both T2DM and GDM (7). Body mass index often exceeds $30 \text{ kg} \cdot \text{m}^{-2}$ and abdominal girth is large (men ≥ 102 cm or 40 in; women ≥ 88 cm or 35 in) in those with T2DM and GDM, placing many individuals at high risk for cardiovascular disease and cancer (11,127). Therefore, weight loss is a primary treatment goal to improve insulin action and reduce disease risk in T2DM. A 7%–10% reduction in body weight is recommended for important health outcomes related to BP, glucose control, and cardiovascular disease risk (11,148). For those with T1DM, insulin use and intensive therapy can lead to weight gain and to the deposition of visceral (central) abdominal fat in particular (28,45,88); in such cases, weight management goals should likely follow recommendations for T2DM.

ACUTE AND CHRONIC EXERCISE-RELATED PHYSIOLOGIC RESPONSES IN DIABETES

An acute bout of PA/exercise improves insulin sensitivity, facilitates glucose uptake, and aids in glucose homeostasis (37,38), with effects that lower blood glucose for 24–72 h postexercise (24,91,131). Thus, acute effects of exercise are transient and short lived. Individuals with diabetes should regularly participate in PA to maximize these benefits.

Chronic benefits of regular, long-term participation in PA/exercise have been reported for individuals with T1DM (18) and T2DM (37,38,159) (*Table 40-3*). Regular aerobic and resistance training, combined with dietary improvements, promotes improved cardiovascular function, along with favorable changes in lipids and lipoproteins, BP, body mass, fat-free mass (maintain or increase), fat mass, body fat distribution, insulin sensitivity, glucose control and metabolism, and postprandial thermogenesis (37,38). These physiologic changes usually result in a lowering of the daily medication dose (*e.g.*, insulin or oral agents) needed to manage glucose levels in T1DM and T2DM and in some women with GDM. In addition, higher levels of PA before pregnancy or in early pregnancy significantly lower the risk of developing GDM (174).

Regular exercise training improves glucose control in T2DM primarily through increased insulin sensitivity

TABLE 40-3. Effects of Exercise/Physical Activity in Diabetes

Parameter	Type 1	Type 2
Cardiovascular		
Aerobic capacity or fitness level	⇑	⇑/⇔
Resting pulse rate and rate–pressure product	⇓	⇓
Resting systolic BP (in mild-to-moderate hypertension)	⇓	⇓
HR at submaximal loads (aerobic only)	⇓	⇓
Lipid and Lipoprotein Alterations		
HDL-C	⇑	⇑
LDL-C	⇓/⇔	⇓/⇔
VLDL-C	⇓	⇓
Total cholesterol	⇔	⇔
Cardiovascular risk ratio (total cholesterol/HDL)	⇓	⇓
Anthropometric Measures		
Body mass (aerobic exercise in particular)	⇓/⇔	⇓
Fat mass (including visceral fat)	⇓	⇓
Fat-free mass (resistance exercise mainly)	⇑	⇑/⇔
Metabolic Parameters		
Insulin sensitivity and glucose/fat metabolism	⇑	⇑
HbA1C (overall glycemic control)	⇓/⇔	⇓
Postprandial thermogenesis or thermic effect of food	⇑	⇑
Presumed Psychological Outcomes		
Self-concept and self-esteem	⇑	⇑
Depression and anxiety	⇓	⇓
Stress response to psychological stimuli	⇓	⇓

BP, blood pressure; HR, heart rate; HDL-C, high-density lipoprotein cholesterol; LDL-C, low-density lipoprotein cholesterol; VLDL-C, very low–density lipoprotein cholesterol; HbA1C, glycated hemoglobin; ⇑, increase; ⇓, decrease; ⇔, no change.

(22,24,37,38). Improved glucose uptake through increased insulin sensitivity following both aerobic and resistance training has also been demonstrated in GDM (8,13,26). Although exercise improves insulin sensitivity in T1DM as well, little or no improvement in glucose control has been demonstrated after regular exercise training among these individuals, even though insulin doses generally decrease (147,150). Blood glucose responses to exercise can vary with each exercise session. The individual will need to use self-monitoring of blood glucose to better understand his or her glucose response to a specific exercise bout and make appropriate regimen changes that effectively manage blood glucose levels, keeping in mind that exercise adaptations are specific to the type of training, as is the blood glucose response.

Both acute bouts of PA and regular exercise training may also favorably alter stress-related psychological factors like well-being (96), as well as cognitive function in individuals with diabetes (39). Depression is common with diabetes, and regular PA/exercise may assist in overcoming mild-to-moderate depression (114). Overall, regular PA/exercise may offer quality-of-life improvements for individuals with diabetes that other therapies frequently fail to fully achieve.

EXERCISE PRESCRIPTION IN DIABETES

Comprehensive diabetes therapy includes participation in regular PA and intentional exercise (11,68). Identifiable limitations (*e.g.*, presence of disease complications) and precautions must be addressed while developing an appropriate exercise program for all persons with diabetes.

SCREENING

A thorough preactivity screening of the individual's clinical status is recommended to ensure safe and effective participation (37,38,159). The presence of comorbidities may affect an individual's clinical status and ability to safely engage in exercise, as well as the level of supervision/monitoring needed. For anyone desiring to participate in low-intensity PA like walking, however, health care providers should use their clinical judgment in deciding whether to recommend or require preexercise testing (37,38). Conducting exercise stress testing prior to beginning a program consisting solely of walking is not routinely necessary as a cardiovascular disease diagnostic tool and very likely creates barriers to PA/exercise participation.

For PA is more vigorous than brisk walking or exceeding the demands of everyday living, sedentary and older individuals with diabetes may benefit from being assessed for conditions that are associated with a higher risk of cardiovascular disease, contraindications to exercise, or diabetes-related factors that may predispose them to injury (*e.g.*, severe peripheral neuropathy, severe autonomic neuropathy, and preproliferative or proliferative retinopathy) (160). Preexercise assessments may include a symptom-limited exercise test depending on the age of the person, diabetes duration, and the presence of additional cardiovascular disease risk factors (37,38).

Although a symptom-limited exercise test may be done on anyone, it may not be necessary in young individuals with diabetes and those with a low cardiovascular disease risk. Specific indications for a symptom-limited exercise test are shown in *Box 40-1*. Following these criteria will avoid automatic inclusion of lower risk individuals with diabetes and advise such testing primarily for previously sedentary individuals who plan to engage in more intense PA. Although a symptom-limited exercise test may be

BOX 40-1	**Indications for Symptom-Limited Exercise Testing Prior to Vigorous Physical Activity/Exercise Participation (37,38)**

Individuals with diabetes and at least one of the following:

- Age >35 yr
- Type 1 for >10 yr duration or Type 2 diabetes for >15 yr duration
- Any additional cardiovascular risk factor (see *GETP, Table 2.3*)
- Microvascular disease evidenced by proliferative retinopathy or nephropathy including microabluminuria
- Autonomic dysfunction

Any of the following, regardless of age:
- Diagnosed cardiovascular disease including prior coronary and peripheral vascular atherosclerotic disease
- New or changing symptoms suggestive of cardiovascular disease as detected by Physical Activity Readiness-Questionnaire (PAR-Q)
- End-stage renal disease
- Patients with symptomatic or diagnosed pulmonary disease

used for exercise prescription and risk stratification, its comprehensive use to diagnose myocardial ischemia in asymptomatic individuals is not recommended. A recent meta-analysis suggested that systematic detection of silent ischemia in high-risk, asymptomatic patients with diabetes is unlikely to provide any major benefit in individuals whose cardiovascular risk is controlled by an optimal medical treatment (108).

The need for a symptom-limited exercise test prior to starting a resistance training program remains untested. Maximal stress testing is common, but an alternate form of testing involving resistance exercise is not. Coronary ischemia is less likely to occur during resistance compared to aerobic exercise eliciting the same heart rate (HR), and resistance exercise may not easily induce ischemia (64,187). Procedures for general exercise testing and testing in persons with diabetes are discussed in *Chapters 23* and *26*.

AEROBIC EXERCISE PRESCRIPTION

In general, aerobic exercise programming for individuals without complications follows the frequency, intensity, time (duration), and type (mode) of activities presented in *Table 40-4*. Each exercise session is composed of

TABLE 40-4. Recommended FITT Program for Aerobic Training in Diabetes

Variable	T1DM	T2DM
Frequency	3–7 d · wk^{-1} (3 d of vigorous or 5 d of moderate intensity; greater regularity may facilitate diabetes management)	3–7 d · wk^{-1} (no more than two consecutive days without PA/exercise)
Intensity	40%–85% HRR RPE = 12–16 (6–20 scale)	40%–85% HRR RPE = 12–16 (6–20 scale)
Time	20–30 min per session At least 150 min · wk^{-1} of moderate intensity (3.0–6.0 METs), 60 min · wk^{-1} at vigorous intensity (>6.0 METs), or a combination	30–60 min per session At least 150 min · wk^{-1} of moderate-to-vigorous (3.0 METs and higher) intensity
Type[a]	Walk, jog, cycle, row, swim, aquatic activities, seated exercises, team sports	

FITT, frequency, intensity, time, and type; T1DM, Type 1 diabetes mellitus; T2DM, Type 2 diabetes mellitus; PA, physical activity; HRR, heart rate reserve; RPE, rating of perceived exertion; MET, metabolic equivalent (1 MET = resting metabolism).

[a]Some individuals may choose to engage in non–weight-bearing activities or alternate them with weight-bearing activities because of orthopedic limitations, peripheral neuropathy, the presence of unhealed foot ulcers, and/or peripheral arterial disease.

a warm-up, aerobic-based exercise, and a cool-down phase. Appropriate exercise prescription is critical for preventing compliance issues related to the development of overuse injuries and motivational factors (146).

For individuals with T1DM, exercise recommendations are closely aligned with those for apparently healthy persons (54,74), whereas recommendations for individuals with T2DM are more closely aligned with guidelines for individuals with obesity, hypertension, and sedentary lifestyles (32,159). Nearly 80% of adults with diabetes are obese (7), and most with T2DM have low aerobic capacity (23).

Warm-up

At least a 5- to 10-min period of warm-up of a less-intense activity is recommended before progressing to moderate- (or higher) intensity exercise. Warming up before the conditioning phase (a) facilitates transition from rest to exercise via increasing blood flow, body temperature, oxygen disassociation, and metabolism; (b) may reduce susceptibility to muscular injury, improves joint range of motion (ROM), and improves muscular performance; and (c) decreases occurrence of myocardial ischemia, angina onset, ventricular arrhythmias, and transient left ventricular dysfunction (140). Thus, performing a warm-up improves physiologic function, reduces risk associated with sudden strenuous exercise, and enhances overall safety.

Frequency

A minimum of 3 d of PA per week is recommended for all individuals with diabetes, and ideally no more than 2 d should lapse between bouts of activity in order to maintain a heightened insulin action (24,37,38,131). For individuals with T1DM, engaging in daily PA may improve the balance between insulin dose and caloric needs and make blood glucose management easier (33). For long-term weight loss and maintenance, larger volumes of exercise (7 h · wk^{-1} of moderate or vigorous activity) for overweight individuals with T1DM or T2DM are recommended (56,107).

Volume

In uncomplicated T1DM, following the American College of Sports Medicine/American Heart Association guidelines to promote and maintain health for healthy adults aged 18–65 yr is likely appropriate (74), that is, engaging in moderate-intensity aerobic physical activity for a minimum of 30 min on 5 d each week, vigorous-intensity aerobic activity for a minimum of 20 min on 3 d each week, or combinations of moderate- and vigorous-intensity activity weekly. The U.S. federal guidelines (141) recommend 150 min of moderate or 75 min of vigorous PA, assuming that an exercise volume of 500–1,000 MET-minutes per week (METs × number of minutes) can be achieved with 150 min · wk^{-1} of walking at 6.4 km · h^{-1} (4 mph; intensity of 5 METs) or 75 min of jogging at 9.6 km · h^{-1} (6 mph; 10 METs).

For T2DM, the current ACSM/American Diabetes Association recommendation is 150 min · wk^{-1} of moderate- to vigorous-intensity exercise, with no lesser amount given for the latter (37,38). Although around 150 min · wk^{-1} of moderate-intensity exercise is associated with reduced morbidity and mortality (23,165), most with T2DM do not have sufficient aerobic capacity to jog at a higher intensity for the recommended weekly duration of 60–75 min (23), and they may have orthopedic or other limitations. In a study by Boule et al. (23), the mean maximal aerobic capacity in individuals with T2DM was only 22.4 mL · kg^{-1} · min^{-1} (6.4 METs), making 4.8 METs (a moderate level in absolute terms but a vigorous level [70% of $\dot{V}O_2$ reserve] in relative terms) the highest sustainable intensity and requiring at least 150 min of moderate-to-vigorous aerobic exercise per week to achieve optimal cardiovascular risk reduction.

By way of contrast, new guidelines from Exercise & Sports Science Australia recommend that patients with T2DM or prediabetes accumulate a minimum of 210 min · wk^{-1} of moderate-intensity exercise or 125 min · wk^{-1} of vigorous exercise, with no more than two consecutive days without training. These individuals should also include two or more days each week of resistance training (2–4 sets of 8–10 repetitions) (79). A recent meta-analysis suggested that structured exercise training that consists of aerobic exercise, resistance training, or both combined is associated with HbA1C reduction in T2DM and that total training (of all types) of more than 150 min $\cdot$ wk^{-1} is associated with greater declines than that of 150 min or less per week (177).

Brisk walking qualifies as a moderate-intensity exercise (in absolute terms, but may be vigorous in relative terms for low fit individuals), one that is equally as effective as other training programs (146). Beginning exercisers should be encouraged to start at a moderate pace; however, for individuals already exercising moderately, undertaking more vigorous PA will likely result in additional blood glucose and cardiovascular benefits (23). Doing interspersed, faster intervals during an aerobic training session may increase fitness gains in T2DM (86), as well as lower risk for nocturnal hypoglycemia in T1DM (84). In GDM, moderate physical exercise (aerobic and/or resistance) is warranted in women who have obtained medical approval (26,132), particularly because of its glucose-lowering effects (8,13).

Exercise intensity can be objectively derived from HR, most appropriately as a target HR derived as a percentage of HR reserve (HRR). Recommended exercise intensity ranges from 40% to 85% of HRR (where HRR = maximal HR [HR$_{max}$] $-$ resting HR [HR$_{rest}$]). This range is broad because previously sedentary individuals can improve fitness at lower intensities and may be unable to sustain higher workloads, whereas more fit individuals will likely be able to maintain them. Intensity, therefore, should be prescribed based on initial fitness level, diabetes duration, presence and degree of complications, and individual goals (37,38). It can also be prescribed and monitored using subjective ratings of perceived exertion (RPE) (140). In reflecting exercise effort, individuals must be familiarized with the scale used for RPE determination.

In summary, individuals with T1DM should engage in a minimum of 30 min of moderate-intensity aerobic PA, 20 min of vigorous-intensity PA, or combinations of moderate- and vigorous-intensity activity at least 5 d $\cdot$ wk^{-1}. In addition, daily bouts of 10 or more minutes should be encouraged (33,74). Individuals with T2DM should aim for at least 150 min of moderate- to vigorous-intensity aerobic exercise, with no more than two sedentary days between bouts of activity (37,38).

Type

Training modalities selected for the exercise prescription are commonly predicated on individual goals, preferences, and abilities, along with fitness level and orthopedic limitations. The type, or mode, of exercise prescribed and potential equipment used should be considered carefully, particularly for individuals who are physically disabled or have weight management/obesity issues, low back concerns, peripheral neuropathy, or low fitness levels. Whereas general mode recommendations for individuals

with uncomplicated T1DM are similar to advice for adults without diabetes (74,141), walking is a preferred low-impact PA that lessens joint loading (compared to jogging or running) for those with T2DM and GDM (8,37,38,41,86). Non–weight-bearing or low-impact activities (*e.g.*, cycle ergometer, aquatic exercise classes, elastic bands, yoga, tai chi) may be useful alternatives to lessen joint stress (2,82,103). In GDM, activities performed lying on the back or belly are contraindicated (see *Chapter 36*) after the first trimester of pregnancy (8), and PA that is more vigorous than walking may require physician approval to lower risk for complicating outcomes.

Cool-down

The cool-down after exercise should be an active, low-level recovery period at a reduced exercise intensity to prevent sudden reduction in venous return, thereby reducing the possibility of postexercise hypotension or syncope. Medication for hypertension, or other vasodilators, may require individuals to participate in a longer period of active cool-down (32,140).

Precautions for Aerobic Training

Supervised exercise for uncomplicated diabetes is frequently recommended and encouraged during initial phases of an exercise program to aid in monitoring signs/symptoms, response to exercise, and glucose levels. In individuals who recently experienced a cardiac-related event (*e.g.*, myocardial infarction, percutaneous coronary intervention), supervision during exercise may be indicated (4,75). Supervision may include monitoring HR, electrocardiogram (ECG), and symptoms (*e.g.*, dyspnea, claudication, and angina scales) in order to ensure the safety of exercise in individuals with diabetes (140).

Poorly controlled diabetes increases the likelihood of dehydration (176). Ensuring proper hydration in any environmental condition is important for the exercise professional to convey (6). Exercising in a thermally challenging environment (*e.g.*, hot and/or humid) can pose difficulties for those with diabetes because of hydration issues and heightened glucose metabolism. Exercise professionals should offer precautionary measures and prevention strategies to avoid dehydration and/or hypoglycemia in those with diabetes (6,55,77). In some instances, outdoor exercise should be postponed to ensure a safe environment in which to participate. Exercise professionals should apprise individuals of risks and educate them on the management of expected environmental challenges.

RESISTANCE TRAINING EXERCISE PRESCRIPTION

The goal of resistance training is increased muscular fitness, both muscular strength and endurance. *Muscle strength* is the ability of the muscle to exert force, whereas *muscle endurance* is the ability of the muscle to continue to perform without fatigue (73). Resistance training is recommended for persons with diabetes and follows guidelines for apparently healthy individuals, with age and experience as prime considerations in program development (*Table 40-5*). Such training has been shown to improve musculoskeletal health, maintain independence in performing daily activities, and reduce the possibility of injury (5). Properly designed resistance programs may improve cardiovascular function, glycemic control, strength, and body composition in individuals with diabetes (57,72,83,169,188).

Frequency

Resistance exercise should be undertaken at least twice weekly on nonconsecutive days (37,38,74,141) but more ideally three times a week (57,165) as part of a PA program for both T1DM and T2DM, along with regular aerobic activities. Adequate rest periods between sets during a workout session are needed to successfully complete all sets on each exercise. Typically, lower intensity training requires 15 s to 1 min of rest, whereas higher intensity training may necessitate up to 2–3 min of rest between sets.

Intensity

Using one repetition maximum (1-RM) to define the amount of weight that an individual can successfully lift one time, resistance training should be moderate (50% of 1-RM) or vigorous (75%–80% of 1-RM) in intensity to optimize gains in strength and insulin action (54,72). Higher intensity resistance exercise is safe and effective in lowering HbA1C (57,188). Home-based resistance training is adequate for maintaining muscle mass and strength but less effective than supervised, gym-based training for improving blood glucose control (58). Thus, using heavier weights or resistance may be needed to optimize insulin action (188).

Time

Resistance exercises should ideally be performed to fatigue during a given set and consist of 10–15 repetitions to near fatigue per set early in training, progressing over time to heavier weights or resistance that limit sets to 8–12 repetitions (74,141). A minimum of one set of repetitions to near fatigue is recommended for strength gains, and some individuals may benefit from as many as three to four sets. Resistance exercise should progress over 6 mo or so to thrice weekly sessions of three sets of 8–12 repetitions done at 75%–80% of 1-RM on 8–10 exercises as an optimal goal (57).

Resistance programs should include at least 8–10 exercises encompassing all of the major muscle groups, including the back, legs, hips, chest, shoulders, arms, and abdomen (141). To maximize gains and avoid injury, exercise large muscle groups before smaller ones (*e.g.*, chest exercises before specific arm exercises). Exercises involving multiple joints should also be done before those that involve a single joint, such as doing leg presses before leg extensions or leg curls, with abdominal and core muscle exercises at the end of training sessions.

Type

Exercises should reflect individual goals, preferences, and skill level. Specific muscle groups may also be targeted to enhance aerobic components of the activity program, such as cycling or swimming. Muscular fitness can be improved by including free weights (dumbbells and barbells), weight or resistance machines, or resistance bands and doing isometric exercises or calisthenics using body weight as resistance (*e.g.*, push-ups). Resistance machines and free weights result in fairly equivalent gains in strength and mass of targeted muscles (57), although no research has specifically evaluated the use of resistance bands or body-weight resistance only. Typically, heavier weights or resistance are needed for optimization of insulin action and blood glucose control (58,188).

TABLE 40-5. Recommended FITT Program for Resistance Training in Diabetes	
Variable	**T1DM and T2DM**
Type of exercise	All major muscle groups Upper body: 4–5 exercises Lower body/core: 4–5 exercises
Frequency	2–3 d · wk^{-1a}
Intensity[b]	60%–80% 1-RM (lower intensity to start) RPE ~11–15 (6–20 scale)
Time	8–12 repetitions/exercise (10–15 to start) 1–3 sets/exercise

FITT, frequency, intensity, time, and type; T1DM, Type 1 diabetes mellitus; T2DM, Type 2 diabetes mellitus; 1-RM, one repetition maximum; RPE, rating of perceived exertion.

[a]3 d · wk^{-1} is strongly encouraged.

[b]Individuals may need to lower their intensity (*i.e.*, use less resistance and do more repetitions) when diabetic retinopathy, hypertension, or orthopedic limitations are comorbid conditions.

Precautions for Resistance Training

For safe and effective exercise participation, it is imperative that glucose levels are carefully managed (83,162,190). Appropriate attention to modifying the intensity of the lifting session may reduce the risk for elevations in BP, glucose, and onset of musculoskeletal injury.

Resistance training should progress slowly enough to prevent injury and motivational issues. Increases in weight or resistance used should be undertaken only once the target number of repetitions per set can consistently be exceeded, followed by a greater number of sets, and lastly by increased training frequency (5,67). Individuals with joint limitations or other health complications should complete one set of exercises for all major muscle groups, starting with 10–15 repetitions and progressing to 15–20 repetitions before additional sets are added (170).

Although studies have found that moderate- to high-intensity resistance training provoked no evidence of ischemia, resistance exercises should be dynamic and undertaken at a moderate intensity to ensure a safe and effective program. Individuals should avoid the Valsalva maneuver and breathe on effort to avoid untoward outcomes of resistance training, particularly with respect to increased BP that may contribute to retinal damage (19). In cases of untreated, severe diabetic retinopathy, intense resistance training may be contraindicated.

COMBINED AEROBIC AND RESISTANCE AND ALTERNATE TRAINING

Prescribing both aerobic and resistance exercise training is recommended for individuals with T1DM and T2DM. Combined training thrice weekly in individuals with T2DM may be of greater benefit to glycemic control than either aerobic or resistance exercise alone (35,49,117,158), even when caloric expenditure is held constant for the combination (35). Similar training in individuals with T1DM results in significantly lower insulin requirements, with unchanged HbA1C values (54). At present, it is unknown whether daily, but alternating, training is more effective than both types undertaken on the same day. Alternate types of PA, such as yoga and tai chi, may bestow some benefits with regard to short- and long-term control of blood glucose levels, flexibility, and balance, but more research is needed (2,82,103).

FLEXIBILITY EXERCISE PRESCRIPTION

Flexibility training may be included as part of a PA program but not in place of other training. Individuals should perform exercises that maintain or improve balance (129), which may include some flexibility training, particularly for older individuals with T2DM with a higher risk of falling (122). Although frequently recommended as a means of increasing joint ROM and lowering the risk of injury, flexibility exercise likely does not reduce the risk of exercise-induced injury (157,189). ROM exercises may modestly decrease peak plantar pressures (71), but the impact of such training on risk of ulceration or injury in T2DM remains to be studied. Flexibility exercise combined with resistance training can increase ROM in individuals with T2DM (78) and allow individuals to more easily engage in activities that require greater ROM around joints.

DAILY MOVEMENT AND OTHER PHYSICAL ACTIVITY

Individuals with diabetes should be encouraged to engage in other types of PA outside of scheduled exercise sessions (*i.e.*, more daily movement). Individuals with T2DM, who are frequently physically deconditioned and sedentary, should incorporate more unstructured PA into daily living to initially increase their daily activity level and build a fitness base (107,178). Once these individuals have successfully implemented more PA into their daily lifestyle, they may feel more confident, willing, and able to initiate structured forms of activity (51,142). Energy expended during activities of daily living can create a large daily caloric deficit to cause weight loss or prevent excessive weight gain (106,107). In addition, a single bout of low-intensity, as opposed to high-intensity, exercise substantially reduces the prevalence of hyperglycemia throughout the subsequent 24-h postexercise period in individuals with T2DM (116).

Use of step counters (pedometers) may aid individuals in reaching daily movement goals. Pedometers provide immediate feedback, build confidence, and enhance enjoyment of daily PA (12). Moreover, pedometer users increase their overall physical activity by 27% over baseline in studies having an average intervention of 18 wk, particularly when combined with a goal like taking 10,000 steps per day (27). Pedometers are most suitable for walking-based activities and cannot detect changes in type, intensity, or pattern of activity. Accelerometers and global positioning system devices may alternately be used to detect such movements (186).

EXERCISE RECOMMENDATIONS FOR DIABETES-RELATED COMPLICATIONS

Although favorable changes occur in cardiovascular and hemodynamic function — insulin action and sensitivity, glucose metabolism, weight management, and cardiovascular disease risk — these benefits must be weighed against potential acute risks of exercise for individuals with diabetes. A safe and effective exercise program for diabetes minimizes the acute risks and long-term complications while maximizing the benefits (8,37,38,155).

ACUTE BLOOD GLUCOSE LIMITATIONS AND CONTRAINDICATIONS

Acutely uncontrolled diabetes is a relative contraindication to exercise participation. Self-monitoring of blood glucose before and after exercise is essential, especially in insulin users, to allow individuals to make appropriate adjustments in insulin or other medications and food intake (63,167). Although exercise done at a mild intensity will expend calories and assist with weight maintenance, it will likely lower blood glucose levels less than moderate-intensity workouts. Conversely, very vigorous exercise may result in transient hyperglycemia because glucose production tends to increase more than glucose use particularly just after cessation of exercise (161). Thus, two common risks associated with exercise in individuals with diabetes are hypoglycemia and hyperglycemia; however, practical precautions can be taken to reduce the risk or avoid their onset (*Table 40-6*).

Hypoglycemia

In individuals managing T2DM with diet and exercise alone, the risk of developing hypoglycemia during or after PA is minimal, even though undertaking longer duration and lower intensity PA generally reduces glycemic levels (14,61,80,101). More intense activities can cause transient blood glucose elevations in all individuals with diabetes (97,161,171,172), but intermittent high-intensity exercise done immediately after breakfast in individuals treated with diet only reduces blood glucose levels and insulin secretion (100). As a precaution, though, glucose monitoring can be performed before and after PA to assess its individualized effect.

When patients use insulin or insulin secretagogues, PA may complicate diabetes management (90,123,151). In the presence of excess peripheral insulin, hepatic glucose production is blunted and glucose uptake into exercising muscle is heightened (101,184). If starting exercise with blood glucose levels of less than 100 mg $\cdot$ dL^{-1} (5.5 mmol $\cdot$ L^{-1}), the American Diabetes Association recommends carbohydrate consumption preexercise (9), but doing so may only be necessary in individuals taking insulin or the secretagogues shown in *Table 40-2* that are more likely to cause hypoglycemia (101,151). If controlled with diet or other oral medications, most individuals will not need supplemental carbohydrate for exercise lasting less than an hour or for short, intense workouts because of the release of glucose-raising hormones (97). Insulin users should likely consume up to 15 g of carbohydrate preexercise for starting blood glucose levels of 100 mg $\cdot$ dL^{-1} (5.5 mmol $\cdot$ L^{-1}) or lower depending on injected insulin doses and planned exercise duration and intensity (33).

TABLE 40-6. Practical Recommendations for Exercise with Diabetes

Perform SMBG	Check before and after each exercise session. Allows the individual to understand glucose response to PA. It is important to ensure that glucose is in relatively good control before beginning exercise. If blood glucose is: >250–300 mg $\cdot$ dL^{-1} plus ketones, exercise should be postponed. >250–300 mg $\cdot$ dL^{-1} without ketones, exercise is okay but use caution; <100 mg $\cdot$ dL^{-1}, consider eating a snack consisting of easily absorbed carbohydrates (~20–30 g) based on insulin regimen and circulating insulin levels during PA; 100–250 mg $\cdot$ dL^{-1}, exercise is recommended.
Keep a daily log	Record the time of day the SMBG values are obtained and the amount of any pharmacologic agent (*e.g.*, oral drugs, insulin). Also, approximate the duration (min), intensity (HR or perceived exertion), and distance (miles or meters) of exercise session. Over time, this aids the individual in understanding the type of glucose response to anticipate from an exercise bout.
Plan for exercise sessions	How much (*e.g.*, duration and intensity) exercise is anticipated allows adjusting insulin or oral drugs. If needed, carry extra carbohydrate feedings (~10–15 g $\cdot$ 30 min^{-1}) to limit hypoglycemia. Hydrate before and rehydrate after each exercise session to prevent dehydration.
Modify caloric intake accordingly	Through frequent SMBG, caloric intake can be regulated more carefully on days of and after exercise.
Adjust insulin accordingly	If using insulin, reduce rapid- or short-acting insulin dosage by 50% to limit hypoglycemia episodes.
Exercise with a partner	This affords a support system for the exercise habit. Initially, individuals with diabetes should exercise with a partner until their glucose response is known.
Wear a diabetes identification tag	A diabetes necklace or shoe tag with relevant medical information should always be worn. Hypoglycemia and other problems can arise that require immediate attention.
Wear good shoes	Always wear proper-fitting and comfortable footwear with socks to minimize foot irritations and limit orthopedic injury to the feet and lower legs.
Practice good hygiene	Always take extra care to inspect feet for any irritation spots to prevent possible infection. Tend to all sores immediately and limit any irritations.

SMBG, self-monitoring of blood glucose; PA, physical activity; HR, heart rate.

Hypoglycemia is relative, and the exercise professional should not focus only on the blood glucose level (37,38). Rapid drops in blood glucose may occur with exercise and cause symptoms even when blood glucose is well above 70 mg $\cdot$ dL^{-1} or occur without generating noticeable symptoms. Common symptoms associated with hypoglycemia include shakiness, weakness, abnormal sweating, nervousness, anxiety, tingling of the mouth and fingers, and hunger. Neuroglycopenic symptoms may include headache, visual disturbances, mental dullness, confusion, amnesia, seizures, and coma. Any incidences of hypoglycemia should be treated with ingestion of rapidly absorbed carbohydrate sources, such as glucose tablets or gels, hard candy, regular soda, skim milk, or juice (33,149,173). Severe hypoglycemia resulting in an inability to self-treat or unconsciousness may require the use of a glucagon injection.

Self-monitoring of blood glucose should be used to look for possible declines in blood glucose, particularly when hypoglycemia unawareness is present. Hypoglycemia unawareness is thought to be largely the result of reduced sympathetic neural responses to falling glucose levels (48). Recent hypoglycemia or prior exercise can result in defective glucose counterregulation (by reducing epinephrine responses to subsequent hypoglycemia) and hypoglycemia unawareness (50,153,154). It is now known to be largely reversible by as little as 2–3 wk of scrupulous avoidance of hypoglycemia.

Importantly, hypoglycemia may be delayed and can occur up to 12 h (or more) postexercise, even with reductions in insulin doses (1), although inclusion of intermittent high-intensity work may lower the risk (84). Reliance on the use of blood glucose appears to be elevated during and shortly following 45 min of moderate aerobic exercise and again from 7–11 h afterward, suggesting a biphasic glycemic response to PA (120). Consumption of either whole milk and sports drinks before, during, and after 1 h of moderate exercise may lower the risk of later-onset hypoglycemia in T1DM (77). Similarly, the risk of nocturnal hypoglycemia following PA may be lowered with ingestion of a bedtime snack and/or reduced basal rates of insulin overnight (52,89,173). Finally, some preliminary studies have also investigated the use of terbutaline, a β_2-adrenergic agonist, at bedtime, which appears to prevent most nocturnal hypoglycemia but may cause morning hyperglycemia in individuals with T1DM (46,173).

Hyperglycemia

In the presence of low insulin levels, insulin-stimulated glucose uptake in skeletal muscle is reduced and exercise-induced hepatic glucose output is increased, frequently resulting in hyperglycemia (162). In T1DM and other very insulin deficient states, after glucose levels exceed 250–300 mg $\cdot$ dL^{-1}, urinary ketones begin to form as a result of ineffective fat metabolism and contribute to **diabetic ketoacidosis (DKA)** if hyperglycemia persists (92,176). This scenario requires insulin to be administered to lower the glucose level and reestablish euglycemia prior to the initiation of PA. If blood glucose is elevated (*e.g.*, >250–300 mg $\cdot$ dL^{-1}) before exercise, an acute bout may cause further elevation in blood glucose (hyperglycemia) if moderate or higher levels of ketones are evident. Poor glycemic control in athletes with T1DM may negatively impact their exercise training adaptations, such as maximal oxygen consumption, workload, HR, stroke volume, and cardiac output (16).

Because most persons with T2DM and GDM still produce endogenous insulin, they generally do not need to postpone exercise because of hyperglycemia, assuming that they feel well (13,116). If they undertake strenuous PA with glucose levels more than 300 mg $\cdot$ dL^{-1} (16.7 mmol $\cdot$ L^{-1}), they should make certain that they are adequately hydrated (37,38) given that dehydration resulting from polyuria (a common occurrence of hyperglycemia) may contribute to a compromised thermoregulatory response (180). Even if individuals are transiently hyperglycemic after eating, mild- to moderate-intensity aerobic work will likely reduce glycemic levels given that circulating insulin levels are typically higher postmeal (41,144), although persistent postexercise hyperglycemia will likely require an increase in insulin levels to return resting blood glucose levels to normal (162). In individuals with T2DM, a single bout of mild exercise may lower blood glucose levels during the 24-h period following the activity better than intense exercise (116).

CHRONIC DIABETES-RELATED COMPLICATIONS

Diabetes poses challenges for exercise/PA participation because of the increased morbidity and mortality associated with many diabetes-related complications, particularly vascular and neurologic diseases. The presence of diabetes-related complications is usually not an absolute contraindication to PA, and the benefits of low- to moderate-intensity exercise generally outweigh the risks presented by diabetes (110). Although precautions and limitations must be recognized with prudent modifications, a safe exercise plan can be achieved when the clinical status and existing complications are thoroughly assessed in the screening process. Exercise considerations and precautions for individuals with complicated diabetes are summarized in *Table 40-7*.

Assessment of overall health, especially identification and prevention of cardiovascular disease risk factors and other diabetes-related complications, are essential components of effective diabetes care (11). Macrovascular (*e.g.*, coronary, cerebrovascular, and peripheral) and microvascular (*e.g.*, peripheral and autonomic nerves,

TABLE 40-7. Special Precautions for Diabetes-Related Complications

Complication	Precaution
Autonomic neuropathy[a]	Likelihood of hypoglycemia, abnormal BP ($\Uparrow$/$\Downarrow$), and impaired thermoregulation; abnormal resting HR ($\Uparrow$) and maximal HR ($\Downarrow$); impaired SNS or PNS nerves yield abnormal exercise HR, BP, and SV; use of RPE is suggested; prone to dehydration and hyperthermia/hypothermia.
Peripheral neuropathy	Check feet daily and minimize participation in exercise that may cause trauma to the feet (*e.g.*, prolonged hiking, jogging, or walking on uneven surfaces). Non–weight-bearing exercises (*e.g.*, cycling, chair exercises, swimming) may be more appropriated in some cases, although risk of reulceration is not increased by walking if ulcers are fully healed. Aquatic exercises are not recommended if active ulcers are present. Regular assessment of the feet is recommended. Keep feet clean and dry. Choose shoes carefully for proper fit. Avoid activities requiring a great deal of balance.
Nephropathy	Avoid exercise that increases BP (*e.g.*, weightlifting, high-intensity aerobic exercise) excessively and refrain from breath holding. High BP is common. Lower PA intensity is recommended.
Retinopathy[a,b]	With proliferative and severe stages of retinopathy, avoid vigorous, high-intensity activities that involve breath holding (*e.g.*, weightlifting and isometrics) or overhead lifting. Avoid activities that lower the head (*e.g.*, yoga, gymnastics) or that risk jarring the head. Consult an ophthalmologist for specific restrictions and limitations. In the absence of peak HR identified through a maximal exercise test, use of RPE is recommended (10–12 on 6–20 scale).
Hypertension	Avoid heavy weightlifting or breath holding. Perform dynamic exercises using large muscle groups, such as walking and cycling at a low-to-moderate intensity. Follow BP guidelines. In the absence of peak HR identified through a maximal exercise test, use of RPE is recommended (10–12 on 6–20 scale).
All individuals	Carry identification with diabetes information. Maintain hydration (drink fluids before, during, and after exercise). Avoid exercise in the heat of the day and in direct sunlight (wear hat and sunscreen when in the sun). Carry rapid-acting carbohydrate sources with you during all PA and consider packing a glucagon kit in your workout bag to treat severe hypoglycemia.

BP, blood pressure; HR, heart rate; SNS, sympathetic nervous system; PNS, parasympathetic nervous system; SV, stroke volume; RPE, rating of perceived exertion; PA, physical activity; $\Uparrow$, increase; $\Downarrow$, decrease.

[a]Submaximal exercise testing is recommended for individuals with proliferative retinopathy and autonomic neuropathy.

[b]If individual has proliferative retinopathy and has recently undergone photocoagulation or surgical treatment or is not properly treated, exercise is contraindicated.

kidney, and eye) diseases are common and constitute the diabetes-related complications that develop and worsen with inadequate blood glucose control (10,21). The onset and progression of vascular and neural complications of diabetes often cause physical limitation and varying levels of disability and are linked with depression and cognitive deficits (39,60,112,114,137). Thus, the quality of life in those with diabetes can be adversely affected without aggressive management of these health issues. For those who have difficulty managing blood glucose levels, it is prudent to refer them to allied health professionals (*e.g.*, diabetes educator, diabetes nurse, registered dietician) to assist them in improving their diabetes management and care (11).

Cardiovascular Disease

Current recommendations focus on aggressive management of cardiovascular disease risk factors (21,29,164). Glucose-lowering agents used in diabetes management are frequently supplemented by medications that target cardiovascular disease, such as antihypertensive drugs, lipid-lowering agents, and antiplatelet medications (11). Lifestyle management is also effective in lowering cardiovascular risk (110). Adherence to home-based and other

exercise programs is associated with a reduced incidence of cardiovascular disease in persons with T2DM (118,156) and improved lipids and cardiovascular risk factors in T1DM (76,99). Aerobic exercise training done alone or combined with resistance training improves cardiovascular risk factors (*i.e.*, glycemic control, systolic BP, triglycerides, and waist circumference), whereas the impact of resistance exercise alone on these risk markers is also likely significant in T2DM (169) but less well defined (34).

Diabetes is a major risk factor for many cardiovascular diseases. Individuals with T2DM have a lifetime risk of coronary artery disease that includes 67% of women and 78% of men (21,65). Individuals experiencing an acute myocardial infarction may not experience chest pain, and up to a third may have silent myocardial ischemia (115). For individuals with peripheral arterial disease, with and without intermittent claudication in the extremities during exercise, low-to-moderate walking, arm ergometer, and leg ergometer exercise can enhance mobility, functional capacity, exercise pain tolerance, and quality of life (138). Home-based walking interventions may not increase walking distance, but they have been shown to improve walking speed and quality of life in people with diabetes and peripheral artery disease (43). Lower-extremity resistance training also improves functional performance (119). Individuals at very high risk for cardiovascular disease (*e.g.*, those with known coronary disease and exercise-induced ischemia) should exercise in a supervised cardiac rehabilitation program, at least initially (164).

Peripheral Neuropathy

Up to 40% of individuals with diabetes may experience peripheral neuropathy, and 60% of lower-extremity amputations in Americans are related to poor blood glucose management (104,126). Distal symmetric poly-neuropathy is the most common form of diabetic neuropathy and typically involves small and large nerve fibers (30). Small-nerve fiber neuropathy, a component of impaired glucose tolerance and the metabolic syndrome, often presents with pain and loss of intraepidermal nerve fibers but without objective signs or evidence of nerve damage. The greatest risk from small-nerve fiber neuropathy is foot ulceration and subsequent gangrene and amputation (127). Large-nerve fiber neuropathy produces numbness, ataxia, and incoordination, thus impairing activities of daily living and causing falls and fractures.

Mild-to-moderate exercise may help prevent the onset of peripheral neuropathy (17). Individuals without acute foot ulcers can undertake moderate weight-bearing exercise using proper foot ware, including appropriate socks (synthetic/cotton blends that keep feet drier) and shoes; although a foot injury or open sore or ulcer requires participation in non–weight-bearing PA. Daily inspection of the feet can prevent or detect sores or ulcers early. Moderate walking is not likely to increase risk of foot ulcers or reulceration with peripheral neuropathy (104,105).

Autonomic Neuropathy

The development of autonomic neuropathy broadly affects the involuntary functions of the body, including the cardiac, vascular, gastrointestinal, and genitourinary systems. When affecting the innervation of the heart, it is referred to as *cardiac autonomic neuropathy* (CAN), and its presence is linked with poor prognosis and premature mortality (182). Almost a quarter of individuals with diabetes have CAN, but most exhibit some alterations in autonomic function (191).

Clinical features of CAN include silent ischemia and infarction, tachycardia at rest and early in exercise, reduced HR_{max} and exercise intolerance, exercise-induced hypotension after strenuous activity, thermoregulatory dysfunction, a tendency to dehydrate, and reduced HR variability, which is caused by a shift in cardiac autonomic balance toward sympathetic dominance (181). The presence of CAN doubles the risk of mortality (182) and results in more frequent silent myocardial ischemia,

orthostatic hypotension, or resting tachycardia (62). CAN also impairs exercise tolerance, lowers HR_{max}, and increases mortality risk when slower HR recovery after PA is present (31,182). Given their likelihood of silent ischemia and HR abnormalities, individuals with CAN should have physician approval and possibly undergo symptom-limited exercise testing before commencing exercise.

Moderate-intensity aerobic training can improve autonomic function in individuals with and without CAN (81,109,134,166,181). However, if postural hypotension is present, inadequate HR and BP responses are observed with incremental work; therefore, these individuals should focus on lower intensity activities in which mild changes in HR and BP are more easily tolerated and lessen ventricular ectopy. Exercise intensity when CAN is present may be accurately prescribed using the HRR method with HR_{max} directly measured, rather than estimated, for better accuracy; RPE may also be used (40).

Nephropathy and Microalbuminuria

Diabetic nephropathy develops in 30% of individuals with diabetes (20,36). *Microalbuminuria*, or minute amounts of albumin in the urine, is a common risk factor for overt nephropathy (36) and cardiovascular mortality (69). Although an acute bout of exercise has been shown to transiently increase postexercise levels of urinary albumin even in normoalbuminuric individuals with no evidence of kidney disease (130), PA does not appear to worsen kidney function otherwise (94). Smoking cessation in newly diagnosed individuals with T2DM, patients is associated with amelioration of metabolic parameters, BP, and the reduction of microalbuminuria (183). Use of current therapies to maintain good glycemic control, adequate BP and lipid levels, along with adoption of lifestyle measures such as regular exercise, optimization of diet, and smoking cessation, may help to reduce oxidative stress and endothelial cell dysfunction and retard the progression of diabetic nephropathy (163).

Both aerobic and resistance training improve physical function and quality of life in individuals with kidney disease (85,135,136). Resistance exercise training is especially effective in improving muscle function and activities of daily living, which are normally severely impacted by later-stage kidney disease (85). Individuals with overt nephropathy should be screened, have physician approval, and possibly undergo symptom-limited exercise testing to detect cardiovascular disease and abnormal exercise responses (25). Exercise should begin at a low intensity and volume, and breath holding and high-intensity exercise should be avoided to prevent large increases in BP. Doing supervised, moderate aerobic PA undertaken during dialysis sessions may be beneficial and increase compliance (95).

Retinopathy

The main cause of blindness in developed countries, diabetic retinopathy is associated with increased cardiovascular mortality (87,93). It occurs in varying degrees of severity as nonproliferative diabetic retinopathy or proliferative diabetic retinopathy (PDR) (93). BP and glucose control are essential in limiting progression of retinopathy. However, in cases where PDR results in blindness, the perceived loss of independence and mobility may result in a need for support in managing the lifestyle changes necessary for good blood sugar control, particularly regarding exercise (53).

Research has shown that low-intensity training in persons with T1DM and T2DM with PDR improved cardiovascular function by 15% without adverse retinal outcomes (19). Although PA/exercise increases systemic and retinal BP, few studies have shown a worsening of retinopathy with exercise (19). Individuals with retinopathy have a higher risk for retinal detachment and vitreous hemorrhage associated with vigorous-intensity exercise; thus, in anyone with preproliferative retinopathy or macular degeneration, careful screening and physician approval are recommended before initiating an exercise program. High-intensity aerobic or resistance exercise and head-down activities that increase intraocular pressures are neither advised with uncontrolled proliferative disease nor are jumping or jarring activities because of increased hemorrhage risk (37,38). Recommended precautions for exercise in individuals with varying severity of retinopathy are shown in *Table 40-8* (16).

IMPLEMENTATION OF SUPERVISED AND OTHER EXERCISE PROGRAMS

Greater effort needs to be focused on the promotion of regular exercise among individuals with and at risk for developing T2DM and GDM in particular because lifestyle choices largely influence its onset, although health behavior change interventions benefit glycemic control in T1DM as well (44). Several factors influence PA participation, including self-efficacy (a person's belief in his or her ability to succeed), enjoyment, perceived barriers, beliefs about the benefits of PA, support from others, and cultural beliefs and practices. In individuals with T2DM in particular, exercise interventions should focus on self-efficacy, problem solving and goal setting, social-environmental support to improve self-management (including PA, dietary, and medication behaviors), barriers imposed by the built environment, and cultural nuances.

One of the most consistent predictors of greater levels of PA, both aerobic and resistance training, has been higher levels of self-efficacy, which reflect confidence in the ability to exercise (51,59,113,142). Developing realistic activity goals, using appropriate progression of exercise, and getting supportive feedback all increase confidence in individuals with diabetes (113,124). In individuals with diabetes and peripheral artery disease, self-efficacy is also associated with walking ability (42,43). For individuals with T1DM, confidence in the ability to avoid hypoglycemia related to PA is an important determinant in their participation (149), whereas use of continuous glucose monitoring may increase exercise compliance in some individuals with T2DM (3).

When planning to increase PA participation by overcoming potential obstacles or problems, individuals must also set realistic and practical goals (113,124). Goals that are too vague, too ambitious, or too distant do not provide enough self-motivation to maintain long-term interest (*i.e.*, short-term goals). Health care professionals should encourage individuals with diabetes to plan out their exercise participation, track their goals to help see their progress, and identify potential barriers (111).

Social-environmental support has also been associated with greater levels of PA (70). Social dynamics

TABLE 40-8. Diabetic Retinopathy: Considerations for Activity Limitation

Level of DR	Acceptable Activities	Discouraged Activities	Ocular and Activity Reevaluation
No DR	All	None (or dictated by medical status)	12 mo
Mild NPDR	All	None (or dictated by medical status)	6–12 mo
Moderate NPDR	Most	Activities that dramatically increase BP, such as power lifting; Valsalva maneuver	
Severe NPDR	Most	Activities that dramatically increase BP, Valsalva maneuvers, active jarring, boxing, heavy competitive sports	2–4 mo (may require laser surgery)
PDR	Low-impact cardiovascular conditioning activities, swimming, walking, low-impact aerobics, stationary cycling, endurance exercises	Low-impact cardiovascular jarring, weightlifting, jogging, high-impact aerobics, racquet sports, water skiing, head-down activities, strenuous trumpet playing, roller coasters, any activities during retinal hemorrhages	1–2 mo (may require laser surgery)

DR, diabetic retinopathy; NPDR, nonproliferative diabetic retinopathy; BP, blood pressure; PDR, proliferative diabetic retinopathy.

may be exploited to increase the effects of interventions beyond the target individual and potentially can help spread exercise behavior. Likewise, counseling delivered by health care professionals may also be a meaningful and effective source of support (12). On average, physician advice or referral related to exercise occurred at 18% of office visits among patients with diabetes, and 73% of patients reported receiving advice at some point to exercise more, although such advice has clearly not led to widespread adoption of increased PA. In fact, PA advice from is associated with lower A1C values only when combined with dietary advice but not when given alone (177).

The availability of facilities, pleasant places to walk, and economical exercise options (*i.e.*, the built environment) may also be an important predictor of regular PA (66,121). Similarly, exercise intervention studies showing the greatest impact on blood glucose control have all involved supervision of exercise sessions by qualified exercise trainers (128,158). When supervision is absent, both compliance and glycemic control decrease (128). Engaging in supervised training allows individuals to attain benefits beyond those of exercise counseling and increased PA undertaken alone (177).

Finally, health care providers must also be aware of the cultural practices and beliefs that may influence the adoption of PA programs. Activities should not offend or ignore the cultural beliefs of the individual, and suggestions to help tailor a suitable exercise prescription should be culturally appropriate (139). By way of example, in one program focusing Puerto Ricans living in the northeast United States, these individuals were taught in a culturally appropriate way how inactivity increases the risk for diabetes-related complications; what the benefits of exercising for people with diabetes are; and how lifestyle activity (*e.g.*, house or yard work, walking a pet, or walking around town to complete errands) can serve as an alternative to traditional, regimented exercise (133). Likewise, dance and music are a vital part of tradition and celebration for many ethnically diverse groups, including Native, Hispanic, and African Americans, whereas Asian and Middle Eastern groups may have other cultural traditions such as yoga, tai chi, and dance that can be part of an exercise routine that can boost fitness and lower blood glucose levels (67).

SUMMARY

Regular PA/exercise is an essential part of the therapeutic regimen in diabetes management and care. Diabetes presents challenges for the individual and for the exercise professional that require comprehensive evaluation of individual status, assessment of individual ability, and individualizing the exercise prescription to meet the needs and goals of those with any type of diabetes. Careful attention to individuals and their diabetes-related comorbidities is required for safe and effective exercise training.

REFERENCES

1. Admon G, Weinstein Y, Falk B, et al. Exercise with and without an insulin pump among children and adolescents with type 1 diabetes mellitus. *Pediatrics.* 2005;116(3):e348–55.
2. Aljasir B, Bryson M, Al-Shehri B. Yoga practice for the management of type II diabetes mellitus in adults: a systematic review. *Evid Based Complement Alternat Med.* 2010;7(4):399–408.
3. Allen NA, Fain JA, Braun B, Chipkin SR. Continuous glucose monitoring counseling improves physical activity behaviors of individuals with type 2 diabetes: a randomized clinical trial. *Diabetes Res Clin Pract.* 2008;80(3):371–9.
4. American Association of Cardiovascular and Pulmonary Rehabilitation. *AACVPR Cardiac Rehabilitation Resource Manual: Promoting Health and Preventing Disease.* Chicago (IL): Human Kinetics; 2006. 214 p.
5. American College of Sports Medicine. American College of Sports Medicine position stand. Progression models in resistance training for healthy adults. *Med Sci Sports Exerc.* 2009;41(3):687–708.
6. American College of Sports Medicine, Sawka MN, Burke LM, et al. American College of Sports Medicine position stand. Exercise and fluid replacement. *Med Sci Sports Exerc.* 2007;39(2):377–90.
7. American Diabetes Association. Diagnosis and classification of diabetes mellitus. *Diabetes Care.* 2011;34 Suppl 1:S62–9.
8. American Diabetes Association. Gestational diabetes mellitus. *Diabetes Care.* 2004;27 Suppl 1:S88–90.
9. American Diabetes Association. Physical activity/exercise and diabetes mellitus: position statement. *Diabetes Care.* 2003;26(Suppl 1):S73–7.
10. American Diabetes Association. Standards of medical care in diabetes—2007. *Diabetes Care.* 2007;30 Suppl 1:S4–S41.
11. American Diabetes Association. Standards of medical care in diabetes—2011. *Diabetes Care.* 2011;34 Suppl 1:S11–61.
12. Armit CM, Brown WJ, Marshall AL, et al. Randomized trial of three strategies to promote physical activity in general practice. *Prev Med.* 2009;48(2):156–63.
13. Avery MD, Walker AJ. Acute effect of exercise on blood glucose and insulin levels in women with gestational diabetes. *J Matern Fetal Med.* 2001;10(1):52–8.
14. Bajpeyi S, Tanner CJ, Slentz CA, et al. Effect of exercise intensity and volume on persistence of insulin sensitivity during training cessation. *J Appl Physiol.* 2009;106(4):1079–85.
15. Balady GJ, Williams MA, Ades PA, et al. Core components of cardiac rehabilitation/secondary prevention programs: 2007 update: a scientific statement from the American Heart Association Exercise, Cardiac Rehabilitation, and Prevention Committee, the Council on Clinical Cardiology; the Councils on Cardiovascular Nursing, Epidemiology and Prevention, and Nutrition, Physical Activity, and Metabolism; and the American Association of Cardiovascular and Pulmonary Rehabilitation. *Circulation.* 2007;115(20):2675–82.
16. Baldi JC, Cassuto NA, Foxx-Lupo WT, Wheatley CM, Snyder EM. Glycemic status affects cardiopulmonary exercise response in athletes with type I diabetes. *Med Sci Sports Exerc.* 2010;42(8):1454–9.
17. Balducci S, Iacobellis G, Parisi L, et al. Exercise training can modify the natural history of diabetic peripheral neuropathy. *J Diabetes Complications.* 2006;20(4):216–23.
18. Benevento D, Bizzarri C, Pitocco D, et al. Computer use, free time activities and metabolic control in patients with type 1 diabetes. *Diabetes Res Clin Pract.* 2010;88(3):e32–4.
19. Bernbaum M, Albert SG, Cohen JD, Drimmer A. Cardiovascular conditioning in individuals with diabetic retinopathy. *Diabetes Care.* 1989;12(10):740–2.

20. Bo S, Ciccone G, Rosato R, et al. Renal damage in patients with type 2 diabetes: a strong predictor of mortality. *Diabet Med.* 2005;22(3):258–65.

21. Booth GL, Kapral MK, Fung K, Tu JV. Recent trends in cardiovascular complications among men and women with and without diabetes. *Diabetes Care.* 2006;29(1):32–7.

22. Boule NG, Haddad E, Kenny GP, Wells GA, Sigal RJ. Effects of exercise on glycemic control and body mass in type 2 diabetes mellitus: a meta-analysis of controlled clinical trials. *JAMA.* 2001;286(10):1218–27.

23. Boule NG, Kenny GP, Haddad E, Wells GA, Sigal RJ. Meta-analysis of the effect of structured exercise training on cardiorespiratory fitness in Type 2 diabetes mellitus. *Diabetologia.* 2003;46(8):1071–81.

24. Boule NG, Weisnagel SJ, Lakka TA, et al. Effects of exercise training on glucose homeostasis: the HERITAGE Family Study. *Diabetes Care.* 2005;28(1):108–14.

25. Braden C. Nephropathy: advanced. In: Ruderman N, Devlin JT, editor. *The Health Professional's Guide to Diabetes and Exercise.* Alexandria: American Diabetes Association; 1995. p. 177–180.

26. Brankston GN, Mitchell BF, Ryan EA, Okun NB. Resistance exercise decreases the need for insulin in overweight women with gestational diabetes mellitus. *Am J Obstet Gynecol.* 2004;190(1):188–93.

27. Bravata DM, Smith-Spangler C, Sundaram V, et al. Using pedometers to increase physical activity and improve health: a systematic review. *JAMA.* 2007;298(19):2296–304.

28. Brown RJ, Wijewickrama RC, Harlan DM, Rother KI. Uncoupling intensive insulin therapy from weight gain and hypoglycemia in type 1 diabetes. *Diabetes Technol Ther.* 2011;13(4):457–60.

29. Buse JB, Ginsberg HN, Bakris GL, et al. Primary prevention of cardiovascular diseases in people with diabetes mellitus: a scientific statement from the American Heart Association and the American Diabetes Association. *Circulation.* 2007;115(1):114–26.

30. Casellini CM, Vinik AI. Clinical manifestations and current treatment options for diabetic neuropathies. *Endocr Pract.* 2007;13(5):550–66.

31. Cheng YJ, Lauer MS, Earnest CP, et al. Heart rate recovery following maximal exercise testing as a predictor of cardiovascular disease and all-cause mortality in men with diabetes. *Diabetes Care.* 2003;26(7):2052–7.

32. Chobanian AV, Bakris GL, Black HR, et al. The Seventh Report of the Joint National Committee on Prevention, Detection, Evaluation, and Treatment of High Blood Pressure: the JNC 7 report. *JAMA.* 2003;289(19):2560–72.

33. Chu L, Hamilton J, Riddell MC. Clinical management of the physically active patient with type 1 diabetes. *Phys Sportsmed.* 2011;39(2):64–77.

34. Chudyk A, Petrella RJ. Effects of exercise on cardiovascular risk factors in type 2 diabetes: a meta-analysis. *Diabetes Care.* 2011;34(5):1228–37.

35. Church TS, Blair SN, Cocreham S, et al. Effects of aerobic and resistance training on hemoglobin A1c levels in patients with type 2 diabetes: a randomized controlled trial. *JAMA.* 2010;304(20):2253–62.

36. Coccheri S. Approaches to prevention of cardiovascular complications and events in diabetes mellitus. *Drugs.* 2007;67(7):997–1026.

37. Colberg SR, Albright AL, Blissmer BJ, et al. Exercise and type 2 diabetes: American College of Sports Medicine and the American Diabetes Association: joint position statement. Exercise and type 2 diabetes. *Med Sci Sports Exerc.* 2010;42(12):2282–303.

38. Colberg SR, Sigal RJ, Fernhall B, et al. Exercise and type 2 diabetes: the American College of Sports Medicine and the American Diabetes Association: joint position statement. *Diabetes Care.* 2010;33(12):e147–67.

39. Colberg SR, Somma CT, Sechrist SR. Physical activity participation may offset some of the negative impact of diabetes on cognitive function. *J Am Med Dir Assoc.* 2008;9(6):434–8.

40. Colberg SR, Swain DP, Vinik AI. Use of heart rate reserve and rating of perceived exertion to prescribe exercise intensity in diabetic autonomic neuropathy. *Diabetes Care.* 2003;26(4):986–90.

41. Colberg SR, Zarrabi L, Bennington L, et al. Postprandial walking is better for lowering the glycemic effect of dinner than pre-dinner exercise in type 2 diabetic individuals. *J Am Med Dir Assoc.* 2009;10(6):394–7.

42. Collins TC, Lunos S, Ahluwalia JS. Self-efficacy is associated with walking ability in persons with diabetes mellitus and peripheral arterial disease. *Vasc Med.* 2010;15(3):189–95.

43. Collins TC, Lunos S, Carlson T, et al. Effects of a home-based walking intervention on mobility and quality of life in people with diabetes and peripheral arterial disease: a randomized controlled trial. *Diabetes Care.* 2011;34(10):2174–9.

44. Conn VS, Hafdahl AR, Lemaster JW, Ruppar TM, Cochran JE, Nielsen PJ. Meta-analysis of health behavior change interventions in type 1 diabetes. *Am J Health Behav.* 2008;32(3):315–29.

45. Conway B, Miller RG, Costacou T, et al. Temporal patterns in overweight and obesity in type 1 diabetes. *Diabet Med.* 2010;27(4):398–404.

46. Cooperberg BA, Breckenridge SM, Arbelaez AM, Cryer PE. Terbutaline and the prevention of nocturnal hypoglycemia in type 1 diabetes. *Diabetes Care.* 2008;31(12):2271–2.

47. Coughlan MT, Yap FY, Tong DC, et al. Advanced glycation end products are direct modulators of β-cell function. *Diabetes.* 2011;60(10):2523–32.

48. Cryer PE. Mechanisms of hypoglycemia-associated autonomic failure and its component syndromes in diabetes. *Diabetes.* 2005;54(12):3592–601.

49. Cuff DJ, Meneilly GS, Martin A, Ignaszewski A, Tildesley HD, Frohlich JJ. Effective exercise modality to reduce insulin resistance in women with type 2 diabetes. *Diabetes Care.* 2003;26(11):2977–82.

50. Davis SN, Mann S, Briscoe VJ, Ertl AC, Tate DB. Effects of intensive therapy and antecedent hypoglycemia on counter-regulatory responses to hypoglycemia in type 2 diabetes. *Diabetes.* 2009;58(3):701–9.

51. Delahanty LM, Conroy MB, Nathan DM, Diabetes Prevention Program Research Group. Psychological predictors of physical activity in the diabetes prevention program. *J Am Diet Assoc.* 2006;106(5):698–705.

52. Delvecchio M, Zecchino C, Salzano G, et al. Effects of moderate-severe exercise on blood glucose in Type 1 diabetic adolescents treated with insulin pump or glargine insulin. *J Endocrinol Invest.* 2009;32(6):519–24.

53. Devenney R, O'Neill S. The experience of diabetic retinopathy: a qualitative study. *Br J Health Psychol.* 2011;16(4):707–21.

54. D'hooge R, Hellinckx T, Van Laethem C, et al. Influence of combined aerobic and resistance training on metabolic control, cardiovascular fitness and quality of life in adolescents with type 1 diabetes: a randomized controlled trial. *Clin Rehabil.* 2011;25(4):349–59.

55. Diabetes Research in Children Network (DirecNet) Study Group, Tsalikian E, Kollman C, et al. Prevention of hypoglycemia during exercise in children with type 1 diabetes by suspending basal insulin. *Diabetes Care.* 2006;29(10):2200–4.

56. Donnelly JE, Blair SN, Jakicic JM, et al. American College of Sports Medicine position stand. Appropriate physical activity intervention strategies for weight loss and prevention of weight regain for adults. *Med Sci Sports Exerc.* 2009;41(2):459–71.

57. Dunstan DW, Daly RM, Owen N, et al. High-intensity resistance training improves glycemic control in older patients with type 2 diabetes. *Diabetes Care.* 2002;25(10):1729–36.

58. Dunstan DW, Daly RM, Owen N, et al. Home-based resistance training is not sufficient to maintain improved glycemic control following supervised training in older individuals with type 2 diabetes. *Diabetes Care.* 2005;28(1):3–9.

59. Dutton GR, Tan F, Provost BC, Sorenson JL, Allen B, Smith D. Relationship between self-efficacy and physical activity among patients with type 2 diabetes. *J Behav Med.* 2009;32(3):270–7.

60. Egede LE. Diabetes, major depression, and functional disability among U.S. adults. *Diabetes Care.* 2004;27(2):421–8.

61. Evans EM, Racette SB, Peterson LR, Villareal DT, Greiwe JS, Holloszy JO. Aerobic power and insulin action improve in response to endurance exercise training in healthy 77–87 yr olds. *J Appl Physiol.* 2005;98(1):40–5.

62. Ewing DJ, Clarke BF. Diabetic autonomic neuropathy: present insights and future prospects. *Diabetes Care.* 1986;9(6):648–65.

63. Farmer A, Balman E, Gadsby R, et al. Frequency of self-monitoring of blood glucose in patients with type 2 diabetes: association with hypoglycaemic events. *Curr Med Res Opin.* 2008;24(11):3097–104.

64. Featherstone JF, Holly RG, Amsterdam EA. Physiologic responses to weight lifting in coronary artery disease. *Am J Cardiol.* 1993;71(4):287–92.

65. Fox CS, Pencina MJ, Wilson PW, Paynter NP, Vasan RS, D'Agostino RB,Sr. Lifetime risk of cardiovascular disease among individuals with and without diabetes stratified by obesity status in the Framingham heart study. *Diabetes Care.* 2008;31(8):1582–4.

66. Frank LD, Engelke PO, Schmid TL. *Health and Community Design: The Impact of the Built Environment on Physical Activity.* Washington (DC): Island Press; 2003. 253 p.

67. Garber CE, Blissmer B, Deschenes MR, et al. Quantity and quality of exercise for developing and maintaining cardiorespiratory, musculoskeletal, and neuromotor fitness in apparently healthy adults: guidance for prescribing exercise. *Med Sci Sports Exerc.* 2011;43(7):1334–59.

68. Gavi S, Hensley J. Diagnosis and management of type 2 diabetes in adults: a review of the ICSI guideline. *Geriatrics.* 2009;64(6):12–7, 29.

69. Gimeno Orna JA, Boned Juliani B, Lou Arnal LM, Castro Alonso FJ. Microalbuminuria and clinical proteinuria as the main predictive factors of cardiovascular morbidity and mortality in patients with type 2 diabetes. *Rev Clin Esp.* 2003;203(11):526–31.

70. Gleeson-Kreig J. Social support and physical activity in type 2 diabetes: a social-ecologic approach. *Diabetes Educ.* 2008;34(6):1037–44.

71. Goldsmith JR, Lidtke RH, Shott S. The effects of range-of-motion therapy on the plantar pressures of patients with diabetes mellitus. *J Am Podiatr Med Assoc.* 2002;92(9):483–90.

72. Gordon BA, Benson AC, Bird SR, Fraser SF. Resistance training improves metabolic health in type 2 diabetes: a systematic review. *Diabetes Res Clin Pract.* 2009;83(2):157–75.

73. Graves JE, Pollock ML, Bryant CX. Assessment of muscular strength and endurance. In: Roitman JL, Herridge M, editors. *ACSM's Resource Manual for Guidelines for Exercise Testing and Prescription.* 4th ed. Philadelphia: Lippincott Williams & Wilkins; 2001. p. 376–380.

74. Haskell WL, Lee IM, Pate RR, et al. Physical activity and public health: updated recommendation for adults from the American College of Sports Medicine and the American Heart Association. *Med Sci Sports Exerc.* 2007;39(8):1423–34.

75. Heran BS, Chen JM, Ebrahim S, et al. Exercise-based cardiac rehabilitation for coronary heart disease. *Cochrane Database Syst Rev.* 2011(7):CD001800.

76. Herbst A, Kordonouri O, Schwab KO, Schmidt F, Holl RW, DPV Initiative of the German Working Group for Pediatric Diabetology Germany. Impact of physical activity on cardiovascular risk factors in children with type 1 diabetes: a multicenter study of 23,251 patients. *Diabetes Care.* 2007;30(8):2098–100.

77. Hernandez JM, Moccia T, Fluckey JD, Ulbrecht JS, Farrell PA. Fluid snacks to help persons with type 1 diabetes avoid late onset postexercise hypoglycemia. *Med Sci Sports Exerc.* 2000;32(5):904–10.

78. Herriott MT, Colberg SR, Parson HK, Nunnold T, Vinik AI. Effects of 8 weeks of flexibility and resistance training in older adults with type 2 diabetes. *Diabetes Care.* 2004;27(12):2988–9.

79. Hordern MD, Dunstan DW, Prins JB, Baker MK, Singh MA, Coombes JS. Exercise prescription for patients with type 2 diabetes and pre-diabetes: a position statement from Exercise and Sport Science Australia. *J Sci Med Sport.* 2012;15(1):25–31.

80. Houmard JA, Tanner CJ, Slentz CA, Duscha BD, McCartney JS, Kraus WE. Effect of the volume and intensity of exercise training on insulin sensitivity. *J Appl Physiol.* 2004;96(1):101–6.

81. Howorka K, Pumprla J, Haber P, Koller-Strametz J, Mondrzyk J, Schabmann A. Effects of physical training on heart rate variability in diabetic patients with various degrees of cardiovascular autonomic neuropathy. *Cardiovasc Res.* 1997;34(1):206–14.

82. Innes KE, Vincent HK. The influence of yoga-based programs on risk profiles in adults with type 2 diabetes mellitus: a systematic review. *Evid Based Complement Alternat Med.* 2007;4(4):469–86.

83. Irvine C, Taylor NF. Progressive resistance exercise improves glycaemic control in people with type 2 diabetes mellitus: a systematic review. *Aust J Physiother.* 2009;55(4):237–46.

84. Iscoe KE, Riddell MC. Continuous moderate-intensity exercise with or without intermittent high-intensity work: effects on acute and late glycaemia in athletes with Type 1 diabetes mellitus. *Diabet Med.* 2011;28(7):824–32.

85. Johansen KL. Exercise and chronic kidney disease: current recommendations. *Sports Med.* 2005;35(6):485–99.

86. Johnson ST, McCargar LJ, Bell GJ, Tudor-Locke C, Harber VJ, Bell RC. Walking faster: distilling a complex prescription for type 2 diabetes management through pedometry. *Diabetes Care.* 2006;29(7):1654–5.

87. Juutilainen A, Lehto S, Ronnemaa T, Pyorala K, Laakso M. Retinopathy predicts cardiovascular mortality in type 2 diabetic men and women. *Diabetes Care.* 2007;30(2):292–9.

88. Kabadi UM, Vora A, Kabadi M. Hyperinsulinemia and central adiposity: influence of chronic insulin therapy in type 1 diabetes. *Diabetes Care.* 2000;23(7):1024–6.

89. Kalergis M, Schiffrin A, Gougeon R, Jones PJ, Yale JF. Impact of bedtime snack composition on prevention of nocturnal hypoglycemia in adults with type 1 diabetes undergoing intensive insulin management using lispro insulin before meals: a randomized, placebo-controlled, crossover trial. *Diabetes Care.* 2003;26(1):9–15.

90. Kennedy JW, Hirshman MF, Gervino EV, et al. Acute exercise induces GLUT4 translocation in skeletal muscle of normal human subjects and subjects with type 2 diabetes. *Diabetes.* 1999;48(5):1192–7.

91. King DS, Baldus PJ, Sharp RL, Kesl LD, Feltmeyer TL, Riddle MS. Time course for exercise-induced alterations in insulin action and glucose tolerance in middle-aged people. *J Appl Physiol.* 1995;78(1):17–22.

92. Kitabchi AE, Umpierrez GE, Murphy MB, et al. Hyperglycemic crises in diabetes. *Diabetes Care.* 2004;27 Suppl 1:S94–102.

93. Klein R, Klein BE, Moss SE. Epidemiology of proliferative diabetic retinopathy. *Diabetes Care.* 1992;15(12):1875–91.

94. Koh KH, Dayanath B, Doery JC, et al. Effect of exercise on urine albuminuria excretion in diabetic subjects. *Nephrology (Carlton).* 2011;16(8):704–9.

95. Koh KP, Fassett RG, Sharman JE, Coombes JS, Williams AD. Effect of intradialytic versus home-based aerobic exercise training on physical function and vascular parameters in hemodialysis patients: a randomized pilot study. *Am J Kidney Dis.* 2010;55(1):88–99.

96. Kopp M, Steinlechner M, Ruedl G, Ledochowski L, Rumpold G, Taylor AH. Acute effects of brisk walking on affect and psychological well-being in individuals with type 2 diabetes. *Diabetes Res Clin Pract.* 2012;95(1):25–9.

97. Kreisman SH, Halter JB, Vranic M, Marliss EB. Combined infusion of epinephrine and norepinephrine during moderate exercise reproduces the glucoregulatory response of intense exercise. *Diabetes.* 2003;52(6):1347–54.

98. Krentz AJ, Bailey CJ. Oral antidiabetic agents: current role in type 2 diabetes mellitus. *Drugs.* 2005;65(3):385–411.

99. Laaksonen DE, Atalay M, Niskanen LK, et al. Aerobic exercise and the lipid profile in type 1 diabetic men: a randomized controlled trial. *Med Sci Sports Exerc.* 2000;32(9):1541–8.

100. Larsen JJ, Dela F, Madsbad S, Galbo H. The effect of intense exercise on postprandial glucose homeostasis in type II diabetic patients. *Diabetologia.* 1999;42(11):1282–92.

101. Larsen JJ, Dela F, Madsbad S, Vibe-Petersen J, Galbo H. Interaction of sulfonylureas and exercise on glucose homeostasis in type 2 diabetic patients. *Diabetes Care.* 1999;22(10):1647–54.

102. Lee AJ, Hiscock RJ, Wein P, Walker SP, Permezel M. Gestational diabetes mellitus: clinical predictors and long-term risk of developing type 2 diabetes: a retrospective cohort study using survival analysis. *Diabetes Care.* 2007;30(4):878–83.

103. Lee MS, Choi TY, Lim HJ, Ernst E. Tai chi for management of type 2 diabetes mellitus: a systematic review. *Chin J Integr Med.* 2011.

104. Lemaster JW, Mueller MJ, Reiber GE, Mehr DR, Madsen RW, Conn VS. Effect of weight-bearing activity on foot ulcer incidence in people with diabetic peripheral neuropathy: feet first randomized controlled trial. *Phys Ther.* 2008;88(11):1385–98.

105. Lemaster JW, Reiber GE, Smith DG, Heagerty PJ, Wallace C. Daily weight-bearing activity does not increase the risk of diabetic foot ulcers. *Med Sci Sports Exerc.* 2003;35(7):1093–9.

106. Levine JA, Lanningham-Foster LM, McCrady SK, et al. Interindividual variation in posture allocation: possible role in human obesity. *Science.* 2005;307(5709):584–6.

107. Levine JA, McCrady SK, Lanningham-Foster LM, Kane PH, Foster RC, Manohar CU. The role of free-living daily walking in human weight gain and obesity. *Diabetes.* 2008;57(3):548–54.

108. Lievre MM, Moulin P, Thivolet C, et al. Detection of silent myocardial ischemia in asymptomatic patients with diabetes: results of a randomized trial and meta-analysis assessing the effectiveness of systematic screening. *Trials.* 2011;12:23.

109. Loimaala A, Huikuri HV, Koobi T, Rinne M, Nenonen A, Vuori I. Exercise training improves baroreflex sensitivity in type 2 diabetes. *Diabetes.* 2003;52(7):1837–42.

110. Look AHEAD Research Group, Wing RR. Long-term effects of a lifestyle intervention on weight and cardiovascular risk factors in individuals with type 2 diabetes mellitus: four-year results of the Look AHEAD trial. *Arch Intern Med.* 2010;170(17):1566–75.

111. Lubans DR, Plotnikoff RC, Jung M, Eves N, Sigal R. Testing mediator variables in a resistance training intervention for obese adults with type 2 diabetes. *Psychol Health.* 2011. Sep 6. [Epub ahead of print]

112. Lustman PJ, Clouse RE. Depression in diabetic patients: the relationship between mood and glycemic control. *J Diabetes Complications.* 2005;19(2):113–22.

113. Luszczynska A, Schwarzer R, Lippke S, Mazurkiewicz M. Self-efficacy as a moderator of the planning-behaviour relationship in interventions designed to promote physical activity. *Psychol Health.* 2011;26(2):151–66.

114. Lysy Z, Da Costa D, Dasgupta K. The association of physical activity and depression in Type 2 diabetes. *Diabet Med.* 2008;25(10):1133–41.

115. Mamcarz A, Chmielewski M, Braksator W, et al. Factors influencing cardiac complications in patients with type-2 diabetes mellitus and silent myocardial ischaemia: five-year follow-up. *Pol Arch Med Wewn.* 2004;112(6):1433–43.

116. Manders RJ, Van Dijk JW, van Loon LJ. Low-intensity exercise reduces the prevalence of hyperglycemia in type 2 diabetes. *Med Sci Sports Exerc.* 2010;42(2):219–25.

117. Marcus RL, Smith S, Morrell G, et al. Comparison of combined aerobic and high-force eccentric resistance exercise with aerobic exercise only for people with type 2 diabetes mellitus. *Phys Ther.* 2008;88(11):1345–54.

118. Marwick TH, Hordern MD, Miller T, et al. Exercise training for type 2 diabetes mellitus: impact on cardiovascular risk: a scientific statement from the American Heart Association. *Circulation.* 2009;119(25):3244–62.

119. McDermott MM, Ades P, Guralnik JM, et al. Treadmill exercise and resistance training in patients with peripheral arterial disease with and without intermittent claudication: a randomized controlled trial. *JAMA.* 2009;301(2):165–74.

120. McMahon SK, Ferreira LD, Ratnam N, et al. Glucose requirements to maintain euglycemia after moderate-intensity afternoon exercise in adolescents with type 1 diabetes are increased in a biphasic manner. *J Clin Endocrinol Metab.* 2007;92(3):963–8.

121. Michael Y, Beard T, Choi D, Farquhar S, Carlson N. Measuring the influence of built neighborhood environments on walking in older adults. *J Aging Phys Act.* 2006;14(3):302–12.

122. Morrison S, Colberg SR, Mariano M, Parson HK, Vinik AI. Balance training reduces falls risk in older individuals with type 2 diabetes. *Diabetes Care.* 2010;33(4):748–50.

123. Musi N, Fujii N, Hirshman MF, et al. AMP-activated protein kinase (AMPK) is activated in muscle of subjects with type 2 diabetes during exercise. *Diabetes.* 2001;50(5):921–7.

124. Naik AD, Palmer N, Petersen NJ, et al. Comparative effectiveness of goal setting in diabetes mellitus group clinics: randomized clinical trial. *Arch Intern Med.* 2011;171(5):453–9.

125. Narayan KM, Boyle JP, Geiss LS, Saaddine JB, Thompson TJ. Impact of recent increase in incidence on future diabetes burden: U.S., 2005–2050. *Diabetes Care.* 2006;29(9):2114–6.

126. Narayan KM, Boyle JP, Thompson TJ, Sorensen SW, Williamson DF. Lifetime risk for diabetes mellitus in the United States. *JAMA.* 2003;290(14):1884–90.

127. *National Diabetes Fact Sheet, 2011: National Estimates and General Information on Diabetes and Prediabetes in the United States* [Internet]. Atlanta (GA): U.S. Department of Health and Human Services, Centers for Disease Control and Prevention; 2011 [cited 2011 Mar 10]. 12 p. Available from: http://www.cdc.gov/diabetes/pubs/factsheet11.htm

128. Negri C, Bacchi E, Morgante S, et al. Supervised walking groups to increase physical activity in type 2 diabetic patients. *Diabetes Care.* 2010;33(11):2333–5.

129. Nelson ME, Rejeski WJ, Blair SN, et al. Physical activity and public health in older adults: recommendation from the American College of Sports Medicine and the American Heart Association. *Med Sci Sports Exerc.* 2007;39(8):1435–45.

130. Newman DJ, Pugia MJ, Lott JA, Wallace JF, Hiar AM. Urinary protein and albumin excretion corrected by creatinine and specific gravity. *Clin Chim Acta.* 2000;294(1–2):139–55.

131. O'Gorman DJ, Karlsson HK, McQuaid S, et al. Exercise training increases insulin-stimulated glucose disposal and GLUT4 (SLC2A4) protein content in patients with type 2 diabetes. *Diabetologia.* 2006;49(12):2983–92.

132. Oostdam N, van Poppel MN, Eekhoff EM, Wouters MG, van Mechelen W. Design of FitFor2 study: the effects of an exercise program on insulin sensitivity and plasma glucose levels in pregnant women at high risk for gestational diabetes. *BMC Pregnancy Childbirth.* 2009;9:1.

133. Osborn CY, Amico KR, Cruz N, et al. A brief culturally tailored intervention for Puerto Ricans with type 2 diabetes. *Health Educ Behav.* 2010;37(6):849–62.

134. Pagkalos M, Koutlianos N, Kouidi E, Pagkalos E, Mandroukas K, Deligiannis A. Heart rate variability modifications following exercise training in type 2 diabetic patients with definite cardiac autonomic neuropathy. *Br J Sports Med.* 2008;42(1):47–54.

135. Painter P, Carlson L, Carey S, Paul SM, Myll J. Low-functioning hemodialysis patients improve with exercise training. *Am J Kidney Dis.* 2000;36(3):600–8.

136. Painter P, Carlson L, Carey S, Paul SM, Myll J. Physical functioning and health-related quality-of-life changes with exercise training in hemodialysis patients. *Am J Kidney Dis.* 2000;35(3):482–92.

137. Pan A, Lucas M, Sun Q, et al. Bidirectional association between depression and type 2 diabetes mellitus in women. *Arch Intern Med.* 2010;170(21):1884–91.

138. Pena KE, Stopka CB, Barak S, Gertner HR,Jr, Carmeli E. Effects of low-intensity exercise on patients with peripheral artery disease. *Phys Sportsmed.* 2009;37(1):106–10.

139. Pentecost C, Taket A. Understanding exercise uptake and adherence for people with chronic conditions: a new model demonstrating the importance of exercise identity, benefits of attending and support. *Health Educ Res.* 2011;26(5):908–22.

140. Pescatello LS, Arena R, Riebe D, American College of Sports Medicine. *ACSM's Guidelines for Exercise Testing and Prescription.* 9th ed. Philadelphia (PA): Lippincott Williams & Wilkins; 2012. 380 p.

141. Physical Activity guidelines Advisory Committee. *Physical Activity Guidelines Advisory Committee Report, 2008* [Internet]. Washington (DC): U.S. Department of Health and Human Services; 2008. Available from: http://www.health.gov/paguidelines/committeereport.aspx

142. Plotnikoff RC, Trinh L, Courneya KS, Karunamuni N, Sigal RJ. Predictors of physical activity in adults with type 2 diabetes. *Am J Health Behav.* 2011;35(3):359–70.

143. Ploug T, Galbo H, Richter EA. Increased muscle glucose uptake during contractions: no need for insulin. *Am J Physiol.* 1984;247(6 Pt 1):E726–31.

144. Poirier P, Mawhinney S, Grondin L, et al. Prior meal enhances the plasma glucose lowering effect of exercise in type 2 diabetes. *Med Sci Sports Exerc.* 2001;33(8):1259–64.

145. Polster M, Zanutto E, McDonald S, Conner C, Hammer M. A comparison of preferences for two GLP-1 products—liraglutide and exenatide—for the treatment of type 2 diabetes. *J Med Econ.* 2010;13(4):655–61.

146. Praet SF, van Rooij ES, Wijtvliet A, et al. Brisk walking compared with an individualised medical fitness programme for patients with type 2 diabetes: a randomised controlled trial. *Diabetologia.* 2008;51(5):736–46.

147. Ramalho AC, de Lourdes Lima M, Nunes F, et al. The effect of resistance versus aerobic training on metabolic control in patients with type-1 diabetes mellitus. *Diabetes Res Clin Pract.* 2006;72(3):271–6.

148. Ratner R, Goldberg R, Haffner S, et al. Impact of intensive lifestyle and metformin therapy on cardiovascular disease risk factors in the diabetes prevention program. *Diabetes Care.* 2005;28(4):888–94.

149. Realsen JM, Chase HP. Recent advances in the prevention of hypoglycemia in type 1 diabetes. *Diabetes Technol Ther.* 2011;13(12):1177–86.

150. Roberts L, Jones TW, Fournier PA. Exercise training and glycemic control in adolescents with poorly controlled type 1 diabetes mellitus. *J Pediatr Endocrinol Metab.* 2002;15(5):621–7.

151. Rosenstock J, Hassman DR, Madder RD, et al. Repaglinide versus nateglinide monotherapy: a randomized, multicenter study. *Diabetes Care.* 2004;27(6):1265–70.

152. Ross SA, Tildesley HD, Ashkenas J. Barriers to effective insulin treatment: the persistence of poor glycemic control in type 2 diabetes. *Curr Med Res Opin.* 2011.

153. Sandoval DA, Guy DL, Richardson MA, Ertl AC, Davis SN. Acute, same-day effects of antecedent exercise on counterregulatory responses to subsequent hypoglycemia in type 1 diabetes mellitus. *Am J Physiol Endocrinol Metab.* 2006;290(6):E1331–8.

154. Sandoval DA, Guy DL, Richardson MA, Ertl AC, Davis SN. Effects of low and moderate antecedent exercise on counterregulatory responses to subsequent hypoglycemia in type 1 diabetes. *Diabetes.* 2004;53(7):1798–806.

155. Seeger JP, Thijssen DH, Noordam K, Cranen ME, Hopman MT, Nijhuis-van der Sanden MW. Exercise training improves physical fitness and vascular function in children with type 1 diabetes. *Diabetes Obes Metab.* 2011;13(4):382–4.

156. Shinji S, Shigeru M, Ryusei U, Mitsuru M, Shigehiro K. Adherence to a home-based exercise program and incidence of cardiovascular disease in type 2 diabetes patients. *Int J Sports Med.* 2007;28(10):877–9.

157. Shrier I. Stretching before exercise does not reduce the risk of local muscle injury: a critical review of the clinical and basic science literature. *Clin J Sport Med.* 1999;9(4):221–7.

158. Sigal RJ, Kenny GP, Boule NG, et al. Effects of aerobic training, resistance training, or both on glycemic control in type 2 diabetes: a randomized trial. *Ann Intern Med.* 2007;147(6):357–69.

159. Sigal RJ, Kenny GP, Wasserman DH, Castaneda-Sceppa C. Physical activity/exercise and type 2 diabetes. *Diabetes Care.* 2004;27(10):2518–39.

160. Sigal RJ, Kenny GP, Wasserman DH, Castaneda-Sceppa C, White RD. Physical activity/exercise and type 2 diabetes: a consensus statement from the American Diabetes Association. *Diabetes Care.* 2006;29(6):1433–8.

161. Sigal RJ, Purdon C, Bilinski D, Vranic M, Halter JB, Marliss EB. Glucoregulation during and after intense exercise: effects of beta-blockade. *J Clin Endocrinol Metab.* 1994;78(2):359–66.

162. Sigal RJ, Purdon C, Fisher SJ, Halter JB, Vranic M, Marliss EB. Hyperinsulinemia prevents prolonged hyperglycemia after intense exercise in insulin-dependent diabetic subjects. *J Clin Endocrinol Metab.* 1994;79(4):1049–57.

163. Singh DK, Winocour P, Farrington K. Oxidative stress in early diabetic nephropathy: fueling the fire. *Nat Rev Endocrinol.* 2011;7(3):176–84.

164. Smith SC,Jr, Allen J, Blair SN, et al. AHA/ACC guidelines for secondary prevention for patients with coronary and other atherosclerotic vascular disease: 2006 update: endorsed by the National Heart, Lung, and Blood Institute. *Circulation.* 2006;113(19):2363–72.

165. Snowling NJ, Hopkins WG. Effects of different modes of exercise training on glucose control and risk factors for complications in type 2 diabetic patients: a meta-analysis. *Diabetes Care.* 2006;29(11):2518–27.

166. Sridhar B, Haleagrahara N, Bhat R, Kulur AB, Avabratha S, Adhikary P. Increase in the heart rate variability with deep breathing in diabetic patients after 12-month exercise training. *Tohoku J Exp Med.* 2010;220(2):107–13.

167. St. John A, Davis WA, Price CP, Davis TM. The value of self-monitoring of blood glucose: a review of recent evidence. *J Diabetes Complications.* 2010;24(2):129–41.

168. Stewart KJ. Exercise training and the cardiovascular consequences of type 2 diabetes and hypertension: plausible mechanisms for improving cardiovascular health. *JAMA.* 2002;288(13):1622–31.

169. Strasser B, Siebert U, Schobersberger W. Resistance training in the treatment of the metabolic syndrome: a systematic review and meta-analysis of the effect of resistance training on metabolic clustering in patients with abnormal glucose metabolism. *Sports Med.* 2010;40(5):397–415.

170. Swank AM. *Resistance Training for Special Populations: Quick Reference Guide.* Clifton Park (NY): Delmar Pub; 2009. 538 p.

171. Szewieczek J, Dulawa J, Strzalkowska D, Batko-Szwaczka A, Hornik B. Normal insulin response to short-term intense exercise is abolished in Type 2 diabetic patients treated with gliclazide. *J Diabetes Complications.* 2009;23(6):380–6.

172. Szewieczek J, Dulawa J, Strzalkowska D, Hornik B, Kawecki G. Impact of the short-term, intense exercise on postprandial glycemia in type 2 diabetic patients treated with gliclazide. *J Diabetes Complications.* 2007;21(2):101–7.

173. Taplin CE, Cobry E, Messer L, McFann K, Chase HP, Fiallo-Scharer R. Preventing post-exercise nocturnal hypoglycemia in children with type 1 diabetes. *J Pediatr.* 2010;157(5):784–8.e1.

174. Tobias DK, Zhang C, van Dam RM, Bowers K, Hu FB. Physical activity before and during pregnancy and risk of gestational diabetes mellitus: a meta-analysis. *Diabetes Care.* 2011;34(1):223–9.

175. Type 2 diabetes in children and adolescents. American Diabetes Association. *Diabetes Care.* 2000;23(3):381–9.

176. Ugale J, Mata A, Meert KL, Sarnaik AP. Measured degree of dehydration in children and adolescents with type 1 diabetic ketoacidosis. *Pediatr Crit Care Med.* 2012;13(2)e103–7.

177. Umpierre D, Ribeiro PA, Kramer CK, et al. Physical activity advice only or structured exercise training and association with HbA1c levels in type 2 diabetes: a systematic review and meta-analysis. *JAMA.* 2011;305(17):1790–9.

178. Vanhecke TE, Franklin BA, Miller WM, deJong AT, Coleman CJ, McCullough PA. Cardiorespiratory fitness and sedentary lifestyle in the morbidly obese. *Clin Cardiol.* 2009;32(3):121–4.

179. Vinik A. Advancing therapy in type 2 diabetes mellitus with early, comprehensive progression from oral agents to insulin therapy. *Clin Ther.* 2007;29(6 Pt 1):1236–53.

180. Vinik AI, Erbas T. Neuropathy. In: Ruderman N, Devlin JT, Schneider SH, Kriska AM, American Diabetes Association, editors. *Handbook of Exercise in Diabetes.* 2nd ed. Alexandria: American Diabetes Association; 2002. p. 463–496.

181. Vinik AI, Maser RE, Ziegler D. Autonomic imbalance: prophet of doom or scope for hope? *Diabet Med.* 2011;28(6):643–51.

182. Vinik AI, Ziegler D. Diabetic cardiovascular autonomic neuropathy. *Circulation.* 2007;115(3):387–97.

183. Voulgari C, Katsilambros N, Tentolouris N. Smoking cessation predicts amelioration of microalbuminuria in newly diagnosed type 2 diabetes mellitus: a 1-year prospective study. *Metabolism.* 2011;60(10):1456–64.

184. Wahren J, Ekberg K. Splanchnic regulation of glucose production. *Annu Rev Nutr.* 2007;27:329–45.

185. Want LL. Optimizing treatment success with an amylin analogue. *Diabetes Educ.* 2008;34 Suppl 1:11S–7S.

186. Webber SC, Porter MM. Monitoring mobility in older adults using global positioning system (GPS) watches and accelerometers: a feasibility study. *J Aging Phys Act.* 2009;17(4):455–67.

187. Wenger NK, Froelicher ES, Smith LK, et al. Cardiac rehabilitation as secondary prevention. Agency for Health Care Policy and Research and National Heart, Lung, and Blood Institute. *Clin Pract Guidel Quick Ref Guide Clin.* 1995;17:1–23.

188. Willey KA, Singh MA. Battling insulin resistance in elderly obese people with type 2 diabetes: bring on the heavy weights. *Diabetes Care.* 2003;26(5):1580–8.

189. Yeung EW, Yeung SS. Interventions for preventing lower limb soft-tissue injuries in runners. *Cochrane Database Syst Rev.* 2001(3):CD001256.

190. Younk LM, Mikeladze M, Tate D, Davis SN. Exercise-related hypoglycemia in diabetes mellitus. *Expert Rev Endocrinol Metab.* 2011;6(1):93–108.

191. Ziegler D, Gries FA, Spuler M, Lessmann F. The epidemiology of diabetic neuropathy. Diabetic Cardiovascular Autonomic Neuropathy Multicenter Study Group. *J Diabetes Complications.* 1992;6(1):49–57.

SELECTED REFERENCES FOR FURTHER READING

American Diabetes Association. Physical activity/exercise and diabetes. *Diabetes Care.* 2004;27:S58–62.

Colberg SR. *Diabetic Athlete's Handbook: Your Guide to Peak Performance.* Champaign (IL): Human Kinetics, 2009. 284 p.

Colberg SR. *The 7 Step Diabetes Fitness Plan: Living Well and Being Fit with Diabetes, No Matter Your Weight.* New York (NY): Marlowe & Company, 2007. 272 p.

Colberg SR, Sigal RJ, Fernhall B, et al. Exercise and type 2 diabetes: the American College of Sports Medicine and the American Diabetes Association: joint position statement. *Diabetes Care.* 2010;33:e147–67.

INTERNET RESOURCES

- American College of Sports Medicine: http://www.acsm.org
- American Diabetes Association: http://www.diabetes.org
- National Institute of Diabetes and Digestive and Kidney Diseases: http://www2.niddk.nih.gov
- American Society of Diabetes Educators: http://www.aadenet.org
- Centers for Disease Control and Prevention, National Center for Chronic Disease Prevention and Health Promotion (Diabetes Public Health Resource): http://www.cdc.gov/diabetes/index.htm

Exercise Prescription for Patients with Comorbidities and Other Chronic Diseases

Current trends show that Americans are living longer although the number of U.S. citizens with chronic diseases continues to increase. In the past 100 yr, life expectancy at birth in the United States increased from less than 50 yr to more than 76 yr (2,85). In 2011, the "baby boomers" began to turn 65 yr old, which is expected to start a dramatic increase in the older population through 2030. According to the Federal Interagency Forum on Aging-Related Statistics, the older population in 2030 will be twice as large as in 2000, growing from 35 million to 72 million, which will represent approximately 20% of the U.S. population (75). Concerned health care providers, including exercise professionals, are faced with maintaining quality of life, limiting the impact and progression of chronic diseases, and reducing the number of disabilities in this aging population (65).

Chronic diseases and disabilities associated with a sedentary lifestyle are important because maintaining a physically active lifestyle does affect health. In 2005, approximately 63 million Americans (21%) had more than one chronic condition or multiple illnesses/impairments expected to last 1 yr or longer (110). Approximately 80% of individuals aged 65 yr or older are living with at least one chronic health problem, and another 50% are living with two (7,35,86). Currently, the American Heart Association (AHA) and the American College of Sports Medicine (ACSM) list sedentary lifestyle as a controllable risk factor for many chronic health problems. Notably, lifestyle, not just aging, is a leading cause for many chronic diseases and disabilities. As the aging process occurs, many physiologic changes take place. For example, as individuals age, they tend to have less ability to maintain their balance, they have slower reaction time, they tend to lose flexibility or joint range of motion, they tend to lose lean body mass (*i.e.*, sarcopenia), they tend to increase interstitial fat, and they have reduced blood levels of estrogen and androgen, and their muscle strength and endurance decrease (7,25).

Discouraging as these aging effects sound, the deterioration of physiologic and functional changes can be delayed by a lifestyle that emphasizes increased daily physical activity and/or planned regular exercise. Regular physical activity and/or planned exercise programming helps to favorably alter body composition, resting blood pressure (BP), and resting heart rate while improving cognitive and cardiopulmonary function and sleep quality (115). Physical activity aids in maintaining muscle mass, joint flexibility, and bone mineralization despite advancing age. An active lifestyle increases neuromuscular coordination, balance, and agility, all of which can be important in the prevention of falls. This may reduce the likelihood of a disability while increasing the ability of independence as aging occurs. Thus, a lifestyle that incorporates a lifetime of increased daily physical activity and planned exercise results in reduced chronic disease risk for coronary heart disease (CHD), diabetes, and other debilitating conditions, such as arthritis and osteoporosis (6,7,25,50,65,70,71,86,89,112).

KEY TERMS

Apraxia: Inability to make purposeful bodily motions or movements.

Claudication: Painful sensation in skeletal muscles of the lower extremity, most commonly related to atherosclerosis in the lower extremities.

Dyslipidemia: Abnormal blood levels of triglyceride and/or cholesterol-carrying lipoproteins affecting one or all of the subfractions of blood lipids; characteristically, these levels are abnormally high, although some forms of dyslipidemia can include low values (typically of high-density lipoprotein cholesterol).

Hypertonia: Abnormally increased amount of tension in resting skeletal muscle.

Vertebrobasilar: Pertaining to the part of cerebral circulation that is supplied by the vertebral and basilar arteries in the neck and head.

In this chapter, we discuss strategies for preventing, managing, and improving the functional deterioration brought on by hyperlipidemia, hypertension, obesity, peripheral arterial disease (PAD), and stroke (also known as cerebrovascular accident [CVA]) — all diseases that increase the risk for developing heart disease and cardiovascular complications. These can lead to a difficult downward spiral and deterioration in functional capacity. Exercise management in these populations serves to reduce risk for chronic diseases and secondary conditions or disorders while optimizing functional capacity, ability to perform basic and instrumental activities of daily living, and improve overall quality of life.

EPIDEMIOLOGY AND PATHOPHYSIOLOGY

DYSLIPIDEMIA

Hyperlipidemia or dyslipidemia is primary in determining CHD risk and is formally defined as the consequence of various genetic, environmental, and pathologic factors resulting in elevated blood cholesterol and triglyceride levels. Factors associated with dyslipidemia include sex, age, body fat distribution, cigarette smoking, some medications, genetics, dietary habits, and whether physically activity or regular participation in exercise is built into daily activities.

An estimated 98.8 million Americans have blood cholesterol levels that exceed 200 mg · dL^{-1} (20,102). Current guidelines from the National Cholesterol Education Program Adult Treatment Panel III (NCEP ATP III) state that CHD risk increases dramatically when blood cholesterol level is $\geq$240 mg · dL^{-1} (106). It is estimated that 33.6 million Americans have cholesterol levels exceeding this high-risk cutpoint. The 65.2 million individuals with blood cholesterol levels between 200 mg · dL^{-1} and 239 mg · dL^{-1} are considered to have borderline-high CHD risk (102,106).

Lipids are not soluble in water (i.e., are hydrophobic) and do not mix well with body fluids. In order for these lipids to move around the body, they must combine with proteins (apolipoproteins) to form lipoproteins, or micelle particles. Four principal lipoprotein classes exist and are classified by density (dictated by both lipid and protein content). Chylomicrons are derived from intestinal absorption of exogenous dietary fat. Very low-density lipoproteins (VLDL) are smaller and denser than chylomicrons and are synthesized primarily by the liver; some VLDL particles are also derived from chylomicron breakdown. Liver VLDL is mostly responsible for movement of endogenous triglyceride. Within circulation, VLDL particles liberate fatty acids at the tissue level — known as "delipidation." Through this process, the particle size decreases and density increases, yielding intermediate-density lipoprotein (IDL) particles. Further delipidation leads to the formation of low-density lipoprotein (LDL) particles, which represent the final stage of catabolism of VLDL. LDL particles are the primary carrier of cholesterol in humans. LDL particles are heterogeneous in size; larger, more buoyant particles impose a lower cardiovascular risk, whereas smaller, denser LDL particles impose a greater cardiovascular risk given their greater access into arterial intima. High-density lipoprotein (HDL) particles function to transport cholesterol from all areas in the body back to the liver for degradation and disposal. This process, known as reverse cholesterol transport, is a major cardioprotective function of HDL because it counters the atherogenic effects of LDL within the arterial wall. HDL particles include the subfractions of the larger and less dense HDL subfraction 2 (HDL$_2$) (cardioprotection is associated with HDL$_2$) and the smaller, more dense HDL subfraction 3 (HDL$_3$) particles. The characteristics of HDL and other lipids and lipoproteins are listed in Table 41-1.

Several key enzymes regulate intravascular lipoprotein metabolism: lipoprotein lipase (LPL), hepatic lipase (HL), lecithin-cholesterol acyltransferase (LCAT), and cholesterol ester transfer protein (CETP). Together with plasma lipoproteins, these enzymes foster the movement and exchange of triglyceride and cholesterol between lipoproteins, the intestine, liver, and extrahepatic tissues. Several lipoprotein metabolic pathways exist, but the LDL receptor pathway and reverse cholesterol transport account for most of the cholesterol and triglyceride movement in the blood. When either genetic or unfavorable environmental influences affect the function of these pathways, dyslipidemia results, and CHD risk is increased.

Elevated blood cholesterol, triglycerides, LDL cholesterol (LDL-C), and reduced HDL cholesterol (HDL-C) are linked with clinical manifestations of CHD, but it is well established that the initiation and progression of atherosclerotic CHD depends greatly on the presence of elevated LDL-C. Therefore, LDL-C is the primary lipoprotein target in the NCEP ATP III intervention algorithm (106). The ratio of total cholesterol to HDL-C and apolipoprotein B to apolipoprotein A-I (the primary apolipoproteins in LDL and HDL particles, respectively) may also be important indicators of CHD risk. The evidence in support of elevated triacylglycerol (hypertriglyceridemia) as an independent risk factor for CHD is less clear and appears more strongly associated with CHD risk in women than in men (49,106). Elevated triacylglycerol levels are associated with higher quantities of small, dense LDL particles and with reduced levels of HLD-C; as such, whether hypertriglyceridemia is directly or indirectly implicated in CHD is not clear. Regardless, large amounts of triglyceride are found in all coronary atherosclerotic plaques, and blood triglyceride levels need be determined when assessing an individual's CHD risk (32,49,106). Recommendations

TABLE 41-1. Characteristics of Plasma Lipids and Lipoproteins

Lipid/Lipoprotein	Source	COMPOSITION							
		Protein %	Total Lipid %	Percentage of Total Lipid				Apolipoprotein
				TG	Chol	Phosp	Free Chol	
Chylomicron	Intestine	1–2	98–99	88	8	3	1	Major: A-IV, B-48, B-100, H Minor: A-I, A-II, C-I, C-II, C-III, E
VLDL	Major: Liver Minor: Intestine	7–10	90–93	56	20	15	8	Major: B-100, C-III, E, G Minor: A-I, A-II, B-48, C-II, D
IDL	Major: VLDL Minor: Chylomicron	11	89	29	26	34	9	Major: B-100 Minor: B-48
LDL	Major: VLDL Minor: Chylomicron	21	79	13	28	48	10	Major: B-100 Minor: C-I, C-II, (a)
HDL$_2$	Major: HDL$_3$	33	67	16	43	31	10	Major: A-1, A-II, D, E, F Minor: A-IV, C-I, C-II, C-III
HDL$_3$	Major: Liver and intestine Minor: VLDL and chylomicron remnants	57	43	13	46	29	6	Major: A-1, A-II, D, E, F Minor: A-IV, C-I, C-II, C-III
Chol	Liver and diet		100	70–75	25–30			
TG	Diet and liver		100	100				

VLDL, very low-density lipoprotein; IDL, intermediate-density lipoprotein; LDL, low-density lipoprotein; HDL, high-density lipoprotein; Chol, cholesterol; TG, triglycerides; Phosp, phospholipid.

for classifying levels of blood cholesterol, triglyceride, and LDL-C regarding CHD risk are summarized in *Table 41-2*. The recommended LDL-C goal for high-risk persons is <100 mg · dL^{-1}, but when CHD, or other diseases that further increase risk are present, a more aggressive LDL-C goal of <70 mg · dL^{-1} is recommended (45).

Another lipid condition associated with increased CHD risk is exaggerated postprandial lipemia, which is a prolonged amount of time required for the removal of chylomicrons or their movement into extrahepatic tissue. Exaggerated postprandial lipemia adversely affects endothelial function and contributes to atherosclerotic plaque

formation. In healthy persons, postprandial triglyceride levels return to baseline levels within 8–10 h after consumption of dietary fat (83).

HYPERTENSION

High BP, or hypertension, is a major health concern in western societies. In the United States, an estimated 75 million individuals older than the age of 20 yr have systolic BP >140 mm Hg or a diastolic BP >90 mm Hg (19,29,88). The prevalence of the disease is especially high within the African American population, particularly among females (88). The Joint National Commission VII

TABLE 41-2. Low-Density Lipoprotein Cholesterol Goals and Cutpoints for Therapeutic Lifestyle Changes and Drug Therapy in Different Risk Categories

Risk Category	LDL Goal	LDL Level at which to Initiate Therapeutic Lifestyle Changes	LDL Level at which to Consider Drug Therapy
CHD or CHD risk equivalents (10-yr risk >20%)	<100 mg · dL^{-1}	≥100 mg · dL^{-1}	≥130 mg · dL^{-1} (100–129 mg · dL^{-1}: drug therapy optional)[a]
2+ risk factors (10-yr risk $\geq20\%$)	<130 mg · dL^{-1}	≥130 mg · dL^{-1}	10-yr risk = 10%–20%: ≥130 mg · dL^{-1} 10-yr risk <10%: ≥160 mg · dL^{-1}
0–1 risk factor[b] (10-yr risk <10%)	<160 mg · dL^{-1}	≥160 mg · dL^{-1}	≥190 mg · dL^{-1} (160–189 mg · dL^{-1}: LDL-lowering drug optional)

CHD, coronary heart disease; LDL, low-density lipoprotein.

[a]Some authorities recommend use of LDL-lowering drugs in this category if an LDL cholesterol <100 mg · dL^{-1} cannot be achieved by therapeutic lifestyle changes. Others prefer use of drugs that primarily modify triglycerides and high-density lipoprotein (HDL) (*e.g.*, nicotinic acid or fibrate). Clinical judgment also may call for deferring drug therapy in this subcategory.

[b]Almost all people with zero to one risk factor have a 10-yr risk <10%, thus 10-yr risk assessment in people with zero to one risk factor is not necessary.

TABLE 41-3. Classification of Blood Pressure for Adults

BP Classification	SBP (mm Hg)	DBP (mm Hg)
Normal	<120	and <80
Prehypertension	120–139	or 80–89
Stage 1 hypertension	140–159	or 90–99
Stage 2 hypertension	≥160	or ≥100

BP, blood pressure; SBP, systolic blood pressure; DBP, diastolic blood pressure; mm Hg, millimeters of mercury.

From Chobanian AV, Bakris GL, Black HR, et al. Seventh Blood Pressure Report of the Joint National Committee on Detection, Evaluation, and Treatment of High Blood Pressure. JNC 7—complete version. *Hypertension.* 2003;42:1206–52.

(JNC VII) developed a classification scheme containing the designation prehypertension, which is defined as a systolic BP between 120 and 139 mm Hg and a diastolic BP of 80–89 mm Hg, because the lifetime risk of developing overt disease is high for individuals within this BP range (*Table 41-3*) (19). Hypertension is a disorder with multiple factors contributing to elevated systolic and diastolic pressures. Mean arterial pressure (MAP) is the product of cardiac output ($\dot{Q}$) and systemic vascular resistance (SVR). Therefore, for an individual to have hypertension, either $\dot{Q}$ and /or SVR must be elevated. In most cases of essential hypertension, as individuals age, the SVR increases. Factors influencing BP include genetics, sodium sensitivity, sympathetic nervous system hyperactivity, alterations within the renin-angiotensin system, hyperinsulinemia or insulin resistance, and endothelial cell dysfunction (93,116).

In approximately 90% of the cases of hypertension, the exact cause for the abnormal elevation in BP is not known; a condition referred to as *primary* or *essential hypertension*. In contrast, *secondary hypertension* refers to hypertension that is secondary to some identifiable disorder. Diagnosis of these disorders is beyond the scope of this chapter, other than to note that if the underlying cause for the elevation of BP is identified and treated, the hypertension can be corrected.

Hypertension presents differently in younger than in older individuals. In adults, isolated systolic hypertension (systolic BP >140 mm Hg with diastolic BP <90 mm Hg) is rare before 50 yr of age. Among older adults, however, isolated systolic hypertension is the most common form of hypertension. Another form of hypertension is pulmonary hypertension, an elevation of pulmonary artery pressure that often presents with symptoms of dyspnea and fatigue and may be accompanied by syncope and substernal chest pain. Pulmonary hypertension can accompany other forms of pulmonary disease, as well as heart disease (64,80).

Uncontrolled hypertension contributes to coronary artery disease (CAD), heart failure, atrial fibrillation, cerebrovascular disease, end-stage renal disease, PAD, aortic aneurysm, and retinal disease. Hypertension is one of the four major factors (along with obesity, dyslipidemia and insulin resistance) of the metabolic syndrome that predisposes people to cardiovascular disease and diabetes mellitus (27).

OVERWEIGHT AND OBESITY

Overweight and obesity are major public health concerns for many developed countries throughout the world. In the United States, obesity prevalence rates doubled in adults between 1980 and 2000 (31), and by 2004, almost one-third of U.S. adults were classified as obese (46,74). According to the most recent data from the U.S. Centers for Disease Control and Prevention (CDC), approximately 68% of Americans are overweight or obese; approximately 34% of Americans are obese. In 2008, medical costs associated with obesity were estimated at $147 billion, and the medical costs paid by third-party payers for individuals who are obese were $1,429 higher than for individuals of normal weight (30). Overweight and obesity are linked to numerous chronic diseases, including CAD, diabetes mellitus, many forms of cancer, gallbladder disease, arthritis, poor quality of life, and numerous musculoskeletal problems (96).

Fat is the body's major form of energy storage and is found throughout all regions of the body. Although a positive energy balance is requisite to the overaccumulation of body fat (overweight and obesity), many biological factors affect this energy balance. Several medical conditions exist that promote weight gain. These include endocrine disorders, such as Cushing syndrome or newly discovered hypothyroidism; side effects of some medications; and smoking cessation. However, treatable medical causes for obesity are rare, and overweight and obesity are typically caused by combined inactivity and excess caloric consumption (96).

Excess fat deposition in the abdominal region, commonly referred to as *central obesity* or *abdominal obesity*, is often associated with a condition referred to as *metabolic syndrome*, which is a group of risk factors that correlate with increased risk for cardiovascular disease and Type 2 diabetes mellitus. The following diagnostic criteria for the metabolic syndrome are based on NCEP ATP III (three or more criteria must be present): fasting triglycerides $\geq$150 mg $\cdot$ dL^{-1}, fasting glucose $\geq$110 mg $\cdot$ dL^{-1}, systolic BP $\geq$130 mm Hg or diastolic BP $\geq$85 mm Hg, HDL-C <50 mg $\cdot$ dL^{-1} in women or <40 mg $\cdot$ dL^{-1} in men, waist circumference >88 cm in women or >102 cm in men. The prevalence of metabolic syndrome continues to increase in the United States, affecting approximately 34% of the adult population. The prevalence of metabolic syndrome increases with age; approximately 52% of men and 54% of women aged 60 yr and older have metabolic syndrome (28).

PERIPHERAL ARTERIAL DISEASE

PAD is the manifestation of atherosclerosis in systemic arteries outside of the heart. It more commonly affects the vessels in the lower extremity. Approximately 8 million Americans have PAD, with an estimated prevalence of 12%–20% in people aged 60 yr and older (22,88). Diabetes mellitus, hypertension, and smoking are major PAD risk factors (96). Patients with PAD have a 6.6-fold greater risk of suffering cardiovascular death compared with individuals without PAD (103).

Common signs and symptoms of PAD can include calf pain (usually the primary symptom), pain in the buttocks, leg numbness or weakness, cold legs or feet, sores (ulcers) on lower extremities that won't heal, color change in legs, hair loss on legs, and toenail color change. Whether a patient has some or all of these signs/symptoms depends on the disease severity. As the severity of PAD worsens, the individual typically develops exertional leg pain, known as claudication, which is a burning, painful sensation that may also feel like a muscle cramp. As PAD worsens, the symptoms can become so severe to limit the person's ability to perform activities of daily living (37). Claudication does not go away if the person continues to walk; it is only relieved by rest. The pain, as with ischemia of the heart, is the result of a mismatch between oxygen delivery and metabolic oxygen demand. This occurs in the working tissue, secondary to flow-limiting stenosis upstream in the arterial trunks. Although ischemia of the heart is potentially dangerous, intermittent ischemia of the skeletal muscles, as with PAD, is uncomfortable but not dangerous unless ignored and not evaluated. If the pain progresses to resting pain, the individual will be at risk for gangrene and subsequent tissue loss.

Estimates vary, but claudication is found in less than half (~35%) of persons afflicted with PAD (48,73). Reasons for not having claudication in all persons with PAD are not completely clear. Some patients with PAD may not walk far or fast enough to induce muscle ischemic symptoms because of comorbidities such as pulmonary disease or arthritis, may have neuropathies that deaden nerve endings in the legs as with diabetes, may have atypical symptoms unrecognized as intermittent claudication, may fail to mention their symptoms to their physician, or may have sufficient collateral arterial channels to tolerate their arterial obstruction (8).

CEREBROVASCULAR DISEASE

Stroke ranks third among all causes of death in the United States, only behind CHD and cancer. An estimated 795,000 Americans suffer new (610,000) or recurrent (185,000) strokes each year (88). As a result, stroke accounts for about 1 of every 18 deaths in the United States (88). Approximately 55,000 more women than men have strokes each year (88,107). Stroke death rates are higher in Blacks than in Whites, particularly among the young adult population. Fortunately, the good news is that from 1997 to 2007, the U.S. stroke death rate fell 34.3%, and the actual number of stroke deaths declined by 18.8% (88).

Ischemic and hemorrhagic strokes are the two major types of stroke, with ischemic stroke accounting for approximately 87% of all strokes (88). The following are risk factors for stroke: age, sex, ethnicity, hypertension, impaired glucose tolerance, atrial fibrillation, smoking, diabetes, depression, oral contraceptives, and physical inactivity (88).

A previous transient ischemic attack (TIA) should be considered a strong indicator to intervene with any modifiable or potentially modifiable risk factors for stroke (88). Atherosclerosis is the most common underlying cause of ischemic stroke, and all of the major modifiable CHD risk factors are included in the listing mentioned earlier.

Hemorrhagic strokes account for the remaining 13% of all strokes. Two major hemorrhagic stroke categories are intracerebral hemorrhage and subarachnoid hemorrhage. Most intracerebral hemorrhages (10%) are related to hypertension, whereas a subarachnoid hemorrhage (3%) is most likely a result of a ruptured aneurysm, also often precipitated by hypertension. Hemorrhagic strokes, although less common than ischemic strokes, are more likely to be fatal within 30 d. On the other hand, hemorrhagic stroke survivors are less likely to be severely disabled when compared with survivors of ischemic strokes (41,88).

MEDICAL MANAGEMENT

Because the diseases presented in this chapter very often occur together, they are presented as such here as opposed to separate chapters for each. As comorbidities, medical management is sometimes interconnected, and the lifestyle modification and exercise planning and programming for these conditions are highly interconnected. The following is a cursory discussion of the medical management of these conditions followed by discussion of exercise management and programming.

DYSLIPIDEMIA

The evidence-based medical management of dyslipidemia is well described in the NCEP ATP III recommendations (106). In brief, lipid management is triaged into three cardiovascular disease risk classes: low risk, moderate risk, and high risk. People who are low risk have at most one cardiovascular disease risk factor; those at moderate risk have two or more cardiovascular disease risk factors but do not have known cardiovascular disease. High-risk individuals have a history of CAD, have atherosclerosis in peripheral arteries (most typically carotid, aorta, iliac, femoral, or popliteal), or have diabetes.

The degree of recommended lipid lowering is determined by the level of cardiovascular disease risk. The primary target of lipid lowering recommended in NCEP ATP III is the LDL-C. Secondary targets include the HDL-C and triglycerides. The LDL-C recommended goals of therapy are shown in *Table 41-2*.

Triglycerides are a secondary cardiovascular disease risk factor under NCEP ATP III. A normal fasting triglyceride is considered to be <150 mg · dL^{-1}, borderline high is 150–199 mg · dL^{-1}, high is 200–499 mg · dL^{-1}, and very high is ≥500 mg · dL^{-1}. In the current epidemic of obesity, high triglycerides are common among people with Type 2 diabetes or metabolic syndrome, although high triglycerides can also be an isolated finding (*e.g.*, type V hyperlipidemia, or *familial hypertriglyceridemia*). Evidence is mounting that high triglycerides are an independent risk factor for atherosclerosis (11,72). Specific pharmacological treatment to lower triglyceride levels (usually with fibric acid derivatives) to prevent possible pancreatitis is indicated when they are ≥500 mg · dL^{-1}.

HDL-C levels are considered low when they are <40 mg · dL^{-1} in men and <50 mg · dL^{-1} in women. NCEP ATP III does not make recommendations about raising the HDL-C, but many experts feel that HDL-C should also be treated if the value is low, particularly if it is <30 mg · dL^{-1} or if the ratio of total cholesterol to HDL-C is >5. In spite of this, data from clinical trials that specifically target raising HDL-C are lacking.

Lifestyle factors are very important in managing dyslipidemia (69). The core of lifestyle recommendations in NCEP ATP III is the therapeutic lifestyle change (TLC) diet (106). This recommended nutritional composition is outlined in *Table 41-4* (106). However, the team of professionals involved in the prevention and treatment of cardiovascular disease should carefully assess each patient individually. Although the TLC approach has been successful at reducing LDL-C levels, only modest improvements in triglycerides are expected, and many patients will experience reductions in HDL-C. Dietary strategies that reduce carbohydrates have been consistently shown to significantly reduce fasting and postprandial triglycerides, to favorably alter the LDL particle pattern, and to often increase HDL-C (111).

These nutritional recommendations are reasonably similar in all chronic conditions requiring lifestyle intervention as an integral part of medical management. In addition, physical activity recommendations that are in line with the ACSM/CDC guidelines on exercise are recommended (32).

When people do not achieve the recommended lipid levels within 12 wk of diet and exercise, drug therapy is recommended. Multiple randomized controlled trials now unequivocally show that 3-hydroxy-3-methylglutaryl coenzyme A (HMG CoA) reductase inhibitors (statins) prevent cardiovascular events and death from myocardial infarctions. Accordingly, statins

TABLE 41-4. Nutrient Composition of the Therapeutic Lifestyle Changes Diet

Nutrient	Recommended Intake
Saturated fat^a	<7% of total calories
Polyunsaturated fat	Up to 10% of total calories
Monounsaturated fat	Up to 20% of total calories
Total fat	25%–35% of total calories
Carbohydrate^b	50%–60% of total calories
Fiber	20–30 g · d^{-1}
Protein	Approximately 15% total calories
Cholesterol	<200 mg · d^{-1}
Total calories (energy)^c	Balance energy intake and expenditure to maintain desirable body weight/prevent weight gain

^{a}Trans fatty acids are another low-density lipoprotein–raising fat that should be kept at a low intake.

^{b}Carbohydrate should be derived predominantly from foods rich in complex carbohydrates, including grains, especially whole grains, fruits, and vegetables.

^{c}Daily energy expenditure should include at least moderate physical activity (contributing approximately 200 kcal · d^{-1}).

From National Cholesterol Education Program Expert Panel. *Detection, Evaluation, and Treatment of High Blood Cholesterol in Adults (Adult Treatment Panel III): Executive Summary.* Washington (DC): National Heart, Lung, and Blood Institute, National Institutes of Health; 2001. 36 p.

are considered the first-line therapy for LDL-C lowering. The clinician directing therapy with a particular statin should take into account the current LDL-C level and the recommended therapeutic goal based on the patient's cardiovascular disease risk level. For those requiring ≥50% reduction in LDL-C, a high dose of a potent statin (usually atorvastatin or rosuvastatin) should be chosen. Recent recommendations from the U.S. Food and Drug Administration (FDA) discourage the use of an 80-mg dose of simvastatin (unless the patient has received this therapy for >1 yr without adverse effects) because of an increased risk of muscle injury. When LDL-C goals cannot be met by use of statin therapy alone because of side effects or insufficient reductions of LDL-C, combination therapy (using statin plus binding resins, ezetimibe or niacin) can be considered. The main rationale to use combination therapy is that the interrelated metabolic pathways involved in cholesterol metabolism often adjust by upregulating gene expression and thereby reducing the impact of monotherapy.

Additional classes of lipid-lowering drugs include bile acid sequestrants (resins), fibric acids, nicotinic acid (niacin), and cholesterol absorption blocking agents (ezetimibe). All of these drugs by themselves have good safety profiles, but some combinations are known to increase risk of serious side effects (33). Statins and fibric acid derivatives can cause severe myopathy and rhabdomyolysis, with the potential of kidney failure and death. Nonetheless, some patients who have extremely high cardiovascular disease risk sometimes can be prescribed both classes of drugs (33).

Caution is given with the use of statins and exercise intervention. These drugs are rarely associated with exertional rhabdomyolysis, as reflected by muscle symptoms and blood levels of creatine kinase (69). This is often medically managed by the physician, but the clinical exercise specialist working with patients on a statin should be aware of this possibility. Numerous patients have normal blood levels of creatine kinase but report muscle symptoms that resolve when the statin is stopped (51,84,99,100). In such individuals, it is difficult to discriminate between delayed-onset muscle soreness and statin side effects.

HYPERTENSION

The diagnosis of hypertension requires determination on three separate occasions that the systolic BP is ≥140 mm Hg or the diastolic BP is ≥90 mm Hg (see *Table 41-3*). For those with diabetes mellitus or chronic kidney disease, hypertension is considered to exist when the BP is ≥130/80 mm Hg. Measurement of BP should be obtained after the subject has been seated quietly for at least 5 min because the exertion of walking is likely to mildly elevate BP.

Once the diagnosis is made, recommendations are to use a trial of lifestyle intervention before the prescription of antihypertensive medications (19,21). Patients with systolic BP >160 mm Hg or diastolic BP >100 mm Hg (stage II hypertension) often require immediate institution of pharmacological therapy (frequently with two agents) in addition to lifestyle modifications to achieve adequate BP control (JNC VII). Typically, a low-sodium diet or a diet such as dietary approaches to stop hypertension (DASH) is prescribed (56). Alcohol can also exacerbate high BP. Although one to two alcoholic beverages a day can reduce cardiovascular mortality, consumption beyond this level increases the risk of poor BP control (114). Thus, people with high BP should be counseled on a low sodium–, vegetable-, and fruit-oriented diet, with only modest alcohol consumption. Such changes in diet can be expected to reduce systolic BP by 2–14 mm Hg. Also, weight loss can yield a 5–20 mm Hg reduction in systolic BP. In addition to dietary changes, exercise can achieve another 5–7 mm Hg reduction in systolic and diastolic BP (81). Many patients are not able to achieve sufficient reductions in BP with lifestyle modification alone and will often require pharmacological therapy. The goal of hypertension medical management for most patients is to achieve a BP <140/90 mm Hg. For those with diabetes mellitus or chronic kidney disease, a more aggressive BP goal of <130/80 mm Hg is recommended. Although some patients can achieve adequate control on only one medication, most patients required two or more medications to achieve their BP goal. Several classes of medications are available to treat hypertension. It is recommended that the initial choice

of drug therapy be guided by consideration of underlying medical conditions (19). Stated another away, if a compelling indication for choice of a particular class of medications exists (*e.g.*, β-adrenergic blocking agents for ischemic heart disease), a member of that class of drugs should be chosen as the initial therapy with agents from other classes added as required to achieve the desired BP goal. For those without such compelling indications, the most common initial medication chosen is a diuretic. In the United States, this is most often hydrochlorothiazide because it is available as an inexpensive generic drug and is well tolerated. Another common drug class used as a first- or second-line agent is an angiotensin converting enzyme inhibitor. Alternatively, a β-blocker can be chosen; however, in contemporary practice, these agents are most often relegated to third- or fourth-line use.

Many physicians prefer to prescribe, as initial therapy, antihypertensive drugs that reduce afterload as a mechanism of action, especially angiotensin converting enzyme inhibitors and angiotensin receptor blockers as well as dihydropyridine-type calcium channel blockers. These classes of medications have an **ergomimetic** profile in that they decrease peripheral vascular resistance, much as occurs with exercise. However, except in persons with diabetes, there is no current research to support that afterload reducers are better than other approaches to hypertensive therapy; in fact, diuretics are known to reduce cardiovascular mortality. Although there is a reason to believe that reduction in cardiovascular mortality is a pressure-related phenomenon, this is not known for certain; thus, there is a good rationale for using diuretics initially, then moving to other classes of medications. One must also consider the potential side effects of medications when choosing therapy, for example, diuretics and β-adrenergic blocking agents in those who are active and athletic (*e.g.*, fatigue-reduced physical performance, decreased libido).

PERIPHERAL ARTERIAL DISEASE

Medical management of PAD is similar to management of CAD. The mainstay of treatment is lifestyle modification to reduce the primary risk factors of PAD, which are hypertension, smoking, and diabetes. The recommended approach to lifestyle modification in this population is similar to that outlined earlier for hypertension and hyperlipidemia.

Surgical management of PAD depends on the severity of circulatory inadequacy. In the most severe cases, in which tissue becomes nonviable, the vascular anatomy cannot be repaired, and amputation is the only choice. In less severe cases, the magnitude of circulatory impairment is often estimated in a vascular lab where an ankle-brachial index (ABI) is obtained (*Table 41-5*). An ABI is the ratio of pressures in the posterior tibial or dorsalis pedis artery and brachial artery and is taken while the

TABLE 41-5. Ankle Brachial Index

≥1.30	Noncompressible vessel
1.00–1.29	Normal
0.91–0.99	Borderline (equivocal)
0.41–0.90	Mild-to-moderate PAD
0.00–0.40	Severe PAD

PAD, peripheral arterial disease.

From Hirsch AT, Haskal ZJ, Hertzer NR, et al. ACC/AHA 2005 guidelines for the management of patients with peripheral arterial disease (lower extremity, renal, mesenteric, and abdominal aortic): executive summary. *J Am Coll Cardiol.* 2006;47:1239–312.

patient is supine. The lower the ratio, particularly when it is <0.9, the more severe of a blood flow limitation exists. Also, one can obtain other images of the vascular anatomy, such as arteriograms or magnetic resonance angiograms. The main purpose of such imaging is to determine whether the arteries can be repaired with bypass grafts or angioplasty with stent placement.

Medical management of PAD is quite similar to that of CAD. Goals are to normalize BP and cholesterol, promote smoking cessation, and provide antiplatelet therapy for all patients, as well as therapy to relieve the symptoms of intermittent claudication.

Smoking cessation success rates improve about two-fold or more when counseling is coupled with nicotine replacement, nicotine receptor blockade, and/or antide-pressant therapy. Nicotine replacement is best achieved not only with transdermal patches but also can be deliv-ered with chewing gum. Nicotine replacement in com-bination with antidepressant therapy, best documented for bupropion, improves successful smoking cessation. Bupropion alone is also helpful. More recently, the nico-tine receptor partial agonist varenicline has been approved by the FDA. Varenicline appears to be superior to bupro-pion, and compared with placebo, varenicline appears to triple the probability of being smoke free at 12 mo (101). Medical management to support smoking cessation is of paramount importance in patients with PAD.

All patients with PAD should receive aspirin therapy unless a contraindication exists. For patients who have had a stent placed, the antiplatelet agent clopidogrel, along with aspirin, is used to prevent thrombosis. Clopidogrel can be used instead of aspirin in patients with intermittent claudication who do not receive a stent. Cilostazol, a drug from a different class of anti-platelet agents, is indicated specifically for intermittent claudication. These drugs, despite being approved for similar mechanisms of action, have different clinical benefits. Clopidogrel is primarily beneficial in prevent-ing restenosis and/or thrombosis. Cilostazol is indicated for the symptom of intermittent claudication and is used specifically to reduce pain and increase walking distance. These medications can also be combined in patients without a stent, but this is an uncommon practice.

OVERWEIGHT AND OBESITY

Chapter 35 reviews the techniques of weight management in detail. The cornerstone of management for overweight and obesity is lifestyle modification that is emphasiz-ing diet and exercise. In some patients for whom life-style modification is insufficient, FDA-approved weight loss medications or bariatric surgery (for patients who are morbidly obese with a body mass index ≥40 or ≥35 kg · m^{-2} with comorbid conditions) may be consid-ered. Recent evidence demonstrated a beneficial mortal-ity effect following bariatric surgery (101).

CEREBROVASCULAR DISEASE

Medical management of carotid and vertebrobasilar atherosclerosis is similar to CAD and PAD; the main difference is that cilostazol has not been approved for use in cerebrovascular disease. Medical management of patients who have had a stroke is an extensive and highly complex problem that would require several chapters to address the many kinds of disabilities that result from strokes. In this chapter, we confine our comments to a few major points. First, patients who have had a stroke often die from cardiovascular disease. It is therefore important that people who have suffered a stroke receive appropriate and intensive cardiovascular risk-reduction interventions. Second, some strokes may resolve and have minimal residual impact, and others may leave the patient in a permanent hemiplegic state and with ataxia. The medical needs will be dramatically different depend-ing on the severity of the disability, and exercise pro-gramming will need to be appropriately individualized. Third, all lifestyle modification intervention program-ming rely on cognitive therapy, and the cognitive decline associated with cerebrovascular disease needs to be fac-tored into the design of the lifestyle/exercise program. Unfortunately, this remains an uncommon skill, and more knowledge is needed to better understand how to work with individuals who are cognitively impaired (14).

EXERCISE RESPONSES AND ADAPTATIONS

In this section, we consider the acute exercise response and the adaptations to chronic exercise training.

DYSLIPIDEMIA

Generally, the exercise response to a single exercise ses-sion will not be altered as a result of dyslipidemia alone. After a single exercise session, blood triglycerides and postprandial lipemia are reduced, and HDL-C is usually, but not always, increased (23,44). Typically, these effects have no discernable symptoms. However, dyslipidemia can lead to secondary illness, such as angina or clau-dication, and these secondary problems often alter the exercise response in accordance with that problem. In these cases, attention is given to the exercise response in view of these other secondary conditions.

Exceptions to this rule include individuals with genetic disorders. For example, individuals who have an extremely high triglyceride or cholesterol level can have inadequate oxygen supply to vital tissues, such as the heart or brain, and are at greater risk for stroke and/or myocardial infarctions. It is best to gain control of the dyslipidemia with medical management before the patient begins exercising. Because patients who have familial (or genetic) dyslipidemia are usually prescribed various medications for other conditions, the type and dosage of their medications should be noted before undergoing exercise testing or training.

Regular participation in physical activity is shown to cause beneficial changes in people with normal lipid and lipoprotein concentrations as well as in most persons with dyslipidemia. Beneficial changes include the following: decreased triglyceride (58), increased HDL-C (but not always) (61,62), and increased lipoprotein enzyme activity (LPL, LCAT, and CETP) (61,62). These exercise training changes enhance reverse cholesterol transport and are augmented further by weight loss and reduction in adiposity. Thus, exercise training can directly (*e.g.*, by increased LPL activity) and indirectly (*e.g.*, by reductions in body weight and body fat) improve blood lipid and lipoprotein profiles. Work by Kraus et al. (59) demonstrates that the volume of exercise completed on a weekly basis is more important than the exercise intensity for affecting favorable blood lipid and lipoprotein changes. They showed that regular aerobic exercise can induce favorable changes in LDL subfractions (*e.g.*, converting smaller, denser LDLs to larger, less dense LDLs) thus reducing cardiovascular disease risk.

Abnormal blood lipid and lipoprotein profiles can result from congenital deficiencies, and patients having these deficiencies have substantially different lipid and lipoprotein responses to routine physical activity from that seen in healthy individuals. For example, LPL activity is not increased by exercise training in those with LPL deficiency; nor does HDL-C concentration increase in individuals with low HDL-C (hypoalphalipoprotein syndrome). The mechanisms responsible for changes in dyslipidemic conditions as a consequence of exercise training are unclear and, in many cases, are likely to be different from those reported for healthy subjects.

HYPERTENSION

A single dynamic exercise session usually induces a normal rise in systolic BP from baseline in persons with hypertension who are not on medications. Often, the slope of the pressor response is either exaggerated or diminished. On the other hand, when the baseline BP level is elevated, the absolute level of systolic BP attained during dynamic exercise is usually higher in persons with hypertension compared to healthy individuals. Furthermore, diastolic BP typically stays constant or is slightly higher during dynamic exercise. Rarely does the diastolic BP decrease. A rise in diastolic BP during dynamic exercise is likely the result of an impaired vasodilatory response (77).

Aerobic or endurance exercise usually produces immediate decreases in BP of similar magnitude to exercise training programs and may persist up to 22 h after the exercise (81,82). After 30–45 min of moderate-intensity dynamic exercise in persons with hypertension, there can be reductions of 10–20 mm Hg in systolic BP during the initial 1–3 h postexercise (25). Researchers have found evidence to indicate that a higher baseline reading prior to an acute bout of exercise is linked to a greater reduction in BP following exercise (81).

Exercise training has also been shown to reduce 24-h ambulatory BP by about 3 mm Hg for both systolic and diastolic BP (81). Ambulatory BP readings are better correlated to cardiovascular outcomes than resting BP readings (81). Mechanisms for the decrease in resting or ambulatory BPs after exercise training are not well understood. Decreased plasma norepinephrine levels, increases in circulating vasodilator substances, improvements in hyperinsulinemia, and altered renal function are all possible explanations. It is also important to note that approximately 25% of the hypertensive population is resistant to the BP lowering effects of exercise training (81). Specific gene polymorphisms (*e.g.*, α-adducin) have been associated with some of this variability in response to exercise (4,81). Hypertension that goes untreated is often accompanied by limitations in exercise tolerance. In addition, some antihypertensive drugs impair exercise performance (see *Appendix A* in *GETP9*). Nevertheless, when hypertension is controlled with lifestyle modification and well-tolerated antihypertensive medications, exercise tolerance typically improves over the long term.

Resistance training is commonly advised today, but the cardiovascular responses to a single resistance exercise session are quite different from a session of endurance exercise. Heavy resistance exercise in particular elicits a pressor response causing only moderate heart rate and cardiac output increases, relative to those seen with dynamic endurance exercise. However, systolic and diastolic BP can increase dramatically more than that seen in endurance exercise. Researchers have reported a 3-mm Hg reduction in systolic BP and diastolic BP following a period of resistance training (81). The 2004 ACSM position stand on exercise and BP recommends aerobic exercise as an indicated intervention in hypertension, with resistive training as an *adjunct* (81). Based on current data, dynamic resistive exercise training is recommended because there are no data to suggest that static (isometric) exercise has any benefit. Resistance training is therefore recommended for overall fitness, but in a person with hypertension, the clinical exercise specialist should monitor the BP to make sure that the individual does not have an exaggerated pressor response.

PERIPHERAL ARTERIAL DISEASE

The primary effect of PAD on a single exercise session is the development of claudication pain (*i.e.*, pain that develops with walking that is relieved by about 10 min of rest) (63). Prospective exercise training studies demonstrate beneficial improvement in exercise tolerance in patients with claudication (38,60,87,108). Exercise-induced improvements in walking ability are well established, but the degree of exercise training is varied across studies. Clinical benefits are reported after 4 wk of exercise training and continue to accrue with 6 mo of regular exercise participation (38,40). Thus, exercise training is important, but the dose-response relationship is not clear.

Symptoms of intermittent claudication are improved by exercise training. Possible mechanisms for this increased exercise tolerance include improved endothelial function, better redistribution of blood flow, improved hemorheologic and fibrinolytic properties of blood (*e.g.*, reduced viscosity), greater reliance on aerobic metabolism because of a higher concentration of oxidative enzymes, less reliance on anaerobic metabolism, an improvement in the efficiency of walking economy, improved oxygen uptake kinetics, a reduction of inflammatory markers, and an increased free-living daily energy expenditure (25,63,104). Changes in hemodynamic variables, as assessed by the ABI, do not seem to be related to the improvements observed with exercise training (78).

OVERWEIGHT AND OBESITY

A single exercise session has little impact on body weight. Obesity increases the load on weight-bearing joints and spine and can impair thermoregulation in hot environmental conditions. Exercise is often a very uncomfortable experience for persons with obesity. Thus, exercise training for the obese must be undertaken with care. Nonetheless, exercise training is a key component for success in long-term lifestyle management of obesity. Although exercise training is modestly effective in reducing body weight 5%–10% in moderate obesity, there are some questions as to its effectiveness in morbid obesity.

The exact exercise training dose necessary to control weight is not yet defined. Emerging evidence suggests that exercise time ranging from 45 to 60 min $\cdot$ d^{-1} on most days of the week is most effective for preventing weight regain in adults who are overweight and obese (24,53,57,95). For weight control, ACSM recommends approximately 60 min $\cdot$ d^{-1} on most days of the week (52), whereas the International Association for the Study of Obesity recommends 60–90 min $\cdot$ d^{-1} on most days of the week (94). Recent research concerning exercise intensity supports the view that moderate (40%–59% of volume of oxygen consumed per unit time reserve [$\dot{V}O_2R$]) intensity exercise has a positive impact on health parameters (109) and is likely as effective for weight control as vigorous-intensity exercise (53). Consequently, a sensible recommendation is for patients who are obese to work toward weight loss and continue long-term exercise training for weight maintenance. A logical approach to this goal is a moderate-intensity exercise regimen for 60 min or more on most days of the week for a total of 240 min $\cdot$ wk^{-1} or more (66).

Physical activity is believed to affect body fat distribution by promoting visceral fat loss in the abdomen. This reduction of abdominal fat decreases the risk of the diseases associated with visceral body fat distribution. The effects of exercise training on metabolism are not well established. Metabolic rate, including the caloric cost of physical activity, is shown to decline with weight reduction via caloric restriction (10,47). In the starvation state, however, the maintenance of metabolic rate through exercise may not always counteract the reduction mediated by food restriction. Despite this, exercise training has positive effects on glucose metabolism in both the moderately obese and the morbidly obese. These benefits of exercise include decreasing fasting glucose, decreasing fasting insulin, increasing glucose tolerance, and decreasing insulin resistance/increasing insulin sensitivity. These changes are achieved, in some instances, without changes in body weight or body fat. Other reports show that the more dramatic changes in glucose metabolism occurred in those who exhibited the greatest reduction in deep abdominal fat (12,39,55,67,76,90–92).

CEREBROVASCULAR STROKE/TRANSIENT ISCHEMIC ATTACK

The severity of neurologic involvement and existing comorbidities that occur in those with stroke greatly affects one's ability to perform bodily movements, including exercise. The following items are examples of potential effects of neurologic deficits on exercise.

- Muscle weakness, limited range of motion, and impaired sensation may limit independent ambulation or ability to exercise in the standing position.
- Lack of adequate balance may interfere with the ability to perform stationary cycle exercise.
- Weakness or limited range of motion of the arm or leg may also interfere with a person's ability to maintain desired pedal speed during ergometry.
- Receptive aphasia, mental confusion, and/or apraxia may interfere with the ability to understand and follow directions during exercise testing or training sessions.

Cognitive and behavioral sequelae may influence compliance with and retention of an exercise program.

Involvement of the frontal lobe can result in lack of initiation, apathy, easy frustration, loss of inhibition, and impaired cognitive and executive functions. Lesions in the temporal lobe may cause difficulties with new learning, memory deficits, and possible outbursts of aggression. Involvement of the areas of the brain mediating perception and arousal may lead to difficulty screening irrelevant sensory input in the environment and focusing on important cues.

Because most strokes occur in elderly individuals, participation in aerobic exercise may be further complicated by the arthritic, orthopedic, and cardiovascular problems common in this population. Motor function deficits may interfere with exercise performance. In studies, only 20%–34% of individuals with stroke were able to achieve 85% of age-predicted maximal heart rate (25).

Most individuals with a recent history of stroke are highly deconditioned, exhibiting a peak oxygen consumption ($\dot{V}O_{2peak}$) that is about half that achieved by age-matched individuals without a previous CVA (54). This deconditioned state, however, leaves tremendous room for improvement. If a person with CVA recovers enough motor function to take part in a leg cycle exercise program, aerobic training studies suggest that 60% increases in $\dot{V}O_{2peak}$ might be expected (43). Endurance training not only has the potential to increase aerobic capacity but may also increase self-selected walking speed, decrease reliance on assistive devices during ambulation, and increase functional mobility scores.

Resistance training also has positive effects in those who suffered from a CVA. In particular, several studies have shown strong associations between paretic knee extension torque and locomotion ability and between both hip flexor and ankle plantar flexor strength of the paretic limb and walking speed after stroke (42). These data suggest that a carefully planned resistance training regimen might be beneficial for some selected individuals who have suffered a CVA.

EXERCISE PRESCRIPTION FOR CHRONIC CONDITIONS

The exercise prescription for an apparently healthy individual is described in *Chapters 30* and *31*. This prescription can be modified for the individual with a chronic condition. Remember that each person has individual signs and symptoms, needs, and goals related to his or her diagnosis. The exercise prescription should focus on these specific needs and be updated continuously as the individual progresses.

DYSLIPIDEMIA

Assuming no other chronic conditions are present, the same exercise prescription that is used for a healthy adult is commonly used for the individual with dyslipidemia

with several considerations. In order for these individuals to affect lipid and lipoprotein levels, they must expend a large quantity of calories (26). Thus, the upper end of the frequency (at least 5 d $\cdot$ wk^{-1}) and duration (30–60 min but can be more) are emphasized along with an intensity ranging from moderate to somewhat vigorous, that is, 40%–75% of $\dot{V}O_2R$ or heart rate reserve (HRR) (*Chapter 10* of *GETP9*). Not only are large quantities of energy expenditure required for lipid and lipoprotein change but also different energy expenditure thresholds for different lipids and lipoproteins exist. For example, triglyceride concentrations are lower in hypertriglyceridemic men after 2 wk of aerobic exercise when at least 45 min of exercise per day is performed on consecutive days, whereas total plasma cholesterol concentration usually remains unchanged even after 1 yr of exercise training unless body weight is concomitantly reduced (26). On the other hand, HDL-C concentrations are frequently increased by exercise regimens requiring 1,000–1,200 kcal of energy expenditure per week for a minimal training period of 12 wk (26). Inactive subjects may also have a lower exercise threshold than physically active persons for HDL-C change. In any case, inactive persons can expect a favorable change in blood lipids within several months when an exercise threshold is met.

HYPERTENSION

Individuals with stage 1 hypertension (systolic BP is 140–159 mm Hg or diastolic BP is 90–99 mm Hg) should be under a physician's care to bring the BP under control. However, hypertension is only one risk factor for ACSM screening purposes, and these individuals may engage in low-to-moderate intensity aerobic exercise (up to 59% of $\dot{V}O_2R$ or HRR) without physician clearance. Individuals with stage 2 hypertension (BP $\geq$160/100 mm Hg) should obtain a medical evaluation and medical clearance before beginning an exercise program. Individuals with stage 2 hypertension who have medical clearance to exercise may be allowed to exercise as long as their preexercise BP is below 200/110 mm Hg. The exercise program for an individual with hypertension is similar to that for healthy adults (36). Individuals with hypertension should include aerobic exercise on most, and preferably all, days per week. The exercise duration ranges from 30 to 60 min at an exercise intensity of 40%–59% of $\dot{V}O_2R$. Interestingly, exercise training at these somewhat lower intensities appears to lower BP as much as exercise at higher intensities (81). The latter is especially important in certain specific populations of persons with hypertension such as those who are elderly or who have chronic diseases in addition to hypertension.

Strength or resistance training is recommended for individuals with hypertension, but endurance (aerobic) exercise training should be the focus of the exercise program. With the exception of circuit weight training, resistance training has not consistently been shown to lower BP. A resistance training regimen of 8–10 different exercises at 60%–80% of the one repetition maximum and targeting major muscle groups is recommended.

Resting systolic BP >200 mm Hg or diastolic BP >110 mm Hg is a relative contraindication to exercise testing and, therefore, is a useful reference for exercise training. Consider occasional BP assessments during exercise in individuals who present with values near 200/110 mm Hg and avoid systolic BP >220 mm Hg and or diastolic BP >105 mm Hg.

PERIPHERAL ARTERIAL DISEASE

Exercise programs for patients with PAD are designed with a goal of improving claudication pain symptoms and reducing cardiovascular risk factors (113).There is evidence to show that exercise rehabilitation programs lead to a 179% improvement in pain-free walking distance and a 122% improvement in maximal walking distance (63). Most patients with PAD should perform interval walking or stair climbing (i.e., weight-bearing activities) three to five times a week at an intensity that causes pain to reach a 3 on a 4-point claudication pain scale (see GETP9, Fig. 5.4) (37). The onset of claudication will usually occur in approximately 3–5 min, and exercise is stopped when the pain reaches the 3 on the 4-point claudication pain scale. Full pain-free recovery is encouraged between intervals. This type of program may start with 10–20 min of total exercise (not exercise plus rest) per session at 40% of $\dot{V}O_2R$ or HRR, and gradually progress to 30–60 min $\cdot$ d^{-1} at 60% of $\dot{V}O_2R$ or HRR over a period of about 6 mo. Non–weight-bearing tasks (e.g., cycling) are recommended for warm-up and cooldown. Although the walking protocol described earlier is currently the standard for exercise training in patients with PAD, interest in the benefits of non–weight-bearing exercise (e.g., arm or leg ergometry) and resistance training has been developing and may provide adjuvant benefits. Medical clearance should include a physical exam, blood screening, and assessment and treatment of any potentially hazardous or exercise-limiting comorbid medical condition. Because patients with PAD are classified as high risk, ACSM recommends exercise testing with medical supervision prior to starting an exercise program. A graded exercise test before and after several weeks of exercise training is completed can be useful to detect myocardial ischemia and to quantify exercise tolerance. The presence of PAD increases the risk that other vascular abnormalities exist.

Special considerations exist for individuals with PAD, including the need for an aggressive lifestyle and lipid management. With an exercise training program, repeated submaximal treadmill tests to evaluate time to pain and maximum walking distance or 6-min walk tests are helpful to objectively gauge progress. Unfortunately, these are typically not available because of insufficient third-party reimbursement, and many patients are not willing to pay for the cost of these tests. Remember that improvements in walking ability may unmask signs and symptoms of angina pectoris and the presence of CHD. Also, cold weather may exacerbate symptoms, requiring the need for longer warm-ups (17). These patients often do better in a controlled environment, and results are better under the supervision of an exercise professional (63). Finally, a quality of life questionnaire (e.g., Short Form 36) and watching for changes in comorbid conditions can be extremely useful in both designing and measuring individual progress.

OVERWEIGHT AND OBESITY

Although the primary objective of exercise in the treatment of obesity is to expend more calories, the optimal approach to increase energy expenditure is debatable. The exercise prescription must optimize energy expenditure yet minimize potential for injury. The energy expenditure of the actual exercise as well as that of the recovery period, otherwise known as excess postexercise oxygen consumption (EPOC), is considered in the total energy expenditure for a single exercise session. There is considerable debate on whether two or more short sessions a day will produce a higher total energy expenditure (exercise + EPOC) than one longer session of the same intensity. The use of two or more shorter sessions has been suggested by some because of the potential benefits of elevated energy expenditure following exercise that is sustained for a longer period of time than after a single exercise session. On the other hand, a single longer exercise session provides an advantage in substrate utilization and for ease of incorporation into some individuals' lifestyles.

Whether substrate utilization is important for weight reduction is not clear. Total calories expended are the primary goal for body fat reduction. In this regard, certain considerations and recommendations for the exercise prescription include increases in daily living activities such as walking; the incorporation of resistance training as part of the exercise regimen; daily exercise or at least 5 or more days per week, with a goal of maximizing the amount of daily/weekly caloric expenditure; sessions of 30–60 min $\cdot$ d^{-1} performed continuously or in bouts no shorter than 10 min; and exercise intensity at 40%–60% of $\dot{V}O_2R$ or HRR with progression to 60%–89% of $\dot{V}O_2R$ or HRR (5,46,109).

Exercise programs that include resistance training can lead to preferential retention of lean body weight. However, aerobic activity has more potential to decrease fat weight than does resistance training because the aerobic exercises can be sustained for a longer time, allowing more energy to be expended.

Injury prevention is an important consideration in exercise for adults who are obese. Physical injury is a principle reason for discontinuation of exercise. Excess body weight may accelerate joint deterioration secondary to osteoarthritis. Another important concern in individuals who are obese is thermoregulation. Other considerations may be dependent on associated diseases that coexist with obesity. Further information about exercise training for the individuals who are overweight and obese can be found in *Chapter 35*.

CEREBROVASCULAR DISEASE

Overall medical management and exercise program design for the patient following a stroke is highly individualized and is in accordance with the severity of the stroke. Before exercise training is started, all other conditions resulting from the stroke and the factors associated with stroke must be taken into consideration. Hypertension is one of the primary risk factors for stroke, and uncontrolled hypertension must be controlled before exercise training begins. Exercise training programs for individuals with stroke should focus at increasing the level of physical fitness and reducing CHD risk factors. Aerobic conditioning can positively alter many of the risk factors associated with stroke, including hypertension, glucose regulation, blood lipid profile, and body fat.

Patients who have experienced a stroke are at risk for sustaining permanent cognitive and behavioral sequelae that might interfere with their ability to follow directions for exercise testing and training. Cognitive deficits include memory loss and decreased rate of information processing, whereas behavioral problems include loss of impulse control, increased agitation, and impaired mood control. Many of these deficits can be addressed using cognitive retraining, behavioral management, and medication. Ideally, these should take place before beginning an exercise training program.

Aerobic exercise training mode depends on the individual's ability and choice, but the various modes used for exercise testing are also used for exercise training. Suggested exercise frequency is at least 3 d · wk⁻¹ and preferable most days of the week, with the exercise intensity based on the subject's initial fitness level (40%–80% HRR). A very unfit individual, or one who is limited because of consequences of the stroke, will likely have to begin at exercise intensities equivalent to 40%–50% HRR (77). Exercise duration also depends on the subject's initial fitness level. Intermittent (interval training) protocols are often employed during the initial weeks of training because of the extremely deconditioned level of many patients after a stroke. The exercise prescription for the person who has experienced a stroke parallels recommendations for those with CVD. Exercise professionals should aim for at least a 20-min exercise duration, which can be accomplished with several 5–10 min bouts (or shorter if needed). The goal is 20–60 min of continuous exercise.

Previously, resistance exercise was thought to cause further increases in muscle tone in those individuals demonstrating hypertonia and/or spasticity. Therefore, resistance exercise training programs were often not included in the rehabilitation programs of many individuals following stroke. These fears have proven unfounded, and resistance exercises are often prescribed to address muscle weakness identified during the fitness assessment (3,79,105). Use of resistance exercise in persons with stroke has not, however, been demonstrated to be universally effective in improving functional capacity. In large part, this is related to complexity of studying such individuals and in designing a representative control group. Some data suggest that progressive resistance exercise training does not improve clinical outcomes (68). Clarification of the role of resistance exercise training will likely involve timing of the program relative to the brain injury/stroke, nature/severity of the neurologic deficits, and careful study design that examines the role of resistance exercise not only as specific therapy but also as additional therapy to a standard rehabilitation regimen.

Individuals with neurologic impairments may have difficulty with preparatory postural adjustments and recruiting strength quickly enough to combat a loss of balance. Thus, some of the positions typically used for resistance training may need modification. For example, many healthy individuals perform dumbbell exercises while standing to increase upper-body strength. A person who has difficulty maintaining standing balance should perform these exercises unilaterally while holding onto a bar or other stationary object. They could also perform these exercises from a seated position.

EXERCISE TRAINING SUPERVISION

Individuals with chronic diseases can benefit from a supervised exercise program. This supervision can be in various forms, such as cardiac or a medical fitness center. The need to be in a supervised environment is dependent on the individual's ability to exercise independently and their risk for a cardiac event or injury (*e.g.*, fall). Some individuals may do well in a supervised environment, such as a fitness center or at home. Participation in a supervised environment is believed to improve long-term outcomes and adherence to a more active lifestyle (9,13,15,16,34,97,98).

For those taking part in a medically supervised program, the highest level of supervision is usually offered. However, for most chronic diseases, a third-party reimbursement is not available, and medically supervised exercise can become quite expensive over time. The next choice is a public gym. In this setting, the supervision level varies based on the level of expertise of those operating the facility. Here again, no reimbursement is readily available except possibly from work as a health incentive. This too can be quite expensive but is usually less than that of the medical model. The final choice of home exercise is the least expensive. However, it is also the one with the least supervision. In this situation, it is important to have communication between the individual and his or her physician or clinical exercise professional in developing the correct exercise program. All choices can provide equal benefits. The main difference is the level and expertise of supervision. This choice is best made by the individual after discussing all options with their physician and/or a clinical exercise specialist.

ECONOMIC BURDEN OF CHRONIC DISEASES

The diseases discussed in this chapter place heavy economic burdens on society. Hypertension is a prime example of this burden. The current direct and indirect costs of hypertension are $76.6 billion (USD), underscoring the social and economic burden of the problem (18). Hypertension is the most common primary diagnosis in America and is a major contributor to the metabolic syndrome (27). High cholesterol (*i.e.*, levels >240 mg $\cdot$ dL^{-1}) is estimated to affect approximately 16.3% of the U.S. adult population (18). As previously stated, PAD affects approximately 8 million American adults (18,103). Based on data from 2008, the estimated medical cost associated with the treatment of obesity in the United States is $147 billion (18). This is because an estimated 68% of adults are categorized as overweight or obese, with 33.8% obese (30). In the United States, 795,000 individuals have a stroke each year with approximately 610,000 of these occurring for the first time. Based on 2009 data, the economic cost of treating strokes in the United States is estimated to be $68.9 billion (18).

CONSEQUENCES OF PHYSICAL INACTIVITY

Considerable data are available on the detrimental physiologic effects of bed rest and restricted physical activity on health. Most individuals with a chronic disease become less active. This, in turn, leads to a cycle of deconditioning that results in the impairment of multiple physiologic systems. Some specific consequences of inactivity for individuals with a chronic disease include reduced cardiorespiratory fitness, osteoporosis, impaired circulation to the lower extremities, diminished self-concept, greater dependence on others for normal activities of daily living, and reduced ability for normal social interactions. As with any disease, the physical abilities and response to exercise, or lack thereof, varies tremendously among individuals. These variations are largely determined by one or more of the following: the severity and/or progression of the disease, response to treatments, and presence of concomitant illnesses. Large variations

between individuals make expected health benefits from increased physical activity less predictable. However, the majority of the diseases discussed in this chapter do have generalized benefits from increased physical activity.

BENEFITS OF EXERCISE REVIEW

As outlined in the National Physical Activity Guidelines for Americans, there are substantial benefits to be gained from the judicious use of physical activity programs (1). These benefits are often related to improved functional capacity and quality of life, but some patient groups also benefit from decreased morbidity and mortality (1). Furthermore, it is sometimes possible to decrease the intensity of pharmacological therapy as a result of the adoption of a physically active lifestyle.

Programs consisting of moderate-intensity exercise are typically used to treat the conditions described in this chapter because the risk-to-benefit ratio is low. Recently, there has been speculation about the benefits of high-intensity interval training in diseased populations, but this approach needs to be more widely tested before adoption can be recommended. The exact intensity, duration, and frequency of physical activity are still not clear for most diseases because of the highly individualized nature of each of these chronic diseases and the variable response to treatments (pharmacological and behavioral) often observed between individuals.

REFERENCES

1. 2008 Physical Activity Guidelines for Americans [Internet]. Washington (DC): U.S. Department of Health and Human Services; [cited 2011 Sept 2]. Available from: http://www.health.gov/paguidelines/pdf/paguide.pdf
2. Accreditation Counsel for Graduate Medical Education [Internet]. SeniorJournal.com; [cited 2011 Mar 15]. Available from: http://www.seniorjournal.com/NEWS/Eldercare/5-02-27MedicalTraining.htm
3. Ada L, Dorsch S, Canning CG. Strengthening interventions increase strength and improve activity after stroke: a systematic review. *Aust J Physiother*. 2006;52(4):241–8.
4. Alioğlu E, Ercan E, Tengiz I, et al. The influence of α-adducin gene polymorphism on response of blood pressure to exercise in patients with hypertension. *Anadolu Kardiyol Derg*. 2010;10(5):400–5.
5. American College of Sports Medicine Position Stand. The recommended quantity and quality of exercise for developing and maintaining cardiorespiratory and muscular fitness, and flexibility in healthy adults. *Med Sci Sports Exerc*. 1998;30(6):975–91.
6. American College of Sports Medicine Position Stand. The recommended quantity and quality of exercise for developing and maintaining cardiorespiratory and muscular fitness in healthy adults. *Med Sci Sports Exerc*. 1990;22(2):265–74.
7. American Heart Association Web site [Internet]. Dallas (TX): American Heart Association; [cited 2011 Mar 15]. Available from: http://www.heart.org/HEARTORG/
8. Aronow WS. Management of peripheral arterial disease. *Cardiol Rev*. 2005;13(2):61–8.
9. Ashworth NL, Chad KE, Harrison EL, Reeder BA, Marshall SC. Home versus center based physical activity programs in older adults. *Cochrane Database Syst Rev*. 2005(1):CD004017.
10. Atkinson RL, Walberg-Rankin J. Physical activity, fitness, and severe obesity. In: Bouchard C, Shephard RJ, editors. *Physical*

Activity, Fitness, and Health: International Proceedings and Consensus Statement. Champaign: Human Kinetics Publishers; 1994. p. 696–711.

11. Bansal S, Buring JE, Rifai N, Mora S, Sacks FM, Ridker PM. Fasting compared with nonfasting triglycerides and risk of cardiovascular events in women. *JAMA.* 2007;298(3):309–16.

12. Bell LM, Watts K, Siafarikas A, et al. Exercise alone reduces insulin resistance in obese children independently of changes in body composition. *J Clin Endocrinol Metab.* 2007;92(11):4230–5.

13. Bock BC, Albrecht AE, Traficante RM, et al. Predictors of exercise adherence following participation in a cardiac rehabilitation program. *Int J Behav Med.* 1997;4(1):60–75.

14. Bowen A, Lincoln NB. Cognitive rehabilitation for spatial neglect following stroke. *Cochrane Database Syst Rev.* 2007(2):CD003586.

15. Burke LE, Dunbar-Jacob JM, Hill MN. Compliance with cardiovascular disease prevention strategies: a review of the research. *Ann Behav Med.* 1997;19(3):239–63.

16. Carlson JJ, Norman GJ, Feltz DL, Franklin BA, Johnson JA, Locke SK. Self-efficacy, psychosocial factors, and exercise behavior in traditional versus modified cardiac rehabilitation. *J Cardiopulm Rehabil.* 2001;21(6):363–73.

17. Castellani JW, Young AJ, Ducharme MB, et al. American College of Sports Medicine position stand: prevention of cold injuries during exercise. *Med Sci Sports Exerc.* 2006;38(11):2012–29.

18. Centers for Disease Control and Prevention Web site [Internet]. Atlanta (GA): Centers for Disease Control and Prevention; U.S. Department of Health and Human Services; [cited 2011 Mar 15]. Available from: http://www.cdc.gov/

19. Chobanian AV, Bakris GL, Black HR, et al. Seventh report of the Joint National Committee on Prevention, Detection, Evaluation, and Treatment of High Blood Pressure. *Hypertension.* 2003;42(6):1206–52.

20. Cholesterol Statistics [Internet]. Dallas (TX): American Heart Association; [cited 2011 Mar 15]. Available from: http://216.185.112.5/presenter.jhtml?identifier=4506

21. Clinical guidelines on the identification, evaluation, and treatment of overweight and obesity in adults—The evidence report. National Institutes of Health. *Obes Res.* 1998;6 Suppl 2:51–209S.

22. Criqui MH. Peripheral arterial disease—epidemiological aspects. *Vasc Med.* 2001;6(3 Suppl):3–7.

23. Crouse SF, O'Brien BC, Grandjean PW, Lowe RC, Rohack JJ, Green JS. Effects of training and a single session of exercise on lipids and apolipoproteins in hypercholesterolemic men. *J Appl Physiol.* 1997;83(6):2019–28.

24. Duncan JJ, Gordon NF, Scott CB. Women walking for health and fitness. How much is enough? *JAMA.* 1991;266(23):3295–9.

25. Durstine JL, Moore GE, American College of Sports Medicine. *ACSM's Exercise Management for Persons with Chronic Diseases and Disabilities.* 2nd ed. Champaign (IL): Human Kinetics; 2003. 374 p.

26. Durstine JL, Peel JB. Dyslipidemia. In: Durstine JL, editor. *Pollock's Textbook of Cardiovascular Disease and Rehabilitation.* Leeds: Human Kinetics; 2008. p. 219–228.

27. Ehrman JK. *Clinical Exercise Physiology.* 2nd ed. Champaign (IL): Human Kinetics; 2008. 712 p.

28. Ervin RB. Prevalence of metabolic syndrome among adults 20 years of age and over, by sex, age, race and ethnicity, and body mass index: United States, 2003–2006. *Natl Health Stat Report.* 2009;13:1–7.

29. Fields LE, Burt VL, Cutler JA, Hughes J, Roccella EJ, Sorlie P. The burden of adult hypertension in the United States 1999 to 2000: a rising tide. *Hypertension.* 2004;44(4):398–404.

30. Flegal KM, Carroll MD, Ogden CL, Curtin LR. Prevalence and trends in obesity among US adults, 1999–2008. *JAMA.* 2010;303(3):235–41.

31. Flegal KM, Carroll MD, Ogden CL, Johnson CL. Prevalence and trends in obesity among US adults, 1999–2000. *JAMA.* 2002;288(14):1723–7.

32. Fletcher B, Berra K, Ades P, et al. Managing abnormal blood lipids: a collaborative approach. *Circulation.* 2005;112(20):3184–209.

33. Fletcher GF, Bufalino V, Costa F, et al. Efficacy of drug therapy in the secondary prevention of cardiovascular disease and stroke. *Am J Cardiol.* 2007;99(6 Suppl 3):S1–35.

34. Forkan R, Pumper B, Smyth N, Wirkkala H, Ciol MA, Shumway-Cook A. Exercise adherence following physical therapy intervention in older adults with impaired balance. *Phys Ther.* 2006; 86(3):401–10.

35. Franklin BA, Whaley MH, Howley ET, Balady GJ, American College of Sports Medicine. *ACSM's Guidelines for Exercise Testing and Prescription.* 6th ed. Philadelphia (PA): Lippincott Williams & Wilkins; 2000. 368 p.

36. Garber CE, Blissmer B, Deschenes MR, et al. Quantity and quality of exercise for developing and maintaining cardiorespiratory, musculoskeletal, and neuromotor fitness in apparently healthy adults: guidance for prescribing exercise. *Med Sci Sports Exerc.* 2011; 43(7):1334–59.

37. Gardner AW, Montgomery PS, Flinn WR, Katzel LI. The effect of exercise intensity on the response to exercise rehabilitation in patients with intermittent claudication. *J Vasc Surg.* 2005;42(4): 702–9.

38. Gardner AW, Poehlman ET. Exercise rehabilitation programs for the treatment of claudication pain. A meta-analysis. *JAMA.* 1995;274(12):975–80.

39. Giannopoulou I, Fernhall B, Carhart R, et al. Effects of diet and/or exercise on the adipocytokine and inflammatory cytokine levels of postmenopausal women with type 2 diabetes. *Metabolism.* 2005;54(7):866–75.

40. Gibellini R, Fanello M, Bardile AF, Salerno M, Aloi T. Exercise training in intermittent claudication. *Int Angiol.* 2000;19(1):8–13.

41. Gordon NF, Contractor A, Leighton RF. Resistance training for hypertension and stroke patients. In: Franklin BA, Graves JE, editors. *Resistance Training for Health and Rehabilitation.* Champaign (IL): Human Kinetics; 2001. p. 237–52.

42. Gordon NF, Gulanick M, Costa F, et al. Physical activity and exercise recommendations for stroke survivors: an American Heart Association scientific statement from the Council on Clinical Cardiology, Subcommittee on Exercise, Cardiac Rehabilitation, and Prevention; the Council on Cardiovascular Nursing; the Council on Nutrition, Physical Activity, and Metabolism; and the Stroke Council. *Circulation.* 2004;109(16):2031–41.

43. Gordon WA, Sliwinski M, Echo J, McLoughlin M, Sheerer MS, Meili TE. The benefits of exercise in individuals with traumatic brain injury: a retrospective study. *J Head Trauma Rehabil.* 1998;13(4):58–67.

44. Grandjean PW, Crouse SF, Rohack JJ. Influence of cholesterol status on blood lipid and lipoprotein enzyme responses to aerobic exercise. *J Appl Physiol.* 2000;89(2):472–80.

45. Grundy SM, Cleeman JI, Merz CN, et al. Implications of recent clinical trials for the National Cholesterol Education Program Adult Treatment Panel III guidelines. *Circulation.* 2004;110(2):227–39.

46. Haskell WL, Lee IM, Pate RR, et al. Physical activity and public health: updated recommendation for adults from the American College of Sports Medicine and the American Heart Association. *Med Sci Sports Exerc.* 2007;39(8):1423–34.

47. Hill JO, Drougas HJ, Peters JC. Physical activity, fitness, and moderate obesity. In: Bouchard C, Shephard RJ, editors. *Physical Activity, Fitness, and Health: International Proceedings and Consensus Statement.* Champaign (IL): Human Kinetics Publishers; 1994. p. 684–95.

48. Hirsch AT, Haskal ZJ, Hertzer NR, et al. ACC/AHA 2005 guidelines for the management of patients with peripheral arterial disease (lower extremity, renal, mesenteric, and abdominal aortic): executive summary a collaborative report from the American Association for Vascular Surgery/Society for Vascular Surgery, Society for Cardiovascular Angiography and Interventions, Society

for Vascular Medicine and Biology, Society of Interventional. *J Am Coll Cardiol*. 2006;47(6):1239–312.

49. Hokanson JE, Austin MA. Plasma triglyceride level is a risk factor for cardiovascular disease independent of high-density lipoprotein cholesterol level: a meta-analysis of population-based prospective studies. *J Cardiovasc Risk*. 1996;3(2):213–9.

50. Hui EK, Rubenstein LZ. Promoting physical activity and exercise in older adults. *J Am Med Dir Assoc*. 2006;7(5):310–4.

51. Hyman MH, Torgovnick J, Arsura E, et al. Statin-associated myopathy with normal creatine kinase levels [2] (multiple letters). *Ann Intern Med*. 2003;138(12):1007–9.

52. Jakicic JM, Clark K, Coleman E, et al. American College of Sports Medicine position stand. Appropriate intervention strategies for weight loss and prevention of weight regain for adults. *Med Sci Sports Exerc*. 2001;33(12):2145–56.

53. Jakicic JM, Winters C, Lang W, Wing RR. Effects of intermittent exercise and use of home exercise equipment on adherence, weight loss, and fitness in overweight women: a randomized trial. *JAMA*. 1999;282(16):1554–60.

54. Jankowski LW, Sullivan SJ. Aerobic and neuromuscular training: effect on the capacity, efficiency, and fatigability of patients with traumatic brain injuries. *Arch Phys Med Rehabil*. 1990;71(7):500–4.

55. Janssen I, Fortier A, Hudson R, Ross R. Effects of an energy-restrictive diet with or without exercise on abdominal fat, intermuscular fat, and metabolic risk factors in obese women. *Diabetes Care*. 2002;25(3):431–8.

56. Karanja N, Lancaster KJ, Vollmer WM, et al. Acceptability of sodium-reduced research diets, including the dietary approaches to stop hypertension diet, among adults with prehypertension and stage 1 hypertension. *J Am Diet Assoc*. 2007;107(9):1530–8.

57. Klem ML, Wing RR, McGuire MT, Seagle HM, Hill JO. A descriptive study of individuals successful at long-term maintenance of substantial weight loss. *Am J Clin Nutr*. 1997;66(2):239–46.

58. Kokkinos PF, Holland JC, Narayan P, Colleran JA, Dotson CO, Papademetriou V. Miles run per week and high-density lipoprotein cholesterol levels in healthy, middle-aged men. A dose-response relationship. *Arch Intern Med*. 1995;155(4):415–20.

59. Kraus WE, Houmard JA, Duscha BD, et al. Effects of the amount and intensity of exercise on plasma lipoproteins. *N Engl J Med*. 2002;347(19):1483–92.

60. Leng GC, Fowler B, Ernst E. Exercise for intermittent claudication. *Cochrane Database Syst Rev*. 2000(2):CD000990.

61. Leon AS, Gaskill SE, Rice T, et al. Variability in the response of HDL cholesterol to exercise training in the HERITAGE Family Study. *Int J Sports Med*. 2002;23(1):1–9.

62. Leon AS, Rice T, Mandel S, et al. Blood lipid response to 20 weeks of supervised exercise in a large biracial population: the HERITAGE Family Study. *Metabolism*. 2000;49(4):513–20.

63. Mangiafico RA, Fiore CE. Current management of intermittent claudication: the role of pharmacological and nonpharmacological symptom-directed therapies. *Curr Vasc Pharmacol*. 2009;7(3):394–413.

64. Mason RJ, Broaddus VC, Murray JF, Nadel JA. *Murray and Nadel's Textbook of Respiratory Medicine*. 4th ed. Oxford: Elsevier; 2005. 2432 p.

65. McDermott AY, Mernitz H. Exercise and older patients: prescribing guidelines. *Am Fam Physician*. 2006;74(3):437–44.

66. Miller WM, McCullough PA. Obesity. In: Durstine JL, editor. *Pollock's Textbook of Cardiovascular Disease and Rehabilitation*. Leeds: Human Kinetics; 2008. p. 209–18.

67. Miyatake N, Nishikawa H, Morishita A, et al. Daily walking reduces visceral adipose tissue areas and improves insulin resistance in Japanese obese subjects. *Diabetes Res Clin Pract*. 2002;58(2):101–7.

68. Moreland JD, Goldsmith CH, Huijbregts MP, et al. Progressive resistance strengthening exercises after stroke: a single-blind randomized controlled trial. *Arch Phys Med Rehabil*. 2003;84(10):1433–40.

69. National Heart Lung Blood Institute Web site [Internet]. Bethesda (MD): National Institutes of Health; National Heart, Lung, and Blood Institute; [cited 2011 Mar 15]. Available from: http://www.nhlbi.nih.gov/

70. Nied RJ, Franklin B. Promoting and prescribing exercise for the elderly. *Am Fam Physician*. 2002;65(3):419–26.

71. Nimalasuriya K, Frank E. A new key to improving the health of patients and of the whole population: physicians preach what we practice. *Medscape Public Health & Prevention*. 2006;47(1). Available from: http://www.medscape.com/viewarticle/522907

72. Nordestgaard BG, Benn M, Schnohr P, Tybjaerg-Hansen A. Nonfasting triglycerides and risk of myocardial infarction, ischemic heart disease, and death in men and women. *JAMA*. 2007; 298(3):299–308.

73. Norgren L, Hiatt WR, Dormandy JA, et al. Inter-society consensus for the management of peripheral arterial disease (TASC II). *Eur J Vasc Endovasc Surg*. 2007;33 Suppl 1:S1–75.

74. Ogden CL, Carroll MD, Curtin LR, McDowell MA, Tabak CJ, Flegal KM. Prevalence of overweight and obesity in the United States, 1999–2004. *JAMA*. 2006;295(13):1549–55.

75. Older Americans 2010: Key Indicators of Well-Being [Internet]. Washington (DC): Federal Interagency Forum on Aging-Related Statistics; [cited 2011 Nov 21]. Available from: http://www.agingstats.gov/agingstatsdotnet/Main_Site/Data/2010_Documents/Docs/OA_2010.pdf

76. O'Leary VB, Marchetti CM, Krishnan RK, Stetzer BP, Gonzalez F, Kirwan JP. Exercise-induced reversal of insulin resistance in obese elderly is associated with reduced visceral fat. *J Appl Physiol*. 2006;100(5):1584–9.

77. Palmer-McLean K, Harbst KB. Stroke and brain injury. In: American College of Sports Medicine, editor. *ACSM's Exercise Management for Persons with Chronic Diseases and Disabilities*. 2nd ed. Champaign: Human Kinetics; 2003. p. 238–246.

78. Parmenter BJ, Raymond J, Fiatarone Singh MA. The effect of exercise on haemodynamics in intermittent claudication: a systematic review of randomized controlled trials. *Sports Med*. 2010; 40(5):433–47.

79. Patten C, Lexell J, Brown HE. Weakness and strength training in persons with poststroke hemiplegia: rationale, method, and efficacy. *J Rehabil Res Dev*. 2004;41(3A):293–312.

80. Pescatello LS. Hypertension. In: Durstine JL, editor. *Pollock's Textbook of Cardiovascular Disease and Rehabilitation*. Leeds: Human Kinetics; 2008. p. 191–98.

81. Pescatello LS, Franklin BA, Fagard R, et al. American College of Sports Medicine position stand. Exercise and hypertension. *Med Sci Sports Exerc*. 2004;36(3):533–53.

82. Pescatello LS, Guidry MA, Blanchard BE, et al. Exercise intensity alters postexercise hypotension. *J Hypertens*. 2004;22(10):1881–8.

83. Petitt DS, Cureton KJ. Effects of prior exercise on postprandial lipemia: a quantitative review. *Metabolism*. 2003;52(4):418–24.

84. Phillips PS, Haas RH, Bannykh S, et al. Statin-associated myopathy with normal creatine kinase levels. *Ann Intern Med*. 2002; 137(7):581–5.

85. Physical Activity and Older Americans: Benefits and Strategies [Internet]. Rockville (MD): Agency for Healthcare Research and Quality, Centers for Disease Control and Prevention; [cited 2011 Mar 15]. Available from: http://www.ahrq.gov/ppip/activity.htm

86. Pratt M, Macera CA, Wang G. Higher direct medical costs associated with physical inactivity. *Phys Sportsmed*. 2000;28(10):63–70.

87. Regensteiner JG. Exercise in the treatment of claudication: assessment and treatment of functional impairment. *Vasc Med*. 1997;2(3): 238–42.

88. Roger VL, Go AS, Lloyd-Jones DM, et al. Heart disease and stroke statistics—2012 update: a report from the American Heart Association. *Circulation*. 2012;125(1):e2–e220.

89. The Role of Midlife and Older Consumers in Promoting Physical Activity through Healthcare, 2002 [Internet]. College Station (TX):

Active for Life; [cited 2011 Mar 15]. Available from: http://www.activeforlife.info/resources/files/CDC%20Final%20Paper.pdf

90. Ross R, Dagnone D, Jones PJ, et al. Reduction in obesity and related comorbid conditions after diet-induced weight loss or exercise-induced weight loss in men. A randomized, controlled trial. *Ann Intern Med.* 2000;133(2):92–103.

91. Ross R, Janssen I, Dawson J, et al. Exercise-induced reduction in obesity and insulin resistance in women: a randomized controlled trial. *Obes Res.* 2004;12(5):789–98.

92. Ryan AS, Nicklas BJ, Berman DM. Aerobic exercise is necessary to improve glucose utilization with moderate weight loss in women. *Obesity (Silver Spring).* 2006;14(6):1064–72.

93. Saltin B. *Exercise and Circulation in Health and Disease.* Champaign (IL): Human Kinetics; 2000.

94. Saris WH, Blair SN, van Baak MA, et al. How much physical activity is enough to prevent unhealthy weight gain? Outcome of the IASO 1st Stock Conference and consensus statement. *Obes Rev.* 2003;4(2):101–14.

95. Schoeller DA, Shay K, Kushner RF. How much physical activity is needed to minimize weight gain in previously obese women? *Am J Clin Nutr.* 1997;66(3):551–6.

96. The Seventh Report of the Joint National Committee on Prevention, Detection, Evaluation, and Treatment of High Blood Pressure [Internet]. Bethesda (MD): National Institutes of Health; National Heart, Lung, and Blood Institute; [cited 2011 Jan 19]. Available from: http://www.nhlbi.nih.gov/guidelines/hypertension/

97. Shaughnessy M, Resnick BM, Macko RF. Testing a model of poststroke exercise behavior. *Rehabil Nurs.* 2006;31(1):15–21.

98. Shepich J, Slowiak JM, Keniston A. Do subsidization and monitoring enhance adherence to prescribed exercise? *Am J Health Promot.* 2007;22(1):2–5.

99. Sinzinger H. Statin-induced myositis migrans. *Wien Klin Wochenschr.* 2002; 114(21–2):943–4.

100. Sinzinger H, Schmid P, O'Grady J. Two different types of exercise-induced muscle pain without myopathy and CK-elevation during HMG-Co-enzyme-A-reductase inhibitor treatment. *Atherosclerosis.* 1999;143(2):459–60.

101. Sjöström L, Narbro K, Sjöström CD, et al. Effects of bariatric surgery on mortality in Swedish obese subjects. *N Engl J Med.* 2007;357(8):741–52.

102. Statistical Fact Sheet—Risk Factors 2011 Update [Internet]. Dallas (TX): American Heart Association; [cited 2011 Nov 19]. Available from: http://www.heart.org/HEARTORG/General/Risk-Factors_UCM_319118_Article.jsp#.Ts04HXI4RBk

103. Stein R, Hriljac I, Halperin JL, Gustavson SM, Teodorescu V, Olin JW. Limitation of the resting ankle-brachial index in symptomatic patients with peripheral arterial disease. *Vasc Med.* 2006;11(1):29–33.

104. Stewart KJ, Hiatt WR, Regensteiner JG, Hirsch AT. Exercise training for claudication. *N Engl J Med.* 2002;347(24):1941–51.

105. Taylor NF, Dodd KJ, Damiano DL. Progressive resistance exercise in physical therapy: a summary of systematic reviews. *Phys Ther.* 2005;85(11):1208–23.

106. Third Report of the National Cholesterol Education Program (NCEP) Expert Panel on Detection, Evaluation, and Treatment of High Blood Cholesterol in Adults (Adult Treatment Panel III) Executive Summary [Internet]. Bethesda (MD): National Cholesterol Education Program; [cited 2011 Mar 15]. Available from: http://purl.access.gpo.gov/GPO/LPS15056

107. Thom T, Haase N, Rosamond W, et al. Heart disease and stroke statistics—2006 update: a report from the American Heart Association Statistics Committee and Stroke Statistics Subcommittee. *Circulation.* 2006;113(6):e85–151.

108. Tsai JC, Chan P, Wang CH, et al. The effects of exercise training on walking function and perception of health status in elderly patients with peripheral arterial occlusive disease. *J Intern Med.* 2002;252(6):448–55.

109. U.S. Department of Health and Human Services, Centers for Disease Control and Prevention, National Center for Chronic Disease Prevention and Health Promotion, The President's Council on Physical Fitness and Sports. *Physical Activity and Health: A Report of the Surgeon General.* Atlanta (GA): President's Council on Physical Fitness and Sports; 1996. 278 p.

110. Vogeli C, Shields AE, Lee TA, et al. Multiple chronic conditions: prevalence, health consequences, and implications for quality, care management, and costs. *J Gen Intern Med.* 2007;22 Suppl 3:391–5.

111. Volek JS, Feinman RD. Carbohydrate restriction improves the features of Metabolic Syndrome. Metabolic Syndrome may be defined by the response to carbohydrate restriction. *Nutr Metab (Lond).* 2005;2:31.

112. Wenger NK, Scheidt S, Weber MA, US Agency for Health Care Policy and Research, National Heart, Lung, and Blood Institute. Exercise and elderly persons. *Am J Geriatr Cardiol.* 2001;10(5):241–2.

113. Womack CJ, Gardner AW. Peripheral arterial disease. In: American College of Sports Medicine, editor. *ACSM's Exercise Management for Persons with Chronic Diseases and Disabilities.* 2nd ed. Champaign: Human Kinetics; 2003, p. 81–5.

114. Xin X, He J, Frontini MG, Ogden LG, Motsamai OI, Whelton PK. Effects of alcohol reduction on blood pressure: a meta-analysis of randomized controlled trials. *Hypertension.* 2001;38(5):1112–7.

115. Youngstedt SD. Effects of exercise on sleep. *Clin Sports Med.* 2005;24(2):355–65.

116. Zipes DP, Braunwald E. Heart disease. *Braunwald's Heart Disease: A Textbook of Cardiovascular Medicine.* 7th ed. Philadelphia (PA): W.B. Saunders; 2005.

SELECTED REFERENCES FOR FURTHER READING

2008 Physical Activity Guidelines for Americans [Internet]. Washington (DC): U.S. Department of Health and Human Services; [cited 2011 Sep 2]. Available from: http://www.health.gov/paguidelines/pdf/paguide.pdf

Chobanian AV, Bakris GL, Black HR, et al. Seventh report of the Joint National Committee on Prevention, Detection, Evaluation, and Treatment of High Blood Pressure. *Hypertension.* 2003;42(6): 1206–52.

Gordon NF. *Stroke: Your Complete Exercise Guide.* Champaign (IL): Human Kinetics; 1993. 126 p.

Gordon NF, Gulanick M, Costa F, et al. Physical activity and exercise recommendations for stroke survivors: an American Heart Association scientific statement from the Council on Clinical Cardiology, Subcommittee on Exercise, Cardiac Rehabilitation, and Prevention; the Council on Cardiovascular Nursing; the Council on Nutrition, Physical Activity, and Metabolism; and the Stroke Council. *Circulation.* 2004;109(16):2031–41.

Older Americans 2010: Key Indicators of Well-Being [Internet]. Washington (DC): Federal Interagency Forum on Aging-Related Statistics; [cited 2011 Nov 21]. Available from: http://www.agingstats.gov/agingstatsdotnet/Main_Site/Data/2010_Documents/Docs/OA_2010.pdf

Physical Activity and Older Americans: Benefits and Strategies [Internet]. Rockville (MD): Agency for Healthcare Research and Quality, Centers for Disease Control and Prevention; [cited 2011 Mar 15]. Available from: http://www.ahrq.gov/ppip/activity.htm

INTERNET RESOURCES

- National Heart, Lung and Blood Institute: http://www.nhlbi.nih.gov
- National Hypertension Association: http://www.nathypertension.org
- National Lipid Association: http://www.lipid.org
- National Stroke Association: http://www.stroke.org
- North American Association for the Study of Obesity (NAASO): http://www.naaso.org

CHAPTER

42

Exercise Prescription for Patients with Osteoporosis

EPIDEMIOLOGY

Osteoporosis is a skeletal disorder characterized by compromised bone strength that results in an increased susceptibility to fracture (41,86). It is estimated that approximately 200 million women worldwide currently have osteoporosis (50), and the prevalence among all adults is expected to rise with the increase in life expectancy and aging population (17).

The clinical relevance of osteoporosis is the dramatic increase in risk of fracture. More than 1.5 million fractures are associated with osteoporosis each year. **Osteoporotic fractures** are low-trauma fractures that occur with forces generated by a fall from a standing

height or lower and are most common at the spine, hip, and wrist. Regardless of the initial fracture site, adults who fracture have a much greater risk of fracturing again at any location (28). After the age of 50 yr, it is estimated that approximately one in three women and one in five men will suffer from an osteoporotic-related fracture in their lifetime (53,78,79). To put this in perspective, the combined lifetime risk for hip, forearm, and vertebral fractures is equal to the risk of developing cardiovascular disease (49).

Hip fractures are considered to be the most devastating consequences of osteoporosis because they are associated with severe disability and increased mortality (80). Furthermore, the economic burden of hip

KEY TERMS

Bone balance: The amount of bone formed in a remodeling pit compared to the amount resorbed. When the bone balance is zero, no bone is lost. With menopause and advancing age, bone balance becomes negative, and bone is lost.

Bone mineral density (BMD): A surrogate measure of bone strength that is typically measured by dual-energy X-ray absorptiometry (DXA). It represents the amount of mineralized tissue per area of bone expressed in $g \cdot cm^{-2}$.

Cortical bone: Dense bone that constitutes the shaft of long bones and provides a protective shell around the ends of long bones and vertebrae.

Modeling: Formation or resorption of bone along a surface that changes the size and shape of bones.

Mechanotransduction: The process by which bone cells convert mechanical stimuli (*e.g.*, load from physical activity) into a chemical response.

Osteoblasts: Cells involved in the formation and mineralization of new bone.

Osteoclasts: Multinucleated cells involved in resorbing old, damaged, or excess bone.

Osteocytes: Osteoblasts that become entombed in the matrix they helped secrete. These are thought to be the main cells in the skeleton that can sense physical activity.

Osteopenia: Low bone mass; designated as a bone density between 1.0 and 2.5 standard deviations less than the mean peak value for young normal adults.

Osteoporosis: A skeletal disorder characterized by compromised bone strength that results in an increased susceptibility to fracture; diagnosed by a BMD more than 2.5 standard deviations below the mean peak value for young normal adults.

Osteoporotic fracture: A low-trauma fracture that occurs from forces generated by a fall from a standing height or lower; most common at the spine, hip, and wrist.

Remodeling: A dynamic process of bone resorption and subsequent formation that results in turnover of small pits of bone material.

Strain: The deformation of a material; refers to the relative change in bone length in response to an applied load.

Trabecular bone: Porous bone found in flat bones, the ends of long bones, and in cuboidal bones (*e.g.*, vertebrae).

699

fractures is substantial, with an estimated worldwide annual cost of $131.5 billion (48). The combination of all osteoporotic fractures cost the U.S. health care system approximately $17 billion per year, and these annual costs are expected to nearly double to $25 billion by the year 2025 (17).

Osteoporosis is a silent disease, i.e., typically without symptoms. It is first detected by clinical screening or by experiencing an osteoporotic fracture. This is why much attention is focused on early prevention, detection, and treatment of osteoporosis. This chapter will provide a brief overview of the pathogenesis, diagnosis, risk assessment, prevention, and treatment of osteoporosis — with special emphasis placed on the role of exercise in building and maintaining a strong skeleton.

OSTEOPOROSIS AMONG MEN AND WOMEN

Women are much more likely than men to have low bone mass (27) and are at greater risk of experiencing a fracture in their lifetime (88). Therefore, osteoporosis is often perceived as a disease that affects only women, and men often go undiagnosed and untreated (90). However, it is estimated that 17% of men older than the age of 50 yr meet the criteria for osteoporosis, and like women, men experience an increase in the prevalence of osteoporosis with age; although the prevalence in men remains low until later in life (80 yr and beyond) (27). With the aging population, it is estimated that the prevalence of osteoporosis in men will increase by 50% in the next 15 yr (82).

With an increase in low bone mass comes an increase in risk of fracture. It is estimated that one in five men will experience a fracture in their lifetime. Research shows that when men experience a hip fracture, they do not fare as well as women. In a large study, researchers found that 32% of men died within 1 yr of a hip fracture (9). Men are also at greater risk than woman for experiencing a subsequent hip fracture (12). Given the increasing prevalence of osteoporosis and related fractures in men, coupled with susceptibility to greater consequences following fractures, increased attention should be paid to preventing, diagnosing, and treating osteoporosis in men.

BASIC BONE PHYSIOLOGY

Bone is a tissue that is composed of two main materials — inorganic hydroxyapatite (calcium phosphate) crystals and an organic collagen matrix. The collagen gives bone flexible properties, whereas the mineral adds stiffness. Bone tissue is fashioned into two main types of bone. Cortical bone (also referred to as compact bone) is dense and stiff and comprises the shaft of long bones as well as provides a shell of protection

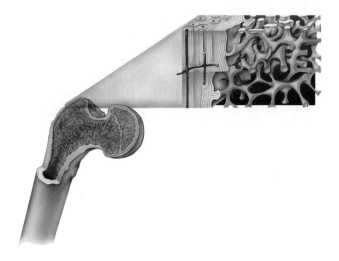

FIGURE 42-1. Bone is a dynamic tissue that is vascularized and innervated. *Cortical* bone is dense and stiff and makes up the shaft of long bones. Cortical bone also provides a shell of protection around *trabecular* bone, which is more porous and flexible and is found at the ends of long bones and in vertebrae.

around trabecular bone (*Fig. 42-1*). Trabecular bone (also referred to as cancellous or spongy bone) is more porous and flexible and is found in flat bones, the ends of long bones, and in cuboidal bones (*e.g.*, vertebrae). In trabecular bone, the bone material is in the form of plates and struts called trabeculae.

The characteristics of bone that determine its strength include the quantity of bone material present, the quality of the material, and the distribution of the material in space (the *structure of the bone*). These factors are determined by the dynamic cellular activities known as bone modeling and remodeling, which are regulated by bone's hormonal and mechanical environments. Modeling is the *independent* action of osteoclasts (bone-resorbing cells) and osteoblasts (bone-forming cells) on the surfaces of bone, whereby new bone is added along some surfaces and removed from others. Modeling affects the size and shape of bones and is especially important for reshaping long bones as they grow in length during adolescence or in response to changing mechanical load throughout life. Remodeling (*Fig. 42-2*) is a localized process that involves the *coupled* action of osteoclasts and osteoblasts, in which osteoclasts first resorb a pit of older bone, and osteoblasts are subsequently recruited to the site to form and mineralize new bone. This process happens throughout the lifespan and occurs diffusely throughout the skeleton. An important role of remodeling is to replace damaged bone with new healthy bone. Like any material subjected to repetitive loading, bone experiences fatigue damage in the form of very small cracks. However, unlike inert materials, bone is able to replace damaged bone with new bone through the process of resorption and formation (*i.e.*, remodeling) (92).

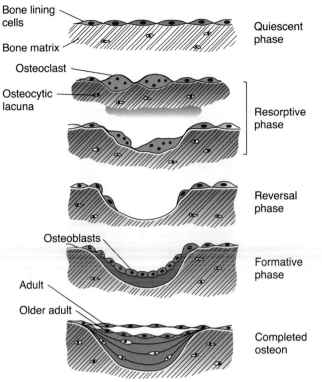

FIGURE 42-2. Bone remodeling is the *coupled* actions of osteoclasts and osteoblasts whereby a portion of older bone is resorbed by osteoclasts and replaced with newly formed bone by osteoblasts. The new bone begins as osteoid (unmineralized matrix). Eventually, the osteoid incorporates mineral.

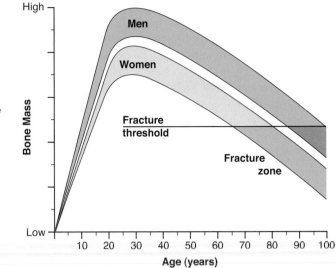

FIGURE 42-3. Normal pattern of bone mineral accretion and loss throughout the lifespan in men and women.

OSTEOPOROSIS PATHOPHYSIOLOGY

Osteoporotic fractures occur when the magnitude of a load on a bone is greater than the strength of a bone. Therefore, although osteoporosis denotes skeletal fragility, osteoporotic fractures are the result of *both* skeletal fragility and overload that result primarily from a fall. Because most hip and wrist fractures occur as a consequence of falling, factors influencing both bone fragility *and* risk of falling are important to consider for fracture prevention.

SKELETAL FRAGILITY

Many skeletal characteristics contribute to bone strength and, consequently, bone fragility, including the quantity of bone material present, the quality of the material, and the distribution of the material. It is important to understand how each of these features of bone strength change with age in order to understand why our bones become weaker and are more susceptible to fracture in later life.

Bone Quantity

Bone "quantity" refers to the amount of bone material present. The average pattern of change in bone mass across the lifespan is displayed graphically in *Figure 42-3,*

although the actual pattern of bone mass change is more dynamic than shown both during growth and in later life. For example, approximately 26% of total adult bone mass is accrued in a 2-yr period during adolescence (7). This is approximately equivalent to the entire amount of bone lost in later life (31). Overall, global bone formation continues at a faster pace than bone resorption until peak bone mineral accretion is attained sometime in the second or third decade of life (depending on site, region, and sex). In later life, the process of bone formation in each remodeling site no longer equals the bone that was resorbed, and thus, a small amount of bone is lost with each new remodeling cycle. This is referred to as a negative bone balance.

In later life, gonadal hormones (*e.g.*, testosterone and estrogen) decrease in both men and women. Estrogen, in particular, suppresses activation of new remodeling cycles, and thus, low estrogen levels partially contribute to an increased rate of remodeling (112). As resorption precedes formation in the process of remodeling, and formation and subsequent mineralization are time-intensive processes, an increase in the rate of remodeling results in temporary decreases in bone mass. Although temporary losses in bone mass lead to a transient increase in bone fragility, increased rates of remodeling with a negative bone balance lead to sustained bone loss of approximately 9%–13% during the first 5 yr after menopause (93). Bone turnover eventually slows to a rate similar to premenopausal years. Men also experience age-related bone loss but usually not until their eighth decade of life (18).

Bone Material Quality

Although the amount of bone in the human skeleton decreases with menopause and advancing age, there is evidence that properties of the remaining bone material may change with age in a way that increases susceptibility to fracture. Bone material from older individuals is less able to absorb energy before failure likely because of an increase in the amount of mineral in bone tissue compared to collagen as well as changes in collagen properties that are associated with advancing age (25). Also, with advancing age comes susceptibility to fatigue damage. Microcracks have been shown to increase in number and length with age (116). This microdamage accumulation is associated with reduced bone strength (85).

Bone Structure

Another important component of bone strength is the structure of bone — that is, how the material is distributed in space. Subtle changes in cross-sectional geometry can markedly increase bone strength with little or no changes in bone mass or density. Structural differences in cortical bone geometry may partially explain some of the differences in fracture rates between men and women. During growth, the long bones of boys have greater gains in periosteal (outer) diameter, resulting in a greater overall bone size in boys that remains throughout life, whereas girls have a narrowing of the endocortical (inner) surface (39,101). In later life, bone is lost primarily from the endosteal surfaces (inner surface of long bones and intracortical surfaces within the cortex). Thus, the cortex becomes more porous, and the cortices become thinner and more fragile. To offset these losses, bone may be added to the periosteum (outside surface of bone), thereby increasing the diameter of bone and maintaining the strength of the structure in bending (11,102,103). However, as more bone is resorbed from the endocortical surface than is formed on the periosteal surface, the cortices continue to thin, becoming fragile and more likely to fracture.

Microarchitecture of trabecular bone is also an important contributor to skeletal fragility (56). For example, if the resorption phase of remodeling is too aggressive, as is seen at menopause and thereafter, trabeculae may be penetrated, and the entire trabecular elements may be lost (*Fig. 42-4*). In these cases, the loss in structural strength disproportionately exceeds the amount of bone lost (94). Furthermore, trabeculae that remain intact may be thinned by excessive remodeling, creating a weakness in the ability to bear loads.

FALLS

Although skeletal fragility increases susceptibility to fracture, it would be of little concern if damaging loads, such as those generated in a fall, were prevented. Most hip fractures occur after a sideways fall and landing on the hip (42,114). The incidence of falls increases with age because several sensory systems that control posture (vestibular, visual, and somatosensory) become compromised with advancing age. Furthermore, muscle mass and strength, which prevent instability and correct

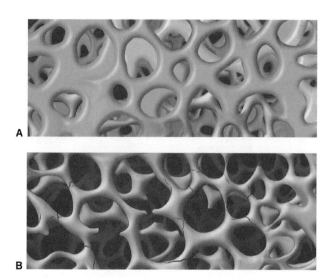

FIGURE 42-4. Slice of trabecular bone in a normal **(A)** and an individual with osteoporosis **(B)** showing loss of trabecular connectivity and increased microdamage with ageing.

imbalance, decline 30%–50% between the ages of 30 and 80 yr (57).

DIAGNOSIS OF OSTEOPOROSIS

There is currently no method for diagnosing osteoporosis based on measuring bone strength. Therefore, identification of individuals with osteoporosis relies on the use of noninvasive technology to measure surrogates of bone strength. A measurement of bone mineral density (BMD) by DXA is the primary factor involved in the diagnosis of osteoporosis (109). BMD represents the amount of bone per unit area and is currently the most commonly used surrogate of bone strength in clinical settings. The World Health Organization (WHO) has defined osteopenia (low bone mass) as a site-specific bone density between 1.0 and 2.5 standard deviations less than the mean for young white adult women, and osteoporosis as a bone density that is more than 2.5 standard deviations less than the mean for young white adult women (86,115). Expressing an individual's BMD relative to the young adult mean is referred to as a *T*-score (i.e., $T \leq 2.5$ = osteoporosis). These criteria were developed based on population data of primarily white women. Controversy exists among experts as to how this criterion applies to men, children, and various ethnic groups (4,86). Furthermore, as these categories were derived from BMD data at the hip, the application of these criteria to other skeletal sites has been questioned (49,51). Despite these issues, BMD measurements have been shown to predict 60%–70% of a patient's risk for fracture (84), therefore making them better predictors of fracture than the measurement of lipids in predicting heart disease (49,84,115).

New software such as the hip structure analysis program and new technology such as quantitative computed tomography (QCT), peripheral QCT (pQCT), and magnetic resonance imaging (MRI) are used to better assess important components of bone strength such as bone geometry and cortical and trabecular volumetric density and, therefore, provide better estimates of bone strength. However, these technologies are currently used primarily in research settings, and their clinical use has not been clearly established.

RISK FACTORS FOR OSTEOPOROTIC FRACTURE

Despite the appreciable capabilities of BMD measurements in predicting fracture, combining multiple risk factor assessment with a measure of BMD may more accurately determine overall fracture risk (49,84,115). This notion is strengthened by the observation that the presence of multiple risk factors is a better predictor of hip fracture than low bone density alone (49). Many risk factors for osteoporosis and fracture have been identified, including age, family history of fracture, previous fracture, physical inactivity, and medication use (*Table 42-1*). Advancing age is perhaps one of the best predictors of fracture because the risk of a hip fracture increases three to six times from 50 to 80 yr of age, independent of BMD status (24,52).

Because of estrogen's effect on suppression of remodeling, hypogonadism is an important risk factor in both men and women. In men, hypogonadism can be caused by several conditions including hypopituitarism, hyperprolactinemia, overtraining, and inadequate energy intake. In young women, hypogonadism secondary to amenorrhea may be associated with inadequate energy intake (69). When taken to the extreme, the female athlete triad syndrome (amenorrhea, disordered eating, and low bone mass) is associated with increased risk for osteoporosis (91), although the prevalence of all three components of the triad is low (58). Menopause, whether spontaneous or caused by surgery, chemotherapy, or radiotherapy, is also associated with increased risk of osteoporosis and fracture.

History of fracture is another important risk factor for subsequent fragility fractures, with a twofold increase in risk of hip fracture following a previous hip or spinal fracture (59). Several medications can increase risk of osteoporosis, including glucocorticoids, which result in greater losses in spine bone mass. However, bone loss can be reduced by use of inhaled glucocorticoid therapy (111). Medications such as anticonvulsants, gonadotropin-releasing hormone agonists, immunosuppressants, and heparin have also been associated with osteoporosis and fracture risk (87). Furthermore, several conditions are associated with secondary osteoporosis, including hyperthyroidism and bariatric surgery (see the following section).

As discussed previously, factors related to risk of falls have important considerations. Exercise professionals should pay close attention to neuromuscular deficits, balance, and coordination in older individuals, particularly those with osteopenia or osteoporosis, who would be at increased risk of fracture in the case of a fall. Improving these deficits is equally (if not more) important in older individuals than attempting to increase bone integrity.

Physiological impairments associated with aging such as slow reaction time, loss of balance, and muscular weakness can contribute to the likelihood of falling (20,68). Psychological factors, such as fear of falling, are also associated with falls (20). Other risk factors associated with fall risk include orthostatic hypotension (low blood pressure with standing), Parkinson disease, stroke, depression, epilepsy, eye diseases, osteoarthritis, peripheral neuropathy, delirium, anemia, diabetes mellitus, depression, cognitive impairment, vitamin D deficiency, and syncope. Therefore, these factors should all be considered when determining risk, treatment, and preventative strategies for osteoporotic fracture (57).

BARIATRIC SURGERY: A RISK FACTOR FOR OSTEOPOROSIS?

In the United States, 68% of adults are overweight or obese, and approximately 6% are morbidly obese (BMI ≥ 40 kg $\cdot$ m^{-2}) (32). Obesity is directly associated with cardiovascular disease and related comorbidities, including Type 2 diabetes and obstructive sleep apnea (98). Bariatric surgery has become an increasingly popular therapeutic approach to treat morbid obesity. The number of bariatric surgical procedures performed in the United States increased 114% from 103,000 in 2003 to 220,000 in 2008 (16). People who undergo bariatric surgery lose substantial weight (up to 62% of their excess

TABLE 42-1. Risk Factors for Osteoporotic Fractures

Age	**Neuromuscular disorders**	Excessive alcohol consumption
Previous fragility fracture	**Cigarette smoking**	Long-term immobilization
Glucocorticoid therapy	**Low body weight**	Low dietary calcium intake
High bone turnover	Premature menopause	Vitamin D deficiency
Family history of hip fracture	Primary or secondary amenorrhea	Female sex
Poor visual acuity	Primary or secondary hypogonadism in men	Asian or White ethnic origin

Bold text indicates characteristics that capture aspects of fracture risk over and above that provided by bone mineral density.

Adapted from Kanis JA. Diagnosis of osteoporosis and assessment of fracture risk. *Lancet.* 2002;359(9321):1929–36.

weight) and resolve or attenuate comorbidities within 2 yr of surgery (44). There are numerous side effects associated with this surgery, including vomiting, "dumping syndrome" (malaise associated with sugars reaching the large intestine), excessive skin resulting in sores and infections requiring plastic surgery, weight regain, and nutritional deficiencies.

With rapid and dramatic weight loss, there is an increasing concern that bariatric surgery may negatively affect the skeleton by accelerating bone loss and increasing bone fragility (44). Several large studies have shown increased rates of hip bone loss in older individuals (29,30) and an increased risk for hip fracture in middle-aged and older women (64) among people who lose weight without surgery. A recent review showed that BMD loss may be as high as 15% at the hip 1 yr following gastric bypass procedures (100). BMD is a strong predictor of fracture risk, and a 10% loss of bone mass at the hip more than doubles the risk of hip fracture (59). Given the rise in popularity of surgery-associated weight loss and the evidence for

accompanying bone loss, there is a potential concern for risk for osteoporosis with weight loss surgery. Therefore, long-term studies are needed to determine if bariatric surgery may have negative consequences for skeletal health.

CLINICAL MANAGEMENT

Although prevention of osteoporosis is important, once an individual is diagnosed with the disease, attention is turned to treatment to offset initial and subsequent fractures. Management strategies involve both pharmacological therapy and lifestyle modifications.

PHARMACOLOGICAL THERAPY

Several pharmacological agents (listed in *Table 42-2*) are currently prescribed for the treatment of osteoporosis. These agents can be categorized according to whether they act by suppressing bone resorption (antiresorptive agents) or by promoting bone formation (anabolic

TABLE 42-2. Medical Therapies Available for the Treatment or Prevention of Osteoporosis

Class	Generic Name	Brand Name
Estrogens	Conjugated estrogens	Premarin
	Estradiol transdermal	Estraderm
	Estropipate	Ogen, Ortho-Est
	Esterified estrogens	Estratab
	Conjugated estrogens, medroxyprogestrone	Premphase Prempro
	Estradiol, Norethindrone	Activella
Bisphosphonates	Alendronate	Fosamax
	Risedronate	Actonel
	Etidronate	Didronel
	Ibandronate	Boniva
	Zoledronic acid	Reclast
	Pamidronate	Aredia
	Tiludronate	Skelid
RANKL Inhibitor	Denosumab	Prolia Xgeva
Anabolic agent	Teriparatide	Forteo
Antiresorptive and anabolic	Strontium	Protelos Prolos
SERMs	Raloxifene	Evista
	Tamoxifen	Nolvadex
Others		
Calcitonin	Calcitonin-salmon	Miacalcin
	Calcitriol or other vitamin D metabolites	
	Sodium fluoride	

RANKL, receptor activator of nuclear factor kappa-B ligand; SERM, selective estrogen receptor modulator.

agents). Antiresorptive agents include bisphosphonates, salmon calcitonin, hormone replacement therapy (HRT), selective estrogen receptor modulators (SERMs), and receptor activator of nuclear factor kappa-B ligand (RANKL) inhibitors. These medications act by suppressing the resorption of bone. In the remodeling cycle, when bone resorption is suppressed, existing remodeling cavities are allowed to fill with new bone while subsequent remodeling cavities are prevented from forming, resulting in an increase in bone density. Also, by suppressing resorption, these agents can prevent trabecular thinning and loss of trabecular connectivity associated with menopause and aging.

Other pharmacologic agents act on promoting bone formation. One of the major hormones regulating calcium homeostasis is parathyroid hormone (PTH), which is secreted in response to falling serum calcium levels. PTH helps to regulate serum calcium levels by (a) stimulating bone resorption in the presence of adequate vitamin D, (b) increasing intestinal calcium absorption, and (c) enhancing reabsorption of calcium in the kidney (57). Although PTH can stimulate both bone formation and bone resorption, when administered intermittently, it results in net bone formation and is thus classified as an anabolic agent (87). Recombinant PTH is an anabolic agent that works by stimulating an increase in osteoblastic bone formation. Although some medications inhibit bone resorption, and some promote bone formation, strontium ranelate is a treatment that does both.

Considering the roles of estrogen in the suppression of osteoclast function and progestin in the stimulation of osteoblast activity, HRT has been shown to increase BMD at the spine and hip in women during the postmenopausal years when substantial losses are typically observed. However, approximately 40% of women who begin HRT choose to stop taking the medication because of its many side effects (34). Furthermore, HRT is associated with an increased risk of coronary artery disease, stroke, and breast and ovarian cancer (40). For women unable to take HRT because they are at high risk of ovarian and breast cancer, the SERM raloxifene is a treatment option because it does not stimulate breast or endometrial tissues (63).

Antiresorptive Agents and Increased Risk of Fracture

The importance of bone remodeling can be seen in the increasing reports of atypical femoral fractures with long-term use of antiresorptive treatment and, in particular, use of bisphosphonates. Bisphosphonates are one of several types of medications used to treat osteoporosis through inhibition of bone resorption. Inhibition of bone resorption results in increases in bone mass. Clinical trials have demonstrated that bisphosphonates reduce the incidence of fractures of the spine and hip

and related health care costs (13,22,23). However, as previously mentioned in this chapter, there is more to bone strength than bone mass alone. Recall that bone remodeling plays an important role in maintaining bone material quality by replacing fatigue-damaged and older bone with damage-free and younger (less mineralized) bone. With antiresorptive agents, remodeling is inhibited, and it is possible that if suppression of bone remodeling occurs for an extended period of time, fatigue damage may build up, bone may become hypermineralized, and bones can become brittle. In essence, with long-term use, antiresorptive medications may lose value in preventing fracture, and in some cases, may lead to fracture.

A case series published in 2005 introduced the first connection between long-term use of bisphosphonates and low-energy fractures of the femur (89). Hip fractures commonly occur in the proximal femur (often in the femoral head and the femoral neck). However, these atypical fractures began occurring in the femoral shaft below the trochanteric region. This initial case series was followed by several more case studies and series that reported similar fractures among individuals on long-term bisphosphonate therapy (43,65). Although recent epidemiological studies have also supported an association between long-term bisphosphonate use and atypical femoral fractures (1,113), because these fractures appear to occur infrequently and because there is a lack of strong evidence, long-term bisphosphonate use remains controversial. Nevertheless, the U.S. Food and Drug Administration (FDA) has issued a warning regarding the possible risk of atypical femoral fractures with long-term bisphosphonate use and has recommended extensive discussion and strict surveillance with continued drug usage.

LIFESTYLE MODIFICATIONS

Many of the risk factors for both osteoporosis and falls can be prevented or at least attenuated by lifestyle modifications. All postmenopausal women and older men, regardless of fracture risk, should be encouraged to engage in behaviors that may reduce their risk for osteoporosis and an osteoporotic fracture, including adequate calcium (1,000–1,500 mg $\cdot$ d^{-1}) and vitamin D (600–800 IU $\cdot$ d^{-1}) intake, regular exercise, smoking cessation, avoidance of excessive alcohol intake, and visual correction to decrease risk of falling. Of these lifestyle behaviors, exercise is the only one that can simultaneously ameliorate low BMD, augment muscle mass, promote strength gain, and improve dynamic balance — all of which are independent risk factors for fracture (54). However, there is currently no direct evidence that exercise reduces the risk of osteoporotic fracture. Nevertheless, clinicians and exercise professionals should embrace the theoretical basis behind exercise prescription in osteoporosis prevention and treatment (57). Exercise prescription for individuals diagnosed with osteoporosis is outlined at the end of this chapter.

EXERCISE AND OSTEOPOROSIS

PHYSIOLOGICAL RESPONSES OF BONE TO EXERCISE

The response of bone to exercise can be classified by the initial (or acute) response of bone to exercise as well as the chronic physiologic and anatomical changes that occur in bone because of exercise training.

Acute Physiological Response

Bone is a dynamic tissue that is capable of continually adapting to its changing mechanical environment. When a bone is loaded in compression, tension, or torsion, bone tissue is deformed. Deformation of bone tissue, or the relative change in bone length, is referred to as strain. Bone tissue strain causes movement of fluid within the bone that perturbs bone's resident cells — osteocytes. These bone cells are embedded throughout bone tissue and are connected with one another, to other bone cells, and with the bone marrow through slender dendritic processes. The current prevailing theory is that this fluid flow along the osteocyte and its cell processes causes a release of molecular signals that lead to osteoclast and osteoblast recruitment (47). This process of turning a mechanical signal into a biochemical one is called mechanotransduction. Mechanotransduction causes physiological processes of modeling and remodeling that creates anatomical changes in bone, resulting in a bone that is better suited to its new mechanical environment.

Chronic Physiological Response

It has been suggested that the response of bone to its mechanical environment is controlled by a "mechanostat" that aims to keep bone tissue strain at an optimal level by homeostatically altering bone structure (36). Indeed, when bone is subjected to lower than customary loads (as in space flight and immobilization), bone will adapt by ridding itself of excess mass. Alternately, when bone is subjected to greater loads such as uncustomary exercise, bone will become stronger by altering its structure and increasing in mass. Although mechanotransduction is an acute response to exercise, the adaptation of bone structure through modeling and remodeling takes up to several months to complete. In the case of bone modeling, bone does not respond to exercise by solely adding mass randomly to the skeleton. Rather, from animal studies, it is clear that bone is added where strains are the highest — typically on the periosteal surface in long

bones (97). This has the effect of increasing the diameter of long bones, making them more resistant to strain.

The prevalence of remodeling in bone is also increased with exercise. With the increase in bone tissue strain that occurs with exercise, there is an increase in the number of microcracks in bone. This damage is targeted for removal by osteoclasts, and new bone is formed in its place (19,92). Thus, one of the chronic effects of exercise on the skeleton involves the maintenance of bone tissue quality through targeted remodeling.

OSTEOGENIC ACTIVITIES

Bone responds to exercise in a site-specific manner. That is, bone will be added in locations where adequate strain is generated. Thus, to optimize bone health at the hip, physical activity should be designed to load the hip region. Evidence from animal studies suggests that effective exercise programs for bone health should result in high strain rates and unusual strain distributions (i.e., loading in directions the bone is unaccustomed to). In practical terms, an osteogenic (bone-forming) exercise regimen should generate moderate-to-high mechanical forces at high rates of force application produced in versatile movements (97,108). Research also suggests that inserting rest between loading cycles can optimize the bone response to exercise (96,107). That is, bone cells seem to saturate after a short loading period. In animal studies, bone loses more than 95% of its mechanosensitivity after only 20 loading cycles (97,108). For example, doing 10 jumps three times per day with 2–4 hr of rest between sets should be more effective for bone health than doing 30 jumps all at one time.

Although generally high magnitude and high strain rates lead to an optimal bone response, strain patterns can be altered to stimulate bone adaptation. For example, low-magnitude strains that were otherwise ineffective stimulated an osteogenic response in mature animals if 10 s of rest were inserted between loading bouts (107) or if strains were generated at a very high frequency (>20 Hz) (43,96,97). These novel strain applications have important implications for interventions in individuals with low bone mass such as adults with osteoporosis.

EXERCISE DURING YOUTH: BUILDING A STRONG SKELETON

Although osteoporosis is a disease associated with advancing age, there is almost universal consensus that healthy behaviors in youth are important in reducing the risk of osteoporosis in later life (31). The observation that more than 25% of adult bone mineral is laid down during the 2 yr surrounding the age of peak linear growth emphasizes the importance of the adolescent years in optimizing bone mineral accrual (6). It is estimated that as much bone mineral is laid down during this period as an adult will lose from 50 to 80 yr of age (3,6). Thus, optimizing bone mineral accrual during the growing years is an essential ingredient for the prevention of osteoporosis later in life (26).

Several excellent reviews have all concluded that appropriate physical activity augments bone development (5,8,70,75). Retrospective human studies clearly indicate that bone responds more favorably to physical activity that were undertaken during childhood and adolescence than during adulthood (5,33). Mechanical loading studies using animal models lend strong support to these human studies (33,97).

Numerous randomized controlled intervention studies have been conducted to investigate the change in bone mass and bone strength in children secondary to an exercise intervention. In general, these studies demonstrate a positive effect of physical activity during growth and development. Interventions were diverse, and activities ranged from moderate- to high-impact exercises performed for 10–40 min, two to three times per week. In all studies of prepubertal and early pubertal children, BMD increased more in the intervention group than in controls at various regions of the proximal femur and/or lumbar spine (15,37,46,72,77,83). Generally, the magnitude of the augmented response over 7–10 mo varied from 1% at the trochanteric region of the proximal femur (77) to ~3% at the femoral neck for a high-impact jumping intervention (37,83). When moderate activity was increased through daily physical education, a positive effect on bone accretion in prepubertal girls was noted (110). In a school-based intervention with a 10-min moderate-impact circuit training three times per week, the benefit doubled if the intervention continued for a second school year (71,73). In these studies, bone mass benefits increased from 2% to approximately 4% at the femoral neck and lumbar spine in both boys and girls. These and other studies suggest that the bone response to loading is optimized in prepubertal and early puberty (14,46,55).

Exercise Prescription for Optimizing Bone Development in Youth

The American College of Sports Medicine (ACSM) position stand on physical activity and bone health (60) states that exercise to optimize bone health in children and adolescents should involve 10–20 min, $3 \ d \cdot wk^{-1}$ of impact activities such as plyometrics, jumping, moderate-intensity resistance training, and participation in sports that involve running and jumping (*e.g.*, soccer and basketball). Since the publication of this position stand, a trial of exercise in youth has further elucidated the appropriate anabolic dose of exercise to strengthen the growing skeleton. A pilot study of a simple jumping intervention, "Bounce at the Bell," showed that 10 jumps, three times per day for more than 8 mo was associated with a significant increase in proximal femur

(+2.3%) and intertrochanteric region (+3.2%) BMD (76). To perform their jumps, children simply stood next to their desk and jumped for <1 min, three times per day when the bell rang. The intervention took <3 min · d^{-1} and required no equipment or special training from teachers. Although more work is needed to confirm these results, these data suggest that interventions can be very simple and short and still be effective at improving bone development. They may be excellent adjunctive exercises to those recommended in the ACSM position stand.

EXERCISE DURING ADULTHOOD: MAINTAINING A STRONG SKELETON

The goal of exercise in adulthood should be to gain bone strength and to offset bone loss that is observed during this time in life. Trials of exercise lasting 8–12 mo in premenopausal women generally show increases in BMD of 1%–3% at loaded sites (usually the spine and hip) compared to controls (35,45,67,104–106). Differences between exercisers and controls in the premenopausal cohorts are attributed to gains in bone mineral of exercisers (10,45), attenuation of bone loss in exercisers, or a combination of bone gain in exercisers and bone loss in controls (35). Trials of exercise in premenopausal women (ages 22–49 yr) have shown favorable outcomes as a result of jogging, strength training, aerobics, and jumping exercises (57).

Of the few studies performed in men, most found positive effects of resistance training on BMD at loaded sites. Menkes et al. (81) showed that 16 wk of resistance training in men (mean age = 59 yr) resulted in a 3.8% increase in femoral neck BMD compared with controls. Similarly, Ryan et al. (99) found that 16 wk of resistance training in men (mean age = 61 yr) resulted in a 2.8% increase in femoral neck BMD compared with controls. Overall, studies in adults indicate that exercise, if done with adequate loading such as resistance and impact training, is effective at attenuating bone loss observed with advancing age (57).

Exercise Prescription to Preserve Bone Health during Adulthood

The ACSM position stand on physical activity and bone health states that exercise to preserve bone health during adulthood should involve 30–60 min · d^{-1} of a combination of moderate-to-high intensity weight-bearing endurance activities (three to five times per week), resistance exercise (two to three times per week), and jumping activities (60). Weight-bearing endurance activities include tennis, stair climbing, and jogging at least intermittently during walking. Activities should involve jumping (*e.g.*, volleyball and basketball) and resistance exercises such as weightlifting. It is recommended that these exercises should target all major muscle groups (60).

EXERCISE FOR THE ELDERLY AND INDIVIDUALS WITH OSTEOPOROSIS

Exercise Testing for Those with Osteoporosis

By itself, a diagnosis of osteoporosis is not a contraindication for a symptom-limited exercise test. When exercise tests to assess cardiorespiratory or muscular fitness are performed in individuals with osteoporosis, the following should be considered:

- Use of cycle ergometry as an alternative to treadmill exercise testing to assess cardiovascular function may be indicated in patients with severe vertebral osteoporosis for whom walking is painful.
- Vertebral compression fractures leading to a loss of height and spinal deformation can compromise ventilatory capacity and result in a forward shift in the center of gravity. The latter may affect balance during treadmill walking.
- Maximal muscle strength testing are contraindicated in patients with severe osteoporosis.

The effects of any of the FDA-approved medications for the specific prevention and treatment of osteoporosis (*e.g.*, calcium, vitamin D, calcitonin, bisphosphonates, fluoride, estrogens, and androgens) on acute or chronic exercise responses have not been extensively studied. However, there is no evidence that any of these agents would affect exercise response during testing with the possible exception of estrogen, which has an acute vasodilator effect and may alter electrocardiographic responses to exercise during an exercise test. This effect has been seen in studies using large doses of estrogen but has not been demonstrated in doses used for the treatment of osteoporosis (2,61).

Osteoporosis can preclude detection of abnormal responses associated with heart diseases during an exercise test because performance may be limited by the symptoms of osteoporosis, thus preventing the individual from achieving an adequate heart rate and blood pressure response necessary for an accurate diagnosis. Severe kyphosis (rounding of the upper spine) is one such example unique to osteoporosis that may limit an exercise test because of an imposed mechanical limitation on respiratory muscle function. Ideally, data from a symptom-limited exercise test is available for the calculation of an exercise target heart rate range using the heart rate reserve method. If a maximal exercise test is contraindicated or cannot be performed, ratings of perceived exertion can be used to guide exercise intensity in this population. However, if the participant is at moderate or high risk for cardiovascular disease, it would be prudent to closely assess the patient for indications of ischemia (*e.g.*, angina) or excessive exercise intensity (*e.g.*, excessive heart rate or blood pressure responses).

Exercise Prescription for Individuals with Osteoporosis

Prior to prescribing exercise for someone with osteoporosis, especially an individual who has recently experienced a fracture, an exercise professional should consult with the client's physician. For patients with debilitating osteoporosis and severe pain or recent joint replacement, exercise program options will be limited. These patients should typically work with a physical therapist or rehabilitation specialist until mobility is improved. There is a high prevalence of back pain in patients with osteoporosis, which is related to limited functional ability (66). Thus, pain management may be an important part of the care for individuals with osteoporosis. A warm pool-based program (*e.g.* hydrotherapy) can improve flexibility and muscle strength and be an important part of an exercise program for these individuals. In light of the rapid and profound effects of immobilization and bed rest on bone loss and the poor prognosis for recovery of bone mineral content after remobilization, even the frailest elderly people should remain as physically active as their health permits to preserve skeletal integrity. If a person cannot tolerate active exercises, functional electrical stimulation may improve vital muscle strength in preparation for active strengthening as pain diminishes (57).

As stated in the ACSM position stand on physical activity and bone health (60), "Exercise programs for elderly women and men should include not only weight-bearing endurance and resistance activities aimed at preserving bone mass but also activities designed to improve balance and prevent falls." However, few well-designed trials have tested the efficacy of such programs. A 20-wk strength, posture, and balance program ("Osteofit") improved dynamic balance in females with osteoporosis (21). In a study of females with a history of spinal fracture, a 10-wk balance, strengthening, stretching, and relaxation program resulted in a significant reduction in pain and use of analgesia and increased quality of life (74). In both men and women with osteoporosis, 12 mo of balance and strength training resulted in improved BMD, balance, and aerobic capacity (62). Although these trials indicate that exercise has beneficial effects on surrogates of osteoporotic fracture, well-designed studies with fracture endpoints are needed to further guide exercise prescription in men and women with osteoporosis.

Contraindicated Exercises for Individuals with Osteoporosis

Several general types of exercise are contraindicated for people with osteoporosis because they can generate large forces on relatively weak bone. Twisting movements (*e.g.*, golf swing), dynamic abdominal exercises (*e.g.*, sit-ups), and excessive trunk flexion should all be avoided because they can all result in vertebral fracture. Individuals with osteoporosis should be taught the correct forms for activities of daily living, such as bending to pick up objects to avoid vertebral fractures. Furthermore, exercises that involve abrupt or explosive loading, or high-impact loading, are contraindicated for people with osteoporosis.

Flexibility Training for Individuals with Osteoporosis

A program to increase flexibility can also benefit patients with osteoporosis because decreased flexibility can cause problems with posture. However, many of the commonly prescribed exercises for increasing flexibility, especially of the hamstring muscles, involve spinal flexion and should be avoided. There is little consensus on the optimal training program for increasing flexibility in individuals with osteoporosis, but slow and controlled movements should be the rule with stretching, and ballistic-type stretching should be avoided.

Aerobic Training for Individuals with Osteoporosis

The primary reasons for prescribing aerobic exercise for those with osteoporosis are to increase aerobic fitness and work capacity, decrease cardiovascular disease risk factors, help maintain bone strength, and improve balance. Aerobic exercise for those with osteoporosis should primarily involve weight-bearing modes of exercise such as walking. For those with more significant osteoporosis-induced pain who cannot tolerate weight-bearing activities, cycling, swimming, or water aerobics are possible alternatives. Aerobic exercise for individuals with osteoporosis should be performed 3–5 d · wk^{-1} at an intensity of 40%–59% of heart rate reserve or peak oxygen consumption ($\dot{V}O_2$). An initial goal of 20–30 min per session is reasonable but may be shorter at the beginning of a program in cases of extreme deconditioning. Orthopedic limitations may slow progress or mandate the use of additional supports such as handrails for walking. Once 20–30 min becomes well tolerated, the duration can slowly be increased in much the same fashion as with healthy populations. If the individual is severely limited by pain, his or her physician should be consulted prior to exercise participation.

Resistance Training in Patients with Osteoporosis

Resistance training offers an option to meet both the bone health and fall prevention criteria on an individual basis. Resistance training requires little skill and has the added advantage of being highly adaptable to changes in both magnitude and strain distribution. In addition, increases in strength and muscle size have been demonstrated after resistance training, even in elderly individuals, which has the added benefit of reducing these patients' risk of falls (20,95).

Improving muscle strength helps to conserve bone and muscle mass and enhance dynamic balance. Resistance training with free weights, machines, calisthenics, or elastic bands is recommended for osteoporotic populations with the loads ideally being directed over the long axis of the bone (axial loading). A resistance exercise prescription for individuals *at risk* for osteoporosis should follow the standard adult recommendations of 2–3 d · wk^{-1}, using 8–12 repetitions at an intensity that causes fatigue but not complete exhaustion (60%–80% of 1-repetition maximum) for two to four sets per exercise using a sufficient number of exercises to involve the major muscle groups (38). Additionally, those *with* osteoporosis should avoid any ballistic or jumping activities that are recommended for those who are at risk. The overall goal for the combination of aerobic and resistance training exercises for individuals with osteoporosis is 30–60 min exercise.

SUMMARY

Many of the risk factors for both osteoporosis and falls can be prevented or at least attenuated by lifestyle modifications. In particular, exercise builds bone strength in youth, helps maintain bone strength in adulthood, and prevents the loss of bone strength in old age. Exercise also increases muscle strength, improves posture and balance, and improves overall coordination, which all help to avoid falls. Therefore, there is a critical role for the exercise professional in preventing osteoporotic fractures, and therefore, helping people maintain a high quality of life.

REFERENCES

1. Abrahamsen B, Eiken P, Eastell R. Cumulative alendronate dose and the long-term absolute risk of subtrochanteric and diaphyseal femur fractures: a register-based national cohort analysis. *J Clin Endocrinol Metab.* 2010;95(12):5258–65.

2. American College of Sports Medicine position stand. Osteoporosis and exercise. *Med Sci Sports Exerc.* 1995;27(4):i–vii.

3. Arlot ME, Sornay-Rendu E, Garnero P, Vey-Marty B, Delmas PD. Apparent pre- and postmenopausal bone loss evaluated by DXA at different skeletal sites in women: the OFELY cohort. *J Bone Miner Res.* 1997;12(4):683–90.

4. Bachrach LK. Assessing bone health in children: who to test and what does it mean? *Pediatr Endocrinol Rev.* 2005;2 Suppl 3:332–6.

5. Bailey DA, Faulkner RA, McKay HA. Growth, physical activity, and bone mineral acquisiton. In: Holloszy JO, American College of Sports Medicine, editors. *Exercise and Sport Sciences Reviews.* Baltimore (MD): Williams & Wilkins; 1996. p. 233–66.

6. Bailey DA, Martin AD, McKay HA, Whiting S, Mirwald R. Calcium accretion in girls and boys during puberty: a longitudinal analysis. *J Bone Miner Res.* 2000;15(11):2245–50.

7. Bailey DA, McKay HA, Mirwald RL, Crocker PR, Faulkner RA. A six-year longitudinal study of the relationship of physical activity to bone mineral accrual in growing children: the university of Saskatchewan bone mineral accrual study. *J Bone Miner Res.* 1999;14(10):1672–9.

8. Barr SI, McKay HA. Nutrition, exercise, and bone status in youth. *Int J Sport Nutr.* 1998;8(2):124–42.

9. Bass E, French DD, Bradham DD, Rubenstein LZ. Risk-adjusted mortality rates of elderly veterans with hip fractures. *Ann Epidemiol.* 2007;17(7):514–9.

10. Bassey EJ, Ramsdale SJ. Increase in femoral bone density in young women following high-impact exercise. *Osteoporos Int.* 1994;4(2):72–5.

11. Beck TJ, Oreskovic TL, Stone KL, et al. Structural adaptation to changing skeletal load in the progression toward hip fragility: the study of osteoporotic fractures. *J Bone Miner Res.* 2001;16(6):1108–19.

12. Bischoff HA, Solomon DH, Dawson-Hughes B, Wang PS, Avorn J. Repeat hip fractures in a population-based sample of Medicare recipients in the US: timing and gender differences [abstract]. *J Bone Miner Res.* 2001;16(Suppl 1):S213.

13. Black DM, Cummings SR, Karpf DB, et al. Randomised trial of effect of alendronate on risk of fracture in women with existing vertebral fractures. Fracture Intervention Trial Research Group. *Lancet.* 1996;348(9041):1535–41.

14. Blimkie CJ, Rice S, Webber CE, Martin J, Levy D, Gordon CL. Effects of resistance training on bone mineral content and density in adolescent females. *Can J Physiol Pharmacol.* 1996;74(9):1025–33.

15. Bradney M, Pearce G, Naughton G, et al. Moderate exercise during growth in prepubertal boys: changes in bone mass, size, volumetric density, and bone strength: a controlled prospective study. *J Bone Miner Res.* 1998;13(12):1814–21.

16. Buchwald H, Oien DM. Metabolic/bariatric surgery Worldwide 2008. *Obes Surg.* 2009;19(12):1605–11.

17. Burge R, Dawson-Hughes B, Solomon DH, Wong JB, King A, Tosteson A. Incidence and economic burden of osteoporosis-related fractures in the United States, 2005–2025. *J Bone Miner Res.* 2007;22(3):465–75.

18. Burger H, de Laet CE, van Daele PL, et al. Risk factors for increased bone loss in an elderly population: the Rotterdam Study. *Am J Epidemiol.* 1998;147(9):871–9.

19. Burr DB. Why bones bend but don't break. *J Musculoskelet Neuronal Interact.* 2011;11(4):270–85.

20. Carter ND, Kannus P, Khan KM. Exercise in the prevention of falls in older people: a systematic literature review examining the rationale and the evidence. *Sports Med.* 2001;31(6):427–38.

21. Carter ND, Khan KM, Petit MA, et al. Results of a 10 week community based strength and balance training programme to reduce fall risk factors: a randomised controlled trial in 65–75 year old women with osteoporosis. *Br J Sports Med.* 2001;35(5):348–51.

22. Chrischilles EA, Dasbach EJ, Rubenstein LM, et al. The effect of alendronate on fracture-related healthcare utilization and costs: the fracture intervention trial. *Osteoporos Int.* 2001;12(8):654–60.

23. Cummings SR, Black DM, Thompson DE, et al. Effect of alendronate on risk of fracture in women with low bone density but without vertebral fractures: results from the Fracture Intervention Trial. *JAMA.* 1998;280(24):2077–82.

24. Cummings SR, Melton LJ. Epidemiology and outcomes of osteoporotic fractures. *Lancet.* 2002;359(9319):1761–7.

25. Currey JD. *Bones: Structure and Mechanics.* Princeton (NJ): Princeton University Press; 2002. 436 p.

26. Daly RM, Petit MA. *Optimizing Bone Mass and Strength: The Role of Physical Activity and Nutrition during Growth.* Basel (Switzerland): Karger; 2007. 162 p.

27. Dawson-Hughes B, Looker AC, Tosteson AN, Johansson H, Kanis JA, Melton LJ,3rd. The potential impact of the National Osteoporosis Foundation guidance on treatment eligibility in the USA: an update in NHANES 2005–2008. *Osteoporos Int.* 2012;23(3):811–20.

28. Delmas PD, Genant HK, Crans GG, et al. Severity of prevalent vertebral fractures and the risk of subsequent vertebral and nonvertebral fractures: results from the MORE trial. *Bone.* 2003;33(4):522–32.

29. Ensrud KE, Ewing SK, Stone KL, et al. Intentional and unintentional weight loss increase bone loss and hip fracture risk in older women. *J Am Geriatr Soc.* 2003;51(12):1740–7.

30. Ensrud KE, Fullman RL, Barrett-Connor E, et al. Voluntary weight reduction in older men increases hip bone loss: the osteoporotic fractures in men study. *J Clin Endocrinol Metab.* 2005;90(4):1998–2004.

31. Faulkner RA, Bailey DA. Osteoporosis: a pediatric concern? *Med Sport Sci.* 2007;51:1–12.

32. Flegal KM, Carroll MD, Ogden CL, Curtin LR. Prevalence and trends in obesity among US adults, 1999–2008. *JAMA.* 2010;303(3):235–41.

33. Forwood MR, Burr DB. Physical activity and bone mass: exercises in futility? *Bone Miner.* 1993;21(2):89–112.

34. Friedlander AH, Jones LJ. The biology, medical management, and podiatric implications of menopause. *J Am Podiatr Med Assoc.* 2002; 92(8):437–43.

35. Friedlander AL, Genant HK, Sadowsky S, Byl NN, Gluer CC. A two-year program of aerobics and weight training enhances bone mineral density of young women. *J Bone Miner Res.* 1995;10(4):574–85.

36. Frost HM. Bone's mechanostat: a 2003 update. *Anat Rec A Discov Mol Cell Evol Biol.* 2003;275(2):1081–101.

37. Fuchs RK, Bauer JJ, Snow CM. Jumping improves hip and lumbar spine bone mass in prepubescent children: a randomized controlled trial. *J Bone Miner Res.* 2001;16(1):148–56.

38. Garber CE, Blissmer B, Deschenes MR, et al. Quantity and quality of exercise for developing and maintaining cardiorespiratory, musculoskeletal, and neuromotor fitness in apparently healthy adults: guidance for prescribing exercise. *Med Sci Sports Exerc.* 2011;43(7):1334–59.

39. Garn SM. *The Earlier Gain and the Later Loss of Cortical Bone, in Nutritional Perspective.* Springfield (IL): Thomas; 1970. 146 p.

40. Gass M, Dawson-Hughes B. Preventing osteoporosis-related fractures: an overview. *Am J Med.* 2006;119(4 Suppl 1):S3–11.

41. Genant HK, Cooper C, Poor G, et al. Interim report and recommendations of the World Health Organization Task-Force for Osteoporosis. *Osteoporos Int.* 1999;10(4):259–64.

42. Geusens P, Autier P, Boonen S, Vanhoof J, Declerck K, Raus J. The relationship among history of falls, osteoporosis, and fractures in postmenopausal women. *Arch Phys Med Rehabil.* 2002;83(7):903–6.

43. Goh SK, Yang KY, Koh JS, et al. Subtrochanteric insufficiency fractures in patients on alendronate therapy: a caution. *J Bone Joint Surg Br.* 2007;89(3):349–53.

44. Goldner WS, O'Dorisio TM, Dillon JS, Mason EE. Severe metabolic bone disease as a long-term complication of obesity surgery. *Obes Surg.* 2002;12(5):685–92.

45. Heinonen A, Kannus P, Sievanen H, et al. Randomised controlled trial of effect of high-impact exercise on selected risk factors for osteoporotic fractures. *Lancet.* 1996;348(9038):1343–7.

46. Heinonen A, Sievanen H, Kannus P, Oja P, Pasanen M, Vuori I. High-impact exercise and bones of growing girls: a 9-month controlled trial. *Osteoporos Int.* 2000;11(12):1010–7.

47. Hughes JM, Petit MA. Biological underpinnings of Frost's mechanostat thresholds: the important role of osteocytes. *J Musculoskelet Neuronal Interact.* 2010; 10(2):128–35.

48. Johnell O. The socioeconomic burden of fractures: today and in the 21st century. *Am J Med.* 1997;103(2A):20S,25S; discussion 25S–6S.

49. Kanis JA. Diagnosis of osteoporosis and assessment of fracture risk. *Lancet.* 2002;359(9321):1929–36.

50. Kanis, JA. WHO Technical Report 66: Assessment of Osteoporosis at the Primary Health Care Level. 2007 [Internet]. Sheffield (United Kingdom): University of Sheffield; [cited 2011 Dec 13]. Available from: http://www.shef.ac.uk/FRAX/pdfs/WHO_Technical_Report.pdf

51. Kanis JA, Gluer CC. An update on the diagnosis and assessment of osteoporosis with densitometry. Committee of Scientific Advisors, International Osteoporosis Foundation. *Osteoporos Int.* 2000;11(3):192–202.

52. Kanis JA, Johnell O, Oden A, Dawson A, De Laet C, Jonsson B. Ten year probabilities of osteoporotic fractures according to BMD and diagnostic thresholds. *Osteoporos Int.* 2001;12(12):989–95.

53. Kanis JA, Johnell O, Oden A, et al. Long-term risk of osteoporotic fracture in Malmo. *Osteoporos Int.* 2000;11(8):669–74.

54. Kannus P. Preventing osteoporosis, falls, and fractures among elderly people. Promotion of lifelong physical activity is essential. *BMJ.* 1999;318(7178):205–6.

55. Kannus P, Haapasalo H, Sankelo M, et al. Effect of starting age of physical activity on bone mass in the dominant arm of tennis and squash players. *Ann Intern Med.* 1995;123(1):27–31.

56. Kazakia GJ, Majumdar S. New imaging technologies in the diagnosis of osteoporosis. *Rev Endocr Metab Disord.* 2006;7(1–2):67–74.

57. Khan K, Mckay H, Kannus P, Bailey D, Wark J, Bennel K. *Physical Activity and Bone Health.* Champaign (IL): Human Kinetics; 2001. 288 p.

58. Khan KM, Liu-Ambrose T, Sran MM, Ashe MC, Donaldson MG, Wark JD. New criteria for female athlete triad syndrome? As osteoporosis is rare, should osteopenia be among the criteria for defining the female athlete triad syndrome? *Br J Sports Med.* 2002;36(1):10–3.

59. Klotzbuecher CM, Ross PD, Landsman PB, Abbott TA,3rd, Berger M. Patients with prior fractures have an increased risk of future fractures: a summary of the literature and statistical synthesis. *J Bone Miner Res.* 2000;15(4):721–39.

60. Kohrt WM, Bloomfield SA, Little KD, Nelson ME, Yingling VR, American College of Sports Medicine. American College of Sports Medicine Position Stand: physical activity and bone health. *Med Sci Sports Exerc.* 2004;36(11):1985–96.

61. Kohrt WM, Ehsani AA, Birge SJ,Jr. HRT preserves increases in bone mineral density and reductions in body fat after a supervised exercise program. *J Appl Physiol.* 1998;84(5):1506–12.

62. Kronhed AC, Moller M. Effects of physical exercise on bone mass, balance skill and aerobic capacity in women and men with low bone mineral density, after one year of training—a prospective study. *Scand J Med Sci Sports.* 1998;8(5 Pt 1):290–8.

63. Labovitz JM, Revill K. Osteoporosis: pathogenesis, new therapies and surgical implications. *Clin Podiatr Med Surg.* 2007;24(2):311–32.

64. Langlois JA, Mussolino ME, Visser M, Looker AC, Harris T, Madans J. Weight loss from maximum body weight among middle-aged and older white women and the risk of hip fracture: the NHANES I epidemiologic follow-up study. *Osteoporos Int.* 2001;12(9):763–8.

65. Lenart BA, Lorich DG, Lane JM. Atypical fractures of the femoral diaphysis in postmenopausal women taking alendronate. *N Engl J Med.* 2008;358(12):1304–6.

66. Liu-Ambrose T, Eng JJ, Khan KM, Mallinson A, Carter ND, McKay HA. The influence of back pain on balance and functional mobility in 65- to 75-year-old women with osteoporosis. *Osteoporos Int.* 2002;13(11):868–73.

67. Lohman T, Going S, Pamenter R, et al. Effects of resistance training on regional and total bone mineral density in premenopausal women: a randomized prospective study. *J Bone Miner Res.* 1995;10(7):1015–24.

68. Lord SR, Sambrook PN, Gilbert C, et al. Postural stability, falls and fractures in the elderly: results from the Dubbo Osteoporosis Epidemiology Study. *Med J Aust.* 1994;160(11):684–5, 688–91.

69. Loucks AB, Verdun M, Heath EM. Low energy availability, not stress of exercise, alters LH pulsatility in exercising women. *J Appl Physiol.* 1998;84(1):37–46.

70. MacKelvie KJ, Khan KM, McKay HA. Is there a critical period for bone response to weight-bearing exercise in children and adolescents? a systematic review. *Br J Sports Med.* 2002;36(4):250–7; discussion 257.

71. Mackelvie KJ, McKay HA, Khan KM, Crocker PR. A school-based exercise intervention augments bone mineral accrual in early pubertal girls. *J Pediatr.* 2001;139(4):501–8.

72. MacKelvie KJ, McKay HA, Petit MA, Moran O, Khan KM. Bone mineral response to a 7-month randomized controlled, school-based jumping intervention in 121 prepubertal boys: associations with ethnicity and body mass index. *J Bone Miner Res.* 2002;17(5):834–44.

73. MacKelvie KJ, Petit MA, Khan KM, Beck TJ, McKay HA. Bone mass and structure are enhanced following a 2-year randomized controlled trial of exercise in prepubertal boys. *Bone.* 2004;34(4):755–64.

74. Malmros B, Mortensen L, Jensen MB, Charles P. Positive effects of physiotherapy on chronic pain and performance in osteoporosis. *Osteoporos Int.* 1998;8(3):215–21.

75. McKay HA, Khan KM. Bone mineral acquisition during childhood and adolescence: physical activity as a preventative measure. In: Henderson JE, Goltzman D, editors. *The Osteoporosis Primer.* Cambridge (NY): Cambridge University Press; 2000. p. 170–184.

76. McKay HA, MacLean L, Petit M, et al. "Bounce at the Bell": a novel program of short bouts of exercise improves proximal femur bone mass in early pubertal children. *Br J Sports Med.* 2005;39(8):521–6.

77. McKay HA, Petit MA, Schutz RW, Prior JC, Barr SI, Khan KM. Augmented trochanteric bone mineral density after modified physical education classes: a randomized school-based exercise intervention study in prepubescent and early pubescent children. *J Pediatr.* 2000;136(2):156–62.

78. Melton LJ,3rd, Atkinson EJ, O'Connor MK, O'Fallon WM, Riggs BL. Bone density and fracture risk in men. *J Bone Miner Res.* 1998;13(12):1915–23.

79. Melton LJ,3rd, Chrischilles EA, Cooper C, Lane AW, Riggs BL. Perspective. How many women have osteoporosis? *J Bone Miner Res.* 1992;7(9):1005–10.

80. Melton LJ, Cooper C. Magnitude and impact of osteoporosis and fractures. In: Marcus R, Feldman D, Kelsey JL, editors. *Osteoporosis.* 2nd ed. San Diego (CA): Academic Press; 2001. p. 557–67.

81. Menkes A, Mazel S, Redmond RA, et al. Strength training increases regional bone mineral density and bone remodeling in middle-aged and older men. *J Appl Physiol.* 1993;74(5):2478–84.

82. Morris CA, Cabral D, Cheng H, et al. Patterns of bone mineral density testing: current guidelines, testing rates, and interventions. *J Gen Intern Med.* 2004;19(7):783–90.

83. Morris FL, Naughton GA, Gibbs JL, Carlson JS, Wark JD. Prospective ten-month exercise intervention in premenarcheal girls: positive effects on bone and lean mass. *J Bone Miner Res.* 1997;12(9):1453–62.

84. Moyad MA. Osteoporosis—part I: Risk factors and screening. *Urol Nurs.* 2002;22(4):276–9.

85. Nagaraja S, Couse TL, Guldberg RE. Trabecular bone microdamage and microstructural stresses under uniaxial compression. *J Biomech.* 2005;38(4):707–16.

86. National Institutes of Health (U.S.), Office for Medical Applications of Research. *Osteoporosis Prevention, Diagnosis, and Therapy: NIH Consensus Statement 17; March 27–29, 2000.* Bethesda (MD): U.S. Dept. of Health and Human Services, National Institutes of Health, Office of Medical Applications of Research; 2000.

87. National Osteoporosis Foundation, American Academy of Orthopaedic Surgeons. *Physician's Guide to Prevention and Treatment of Osteoporosis.* 2nd ed. Washington (DC): National Osteoporosis Foundation; 2003. 38 p.

88. Nguyen ND, Ahlborg HG, Center JR, Eisman JA, Nguyen TV. Residual lifetime risk of fractures in women and men. *J Bone Miner Res.* 2007;22(6):781–8.

89. Odvina CV, Zerwekh JE, Rao DS, Maalouf N, Gottschalk FA, Pak CY. Severely suppressed bone turnover: a potential complication of alendronate therapy. *J Clin Endocrinol Metab.* 2005;90(3):1294–301.

90. Orwig DL, Chiles N, Jones M, Hochberg MC. Osteoporosis in men: update 2011. *Rheum Dis Clin North Am.* 2011;37(3):401–14, vi.

91. Otis CL, Drinkwater B, Johnson M, Loucks A, Wilmore J. American College of Sports Medicine position stand. The Female Athlete Triad. *Med Sci Sports Exerc.* 1997;29(5):i–ix.

92. Parfitt AM. Targeted and nontargeted bone remodeling: relationship to basic multicellular unit origination and progression. *Bone.* 2002;30(1):5–7.

93. Ravn P, Hetland ML, Overgaard K, Christiansen C. Premenopausal and postmenopausal changes in bone mineral density of the proximal femur measured by dual-energy X-ray absorptiometry. *J Bone Miner Res.* 1994;9(12):1975–80.

94. Recker RR. Skeletal fragility and bone quality. *J Musculoskelet Neuronal Interact.* 2007;7(1):54–5.

95. Robertson MC, Campbell AJ, Gardner MM, Devlin N. Preventing injuries in older people by preventing falls: a meta-analysis of individual-level data. *J Am Geriatr Soc.* 2002;50(5):905–11.

96. Robling AG, Burr DB, Turner CH. Recovery periods restore mechanosensitivity to dynamically loaded bone. *J Exp Biol.* 2001;204(Pt 19):3389–99.

97. Robling AG, Castillo AB, Turner CH. Biomechanical and molecular regulation of bone remodeling. *Annu Rev Biomed Eng.* 2006;8: 455–98.

98. Roger VL, Go AS, Lloyd-Jones DM, et al. Heart disease and stroke statistics—2012 update: a report from the American Heart Association. *Circulation.* 2012;125(1):e2–e220.

99. Ryan AS, Treuth MS, Rubin MA, et al. Effects of strength training on bone mineral density: hormonal and bone turnover relationships. *J Appl Physiol.* 1994;77(4):1678–84.

100. Scibora LM, Ikramuddin S, Buchwald H, Petit MA. Examining the link between bariatric surgery, bone mineral density, and osteoporosis: a review of bone density studies. *Obes Surg.* 2012;22(4):654–67.

101. Seeman E. From density to structure: growing up and growing old on the surfaces of bone. *J Bone Miner Res.* 1997;12(4):509–21.

102. Seeman E. Pathogenesis of bone fragility in women and men. *Lancet.* 2002;359(9320):1841–50.

103. Seeman E, Delmas PD. Bone quality—the material and structural basis of bone strength and fragility. *N Engl J Med.* 2006;354(21):2250–61.

104. Sinaki M, Wahner HW, Bergstralh EJ, et al. Three-year controlled, randomized trial of the effect of dose-specified loading and strengthening exercises on bone mineral density of spine and femur in nonathletic, physically active women. *Bone.* 1996;19(3):233–44.

105. Snow-Harter C, Bouxsein ML, Lewis BT, Carter DR, Marcus R. Effects of resistance and endurance exercise on bone mineral status of young women: a randomized exercise intervention trial. *J Bone Miner Res.* 1992;7(7):761–9.

106. Snow-Harter C, Marcus R. Exercise, bone mineral density, and osteoporosis. *Exerc Sport Sci Rev.* 1991;19:351–88.

107. Srinivasan S, Agans SC, King KA, Moy NY, Poliachik SL, Gross TS. Enabling bone formation in the aged skeleton via rest-inserted mechanical loading. *Bone.* 2003;33(6):946–55.

108. Turner CH, Robling AG. Designing exercise regimens to increase bone strength. *Exerc Sport Sci Rev.* 2003;31(1):45–50.

109. U.S. Preventive Services Task Force. Screening for osteoporosis in postmenopausal women: recommendations and rationale. *Ann Intern Med.* 2002;137(6):526–8.

110. Valdimarsson O, Linden C, Johnell O, Gardsell P, Karlsson MK. Daily physical education in the school curriculum in prepubertal girls during 1 year is followed by an increase in bone mineral accrual and bone width—data from the prospective controlled Malmo pediatric osteoporosis prevention study. *Calcif Tissue Int.* 2006;78(2):65–71.

111. Van Staa TP, Leufkens HG, Cooper C. Use of inhaled corticosteroids and risk of fractures. *J Bone Miner Res.* 2001;16(3):581–8.

112. Vanderschueren D, Venken K, Ophoff J, Bouillon R, Boonen S. Clinical review: Sex steroids and the periosteum—reconsidering the roles of androgens and estrogens in periosteal expansion. *J Clin Endocrinol Metab.* 2006;91(2):378–82.

113. Wang Z, Bhattacharyya T. Trends in incidence of subtrochanteric fragility fractures and bisphosphonate use among the US elderly, 1996–2007. *J Bone Miner Res.* 2011;26(3):553–60.

114. Wei TS, Hu CH, Wang SH, Hwang KL. Fall characteristics, functional mobility and bone mineral density as risk factors of hip fracture in the community-dwelling ambulatory elderly. *Osteoporos Int.* 2001;12(12):1050–5.

115. World Health Organization. *Assessment of Fracture Risk and its Application to Screening for Postmenopausal Osteoporosis.* Geneva (Switzerland): World Health Organization; 1994. 129 p.

116. Zioupos P. Accumulation of in-vivo fatigue microdamage and its relation to biomechanical properties in ageing human cortical bone. *J Microsc.* 2001;201(Pt 2):270–8.

SELECTED REFERENCES FOR FURTHER READING

Daly RM, Petit MA, editors. Optimizing bone mass and strength: The role of physical activity and nutrition. Vol 51. Basel (Switzerland): Karger; 2007.

Lord S, Sherrington C, Menz HB, Close J. *Falls in Older People: Risk Factors and Strategies for Prevention.* 2nd ed. Cambridge (NY): Cambridge University Press; 2007. 408 p.

Khan K, McKay HA, Kannus P, Bailey D, Wark J, Bennel K. *Physical Activity and Bone Health.* Champaign (IL): Human Kinetics; 2001. 288 p.

Kohrt WM, Bloomfield SA, Little KD, Nelson ME, Yingling VR; American College of Sports Medicine. American College of Sports Medicine Position Stand: physical activity and bone health. *Med Sci Sports Exerc.* 2004;36(11):1985–96.

Howe TE, Shea B, Dawson LJ, et al. Exercise for preventing and treating osteoporosis in postmenopausal women. *Cochrane Database Syst Rev.* 2011;(7):CD000333.

INTERNET RESOURCES

- Action Schools BC: http://www.actionschoolsbc.ca/Content/Home.asp
- American Academy of Physical Medicine and Rehabilitation: How PM&R Physicians Use Exercise to Prevent and Treat Osteoporosis: http://www.aapmr.org/patients/conditions/rheumatology/Pages/osteotreat.aspx
- American Society of Bone and Mineral Research webcasts: "Bone Quality: What Is It and Can We Measure It?" http://app2.capitalreach.com/esp1204/servlet/tc?cn=asbmr&c=10169&s=20292&e=4521&& "Forum on Aging and Skeletal Health" http://www.asbmr.org/TopicalMeetings/Webcasts.aspx
- American Society of Bone and Mineral Research: Bone Curriculum: http://www.asbmr.org/Education/BoneCurriculum.aspx
- International Osteoporosis Foundation: http://www.iofbonehealth.org/
- Mayo Clinic: Exercising with Osteoporosis: http://www.mayoclinic.com/health/osteoporosis/HQ00643
- National Institutes of Health: Osteoporosis and Related Bone Diseases National Resource Center: http://www.niams.nih.gov/bone/
- National Osteoporosis Foundation: http://www.nof.org/
- Osteofit: http://www.osteofit.org/
- Prevention of Falls Network Earth (ProFaNE): http://www.profane.co/
- U.S. Bone and Joint Decade: http://www.usbjd.org/

Exercise Prescription for Patients with Arthritis

More than 100 arthritic diseases and conditions have been identified, with muscle and/or joint involvement being the commonality. The most common types include osteoarthritis (OA), fibromyalgia, and rheumatoid arthritis (RA). An additional group of arthritic diseases that have special exercise needs fall into a category called spondyloarthropathies, of which the most common is ankylosing spondylitis (AS) (4,116). Between 2007 and 2009, almost 50 million Americans reported having physician-diagnosed arthritis (23). This represents more than 22% of the adult population; past the age of 65 yr, the percentage increases to approximately 50% (23).

The economic, social, and psychological costs of arthritis are significant (1). Arthritis is currently the leading cause of disability in the United States, with 21.1 million (9.4% of the U.S. population) reporting limitations in activity because of their arthritis (*Fig. 43-1*) (23). The report from the U.S. Centers for Disease Control and Prevention (CDC) notes that prevalence is greatest in those who are obese, physically inactive, or non-Hispanic blacks. Within the next few decades, the total number with arthritis is projected to increase to 74 million, with an even larger percentage in the 65-and-older age group than in the current population and an estimated 37% or more will have activity limitations because of arthritis (46,65). The estimated total cost attributable to arthritis, both direct and indirect, was $128 billion in 2003 (22).

There are no current estimates of the frequency of each type of arthritis, but earlier studies give some idea of the potential distribution. Osteoarthritis is the most prevalent form of arthritis, with almost 85% of all those affected having this joint-specific problem. Although the other arthritis forms have lower prevalence, their pathologies are systemic. Thus, the resultant impact on the individual is often significant. Fibromyalgia has an estimated prevalence of 2% of the U.S. population (3.7 million) (77), whereas rheumatoid arthritis is now thought to be <1% (1.3 million persons), which is lower than earlier reports (23,62). Ankylosing spondylitis affects roughly 1% of the U.S. population. Its distribution is atypical of the rheumatic diseases, as it is more prevalent in men than women (4). Other forms of arthritis, such as gout, compose the rest of the arthritic population.

OSTEOARTHRITIS

OA, also known as degenerative joint disease, is joint specific. The joints in the hands have the greatest prevalence of arthritis. The most common weight-bearing joints that are affected are the knees, followed by the hips (31,40,77).

KEY TERMS

COX-1: An enzyme that is necessary for normal physiologic function of the stomach, kidney, and platelets.

COX-2: An enzyme involved in the production of prostaglandin, which produces inflammation and contributes to acute pain.

Cyclo-oxygenase (COX): An enzyme found in two main forms, COX-1 and COX-2.

Cytokines: Small proteins that can either step up or step down the immune response.

Fibromyalgia: A rheumatologic syndrome characterized by chronic widespread pain in the muscles, ligaments, and joints.

Osteoarthritis (OA): A degenerative disease that affects the articular cartilage and the underlying subchondral bone.

Rheumatoid arthritis (RA): An inflammatory disease with the major symptoms of pain, swelling, stiffness, and reduced joint mobility.

Spondyloarthropathy: A rheumatic disease that causes inflammation and calcification of joints, especially present in the spine.

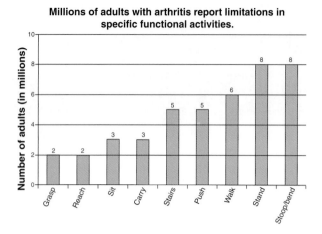

FIGURE 43-1. Specific functional activity limitations for adults with arthritis. (Adapted from the *2002 National Health Interview Survey Arthritis Surveillance Fact Sheet* [Internet]. Atlanta [GA]: U.S. Centers for Disease Control and Prevention; [cited 2012 Oct 2]. Available from: http://www.cdc.gov/arthritis/data_statistics/national_nhis.htm#functional

CLINICAL FEATURES AND DIAGNOSIS

The primary symptom with OA is joint pain and stiffness, usually associated with degeneration of the joint cartilage (*Fig. 43-2*). However, the relationship between radiographic diagnosis of OA and the presence of symptoms is not predictable. Only 25%–50% of people with radiographic evidence of OA have symptoms, whereas others with severe symptoms sometimes have limited medical evidence of OA (1,2,40,77). Thus, diagnosis is based on several different features and can include laboratory and clinical tests, radiographic and clinical results, or purely clinical features. For the knee, the criteria for a clinical diagnosis include age older than 50 yr, stiffness lasting less than 30 min, crepitus (crackling sound), bony tenderness, bony enlargement, and no palpable warmth of the joint (1).

As the joint structure alters, motion becomes limited, and the muscles adjacent to the joint atrophy. Several studies have identified significant weakness in the quadriceps muscles, although it is not known whether this weakness happens before or results from the joint disease (45,67). Another problem which may interact with weakness is knee instability. The complaint associated with this is the sensation of the knee "giving way" and it has been found to be an independent predictor of function (121).

Because of the loss of motion of the joint, muscle atrophy, and instability, physical mobility is decreased. Functional assessment usually reflects difficulties with activities of daily living that require the involved joints. Thus, individuals with arthritis in the upper extremities report problems with lifting, carrying, and dressing, whereas those with lower extremity arthritis have problems with climbing stairs, ambulation, and getting in and out of a chair. Because mobility declines and pain and stiffness increase, loss of independence and quality of life occur (31,40).

ETIOLOGY

The etiology of primary OA has not yet been identified, although numerous factors have been shown to increase the risk of developing OA. Aging used to be considered the cause of OA, however, although it is a risk factor, evidence suggests that aging alone does not cause the changes associated with OA. An examination of other risk factors reveals some of the rationale for proposed etiologies of OA. The most common risk factors include previous injury to the joint, malalignment of the joint, and obesity. Any of these can result in abnormal load distributions in the joint, which alters the accompanying biomechanics. These risk factors have not only been correlated to the development of arthritis, but also to the progression of the disease.

Burr and Radin hypothesize that initial failure to absorb the altered loads results in microcracks in the subchondral tissue and reactivation of the secondary center of ossification (17). These primary changes lead to a cascading cycle that involves thinning of the articular cartilage, leading to increased joint stresses and loads. On radiographs, the progression of arthritis is observed as joint-space narrowing, followed by changes in the subchondral bone and osteophyte (bone spur) formation along the joint line (85). As the cartilage degrades, more stress is transmitted to the underlying bone, resulting in further deformation and decreased shock-absorbing capability (68). Although this proposed etiology of arthritis has yet to be confirmed, others have similarly proposed that an increase of abnormal loads may result in OA (see *Fig. 43-3*). Several studies have found either abnormal external knee adduction or extension moments in individuals with OA (2,89). Furthermore, some have noted an association between altered biomechanics and the severity and progression

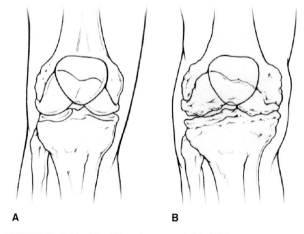

A   **B**

FIGURE 43-2. Healthy **(A)** and osteoarthritic **(B)** knees.

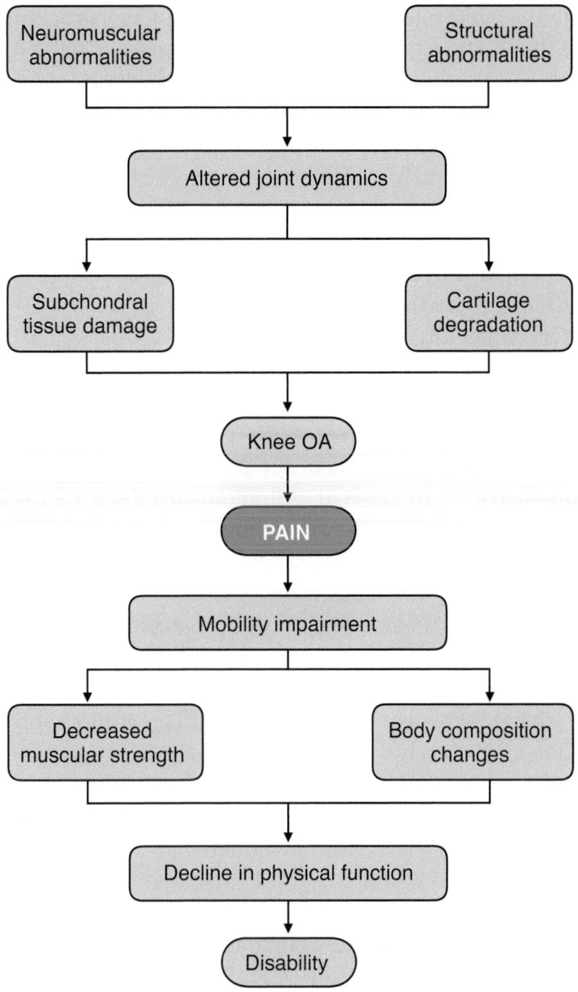
Neuromuscular abnormalities
Structural abnormalities
Altered joint dynamics
Subchondral tissue damage
Cartilage degradation
Knee OA
PAIN
Mobility impairment
Decreased muscular strength
Body composition changes
Decline in physical function
Disability

FIGURE 43-3. Theoretical biomechanical pathways for knee osteoarthritis (OA) and subsequent disability.

of OA (9,89,90,113,126,127). One potential cause of a change in biomechanics and load absorption is injury. A phenomenon that has been identified following injury to the knee is quadriceps activation failure. Individuals with knee OA have been shown to have more quadriceps activation failure than those without OA, regardless of age or sex (67). Fitzgerald et al. suggested that the activation failure moderates the interaction between quadriceps strength and function (45).

Although not necessarily the cause of OA, inflammation is present and appears to be related to progression of the disease. Inflammatory cytokines (interleukin-1 β [IL-1β]) have been found in the joint fluids of patients with OA. Others have found increased serum concentrations of cytokines (interleukin-6 [IL-6], tumor necrosis factor α [TNF-α]) and another inflammatory marker, acute phase reactant C-reactive protein (CRP), in individuals with OA (105,125,129). Several longitudinal studies have shown that elevated serum levels of specific cytokines predicts the progression of knee OA, as determined by radiographic changes in the joint (50,75,106,125,139). Importantly, some of these studies have shown that the level of inflammatory marker in the blood was related to the individual's functional status and severity (both pain and radiographic evidence) of joint disease (106,139). It has been suggested that the cytokines may be one factor affecting cartilage loss observed in OA because the cytokines may stimulate catabolism of the articular cartilage and inhibit chondrocyte formation (108). Another biomarker, which has been related to OA, is serum cartilage oligomeric matrix protein (COMP), which is related to body mass index and age. This marker has been shown to be higher in non–Hispanic Black women as compared to non–Hispanic White women (72).

Although it has been noted that obesity is a risk factor for the development and progression of OA, this relationship has usually been attributed to the increased loads that are transmitted to the lower extremity joints. However, Nicklas et al. note that individuals who are obese have higher concentrations of inflammatory markers than individuals who are not overweight (103). Furthermore, they showed that those who lost weight also had decreases in CRP, IL-6, and TNF-α receptor 1 levels as compared with controls. Thus, inflammation may be an important mediator related to the progression of the disease and function for individuals who are obese (103).

TREATMENTS

Although exercise was initially used to maintain or improve function, many studies have found that it can reduce pain and improve function. The use of supplements has been investigated initially for proposed effects on cartilage and later for potential pain medication. Medical treatment is focused on pain relief, usually through the use of anti-inflammatory medications. When medications are not enough to control pain, orthopedic procedures directed at the joint are used.

Exercise Response

Early studies on individuals with arthritis showed deficits in strength, flexibility, and aerobic capacity as compared with age-matched individuals without arthritis. These deficits are associated with the decreased ability to perform activities of daily living. Much of the difference appears because of a more sedentary lifestyle. Because the joint becomes painful and stiff, the tendency is to decrease activity in an effort not to exacerbate the problem. However, numerous studies have shown that most exercise does not aggravate the symptoms nor increase the progression of the arthritis (38).

The most common aerobic activity that has been used for training is walking. Walking programs ranged from 8 wk to 3 mo, and many of the earlier studies used low-to-moderate intensities. Although the assessment of aerobic capacity varies from study to study, most studies showed improved aerobic capacity and walking time in conjunction with decreases in pain and disability (14,38,75,95). A few studies have looked at jogging from the perspective of impact on the prevalence and progression of arthritis. These studies have shown that jogging neither increases the chances of developing arthritis nor the progression of the disease (15). In fact, longitudinal work has shown that runners with arthritis reported less pain and better function than sedentary individuals with arthritis (15). The use of jogging as a training method for research has been limited to jogging in the water. Although the group that jogged in the water showed improvements in aerobic capacity, endurance, and pain as compared with a control group, the results were mixed when compared with a walking program (95). Cycling has also been used successfully as a training technique in one of the few studies that compared the effect of two different training intensities (84). Patients training for 10 wk at either 40% or 70% of heart rate reserve (HRR) reported decreased pain, which was similar in both groups despite the higher intensity group performing nearly twice as much total work.

Water-based activities have often been promoted for those with arthritis, emphasizing the decreased load on the joints and increased comfort. However, the few studies that have used water-based activities have not focused on aerobic capacity as a measure. In a yearlong study, Cochrane et al. found significant improvement in quality of life measures and physical function for the group that exercised in the water (29).

Resistance training has been examined both as an independent exercise program and in conjunction with aerobic activities. Most programs have focused on lower extremity resistance training and have demonstrated gains in strength and decreased pain. Improvements in strength translate to better function and balance in patients with OA (43,44). Jan et al. (69) compared high-to-low resistance training with individuals with OA. Although both groups demonstrated significant improvements in function and pain, the amount of improvement was consistently greater for the higher resistance group. The authors noted that a few of the subjects were unable tolerate the 80% of one repetition maximum (1-RM) workload, thus reinforcing the need to progress slowly and constantly monitor patient symptoms.

Many studies have combined training modes to have a more traditional exercise program. One study found that strength training resulted in better stair-climbing ability, but the aerobic group reported better quality of life. Importantly, when resistance training was combined with aerobic training, significant improvements in balance, strength, and aerobic capacity — and decreases in disability and pain, as well as body weight — were found (39,91). The Arthritis Foundation developed a program entitled, "People with Arthritis Can Exercise" (PACE), which incorporates education on self-management with a broad-based exercise program (strength, balance,

flexibility, and endurance). After 8 wk of the program, individuals had significant reductions in pain and fatigue, which persisted at a 6-mo follow-up (21). Another combination program that has been established for those with arthritis is the "Fit and Strong!" program (66). Although originally conducted by physical therapists, Seymour et al. (123) showed similar improvements in function and fitness using certified exercise instructors rather than physical therapists, thus decreasing the potential cost to run the program.

A popular alternative form of exercise, particularly with older individuals, is tai chi. A systematic review identified only five studies involving OA and tai chi (58). All showed improvements in pain and self-reported disability, although findings for physical function were inconclusive. Hartman et al. found improved self-efficacy scores for arthritis symptoms following tai chi training (60). Exercise has also been studied for its role in weight control for overweight or obese individuals with arthritis because of the relationship of body weight and arthritis. Although weight loss through diet alone has been shown to improve function (25), there were no noticeable changes in pain with diet alone. The combination of diet and exercise resulted in greater improvements in self-reported function, mobility, and pain than either of those interventions alone or a health education intervention (91,92). The authors noted that subjects who lost between 7.5% and 11.0% of their body weight had significantly better self-reported function than subjects who lost less weight or no weight at all, with an apparent dose-related response.

Exercise Prescription

Although management guidelines for OA of the knee and hip recommend exercise therapy, the specifics — such as frequency, intensity, and mode — have not been addressed. Unfortunately, there is a wide variety in the programs that have been studied. The most common frequency is 3 d · wk^{-1} with 1-h sessions. However, there is no evidence to suggest that individuals with arthritis cannot follow the recommendations for 5 d · wk^{-1} of moderate-intensity aerobic activity. Until recently, the emphasis was on mild intensity, as many feared that higher intensities would exacerbate symptoms. However, several studies have used intensity guidelines defined by the American College of Sports Medicine (ACSM) without detrimental effects (14,39,93,95). As with any patient, the exercise prescription must consider the individual's current level of activity. According to ACSM guidelines, moderate-intensity activity (40%–59% HRR) is appropriate for individuals with arthritis; lower levels (30%–40% HRR) are appropriate for individuals who are deconditioned. Additionally, some researchers have noted that the use of initial durations of 10 min, with several sessions per day, has been shown to improve initial adherence for patients with lower extremity arthritis (95). Progression of intensity and duration should follow ACSM guidelines, with the goal of 30 or more minutes of continuous exercise of moderate intensity.

Resistance training has been shown to be an important component of a training program for those with arthritis (38,93). Resistance training regimens that have been used range from body weight activities, such as partial squats, to the use of specialized equipment (39,69,93). Resistance training should meet the general ACSM guidelines of 2–3 d · wk^{-1}, training multiple muscle groups. Initial intensity may need to be low (10% 1-RM) for individuals with severe arthritis, but loads of 40%–80% of 1-RM, or the 10–15 RM, are otherwise appropriate. Tolerance of load may be related to severity of arthritis, and thus should be monitored. It may be necessary to modify the activity to accommodate reductions in range of motion (ROM) because of the arthritis. Finally, individuals with arthritis often note times of increased joint pain and stiffness, sometimes accompanied by swelling. During these flare-ups, it may be wisest to decrease the intensity of the exercise program.

The third traditional component of an exercise program, flexibility, is a vital part of arthritis treatment. Flexibility and ROM activities address the stiffness and loss of motion that is a primary result of arthritis. Although there is no research on the optimal number of days per week, clinical reports suggest that daily ROM activities are best, which is consistent with the latest ACSM recommendations for arthritis. Movement through the normal, available range, repeated 5–10 times, appears to decrease symptoms of stiffness and may be repeated throughout the day as needed.

Pharmacologic Treatment

The American College of Rheumatology recommends acetaminophen for patients with mild-to-moderate pain (64). Side effects of acetaminophen include the potential for upper gastrointestinal bleeding and liver damage. Anti-inflammatory medications have also become increasingly popular as an initial therapy for OA. The most common of these medications are the nonsteroidal anti-inflammatory drugs (NSAIDs). NSAIDs include aspirin, ibuprofen, and naproxen. They exert anti-inflammatory and usually analgesic actions through their inhibition of the enzyme cyclo-oxygenase (COX), which has two main forms, COX-1 and COX-2. Side effects include an increased chance of gastrointestinal bleeding. COX-2 selective inhibitors (celecoxib; sold as Celebrex or Celebra) decrease the risk of gastrointestinal side effects; however, some have been associated with increased risk of cardiovascular events (*e.g.*, myocardial infarction) (110). Because of some of the rarer but serious side effects, it has been suggested that individuals should be continually monitored for signs of renal toxicity, hypertension, and limb edema (18,122).

Interestingly, although acetaminophen and selective and nonselective NSAIDs are commonly considered the first line of defense for mild-to-moderate OA, Fraenkel et al. (47) reported that many patients with symptomatic knee OA preferred a topical pain medication (capsaicin) because of its negligible side effects. Hence, patients were willing to accept a less effective treatment in exchange for a much lower risk of side effects.

The dietary supplements glucosamine and chondroitin, separately and in combination, have gained widespread use for the treatment of OA. Glucosamine is thought to promote proteoglycan and glycosaminoglycan synthesis, important components of cartilage. Chondroitin is responsible, with collagen and noncollagenous glycoproteins, for giving cartilage its resiliency and inhibiting synovial degradative enzymes (30,80).

Previous clinical trials that compared glucosamine with a placebo suggest that it is moderately effective in reducing pain or improving function for those with hip or knee OA (61,86,87). McAlindon et al. (87) noted in their meta-analysis that many of these studies suffer from methodological problems, but overall, it seems probable that glucosamine and chondroitin have some efficacy in treating the symptoms of OA with few reported side effects (61,87).

Studies of combination therapy of glucosamine and chondroitin have shown reductions in pain in adults with OA, although each study has used supplements in addition to glucosamine and chondroitin (30,111,117,124). Two studies of patients with knee OA found combination therapy along with manganese ascorbate was effective in reducing pain after 4 and 6 mo, respectively (47,78). As with many nonsurgical treatments of OA, the best results occur in patients with mild-to-moderate disease (87). Fish oil has been investigated with patients with RA and found to relieve pain; however, this has not been addressed with the OA population.

Invasive/Surgical Treatment

When noninvasive treatments of knee OA fail to relieve pain and improve function, several surgical treatment options may be considered. Injections of viscosupplementation, specifically hyaluronic acid, have been shown to relieve pain in the knee (116). Although the use of injections into the knee has been approved by the U.S. Food and Drug Administration (FDA), it has not yet been approved for injection into the hip joint, although there is research to suggest that it can effectively decrease pain there as well.

Several surgical methods involve arthroscopic surgery that usually involves a method to "clean out" the joint. Débridement is a method to trim torn and damaged cartilage and may be combined with joint lavage, or "washing" of the joint. Joint lavage may also be performed alone. Lavage and débridement are the most common surgical procedures for mild-to-moderate knee OA, accounting for approximately 650,000 procedures (107). The success of these procedures varies, but approximately 50% of the patients report pain relief from either procedure (98). A randomized, controlled trial comparing arthroscopic débridement with lavage found no difference in clinical, functional, patient overall well-being, and blinded physician global outcomes between the groups. After 1 yr, 44% of the patients who underwent surgery reported improvements in their global assessment versus 58% for the lavage group (24). A randomized, placebo-controlled trial to determine the efficacy of arthroscopic lavage and débridement using a simulated arthroscopic débridement procedure as a placebo surgery found no difference in pain or function between the lavage, débridement, and placebo surgery groups (98).

The second category of surgical procedures commonly used in patients with OA is total knee replacement or arthroplasty. Total knee replacement is most commonly performed in knees with severe OA. The most common age range for total knee replacement is 60–75 yr. Patients younger than 55 yr will increase the stress placed on a total knee replacement, increasing the likelihood of a second procedure. Hence, younger patients are usually considered for alternative procedures, such as unicompartmental knee replacement (partial knee replacement) or osteotomy to improve alignment. Total knee replacement is a safe and effective treatment for end-stage knee OA. The mortality rate is 0.5%, and improvements in pain, function, and health-related quality of life appear rapid and substantial in 90% of the patients (104).

FIBROMYALGIA

Similar to other rheumatologic conditions, fibromyalgia afflicts women more often than men; roughly 80%–90% of individuals with fibromyalgia are women. Fibromyalgia affects about 3.4% of women and 0.5% of men (140).

CLINICAL FEATURES AND DIAGNOSIS

Fibromyalgia is a rheumatologic syndrome characterized by chronic widespread pain in muscles, ligaments, and joints, as well as a heightened tenderness at discrete anatomic locations called *tender points* (Fig. 43-4) (28,141). Historically, fibromyalgia is a diagnosis of exclusion that is reached by the process of elimination. Specifically, fibromyalgia is diagnosed when the subject experiences widespread chronic pain in the absence of other identifiable pathology. Individuals with fibromyalgia have a decreased pain threshold (allodynia) during digital palpation or dolorimetry at these tender points. Besides chronic pain and tender points, individuals with fibromyalgia frequently have additional symptoms, including sleep disturbance, chronic fatigue, psychological distress, morning stiffness, and irritable bowel syndrome (140).

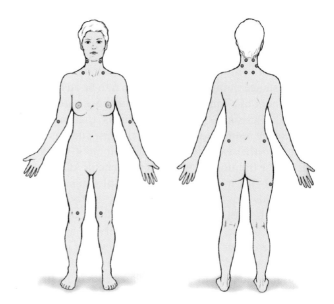

FIGURE 43-4. Tender points for the diagnosis of fibromyalgia. •, tender points.

The American College of Rheumatology (ACR) 1990 Criteria for the Classification of Fibromyalgia (*Table 43-1*) continues to serve as the primary guidelines for the diagnosis of fibromyalgia (141). The main criteria are widespread pain for at least 3 mo, bilateral pain, and pain on palpation with a force of 39 N (*i.e.*, equivalent to 4 kg) at 11 or more of 18 tender-point sites (112,141).

Although the ACR criteria serve as the main diagnostic guidelines, they have received numerous criticisms. Criticisms include heterogeneity of pain attributes, problems with consistency of diagnosis, and the actual validity of tender-points assessment (28). The current definition of fibromyalgia is thought to capture only 20% of individuals with chronic widespread pain.

ETIOLOGY

No definite causal mechanism for fibromyalgia has been identified, but many hypotheses exist. Most of these hypotheses focus on the abnormal levels of nociceptive hormones and neurotransmitters in subjects with fibromyalgia. Particular attention has been paid to the function of the hypothalamic-pituitary-adrenal axis and its associated chemical pain mediators, which include (among others) cortisol, growth hormone, insulin-like growth factor-1, substance P, and serotonin (33). Additionally, genetics and environmental factors (*e.g.*, muscle trauma; certain infections, such as hepatitis C, Lyme disease, Epstein-Barr virus) are possible mechanisms in the development of fibromyalgia (28).

Glucocorticoid deficiency may result in pain, and individuals with fibromyalgia exhibit moderate basal hypocortisolism (16,33). It remains unclear, however, whether low cortisol levels represent a cause or effect of

TABLE 43-1. American College of Rheumatology 1990 Criteria for Fibromyalgia

Criterion	Definition
1. History of widespread pain	Pain is considered widespread when all of the following are present: pain in the left side of the body, pain in the right side of the body, pain above the waist, and pain below the waist. In addition, axial skeletal pain (cervical spine or anterior chest or thoracic spine or low back) must be present. In this definition, shoulder and buttock pain is considered as pain for each involved side. "Low back" pain is considered lower segment pain.
2. Pain in 11 of 18 tender-point sites on digital palpation (Fig. 43-4)	Pain on digital palpation must be present in at least 11 of the following 18 tender-point sites: • Occiput: Bilateral, at the suboccipital muscle insertions • Low cervical: Bilateral, at the anterior aspects of the intertransverse spaces at C5–C7 • Trapezius: Bilateral, at the midpoint of the upper border • Supraspinatus: Bilateral, at origins above the scapula spine near the medial border • Second rib: Bilateral, at the second costochondral junctions, just lateral to the junctions on upper surfaces • Lateral epicondyle: Bilateral, 2 cm distal to the epicondyles • Gluteal: Bilateral, in upper outer quadrants of the buttocks in the anterior folds of muscle • Greater trochanter: Bilateral, posterior to the trochanteric prominence • Knee: Bilateral, at the medial fat pad proximal to the joint line Digital palpation should be performed with an approximate "force" of 4 kg. For a tender point to be considered "positive," the subject must state that palpation was painful. "Tender" is not to be considered "painful."

Reprinted with permission from Wolfe F, Smythe HA, Yunus MB, et al. The American College of Rheumatology 1990 criteria for the classification of fibromyalgia. *Arthritis Rheum.* 1990;33:160–172.

chronic pain. Moreover, low levels of growth hormone in patients with fibromyalgia could be related to sleep disturbances. Growth hormone is secreted primarily during stages 3 and 4 of non–rapid eye movement (REM) sleep (10), and patients with fibromyalgia exhibit an abnormal sleep pattern, particularly for stages 3 and 4 (96).

Substance P is a peptide that may be important in the neurotransmission of pain. Numerous studies have shown twofold to threefold average increases in substance P in the cerebrospinal fluid of subjects with fibromyalgia (12,81,119,134,137). Moreover, a prospective study showed that increases in medication-free substance P concentration were directly related to increased levels of pain and tenderness in patients with fibromyalgia (119). Finally, recent studies have shown a probable reason for the efficacy of antidepressants in the treatment of fibromyalgia. A study of the effects of tricyclic antidepressants (TCAs) on rats showed a downregulation of substance P in the limbic system (128). In a study of human subjects, the antidepressant St. John's wort showed a dose-dependent decrease in substance P (42).

Patients with fibromyalgia have abnormalities in collagen metabolism that are related to increased inflammation. More specifically, Salemi et al. (120) found that abnormalities in collagen metabolism were correlated with increased levels of IL-1β, IL-6, and TNF-α in roughly one-third of patients with fibromyalgia. These data suggest that there is a connection between collagen abnormalities and pain-inducing inflammation in a subset of the fibromyalgia population, which may help explain why some fibromyalgia sufferers experience pain relief from NSAIDs.

TREATMENTS

There is currently no cure for fibromyalgia. Treatment is focused on the management of pain and associated symptoms using nonpharmacologic and pharmacologic therapies separately or in combination (115).

Exercise Response

Exercise therapy is the most common treatment, although much debate still exists regarding the optimal frequency, duration, and intensity of exercise therapy in individuals with fibromyalgia (27). The most effective treatment is a combination exercise along with cognitive behavioral therapy and education carried out by an interdisciplinary team that includes physicians, nurses, clinical exercise specialists, occupational therapists, psychologists, and others.

Short-term aerobic exercise interventions are generally successful in improving function and pain in patients with fibromyalgia. Richards and Scott (118) examined the effects of a 3-mo, 2 d · wk^{-1} aerobic exercise intervention in 136 patients and found significant improvements in self-reported global assessment of well-being compared with a flexibility and relaxation attention control group. Tender-point count was not significantly different at the end of the intervention period; however, a 1-yr follow-up revealed improved pain levels in the aerobic group. Compliance for both groups was low, with only 53% of the participants attending at least one-third of the sessions. Fatigue, pain, and Medical Outcomes Study Questionnaire Short Form (SF-36) scores did not differ between the groups.

Gowans et al. (51,52) randomized 51 patients with fibromyalgia to either a 23-wk aerobic exercise program or a control group and found the exercise group significantly improved mood, 6-min walk distance, and self-efficacy relative to the control group. A meta-analysis of 16 randomized clinical trials that compared various forms of aerobic exercise with control groups found a significant treatment effect with improvements in aerobic performance, tender-point pain threshold, and pain (19,20). A similar systematic review looked at multiple interventions and concluded that definitive evidence exists only for the benefits of aerobic exercise (19). It has been speculated that exercise in the water may reduce pain, thus promoting better adherence to a program. Assis et al. (7) compared deep-water running with land-based exercise and found similar improvements in aerobic measures and depression scores, with fewer reports of pain during the activity.

Strength training may attenuate the accelerated decline in physical function common in patients with fibromyalgia. Jones et al. (70) enrolled 68 women with fibromyalgia into either a 12-wk strength training or a flexibility program. Following training, there were no significant differences between the groups in isokinetic strength, number of tender points, pain, fatigue, sleep, depression, anxiety, or quality of life. In contrast, Hakkinen et al. (55) found significant increases in leg strength in patients with fibromyalgia randomized to a progressive strength training group versus a control group. The trained patients also reported significant decreases in fatigue and depression. The authors concluded that strength training is a safe and effective intervention for patients with fibromyalgia.

Taken together, it appears that aerobic — and to a lesser extent, resistance training — results in short-term improvements in function, mood, self-efficacy, and pain in patients with fibromyalgia. Future investigations need to examine the long-term benefits of aerobic and resistance training in these patients.

Exercise Prescription

The most fundamental rule for recommending exercise for patients with fibromyalgia is to individualize the prescription. Exercise prescription should ideally begin with a detailed assessment that includes both the individual's fitness level and pain and then follows a progression so that severe pain from overexertion is avoided at all times. Many of the exercise clinical trials that reported low adherence indicated that the intervention exacerbated patients' pain. Newcomb et al. (102) found that women with fibromyalgia preferred to exercise at a lower intensity than suggested by exercise guidelines, even though pain was not exacerbated with the higher intensity. The women in their study preferred cycling at approximately 45% of their maximal heart rate. Dawson and Tiidus (32)

suggest beginning at one to two times per week, with a goal of 3–4 d · wk^{-1}. They reported that a training heart rate of <75% of maximum seems to be tolerated more readily, along with shorter durations (10–30 min). Noting that only a limited amount of research has been done with fibromyalgia patients, the ACSM recommends that the frequency of aerobic training should begin at 2–3 d · wk^{-1} and progress to 3–4 d · wk^{-1}; the intensity should begin at 30% of volume of oxygen consumed per unit of time ($\dot{V}O_2$) reserve or HRR and progress to 59% of $\dot{V}O_2$R or HRR; and the duration should begin with 30 min obtained in 10-min increments and progress to 60 min · d^{-1}. Walking and running have been successfully used in several studies, although some have suggested that exercise in the water might not only provide the appropriate cardiovascular stimulus but also result in better compliance (7). Similar to recommendations for other systemic arthropathies, exercise duration may need to be decreased during flare-ups.

Again noting a lack of sufficient research, the ACSM recommends the following resistance training for those with fibromyalgia: a frequency of 2–3 d · wk^{-1}; an intensity of 50%–80% of the 1-RM, provided this does not cause pain; performing three to five repetitions per exercise for strength or 10–20 repetitions for muscular endurance. Up to two to three sets for strength are completed, followed by a 15- to 20-min rest period and then up to two to three sets for muscular endurance.

Pharmacologic Treatment

Antidepressants are a common pharmacologic treatment for fibromyalgia. The most popular include TCAs, selective serotonin reuptake inhibitors, and dual reuptake inhibitors. This class of antidepressants increases neurotransmission and has a positive analgesic effect. TCAs improve sleep, pain, and fatigue, but their effect on mood is less definitive (115). Selective serotonin reuptake inhibitors have proven effective for major depressive disorders, but their effectiveness for patients with fibromyalgia has been inconsistent and appears less than TCAs (6,94,142). Dual reuptake inhibitors are similar pharmacologically to TCAs but have a better analgesic effect and diminished side effects (37).

NSAIDs have also been used to treat fibromyalgia. Goldenberg et al. (49) compared naproxen, amitriptyline (a TCA), and the combination of naproxen and amitriptyline with a placebo in patients with fibromyalgia. The authors found no significant effect of naproxen; however, amitriptyline was significantly better than the placebo on all outcomes, including pain, sleep difficulties, fatigue, and tender-point scores. Several other trials have also failed to find significant improvements in pain using NSAIDs in the treatment of fibromyalgia (76,94). Hence, it appears that NSAIDs are of limited use in the treatment of fibromyalgia.

RHEUMATOID ARTHRITIS

There is a twofold to threefold greater mortality among patients with RA than in the general population. Especially significant is the increased risk of coronary artery disease as compared with age-matched controls (26). This increased risk has been recognized with the recommendation of guidelines related to cardiovascular risk management for individuals with inflammatory arthritis in which it is suggested that cardiovascular risk scores be modified to reflect the presence of inflammatory disease (109). Recently, evidence suggests that the mortality is lower in those that are taking specific medications, although still not equal to age-related cohorts (101). The number of new cases of RA that occur in a population each year has decreased during the past few decades, with a reduction in the prevalence from 61.2 per 100,000 persons (1955–1964) to 32.7 per 100,000 persons (1985–1994) (36,133). More recent findings suggest that this number has decreased even further (62).

CLINICAL FEATURES AND DIAGNOSIS

RA is an inflammatory disease, associated with autoimmune dysfunction, which attacks the joint capsule. The resultant major symptoms are pain, swelling, stiffness, and reduced joint mobility. Inflammatory periods are characterized by an abnormal increase in the cells of the synovial membrane, a thickening of this membrane, and a further increase in joint swelling. As the disease progresses, cartilage and bone that participate in joint articulations are degraded. In severe cases, the bones fuse together, resulting in further loss of function and increased pain and deformity (*Fig. 43-5*).

Diagnosis is based on a combination of at least four signs and symptoms (*Table 43-2*) (5). The rheumatoid

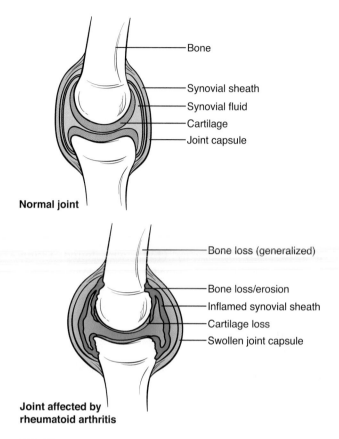

FIGURE 43-5. Normal and rheumatoid arthritic joints. (Adapted from the *Handout on Health: Rheumatoid Arthritis* [Internet]. Bethesda [MD]: National Institutes of Health. Available from: http://www.niams.nih.gov/Health_Info/Rheumatic_Disease/default.asp

factor (RF) is a blood test used to diagnosis RA, although a positive RF test result can also indicate the presence of other diseases, such as Sjögren syndrome, systemic lupus, and systemic sclerosis (63). Approximately 80% of patients with RA have a positive RF test result.

TABLE 43-2. Revised 1987 American Rheumatism Association Criteria for Rheumatoid Arthritis

Criterion[a]	Definition
1. Morning stiffness	Morning stiffness in and around the joints, lasting at least 1 hour before maximal improvement
2. Arthritis of 3 or more joint areas	Swelling of at least 3 joint areas for at least 6 weeks. The 14 possible areas are right or left PIP, MCP, wrist, elbow, knee, ankle, and MTP joints.
3. Arthritis of hand joints	Swelling of the wrist, MCP, or PIP joint for at least 6 weeks
4. Symmetrical arthritis	Simultaneous involvement of the same joint areas (as defined in #2) on both sides of the body (bilateral involvement of PIPs, MCPs, or MTPs is acceptable without absolute symmetry)
5. Rheumatoid nodules	Subcutaneous nodules over bony prominences or extensor surfaces or in juxta-articular regions
6. Serum rheumatoid factor	Abnormal level of serum rheumatoid factor as detected by a method that is positive in <5% of normal control subjects
7. Radiographic changes	Radiographic changes typical of rheumatoid arthritis on posteroanterior hand and wrist radiographs, which must include erosions or unequivocal bony decalcification localized in or most marked adjacent to the involved joints

MCP, metacarpophalangeal; MTP, metatarsophalangeal; PIP, proximal interphalangeal.

[a]At least four criteria must be fulfilled for classification as rheumatoid arthritis.

Reprinted with permission from Arnett FC, Edworthy SM, Bloch DA, et al. The American Rheumatism Association 1987 revised criteria for the classification of rheumatoid arthritis. *Arthritis Rheum.* 1988;31:315–324.

Chronic inflammatory diseases such as RA cause premature aging (132). Diseases that take decades to advance during normal aging — such as atherosclerosis, osteoporosis, muscle wasting, and sleep disorders — change dramatically within a few months in those with RA. Women are affected two to three times more often than men, with the peak incidence occurring between the sixth and seventh decades of life (36).

ETIOLOGY

The development of RA has both genetic and environmental (i.e., nongenetic) determinants. The genetic contribution is estimated at 60% (59,82). Studies that have advanced our understanding of RA genetics include a 1978 study by Stastny (130), who found a link between the human leukocyte antigen system (specifically HLA-DR4) and RA and Gregersen et al. (53) in 1987, who advanced the case for a genetic link by finding a one-in-six chance of developing a higher risk in individuals who are homozygous for a polymorphism of the HLA gene (*HLA-DRB*0408*).

Environmental, or nongenetic, factors linked to the occurrence of RA include age, hormonal factors, infection, smoking, and obesity (73). More specifically, the incidence of RA increases with age, is rare in women before menarche, has declined in women with the increased use of oral contraception, is widely believed to be linked to some type of infection, and is higher in smokers and in individuals with a body mass index of $30 \text{ kg} \cdot \text{m}^{-2}$ or higher. After the onset of RA, the severity of the disease is related to the DR4 alleles, which are alternative forms of the HLA gene; onset after the age of 60 yr; being female; and smoking, which initially decreases pain but ultimately increases the risk for lung and blood vessel involvement (133).

TREATMENTS

Various treatment options for RA, including exercise, medications, and surgery, will be described.

Exercise Response

Patients with RA have reduced muscle strength and compromised joint ROM that decreases mobility and increases pain (54). Initially, the primary concern regarding exercise in patients with RA was that it would exacerbate the chronic inflammation associated with the disease (114). However, numerous studies have demonstrated that exercise does not increase symptoms or physiologic indicators of the disease (71). Furthermore, some of the more recent studies have shown that vigorous, high-intensity workloads result in better fitness gains while still not exacerbating symptoms (100).

Long-term dynamic strength training has a positive effect on muscle strength, self-reported physical function, and physical performance in women with RA (56,114). As little as 1.4 exercise sessions per week for 24 mo provided these positive effects without exacerbating disease activity, as evidenced by inflammatory biomarkers or joint degradation. Importantly, these more recent studies have used workloads that are similar to ACSM guidelines (50%–70% of 1-RM, 10–15 repetitions, three to four sets) (56). Long-term follow-up in a similar study of those who participated in a strength-training program showed continued benefits after 5 yr (57). One study progressed the training group up to 80% of 1-RM, with no adverse events or increase in disease activity. They found significant changes in strength and function as compared to a home exercise group (79).

Aerobic exercise also appears to have a positive effect. A meta-analysis of aerobic training programs found positive effects on quality of life and pain, with a possible associated sparing of the joint. The authors noted that these findings were consistent with mild-to-moderate arthritis, or shorter disease duration, but these improvements were not evident in longer duration or severe arthritis (8). A 12-mo aerobic weight-bearing exercise program significantly improved self-reported function and activity level, and bone mineral density and disease activity remained unchanged (138). One of the few studies to examine the question of intensity used both biking and resistance training. Although the conservative exercise program used isometric exercises with no resistance, the other group did both isometric and isokinetic training using 70% maximal voluntary contractions and biked at 60% of maximal heart rate. The authors found that those participating in the more intense program had fewer swollen joints, less pain, and lower biomarkers with better joint mobility at both 12 and 24 wk (135). In a study that focused on exercise adherence to an intensive program, the authors not only found an adherence rate of 81% after 2 yr but also showed that high adherence was associated with lower disease activity and pain scores (99). Relevant to assessment, one study compared the 6-min walk test to submaximal cycling for exercise testing and found that heart rate and rating of perceived exertion were higher with the cycling test. The authors suggested that the cycling test might be better with individuals with RA, even though they noted that several participants could not complete the cycle test secondary to pain (74).

Exercise Prescription

Although exercise — including joint ROM, resistance exercise, and aerobic conditioning — is recommended for management of RA, specific guidelines regarding type, frequency, and intensity of exercise have not been addressed (3). However, an analysis of 15 randomized clinical trials suggests that aerobic exercises (e.g., walking, aquatics, bicycling) performed three times per week for 30–60 min per session at an intensity of 60%–85% of maximum heart rate successfully improve aerobic capacity and muscle strength. Furthermore, resistance training (*e.g.*, use of weight machines, dumbbells, elastic bands) performed two to three times weekly at 50%–80% of maximal voluntary contraction improves strength and does not have a detrimental effect on pain (131).

Similar to the recommendations for exercise prescription for those with OA, initial intensities should be modified based on previous activity and current joint pain. Joint ROM may be limited and should be considered in activity selection. Flare-ups are more common with RA, thus necessitating the ability to modify the program based on changes in the disease activity. Furthermore, several authors have noted the importance of incorporating behavioral education to improve self-efficacy and self-management arthritis (11,13,34,83).

Pharmacologic Treatment

A mainstay of the treatment of RA is pharmacologic therapy (3,136). Pharmacologic therapy for the treatment of RA includes NSAIDs, disease-modifying antirheumatic drugs (DMARDs), glucocorticoids (steroids), and biologic therapies. NSAIDs reduce swelling, pain, and inflammation, but have some serious side effects, including stomach bleeding and ulcers (management guidelines note a twofold risk for complications as compared with an individual with OA). DMARDs include injectable or oral gold, hydroxychloroquine, penicillamine, sulfasalazine, methotrexate, azathioprine, cyclosporine, and leflunomide. This classification of drugs also works to suppress the immune system and is thought to slow the progression of the disease and reduce cartilage degradation. As noted earlier, not only does this class of medications have a positive effect on the disease itself but has also been linked to a decreased mortality, specifically from cardiovascular disease (101). Possible side effects include liver and kidney damage. Glucocorticoids (steroids), such as prednisone, methylprednisolone, cortisone, and hydrocortisone, reduce inflammation and suppress the immune response. The most serious side effect is the increased risk of infection. Biologic therapies work to suppress joint inflammation that is thought to play a role in cartilage degradation by blocking the action of certain cytokines, specifically, TNF (97). *Table 43-3* lists the general categories of drugs used in the treatment of RA.

Surgical Treatment

Age, disease severity, degree of disability, and the combination of involved joints are important considerations in the timing of orthopedic interventions. Less definitive orthopedic procedures include synovectomy (excision of inflamed synovial tissue), tendon realignment,

TABLE 43-3. Medications Used in the Treatment of Rheumatoid Arthritis

Category	Examples (Trade Names)
NSAIDs	Aspirin Ibuprofen (Advil, Motrin IB) Ketoprofen (Orudis) Naproxen (Naprosyn) Celecoxib (Celebrex)
DMARDs	Gold, injectable or oral Antimalarials (Plaquenil) Penicillamine (Cuprimine, Depen) Sulfasalazine (Azulfidine) Methotrexate (Rheumatrex) Azathioprine (Imuran) Cyclosporine (Sandimmune, Neoral) Leflunomide (Arava)
Glucocorticoids (steroids)	Prednisone (Deltasone, Orasone) Methylprednisolone (Medrol)
Biologic therapy	Etanercept (Enbrel)

NSAIDs, nonsteroidal anti-inflammatory drugs; DMARDs, disease-modifying antirheumatic drugs.

and arthroscopic débridement. These procedures can improve alignment, reduce synovial tissue, control pain, provide stability, and improve function in some patients with RA. These techniques can also prolong periods of good function and delay the need for joint replacement procedures (48). After all other options have been exhausted, joint replacement results in vastly improved function and reduced pain (88).

ADDITIONAL FACTORS

It is important to recognize that there are some other factors that should be considered when prescribing exercise for an individual with arthritis. As OA or RA progresses, joint stability is often compromised. Modifications may be necessary to the activity, such as using a machine versus free weights or modifying a position. For example, increasing seat height and decreasing pedal load reduces joint pain with cycling. With severe joint instability, a brace may be necessary. Improper joint alignment (*e.g.*, excessive knee varus) has been shown to negatively affect progression of the disease and may also warrant activity modification or joint protection. Balance and proprioception have also been shown to be compromised with lower extremity arthritis, and incorporation of balance and kinesthetic activities into a training program has resulted in even greater improvements in some activities, such as stair climbing (35). Knowledge of the type and severity of the arthritis is essential. For example, ankylosing spondylitis results in a loss of joint mobility, especially in the spine. Flexibility exercises are needed on a regular basis to slow the progression of the loss of motion and maintain function (41).

SUMMARY

Arthritis and chronic joint symptoms, both physician diagnosed and undiagnosed, affect more than 50 million Americans and are the leading cause of disability (23). Arthritis increases pain, reduces strength, restricts mobility, and lowers health-related quality of life. Furthermore, it has been shown that individuals with some of the systemic arthropathies have a higher risk for cardiovascular disease and hypertension. There are no known cures for arthritis; however, exercise appears to improve the clinical symptoms of various rheumatic diseases, including OA, fibromyalgia, and RA. Importantly, for many of these groups, psychological factors have also been identified as critical factors in response to both the pain and to treatment. Tailored exercise prescription and programs that promote self-efficacy have been identified as vital to effective exercise participation and adherence (11,34,83).

REFERENCES

1. Altman R, Asch E, Bloch D, et al. Development of criteria for the classification and reporting of osteoarthritis. Classification of osteoarthritis of the knee. Diagnostic and Therapeutic Criteria Committee of the American Rheumatism Association. *Arthritis Rheum*. 1986;29(8):1039–49.

2. Al-Zahrani KS, Bakheit AM. A study of the gait characteristics of patients with chronic osteoarthritis of the knee. *Disabil Rehabil*. 2002;24(5):275–80.

3. American College of Rheumatology Subcommittee on Rheumatoid Arthritis Guidelines. Guidelines for the management of rheumatoid arthritis: 2002 Update. *Arthritis Rheum*. 2002;46(2):328–46.

4. *Ankylosing spondylitis* [Internet]. Atlanta (GA): American College of Rheumatology; [cited 2007 May 22]. Available from: http://www.rheumatology.org/public/factsheets/as.asp

5. Arnett FC, Edworthy SM, Bloch DA, et al. The American Rheumatism Association 1987 revised criteria for the classification of rheumatoid arthritis. *Arthritis Rheum*. 1988;31(3):315–24.

6. Arnold LM, Hess EV, Hudson JI, Welge JA, Berno SE, Keck PE,Jr. A randomized, placebo-controlled, double-blind, flexible-dose study of fluoxetine in the treatment of women with fibromyalgia. *Am J Med*. 2002;112(3):191–7.

7. Assis MR, Silva LE, Alves AM, et al. A randomized controlled trial of deep water running: clinical effectiveness of aquatic exercise to treat fibromyalgia. *Arthritis Rheum*. 2006;55(1):57–65.

8. Baillet A, Zeboulon N, Gossec L, et al. Efficacy of cardiorespiratory aerobic exercise in rheumatoid arthritis: Meta-analysis of randomized controlled trials. *Arth Care Res*. 2010;62:984–92.

9. Baliunas AJ, Hurwitz DE, Ryals AB, et al. Increased knee joint loads during walking are present in subjects with knee osteoarthritis. *Osteoarthr Cartilage*. 2002;10(7):573–9.

10. Bennett RM. Beyond fibromyalgia: ideas on etiology and treatment. *J Rheumatol Suppl*. 1989;19:185–91.

11. Botha-Scheepers S, Riyazi N, Kroon HM, et al. Activity limitations in the lower extremities in patients with osteoarthritis: the modifying effects of illness perceptions and mental health. *Osteoarthr Cartilage*. 2006;14:1104–10.

12. Bradley LA, Alarcon GS. Is Chiari malformation associated with increased levels of substance P and clinical symptoms in persons with fibromyalgia? *Arthritis Rheum*. 1999;42(12):2731–2.

13. Breedland I, van Scheppingen C, Leijsma M, Verheij-Jansen NP, van Weert E. Effects of a group-based exercise and educational program on physical performance and disease self-management in rheumatoid arthritis: A randomized controlled study. *Phys Ther*. 2011;91(6):879–93.

14. Brousseau L, Pelland L, Wells G, et al. Efficacy of aerobic exercises for osteoarthritis (Part II): a meta-analysis. *Phys Ther Rev*. 2004;9(3):125–45.

15. Bruce B, Fries JF, Lubeck DP. Aerobic exercise and its impact on musculoskeletal pain in older adults: a 14 year prospective, longitudinal study. *Arthritis Res Ther*. 2005;7(6):R1263–70.

16. Buchwald D. Fibromyalgia and chronic fatigue syndrome: similarities and differences. *Rheum Dis Clin North Am*. 1996;22(2):219–43.

17. Burr DB, Radin EL. Microfractures and microcracks in subchondral bone: are they relevant to osteoarthrosis? *Rheum Dis Clin North Am*. 2003;29(4):675–85.

18. Burris JE. Pharmacologic approaches to geriatric pain management. *Arch Phys Med Rehabil*. 2004;85(7 Suppl 3):S45,9; quiz S50–1.

19. Busch AJ, Schacter CL, Overend TJ, Peloso PM, Barber KA. Exercise for fibromyalgia: a systematic review. *J Rheumatol*. 2008;35:1130–44.

20. Busch A, Schachter CL, Peloso PM, Bombardier C. Exercise for treating fibromyalgia syndrome. *Cochrane Database Syst Rev*. 2002(3):CD003786.

21. Callahan LF, Mielenz T, Freburger J, et al. A randomized controlled trial of the people with arthritis can exercise program: symptoms, function, physical activity, and psychosocial outcomes. *Arthritis Rheum*. 2008;59:92–101.

22. Centers for Disease Control and Prevention. National and state medical expenditures and lost earnings attributable to arthritis and other rheumatic conditions—United States, 2003. *MMWR Morb Mortal Wkly Rep*. 2007;56(1):4–7.

23. Centers for Disease Control and Prevention. Prevalence of doctor-diagnosed arthritis and arthritis-attributable activity limitation—United States, 2007–2009. *MMWR Morb Mortal Wkly Rep*. 2010;59(39):1261–5.

24. Chang RW, Falconer J, Stulberg SD, Arnold WJ, Manheim LM, Dyer AR. A randomized, controlled trial of arthroscopic surgery versus closed-needle joint lavage for patients with osteoarthritis of the knee. *Arthritis Rheum*. 1993;36(3):289–96.

25. Christensen R, Astrup A, Bliddal H. Weight loss: the treatment of choice for knee osteoarthritis? A randomized trial. *Osteoarthr Cartilage*. 2005;13:20–7.

26. Chung CP, Oeser A, Avalos I, et al. Utility of the Framingham risk score to predict the presence of coronary atherosclerosis in patients with rheumatoid arthritis. *Arthritis Res Ther*. 2006;8(6):R186.

27. Clark SR, Jones KD, Burckhardt CS, Bennett R. Exercise for patients with fibromyalgia: risks versus benefits. *Curr Rheumatol Rep*. 2001;3(2):135–46.

28. Clauw DJ, Crofford LJ. Chronic widespread pain and fibromyalgia: what we know, and what we need to know. *Best Pract Res Clin Rheumatol*. 2003;17(4):685–701.

29. Cochrane T, Davey RC, Matthes Edwards SM. Randomised controlled trial of the cost-effectiveness of water-based therapy for lower limb osteoarthritis. *Health Technol Assess*. 2005;9(31):iii,iv, ix–xi, 1–114.

30. Das AJr, Hammad TA. Efficacy of a combination of FCHG49 glucosamine hydrochloride, TRH122 low molecular weight sodium chondroitin sulfate and manganese ascorbate in the management of knee osteoarthritis. *Osteoarthr Cartilage*. 2000;8(5):343–50.

31. Davis MA, Ettinger WH, Neuhaus JM. The role of metabolic factors and blood pressure in the association of obesity with osteoarthritis of the knee. *J Rheumatol*. 1988;15(12):1827–32.

32. Dawson KA, Tiidus PM. Physical activity in the treatment and management of fibromyalgia. *Critical Reviews in Physical and Rehabilitation Medicine*. 2005;17(1):53–64.

33. Demitrack MA, Crofford LJ. Evidence for and pathophysiologic implications of hypothalamic-pituitary-adrenal axis dysregulation

in fibromyalgia and chronic fatigue syndrome. *Ann N Y Acad Sci.* 1998;840:684–97.

34. Der Ananian C, Wilcox S, Saunders R, Watkins K, Evans A. Factors that influence exercise among adults with arthritis in three activity levels. *Prev Chronic Dis* [Internet]. 2006; [cited 2012 Sep 18] Available from: http://www.cdc.gov/pcd/issues/2006/jul/05_0220.htm

35. Diracoglu D, Aydin R, Baskent A, Celik A. Effects of kinesthesia and balance exercises in knee osteoarthritis. *J Clin Rheumatol.* 2005; 11(6):303–10.

36. Doran MF, Pond GR, Crowson CS, O'Fallon WM, Gabriel SE. Trends in incidence and mortality in rheumatoid arthritis in Rochester, Minnesota, over a forty-year period. *Arthritis Rheum.* 2002;46(3): 625–31.

37. Dwight MM, Arnold LM, O'Brien H, Metzger R, Morris-Park E, Keck PE,Jr. An open clinical trial of venlafaxine treatment of fibromyalgia. *Psychosomatics.* 1998;39(1):14–7.

38. Ettinger WH,Jr, Afable RF. Physical disability from knee osteoarthritis: the role of exercise as an intervention. *Med Sci Sports Exerc.* 1994;26(12):1435–40.

39. Ettinger WH,Jr, Burns R, Messier SP, et al. A randomized trial comparing aerobic exercise and resistance exercise with a health education program in older adults with knee osteoarthritis. The Fitness Arthritis and Seniors Trial (FAST). *JAMA.* 1997;277(1):25–31.

40. Felson DT, Naimark A, Anderson J, Kazis L, Castelli W, Meenan RF. The prevalence of knee osteoarthritis in the elderly. The Framingham Osteoarthritis Study. *Arthritis Rheum.* 1987;30(8): 914–8.

41. Fernandez-de-Las-Penas C, Alonso-Blanco C, Alguacil-Diego IM, Miangolarra-Page JC. One-year follow-up of two exercise interventions for the management of patients with ankylosing spondylitis: a randomized controlled trial. *Am J Phys Med Rehabil.* 2006;85(7): 559–67.

42. Fiebich BL, Hollig A, Lieb K. Inhibition of substance P-induced cytokine synthesis by St. John's wort extracts. *Pharmacopsychiatry.* 2001;34 Suppl 1:S26–8.

43. Fisher NM, Gresham G, Pendergast DR. Effects of a quantitative progressive rehabilitation program applied unilaterally to the osteoarthritic knee. *Arch Phys Med Rehabil.* 1993;74(12):1319–26.

44. Fisher NM, Pendergast DR. Effects of a muscle exercise program on exercise capacity in subjects with osteoarthritis. *Arch Phys Med Rehabil.* 1994;75(7):792–7.

45. Fitzgerald GK, Piva SR, Irrgang JJ, Bouzubar F, Starz TW. Quadriceps activation failure as a moderator of the relationship between quadriceps strength and physical function in individuals with knee osteoarthritis. *Arthritis Rheum.* 2004;51(1):40–8.

46. Fontaine KR, Haaz S, Heo M. Projected prevalence of US adults with self-reported doctor-diagnosed arthritis, 2005 to 2050. *Clin Rheumatol.* 2007;26:772–4.

47. Fraenkel L, Bogardus ST,Jr, Concato J, Wittink DR. Treatment options in knee osteoarthritis: the patient's perspective. *Arch Intern Med.* 2004;164(12):1299–304.

48. Gerber LH, Hicks JE. Surgical and rehabilitation options in the treatment of the rheumatoid arthritis patient resistant to pharmacologic agents. *Rheum Dis Clin North Am.* 1995;21(1):19–39.

49. Goldenberg DL, Felson DT, Dinerman H. A randomized, controlled trial of amitriptyline and naproxen in the treatment of patients with fibromyalgia. *Arthritis Rheum.* 1986;29(11):1371–7.

50. Goldring MB. Osteoarthritis and cartilage: the role of cytokines. *Curr Rheumatol Rep.* 2000;2(6):459–65.

51. Gowans SE, Dehueck A, Voss S, Silaj A, Abbey SE. Six-month and one-year followup of 23 weeks of aerobic exercise for individuals with fibromyalgia. *Arthritis Rheum.* 2004;51(6):890–8.

52. Gowans SE, deHueck A, Voss S, Silaj A, Abbey SE, Reynolds WJ. Effect of a randomized, controlled trial of exercise on mood and physical function in individuals with fibromyalgia. *Arthritis Rheum.* 2001;45(6):519–29.

53. Gregersen PK, Silver J, Winchester RJ. The shared epitope hypothesis. An approach to understanding the molecular genetics of susceptibility to rheumatoid arthritis. *Arthritis Rheum.* 1987;30(11):1205–13.

54. Hakkinen A, Haanonan P, Nyman K, Hakkinen K. Aerobic and neuromuscular performance capacity of physically active females with early or long-term rheumatoid arthritis compared to matched healthy women. *Scand J Rheumatol.* 2002;31(6):345–50.

55. Hakkinen A, Hakkinen K, Hannonen P, Alen M. Strength training induced adaptations in neuromuscular function of premenopausal women with fibromyalgia: comparison with healthy women. *Ann Rheum Dis.* 2001;60(1):21–6.

56. Hakkinen A, Pakarinen A, Hannonen P, et al. Effects of prolonged combined strength and endurance training on physical fitness, body composition and serum hormones in women with rheumatoid arthritis and in healthy controls. *Clin Exp Rheumatol.* 2005;23(4):505–12.

57. Hakkinen A, Sokka T, Hannonen P. A home-based two-year strength training period in early rheumatoid arthritis led to good long-term compliance: a five-year followup. *Arthritis Rheum.* 2004;51(1):56–62.

58. Hall A, Maher C, Latimer J, Ferreira M. The effectiveness of tai chi for chronic musculoskeletal pain conditions: a systematic review and meta-analysis. *Arthritis Rheum.* 2009; 61(6):717–24.

59. Harney S, Wordsworth BP. Genetic epidemiology of rheumatoid arthritis. *Tissue Antigens.* 2002;60(6):465–73.

60. Hartman CA, Manos TM, Winter C, Hartman DM, Li B, Smith JC. Effects of T'ai Chi training on function and quality of life indicators in older adults with osteoarthritis. *J Am Geriatr Soc.* 2000;48(12):1553–9.

61. Hauselmann HJ. Nutripharmaceuticals for osteoarthritis. *Best Pract Res Clin Rheumatol.* 2001;15(4):595–607.

62. Helmick CG, Felson DT, Lawrence RC, et al. Estimates of the prevalence of arthritis and other rheumatic conditions in the United States. *Arthritis Rheum.* 2008;58:15–25.

63. Hess EV. Rheumatoid arthritis: treatment. In: Schumacher HR, Klippel JH, Robinson DR, editors. *Primer on the Rheumatic Diseases.* 9th ed. Atlanta: Arthritis Foundation; 1988. p. 93–96.

64. Hochberg MC, Dougados M. Pharmacological therapy of osteoarthritis. *Best Pract Res Clin Rheumatol.* 2001;15(4):583–93.

65. Hootman JM, Helmick CG. Projections of US prevalence of arthritis and associated activity limitations. *Arthritis Rheum.* 2006;54(1):226–9.

66. Hughes SL, Seymour RB, Campbell RT, et al. Long-term impact of Fit and Strong! on older adults with osteoarthritis. *Gerontologist.* 2006;46(6):801–14.

67. Hurley MV. The effects of joint damage on muscle function, proprioception and rehabilitation. *Man Ther.* 1997;2(1):11–7.

68. Hurwitz DE, Sumner DR, Andriacchi TP, Sugar DA. Dynamic knee loads during gait predict proximal tibial bone distribution. *J Biomech.* 1998;31(5):423–30.

69. Jan M, Lin J, Liau J, Lin Y, Lin D. Investigation of clinical effects of high- and low-resistance training for patients with knee osteoarthritis: a randomized controlled trial. *Phys Ther.* 2008;88(4):427–36.

70. Jones KD, Burckhardt CS, Clark SR, Bennett RM, Potempa KM. A randomized controlled trial of muscle strengthening versus flexibility training in fibromyalgia. *J Rheumatol.* 2002;29(5):1041–8.

71. Jones G, Halbert J, Crotty M, Shanahan EM, Batterham M, Ahern M. The effect of treatment on radiological progression in rheumatoid arthritis: a systematic review of randomized placebo-controlled trials. *Rheumatology (Oxford).* 2003;42(1):6–13.

72. Jordan JM, Luta G, Stabler T, et al. Ethnic and sex differences in serum levels of cartilage oligomeric matrix protein. *Arth Rheum.* 2003;48:675–681.;48:675–81.

73. Kaipiainen-Seppanen O, Aho K, Isomaki H, Laakso M. Shift in the incidence of rheumatoid arthritis toward elderly patients in Finland during 1975–1990. *Clin Exp Rheumatol.* 1996;14(5):537–42.

74. Karlsson A, Opava CH. Cycling or walking? Comparing the Six-minute walk with the cycle ergometer test in patients with rheumatoid arthritis. *Adv Physiotherapy.* 2008;10:203–8.

75. Kovar PA, Allegrante JP, MacKenzie CR, Peterson MG, Gutin B, Charlson ME. Supervised fitness walking in patients with osteoarthritis of the knee. A randomized, controlled trial. *Ann Intern Med.* 1992;116(7):529–34.

76. Lautenschlager J. Present state of medication therapy in fibromyalgia syndrome. *Scand J Rheumatol Suppl.* 2000;113:32–6.

77. Lawrence RC, Helmick CG, Arnett FC, et al. Estimates of the prevalence of arthritis and selected musculoskeletal disorders in the United States. *Arthritis Rheum.* 1998;41(5):778–99.

78. Leffler CT, Philippi AF, Leffler SG, Mosure JC, Kim PD. Glucosamine, chondroitin, and manganese ascorbate for degenerative joint disease of the knee or low back: a randomized, double-blind, placebo-controlled pilot study. *Mil Med.* 1999;164(2):85–91.

79. Lemmey AB, Marcora SM, Chester K, Wilson S, Casanova F, Maddison PJ. Effects of high-intensity resistance training in patients with rheumatoid arthritis: a randomized controlled trial. *Arth Rheum.* 2009;61:1726–34.

80. Lippiello L, Woodward J, Karpman R, Hammad TA. In vivo chondroprotection and metabolic synergy of glucosamine and chondroitin sulfate. *Clin Orthop Relat Res.* 2000;(381):229–40.

81. Liu Z, Welin M, Bragee B, Nyberg F. A high-recovery extraction procedure for quantitative analysis of substance P and opioid peptides in human cerebrospinal fluid. *Peptides.* 2000;21(6): 853–60.

82. MacGregor AJ, Snieder H, Rigby AS, et al. Characterizing the quantitative genetic contribution to rheumatoid arthritis using data from twins. *Arthritis Rheum.* 2000;43(1):30–7.

83. Machado GPM, Gignac MAM, Badley EM. Participation restrictions among older adults with osteoarthritis: a mediated model of physical symptoms, activity limitations, and depression. *Arthritis Rheum.* 2008;59(1):129–35.

84. Mangione KK, McCully K, Gloviak A, Lefebvre I, Hofmann M, Craik R. The effects of high-intensity and low-intensity cycle ergometry in older adults with knee osteoarthritis. *J Gerontol A Biol Sci Med Sci.* 1999;54(4):M184–90.

85. Martin DF. Pathomechanics of knee osteoarthritis. *Med Sci Sports Exerc.* 1994;26(12):1429–34.

86. Mazieres B, Loyau G, Menkes CJ, et al. Chondroitin sulfate in the treatment of gonarthrosis and coxarthrosis. 5-months result of a multicenter double-blind controlled prospective study using placebo]. *Rev Rhum Mal Osteoartic.* 1992;59(7–8):466–72.

87. McAlindon TE, LaValley MP, Gulin JP, Felson DT. Glucosamine and chondroitin for treatment of osteoarthritis: a systematic quality assessment and meta-analysis. *JAMA.* 2000;283(11):1469–75.

88. McCoy TH, Salvati EA, Ranawat CS, Wilson PD,Jr. A fifteen-year follow-up study of one hundred Charnley low-friction arthroplasties. *Orthop Clin North Am.* 1988;19(3):467–76.

89. Messier SP, DeVita P, Cowan RE, Seay J, Young HC, Marsh AP. Do older adults with knee osteoarthritis place greater loads on the knee during gait? A preliminary study. *Arch Phys Med Rehabil.* 2005;86(4):703–9.

90. Messier SP, Loeser RF, Hoover JL, Semble EL, Wise CM. Osteoarthritis of the knee: effects on gait, strength, and flexibility. *Arch Phys Med Rehabil.* 1992;73(1):29–36.

91. Messier SP, Loeser RF, Miller GD, et al. Exercise and dietary weight loss in overweight and obese older adults with knee osteoarthritis: the arthritis, diet, and activity promotion trial. *Arthritis Rheum.* 2004;50(5):1501–10.

92. Messier SP, Loeser RF, Mitchell MN, et al. Exercise and weight loss in obese older adults with knee osteoarthritis: a preliminary study. *J Am Geriatr Soc.* 2000;48(9):1062–72.

93. Messier SP, Thompson CD, Ettinger Jr. WH. Effects of long-term aerobic or weight training regimens on gait in an older, osteoarthritic population. *J Appl Biomech.* 1997;13(2):205–25.

94. Miller LJ, Kubes KL. Serotonergic agents in the treatment of fibromyalgia syndrome. *Ann Pharmacother.* 2002;36(4):707–12.

95. Minor MA, Hewett JE, Webel RR, Anderson SK, Kay DR. Efficacy of physical conditioning exercise in patients with rheumatoid arthritis and osteoarthritis. *Arthritis Rheum.* 1989;32(11):1396–405.

96. Moldofsky H, Scarisbrick P, England R, Smythe H. Musculosketal symptoms and non-REM sleep disturbance in patients with "fibrositis syndrome" and healthy subjects. *Psychosom Med.* 1975;37(4):341–51.

97. Moreland LW, Baumgartner SW, Schiff MH, et al. Treatment of rheumatoid arthritis with a recombinant human tumor necrosis factor receptor (p75)-Fc fusion protein. *N Engl J Med.* 1997;337(3):141–7.

98. Moseley JB, O'Malley K, Petersen NJ, et al. A controlled trial of arthroscopic surgery for osteoarthritis of the knee. *N Engl J Med.* 2002;347(2):81–8.

99. Munneke M, de Jong Z, Zwinderman AH, et al. Adherence and satisfaction of rheumatoid arthritis patients with a long-term intensive dynamic exercise program (RAPIT program). *Arthritis Rheum.* 2003;49(5):665–72.

100. Munneke M, de Jong Z, Zwinderman AH, et al. Effect of a high-intensity weight-bearing exercise program on radiologic damage progression of the large joints in subgroups of patients with rheumatoid arthritis. *Arthritis Rheum.* 2005;53(3):410–7.

101. Naranjo A, Sokka T, Descalzo MA, et al. Cardiovascular disease in patients with rheumatoid arthritis: results from the QUEST-RA study. *Arth Res Ther.* 2008;10:1–10.

102. Newcomb LW, Koltyn KF, Morgan WP, Cook DB. Influence of preferred versus prescribed exercise on pain in fibromyalgia. *Med Sci Sports Exer.* 2011(43):1106–13.

103. Nicklas BJ, Ambrosius W, Messier SP, et al. Diet-induced weight loss, exercise, and chronic inflammation in older, obese adults: a randomized controlled clinical trial. *Am J Clin Nutr.* 2004;79(4):544–51.

104. NIH Consensus Statement on total knee replacement. *NIH Consens State Sci Statements.* 2003;20(1):1–34.

105. Otterness IG, Swindell AC, Zimmerer RO, Poole AR, Ionescu M, Weiner E. An analysis of 14 molecular markers for monitoring osteoarthritis: segregation of the markers into clusters and distinguishing osteoarthritis at baseline. *Osteoarthr Cartilage.* 2000;8(3):180–5.

106. Otterness IG, Weiner E, Swindell AC, Zimmerer RO, Ionescu M, Poole AR. An analysis of 14 molecular markers for monitoring osteoarthritis. Relationship of the markers to clinical end-points. *Osteoarthr Cartilage.* 2001;9(3):224–31.

107. Owings MF, Kozak LJ. Ambulatory and inpatient procedures in the United States, 1996. *Vital Health Stat 13.* 1998;(139):1–119.

108. Pelletier JP, Martel-Pelletier J, Abramson SB. Osteoarthritis, an inflammatory disease: potential implication for the selection of new therapeutic targets. *Arthritis Rheum.* 2001;44(6):1237–47.

109. Peters MJL, Symmons DPM, McCarey D, et al. EULAR evidence-based recommendations for cardiovascular risk management in patients with rheumatoid arthritis and other forms of inflammatory arthritis. *Ann Rheum Dis.* 2010;69:325–31.

110. Psaty BM, Furberg CD. COX-2 inhibitors—lessons in drug safety. *N Engl J Med.* 2005;352(11):1133–5.

111. Pujalte JM, Llavore EP, Ylescupidez FR. Double-blind clinical evaluation of oral glucosamine sulphate in the basic treatment of osteoarthrosis. *Curr Med Res Opin.* 1980;7(2):110–4.

112. Quintner JL, Cohen ML. Fibromyalgia falls foul of a fallacy. *Lancet.* 1999;353(9158):1092–4.

113. Radin EL, Yang KH, Riegger C, Kish VL, O'Connor JJ. Relationship between lower limb dynamics and knee joint pain. *J Orthop Res.* 1991;9(3):398–405.

114. Rall LC, Roubenoff R, Cannon JG, Abad LW, Dinarello CA, Meydani SN. Effects of progressive resistance training on immune response in aging and chronic inflammation. *Med Sci Sports Exerc.* 1996;28(11):1356–65.

115. Rao SG, Bennett RM. Pharmacological therapies in fibromyalgia. *Best Pract Res Clin Rheumatol*. 2003;17(4):611–27.

116. *Recommendations for the Medical Management of Osteoarthritis of the Hip and Knee* [Internet]. Atlanta (GA): American College of Rheumatology; [cited 2011 Oct 12]. Available from: http://www .rheumatology.org/practice/clinical/guidelines/oa-mgmt.asp

117. Reginster JY, Deroisy R, Rovati LC, et al. Long-term effects of glucosamine sulphate on osteoarthritis progression: a randomised, placebo-controlled clinical trial. *Lancet*. 2001;357(9252):251–6.

118. Richards SC, Scott DL. Prescribed exercise in people with fibromyalgia: parallel group randomised controlled trial. *BMJ*. 2002; 325(7357):185.

119. Russell IJ, Fletcher EM, Vipraio GA, Lopez Y, Orr MA. Cerebrospinal fluid (CSF) substance P (SP) in fibromyalgia; changes in CSF SP over time parallel changes in clinical activity [abstract]. *J Musculoskeletal Pain*. 1998;6(Suppl 2):77.

120. Salemi S, Rethage J, Wollina U, et al. Detection of interleukin 1β (IL-1β), IL-6, and tumor necrosis factor-α in skin of patients with fibromyalgia. *J Rheumatol*. 2003;30(1):146–50.

121. Schmitt LC, Fitzgerald GK, Reisman AS, Rudolph KS. Instability, laxity, and physical function in patients with medial knee osteoarthritis. *Phys Ther*. 2008;88:1506–16.

122. Schnitzer TJ. Osteoarthritis management: the role of cyclooxygenase-2-selective inhibitors. *Clin Ther*. 2001;23(3):313, 326; discussion 311–2.

123. Seymour RB, Hughes SL, Campbell RT, Huber GM, Desai P. Comparison of two methods of conducting the Fit and Strong! program. *Arth Rheum*. 2009;61(7):876–84.

124. Shankland WE, 2nd. The effects of glucosamine and chondroitin sulfate on osteoarthritis of the TMJ: a preliminary report of 50 patients. *Cranio*. 1998;16(4):230–5.

125. Sharif M, Shepstone L, Elson CJ, Dieppe PA, Kirwan JR. Increased serum C reactive protein may reflect events that precede radiographic progression in osteoarthritis of the knee. *Ann Rheum Dis*. 2000;59(1):71–4.

126. Sharma L, Hurwitz DE, Thonar EJ, et al. Knee adduction moment, serum hyaluronan level, and disease severity in medial tibiofemoral osteoarthritis. *Arthritis Rheum*. 1998;41(7):1233–40.

127. Sharma L, Song J, Felson DT, Cahue S, Shamiyeh E, Dunlop DD. The role of knee alignment in disease progression and functional decline in knee osteoarthritis. *JAMA*. 2001;286(2):188–95.

128. Shirayama Y, Mitsushio H, Takashima M, Ichikawa H, Takahashi K. Reduction of substance P after chronic antidepressants treatment in the striatum, substantia nigra and amygdala of the rat. *Brain Res*. 1996;739(1–2):70–8.

129. Spector TD, Hart DJ, Nandra D, et al. Low-level increases in serum C-reactive protein are present in early osteoarthritis of the knee and predict progressive disease. *Arthritis Rheum*. 1997;40(4):723–7.

130. Stastny P. Association of the B-cell alloantigen DRw4 with rheumatoid arthritis. *N Engl J Med*. 1978;298(16):869–71.

131. Stenstrom CH, Minor MA. Evidence for the benefit of aerobic and strengthening exercise in rheumatoid arthritis. *Arthritis Rheum*. 2003;49(3):428–34.

132. Straub RH, Scholmerich J, Cutolo M. The multiple facets of premature aging in rheumatoid arthritis. *Arthritis Rheum*. 2003;48(10):2713–21.

133. Symmons DP. Epidemiology of rheumatoid arthritis: determinants of onset, persistence and outcome. *Best Pract Res Clin Rheumatol*. 2002;16(5):707–22.

134. Vaeroy H, Helle R, Forre O, Kass E, Terenius L. Elevated CSF levels of substance P and high incidence of Raynaud phenomenon in patients with fibromyalgia: new features for diagnosis. *Pain*. 1988;32(1):21–6.

135. van den Ende CH, Breedveld FC, le Cessie S, Dijkmans BA, de Mug AW, Hazes JM. Effect of intensive exercise on patients with active rheumatoid arthritis: a randomised clinical trial. *Ann Rheum Dis*. 2000;59(8):615–21.

136. van Schaardenburg D. Rheumatoid arthritis in the elderly. Prevalence and optimal management. *Drugs Aging*. 1995;7(1):30–7.

137. Welin M, Bragee B, Nyberg F, Kristiansson M. Elevated substance levels are contrasted by a decrease in met-enkephalin-arg-phe-levels in CSF from fibromyalgia patients. *J Musculoskelet Pain*. 1995;3(Suppl 1):4.

138. Westby MD, Wade JP, Rangno KK, Berkowitz J. A randomized controlled trial to evaluate the effectiveness of an exercise program in women with rheumatoid arthritis taking low dose prednisone. *J Rheumatol*. 2000;27(7):1674–80.

139. Wolfe F. The C-reactive protein but not erythrocyte sedimentation rate is associated with clinical severity in patients with osteoarthritis of the knee or hip. *J Rheumatol*. 1997;24(8):1486–8.

140. Wolfe F, Ross K, Anderson J, Russell IJ, Hebert L. The prevalence and characteristics of fibromyalgia in the general population. *Arthritis Rheum*. 1995;38(1):19–28.

141. Wolfe F, Smythe HA, Yunus MB, et al. The American College of Rheumatology 1990 Criteria for the Classification of Fibromyalgia. Report of the Multicenter Criteria Committee. *Arthritis Rheum*. 1990;33(2):160–72.

142. Zijlstra TR, van de Laar MA. The lack of a placebo effect in a trial of fluoxetine in the treatment of fibromyalgia. *Am J Med*. 2002;113(7):614; author reply 614–5.

SELECTED REFERENCES FOR FURTHER READING

Brandt KD. *Osteoarthritis* (Rheumatic Disease Clinics of North America). Philadelphia (PA): Elsevier Science Health Science; 2003.

Brent S, Wilk KE. *Clinical Orthopaedic Rehabilitation*. 2nd ed. Philadelphia (PA): Mosby; 2003. 652 p.

Fransen M, McConnell S. Exercise for osteoarthritis of the knee. *Cochrane Database Syst Rev*. 2008;(4):CD004376. doi:10.1002/14651858.

Fransen M, McConnell S, Hernandez-Molina G, Reichenbach S. Exercise for osteoarthritis of the hip. *Cochrane Database Syst Rev*. 2009;(3):CD007912. doi:10.1002/14651858.

Green WB, Snider RK. *Essentials of Musculoskeletal Care*. 2nd ed. Rosemont (IL): American Academy of Orthopaedic Surgeons; 2001. 756 p.

Hakkinen A. Effectiveness and safety of strength training in rheumatoid arthritis. *Curr Opin Rheumatol*. 2004;16:132–37.

Haq I, Murphy E, Dacre J. Osteoarthritis. *Postgrad Med J*. 2003;79:377–83.

Jette AM, Keysor JJ. Disability models: implications for arthritis exercise and physical activity interventions. *Arthritis Rheum*. 2003;49:114–20.

Jordan KM, Arden NK, Doherty M, et al. Standing Committee for International Clinical Studies Including Therapeutic Trials ESCISIT. EULAR Recommendations 2003: An evidence based approach to the management of knee osteoarthritis: report of a Task Force of the Standing Committee for International Clinical Studies Including Therapeutic Trials (ESCISIT). *Ann Rheum Dis*. 2003;62:1145–55.

Krebs D, Herzog W, McGibbon CA, Sharma L. Work group recommendations: 2002 Exercise and Physical Activity Conference. St. Louis. *Arthritis Rheum*. 2003;49:261–62.

O'Dell JR. Therapeutic strategies for rheumatoid arthritis. *N Engl J Med*. 2004;350:2591–602.

Roubenoff R. Exercise and inflammatory disease. *Arthritis Rheum*. 2003;49:263–6.

Sahrmann S. *Diagnosis and Treatment of Movement Impairment Syndromes*. Philadelphia (PA): Mosby; 2001. 384 p.

van Gool CH, Penninx BWJH, Kempen GIJM, et al. Effects of exercise adherence on osteoarthritis-related performance and disability. *Arthritis Care Res*. 2005;53:24–32.

INTERNET RESOURCES

- American College of Rheumatology Practice Guidelines: http://www.rheumatology.org/publications/guidelines/index .asp?aud=prs http://www.rheumatology.org/practice/clinical/ guidelines/oa-mgmt.asp

- Arthritis Foundation (Bulletin on the Rheumatic Diseases): http://www.arthritis.org/research/bulletin/archives.asp
- Arthritis Foundation (Research Update): http://www.arthritis.org/research/ResearchUpdate/archives.asp
- HealthTalk Rheumatoid Arthritis: http://www.healthtalk.com/rheumatoidarthritis/index.cfm
- National Guideline Clearinghouse (Exercise Prescription for Older Adults with Osteoarthritis Pain: Consensus Practice Recommendations): http://www.guideline.gov/summary/summary.aspx? doc_id=3188&nbr=2414&string=arthritis

- National Guideline Clearinghouse (Osteoarthritis: AAOS Clinical Guideline on Osteoarthritis of the Knee): http://www.guideline.gov/summary/summary.aspx?doc_id=3856&nbr=3069&string=arthritis
- National Guideline Clearinghouse (Osteoarthritis: AAOS Clinical Guideline on Osteoarthritis of the Knee [Phase II]): http://www.guideline.gov/summary/summary.aspx?doc_id=4584&nbr=3374&string=arthritis; http://www.rheumatology.org/public/factsheets/as.asp; http://www.cdc.gov/arthritis/data_statistics/national_data_nhis.htm#impact

V

Behavior Change

HEATHER O. CHAMBLISS, PhD, FACSM, *Section Editor*

Theoretical Foundations of Physical Activity Behavior Change

This chapter introduces behavior change theories, gives examples of research applications of each theory, and provides a guide as to how to apply the theoretical principles to working with clients. More in-depth discussion of practical application strategies of behavioral change theories are provided in *Chapters 45 and 46*.

THE IMPORTANCE OF THEORIES

Physical activity is a complex behavior that involves a series of skills to adopt and maintain. It is impossible to consider all influences on physical activity; therefore, psychological theories and models of behavior change can be important to help guide both research and clinical practice (45,80). Theories provide a framework for understanding the process through which a complex behavior, such as physical activity, changes and is sustained over time. Theories can also provide guidance to practitioners in helping people make behavior changes by understanding the connection between theories and results, how to translate theory into practice, and which specific strategies to recommend (45,80). Theories can help provide techniques and shed light on potential pitfalls in becoming more physically active (34,76). This chapter provides an overview of the theories that have been applied to help understand and guide changes in

physical activity behavior in healthy and clinical adult populations (34,76,90).

The theories covered in this chapter include the stages of change for motivational readiness (or the transtheoretical model [TTM]), self-determination theory (SDT), social cognitive theory (SCT), social ecology theory, theories of reasoned action and planned behavior, and relapse prevention (RP). The theories were selected for this chapter based on their clinical and research applications. Each of these theories has been applied to studies of physical activity determinants, as well as in studying other health behavior changes (26). Some of the theories (*e.g.*, SCT) have more predictive use than other theories (*e.g.*, theory of reasoned action [TRA]) (28,29). Although there may be some theories that are not included in this review (*e.g.*, health action process approach) (19,20,81), the theories addressed in this chapter are ones that have been applied most often in relation to physical activity (13,80,90).

INCORPORATING THEORY-BASED TECHNIQUES AND PRINCIPLES

A large body of research addresses the importance of using theory to help guide individuals through behavior changes. Although not all theories or aspects of theories

KEY TERMS

Processes of change: The strategies that individuals use as they are adopting and maintaining behavior changes.

Relapse prevention (RP): The process by which one maintains long-term behavior change by anticipating potentially high-risk situations and devising strategies to cope with these situations.

Self-efficacy: An individual's belief and confidence about his or her ability to make specific behavior changes.

Self-regulation/self-regulatory strategies: Behavior change can be prompted by the use of self-regulation

or self-regulatory strategies, which are ways of exerting self-influence. For behavior change, these include self-monitoring, planning, and goal setting.

Stages of change: A model, also known as the transtheoretical model, which postulates that individuals move through a series of stages that represent increased motivation to be physically active and face common barriers when making a behavior change.

Theory: A theory is a framework that helps to understand, predict, and measure behavior.

can be applied to all individuals at a given time, theories can be helpful in designing an intervention and in selecting evaluation measures for assessing client progress. The approach can incorporate such considerations as one's readiness for change, the environment in which they live, and their social context.

THEORIES OF BEHAVIOR CHANGE

It may be a challenge to directly apply research findings while working in community settings, cardiac rehabilitation facilities, school settings, as a personal trainer, or as an exercise physiologist. Therefore, the last part of each subsection provides a clinical application, which essentially transfers the research findings and applies them to real world examples that a practitioner might encounter in working with different individuals across a variety of settings.

Table 44-1 provides an overview of the theories and key concepts.

THE STAGE OF MOTIVATIONAL READINESS FOR CHANGE MODEL

The stages of motivational readiness for change (SOC) model, or the TTM, consists of numerous components, including the stages of change and processes of change. In addition, components of other theories are used in conjunction with the SOC model including self-efficacy, which is a key concept of SCT (8), will be described in detail in other sections of the chapter.

Stages

The SOC model postulates that individuals move through a series of stages and face common barriers when making behavior changes and that intervention approaches may vary by the individual's identified stage of change (53,75). Several researchers have applied this model to individuals adopting and maintaining physical activity (30,58,69,71,73). The stages include precontemplation, contemplation, preparation, action, and maintenance. The *precontemplation* stage includes individuals who are inactive and not thinking about becoming active. Individuals in the *contemplation* stage are inactive but are thinking about becoming active. The *preparation* stage includes individuals who are physically active but not at the recommended levels (30 min or more of moderate-intensity physical activity on most, preferably all, days of the week) (38,72,90). The *action* stage includes individuals who are physically active at the recommended levels but have been active at this level for fewer than 6 mo. Individuals in the *maintenance* stage are physically active at the recommended levels and have been for more than 6 mo.

The movement across stages may be conceptualized as cyclic rather than linear, given that it takes many individuals numerous attempts before successfully adopting and maintaining physical activity. A self-report four-item questionnaire is available to identify an individual's stage of change, including such statements as, "I intend to become more physically active in the next 6 months," and "I currently engage in regular physical activity" (53,60) (see *Chapter 46* for the recommended questionnaire and scoring information) (94).

Processes of Change

The SOC model also posits that individuals use various processes of change as they progress through the stages. Five behavioral and five cognitive processes have been identified (53,58). The behavioral processes include *rewarding yourself* (*e.g.*, doing something nice for yourself when achieving a physical activity goal), *substituting alternatives* (*e.g.*, participating in physical activity to decrease fatigue and increase energy), *committing yourself* (*e.g.*, making promises to be physically active), *reminding yourself* (*e.g.*, posting reminders to be physically active at work), and *enlisting social support* (*e.g.*, having someone to depend on when having problems sticking with a physical activity program). Cognitive processes include *being aware of risks* (*e.g.*, thinking that physical inactivity can be harmful), *increasing knowledge* (*e.g.*, thinking about physical activity information obtained from articles), *comprehending benefits* (*e.g.*, believing that physical activity would make one healthy), *increasing healthy opportunities* (*e.g.*, awareness of physical activity programs), and *caring about consequences to others* (*e.g.*, wondering how inactivity affects family and

TABLE 44-1. Theories and Key Concepts

Theory	Key Concept
The stage of motivational readiness for change model	Individuals move through a series of stages and face common barriers when making behavior changes.
Self-determination theory	Individuals have three psychological needs including autonomy, competence, and relatedness.
Social cognitive theory	Behavior change is influenced by the interactions between the environment, personal factors, and the behavior itself.
Social ecology theory	Underscores the importance of the interaction between an individual behavior and his or her environment.
The theory of reasoned action/planned behavior	Developed to understand and predict an individual's behavior; such behavior must be clearly specified, volitional in nature, and performed in a specific situation.
Relapse prevention	Goal is to assist individuals in maintaining long-term behavior change by anticipating potentially high-risk situations and devising strategies to cope with these high-risk situations.

friends). The use of cognitive processes typically peaks in the preparation stage, and the use of the behavioral processes typically peaks in the action stage. A self-report 40-item measure has been developed to assess the 10 processes of change (see Marcus and Forsyth [53] and Marcus et al. [58]).

Results from a meta-analysis (63) indicated that all 10 processes of change are used across the stages when individuals are actively making behavior changes. The transition from precontemplation to contemplation and from preparation to action was marked by the sharpest increases in the use of behavioral processes. In a more recent review (76), Rhodes and Pfaeffli reviewed studies examining the importance of SOC-related constructs (*i.e.*, mediators) in physical activity intervention studies. The most consistent support was for self-regulation (*i.e.*, planning, behavior processes), and there was limited support for self-efficacy as a mediator. Studies examining mediators have been limited by inadequate sample sizes, lack of a longitudinal design (*i.e.*, mediators and physical activity measured at the same time), and the use of inappropriate statistical procedures. Therefore, additional research is needed.

Although some of the components of the SOC model can be examined separately, research and practice applications are most effective when combining the different components. Therefore, a summary of the research findings that integrate the different aspects of the model and practice applications for integrating the model are presented later in this chapter.

Research Findings

According to a review of 150 studies applying the SOC model to exercise (85), interventions based on the SOC model appear to be effective for exercise promotion. Additionally, authors from this review highlighted that stage-matched interventions led to forward progression on the stages of change, which is important given the large percentage of individuals who are in precontemplation or contemplation for exercise. The authors also concluded that the measures used to assess constructs related to the SOC model, including measures of the processes of change and decisional balance, appear valid and reliable and have been applied to various populations.

Marcus and colleagues have conducted studies that are excellent examples of research that is guided by the theoretical framework of the SOC. This study used information that was targeted and information that was tailored to the individual. *Targeting* refers to defining and intervening with a subgroup of the population based on one common characteristic (*e.g.*, sex) (46,55). Targeting assumes that individuals have similar enough characteristics to be influenced by the same message (46,55). Alternatively, *tailoring* incorporates a higher level of specificity, and interventions that are tailored

use information on characteristics unique to an individual person (52,55,67). Marcus et al. (54) conducted a randomized controlled trial in which healthy sedentary participants (*n* = 249) were randomly assigned to one of the following three conditions: (a) individually tailored Internet intervention, (b) individually tailored print intervention, or (c) standard Internet comparison arm. Participants in the tailored Internet intervention completed online questionnaires and received immediate tailored feedback based on responses to the questionnaires. The tailored print arm also completed questionnaires and received tailored feedback; however, the questionnaires and feedback were done through the mail. Results indicated that all three groups increased their physical activity from baseline to 6 and 12 mo (54).

Another similar study randomly assigned 239 healthy, sedentary adults to (a) telephone-based, individualized feedback; (b) print-based, individualized feedback; or (c) contact control. Both intervention arms were guided by a motivationally tailored, theoretically driven computer expert system based on SCT and TTM constructs (54). At 6 mo, both the telephone and print arms significantly increased in minutes of moderate-intensity physical activity compared with control, with no differences between the intervention arms. At 12 mo, print participants reported a significantly greater number of moderate-intensity minutes than both telephone and control participants. There were no differences between telephone and control participants. Results suggest that both telephone and print enhance the adoption of physical activity among sedentary adults; however, print interventions may be particularly effective in maintaining physical activity in the longer term.

Practice Applications

To follow is a summary of strategies to help individuals increase or maintain physical activity based on the SOC model. One way to integrate the different components is to provide different types of intervention strategies depending on an individual's stage of change, although there may be some overlap across the stages (see *Table 44-2*).

Precontemplation

The precontemplation stage includes individuals who are not active and are not thinking about becoming active. Therefore, the goal is for the individual to begin thinking about physical activity. The pros and cons of becoming physically active should be discussed with the individual. Specifically, the individual should write down what the benefits of physical activity would be in addition to the disadvantages of physical activity. Specific barriers to physical activity should also be assessed, such as lack of time, lack of energy, environmental constraints (*e.g.*, lack of access to physical activity facilities), and fear of injury.

TABLE 44-2. Stages of Change

Stage of Change	Goals and Strategies
Precontemplation	*Goal*: Help client begin to think about being physically active Strategies: • Assess and discuss pros and cons of activity • Address barriers • Set nonactivity goals (*e.g.*, read about new type of activity)
Contemplation	*Goal*: Increase likelihood that the client will take steps to becoming physically active Strategies: • Consider the pros and cons • Advise how to make physical activity (PA) part of daily life • Set specific goals that are realistic (*e.g.*, think about with whom client would want to exercise)
Preparation	*Goal*: Increase PA to the recommended levels (30 min or more of PA on most, preferably all, days of the week) Strategies • Overcome barriers that prevent client from progressing to regular activity (*e.g.*, problem solve overcoming barrier of bad weather) • Set specific goals that are daily, weekly, and/or monthly • Self-monitor activity
Action	*Goal*: To maintain PA Strategies • Identify risk factors for future relapse (*e.g.*, vacations, stressful life events) • Continue goal setting • Continue self-monitoring
Maintenance	*Goal*: To maintain PA Strategies • Identify additional risk factors for future relapse (*e.g.*, If have relapsed in the past, identify what caused client to stop exercise and what helped getting started again) • Continue goal setting and monitoring progress. • Consider variety and explore ways to enhance enjoyment and prevent boredom

Adapted from Marcus B, Forsyth L. *Motivating People to Be Physically Active.* 2nd ed. Champaign (IL): Human Kinetics; 2009. 200 p.

Another important behavioral strategy for this stage is goal setting. Research indicates that goal setting is important for focusing attention on physical activity behavior change (70). Specifically, a stage-appropriate goal for the precontemplation stage would be to set aside time for reading a pamphlet about physical activity to learn more about the benefits of regular physical activity.

Contemplation

The contemplation stage includes individuals who are not physically active but are thinking about becoming active. The aim is for the individual to begin taking steps to becoming physically active and to think about setting goals. Individuals in this stage should also weigh the pros and cons of physical activity as well as read materials describing how to start a physical activity program. The individual can then make specific physical activity goals after he or she decides on which physical activity he or she would most prefer. Personal preference for specific activities as well as positive experience with certain activities should be considered when developing a program. The individual should also implement a reinforcement program in which he or she rewards himself or herself for meeting his or her specific physical activity goals. Because research indicates that social support is important for becoming physically active (4), individuals might identify one or two people who could be supportive and enlist their support for starting and maintaining a physical activity program.

Preparation

The preparation stage includes individuals who are currently engaging in some physical activity but not at the recommended level (53,58). The goal for this stage is to increase physical activity behavior to the recommended level or beyond. Specifically, the goal is to engage in physical activity of at least moderate intensity on most, preferably all, days of the week for 30 min or more each day (38). Several of the strategies used in the previous stages can also be used in this stage, including weighing the pros and cons of physical activity, choosing an appropriate physical activity program, and implementing a reinforcement schedule. Identifying and overcoming the barriers that prevent the individual from increasing their physical activity to the recommended level is the key for this stage. Goal setting can play an instrumental role in gradually increasing physical activity to the intended level.

Action

The action stage includes individuals who are physically active at the recommended level but have been for fewer than 6 mo. The goal of this stage is to continue to make physical activity a regular part of the individual's life. Important strategies for this stage include setting up a plan for self-monitoring physical activity and making short-term goals (*e.g.*, "I will walk on Monday, Wednesday, and Friday after work with my coworkers and then walk on Saturday and Sunday with my husband"). In addition, it might be helpful to suggest that the individual try a new activity or find a walking or running race that is going to take place in the future for which the individual can train. Talking with the individual about RP (discussed later in this chapter) is also very useful at this stage.

Maintenance

The maintenance stage includes individuals who have been physically active at the recommended level and have been for 6 or more months. The goal for this stage is to prepare for future setbacks and to continue to increase enjoyment for physical activity. Therefore, some of the same suggestions that apply to individuals in the action stage will also apply to individuals in the maintenance phase. It is important to continue to help the individual find ways to avoid boredom, either by trying new activities or by enlisting social support (*e.g.*, walking with a neighbor). Also, it might be helpful to have the individual reflect on the benefits they have already achieved from physical activity because these might be powerful rewards.

SELF-DETERMINATION THEORY

In recent years, SDT has received increased attention for physical activity promotion (21,84). SDT has been used to better understand motivation and psychological well-being (78). According to SDT, individuals have three psychological needs including autonomy, competence, and relatedness. *Autonomy* refers to the individual's perception that he or she initiates and regulates his or her own behavior. Therefore, individuals are more likely to engage in a behavior in a noncontrolling environment. *Competence* refers to the need for particular behavioral outcomes and the ability to achieve the behavioral outcomes. *Relatedness* refers to the need to have satisfying relationships with others (25).

Individuals are more likely to engage in a behavior if he or she is intrinsically motivated. An increased sense of autonomy and competence is believed to lead to higher levels of *intrinsic motivation*. For example, individuals who are intrinsically motivated to engage in physical activity would do so because of the enjoyment of physical activity and/or a sense of accomplishment. On the other hand, *extrinsic motivation* occurs when the individual is motivated by an external reward. Extrinsic motivation can also lead to behavior change depending on the circumstances. For example, individuals who engage in "integrated regulation" believe that physical activity is part of their sense of self and therefore are more likely to engage in physical activity (78).

Research Findings

Silva and colleagues (84) examined an intervention based on SDT designed to increase physical activity and weight control. Specifically, 239 women were randomly assigned to an intervention or health education control each lasting 1 yr. The intervention included 30 sessions in which an autonomy-supportive environment was created. The goal was for participants to gain ownership over their behavior and to increase their intrinsic motivation to be physically active. Results indicated that the intervention group reported higher levels of physical activity and weight loss relative to the control at 12 mo.

Another study examined the efficacy of a school-based physical activity intervention using SDT among 215 students (ages 14–16 yr) (21). Ten schools were randomly assigned to an intervention or control each lasting 10 wk. Physical education teachers in the intervention condition were trained to adopt an "autonomy-supportive interpersonal style" in which the teachers provided positive feedback, acknowledged the challenges for physical education classes, and provided a sense of choice to the students. Results indicated that students in the intervention condition reported a higher intention to exercise and more minute of leisure-time physical activity than the control. These recent studies indicate that SDT may be an important framework for physical activity promotion and further research is needed.

SOCIAL COGNITIVE THEORY

SCT has had more success than other theories in its application to changing physical activity behavior (8,10,89). This theory states that behavior change is influenced by the interactions between the environment, personal factors, and the behavior itself (8,10). This is called the model of *reciprocal determinism* (10) within SCT. Components of this model are shown in *Figure 44-1*.

Self-Efficacy

An important construct of SCT is self-efficacy. *Self-efficacy* is one's beliefs about his or her capabilities to

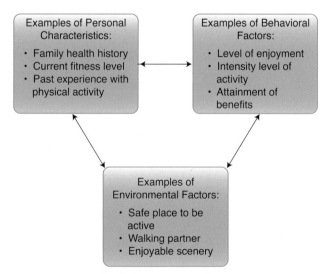

FIGURE 44-1. Components of social cognitive theory. (Adapted with permission from Marcus BH, Forsyth LH. *Motivating People to Be Physically Active.* 2nd ed. Champaign [IL]: Human Kinetics; 2009.)

exercise control over particular or specified life events (7,8). For example, someone with high self-efficacy for physical activity would endorse having the confidence to continue to exercise despite barriers (*e.g.*, feeling tired). Efficacy beliefs influence health behavior choices in that people tend to pursue tasks that they feel competent to perform and avoid those about which they feel incompetent (10,51). The most commonly measured and cited type of self-efficacy, barriers of self-efficacy, is related to the level of effort and persistence expended when faced with adverse situations or barriers to attaining the desired outcome. Self-efficacy to perform the behavior itself (*e.g.*, how confident are you that you can walk 30 min five times per week) has also been measured. Research indicates that self-efficacy level predicts participation in physical activity (18,65).

Differences in self-efficacy have been found for individuals in different stages of change (56,59). Cross-sectional studies indicate that as the stages of change progress from precontemplation to maintenance, a corresponding increase in self-efficacy for physical activity takes place. A five-item self-report measure has been developed to examine self-efficacy for physical activity in different situations (*e.g.*, feeling fatigued, inclement weather) (53,59).

Bandura (10) has listed the four influences on self-efficacy as performance of mastery experiences, vicarious experiences, verbal persuasion regarding one's capabilities, and inferences from physiologic and affective responses. The two that are discussed in this chapter are performance accomplishments and vicarious experience. The sense of efficacy that arises from *performance accomplishments* is based on personal mastery experiences — that is, success increases feelings of mastery, which, in turn, promotes the behavior and increases the likelihood of setting new and more challenging goals. Also, setting smaller, accomplishable goals helps a person feel more confident (or self-efficacious) and helps build more challenging goals. Personal experience is the strongest influence on feelings of self-efficacy. For example, if a person is able to be physically active again after an illness, he or she should have a resulting increase in self-efficacy.

The second influence on self-efficacy, *vicarious experience* or *modeling*, involves improvements in self-efficacy caused by observing others perform the activity (*e.g.*, watching a demonstration or video). Individuals increase their self-efficacy by observing others succeed at being physically active. This type of efficacy expectation is of particular interest in group sessions — if one participant is doing extraordinarily well, this can improve the self-efficacy of the others and further motivate them. For example, in a cardiac rehabilitation setting, if one client is doing well with his or her physical activity program, then this might serve to increase the self-efficacy of others in that setting.

TABLE 44-3. Effective Change Strategies

Self-Regulatory Skill	Tips
Self-monitoring	Find an easy way to monitor, maybe using a monthly calendar or a pedometer
Planning	Add physical activity "appointments" in daily calendar Make a plan for who, what, where?
Goal setting	Be specific Set short- and long-term goals

Self-Regulatory Strategies

Self-regulation is the ability to mobilize oneself to perform a behavior regularly in the face of various personal, situational, or social barriers. Bandura (8) postulates that the major process of self-regulation includes self-monitoring, proximal goal setting, strategy development, and self-motivating incentives. A person's self-regulatory efficacy is crucial for adherence to a behavior such as exercise in that those with low self-regulatory efficacy tend to drop out of programs more quickly and are less able to exercise at the intensity, duration, and frequency needed to accrue health benefits. See *Table 44-3* for examples of effective self-regulation change strategies.

According to Bandura (8), goals do not directly regulate motivation and action. Instead, self-efficacy beliefs influence people's choices of goals and persistence of behavior when they face challenges and obstacles (10). Goals provide direction and reference points against which people can monitor their progress (51). Through self-monitoring, people can develop efficacy beliefs about their current level of competence and expectancies regarding their rate of improvement (50). Bandura (8) states that goal specificity, challenge, and proximity are the most important qualities of goals to enhance motivation and persistence. A recent meta-regression found that interventions that combined self-monitoring with at least one other self-regulation technique (*e.g.*, goal setting) were the most effective (66).

Research Findings

Although studies have examined the efficacy of SCT-based interventions and the surgeon general report on physical activity and health recommends the use of SCT (34,76,80,90), fewer studies have examined different SCT constructs to determine their relationships to physical activity outcomes. Most research focuses on the SCT construct of self-efficacy, which has been recently been shown to relate to exercise session attendance (5). Interestingly, some studies are now showing that self-efficacy predicts physical activity maintenance (65,82), and in one case more so than adoption (96). When self-efficacy was looked at in college freshman it predicted participation in vigorous, but not moderate-intensity physical activity (27).

As already mentioned, SCT incorporates personal influences, cognitions, and environmental factors as variables that influence each other as well as influence behavior (81). Hofstetter et al. (40) investigated correlates of exercise self-efficacy to study the extent to which childhood experience with exercise would affect exercise self-efficacy later in life. They found that environmental variables (*e.g.*, barriers to exercise, the availability of home equipment, facilities), cognitive variables (*e.g.*, benefits and barriers, normative beliefs), and social variables (*e.g.*, social support) all influenced self-efficacy. Therefore, this research supports the notion that self-efficacy is malleable and can be influenced by additional factors, such as the context in which the individual is located.

McAuley et al. (64) conducted a study to examine the effect of walking and stretching on changes in self-efficacy in 184 previously sedentary older adults (mean age = 65.5 yr). Results indicated that there was no change in barriers for self-efficacy from baseline to month 2, but it declined at months 4 and 6. For exercise self-efficacy, there was a reported decline over the four time points (week 2, month 2, month 4, and month 6). It is interesting that efficacy cognitions declined in the context of an exercise intervention rather than increased. These results highlight the temporal relationship of self-efficacy and show that it can vary during the course of an exercise program. The authors conclude that it is important to target different sources of efficacy information (*e.g.*, one's beliefs about exercise, such as "I might become injured if I exercise"; or the barriers related to exercise, such as not having enough time or the weather, which might have implications for the long-term maintenance of physical activity). One area that may be important to target is assessing feelings of confidence and working to build self-efficacy at the end of a program to help individuals maintain their behavior changes. In a recent follow-up study conducted 5 yr following the start of this intervention, McCauley et al. (65) found self-efficacy at 2 yr to be an important predictor of physical activity at 5 yr. This study indicates that self-efficacy may be particularly important for long-term maintenance of physical activity. Similarly, in another study with cardiac and orthopedic rehabilitation participants, structural equation modeling found that self-efficacy for recovery and action planning predicted physical activity adherence after rehabilitation (82).

Several studies have created interventions that targeted social cognitive variables such as self-efficacy, social support, and environmental influences. One such program created a walking program for participants, in which walking leaders delivered a tailored, progressive approach based, in-part, on social cognitive principles that showed nice increase in physical activity (41).

Other examples of programs incorporating SCT (as well as TTM) have done so through non–face-to-face interventions using different delivery channels such as print materials and telephone calls (see also *Chapter 47*). These studies have effectively increased physical activity in adults (43,54,96). In addition to the importance of self-efficacy, two studies examining various SCT constructs suggest that self-efficacy may be an important influence on physical activity in as much as it influences self-regulatory skills (4,77).

Practice Implications

The research findings cited previously underscore the importance of helping clients make intermediate steps toward behavior change. Some of these intermediate steps include increasing social support, increasing self-efficacy, learning how to set goals, receiving feedback on performance and goal attainment, planning for physical activity, and having realistic expectations for behavior change.

Self-efficacy is a powerful component of SCT, and it can be influenced in two primary ways: progressive performance accomplishments and vicarious experience or modeling (9). Thus, one way for SCT to be applied to clinical practice is to assist clients in improving their self-efficacy. Someone who has had a cardiac event might learn to make exercise a part of his or her life by watching others like himself or herself, participate in cardiac rehabilitation (vicarious learning/modeling). Another way to help a person increase his or her self-efficacy is to set small goals and "try out" activities. Therefore, for someone who does not exercise, the strategy might be to have his or her begin to walk for 2 min at a time. As soon as this client begins to feel confident with the short duration of a walking bout, his or her self-efficacy is likely to increase, and then he or she might have the confidence to walk for an even longer distance. For someone who has had a cardiac event or injury, the concept of gaining confidence again might be particularly important so that they are not further derailed (82).

As someone increases their self-efficacy, this in turn, impacts his or her ability to perform the self-regulatory skills of goal setting and planning. The studies including self-regulatory skills (4,77) underscore the importance in targeting self-regulations skills in addition to self-efficacy. Guiding an individual to learn how to set goals, monitor their progress, and plan for modifications when needed could be critical to adopting physical activity. Thus, developing easy-to-use tracking sheets so they can monitor their exercise over the week, setting goals, and reevaluating their goals can be incorporated into weekly sessions.

SOCIAL ECOLOGY AND ECOLOGICAL MODELS

Social ecology underscores the importance of the interaction between an individual behavior and his or her environment. Bronfenbrenner wrote extensively on this topic and described an "ecological paradigm" including a set of nested structures each within the other (16,17). King et al. (12,36,44,87,88) provide specific examples relating to physical activity. *Intrapersonal* (within the individual) *factors* include mood, self-efficacy, and expectancies. Surrounding each individual, there are three levels of factors: (a) *microsystem* (*i.e.*, family, school, work site), (b) *mesosystem* (*i.e.*, reciprocal communication between parent and teacher), and (c) *macrosystem* (*i.e.*, urban design, land use, neighborhood disorder) (12,36,44,87,88). Social ecological models are relevant to physical activity promotion and form a cohesive conceptual approach for this area. These models emphasize multiple influences on behavior, such as sociocultural factors, and suggest that the most successful programs are the ones that combine and target these multiple influences on behavior. *Figure 44-2* is a representation of this model.

Research Findings

Later in this chapter, we describe examples of two studies that were designed to specifically target social ecological factors for promoting physical activity (22,31). The first study was designed to target environmental and peer influences on physical activity (22). Examples of intervention target included community awareness campaigns, walking clubs, and safe walking routes. This study found positive changes in physical activity behavior, with 30.6% of members of the target community becoming more physically active versus 18.3% of individuals in a comparison community. The second study (31) used both the ecological model as well as protection motivation theory to inform the intervention for "CardiACTION," which was an exercise promotion study for at-risk cardiac patients. The intervention targets addressed — both environmental factors and intrapersonal factors, such as self-regulation. Environmental targets followed the social ecological framework and included enhancing an individual's microenvironment context (e.g., providing free access to a fitness facility) and mesoenvironment (e.g., increasing awareness of environmental supports for activity such as a walking path in one's neighborhood). Study results are not yet available but will provide important information about the ways to address the socioecological context in which individuals live.

Vrazel, Saunders, and Wilcox reviewed 43 (25 quantitative and 18 qualitative) studies to highlight themes corresponding to three levels of the social environment

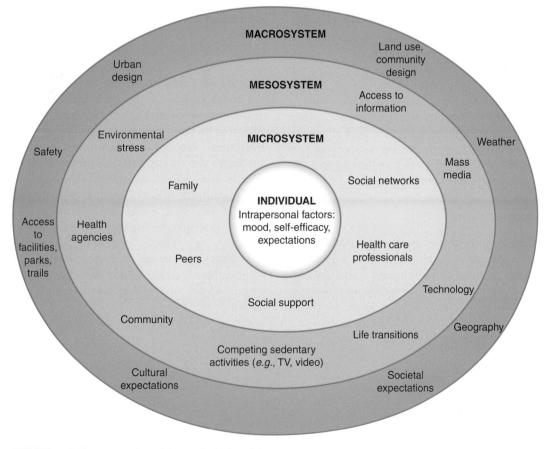

FIGURE 44-2. Representation of the ecological model.

as described by Bronfenbrenner (16,17): the microsystem (*e.g.*, social support and social networks), the mesosystem (*e.g.*, multiple roles and life transitions), and the macrosystem (*e.g.*, cultural standards and societal expectations). Social support and social networks included emotional and tangible support (*i.e.*, child care) and informational support (*i.e.*, having information relevant for women). Multiple roles and life transitions included greater responsibilities because of changing roles, life transitions, and reduced time caused by increased demands. Lastly, cultural standards and societal expectations were a theme for women as they reported (a) feeling guilty for taking time to be physically active, (b) concerns about the cultural appropriateness of engaging in certain types of activities, and (c) lack of active female role models. Each of these different factors has implications for the design and implementation of future physical activity interventions (93), and future interventions based on the social ecological framework are needed that are directly tailored to meet the needs of the women and others in population who are not physically active.

The social ecological model also has implications for understanding school-based physical activity (47). A qualitative study used this model to provide insight on school-based physical activity. Findings suggest that within schools, there are multiple levels of interactions among higher level policies, communities and schools that need to be better understood in relation to providing physical activity programming in schools. For example, policies regarding resource allocation are influenced by societal norms, school-board values, and teachers. As articulated by the participants, schools experience pressure for providing physical activity and health-based opportunities; however, academic achievement is the marker to which they are held accountable, which creates a difficult decision regarding the best allocation of resources. More research is needed in applying this model to assist in developing and evaluating school-based physical activity promotion programs.

Practice Implications

Understanding an individual's social and physical environment is important to better assist them in making behavior change. Aspects of both the social environment (social support, connectedness), as well as the interplay between social and environmental factors can impede as well as assist the adoption of physical activity. For example, if an individual lives within an unsafe area, in which he or she does not feel comfortable walking alone and does not have a "walking buddy," it will be unlikely that he or she will walk outside. Furthermore, if an individual does not have the self-efficacy or confidence that he or she is capable of walking or is embarrassed to be seen trying a new activity within one's neighborhood, this can have a detrimental effect on activity. As clinicians and health care professionals, it is important to assess and understand these factors so that you can best help them toward maximizing their activity. For instance, many people might not recognize that their social and physical environments can function as a facilitator or a barrier to making behavior changes. Therefore, it may be helpful to point out ways that individuals can work within their social structures, such as finding social support to walk in a neighborhood, in a community center, or other safe location within their community.

THE THEORY OF REASONED ACTION AND THEORY OF PLANNED BEHAVIOR

For the purposes of this chapter, the theory of reasoned action (TRA) and theory of planned behavior (TPB) will be combined into one section. The TRA was developed to understand and predict an individual's behavior (32,33); such behavior must be clearly specified, volitional in nature, and performed in a specific situation. According to the TRA, *intention* is the sole and immediate predictor of behavior (32), and intention mediates the effect of attitude toward the behavior and the beliefs about the consequences of the behavior (3,37). The theory of planned behavior (TPB) (49) is an extension of the TRA that includes *perceived behavioral control* as a third exogenous variable. Perceived behavioral control is similar to the concept of self-efficacy (9,11) because it reflects one's belief as to the likelihood of difficulty to be encountered when adopting a particular behavior and the perceived availability of resources and opportunities that may be beneficial in adopting a particular behavior. The methods for helping clients improve their self-efficacy are similar to those that could be used for helping them increase their sense of perceived behavioral control. *Figure 44-3* is a representation of this model.

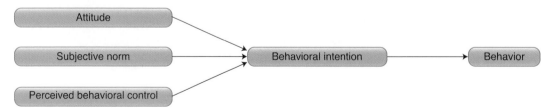

FIGURE 44-3. Representation of the theory of planned behavior.

Research Findings

There has been limited support of the TRA when applied to physical activity (35,80,89). It has been found that the basic variables in this model only account for a fraction of the variance in exercise behavior (35). Also, the TRA has been found to be most useful (1,2) when behaviors are completely under volitional control, meaning no practical constraints or barriers to executing the behavior are present. Research has indicated that the inclusion of perceived behavioral control as an exogenous variable enhances the prediction of intentions and target behaviors (49). Results of previous studies (e.g., [28]) have indicated mixed findings with respect to the usefulness of the TRA or TPB in the area of intervening on exercise behaviors; however, more recent studies (23,28,74) have found greater research applicability of components of these models. A meta-analytic review of 111 exercise studies using the TRA/TPB was conducted (29) to examine the strength of influences of the specific components of the TRA/TPB with exercise behavior. First, this meta-analysis revealed that intention was the strongest predictor of exercise behavior, which is consistent with the TRA/TPB, and other theories (e.g., TTM) as well. Second, perceived behavioral control does not add unique contribution to exercise behavior. Third, attitude is the strongest determinant of exercise intention. Fourth, the intention-behavior relationship was strongest in studies with short-term follow-ups (<1 mo) versus those with longer term follow-ups. Finally, the intention–behavior relationship was strongest for younger (18–25 yr) and older (65–80 yr) adults compared with adults 26–64 yr and children/adolescents. Overall, the utility of the model may be limited when each component is dissected because of the limited scale correspondence among exercise studies. In order to improve the predictive utility of the TRA/TPB, it is important that researchers focus on the measurement issues and aim to examine all the variables (action, target, context, and time) related to the intention-behavior relationship.

In summary, components of the TRA and TPB have provided some theoretical information for understanding health behaviors, such as exercise, and the postulated relationships between the variables have been supported (29,37,39). The theories, however, are limited in their applicability to interventions related to physical activity behavior. Current research has indicated that other factors, such as personal beliefs, attitudes, and ethnicity need to be considered when applying these theories to physical activity interventions (6,14,24,28,42,91). Results from the meta-analysis (29) support the relationship between intention and exercise behavior. Intentions may be an important prerequisite for exercise adoption, but they are not solely sufficient for predicting regular physical activity. In summary, the TRA and TPB intuitively have some merit but have limitations in their application for the field of exercise adoption and maintenance.

Practice Applications

Components of the TRA/TPB may be useful for assisting clients in making changes in their physical activity. The first step in helping a client make a behavior change is to typically understand the framework under which the individual is operating. For example, it is helpful to understand clients' attitudes toward physical activity, the value that they and other people in their lives place on physical activity, and their sense or belief that they have control over the behavior. Discovering the clients' attitudes, values, and beliefs can help determine their motivation to exercise. It is possible that a client may hold certain beliefs toward exercise (e.g., "I have never been athletic, so I can't exercise") or their family members may not understand the importance of being physically active and, therefore, not value it, which may negatively affect your client. Previous experiences with exercise, positive or negative, also impact a client's willingness to begin and maintain an exercise program. By assessing these factors initially, the practitioner can help anticipate potential barriers and help the client problem solve to address those barriers.

Therefore, the role of the practitioner is to first identify the potential barriers that each individual client may have and then formulate strategies of overcoming them. Clients could be encouraged to think about the realistic barriers they might encounter when making behavior changes and about the resources available to them for helping overcome those barriers. An example is a client who thinks he or she does not have a safe place to exercise. The practitioner could help the client think about other options for overcoming this barrier, including finding a walking "buddy," finding a mall in which to walk indoors, or finding other locations (e.g., a YMCA). Another common perceived barrier to exercise is lack of time, which clients may consider to be out of their control. The practitioner could help clients overcome this by asking them to make a schedule of a sample day that is considered to be busy for them. Identify the time gaps when the client could exercise, even if it is only 10–15 min at a time. This can help the client to prioritize the day in order to plan for exercise. The goal is to have the clients believe that exercise is a behavior that is under their volitional control.

Once the perceived barriers are identified, then the focus should be shifted to emphasize the benefits of exercise. Drawing attention to the positive outcomes of exercise will likely contribute to the client forming a more positive attitude. For example, some clients may decide that a benefit of exercise is to socialize with friends, whereas other clients may highlight the health benefits of exercise as a primary reason for participation.

Another strategy that a practitioner could use is to make a decisional balance sheet of the benefits/barriers to exercise. This way, the clients can see written on paper their personal reasons why they should exercise. This can help clients to conclude that the benefits outweigh the barriers, as defined by personal importance, not simply determined by the quantity of reasons. Giving clients the responsibility and accountability of making their decisions about why they should exercise will make it more likely that they will maintain a positive attitude about exercise, and therefore continue to participate. With the focus on the positive aspects, or benefits of exercise, the clients are more likely to adopt exercise. It is important to individualize the goals and desired behavioral outcomes based on each client's beliefs and attitudes.

Allowing the client to identify the benefits and barriers of exercise would not only highlight the importance of physical activity for their physical and mental well-being, but it would also allow the clients to take ownership of their exercise program which may also increase their self-efficacy. By encouraging them to conceptualize the benefits and barriers of exercise, this can create realistic and controllable beliefs about incorporating exercise in their daily lives.

RELAPSE PREVENTION

The RP model was developed to help understand relapse behavior in individuals who were seeking to remain abstinent from a negative health behavior (*e.g.*, smoking, drinking) (62). However, the components of the RP model can be applied to other health behaviors, such as at the beginning of a physical activity program. The overall goal of RP is to assist individuals in maintaining long-term behavior change by anticipating potentially high-risk situations and devising strategies to cope with these high-risk situations (57,62). The RP model is a combination of behavioral skills training, cognitive intervention, and lifestyle change. Therefore, it is an important model for use with physical activity behavior maintenance. The RP model makes two very important distinctions in defining the terms *lapse* and *relapse*. Whereas *lapse* is defined as a slight error or slip (*e.g.*, missing one exercise session), *relapse* is a return to former behavior patterns (*e.g.*, not being physically active for an extended period of time).

The RP model cautions against viewing behavior change as either a complete success or a complete failure. This dichotomous approach ignores the potential influence of situational and psychological factors as determinants in relapse and reinforces the idea that someone who experiences a relapse lacks personal control (62). Furthermore, establishing the dichotomy of success (*e.g.*, exercising 5 d · wk^{-1} for 30 min each time) or failure (*e.g.*, not exercising at all) can also set up an individual

for an "abstinence violation effect," which is one's tendency to give up if even a small slip has occurred. For instance, if someone has missed his or her exercise sessions for the week because of work demands, he or she may think, "Why should I bother now? I am already out of my routine." Instead, the RP model encourages people to view a lapse as a "fork in the road" (62) that could either lead back to successful behavior maintenance or a return to earlier behavior patterns. For example, someone would be using RP strategies if he or she thought in advance about a high-risk situation such as a vacation and devised a plan for exercising during the vacation (*i.e.*, locating a walking path near the hotel).

Research Findings

Although many experts cite the importance of RP strategies for helping individuals maintain behavior changes, little research has focused specifically on RP for physical activity. A large body of literature focuses on RP for weight loss (15,83); however, for physical activity, the focus on RP tends to be incorporated with a variety of other strategies (68,92). One study investigated the use of RP to promote exercise adherence among 120 women who were previously sedentary (61). In this study, subjects were randomly assigned to either a control group or one of two experimental groups (RP or reinforcement/lottery); all groups participated in an 18-wk exercise program. The RP group consisted of focusing on potential high-risk situations, developing coping responses, and using a planned relapse. The reinforcement group consisted of rewarding participants for consistent attendance. Results indicated that compared with the control group, the RP group attended significantly more sessions during the first 9 wk of the program; the reinforcement group was not significantly different from the control group. However, by 18 wk and at the 2-mo posttreatment assessment, there were no differences between the groups. Marcus and Stanton (61) cite some potential considerations when examining the RP approach for physical activity. They state that factors such as the convenience of class schedule, group cohesion, and the strength of the intervention may have been mitigating factors to help explain the lack of longer term efficacy of the RP approach.

One study examined RP strategies among 65 long-term exercisers who identified high-risk situations as bad weather, inconvenient time of day, being alone, negative emotions, and being tired (86). Positive cognitive coping strategies, such as problem solving and positive reappraisal, were employed by 43% of the sample; the positive behavioral coping strategy of having a preexercise ritual was used by 22% of the men, but only 3% of the women. These findings have implications for practice and the suggestion of ways of coping with different types of high-risk situations.

Research has shown a relationship between self-efficacy and RP, such that high levels of self-efficacy were related to high levels of planning (48). A systematic review of physical activity intervention studies examined techniques for changing both physical activity behavior and self-efficacy (95). This review identified 27 studies that reported both self-efficacy and physical activity intervention data. Of note relative to RP was that lower self-efficacy and physical activity behavior levels were found when studies reported using RP as a strategy. This result must be interpreted with caution, however, as neither of the studies reported in this review targeted the RP model as the primary focus nor were there details provided about how the RP coping skills were taught. Many studies may use the term "to prevent relapse" but do not provide adequate coping skills training or problem solving training for planning to prevent slips. Additionally, those who may be at high risk for relapse (i.e., those with low-self efficacy) may be the ones who were given additional RP training; thus, the relationship may not be related to RP per se but related to low self-efficacy or other barriers.

Practice Implications

RP is an important aspect of any behavior change program. Marlatt and Gordon (62) stress the importance of establishing a collaborative relationship with the client and focusing on using a few techniques at a time rather than trying to incorporate all techniques at once. The research of Marcus and Stanton (61) provide an excellent framework for practitioners who are working with clients trying to maintain physical activity behavior change. The RP model has a series of strategies that can be used by clients to learn how to anticipate and cope with the possibility of relapse. In the study conducted by Nies et al. (68), women were asked to identify what they could do to prevent a relapse in their walking program and to consider the use of social support, cognitive restructuring, and identifying personal benefits as potential strategies. The first step in RP helps clients reflect on the importance of regular exercise and the importance of being flexible in their thinking regarding the need to miss a session, if necessary. In addition, the next phase is to work with clients to help them identify situations in which they were able to successfully overcome a potential barrier and the challenges faced when they were not successful. Reflecting on a situation in which the client was successful can help them understand that they have a skill set, or a "toolbox" of skills, that they have successfully engaged in the past.

Next, it is important to teach clients how to identify high-risk situations that may trigger a relapse. It may be helpful in this step to identify some examples of potential relapse situations, which can be combined into two main categories: intrapersonal and interpersonal (79). Examples of intrapersonal determinants include negative emotional states, negative physical states, and positive emotional states. Interpersonal determinants include social pressure and interpersonal conflict. One intrapersonal state that tends to be common is stress. Clients who have difficulty managing stress should be encouraged to take a walk or do some other physical activity. Even if the client only has 10 min between scheduled meetings during a busy day, a brisk walk can help clear the mind, provide some relaxation, and reduce stress. An interpersonal state that clients might identify is having many demands on their time and feeling unable to devote the time to being physically active. One suggestion that might assist clients with these types of high-risk situations is to see if the client might be able to fit in shorter bouts of activity (e.g., 10 min in length three times a day) rather than trying to block out a full 30 min each day. By dividing the time into smaller bouts, this can help clients feel like they have more control over ways to "fit in" the activity.

After identifying high-risk situations, the next step is to anticipate those situations and problem solve around effective coping strategies. Using the example previously, you might suggest to a client who has multiple demands that if he or she is feeling unsure about how to fit in physical activity that he or she can try to do 10 min first thing in the morning, 10 min at lunch, and 10 min right after dinner. By dividing a longer bout into smaller pieces, this can be an effective coping strategy to address a potential high-risk situation and avoid a relapse.

SUMMARY

This chapter has provided an overview of the theories of behavior change that have been applied most successfully to physical activity. This information should be useful for identifying and understanding the factors that influence the complicated process through which individuals decide to begin and maintain a physical activity program. This chapter has provided several theoretical frameworks for understanding the strategies and skills associated with adopting a new behavior such as physical activity and identifying ways to foster maintenance help individuals avoid relapse. As theories are tested through research, scientists and practitioners gain greater understanding of behavior change and provide an evidence-based foundation for application of the concepts derived from theory. The information provided in this chapter should serve as a reference point for practitioners as they assist clients to become and stay physically active to live a healthier lifestyle and prevent disease.

REFERENCES

1. Ajzen I. *Attitudes, Personality, and Behavior*. U.S. ed. Chicago (IL): Dorsey Press; 1988. 175 p.
2. Ajzen I. From intentions to actions: a theory of planned behavior. In: Kuhl J, Beckmann J, editors. *Action Control, from Cognition to Behavior*. New York: Springer-Verlag; 1985. p. 11–39.

3. Ajzen I, Fishbein M. *Understanding Attitudes and Predicting Social Behavior*. Englewood Cliffs, NJ: Prentice-Hall; 1980. 278 p.

4. Anderson ES, Wojcik JR, Winett RA, Williams DM. Social-cognitive determinants of physical activity: the influence of social support, self-efficacy, outcome expectations, and self-regulation among participants in a church-based health promotion study. *Health Psychol*. 2006;25(4):510–20.

5. Annesi JJ, Unruh JL, Marti CN, Gorjala S, Tennant G. Effects of the coach approach intervention on adherence to exercise in obese women: assessing mediation of social cognitive theory factors. *Res Q Exerc Sport*. 2011;82(1):99–108.

6. Armitage CJ. Can the theory of planned behavior predict the maintenance of physical activity? *Health Psychol*. 2005;24(3):235–45.

7. Bandura A. Exercise of personal agency through the self-efficacy mechanism. In: Schwarzer R, editor. *Self-Efficacy: Thought Control of Action*. Washington: Hemisphere Publishing; 1992. p. 3–38.

8. Bandura A. *Self-Efficacy: The Exercise of Control*. New York (NY): W.H. Freeman; 1997. 604 p.

9. Bandura A. Self-efficacy: toward a unifying theory of behavioral change. *Psychol Rev*. 1977;84(2):191–215.

10. Bandura A. *Social Foundations of Thought and Action: A Social Cognitive Theory*. Englewood Cliffs (NJ): Prentice-Hall; 1986. 617 p.

11. Bandura A. *Social Learning Theory*. Englewood Cliffs (NJ): Prentice Hall; 1977. 247 p.

12. Baranowski T, Cullen KW, Nicklas T, Thompson D, Baranowski J. Are current health behavioral change models helpful in guiding prevention of weight gain efforts? *Obes Res*. 2003;11 Suppl: 23S–43S.

13. Biddle SJH, Nigg NR. Theories of exercise behavior. *Int J Sport Psychol*. 2000;31(2):290–304.

14. Blanchard C, Fisher J, Sparling P, et al. Understanding physical activity behavior in African American and Caucasian college students: an application of the theory of planned behavior. *J Am Coll Health*. 2008;56(4):341–6.

15. Bray SR. Self-efficacy for coping with barriers helps students stay physically active during transition to their first year at a university. *Res Q Exerc Sport*. 2007;78(2):61–70.

16. Bronfenbrenner U. Developmental ecology through space and time: a future perspective. In: Moen P, Elder GH, editors. *Perspectives on the Ecology of Human Development*. Washington: American Psychological Association; 1995. p. 619–647.

17. Bronfenbrenner U. Ecological models of human development. In: *International Encyclopedia of Education*. 2nd ed. Oxford: Elsevier Sciences; 1994. p. 1643–1647.

18. Brownell KD, O'Neil PM. Obesity. In: Barlow DH, editor. *Clinical Handbook of Psychological Disorders: A Step-by-Step Treatment Manual*. 2nd ed. New York: Guilford Press; 1993. p. 318–361.

19. Cao D, Xie G. From intention to health behavior: an overview on health action process approach. *Chinese J Clin Psychol*. 2010;18(6): 809–12.

20. Caudroit J, Stephan Y, Le Scanff C. Social cognitive determinants of physical activity among retired older individuals: an application of the health action process approach. *Br J Health Psychol*. 2011;16(2):404–17.

21. Chatzisarantis NLD, Hagger MS. Effects of an intervention based on self-determination theory on self-reported leisure-time physical activity participation. *Psychol Health*. 2009;24(1):29–48.

22. Cochrane T, Davey RC. Increasing uptake of physical activity: a social ecological approach. *J R Soc Promot Health*. 2008;128(1): 31–40.

23. Conner M, Sandberg T, Norman P. Using action planning to promote exercise behavior. *Ann Behav Med*. 2010;40(1):65–76.

24. Darker CD, French DP, Eves FF, Sniehotta FF. An intervention to promote walking amongst the general population based on an 'extended' theory of planned behaviour: a waiting list randomised controlled trial. *Psychol Health*. 2010;25(1):71–88.

25. Deci EL, Ryan RM. *Intrinsic Motivation and Self-Determination in Human Behavior*. New York (NY): Plenum; 1985. 371 p.

26. DiClemente RJ, Crosby RA, Kegler MC, editors. *Emerging Theories in Health Promotion Practice and Research*. 2nd ed. San Francisco (CA): Jossey-Bass; 2009. 624 p.

27. Doerksen SE, Umstattd MR, McAuley E. Social cognitive determinants of moderate and vigorous physical activity in college freshmen. *J Appl Soc Psychol*. 2009;39(5):1201–13.

28. Downs DS. Understanding exercise intention in an ethnically diverse sample of postpartum women. *J Sport Exercise Psychol*. 2006;28(2):159–70.

29. Downs DS, Hausenblas HA. The theories of reasoned action and planned behavior applied to exercise: a meta-analytic update. *J Phys Act Health*. 2005;2(1):76–97.

30. Dunn AL, Marcus BH, Kampert JB, Garcia ME, Kohl HW,3rd, Blair SN. Reduction in cardiovascular disease risk factors: 6-month results from Project Active. *Prev Med*. 1997;26(6):883–92.

31. Estabrooks PA, Glasgow RE, Xu S, et al. Building a multiple modality, theory-based physical activity intervention: the development of CardiACTION. *Psychol Sport Exerc*. 2011;12(1):46–53.

32. Fishbein M. A theory of reasoned action: some applications and implications. *Nebr Symp Motiv*. 1980;27:65–116.

33. Fishbein M, Ajzen I, Joint Author. *Belief, Attitude, Intention, and Behavior: An Introduction to Theory and Research*. Reading (MA): Addison-Wesley Pub. Co; 1975. 578 p.

34. Foster C, Hillsdon M, Thorogood M. Interventions for promoting physical activity. *Cochrane Database Syst Rev*. 2009;(1):CD003180.

35. Godin G. Theories of reasoned action and planned behavior: usefulness for exercise promotion. *Med Sci Sports Exerc*. 1994;26(11): 1391–4.

36. Grzywacz JG, Fuqua J. The social ecology of health: leverage points and linkages. *Behav Med*. 2000;26(3):101.

37. Hagger MS, Chatzisarantis NLD, Biddle SJH. A meta-analytic review of the theories of reasoned action and planned behavior in physical activity: predictive validity and the contribution of additional variables. *J Sport Exercise Psychol*. 2002;24(1):3–32.

38. Haskell WL, Lee I, Pate RR, et al. Physical activity and public health: updated recommendation for adults from the American College of Sports Medicine and the American Heart Association. *Circulation*. 2007;116(9):1081–93.

39. Hausenblas HA, Carron AV, Mack DE. Application of the theories of reasoned action and planned behavior to exercise behavior: a meta-analysis. *J Sport Exercise Psychol*. 1997;19(1):36–51.

40. Hofstetter CR, Hovell MF, Sallis JF. Social learning correlates of exercise self-efficacy: early experiences with physical activity. *Soc Sci Med*. 1990;31(10):1169–76.

41. Jancey JM, Clarke A, Howat PA, Lee AH, Shilton T, Fisher J. A Physical activity program to mobilize older people: a practical and sustainable approach. *Gerontologist*. 2008;48(2):251–7.

42. Jung T, Heald GR. The effects of discriminate message interventions on behavioral intentions to engage in physical activities. *J Am Coll Health*. 2009;57(5):527–35.

43. King AC, Friedman R, Marcus B, et al. Ongoing physical activity advice by humans versus computers: the Community Health Advice by Telephone (CHAT) Trial. *Health Psychol*. 2007;26(6): 718–27.

44. King AC, Stokols D, Talen E, Brassington GS, Killingsworth R. Theoretical approaches to the promotion of physical activity: forging a transdisciplinary paradigm. *Am J Prev Med*. 2002;23(2): 15–25.

45. Kinzie MB. Instructional design strategies for health behavior change. *Patient Educ Couns*. 2005;56(1):3–15.

46. Kreuter MW, Skinner CS. Tailoring: what's in a name? *Health Educ Res*. 2000;15(1):1–4.

47. Langille JD, Rodgers WM. Exploring the influence of a social ecological model on school-based physical activity. *Health Educ Behav*. 2010;37(6):879–94.

48. Luszczynska A, Schwarzer R, Lippke S, Mazurkiewicz M. Self-efficacy as a moderator of the planning-behaviour relationship in interventions designed to promote physical activity. *Psychol Health.* 2011;26(2):151–66.

49. Madden TJ, Ellen PS, Ajzen I. A comparison of the theory of planned behavior and the theory of reasoned action. *Person Soc Psychol Bull.* 1992;18(1):3–9.

50. Maddux JE. *Self-Efficacy, Adaptation, and Adjustment: Theory, Research, and Application.* New York (NY): Plenum Press; 1995. 395 p.

51. Maibach EW, Cotton D. Moving people to behavior change: a staged social cognitive approach to message design. In: Maibach E, Parrott R, editors. *Designing Health Messages: Approaches from Communication Theory and Public Health Practice.* Thousand Oaks (CA): Sage Publications; 1995. p. 41–64.

52. Marcus BH, Emmons KM, Simkin-Silverman LR, et al. Evaluation of motivationally tailored vs. standard self-help physical activity interventions at the workplace. *Am J Health Promot.* 1998;12(4):246–53.

53. Marcus B, Forsyth L. *Motivating People to Be Physically Active.* 2nd ed. Champaign (IL): Human Kinetics; 2009. 200 p.

54. Marcus BH, Lewis BA, Williams DM, et al. Step into motion: a randomized trial examining the relative efficacy of Internet vs. print-based physical activity interventions. *Contemp Clin Trials.* 2007;28(6):737–47.

55. Marcus BH, Nigg CR, Riebe D, Forsyth LH. Interactive communication strategies: implications for population-based physical-activity promotion. *Am J Prev Med.* 2000;19(2):121–6.

56. Marcus BH, Owen N. Motivational readiness, self-efficacy and decision-making for exercise. *J Appl Soc Psychol.* 1992;22(1):3–16.

57. Marcus BH, Rakowski W, Rossi JS. Assessing motivational readiness and decision making for exercise. *Health Psychol.* 1992; 11(4):257–61.

58. Marcus BH, Rossi JS, Selby VC, Niaura RS, Abrams DB. The stages and processes of exercise adoption and maintenance in a worksite sample. *Health Psychol.* 1992;11(6):386–95.

59. Marcus BH, Selby VC, Niaura RS, Rossi JS. Self-efficacy and the stages of exercise behavior change. *Res Q Exerc Sport.* 1992;63(1): 60–6.

60. Marcus BH, Simkin LR. The stages of exercise behavior. *J Sports Med Phys Fitness.* 1993;33(1):83–8.

61. Marcus BH, Stanton AL. Evaluation of relapse prevention and reinforcement interventions to promote exercise adherence in sedentary females. *Res Q Exerc Sport.* 1993;64(4):447–52.

62. Marlatt GA, Gordon JR. *Relapse Prevention: Maintenance Strategies in the Treatment of Addictive Behaviors.* New York (NY): Guilford Press; 1985. 558 p.

63. Marshall SJ, Biddle SJ. The transtheoretical model of behavior change: a meta-analysis of applications to physical activity and exercise. *Ann Behav Med.* 2001;23(4):229–46.

64. McAuley E, Jerome GJ, Marquez DX, Elavsky S, Blissmer B. Exercise self-efficacy in older adults: social, affective, and behavioral influences. *Ann Behav Med.* 2003;25(1):1–7.

65. McAuley E, Morris KS, Motl RW, Hu L, Konopack JF, Elavsky S. Long-term follow-up of physical activity behavior in older adults. *Health Psychol.* 2007;26(3):375–80.

66. Michie S, Abraham C, Whittington C, McAteer J, Gupta S. Effective techniques in healthy eating and physical activity interventions: a meta-regression. *Health Psychol.* 2009;28(6):690–701.

67. Neville LM, O'Hara B, Milat A. Computer-tailored physical activity behavior change interventions targeting adults: a systematic review. *Int J Behav Nutr Phys Act.* 2009;6:30.

68. Nies MA, Reisenberg CE, Chruscial HL, Artibee K. Southern women's response to a walking intervention. *Public Health Nurs.* 2003;20(2):146–52.

69. Nigg CR, Geller KS, Motl RW, Horwath CC, Wertin KK, Dishman RK. A research agenda to examine the efficacy and relevance of the transtheoretical model for physical activity behavior. *Psychol Sport Exerc.* 2011;12(1):7–12.

70. Nothwehr F, Yang J. Goal setting frequency and the use of behavioral strategies related to diet and physical activity. *Health Educ Res.* 2007;22(4):532–8.

71. Parker PD, Martin AJ, Martinez C, Marsh HW, Jackson SA. Stages of change in physical activity: a validation study in late adolescence. *Health Educ Behav.* 2010;37(3):318–29.

72. Pate RR, Pratt M, Blair SN, et al. Physical activity and public health. A recommendation from the Centers for Disease Control and Prevention and the American College of Sports Medicine. *JAMA.* 1995;273(5):402–7.

73. Plotnikoff RC, Brunet S, Courneya KS, et al. The efficacy of stage-matched and standard public health materials for promoting physical activity in the workplace: the Physical Activity Workplace Study (PAWS). *Am J Health Promot.* 2007;21(6): 501–9.

74. Presseau J, Sniehotta FF, Francis JJ, Gebhardt WA. With a little help from my goals: integrating intergoal facilitation with the theory of planned behaviour to predict physical activity. *Br J Health Psychol.* 2010;15(4):905–19.

75. Prochaska JO, DiClemente CC. Stages and processes of self-change of smoking: toward an integrative model of change. *J Consult Clin Psychol.* 1983;51(3):390–5.

76. Rhodes RE, Pfaeffli LA. Mediators of physical activity behaviour change among adult non-clinical populations: a review update. *Int J Behav Nutr Phys Act.* 2010;7:37.

77. Rovniak LS, Anderson ES, Winett RA, Stephens RS. Social cognitive determinants of physical activity in young adults: a prospective structural equation analysis. *Ann Behav Med.* 2002;24(2):149.

78. Ryan RM, Deci EL. Self-determination theory and the facilitation of intrinsic motivation, social development, and well-being. *Am Psychol.* 2000;55(1):68–78.

79. Sallis JF, Owen N. Ecological models of health behavior. In: Glanz K, Rimer BK, Lewis FM, editors. *Health Behavior and Health Education: Theory, Research, and Practice.* 3rd ed. San Francisco: Jossey-Bass; 2002. p. 462–484.

80. Sallis JF, Owen N. *Physical Activity & Behavioral Medicine.* Thousand Oaks (CA): Sage Publications; 1999. 210 p.

81. Schwarzer R. Self-efficacy in the adoption and maintenance of health behaviors: theoretical approaches and a new model. In: Schwarzer R, editor. *Self-Efficacy: Thought Control of Action.* Washington: Hemisphere Publishing; 1992. p. 218–242.

82. Schwarzer R, Luszczynska A, Ziegelmann JP, Scholz U, Lippke S. Social-cognitive predictors of physical exercise adherence: three longitudinal studies in rehabilitation. *Health Psychol.* 2008;27(1): S54–63.

83. Sherwood NE, Crain AL, Martinson BC, et al. Keep it off: a phone-based intervention for long-term weight-loss maintenance. *Contemp Clin Trials.* 2011;32(4):551–60.

84. Silva M, Vieira P, Coutinho S, et al. Using self-determination theory to promote physical activity and weight control: a randomized controlled trial in women. *J Behav Med.* 2010;33(2):110–22.

85. Spencer L, Adams TB, Malone S, Roy L, Yost E. Applying the transtheoretical model to exercise: a systematic and comprehensive review of the literature. *Health Promot Pract.* 2006;7(4): 428–43.

86. Stetson BA, Beacham AO, Frommelt SJ, et al. Exercise slips in high-risk situations and activity patterns in long-term exercisers: an application of the relapse prevention model. *Ann Behav Med.* 2005;30(1):25–35.

87. Stokols D. Establishing and maintaining healthy environments. Toward a social ecology of health promotion. *Am Psychol.* 1992; 47(1):6–22.

88. Stokols D. Social ecology and behavioral medicine: implications for training, practice, and policy. *Behav Med.* 2000;26(3):129.

89. Trost SG, Owen N, Bauman AE, Sallis JF, Brown W. Correlates of adults' participation in physical activity: review and update. *Med Sci Sports Exerc.* 2002;34(12):1996–2001.

90. U.S. Department of Health and Human Services, Centers for Disease Control and Prevention, National Center for Chronic Disease Prevention and Health Promotion, The President's Council on Physical Fitness and Sports. *Physical Activity and Health: A Report of the Surgeon General*. Atlanta (GA): President's Council on Physical Fitness and Sports; 1996. 278 p.

91. Vallance JKH, Courneya KS, Plotnikoff RC, Mackey JR. Analyzing theoretical mechanisms of physical activity behavior change in breast cancer survivors: results from the activity promotion (ACTION) Trial. *Ann Behav Med*. 2008;35(2):150–8.

92. Vickers KS, Nies MA, Patten CA, Dierkhising R, Smith SA. Patients with diabetes and depression may need additional support for exercise. *Am J Health Behav*. 2006;30(4):353–62.

93. Vrazel J, Saunders RP, Wilcox S. An overview and proposed framework of social-environmental influences on the physical-activity behavior of women. *Am J Health Promot*. 2008;23(1):2–12.

94. Whitely JA, Lewis BA, Napolitano MA, Marcus BH. Health behavior counseling skills. In: Ehrman JK, editor. *ACSM's Resource Manual for Guidelines for Exercise Testing and Prescription*. 6th ed. Philadelphia (PA): Lippincott Williams & Wilkins; 2009. p. 723–733.

95. Williams SL, French DP. What are the most effective intervention techniques for changing physical activity self-efficacy and physical activity behaviour—and are they the same? *Health Educ Res*. 2011;26(2):308–22.

96. Williams DM, Papandonatos GD, Jennings EG, et al. Does tailoring on additional theoretical constructs enhance the efficacy of a print-based physical activity promotion intervention? *Health Psychol*. 2011;30(4):432–41.

SELECTED REFERENCES FOR FURTHER READING

King AC, Stokols D, Talen E, Brassington GS, Killingsworth R. Theoretical approaches to the promotion of physical activity: forging a transdisciplinary paradigm. *Am J Prev Med*. 2002;23(2):15–25.

Marcus B, Forsyth L. *Motivating People to be Physically Active*. 2nd ed. Champaign (IL): Human Kinetics; 2009. 200 p.

Doshi A, Patrick K, Sallis JF, Calfas K. Evaluation of physical activity web sites for use of behavior change theories. *Ann Behav Med*. 2005;25:105–11.

Rhodes RE, Pfaeffli LA. Mediators of physical activity behavior change among adult non-clinical populations: a review update. *Int J Behav Nutr Phys Act*. 2010;7:37.

INTERNET RESOURCES

- Centers for Disease Control and Prevention. Understanding and promoting physical activity. In: *Physical Activity and Health*: http://www.cdc.gov/nccdphp/sgr/chap6.htm
- Edwards P. Evidence-based strategies for increasing participation in physical activity in community recreation, fitness and sport: http://www.lin.ca/Files/6703/mm83.htm
- Grizzell J. Behavior Change Theories and Models: http://www.csupomona.edu/~jvgrizzell/best_practices/bctheory.html
- Marcus BH, Lewis BA. Physical activity and the stages of motivational readiness for change model. *Research Digest*: http://www.fitness.gov/Reading_Room/Digests/march2003digest.pdf
- Sallis JF, Kerr J. Physical activity and the built environment. *Research Digest*: http://www.fitness.gov/digests/December2006Digest.pdf

Principles of Behavior Change: Skill Building to Promote Physical Activity

Sedentary lifestyles contribute to the leading causes of death in the United States (34) and the world (42). According to the World Health Organization (WHO), 60%–85% of the world's population receives insufficient physical activity. Physical inactivity is one of the most serious yet inadequately addressed public health problems and is a growing burden on the global economy (42). Sedentary lifestyles are in part caused by passive modes of transportation, sedentary occupational and domestic activities, and changes in leisure-time behaviors. Despite increased interest and support of regular physical activity and exercise, evidence indicates that close to half of Americans do not exercise regularly (*i.e.*, on 4 or more days per week), and one-fourth or more do not exercise at all (15,55). Of the 10% (or less) of initially sedentary adults who begin regular physical activity in a year, as many as 50% may drop out within 3–6 mo, and the recidivism rates are similar among those who were already active. Assisting individuals to stay

physically active is a challenge that requires creativity and patience.

Health behavior change theories and models have been applied in systematic attempts to change physical activity behavior, with varying results (57). There are several factors and practical skills necessary for increasing daily physical activity across a person's lifespan. This chapter provides general information on practical skills for physical activity behavior change and motivational considerations. These practical skills and motivational considerations focus on adoption, early adherence, maintenance, and relapse prevention with consideration of the different psychological and environmental determinants that influence intervention strategies. A summary of behavioral skills and strategies to promote physical activity is given in *Box 45-1*. Internet resources to assist the practitioner in implementing these strategies are presented in *Table 45-1*.

KEY TERMS

Intervention strategies: Any technique or approach that aims at enhancing physical activity participation; these strategies can span a range of domains from individual to policy level.

Physical activity: Any form of repetitive movement, typically involving large muscle groups, that results in energy expenditure.

Physical activity adherence: The percent of physical activity participation, derived by comparing the amount of physical activity engaged in (numerator) with the amount of physical activity recommended or prescribed (denominator).

Physical activity adoption: The initiation or initial increases in physical activity that often accompany an intervention or that can occur naturally by an individual.

Often, the adoption period is considered the initial 3–6 mo of an intervention or program, although there are no definitive or agreed-upon definitions of the length of this period. In fact, the length of the adoption period is likely to differ depending on the experiences and characteristics of the populations under study. Behavioral indicators of successful physical activity adoption are recommended over often arbitrarily set time periods.

Physical activity maintenance: Sustained physical activity participation that occurs over extended periods of time (*i.e.*, 1 yr or longer).

Physical activity participation: The amount of physical activity engaged in, including structured and unstructured (*e.g.*, routine) forms of physical activity.

BOX 45-1   **Behavioral Skills and Strategies to Promote Physical Activity**

- *Decisional balance*: Identify personal benefits of physical activity and evaluate barriers for change; use benefits for motivation and teach problem-solving skills for overcoming barriers.
- *Self-monitoring*: Record type of activity, intensity, minutes, and calories expended as well as sedentary behaviors, such as time spent sitting, watching television, or computer use. Use step counters, particularly for individuals who have not begun structured exercise or find it difficult to keep written logs.
- *Goal setting*: Set realistic short-term and long-term goals for physical activity behaviors. Goals should target specific behaviors, be measurable to monitor progress, be realistic, and occur in a reasonable time frame.

- *Commitment*: Make a commitment to healthy behaviors; use behavioral contracts and incentives to enhance motivation.
- *Social support*: Identify and enlist social support to allow participants to share concerns, gain knowledge, receive encouragement, and practice new behaviors. Identify potential saboteurs who could hinder physical activity efforts, then develop strategies and assertiveness skills to deal with them.
- *Stimulus control*: Recognize and control physical, psychological, environmental, and social cues for physical activity behaviors.
- *Relapse prevention*: Identify high-risk situations and plan for potential lapses in physical activity. Practice cognitive restructuring to overcome unhelpful or negative thought patterns (*e.g.*, all-or-none thinking).

PRACTICAL SKILLS FOR BEHAVIOR CHANGE

KNOWLEDGE, EXPECTATIONS, AND ATTITUDES

Understanding individuals' knowledge, expectations, and attitudes associated with physical activity can be helpful prior to initiating behavior change (24). Knowledge and past exercise experience will likely influence expectations and perceptions. A simple questionnaire or checklist regarding expectations can provide exercise professionals with early clues to individual expectations and areas for important problem solving and planning (37). It may also be helpful to assess and explore physical activity history, both recent and lifetime, as a method to better understand knowledge, expectations, and attitudes. This can be done using interviews, questionnaires, or personal timeline methods as part of formal or informal assessment.

DECISIONAL BALANCE

Discussing the actual and perceived advantages and disadvantages of new physical activity habits may help to (a) establish the reasons and motives for behavior change, (b) set specific goals and avoid future pitfalls, and (c) identify the activities and behaviors needed for adoption and maintenance. A decisional balance is at the core of many theoretical approaches designed to change or challenge current behaviors (*e.g.*, transtheoretical model [TTM]) (40). Advantages ("pros") can be emphasized for motivation, whereas identified disadvantages ("cons") can provide opportunities to learn more about the activity, tailor recommendations to individual

barriers, and assist in developing coping strategies or learning problem-solving skills. *Figure 45-1* presents a sample decisional balance worksheet.

Benefits

Although there are numerous physiological and psychological benefits to regular physical activity, it is worthwhile to consider the importance of each potential benefit as possible motivating factors for adopting and maintaining an effective exercise program (27). Considerations of personal relevance and priorities in evaluating benefits are important to tailor benefits to the individual.

Identified benefits of physical activity include the following:

- Decreases morbidity and mortality rates
- Reduces risk of developing diabetes, hypertension, colon cancer, and heart disease
- Helps control weight
- Promotes and maintain healthy bones, muscles, and joints
- Diminishes feelings of depression, anxiety, and general negative mood states
- Improves body image, self-esteem, and self-concept
- Enhances ability to perform activities of daily living (ADLs)
- Provides opportunities to develop social contacts and relationships with others

In general, the benefits include improved physiological health and physical fitness, enhanced physical appearance, improved psychological and emotional health and cognitive functioning, and enhanced social relations. Although people may acknowledge or experience multiple benefits

TABLE 45-1. Resources for Behavior Strategies

Strategy	Resource
Decisional balance: benefits and barriers of physical activity	• ACSM — Barriers to Exercise Assessment http://www.myexerciseplan.com/assessment/barriers.php • ACSM — Decisional Balance http://www.myexerciseplan.com/assessment/DecisionalBalance.pdf • Eat Smart, Move More NC — Barriers to Being Active http://www.eatsmartmovemorenc.com/NCHealthSmartTlkt/Texts/MM_AppM%20Barriers.pdf
Accessibility and convenience	• ACSM — Exercise Time Finder & Create A Ritual http://www.myexerciseplan.com/assessment/ExerciseTimeFinder.pdf • American Heart Association — MyStart! Walking Plan http://www.startwalkingnow.org/ • Environmental Supports for Physical Activity http://www.prevention.sph.sc.edu/tools/environmental.htm
Goal setting, rewards, and reinforcement	• ACSM — Self-Assessment http://www.myexerciseplan.com/assessment/SelfAssessment.pdf • CDC — Growing Stronger — Define Your Goals http://www.cdc.gov/physicalactivity/growingstronger/motivation/define.html • The President's Challenge http://www.presidentschallenge.org/index.shtml
Self-monitoring	• MyPyramidTracker http://www.mypyramidtracker.gov/Default.htm • 2008 Physical Activity Guidelines — Be Active Your Way http://www.health.gov/paguidelines/adultguide/keepingtrack.pdf • SparkPeople Tracker http://www.sparkpeople.com/myspark/start-now.asp
Self-management and problem solving	• ACSM — The Power of Positive Rituals http://www.myexerciseplan.com/assessment/Rituals.pdf • CDC — National Diabetes Prevention Program — Problem Solving http://www.cdc.gov/diabetes/prevention/pdf/curriculum_session9.pdf
Building confidence	• CDC — National Diabetes Prevention Program — Talk Back to Negative Thoughts http://www.cdc.gov/diabetes/prevention/pdf/curriculum_session11.pdf
Social support	• Be Active E-cards http://www.healthfinder.gov/ecards/cards.aspx?jscript=1 • National Institute on Aging Go4Life program http://go4life.niapublications.org/about/family-and-friends/cheering • CDC — National Diabetes Prevention Program — Make Social Cues Work For You http://www.cdc.gov/diabetes/prevention/pdf/curriculum_session14.pdf
Stimulus control	• CDC — National Diabetes Prevention Program — Taking Charge of What's Around You http://www.cdc.gov/diabetes/prevention/pdf/curriculum_session8.pdf • CDC StairWELL to Better Health Toolkit http://www.cdc.gov/nccdphp/dnpao/hwi/toolkits/stairwell/index.htm
Making a commitment	• My Exercise Plan — Self-Assessment http://www.myexerciseplan.com/assessment/SelfAssessment.pdf • Eat Smart, Move More NC — Move More Pledge Card http://www.eatsmartmovemorenc.com/NCHealthSmartTlkt/Texts/MM_AppG%20Pledge.pdf
Motivational readiness for change	• Exercise Is Medicine — Health Care Providers' Action Guide http://exerciseismedicine.org/documents/HCProActionGuide_HQ.pdf • Lifespan Healthy Living Video Series — Physical Activity Stages of Change http://www.lifespan.org/staywell/healthyvideos/exercise/handout_1.pdf
Avoiding boredom and maximizing enjoyment	• National Institute on Aging's *Go4Life* http://go4life.niapublications.org/try-these-exercises • Compendium of Physical Activities http://sites.google.com/site/compendiumofphysicalactivities/ • CDC — National Diabetes Prevention Program — Jump Start Your Activity Plan http://www.cdc.gov/diabetes/prevention/pdf/curriculum_session13.pdf

(continued)

TABLE 45-1. Resources for Behavior Strategies (*Continued*)

Strategy	Resource
Relapse prevention	• CDC — National Diabetes Prevention Program — The Slippery Slope of Lifestyle Change http://www.cdc.gov/diabetes/prevention/pdf/curriculum_session12.pdf
Helping people reach recommended activity levels	• Physical Activity Guidelines for Americans http://www.health.gov/paguidelines/ • Youth Physical Activity Guidelines Toolkit http://www.cdc.gov/Healthyyouth/physicalactivity/guidelines.htm#1 • Compendium of Physical Activities http://sites.google.com/site/compendiumofphysicalactivities/ • CDC: National Diabetes Prevention Program — Being Active — A Way of Life http://www.cdc.gov/diabetes/prevention/pdf/curriculum_session6.pdf

of physical activity, it is likely that certain benefits hold motivational influence or salience for an individual.

Barriers

Although many people recognize the benefits of regular exercise or physical activity, these pros are often balanced or outweighed by the numerous disadvantages, barriers, risks, or cons that exist (see *GETP9, Table 11-1*). These cons can be real or perceived and may be influenced by factors such as age, ethnicity, socioeconomics, and behavior change stage. For example, health-related barriers and concerns about risks are particularly important among older individuals who may have fears of physical activity–related injury (22). Individuals in groups at risk for physical inactivity may benefit from an emphasis on moderate-intensity activities that can be readily adapted for various fitness levels and abilities and incorporated into their daily routines.

Common barriers to adopting and maintaining a regular exercise program relate to

• individual physical and mental limitations,
• accessibility and convenience of safe facilities and equipment,
• environmental and ecological factors (*e.g.*, geographical location, climate),
• lack of time,
• lack of enjoyment and/or boredom, and
• insufficient encouragement and social support.

Individuals in the early stages of exercise adoption typically report fewer benefits and more barriers than those in the latter stages (36). Other factors such as gender and type of activity may also influence how benefits and barriers are perceived. Fitness professionals can help clarify participant expectations concerning physical activity (what can and cannot be accomplished and when

	ACTIVITY	INACTIVITY
"Pros"		
"Cons"		

FIGURE 45-1. Decisional balance sheet. This is an example of a decision balance sheet that can be used to help clients weigh the advantages and disadvantages of being physically active. In the "pros" category, ask clients to list the perceived benefits of being physically active (*e.g.*, feeling better, losing weight) and the benefits of being inactive (*e.g.*, more free time). Then ask clients to consider the "cons" or the costs that might be associated with being active (*e.g.*, getting up early to exercise) and being inactive (*e.g.*, feeling stressed, gaining weight). It will be important to help clients achieve a "tipping point" where the perceived pros of activity outweigh the perceived cons.

results should be expected) and address individuals' perceived benefits and barriers. The many benefits of making positive physical activity changes should be stressed.

ACCESSIBILITY AND CONVENIENCE

In addition to knowledge of the benefits and barriers of physical activity, several other practical factors can influence initial participation as well as longer term adherence (49,51). These include proximity, access to, and affordability of facilities (for those who prefer facility-based activities); weather; regimen flexibility (type of activity, intensity, location, timing, frequency); convenience and ease of scheduling of the activity (real or perceived); immediate visual or auditory cues and prompts in the environment promoting physical activity (*e.g.*, reminders to exercise); immediate consequences of physical activity for the individual (*e.g.*, discomfort); and social influences and support (*e.g.*, individuals reporting spouses to be neutral or unsupportive of physical activity are more likely to drop out).

Physical activity that is easily accessible and convenient improves the likelihood of adoption and maintenance. Three factors related to convenience are important to successful initiation and maintenance of an exercise program. First, it is clear that the greater the effort required to prepare for physical activity (*i.e.*, location issues such as a long drive to the exercise facility, having to change clothes for activity), the greater the potential for dropping out (37). Encouraging various methods of being physically active in or around the home (the place where many people prefer to exercise) or workplace can make convenience less of a deterrent.

Second, time is often the main factor leading to perceptions of inconvenience. If a physical activity program is offered within a class structure, having several time options may be helpful. For some people with extreme time constraints, alternatives to a class format are often necessary. A practical alternative is to emphasize ways that individuals can build regular physical activity into their daily routines, such as through using more active transportation modes that may facilitate more walking, bicycling, or taking stairs. Participating in both structured, as well as lifestyle physical activity, is important for many people to optimize benefits. Although lack of time is a common barrier to activity, regular exercisers complain as much as persons who are not regularly active about time constraints. Thus, perceived available time may reflect, in large part, one's current priorities related to being active or time management skills rather than actual time limitations. Encouraging short bouts, such as accumulating activity in 10-min segments, may assist people in minimizing the perceived time burden.

Third, modes of physical activity that require special, costly, or time-consuming preparation (*e.g.*, skiing, swimming) may adversely affect adoption and adherence. Thus, location, time, and mode can be critical factors during early stages of acquisition. Both the participant and the physical activity professional should carefully evaluate choices before initiating a physical activity program to help mitigate the negative impact of such factors (56). *Figure 45-2* provides a sample time study worksheet to assist clients in identifying their usual daily routines and finding opportunities for physical activity.

SETTING GOALS, SHAPING BEHAVIORS, AND REWARDING EFFORT

Once the benefits, barriers, and potential risks associated with adopting and maintaining regular physical activity

	Early morning	Mid-morning	Midday	Early afternoon	Evening	Night
Monday						
Tuesday						
Wednesday						
Thursday						
Friday						
Saturday						
Sunday						

FIGURE 45-2. Finding time worksheet. This worksheet can be used with clients to help them assess their time and identify time for activity. Ask clients to fill in the worksheet with their typical schedule. Then discuss where they could add more activity into their day.

are recognized, short- and long-term goals can be established. Physical activity behaviors can be shaped and rewarded appropriately. **Goal setting** is a stepwise process that involves assessing an individual's current level of fitness or physical activity level, evaluating the individual's expected outcome, and considering best practices for physical activity guidelines.

For sedentary persons, the major objective is to establish a successful physical activity habit that targets their goals while decreasing the likelihood for failure. The initial activity prescription should be well within the capabilities of the individual. Additionally, individual preferences, motivation, skills, and life circumstances should be taken into account. For some individuals, shaping may translate into a simple initial increase in ADLs. For example, walking more at work and home, or taking stairs, may be recommended. For others, the initial prescription may involve less frequent structured endurance activity with a concomitant increase in routine activity until more vigorous activity is indicated.

A key consideration in all physical activity program planning should be gradual **shaping** of the physical activity behavior toward the established goal(s) set forth by the client and exercise professional. When physical activity progresses too quickly, adherence is almost always negatively affected. The rate of injury and dropout increases significantly when beginning exercisers are exposed to physical activities of an intensity too high for their fitness level or exposed to very high initial frequency (e.g., $5\,\text{d} \cdot \text{wk}^{-1}$ or more) or duration (e.g., 45 min or more per session). In contrast, after an individual is beyond the initial stages of his or her program, higher intensity, frequency, and duration are often appropriate.

A physical activity regimen should be initially easy to undertake and gradually incremented, ensuring success at each stage. Exercise professionals (and beginning exercisers) should focus primarily on shaping and maintaining the initial physical activity habit for approximately 6–12 wk. This approach emphasizes first establishing behavioral control of the physical activity habit so that beginners are encouraged to simply show up (e.g., "No matter how little you may feel like doing or

are able to do, we are working on reinforcing the habit of regular physical activity; the benefits will come, if you can first form the habit"). Finding immediate or short-term benefits of value to the individual will increase the likelihood of adherence and progression to attain other longer term benefits.

SMART Goal Setting

The success of behavioral shaping is based on the determination of realistic goals. Such goals provide the individual with a modest challenge, leading to increased self-efficacy when achieved. Using the following "SMART" principles as a reminder may help reinforce the keys to goal setting success (30):

- *Specific*: The physical activity behavior should be clearly and precisely established (*e.g.*, mode, frequency, intensity, and duration of physical activity).
- *Measurable*: The behavior should be something that can be readily monitored (*e.g.*, tracked using logs or body monitors).
- *Adjustable*: The physical activity behavior should be adjustable (*e.g.*, intensity level, time frame, weight amount, plan for relapse if injury should occur, or other major life events happen, etc.).
- *Realistic*: The behavior should be somewhat challenging but within the individual's capabilities and readily achievable (*e.g.*, step goal moderately above baseline, graduated exercise prescription).
- *Time-frame specific*: The behavior should be accomplished within a specified period (*e.g.*, 1 mo, 6 mo).

Especially in the beginning, people should set goals that are simple and easy to remember. That is, an attempt should be made to "Keep It Simple and Smart" (the positive "KISS" principle) (30). Devise an action plan associated with the targeted goals, and develop specific strategies for achieving them. Keeping the goals, timeline, steps, and strategies in plain sight (*e.g.*, on a worksheet or calendar, in a journal, or on a poster) can serve as a friendly reminder. See *Figure 45-3* and *GETP9, Box 11-4* for an outline of goal setting methods.

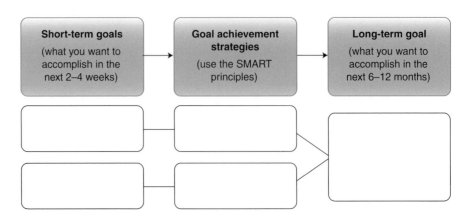

FIGURE 45-3. Goal setting outline. This document can be used to help clients outline their goals, their achievement strategies, and consider how their short-term goals can facilitate achievement of long-term goals.

Rewards and Reinforcement

The initial steps involved in becoming more physically active may not be pleasant or intrinsically rewarding. Often, it is not until several months into a regular physical activity program that participants begin to report positive benefits from physical activity. In fact, the longer the period of inactivity and the more unfit the individual, the longer it may be before physical activity becomes intrinsically reinforcing (*i.e.,* feels good). Therefore, beginners may need external rewards early in the program for encouragement and motivation. Use of such rewards is consistent with the process of behavioral shaping in which early approximations of target behaviors require reinforcement or rewards for optimal acquisition.

For highly unfit or inactive individuals, beginner status might extend to 6 mo or 1 yr, and special external incentives may need to be programmed throughout that time. For more fit persons, the beginner phase may last for only a short time, perhaps as little as 2–3 wk. Generally, the choice of rewards or incentives should reside with the participant. The incentives people find motivating vary from person to person. It is important to help participants identify rewards that will not be counterproductive to desired health goals (*e.g.,* discourage use of high-fat snacks or days off from exercise as rewards). For some individuals, using external rewards or incentives may be unfamiliar, unpalatable, or counterproductive; thus, reinforcement should be tailored to the individual. Smaller rewards for short-term goals (*e.g.,* bubble bath, magazine subscription, movie) and larger rewards for long-term goals (*e.g.,* new running shoes, massage, vacation) can help the individual focus on the steps of the goal setting process and provide incentives for sustained motivation.

In addition to the behavioral skill of rewarding oneself for meeting physical activity goals, exercise professionals should consider program-based incentives as a form of extrinsic motivation. Ideas include the use of point systems, competitions, and recognition, which should be based on readily achievable physical activity goals (*e.g.,* attendance or participation) during the early stages of physical activity adoption. Reward systems may include points accumulated as exercise continues to be maintained. Points may then be redeemed for material rewards (*e.g.,* exercise equipment, gift certificate, training session). Other examples are requiring a monetary deposit that is returned contingent upon achievement of goals (especially behavioral goals such as attendance and participation) or reducing program fees based on program adherence. Because some individuals spend significant time restarting physical activity, strategies for maintenance should be an integral component of programming.

Preparation for maintenance should also focus on maximizing the rewarding aspects of the physical activity (*e.g.,* enjoyment, increased energy, opportunities to socialize or "get away") so less dependence is needed on external rewards and there is increased reliance on intrinsic motivation (*i.e.,* internal desires for achievement). Importantly, self-motivation or intrinsic motivation may be learned when an individual finds personal, self-identified rewards for behavior (*e.g.,* personal achievement, the satisfaction obtained in reaching one's physical activity goals) independent of extrinsic or external reinforcements available for that behavior (21). Self-determination theory and similar perspectives (10,35) indicate that intrinsic motivation may be positively related to continued participation in physical activity. These approaches encourage self-directed and sustained physical activity by exploring the individual's feelings about the proposed change, encouraging a personal rationale for the change, providing a choice of alternative behaviors to reduce conflicts, and recognizing the importance of individual preferences and experiences (11).

SELF-MONITORING

Another important aspect of self-management for behavioral success is identifying physical activity patterns and receiving feedback regarding progress. This can be accomplished through self-monitoring by recording personal thoughts, feelings, and physical activity behavior patterns and gauging them against established standards (see 2008 Physical Activity Guidelines, http://www.health.gov/paguidelines/). Feedback, especially self-monitored feedback, can stimulate a positive reactive effect on a wide variety of behaviors. For example, short-term reduction of caloric intake usually results when it is monitored. Similarly, physical activity habits are frequently enhanced when attendance, general physical activity adherence or performance, or the results of the physical activity program are systematically monitored. Self-monitoring can be used to identify unhelpful patterns or sedentary activities, set goals, monitor progress and identify barriers, as well as prompt physical activity choices. One simple method, especially for those having difficulty engaging in a systematic physical activity, is to provide an inexpensive pedometer or step counter to track walking and related physical activities. Pedometers have been found to be a cost-efficient, valid, and reliable means for providing motivational feedback across various populations (5).

Feedback can also be obtained through use of self-recorded monitoring sheets, an activity journal or diary, computerized applications, and automated body monitors. Graphs showing progress in one or more variables (*e.g.,* attendance, steps, mileage, minutes, plotted heart rates, intensity levels, or attendance) can be used to monitor progress and provide feedback. Computer-generated feedback letters that summarize progress made in the program over time show promise as an efficient, systematic method for providing personalized feedback on a regular basis; several programs are available to allow oversight by fitness professionals. Self-administered fitness tests (*e.g.,* field tests) or professional fitness assessments can be monitored and used as a gauge to compare current measures with past levels of fitness. These assessments can guide setting of future goals. When used in conjunction with short- and long-term goals that are personally relevant and SMART, feedback can be a powerful motivating factor.

Self-monitoring and other forms of feedback are useful for noting progress and enhancing motivation. Research in the field continues to support the usefulness of regular self-monitoring of physical activity for long-term maintenance. However, few behavioral strategies evoke more resistance from participants than the prospect of long-term self-monitoring. As with any goal setting strategy, individuals should fully participate in designing the self-monitoring strategies that will be the easiest and most convenient for them to maintain.

SELF-MANAGEMENT AND PROBLEM SOLVING

Successful behavior change often correlates with self-management strategies coupled with an understanding of the importance of personal responsibility and accountability. Individuals must recognize the importance of physical activity as a lifelong goal rather than as something that ends when a 12-wk class or program is over. Early in all programs, methods to successfully engage participants in alternate forms of physical activity in various settings and under various circumstances should be outlined, along with relevant relapse prevention tips. Forming a partnership with each individual that fosters the individual's feelings of autonomy and control with respect to the physical activity program is important for facilitating long-term participation (21). Thus, participants should be encouraged to take a self-directed approach to all aspects of physical activity (*e.g.*, goal setting, planning) rather than relying on the professional.

Knowledge and use of behavioral and psychological strategies that assist the individual in the negotiation of barriers to physical activity are needed. A useful behavioral skill is the practical and systematic problem solving of specific barriers that the individual is likely to face (See *Box 45-2*).

BUILDING CONFIDENCE

Self-efficacy appears to be a particularly potent predictor of physical activity participation in the early stages (39). **Self-efficacy** is the extent to which individuals feel they will be successful in performing desired behaviors, given the abilities they possess in the particular situation they find themselves (see *GETP9, Box 11-1*). It is important to focus on individuals' initial feelings of self-efficacy and to help them increase their outcome expectations through shaping early successes. This can be accomplished by setting realistic, personally tailored physical activity goals (see SMART goals); encouraging regular positive feedback; receiving social support; and self-monitoring their physical activity levels as a way of measuring

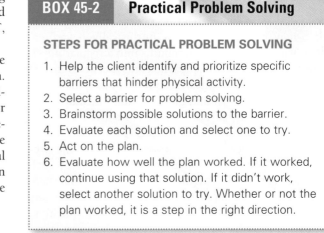

BOX 45-2 **Practical Problem Solving**

STEPS FOR PRACTICAL PROBLEM SOLVING

1. Help the client identify and prioritize specific barriers that hinder physical activity.
2. Select a barrier for problem solving.
3. Brainstorm possible solutions to the barrier.
4. Evaluate each solution and select one to try.
5. Act on the plan.
6. Evaluate how well the plan worked. If it worked, continue using that solution. If it didn't work, select another solution to try. Whether or not the plan worked, it is a step in the right direction.

progress. Self-efficacy and perceived behavior control can be improved using these strategies. Helping clients or patients take charge of their physical activity behaviors and exercise programs leads to improved confidence in maintaining physical activity.

With respect to self-efficacy, previous experience with physical activity should be explored, along with unreasonable beliefs and misconceptions about physical activity (*e.g.*, the "no pain, no gain" fallacy, or myths that older individuals need to "conserve their energy"). For example, many inactive individuals believe that exercise is inherently painful or aversive; sedentary individuals are often unaware of the benefit of moderate activities (*e.g.*, brisk walking) that may be more appealing and comfortable than more vigorous activity regimens (*e.g.*, high-impact aerobics, running). Professionals can provide specific instruction on appropriate ways of performing specific activities at a safe, beneficial intensity to obtain health-related benefits while avoiding injury (16).

A physical activity program should be personally relevant, both in terms of type of activity and goals, both short and long term. For example, if stress reduction is a motivating factor, activities that can be helpful in reducing stress (*i.e.*, not overly competitive, noisy, or demanding) should be targeted. Examples of such activities may include brisk walking, jogging, or bicycling conducted outdoors in pleasant surroundings that allow time to get away. Activities that are performed in a noncompetitive manner or that incorporate relaxation techniques, such as yoga, also would be appropriate. Targeting an individual's specific interests and goals increases the likelihood for enjoyment and sustained motivation for physical activity. *Table 45-2* presents different types of strategies for increasing physical activity self-efficacy.

SOCIAL SUPPORT

One valuable and reinforcing form of reward is social support. Social support is a powerful motivator for many

TABLE 45-2. Suggested Strategies for Increasing Physical Activity Self-Efficacy

Information Sources	Strategies
Past performance	Set goals and activity prescriptions with clients Rehearse activity behaviors (e.g., guided walks) Self-monitoring with pedometers and/or activity logs
Vicarious experience	Use videotapes of peer role models who are exercising Have peer role models conduct group physical activity sessions
Verbal persuasion	Emphasize physiological benefits of physical activity Praise client for any progress Attribute all successes to the client's own efforts Encourage family and friends to support and reinforce the activity behavior
Physiological cues	Help clients anticipate and positively interpret physical discomforts related to physical activity (e.g., fatigue and muscle aches) Relaxation training to decrease anxiety

Reprinted with permission from Pekmezi D, Jennings E, Marcus B. Evaluating and enhancing self-efficacy for physical activity. *ACSM's Health Fitness J.* 2009;13(2):16–21.

people (33,38,52). It can be delivered in various forms, including through a fitness instructor, exercise partners, family members, coworkers, or neighbors who encourage increased activity. Telephone contacts, letters or e-mail prompts from a health professional are other options. Praise is a critical component of social support, especially for inexperienced, beginning exercisers, and completely relapsed former exercisers. To be most effective, encouragement should be both immediate (during or very shortly after the physical activity episode, if possible) and specific. Friends and family members can also be encouraged to participate in physical activity to enhance support. However, others' physical activity pace must be appropriate for the beginner. When support from significant others is active and ongoing, individuals are more likely than those with little or no social support to persist in a physical activity program (50,53).

Professionals, family members, and helpers should all be cautioned against even well-intentioned nagging or use of other aversive procedures (e.g., using guilt) to induce a person to become more physically active. These counterproductive actions almost inevitably increase the punishing characteristics of physical activity as well as potentially impairing the partnership between the individual and the supportive agent, further upsetting the often delicate balance between the motivation to become physically active and remaining inactive.

The use of social support can be extended and formalized using written contracts between the individual and a significant person. Contracts are written, signed agreements that specify the physical activity–related goals in a public format and for which there is value exchange, much like a legal contract. They typically specify short-term, concrete goals and the types of positive consequences that occur upon reaching the goals. The contract should be flexible and avoid rigid daily goals that may be difficult or impossible to meet. In the earlier stages of a program, an appropriate goal might be related to attendance or participation rather than performance. These goal setting contracts often work best if developed in tandem with an interested person or helper. Such contracts can help to increase personal responsibility and commitment. Those managing physical activity programs should also consider using contingency management, in which more highly rewarding or preferred activities are made contingent on achieving a particular goal (e.g., watching a favorite television program only after a physical activity session is completed). Another alternative is a written agreement through which the participant agrees in writing to perform or complete certain behaviors or activities that can be useful for persons who are reluctant to sign a behavioral contract. *Figure 45-4* presents a sample behavioral contract for physical activity.

The use of appropriate and consistent physical activity role models in the environment can also motivate people to begin and continue exercise. These models should be as similar as possible to the targeted individuals (e.g., some programs use successful graduates as future participant assistants for maximal effectiveness) (27,31). When possible, the physical activity professional should set an appropriate example by exercising with participants and displaying other behaviors that are consistent with an active lifestyle (e.g., taking stairs, walking to accomplish errands, adhering to appropriate exercise safeguards such as stretching and hydration).

Continued use of various social support mechanisms is valuable for continued physical activity maintenance (See *Box 45-3*). For instance, if the format is a class or group situation, the leader can call participants who miss two classes in a row (one class in high-risk participants). The purpose of such calls is to let individuals know that they are missed and that others notice and care. Other individuals in the class can assume this type of responsibility as well (i.e., a "buddy system"). If physical activity is conducted outside of a formal setting, the physical activity professional may continue support in the form of periodic telephone calls, letters, e-mails, or newsletters (8). Family members, coworkers, neighbors, and friends should continue to encourage and support the physical activity program. It may be helpful to include support persons in education efforts to train them in providing continuing support through prompting, modeling, and reinforcing physical activity. Most importantly, individuals should be encouraged to be proactive about seeking out and identifying their own meaningful sources of support; this increases their feeling of ownership and their role in sustaining their physical activity regimen and resources.

Date: _____

Client Responsibilities:

1. Over the next 4 weeks, I will walk at least 4 days per week, for a total of at least 30 minutes per day. (I understand that I can break the 30 minutes up into two 15-minute episodes or walk continuously for 30 minutes).

2. For each week that I attain the above set of goals, I will reward myself by putting aside $5 to be used to treat myself to an article of clothing, a movie, or a similar reward.

3. For each week that I don't meet the above set of goals, I will forego watching a favorite TV show (and I will use that time to walk, if possible).

4. I will record my data on my physical activity calendar at the end of each day, and I will evaluate the success of this set of goals (and revise if necessary) on _____ (date) _____ .

My helper in supporting and reminding me about my goals is:

_____

My signature: _____   Date: _____

Helper signature: _____   Date: _____

FIGURE 45-4. Sample behavioral contract.

STIMULUS CONTROL

Stimulus control or structuring the immediate environment to remind or encourage one to be physically active (*e.g.*, through the use of visual or auditory reminders or prompts) can positively impact physical activity behaviors (3,6,14,17,18,32,48,49). Experimental studies on the use of environmental changes to encourage the use of stairs instead of escalators and elevators in public buildings consistently find that the placement of prompts increases rate of stairway use. Research also indicates that making environments more pleasant through use of art and music further increase the rate of stairway use (6). Friendly reminders, whether at home, work, or in public places seem to inspire some individuals to take action. Thus, people should use these types of strategies (post cartoons, sticky notes, inspiration quotes, e-mail, tweet, etc.) to prompt an exercise break. Because adolescents and young adults spend a great portion of their personal time on computer devices for communication, social media, education, and entertainment, they may be more receptive to Internet-based and computer-aided interventions (13,26). These electronic interventions can be more cost-efficient than print media in some circumstances, especially if a large portion of individuals are involved in a similar exercise program (25,41).

MAKING A COMMITMENT

Behavioral modification and cognitive behavioral techniques such as written agreements or writing down daily and future goals, and acknowledging them to others, help make people responsible for their behaviors and

---

BOX 45-3   Types of Social Support

TYPES OF SOCIAL SUPPORT

Encourage the participant to identify different people who can provide different types of support.

- *Knowledge* — provide information and assist in practical advice about exercise and physical activity (*e.g., fitness professional provides instruction on technique*)
- *Participatory* — participate in physical activity with the individual (*e.g., friend acts as a workout buddy*)
- *Motivational* — provide encouragement support and accountability (*e.g., family member provides positive feedback and acts as a "cheerleader"*)
- *Practical* — assist in logistical arrangements to enable the participant to make and complete exercise plans (*e.g., spouse watches the kids*)

actions. Behaviors that are acknowledged and written down prior to starting a program seem to result in habit formation (adherence). Personal contracts should be regularly updated, and if necessary, changed. The goals established in the personal contracts should be based on the SMART goal principles. Personal contracts that include easy or unspecific goals typically do not provide the challenge necessary to motivate individuals to maintain their focus and accomplish the tasks. In contrast, personal contracts that include goals that are too difficult or involve too many goals often lead to frustration, discouragement, and may increase risk for injury.

Incentivizing physical exercise by using rewards has received increased interest because of the rising prevalence of obesity and the growing concerns about health care costs. Providing people with initial incentives to exercise has been shown to increase attendance rates in the subsequent weeks, even when the incentives are later removed (9). Training individuals in simple field methods for evaluating changes in their own fitness or physical functioning levels can serve as a powerful motivator for continued physical activity participation (46,54). Combining incentives and self-administered rewards seem particularly motivational. For example, using a performance or scorecard to keep track of activities that are monitored by another person, and when completed, can be redeemed for prizes or enjoyable activities, can motivate participants to engage in physical activity (2). Likewise, providing contingent and sincere feedback and support from others should further reinforce the health-related behaviors.

MOTIVATIONAL CONSIDERATIONS

STAGES OF CHANGE: MATCHING SKILLS TO MOTIVATIONAL READINESS

Social cognitive theory and related approaches to understanding physical activity behavior have been supplemented in recent years with an increased appreciation for the role of motivational readiness in changing and maintaining physical activity patterns (28,44,57). The need for regularity in performing physical activity to obtain benefits throughout life calls for innovative methods to encourage habitual physical activity. Factors or correlates that influence initial adoption and early participation in physical activity may differ from those that affect subsequent long-term maintenance. Stage-of-change models that take into account **motivational readiness for change** (*e.g.*, the TTM [4,45]) may better identify strategies that work for individuals in different stages and at different levels of physical activity participation (*e.g.*, sedentary persons contemplating joining a physical activity program, those in the early stage of physical activity adoption, those committed to maintaining a program across the long term).

The TTM is the only process-oriented model that is consistently used in exercise environments. This model proposes that individuals move through five stages of readiness for changing health behaviors (4,44): **precontemplation** (not thinking about changing physical activity), **contemplation** (thinking about changing physical activity), **preparation** (making small changes in physical activity but not to a sufficient level), **action** (meeting physical activity goals but for fewer than 6 mo), and **maintenance** (being physically active at the desired level for at least 6 mo). However, movement through the stages may not progress in a linear fashion. Individuals often move back and forth through the stages. By understanding and assessing readiness for change, professionals can tailor physical activity interventions and programs to meet a participant's current needs and level of motivation. Several questionnaires are available to assist exercise professionals in evaluating a participant's motivational readiness to change physical activity behavior (see *GETP9, Fig. 11-1* and *Box 11-3*).

These behavior change theories (*i.e.*, social cognitive theory, TTM) focus on the dynamic relationship between personal attributes and resources, the behavior targeted for change, and influences of the physical and social environment in shaping the adoption and maintenance of the targeted behavior. Along with similar conceptual approaches, these theories provide a framework for development of physical activity intervention strategies. However, theoretical approaches have not often been applied in a comprehensive fashion in physical activity intervention research. When TTM has been applied to specific situations, it appears useful with facilitating adoption and early adherence; it may not be as useful with individuals maintaining regular exercise or in identifying someone at risk of relapse (1,7). See *Table 45-3* for suggested strategies by stage of readiness for change.

AVOIDING BOREDOM AND MAXIMIZING ENJOYMENT

For most individuals, it is critically important for adherence that the activity be enjoyable. The physical discomfort that often accompanies early stages of increased activity should be minimized, or at least moderated, by positive factors and normalized with respect to the individual's expectations. Methods for enhancing enjoyment include tailoring of the mode (or type, *e.g.*, running, skiing, etc.), intensity, duration, format (group or individual, instructor led or videotaped), and location (outside or inside). One method of assessing enjoyment is to ask participants to note their level of enjoyment on a range of values from "very unenjoyable" to "very enjoyable" (*e.g.*, scale of 1–5). If two or more sessions are "unenjoyable," the exercise regimen should be modified and accompanied, if appropriate for the individual, by additional rewards or incentives.

TABLE 45-3. Suggested Strategies by Stage of Motivational Readiness for Change

Stage of Change	Goal	Specific Strategies
Precontemplation	To get your client thinking about physical activity	• Encourage your client to learn more about physical activity • Read articles, watch videos, and talk to others (physician) about physical activity • Make a list of potential benefits to becoming physically active then assess how important these benefits are to him or her
Contemplation	To encourage your client to start being physically active	• Have client observe an aerobics class or take a tour of a gym to build familiarity and confidence • Identify barriers to getting started (lack of time) and strategies for overcoming them (walking during lunch break) • Develop a plan for getting started (when, where, what activity, with whom?) • Set a small goal (5 minutes of walking) and commit to it
Preparation	To encourage your client to be regularly physically active	• Have client use a pedometer and/or activity logs to self-monitor physical activity and track progress toward goals • Encourage client to reward him/herself for meeting the goal of increased physical activity • Leave reminders to exercise everywhere (walking shoes by the door)
Action	To help your client maintain this physical activity habit over time	• Identify any obstacles that might interfere with being active in the future, then develop a plan for how to overcome them • Help client train for an event in the future (fun walk, 5K)
Maintenance	To help the client prepare for any future setbacks and increase enjoyment of physical activity	• Discuss how to get back on track after a break in physical activity • Make physical activity fun: try new activities (kickboxing!); listen to music or watch TV while on treadmill; walk with a friend • Encourage your client to mentor someone else who is interested in becoming more physically active

Reprinted with permission from Pekmezi D, Brooke B, Marcus B. Using the transtheoretical model to promote physical activity. *ACSM's Health Fitness J.* 2010;14(4):8–13.

The mode, intensity, duration, format, and location of physical activity must meet the needs and preferences of differing groups of individuals. For example, women generally report a stronger preference for videotaped exercise and aerobic dance than men. Similarly, the workplace has been shown to be a preferred location for undertaking physical activity in some groups, although not in others (19,23). Physical activity professionals can help individuals develop tailored action plans (*e.g.*, through helping identify new activities, environments, goals, or partners) that increase motivation and adherence.

For many individuals, boredom is a barrier to long-term maintenance. With a wide variety of physical activities, and a diversity of settings in which to conduct activities, the "I'm bored" response can be minimized. Individuals who have achieved improvements in their cardiorespiratory fitness may renew their motivation by trying activities or intensities with a higher level of physical challenge. For some individuals, boredom may be resolved through a regimen involving various activities. For others, a preferred physical activity conducted in varied settings and formats may be more appropriate. Pairing physical activity with another enjoyable activity (*e.g.*, music, reading, or watching TV while on stationary equipment, talking with a friend) can serve as a distraction and increase enjoyment of the exercise session. Often, enjoyable competition (*e.g.*, walkathons) can help to stimulate maintenance and reinvigorate a stale program or regimen.

RELAPSE PREVENTION

Anticipating potential barriers and planning ahead for unforeseen events and inevitable lapses in physical activity participation (*i.e.*, relapse prevention) is another means of maintaining motivation and enhancing self-efficacy levels (20,27). Often, individuals stop exercising completely after an inevitable break because of illness or injury, travel, holidays, inclement weather, or increased work demands. Barriers and interruptions to physical activities have less impact when habits become established. Individuals high in resiliency, cognitive coping skills, and behavioral strategies have fewer relapses. An occasional lapse is to be expected; people can learn to overcome them, thereby developing greater perceived behavioral control.

PLANNING AHEAD TO PREVENT RELAPSE

One useful step is to prepare in advance (both psychologically and behaviorally) for breaks or lapses in activity that may lead to a full-blown relapse (and a return to the previous sedentary lifestyle) (20,27,29). People can be trained to understand and handle lapses before they happen, with the intention of increasing their self-efficacy for returning after the lapse and reducing the risk of a complete relapse. For example, keeping a journal or diary of thoughts, feelings, and events that cause individuals to miss, or even tempt them to miss an exercise session, can be helpful to plan for high-risk situations

Methods for Engaging Participants in Physical Activity

METHODS FOR ENGAGING PARTICIPANTS IN PHYSICAL ACTIVITY

- Carry exercise clothes or walking shoes in the car, place a pair of walking shoes at work, pack a bag with a set of exercise clothes and shoes so it will be ready when needed.
- Leave exercise clothes or shoes by the bed or the front door.
- Formally schedule physical activity into a weekly planner or calendar.
- Spend time with other physically active people.
- Park the car and walk; take stairs whenever possible.
- Only make decisions concerning whether or not to be physically active or how much to exercise *after* arriving at the designated physical activity site or locale.

- Develop a plan or program for high-risk situations (*e.g.*, travel, holidays) to assist with maintaining physical activity.

SUGGESTIONS FOR A MISSED SESSION (RELAPSE PREVENTION)

- Admit responsibility for the slip.
- Develop a restart plan, including appropriate goals.
- Call a physical activity "buddy" for support and motivation.
- Arrange reinforcements or rewards to help restart the activity.
- Simplify or change the routine to accommodate temporary changes in availability or time.
- Begin by simply visiting the usual physical activity place or locale.

that may lead to inactivity. It should also be emphasized that breaks or lapses are inevitable and do not indicate laziness or failure. Strategies to prepare for lapses and for restarting physical activity include identification of alternate activities that can be done in place of the usual activity, planning to exercise as soon as possible after a break, arranging to exercise with someone else, and modifying goals to avoid discouragement (*Box 45-4*).

REMINDERS OF BENEFITS

It is important to provide continued evidence of relevant personal benefits (physical, social, and psychological) from being regularly active. Physical activity professionals should regularly inquire about benefits and positive outcomes experienced from the current physical activity program. For persons at risk for dropping out, these questions should be posed frequently (*e.g.*, one or more times per month). If an individual cannot define the positive aspects of physical activity or, alternatively, provides several negatives, there is serious risk of dropout. Such participants should be targeted for increased attention and support. Having participants regularly revisit their cost-benefits or decisional balance sheet can be useful for reinforcing their personal commitments to be active, as well as revising the physical activity plan to increase the benefits portion of the equation.

GENERALIZATION TRAINING

As individuals adjust physical activity routines and enter into maintenance, it is important to consider the translation of behavioral aspects of the current program into new environments and avoid discontinuing physical

activity programs, especially if no generalization training has been provided. **Generalization training** involves expanding the behavior to a different setting to link the behavior with cues or stimuli in the second setting that may help to facilitate ongoing participation. To ensure adherence, the physical activity habit must be generalized or reestablished in new environments (*e.g.*, self-initiated, home-based) before discontinuing supervised or programmed, facility-based sessions (45). Generalization may be accomplished in several ways, including requiring off-site, home exercise sessions at an early stage of the program; involving family or significant others in physical activity sessions; and adding additional exercises before graduation that are easily maintained in the new environment. Ideally, the responsibility for session supervision, reinforcement, and feedback should be gradually transferred from the instructor to the participant, as well as to helpers in the new environment as the change date approaches. This more closely approximates the conditions likely to be experienced in the maintenance setting.

REASSESSMENT OF GOALS

Regular reassessment of physical activity goals provides an opportunity to verify that they are relevant, realistic, and motivating. Goals that are too long term (*e.g.*, several months) or vague (*e.g.*, "I will exercise more") do not provide sufficient motivation to maintain behavior through difficult periods. During the early stages of a physical activity program (*i.e.*, 1–6 mo), goals should be adjusted as frequently as necessary (*i.e.*, once every 2 wk) to maintain physical activity behavior. For maintenance of physical activity, participants should be taught proper goal setting techniques and convinced of the importance of continuing to set goals to enhance long-term motivation.

HELPING PEOPLE REACH RECOMMENDED ACTIVITY LEVELS

It is helpful for physical activity professionals to consider the application of specific behavioral skills and exercise prescription within the context of an overall lifestyle approach to physical activity. Applying basic counseling strategies can promote an atmosphere that increases the likelihood of success by facilitating self-directed planning for physical activity.

EMPHASIZE THE IMPORTANCE OF ROUTINE ACTIVITIES

Increasing physical activity throughout one's daily routine can help individuals maintain fitness, especially during times when more structured or vigorous activity is not performed. Current public health guidelines recommend that adults engage in at least 150 min or more of moderate-intensity activities weekly (see http://www.health.gov/paguidelines/). An important aspect to these recommendations is accumulated activity, which can be accomplished through various structured and lifestyle physical activities. It is important for individuals to understand that health benefits can be more effectively realized by being active in various ways, both within and outside of formal exercise programs. One method of doing this is to help individuals become aware of times in their daily routines when sedentary activities are performed with little thought or planning (*e.g.*, indiscriminate television viewing). After such time periods are identified, more physically active alternatives can be devised (*e.g.*, going for a walk with family members or dog). Behavior-based interventions have demonstrated that decreasing sedentary activities and increasing lifestyle physical activity can help individuals increase physical activity and fitness (12).

MOTIVATIONAL AND CLIENT-CENTERED COUNSELING TECHNIQUES

In recent years, attention has been given to the application of brief motivational interviewing approaches for health behaviors such as physical activity (47). Motivational interviewing was initially developed as a brief and effective method of helping those with addictive behaviors (primarily alcohol abuse and smoking) increase their motivational readiness to make positive behavior changes. Key components of this approach include acknowledging, normalizing, and gently working through the person's ambivalence concerning physical activity participation; stressing the individual's freedom to choose not to be physically active; encouraging personal responsibility for change and the consequences of not changing; developing an internal discrepancy for remaining inactive through strategic reflections, feedback, and questions from the counselor; and encouraging the participant to evaluate the pros and cons (*i.e.*, decisional balance) of remaining inactive versus becoming more active (47).

The **Five-A's Model** has also been used in client-centered counseling for physical activity (43). This model outlines five elements for professionals to use to engage participants in developing a plan for physical activity:

1. Address the agenda; why the participant is there.
2. Assess relevant aspects of current health and activity level, including readiness for change, physical activity history, and expectations.
3. Advise participants of the importance of behavior change, including risks and benefits.
4. Assist individuals in developing a plan for physical activity and overcoming barriers to change.
5. Arrange for follow-up after the plan is implemented.

This model is useful to structure the physical activity counseling session, assess motivational readiness to be active, and tailor recommendations based on the individual's current physical activity level, goals, and stage of change (see *GETP9, Box 11.2*).

SUMMARY

The variety of personal, social, and environmental factors that influence physical activity and sedentary behavior demonstrate the importance of incorporating behavioral strategies to positively influence successful adoption of physical activity, as well as promote long-term maintenance.

Behavior (including physical activity) is strongly influenced by its immediate consequences rather than distal, long-term consequences. Increasing the immediately rewarding aspects of physical activity, and decreasing the negative aspects, enhances the likelihood that the behavior will occur. Expectations concerning physical activity–related benefits and outcomes should be addressed during the initial stage of a program. Exploring beliefs, attitudes, and barriers early in the program sets the stage for realistic goal setting and minimizes disappointment and frustration. To facilitate sustained participation over time, behavioral self-management strategies should be encouraged. Tools to improve adherence include self-monitoring, goal setting, problem solving, decisional balance, behavioral commitment, self-assessment, reward systems, stimulus control, relapse prevention, social support, and other strategies. When appropriate, motivational interviewing strategies and other client-centered approaches can be used. Finally, it is advisable to encourage self-directed planning as a means of tailoring physical activity programs to fit the needs and preferences of participants and promote personal control and autonomy. Behavioral strategies are critical in providing individuals the skills needed to adopt physical activity and maintain physical activity long term. Professionals should incorporate principles of behavior change when planning and implementing fitness programs for individuals, groups, and communities.

REFERENCES

1. Adams J, White M. Are activity promotion interventions based on the transtheoretical model effective? A critical review. *Br J Sports Med*. 2003;37(2):106–14.

2. Alfonso ML, McDermott RJ, Thompson Z, et al. Vigorous physical activity among tweens, VERB Summer Scorecard program, Lexington, Kentucky, 2004–2007. *Prev Chronic Dis*. 2011;8(5): A104:1–11.

3. Andersen RE, Franckowiak SC, Snyder J, Bartlett SJ, Fontaine KR. Can inexpensive signs encourage the use of stairs? Results from a community intervention. *Ann Intern Med*. 1998;129(5):363–9.

4. Bandura A. The anatomy of stages of change. *Am J Health Promot*. 1997;12(1):8–10.

5. Bassett DR,Jr, Ainsworth BE, Leggett SR, et al. Accuracy of five electronic pedometers for measuring distance walked. *Med Sci Sports Exerc*. 1996;28(8):1071–7.

6. Boutelle KN, Jeffery RW, Murray DM, Schmitz MK. Using signs, artwork, and music to promote stair use in a public building. *Am J Public Health*. 2001;91(12):2004–6.

7. Brug J, Conner M, Harre N, Kremers S, McKellar S, Whitelaw S. The Transtheoretical Model and stages of change: a critique: observations by five commentators on the paper by Adams, J. and White, M. (2004) why don't stage-based activity promotion interventions work? *Health Educ Res*. 2005;20(2):244–58.

8. Castro CM, King AC. Telephone-assisted counseling for physical activity. *Exerc Sport Sci Rev*. 2002;30(2):64–8.

9. Charness G, Gneezy U. Incentives to exercise. *Econometrica*. 2009; 77(3):909–31.

10. Deci EL, Ryan RM. *Intrinsic Motivation and Self-Determination in Human Behavior*. New York (NY): Plenum; 1985. 371 p.

11. Deci EL, Ryan RM. The support of autonomy and the control of behavior. *J Pers Soc Psychol*. 1987;53(6):1024–37.

12. Dunn AL, Marcus BH, Kampert JB, Garcia ME, Kohl HW,3rd, Blair SN. Comparison of lifestyle and structured interventions to increase physical activity and cardiorespiratory fitness: a randomized trial. *JAMA*. 1999;281(4):327–34.

13. Fotheringham MJ, Wonnacott RL, Owen N. Computer use and physical inactivity in young adults: public health perils and potentials of new information technologies. *Ann Behav Med*. 2000;22(4): 269–75.

14. French SA, Story M, Jeffery RW. Environmental influences on eating and physical activity. *Annu Rev Public Health*. 2001;22: 309–35.

15. *Healthy People 2010* [Internet]. Washington (DC): U.S. Department of Health and Human Services; [cited 2011 Mar 22]. Available from: http://www.healthypeople.gov/2010/

16. Jackson D. How personal trainers can use self-efficacy theory to enhance exercise behavior in beginning exercisers. *Strength Cond J*. 2010;32(3):67–71.

17. Kahn EB, Ramsey LT, Brownson RC, et al. The effectiveness of interventions to increase physical activity. A systematic review. *Am J Prev Med*. 2002;22(4 Suppl):73–107.

18. Kerr J, Eves F, Carroll D. Encouraging stair use: stair-riser banners are better than posters. *Am J Public Health*. 2001;91(8):1192–3.

19. King AC, Carl F, Birkel L, Haskell WL. Increasing exercise among blue-collar employees: the tailoring of worksite programs to meet specific needs. *Prev Med*. 1988;17(3):357–65.

20. King AC, Frederiksen L. Low-cost strategies for increasing exercise behavior: relapse preparation training and social support. *Behav Modif*. 1984;8(1):3–21.

21. King AC, Friedman R, Marcus B, et al. Harnessing motivational forces in the promotion of physical activity: the Community Health Advice by Telephone (CHAT) project. *Health Educ Res*. 2002;17(5):627–36.

22. King AC, Rejeski WJ, Buchner DM. Physical activity interventions targeting older adults. A critical review and recommendations. *Am J Prev Med*. 1998;15(4):316–33.

23. King AC, Taylor CB, Haskell WL, DeBusk RF. Identifying strategies for increasing employee physical activity levels: findings from the Stanford/Lockheed Exercise Survey. *Health Educ Q*. 1990;17(3): 269–85.

24. Lewis BA, Marcus BH, Pate RR, Dunn AL. Psychosocial mediators of physical activity behavior among adults and children. *Am J Prev Med*. 2002;23(2 Suppl):26–35.

25. Lewis BA, Williams DM, Neighbors CJ, Jakicic JM, Marcus BH. Cost analysis of Internet vs. print interventions for physical activity promotion. *Psychol Sport Exerc*. 2010;11(3):246–9.

26. Marcus BH, Ciccolo JT, Sciamanna CN. Using electronic/computer interventions to promote physical activity. *Br J Sports Med*. 2009; 43(2):102–5.

27. Marcus BH, Dubbert PM, Forsyth LH, et al. Physical activity behavior change: issues in adoption and maintenance. *Health Psychol*. 2000;19(1 Suppl):32–41.

28. Marcus BH, Simkin LR. The transtheoretical model: applications to exercise behavior. *Med Sci Sports Exerc*. 1994;26(11):1400–4.

29. Marcus BH, Stanton AL. Evaluation of relapse prevention and reinforcement interventions to promote exercise adherence in sedentary females. *Res Q Exerc Sport*. 1993;64(4):447–52.

30. Martin JE, Dubbert PM, Katell AD, et al. Behavioral control of exercise in sedentary adults: studies 1 through 6. *J Consult Clin Psychol*. 1984;52(5):795–811.

31. Martin SB. Mental training for success. *American College of Sports Medicine FIT Society Page*. 2007(Fall): p. 3.

32. Matson-Koffman DM, Brownstein JN, Neiner JA, Greaney ML. A site-specific literature review of policy and environmental interventions that promote physical activity and nutrition for cardiovascular health: what works? *Am J Health Promot*. 2005;19(3):167–93.

33. McAuley E, Blissmer B, Marquez DX, Jerome GJ, Kramer AF, Katula J. Social relations, physical activity, and well-being in older adults. *Prev Med*. 2000;31(5):608–17.

34. McGinnis JM, Foege WH. The immediate vs the important. *JAMA*. 2004;291(10):1263–4.

35. Mullan E, Markland D, Ingledew D. A graded conceptualisation of self-determination in the regulation of exercise behavior: development of a measure using confirmatory factor analytic procedures. *Person Individ Diff*. 1997;23(5):745–52.

36. Myers RS, Roth DL. Perceived benefits of and barriers to exercise and stage of exercise adoption in young adults. *Health Psychol*. 1997;16(3):277–83.

37. Neff KL, King AC. Exercise program adherence in older adults: the importance of achieving one's expected benefits. *Med Exerc Nutr Health*. 1995;4(6):355–62.

38. Oka RK, King AC, Young DR. Sources of social support as predictors of exercise adherence in women and men ages 50 to 65 years. *Womens Health*. 1995;1(2):161–75.

39. Oman RF, King AC. Predicting the adoption and maintenance of exercise participation using self-efficacy and previous exercise participation rates. *Am J Health Promot*. 1998;12(3):154–61.

40. Pekmezi D, Barbera B, Marcus BH. Using the transtheoretical model to promote physical activity. *ACSM's Health Fit J*. 2010;14(4):8–13.

41. Pekmezi DW, Williams DM, Dunsiger S, et al. Feasibility of using computer-tailored and internet-based interventions to promote

physical activity in underserved populations. *Telemed J E Health.* 2010;16(4):498–503.

42. *Physical Inactivity: A Global Public Health Problem* [Internet]. Geneva (Switzerland): World Health Organization; [cited 2011 Jun 28]. Available from: http://www.who.int/dietphysicalactivity/ factsheet_inactivity/en/index.html

43. Pinto BM, Goldstein MG, Marcus BH. Activity counseling by primary care physicians. *Prev Med.* 1998;27(4):506–13.

44. Prochaska JO, Di Clemente CC. Transtheoretical therapy: toward a more integrative model of change. *Psychotherapy.* 1982;19(3):276–88.

45. Rejeski WJ, Brawley LR. Shaping active lifestyles in older adults: a group-facilitated behavior change intervention. *Ann Behav Med.* 1997;19(suppl):S106.

46. Rikli RE, Jones CJ. Development and validation of a functional fitness test for community-residing older adults. *J Aging Phys Activity.* 1999;7(2):129–61.

47. Rollnick S, Mason P, Butler C. *Health Behavior Change: A Guide for Practitioners.* New York (NY): Churchill Livingstone; 1999. 225 p.

48. Russell WD, Dzewaltowski DA, Ryan GJ. The effectiveness of a point-of-decision prompt in deterring sedentary behavior. *Am J Health Promot.* 1999;13(5):257–9, ii.

49. Sallis JF, Bauman A, Pratt M. Environmental and policy interventions to promote physical activity. *Am J Prev Med.* 1998;15(4):379–97.

50. Sallis JF, Owen N. Ecological models of health behavior. In: Glanz K, Rimer BK, Lewis FM, editors. *Health Behavior and Health Education: Theory, Research, and Practice.* 3rd ed. San Francisco: Jossey-Bass; 2002. p. 462–484.

51. Sallis JF, Owen N. *Physical Activity & Behavioral Medicine.* Thousand Oaks (CA): Sage Publications; 1999. 210 p.

52. Treiber FA, Baranowski T, Braden DS, Strong WB, Levy M, Knox W. Social support for exercise: relationship to physical activity in young adults. *Prev Med.* 1991;20(6):737–50.

53. Trost SG, Owen N, Bauman AE, Sallis JF, Brown W. Correlates of adults' participation in physical activity: review and update. *Med Sci Sports Exerc.* 2002;34(12):1996–2001.

54. Tudor-Locke C, Lutes L. Why do pedometers work?: a reflection upon the factors related to successfully increasing physical activity. *Sports Med.* 2009;39(12):981–93.

55. U.S. Department of Health and Human Services, Centers for Disease Control and Prevention, National Center for Chronic Disease Prevention and Health Promotion, The President's Council on Physical Fitness and Sports. *Physical Activity and Health: A Report of the Surgeon General.* Atlanta (GA): President's Council on Physical Fitness and Sports; 1996. 278 p.

56. Writing Group for the Activity Counseling Trial Research Group. Effects of physical activity counseling in primary care: the Activity Counseling Trial: a randomized controlled trial. *JAMA.* 2001;286(6): 677–87.

57. Young DR, King AC. Exercise adherence: determinants of physical activity and applications of health behavior change theories. *Med Exerc Nutr Health.* 1995;4(6):335–48.

SELECTED REFERENCES FOR FURTHER READING

American College of Sports Medicine. *ACSM FIT Society Page.* Behavior change and exercise adherence. 2011.

Anshell MH. *Applied Exercise Psychology: A Practitioner's Guide to Improving Client Health and Fitness.* New York (NY): Springer Publishing; 2006. 241 p.

Blair SN, Dunn AL, Marcus BH, Carpenter RA, Jaret P. *Active Living Every Day.* 2nd ed. Champaign (IL): Human Kinetics; 2011. 174 p.

Haugen K. Creating incentive campaigns. *ACSM's Health Fitness J.* 2009;13(2):22–6.

Marcus BH, Forsyth LH. *Motivating People to be Physically Active.* 2nd ed. Champaign (IL): Human Kinetics; 2009. 200 p.

INTERNET RESOURCES

American Heart Association. Better U Program: http://www.gored forwomen.org/betteru/index.aspx

Centers for Disease Control and Prevention. Division of Nutrition, Physical Activity and Obesity: http://www.cdc.gov/nccdphp/dnpao/ index.html

Centers for Disease Control and Prevention. Understanding and promoting physical activity. In: *Physical Activity and Health*: http://www.cdc.gov/nccdphp/sgr/chap6.htm

Exercise Is Medicine. http://www.exerciseismedicine.org/

Guide to Community Preventive Services. Behavioral and Social Approaches to Increase Physical Activity: Individually-Adapted Health Behavior Change Programs: http://www.thecommunity guide.org/pa/behavioral-social/individuallyadapted.html

U.S. Department of Health & Human Services. 2008 Physical Activity Guidelines for Americans: http://www.health.gov/paguidelines/

Counseling Physical Activity Behavior Change

This chapter discusses fundamental health counseling skills and describes methods for applying them with clients. In doing so, this chapter borrows from several of the theoretical principles described in *Chapter 44* and builds upon the specific skills discussed in *Chapter 45*. Practical application strategies are provided in more detail for the transtheoretical model (29), social cognitive theory (2,3), and the relapse prevention model (22). In addition, this chapter introduces some strategies from motivational interviewing, a counseling technique in which motivation for change is elicited and enhanced from the client, rather than imposed upon externally by the health professional (4,7,14,25,30). The intention is to teach strategies that will help practitioners to better understand how to communicate with their clients by applying the theoretical strategies and behavior

change skills presented in *Chapters 44* and *45*. The communication techniques discussed in this chapter will blend a client-centered approach (12,14,31,32), in which the practitioner listens and follows what the clients say, and a directive approach, in which the practitioner leads constructive discussions regarding behavior change (32). The strategies provided in this chapter do not highlight giving direct advice. Advice giving, although effective in some instances, can be detrimental to behavior change in others (11,32). Some clients may perceive advice giving as condescending or presumptuous, in that the client might perceive that he or she is being told what to do, thereby undermining his or her autonomy and possibly generating resistance (32). Instead, this chapter focuses on a client-centered approach that incorporates the counseling skills of rapport building, active listening, reflective

KEY TERMS

Active listening: A process whereby a practitioner tries to understand the underlying meaning of what a client is saying.

Client-centered approach: A counseling style that takes the client's perspective into account, features collaboration between the client and the practitioner, and includes genuine respect for the client's opinions.

Decisional balance: The comparison of the benefits versus the costs of making a behavior change.

Empathy: The understanding that is conveyed by a practitioner to a client.

Motivational interviewing: A client-centered counseling method in which the client's own motivation for change is elicited and enhanced by exploring and resolving ambivalence to change.

Open-ended questions: Questions that allow the client to provide expansive responses beyond a simple yes or no in which he or she can explore his or her thoughts and feelings.

Processes of change: The strategies that individuals use as they are adopting and maintaining behavior

changes; five behavioral (*e.g.*, obtaining social support) and five cognitive processes (*e.g.*, increasing knowledge) have been identified.

Rapport: The positive relationship that practitioners establish with their clients.

Reflective statements: Statements that repeat back to the client what the practitioner has heard and understood what the client has to say. If done in conjunction with active listening, these statements reflect the underlying meaning and/or feeling of what the client is saying.

Relapse prevention: The process by which one maintains long-term behavior change by anticipating potentially high-risk situations and devising strategies to cope with these situations.

Self-efficacy: An individual's belief and confidence about his or her ability to make specific behavior changes.

Stages of change: A model that postulates that individuals move through a series of stages and face common barriers when making a behavior change.

listening, and empathy, all of which are motivational interviewing skills (25,32). These counseling skills can then be the tools that are used with a directive approach in which discussions regarding self-monitoring, benefits and barriers, confidence, feedback, and relapse prevention can take place. Ultimately, the strategies decided on for guiding clients to increase physical activity levels are determined by a mutual working relationship between client and practitioner. This chapter assumes that the counseling techniques described are applied in the context of a relationship between a practitioner functioning as a health/wellness coach and a client or clients with the intent to encourage physical activity behavior.

HEALTH COUNSELING TECHNIQUES

The client-centered approach (6,11–14,31,32,38) takes the client's perspective into account when making decisions about behavior change. *Box 46-1* lists what Stewart et al. (38) have described as several of the key elements of the client-centered approach. This approach, when used by practitioners, has been shown to be related to higher client satisfaction, increased medication compliance, a reduction in clients' concerns, and a reduction in actual symptoms, such as raised blood pressure (38).

Rollnick et al. (32) summarize the goals of the client-centered approach as encouraging clients to express concerns, helping them to be more active in the consultation, allowing them to state what information they need, giving them more control of the decision making, and reaching joint decisions. One caveat to this approach is that there is typically a very limited amount of time with a client (*e.g.*, one 15-min consultation), which makes the client-centered approach more difficult. However, studies have indicated that even brief counseling can have impact on changes in physical activity behaviors (8). Therefore, the five A's of health behavior change will be reviewed at the end of this chapter to describe how the techniques and strategies illustrated throughout this manual can assist practitioners in delivering brief, specifically tailored messages for improving physical activity levels. To achieve the goals of the client-centered approach, practitioners need to be nonjudgmental and create a collaborative and cooperative partnership with their clients. Practitioners should establish rapport, be encouraging, be interested in the client's perspective, ask open-ended questions, and be good active listeners.

ESTABLISHING RAPPORT

The first important aspect in using the client-centered approach in working with clients is establishing rapport. Rapport is the relationship established with a client. It is built on trust and mutual respect. Practitioners need to be aware that rapport is usually necessary for a working relationship and is often perceived by the client in the initial meeting (33). If a strong therapeutic relationship is established from the beginning, the behavior change process is more likely to succeed. One strategy for establishing rapport is to ask the client open-ended questions. Open-ended questions give the client the opportunity to identify what is important to him or her. The information gathered from open-ended questions gives the practitioner useful information that can be used as leverages for change. For example, Rollnick et al. (32) suggest asking clients, "Can you please describe what a typical day is like for you?" This question is also part of the dialogue presented in *Box 46-2*.

This is meant to allow clients to tell about activities that occur throughout their day while providing several facts regarding how they spend their time. Practitioners should actively listen to the information being offered and observe the client's nonverbal behavior (*e.g.*, eye contact, body posture). This may be helpful in identifying client's thinking patterns, motivations, strengths, barriers, and, ultimately, opportunities for decreasing sedentary behavior and increasing active behavior. The practitioner should be aware that asking thoughtful and effective questions is the foundation of guiding the client to health behavior change. Rollnick et al. (33) state that practitioners need to be cognizant of what questions will elicit "change talk." Change talk represents the client's intentions on following through on the strategies discussed.

INTEREST AND EMPATHY

Conveying interest and empathy also helps to establish rapport (32). The process of listening and conveying understanding, or empathy, is not a passive process. When listening carefully to a client, one can convey what

| BOX 46-1 | Key Elements of the Client-Centered Approach |

- Approach the client with unconditional positive regard.
- Behavior change is based on a genuine, respectful relationship.
- Assessment of the client occurs when the practitioner seeks to enter the world of the client to understand his or her unique perspective.
- The client and the practitioner work together to define the problem and to establish the goals and the roles of the client and the practitioner.
- Each contact between the practitioner and the client is an opportunity to build the therapeutic relationship for health promotion.

Adapted from Rollnick S, Miller WR, Butler C. *Motivational Interviewing in Health Care: Helping Patients Change Behavior.* New York (NY): Guilford Press; 2008. 210 p.

BOX 46-2   Case Study

Case: A 43-yr-old woman has come to your fitness facility looking to get in shape. From her initial paperwork, you learn that she was active in sports as a child but has not had the time to fit regular activity into her daily life. She has a part-time job and is a mother of three children.

DIALOGUE	HEALTH BEHAVIOR COUNSELING SKILLS
Fitness Professional: Hello, Jane. It's great to meet you. Why don't you tell me a little bit about why you are here today?	Rapport building and an open-ended question
Client: Well, I need to lose a little weight, and I would like to be fit again.	
Fitness Professional: Okay, so, you would like to get in shape and lose weight. Can you tell me more about that?	Active listening with a reflective statement, open-ended question
Client: Sure. I used to be very active in high school. I played sports and loved it. Now I just can't seem to find the time to exercise. Yes, I have three kids and I work part time. I am always running them to after school activities and feel like a chauffeur more than anything most days [*sighs and slumps her shoulders*]. It's been so long since I was active. I'm not sure I'll be good at it or enjoy it, and I'm also not sure I can find the time to exercise.	
Fitness Professional: It sounds like you are a little apprehensive about exercising right now. This is common when you haven't been active in a while. Let me just make sure I am following you, Jane. You played sports as a child, but as you have gotten older and have more responsibilities with your job and family, you have had less time to be active. It also sounds like you aren't sure if you will enjoy it anymore. Is that right?	Active listening, reflective statement, empathetic statement, summary statement, verification
Client: That pretty much sums it up.	
Fitness Professional: Okay, well I can see that you are a very busy woman and that your schedule changes from day to day. But it would help if we have a starting point. So let's try to capture a typical day the best that we can. What would this look like for you?	Reflection with an open-ended question to build rapport and gather information

is heard by either reflecting or repeating the information, summarizing his or her statements, or asking questions for clarification. People want to feel heard and understood by others. An example of empathy is provided in the dialogue in *Box 46-2*. Using empathy demonstrates listening and gives a chance to make sure all is understood. Having empathy requires verbal and nonverbal acknowledgment of the other person's thoughts and feelings. This helps to build rapport with a client.

ACTIVE LISTENING

Another client-centered technique is called active listening (11,32). *Active listening* is a process wherein the practitioner tries to understand the *underlying meaning* of what the client is saying. The practitioner then makes reflective statements to convey that he or she has heard and understood this underlying meaning. This is a more advanced counseling skill and typically

takes some practice to use naturally. Reflecting back the underlying meaning can help to establish rapport and empathy in that it demonstrates understanding of the client's perspective. **Summarizing statements** can also be used to summarize content over a longer period of time, and elucidating themes of which the client might not be aware can also demonstrate an understanding of the client's perspective as well as help to keep the session focused (11). Open-ended questions permit an expansion of the dialogue by allowing clients to continue the conversation and clarify their thoughts or meaning (11). Attending to the client's nonverbal communications, such as his or her posture and facial expressions, can also be important to fill in the gaps between what the client might be saying and what he or she is feeling (11). The dialogue in *Box 46-2* illustrates how reflective statements, summarizations, open-ended questions, and attendance to verbal cues allow for an understanding of the client's motives and barriers to change.

SUMMARY OF HEALTH COUNSELING TECHNIQUES

Through the use of a few client-centered counseling techniques, one can increase satisfaction and compliance with clients. Rollnick et al. (32) summarize these techniques found in *Box 46-3*. To determine whether you are performing client-centered approach techniques properly, review the checklist summarized in *Box 46-4* (32).

BEHAVIOR CHANGE STRATEGIES TO INCREASE PHYSICAL ACTIVITY

The health counseling skills described previously can be used within the framework of behavior change strategies. These strategies are more direct but can be accomplished through conversations using the client-centered techniques of summarizing, clarifying, active listening, reflective statements, summarizing statements, and empathy. The following behavior change strategies offer methods to work with clients to assess readiness for behavior change, determine strategies appropriate for a given stage of change, identify socioecological factors related to behavior, track progress, and set goals.

STAGES OF CHANGE

As is described in *Chapter 44*, the transtheoretical model offers both a means of assessing readiness to change as well as several cognitive and behavioral processes to promote behavior change with your clients. In brief, the transtheoretical model postulates that individuals move through a series of stages as they become physically active (18,29,36). As participants move through

BOX 46-4	How You Know When You Are Using the Client-Centered Approach

- You are speaking slowly.
- The client is talking more than you.
- The client is talking about behavior change.
- You are listening intently and directing the conversation when appropriate.
- The client appears to be making realizations and connections that he or she had not previously considered.
- The client is asking you for information or advice.

Adapted from Rollnick S, Mason P, Butler C. *Health Behavior Change: A Guide for Practitioners.* New York (NY): Churchill Livingstone; 1999. 225 p.

the stages of change, they actively engage in cognitive and behavioral processes that allow them to reach the next level.

Although there are a few different versions of how to assess the stages of change, we recommend using the version in *Box 46-5* (18). First, moderate-intensity physical activity is defined for the individuals. Then, clients indicate a "yes" or "no" to four statements about their physical activity behavior and intentions. The algorithm shown in *Box 46-5* is used to identify the stage for a specific individual. In working with clients, you could ask these questions conversationally to assess the client's motivational readiness or you might have the client fill out the questionnaire.

Knowing a person's stage of change suggests different strategies for working with that particular person. It is possible to target an intervention to an individual's stage of change (17,19–21). It has been shown that individuals who are in the earlier stages of change — precontemplation and contemplation — are more likely to use the cognitive processes of change, such as increasing knowledge and comprehending the benefits. As people move into the later stages, they start to use more behavioral processes of change, such as enlisting social support and substituting alternatives. Matching the change processes to the client's stage is another important component of a client-centered approach. In addition, knowing the client's stage of change and being aware of change talk allow the practitioner to use strategies to help motivate the client to transition to the next stage (33). *Change talk* refers to comments that the client makes that portrays his or her willingness and commitment to make changes (34). Examples include the client saying, "I hope that I will exercise more this year" versus "I will exercise more this year." Being able to evaluate change talk conveys that you understand how ready a client is to change.

BOX 46-3	Summary of Client-Centered Techniques

- Ask simple, open-ended questions (*i.e.*, questions that elicit details, not simple yes-or-no responses).
- Listen and encourage with verbal and nonverbal prompts.
- Clarify and summarize. Check your understanding of what the client said and check to see that the client understood what you said.
- Use reflective listening. This involves making statements that aim to bridge the gap between what that client is saying and the meaning behind the statements.

Adapted from Rollnick S, Mason P, Butler C. *Health Behavior Change: A Guide for Practitioners.* New York (NY): Churchill Livingstone; 1999. 225 p.

BOX 46-5   Assessing Physical Activity Stages of Change

PHYSICAL ACTIVITY STAGES OF CHANGE

INSTRUCTIONS: For each question below, please circle Yes (Y) or No (N). Please be sure to follow the instructions carefully.

	Yes	**No**
1. I am currently physically active.	Y	N
2. I intend to become more physically active in the next 6 mo.	Y	N

For activity to be regular, it must add up to a total of 30 or more minutes per day and be done at least 5 d · wk^{-1}. For example, you could take one 30-min walk or three 10-min walks each day.

	Yes	**No**
3. I currently engage in regular physical activity.	Y	N
4. I have been regularly physically active for the past 6 mo.	Y	N

Stage	ITEM			
	1	2	3	4
Precontemplation	No	No	—	—
Contemplation	No	Yes	—	—
Preparation	Yes	—	No	—
Action	Yes	—	Yes	No
Maintenance	Yes	—	Yes	Yes

Modified with permission from Marcus B, Forsyth L. *Motivating People to be Physically Active.* 2nd ed. Champaign (IL): Human Kinetics; 2009. 200 p.

SOCIOECOLOGICAL FACTORS

Understanding the relationships among socioecological factors (*i.e.*, the interpersonal, intrapersonal, community, and organizational factors) and physical activity is essential to successful behavior changes for your clients (23,35). The practitioner uses appropriate health coaching skills to elicit information on the multiple factors that contribute to client inactivity. The practitioner should focus on how the behavior makes sense for each particular client. For example, a child might not be getting the recommended amount of physical activity for several reasons. Some of these reasons might be because the child attends a school that does not have physical education classes nor recess (organizational), he is not allowed to participate in team sports because of transportation problems (intrapersonal), his family lives in an unsafe neighborhood (community), and he feels embarrassed because he is overweight (interpersonal). Using a client-centered approach, the practitioner conceptualizes the multiple determinants of physical inactivity by assisting the client in identifying these multileveled factors, verbalizing unused opportunities, and outlining the most appropriate starting point for intervention. Moreover, the practitioner would guide

the client in identifying strengths in each of the multiple levels, which can create leverages for change. To follow up on the example given, if not being able to participate in team sports because of transportation is deemed a significant barrier and the caregiver's relationships with her neighbors is a strength, then the practitioner can use a client-centered approach to guide the caregiver in developing an appropriate solution. A potential solution could be that the caregiver makes arrangements to carpool with a neighbor and has the child attend an afterschool basketball program that practices three times per week.

In summary, the practitioner evaluates the multiple socioecological factors that are sustaining sedentary behaviors and uses client strengths as the catalyst for change. The evaluation is ongoing and responsive to client progress. It is important to note that if the client is not meeting his or her goals, then the practitioner needs to assess "why" and reformulate more appropriate goals. *Box 46-6* provides a conceptualization tool for the practitioner.

TRACKING ACTIVITY

Another strategy to assess daily activities is to have clients track their daily behaviors on self-monitoring forms

BOX 46-6	**Conceptualization Tool for Current Behavior**

Current Behavior: _____

Current Behavior: (<u>Example: Physical inactivity of a 14-yr-old girl</u>)

INSTRUCTIONS: Identify reasons for physical inactivity per socioecological level and potential strengths, which can be used as leverages for change. (See examples in gray.)

	INFLUENCES THAT LIMIT PHYSICAL ACTIVITY	**INFLUENCES THAT SUPPORT PHYSICAL ACTIVITY**
Interpersonal	1. *Low self-efficacy* 2. 3. 4. 5.	1. *Intelligent* 2. 3. 4. 5.
Intrapersonal	1. *Mother is at work and cannot drive to extracurricular activities.* 2. 3. 4. 5.	1. *Aunt just ran 5 km.* 2. 3. 4. 5.
Community	1. *Neighborhood is not safe.* 2. 3. 4. 5.	1. *Neighbor has child in track and willing to carpool.* 2. 3. 4. 5.
Organizational	1. *Physical education classes are only required once per week for 20 min.* 2. 3. 4. 5.	1. *Church has recreational sports leagues.* 2. 3. 4. 5.

(9,15,20,21). There are many ways to do this, and you can tailor the tracking form to an individual's needs. For example, if a client is in contemplation, she may need to track how she spends her time on a daily basis. This means writing down her activities, including sedentary activities (*e.g.*, time spent watching television, driving, sitting while eating, sitting at the computer) and the time spent at each activity. *Box 46-7* provides an example of a self-monitoring log.

If the client keeps track of this for several days over the course of the week, you can review the monitoring form together the following week. This provides a directive framework for your discussion while still using client-centered counseling strategies. It is important to identify opportunities for decreasing sedentary behavior and increasing physical activity and what the benefits

and barriers might be for both. For instance, if the client is sitting at a computer for many hours at a time, it may be possible to encourage incorporating short walks to break up this computer time. From a client-centered perspective, you would initiate a conversation about how computer time exemplifies physical inactivity that may lead the client to recognize this as an opportunity for change. Finding small instances for the client to become less sedentary can provide the first building block of activity for an individual who has been inactive.

In contrast, if a person is in the preparation stage, the tracking might be quite different. Individuals in the preparation stage may not need to record their activity throughout the day but may focus instead on their bouts of moderate or vigorous activity and identify opportunities for increasing these behaviors. This self-monitoring

BOX 46-7	Tracking Form

EXAMPLE

Date: _____

TIME	ACTIVITY	MINUTES SPENT DOING	NOTES
7:00 a.m.	Got ready for work	60	
8:00 a.m.	Drove to work	45	
8:45 a.m.	Walked in to work	3	Walked slowly
8:50 a.m.	At my desk for computer work	180	Wow!

form would be used to log the type of activity, days and times performed, perceived intensity, and even their enjoyment level during the physical activity bouts. Again, the self-monitoring form can provide the framework for a discussion regarding physical activity. You can review with your client any patterns of behavior that may arise and work with him or her to think of ways to increase his or her activity level. For instance, in tracking his activity, a client may have 2 d when he was physically active. In an attempt to clarify and understand this, you may ask, "How were you able to exercise those two days?" This is a strength-focused question that allows the client to figure out how he was able to exercise those two days compared to the other days he wasn't able to exercise. The client may then describe that on the days when he was inactive, he had planned to go to the fitness facility *after work* rather than before work. However, he often found that he was too tired and went home instead. Thus, he may recognize that he was more successful going to the fitness center before work. The natural tendency is to advise the client based on this information. However, using the client-centered approach, it would be important for the client to come to his own realizations about changing his behavior. By listening carefully, reflecting, and emphasizing the positive, the client might make the connections that you hope he will make (*i.e.*, "I should be physically active in the mornings or make a plan to go the gym even if I am tired"). In some cases, the client may understand what is not working but is unsure of what to do to change the situation. In these situations, the technique of problem solving, as described later, may be used.

DECISIONAL BALANCE

Another strategy for motivating behavior change is to have clients identify the benefits and barriers of being physically active that reflect decisional balance (20,21). To do this, you might have an open-ended conversation about this or you can have your client list his or her

perceived benefits (pros) and perceived barriers (cons) for physical activity. The list must reflect what is important to the client and not just a list of general benefits of physical activity. For example, a client may know that one of the benefits of physical activity is decreasing the risk of osteoporosis, but this might not be personally important. However, feeling less fatigued may be a more motivating factor for this particular client. Information obtained from this list can provide the framework for another conversation about behavior change while continuing to use your counseling techniques. Another resource for a similar measure is the decisional balance questionnaire, which is found in Marcus and Forsyth (18).

Benefits

This list of benefits, or pros, can be important to discuss as a means of affirming the reasons why the client is interested in behavior change (9,20,21,26). This list can also be important to keep in mind when working with your client if his motivation or behavior is low in the future. You can ask your client to recount why he would like to be physically active. For a client who feels tired after work, remembering that one of the pros he listed was increased energy and that he will feel more energetic after exercising may give him the motivation he needs to make that decision in the moment. In addition, if you are working with a client over time, you can emphasize progress with positive statements that will help to reinforce or increase the behavior. For example, if you see the client looking less fatigued, you might comment, "It looks like you have more energy these days." This helps to reaffirm the benefits of his activity that you knew were important to him from his initial list of pros and cons. Observing how a client is readily able or not able to identify his or her personal benefits of being physically active also allows you as the practitioner to understand how the client problem solves. For example, if the client can easily identify three to five personal benefits of being physically active, then he or she might have an easier time overcoming barriers than someone who has a difficult time personalizing the benefits. As a practitioner, this gives you additional information on where you might need to intervene. The practitioner might need to take a step back with the client who is having a hard time identifying and personalizing the benefits of being physically active and help her reevaluate her reasons for wanting to make this health behavior change.

Barriers

The list of barriers, or cons, is important to address to determine the obstacles that may stand in the way of your client's making progress (9,20,21). If your client is having difficulty identifying her barriers or it seems the list is incomplete, you may find that self-monitoring provides insight into the client's barriers. For example, if the client takes a walk only on the days her neighbor is available to walk with her but not on the days when she would need to walk alone, you might have a discussion about this. As mentioned earlier, you should find a way to allow the client to come to her own conclusion. Examples of what you might say include "It seems as though you really enjoy walking with your neighbor" or "What do you enjoy about your walks with your neighbor?" In this way, you may be able to gently direct the client to realize that walking alone is a barrier and having someone to walk with is a facilitator to being active. The goal is to work with your client to determine her unique barriers to increase physical activity. In doing so, you may need to refer to the self-monitoring form, and you may need to help the client determine which barriers are more or less difficult to overcome. It is particularly important to be nonjudgmental in this process so that the client feels comfortable and confident to problem solve solutions to the barriers.

PROBLEM SOLVING

After the barriers have been determined, an important skill to help your client develop is problem solving. Problem solving can be done to determine solutions for the barriers that your client has identified (9,16,18). The *process* of problem solving is more important to learn than a set of solutions for any one barrier so that the client will know *how* to tackle barriers in the future. Problem solving, therefore, fosters independent thinking and self-confidence in one's abilities to remain physically active. Problem solving involves several different steps (18). The acronym IDEA has been developed to identify the four steps of *I*dentifying the problem, *D*eveloping a list of solutions, *E*valuating the solutions, and *A*nalyzing how well the plan worked. *Box 46-8* provides an example of this problem-solving technique.

The first step involves identifying the problem. From the list of barriers that your client has been able to identify, have your client pick one that is most pressing. In identifying the problem, it will be important to think through the problem fully to determine the key element or elements. In our example earlier of the woman who only walked when her neighbor was available, you should ask her to identify why this occurred. As the client starts to talk about this, she may realize that she needs social support to be active. There are often many layers to any one problem, and it may be necessary to probe further to determine what about obtaining social support is important. In doing so, you may learn that walking with her neighbor is enjoyable, the time passes quickly, she feels safer, and she feels more motivated because she knows her friend is going to be meeting her.

The second step is to develop a list of solutions. This is a brainstorming session in which the client thinks of any and all solutions while withholding any evaluation of them until later. This is a time to be creative. You may help your client with a few if he or she is having trouble getting started. It is likely that you will need to remind your client that you do not evaluate the ideas at this stage. Have the client write down all of the solutions that are generated. Possible solutions for the female walker include seeing if her neighbor can walk more often, joining a class at a gym, walking with her spouse, starting a walking club, or finding other friends who are available on other days.

The third step is to evaluate the solutions. Some solutions will be more realistic and address more of the details of the problems than others. You can work with your client to determine which of the solutions seem most appropriate. It may be that starting a walking club is too daunting, but asking her neighbor to walk more often seems feasible. Whatever the solutions, work with your client to set goals and make a concrete plan about how the solution will be implemented. This step is very important, and the practitioner needs to be aware of how the behavior makes sense for that client and not simply give a "laundry list" of solutions that are not personalized. The practitioner might have to ask probing questions that will allow the client to realize how some solutions are more appropriate than others.

The final step is to analyze how well the plan worked. If a plan worked well, then praise the client for a job well done. Many times, however, the plan will not have worked as was intended. It is important to emphasize that problem solving is a process that allows for learning, and it is not uncommon to fine-tune the solution. In some cases, attempts to implement a solution elicit new details regarding the problem or new barriers. This information is critical to correctly identifying all of the important aspects of a problem and searching for a solution that addresses these aspects. Clients may be discouraged with their progress. It is important to emphasize the positive of what the client did

BOX 46-8   Problem-Solving Worksheet Idea

1. Identify the problem.
2. Develop solutions.
3. Evaluate the solutions.
4. Analyze the plan.

EXAMPLE

1. Identify the problem: Don't want to exercise by myself.
   Details of the problem: Prefer the company, need the accountability, and feel safer.
2. Develop solutions.

SOLUTIONS	EVALUATION	SELECT
Walk with my neighbor.		
Walk with other friends.		
Join an aerobics class.		

3. Evaluate the solutions.

SOLUTIONS	EVALUATION	SELECT
Walk with my neighbor.	She is too busy.	
Walk with other friends.	Offers company, safety, and accountability	X
Join an aerobics class.	Offers company, safety, and accountability but is too expensive	

4. Analyze the solution: Two friends agreed, and I went on one walk with one friend and two walks with another friend. Seems to be working. _____

YOUR TURN:

1. Identify the problem:_____
   Details of the problem:_____
   _____

2. Develop solutions.
3. Evaluate solutions.

SOLUTIONS	EVALUATION	SELECT

4. Analyze plan:_____

Modified with permission from Marcus B, Forsyth L. *Motivating People to be Physically Active*. 2nd ed. Champaign (IL): Human Kinetics; 2009. 200 p.

accomplish, emphasize the importance of learning from what does not work, and work together to generate new solutions and plans.

GOAL SETTING

Another important skill for clients to develop is the ability to set goals (1,26,27,36). It is important to identify several characteristics of goal setting, including setting goals that are specific, short term, and challenging yet realistic (2). It is also important to make goals measurable, develop a way to track goals through self-monitoring, and provide feedback regarding success or failure to achieve goals. A popular model for framing a client's goal is provided by the acronym SMART — goals that are *Specific, Measurable, Action-oriented, Realistic,* and *Timely* (36). In the context of the stages of change, the goals that are appropriate for clients vary by stage. For example, a person in precontemplation may read about the benefits of physical activity over the coming week, whereas a person in preparation may set a physical activity goal of walking four times per week for 30 min each time.

Setting goals that are specific is the first important characteristic of a goal. This might initially require some coaching. Clients may set a goal of "I will try to be more physically active." Although this is a good start and should be reinforced, getting the client to fill in the details increases the likelihood of success. Therefore, work with your client to establish specific and realistic goals related to physical activity that includes frequency, intensity, time, and type of activity. Consider individual circumstances and possible physical limitations. Help your client set a short-term goal that is limited to the following week and realistic to achieve. For example, if a client knows that a travel for business is scheduled in the following week, it may not be realistic to set a goal that is more achievable during a routine week at home. Accomplishing goals increases self-confidence and the likelihood that a client will set more challenging goals in the future. On the other hand, it is also important to make sure that the goal is challenging and not too easy to accomplish because more difficult goals can provide increased motivation.

Writing down the goal and then recording activity is an important way for the client to see his or her progress and to continue to identify barriers. The monitoring sheets provide feedback to the client (see *Box 46-7*) and an opportunity to reinforce any positive changes that the client was able to make, even if all of the established goals were not met. Ideally, clients will learn how to give themselves feedback and feel proud of their accomplishments. In addition, the monitoring forms can provide opportunities for identifying barriers and problem-solving opportunities and serve as cues, or reminders, to be active.

CONFIDENCE

Self-efficacy, or confidence in one's abilities to be physically active, is very important for behavior change (1,2,5,9,16,24,26). Confidence can be increased in several ways: (a) through verbal praise and reinforcement, (b) by watching others become successful at the behavior, (c) by correctly interpreting the body's physiologic reaction to physical activity, and (d) through guided mastery experiences (2). The practitioner can help clients with all of these components by encouraging their successes and by having them think of others who were successful. Additionally, the practitioner can encourage clients to think about other areas in their lives in which they are successful and about how information from these experiences can help them with this new behavior change by guiding them to self-monitor, problem solve, set goals, and receive feedback. In this way, clients increase their confidence and become better equipped to problem solve new obstacles. The use of a client-centered approach and matching the activity to clients' particular stages of change also help in increasing clients' confidence in being physically active. See Marcus and Forsyth (18) for a self-efficacy assessment and Brehm's and Griffin's books listed in the Selected References at the end of this chapter for more information about implementing strategies to improve your clients' self-efficacy.

RELAPSE PREVENTION

Another area that can be helpful in working with your clients is that of relapse prevention (9,22,26,37). Relapse prevention should be conducted with every client because we all have times when our activity levels tend to decrease or stop. Preventing relapse (*i.e.,* reverting to inactivity) is a proactive approach to problem solving future obstacles or for managing temporary lapses (*i.e.,* temporary periods of inactivity). If you have a client who has a life event coming up during which it will be difficult to remain active, you can identify the problem and engage in problem solving just as you would any other barrier. These times are often referred to as *high-risk situations.* Examples include times of bad weather, injury, losing an exercise partner, vacations, visitors, holiday gatherings, or other situations that might make it difficult to engage in physical activity. There may also be times when you notice that your client's activity level has dropped. Helping your client see this as a temporary lapse and not a relapse can be helpful in getting the client back into a routine of activity. To do this, you can problem solve and set goals but also let the client know that although it is not unusual to have times of decreased activity, it is important to get back on track as soon as possible.

There may be times, however, when a client is experiencing difficulties that are making physical activity difficult to accomplish. In some cases, a person may be experiencing depression, anxiety, or other mental health issues. Some of the symptoms of depression and anxiety are lack of energy and difficulty concentrating, both of which make attending to physical activity difficult. In these cases, it may be important to determine if there is a need to refer the person for additional help. For suspected depression, simply ask, "Are you feeling so sad or down that it is making it difficult to perform your daily activities?" For anxiety, the question "Are you feeling so nervous or anxious that it is making it difficult to perform your daily activities?" is appropriate. If the client answers yes, then it is appropriate to recommend seeking help from a physician or a mental health professional.

FIVE A'S OF HEALTH BEHAVIOR CHANGE

Because of the inherent time constraints in coaching clients, we would like to review the five A's of health behavior change to assist practitioners in delivering brief, specifically tailored messages to their clients. Research has shown that it can take less than 3 min to successfully intervene with a client on promoting physical activity in a primary care setting (8,10,28,39). The various counseling techniques and strategies discussed in this chapter can be incorporated into implementing the five A's of health behavior change for improving physical activity levels. The five A's are assess, advise, agree, assist, and arrange.

The practitioner should first *assess* the client's type, frequency, intensity, and duration of current physical activity, as well as any contraindications to physical activity. In addition, the practitioner should also evaluate the client's stage of change, benefits and barriers of physical activity, and the client's self-efficacy and social support system. Next, the practitioner uses this evaluation to *advise* the client based on his or her stage of change. This advice is client centered and includes an individually tailored counseling message. For example, the practitioner might review the national recommendations for physical activity but will modify this based on how it makes sense for the client. Thus, the practitioner and client will *agree* on the type and level of intervention. Clients who are not contemplating a change to become more active should not necessarily receive an active plan for increasing physical activity levels. Instead, practitioners should continue to advise these clients at subsequent visits regarding benefits of increasing their physical activity level. But if the client is in the preparation stage, the practitioner can *assist* the client in outlining specific goals of intervention dependent on the client's stage of change. For example, the client could receive a tracking form to write down the number of times he or she is moderately or vigorously active for 30 min with a weekly goal of four times. Other resources that can assist clients are printed support materials; a pedometer, calendar, and other self-monitoring tools; and Internet-based resources. Lastly, the practitioner *arranges* the next steps for the client.

This could include a follow-up visit; reminder phone calls, e-mails, or messages; and/or referrals to a specialist (17,18,20,21).

GROUP COUNSELING

The skills and techniques described thus far can be easily integrated into a group setting. The major advantage of groups is the natural support system that it provides to the clients. Other advantages of a group setting include the client's ability to (a) provide feedback to each other based on experiences, (b) emulate others' successful techniques, (c) evaluate the practicality of desired goals and objectives, (d) encourage commitment, (e) realize that problems are solvable, and (f) provide additional resources.

To maximize effectiveness of group programs and interventions, the practitioner needs to be able to positively manage the group dynamics. Effective groups generally require that the practitioner provides purpose and structure for the group so each member of the group is successful individually and collectively. For example, it is important that the practitioner guides the group participants in identifying the purpose, objectives, and goals of the group together. This will provide ownership to each individual client as well as a unified purpose of the group. An effective group facilitator also guides and controls the group process to ensure participation, mutual understanding, and shared responsibility for the outcomes. This is done through the practitioner's use of ongoing rapport building, active and reflective listening, and empathy to understand the big picture and use of behavior change techniques to improve motivation and ultimately increase levels of physical activity.

SUMMARY

Health practitioners have the opportunity to develop rapport and facilitate behavior change with their clients. This chapter discussed the client-centered approach, which emphasizes techniques such as empathy, active listening, and reflective statements (4,6,7,11–14,30–32,38). These skills can be used by practitioners to understand the perspective of their clients across socioecological factors. These coaching techniques can also be used when using behavior change techniques, such as tracking progress, solving problems, increasing confidence, setting goals, and providing feedback. Long-term success for clients will be enhanced as they become increasingly self-sufficient with these behavior change strategies. It is important to remember that the more the practitioner learns about clients' attitudes, beliefs, motivations, and behaviors, the more information one will have to guide clients in increasing their physical activity levels.

REFERENCES

1. Anderson ES, Wojcik JR, Winett RA, Williams DM. Social-cognitive determinants of physical activity: the influence of social support, self-efficacy, outcome expectations, and self-regulation among participants in a church-based health promotion study. *Health Psychol.* 2006;25(4):510–20.

2. Bandura A. *Self-Efficacy: The Exercise of Control.* New York (NY): W. H. Freeman; 1997. 604 p.

3. Bandura A. *Social Foundations of Thought and Action: A Social Cognitive Theory.* Englewood Cliffs (NJ): Prentice-Hall; 1986. 617 p.

4. Bennett JA, Lyons KS, Winters-Stone K, Nail LM, Scherer J. Motivational interviewing to increase physical activity in long-term cancer survivors: a randomized controlled trial. *Nurs Res.* 2007;56(1):18–27.

5. Bray SR. Self-efficacy for coping with barriers helps students stay physically active during transition to their first year at a university. *Res Q Exerc Sport.* 2007;78(2):61–70.

6. Brehm BA. *Successful Fitness Motivation Strategies.* Champaign (IL): Human Kinetics; 2004. 188 p.

7. Carels RA, Darby L, Cacciapaglia HM, et al. Using motivational interviewing as a supplement to obesity treatment: a stepped-care approach. *Health Psychol.* 2007;26(3):369–74.

8. Carroll JK, Fiscella K, Epstein RM, et al. Getting patients to exercise more: a systematic review of underserved populations. *J Fam Pract.* 2008;57(3):170–6, E1–3, 1 p following E3.

9. Dunn AL, Marcus BH, Kampert JB, Garcia ME, Kohl HW,3rd, Blair SN. Reduction in cardiovascular disease risk factors: 6-month results from Project Active. *Prev Med.* 1997;26(6):883–92.

10. Eden KB, Orleans CT, Mulrow CD, Pender NJ, Teutsch SM. Does counseling by clinicians improve physical activity? A summary of the evidence for the U.S. Preventive Services Task Force. *Ann Intern Med.* 2002;137(3):208–15.

11. Gavin J. *Lifestyle Fitness Coaching.* Champaign (IL): Human Kinetics; 2005. 282 p.

12. Griffin JC. *Client-Centered Exercise Prescription.* 2nd ed. Champaign (IL): Human Kinetics; 2006. 339 p.

13. Grueninger UL, Duffy FD, Goldstein MG. Patient education in the medical encounter: how to facilitate learning, behavior change, and coping. In: Lipkin M, Putnam SM, Lazare A, editors. *The Medical Interview: Clinical Care, Education, and Research.* New York: Springer-Verlag; 1995. p. 122–133.

14. Hardcastle S, Taylor A, Bailey M, Castle R. A randomised controlled trial on the effectiveness of a primary health care based counselling intervention on physical activity, diet, and CHD risk factors. *Patient Educ Couns.* 2008;70(1):31–9.

15. Heesch KC, Masse LC, Dunn AL, Frankowski RF, Mullen PD. Does adherence to a lifestyle physical activity intervention predict changes in physical activity? *J Behav Med.* 2003;26(4):333–48.

16. Hughes SL, Seymour RB, Campbell RT, et al. Long-term impact of Fit and Strong! on older adults with osteoarthritis. *Gerontologist.* 2006;46(6):801–14.

17. Marcus BH, Emmons KM, Simkin-Silverman LR, et al. Evaluation of motivationally tailored vs. standard self-help physical activity interventions at the workplace. *Am J Health Promot.* 1998;12(4):246–53.

18. Marcus B, Forsyth L. *Motivating People to be Physically Active.* 2nd ed. Champaign (IL): Human Kinetics; 2009. 200 p.

19. Marcus BH, Lewis BA. Stages of motivational readiness to change physical activity behavior. *Pres Counc Phys Fit Sports Res Dig.* 2003; 47:1–8.

20. Marcus BH, Lewis BA, Williams DM, et al. Step into motion: a randomized trial examining the relative efficacy of Internet vs. print-based physical activity interventions. *Contemp Clin Trials.* 2007; 28(6):737–47.

21. Marcus BH, Napolitano MA, King AC, et al. Telephone versus print delivery of an individualized motivationally tailored physical activity intervention: Project STRIDE. *Health Psychol.* 2007; 26(4):401–9.

22. Marlatt GA, Gordon JR. *Relapse Prevention: Maintenance Strategies in the Treatment of Addictive Behaviors.* New York (NY): Guilford Press; 1985. 558 p.

23. Maziak W, Ward KD, Stockton MB. Childhood obesity: are we missing the big picture? *Obes Rev.* 2008;9(1):35–42.

24. McAuley E, Morris KS, Motl RW, Hu L, Konopack JF, Elavsky S. Long-term follow-up of physical activity behavior in older adults. *Health Psychol.* 2007;26(3):375–80.

25. Miller WR, Rollnick S. *Motivational Interviewing: Preparing People to Change Addictive Behavior.* New York (NY): Guilford Press; 1991. 348 p.

26. Nies MA, Reisenberg CE, Chruscial HL, Artibee K. Southern women's response to a walking intervention. *Public Health Nurs.* 2003; 20(2):146–52.

27. Nothwehr F, Yang J. Goal setting frequency and the use of behavioral strategies related to diet and physical activity. *Health Educ Res.* 2007; 22(4):532–8.

28. Pinto BM, Lynn H, Marcus BH, DePue J, Goldstein MG. Physician-based activity counseling: intervention effects on mediators of motivational readiness for physical activity. *Ann Behav Med.* 2001; 23(1):2–10.

29. Prochaska JO, DiClemente CC. Stages and processes of self-change of smoking: toward an integrative model of change. *J Consult Clin Psychol.* 1983;51(3):390–5.

30. Resnicow K, Jackson A, Blissett D, et al. Results of the healthy body healthy spirit trial. *Health Psychol.* 2005;24(4):339–48.

31. Rogers CT. A theory of therapy, personality, and interpersonal relationships as developed in the client-centered framework. In: Koch S, editor. *Psychology: A Study of a Science.* New York: McGraw-Hill; 1959. p. 184–256.

32. Rollnick S, Mason P, Butler C. *Health Behavior Change: A Guide for Practitioners.* New York (NY): Churchill Livingstone; 1999. 225 p.

33. Rollnick S, Miller WR, Butler C. *Motivational Interviewing in Health Care: Helping Patients Change Behavior.* New York (NY): Guilford Press; 2008. 210 p.

34. Rosengren DB. *Building Motivational Interviewing Skills: A Practitioner Workbook.* New York (NY): Guildford Press; 2009. 335 p.

35. Sallis JF, Owen N. Ecological models of health behavior. In: Glanz K, Rimer BK, Lewis FM, editors. *Health Behavior and Health Education: Theory, Research, and Practice.* 3rd ed. San Francisco: Jossey-Bass; 2002. p. 462–484.

36. Shilts MK, Horowitz M, Townsend MS. Goal setting as a strategy for dietary and physical activity behavior change: a review of the literature. *Am J Health Promot.* 2004;19(2):81–93.

37. Stetson BA, Beacham AO, Frommelt SJ, et al. Exercise slips in high-risk situations and activity patterns in long-term exercisers: an application of the relapse prevention model. *Ann Behav Med.* 2005;30(1):25–35.

38. Stewart M, Brown JB, Weston WW, McWhinney IR, McWilliam CL, Freeman TR. *Patient-Centered Medicine: Transforming the Clinical Method.* Thousand Oaks (CA): Sage Publications; 1995. 267 p.

39. Whitlock EP, Orleans CT, Pender N, Allan J. Evaluating primary care behavioral counseling interventions: an evidence-based approach. *Am J Prev Med.* 2002;22(4):267–84.

SELECTED REFERENCES FOR FURTHER READING

American College of Sports Medicine. *ACSM Fitness Book.* 3rd ed. Champaign (IL): Human Kinetics; 2003. 184 p.

Brehm BA. *Successful Fitness Motivation Strategies.* Champaign (IL): Human Kinetics; 2004. 200 p.

Gavin J. *Lifestyle Fitness Coaching.* Champaign (IL): Human Kinetics; 2005. 282 p.

Griffin JC. *Client-Centered Exercise Prescription.* 2nd ed. Champaign (IL): Human Kinetics; 2006. 339 p.

Marcus BH, Forsyth LH. *Motivating People to be Physically Active*. 2nd ed. Champaign (IL): Human Kinetics; 2009. 200 p.

Marcus BH, Lewis BA. Stages of motivational readiness to change physical activity behavior. *Pres Counc Phys Fit Sports Res Dig*. 2003; 4:1–8.

Rollnick S, Mason P, Butler C. *Health Behavior Change: A Guide for Practitioners*. New York (NY): Churchill Livingstone; 1999. 225 p.

Stewart M, Brown JB, Weston WW, McWhinney IR, McWilliam CL, Freeman TR. *Patient-Centered Medicine: Transforming the Clinical Method*. Thousand Oaks (CA): Sage Publications; 1995. 267 p.

INTERNET RESOURCES

- American Heart Association (exercise [physical activity] counseling): http://www.americanheart.org/presenter.jhtml?identifier=4534
- Cancer Control Planet (Physical Activity: 5 Steps to Effective Cancer Control Planning): http://www.cancercontrolplanet.cancer.gov/physical_activity.html
- Centers for Disease Control and Prevention, National Center for Chronic Disease Prevention and Health Promotion (Nutrition and Physical Activity): http://www.cdc.gov/nccdphp/dnpa/physical/index.htm

INTRODUCTION

Chapter 44 covered theoretically based physical activity interventions delivered to individuals. Such interventions are typically done face-to-face. This chapter will focus on various approaches, or delivery channels, which can be useful in reaching individuals through means other than face-to-face interventions. When the mode of delivering an intervention, or delivery channel, is not face-to-face, this has been referred to as mediated interventions (28). Examples of mediated interventions include the mediums of printed materials, telephone and cell phones, the Internet, television, and other media outlets. Most fitness professional are accustomed to working with individuals or groups. However, there may be utility in using mediated interventions if the fitness professional is interested in

- reaching larger groups and
- effective approaches to supplement the face-to-face work done in a fitness facility.

The advantage of mediated interventions and electronic health, or eHealth technologies, is that they have the potential to reach large numbers of people without the typical barriers of transportation, expense, and time (27,32). In this chapter, there will be an emphasis on health communications channels using social change approaches for delivering physical activity programs, especially where technology is used as either an adjunct or the primary delivery modality. Several practical, evidence-based examples will be provided to highlight fitness professionals' opportunities and roles in this area.

BACKGROUND IN HEALTH COMMUNICATIONS

Before describing the specific channels and strategies for communicating physical activity messages, it is helpful to have an understanding of general communication principles. With advances in technology and interactive

KEY TERMS

Advocacy: Communication directed at policy makers to promote policies and programs to support (health behavior) change.

Audience: The intended receiver of a communication or health program.

Channel: A mode of communication or access for delivering a health program.

Context: The setting where people may be reached with communications or programs.

Formative research: Research that is conducted to better understand the characteristics, needs, and behaviors that influence the decisions and actions of your target population (15).

Mediated interventions: Programs that are delivered to individuals through means other than a face-to-face format such as print, telephone, and Internet (28).

Message: Information that is intended to be communicated.

Policy: An organizational statement or rule meant to influence behavior.

Reach: The extent to which a message or program is delivered to the target population.

Social marketing: Commercial marketing technologies applied to the analysis, planning, execution, and evaluation of programs designed to influence your target audience's behavior with the aim of improving personal welfare and society (3).

Social movement: A large informal grouping of individuals and/or organizations that use political and social forces to create social change in which physical activity becomes a social and cultural norm (34).

Tailoring: Aiming a program at one specific individual based on characteristics that are unique to that individual (23).

Targeting: Aiming an intervention at a particular population that has a common characteristic. Targeting is less precise than tailoring (23).

communications, a multitude of channels for delivering health messages (*e.g.*, personal, print, or electronic media) are available. A communication framework can help users select the most effective channel in delivering a message when considering important factors. Factors that influence the choice of channel delivery include the message and program objectives, the source, the target audience, and the context or setting.

The *message* may focus on health-supporting (*e.g.*, walking, aerobic activity, strength training, stretching) or potentially health-compromising (*e.g.*, excessive sedentary behaviors associated with television watching, video gaming) behavior. The *source* of the message may be an authoritative voice (*e.g.*, exercise professional, teacher, physician) or organization (*e.g.*, American College of Sports Medicine [ACSM], Centers for Disease Control and Prevention [CDC]), a famous figure (*e.g.*, athlete, actor), or a layperson (*e.g.*, peer). The *target audience* is the receiver of the message and may be defined by demographic (*e.g.*, age, sex), geographic, social, cultural, or psychological factors. The message or program may occur in various *contexts* or settings, such as a school, home, or work.

Characteristics of each factor influence the strategies chosen in delivering behavioral programs. Ideally, the selected channel should reflect the target audience's preferred format and context. It should also provide a feasible medium for delivering the message or program. For example, a program to increase vigorous physical activity (message) among adolescents (target audience) at school (context) might be delivered via the Internet, a text message, or an after-school program (channels). But a program developed for older adults with disabilities (target audience) to promote strength training (message) in assisted living programs (context) may select a very different delivery channel (*e.g.*, individualized personal training, video). Repeated presentations of information and behavior change strategies are often key for the adoption and maintenance of physical activity, and a multilevel approach is recommended. As much as possible, the strategies presented in this chapter are evidence based — that is, they are drawn from the research literature.

CHANNELS OF COMMUNICATION

There are many methods, or *channels of communication*, to deliver information to a target audience. Choosing applicable channels of communication depends on the audience's availability, setting, and access to the content. Inclusion of several channels may be needed to deliver the message. For example, in addition to weekly one-on-one sessions with a fitness professional, a client might access a Web site for general information and be a member of a monthly group support

network to provide accountability for sustaining behavioral change (4). Various channels of communication are shown in *Table 47-1*. Some channels are straightforward where only information is made available. Other channels are interactive and may require feedback, discussion, and multiple contacts over time.

FACE-TO-FACE DELIVERY CHANNELS

The first channel of communication is individual or the *face-to-face approach* to deliver a message. This is the type of contact that most fitness professionals currently use but can also be used by a physician, wellness coordinator, or others who understand the benefits and mechanics of physical activity. Feedback from the client is important when evaluating which type and how much physical activity is feasible or within his or her ability. Usually, at least one follow-up meeting is necessary to gauge the client's progress. Individual-based programs seem to be successful overall (4), and interventions that include risk appraisal, activity counseling, and behavioral strategies have shown increases in physical activity levels (37); see *Chapter 44* for a review of effective, theory-based individual interventions.

Face-to-face group-based sessions have shown positive effects for weight loss groups and physical activity promotion. These use behavioral aspects of social support for participants to learn about being active and use combinations of different theories to develop skills, problem solve barriers, set behavioral goals, and maintain accountability. This could entail groups using a booklet or manual as a guide for a program, or to learn other practical skills. Groups can meet at any venue including fitness facilities, churches, conference rooms in the workplace, recreational centers, or other similar areas.

MEDIATED INTERVENTIONS

Various options are available to fitness professionals to assist in the delivery of physical activity interventions beyond face-to-face contact. Mediated interventions include printed materials, telephone communication, and other technology-assisted interventions, and these methods may be used as a stand-alone or adjunctive approach to physical activity promotion.

Print Materials

Print materials and media include any information that is printed or posted. Print materials can take several forms. One common use of printed materials such as pamphlets and training manuals are to impart information about a topic for educational purposes. Other printed materials promote discussions or raise awareness of the campaign, issue, or program. This would include billboards, leaflets, flyers, posters, and even bus and car wraparounds. The purpose of the material is to expand on a specific

TABLE 47-1. Channels of Communication for Physical Activity

Channels	Examples	Tools Used	Settings
Face-to-face Interventions			
Individual	Personal training Wellness coaching Counseling Physician contact	• Exercise prescription • Lifestyle assessments • Open discussion • Individualized feedback	Gym/wellness centers Doctor's offices
Group based	Seminar or classroom Peer groups Public health activities	• Booklets or worksheets to increase physical activity • Hands-on experience or modeling activity • Q&A sessions to discuss topics • Speaking about past experiences • Accountability	Fitness centers Medical settings Classrooms/schools Activity centers Churches Assisted living
Mediated Interventions			
Print materials and media	Pamphlets and flyers Manuals Posters and signs Billboards Tailored feedback reports	• Targeted adds • Slogans • Contextual pictures • Expert systems	Businesses Information booths Physicians' offices
Telephone	Automated Calling centers Personal coaching	• Phone surveys • Assessments • Individualized feedback	Home Place of work
Electronic Media	Web sites and blogs Podcasts Texting E-mail Television Mobile apps Social media	• Computers • Mobile phones/smartphones • Personal music players (*e.g.*, iPod) • Tablet computers • Televisions	Home Work Electronic devices
Self-monitoring feedback devices	Pedometers Accelerometers Armbands PDA/mobile device applications	• Pedometers • Accelerometers • Armbands • PDA/mobile device applications	Anywhere Real-time feedback Computers

message from a slogan to a more detailed explanation (24). If the target audience is people with diabetes, then placement of materials at clinics or doctor's offices would be appropriate. If the target audience includes Hispanic clients, then a brochure that includes a Spanish translation may be needed.

Print materials also have the ability to target or tailor the physical activity interventions to individuals. Targeted messages and materials are directed at a specific segment of the population, usually defined by one or more demographic or other shared characteristics such as age, sex, race or ethnicity, or disease group. Tailored communications, on the other hand, are designed to reach specific individuals based on an assessment of their unique characteristics. As one moves from print mass media to targeted and tailored print communications, the message salience and relevance increases along with the program complexity and associated costs. Although tailored communications can be delivered as print media — a personalized handwritten prescription is a simple example (*Fig. 47-1*) — the advance of interactive technologies has made tailoring of health messages more feasible and cost-effective.

In several studies, interventions that were targeted to an individual's stage of change were found to increase physical activity with no face-to-face contact (25). Similarly, printed reports using computerized algorithms, called expert systems, can be used to create tailored feedback reports that also can influence behavior that increases physical activity (26) without any face-to-face contact.

Print Materials Applied

As a fitness professional, there are many ways to supplement face-to-face contact with printed materials. For example, ACSM's Exercise is Medicine (http://www.exerciseismedicine.org) campaign has downloadable *Prescription for Health* tip sheets on various topics that can be matched to patient needs (diabetes, arthritis, asthma, hypertension, etc.) (14). As clients better understand the connection between their health and physical activity, they become more invested in engaging in physical activity. Other examples include signs for the workplace to encourage taking the stairs or pamphlets on the benefits of physical activity distributed at health fairs.

EXERCISE PRESCRIPTION & REFERRAL FORM

Your Prescription for Health

Exe℞cise is Medicine®
www.ExerciseisMedicine.org

PATIENT'S NAME: _____ DOB: _____ DATE: _____

HEALTH CARE PROVIDER'S NAME: _____ SIGNATURE: _____

PHYSICAL ACTIVITY RECOMMENDATIONS

Type of physical activity:	Aerobic	Strength
Number of days per week:		
Minutes per day:		
Total minutes per week*:		

*PHYSICAL ACTIVITY GUIDELINES
Adults aged 18-64 with no chronic conditions: Minimum of 150 minutes of moderate physical activity a week (for example, 30 minutes per day, five days a week) *and* muscle-strengthening activities on two or more days a week (2008 Physical Activity Guidelines for Americans). For more information, visit www.acsm.org/physicalactivity.

REFERAL TO HEALTH & FITNESS PROFESSIONAL

Name: _____

Phone: _____

Address: _____

_____

Web Site: _____

Follow-up Appointment Date: _____

Notes: _____

_____

_____

_____

FIGURE 47-1. Exercise is medicine exercise prescription and referral form.

Telephone Interventions

The telephone is another way to communicate information, especially if the clients are out of town or have difficult work schedules and cannot meet face-to-face. There are several ways that the telephone has been used to deliver physical activity interventions. Routine telephone calls for ongoing assessments after a group-based program have been used to increase accountability to program protocols (5). Fitness professionals can use a telephone call to assess client progress or engage the client in additional programming for physical activity or other health-related behaviors. In addition to the telephone being used as an adjunct to face-to-face sessions, telephone-only interventions, where individuals were counseled on theoretically based strategies from the transtheoretical model and social cognitive theory, have also been tested and found to increase physical activity in the short term, particularly when the contact was regular (11,26). More recently, interactive voice response (IVR) has been used in physical activity interventions. Here, a complex series of messages are prewritten and recorded, and through voice recognition or use of the touch pad, the participant is lead through a physical activity session that might include an assessment of their progress, some theory-based strategies for improvement, and goal setting (6). These systems can then be targeted and tailored to different populations such as those with high blood pressure, diabetes, or in different age groups.

Telephone Interventions Applied

Fitness professionals often use telephone calls to supplement work with clients. As a fitness professional, you do have to be mindful about how and when you use additional services in terms of pay and reimbursement. Options may include offering different packages or levels of intervention to clients. Clients could opt for a certain frequency of face-to-face sessions supplemented by a certain number of telephone calls. The length and structure of the calls should be discussed in advance. Theory and evidence-based techniques should be used to guide contact with clients; components may include a reviewing goal progress; exploring and problem-solving barriers; determining if social support, cues, reminders, or other behavioral strategies are needed; and ultimately, setting new goals.

Electronic Media

Electronic media is a channel of communication that changes rapidly as technology evolves. Obtaining the message through this channel is also dependent on the access capabilities of the population. Many of the messages in large mass media campaigns use radio and television commercials, but these can be expensive to produce. Current common delivery methods include e-mail, text-based/SMS messaging (7), Web sites or blogs, podcasting, mobile applications (apps), and various forms of social media (*e.g.*, Facebook, Twitter, YouTube). The biggest advantage of electronic media is the potential for mass distribution to maximize reach. Interactive media also allows for dynamic tailoring of messages based on assessment of the target audience's characteristics and individual needs.

Internet-based information that is displayed as an online pamphlet can be described as *Web 1.0 type sites*, where there is no interaction with the user. *Web 2.0 channels* include user-centered apps, blogs, Web sites, and social media where the users interact and contribute to the content. *Web 3.0* is similar to Web 2.0 but also incorporates application-to-application communication such as multiple search engines that communicate with each other to tailor messaging to the particular user. In a recent review of Web-based interventions, interaction with the program materials was found to be an important component for weight loss. Only four of the seven studies were found to be effective, and it was noted that the Web-based interventions were as effective as face-to-face programs (29).

Electronic Media Applied

There are many ways to use electronic media, and it is important to assess the client's preference. Texting could be used to communicate quick reminders, provide encouragement, or to increase accountability. However, a client that does not know how to receive texts or is charged by the text may prefer another form of communication. Similarly, client's experience and comfort with blogs, apps, and the Internet will vary.

The Internet can be used for several purposes. It has been suggested that a "hybrid model" for online use could be to combine (a) human-to-human interactions (support groups), (b) expert systems that provide tailored health feedback, and (c) user navigation (information libraries) (32). Fitness professionals should be aware of various evidence-based Web sites that allow clients to do one or all three of these options. Various free Web sites offer online tracking of physical activity. Some fitness facilities are now posting daily workouts that are done with minimal equipment so that clients could do a different workout at home on the days that they are not at the gym. This online format also allows for discussions and comments from clients.

To evaluate a Web site or mobile application (see *Box 47-1*), fitness professionals may want to use it first before recommending it to a client. Take note of the type of information it is providing and whether it is from a trustworthy source. If the site is informational only, it is best considered as an adjunctive source but would not, in and of itself, promote behavior change. Web sites or apps with increased interactivity that allow the client to personalize goals, receive feedback, create their own profile, and monitor their progress will be more likely to promote behavior change. *Chapter 45* details the kinds of theoretically based strategies that promote health behavior change.

Physical Activity Monitoring

The last channel involves devices that are used for physical activity monitoring. These devices include pedometers, accelerometers, activity armbands, and mobile phone devices. They rely on concepts of self-regulatory strategies described in *Chapter 45*, such as tracking behavioral compliance and setting goals for that behavior. These devices give the user feedback on their physical activity so individuals can make changes to their behavior to reach their goals. This has been done with pedometers in many studies using a goal of 10,000 steps a day (35). Some accelerometers measure steps but can also be used to identify the amount of time in light, moderate, and vigorous activity. A study in the United Kingdom using wrist-worn accelerometers with an Internet/mobile phone program showed increases and maintenance in physical activity over a 9-wk period (19). Some armband devices can estimate the amount of energy expenditure and, when used along with diet tracking, can determine the energy balance of the individual for weight loss. Some devices may need a computer to display their information, whereas others use real-time feedback on the device to inform the user of their current activity status. With the advancement

---

| **BOX 47-1** | **Tips on Identifying Evidence-Based Physical Activity Web Sites** |

- Determine that the source of the information is legitimate and the content providers are qualified. Go to *About Us* or similar sections of the Web site for this information.
- Is the information given accurate? Do the recommendations for physical activity follow the ACSM guidelines? Does it recommend consulting a physician before beginning an exercise program?
- Is there information on the benefits of physical activity?

- How many of the following features are present?
  — Tracking of physical activity
  — Feedback or graphs of physical activity
  — Goal setting
  — Social support or networking
  — Targeted or tailored exercise plan
  — Targeted or tailored motivational plan (*i.e.*, Are decisional balance, self-efficacy, and other psychosocial constructs measured and tailored feedback provided for them?)

of smartphones and personal digital assistants (PDAs), users can also record exercise and diet information to the devices and call up reports through downloadable apps. Trainers can use apps for clients to assess their activity and diet by forming a coaching group, thereby maintaining contact when the client is away from the facility.

Physical Activity Monitoring Applied

Having clients wear pedometers or accelerometers can be helpful for tracking their activity during structured exercise and daily routines. The devices also provide feedback that the client can use to self-correct. For example, an individual may set a daily step goal of 8,000 steps; if she looks at her pedometer at 5 p.m. and realizes that she is only up to 5,000 steps, she might still have time to take a 30-min walk to meet her daily goal. Although there are many apps to track physical activity and diet, to our knowledge, they have not been scientifically evaluated. Thus, understanding the theoretical principles of behavior change (*Chapter 44*) can be important for you to informally evaluate the potential of an application. As stated previously, if the application has monitoring, feedback, and goal setting, it could be a nice adjunct to in-person sessions with clients.

Special considerations such as reach, cost, accessibility, and setting are important when considering the use of specific channels. Creativity using multiple channels in a program may deliver the best results.

POPULATION-BASED PHYSICAL ACTIVITY PLANS AND POLICIES

This section will define, identify, and provide examples of several strategies for physical activity health promotion to communicate with large populations. As a fitness professional, it is important to be familiar with several physical activity campaigns as well as the techniques used to improve physical activity. This includes campaigns clients might have already been exposed to. With this knowledge, fitness professionals can initiate advocacy work within fitness facilities, work sites, or community that could expand reach beyond current clientele and promote societal changes that will encourage and support physical activity — for everyone.

NATIONAL PHYSICAL ACTIVITY PLAN

The main purpose of many physical activity campaigns is to initiate social change by increasing awareness of the risks of inactivity, to provide education, and to provide opportunities to be active. One recent example of a campaign is the U.S. National Physical Activity Plan (36). The National Physical Activity Plan is a set of policies, programs, and initiatives that aim to increase physical activity in all segments of the U.S. population. The plan is based on organizing the country by sectors (health care, schools, business and industry, etc.) to implement large-

scale policy and program changes to increase physical activity. Members are working together with hundreds of organizations to enable every American to reach beneficial levels of physical activity stated in the 2008 Physical Activity Guidelines for Americans (1). The guidelines were created to educate the general public about the level of physical activity needed to live healthy lives and minimize their risk of chronic diseases. The United States joins 24 other countries in the European Union including Sweden, Portugal, Poland, Netherlands, and Germany that have national health plans that include physical activity (30).

The U.S. National Physical Activity Plan (36) is a good example of a reputable resource available to fitness professionals interested in promoting physical activity for all. For example, on the Web site, there is a section entitled "Parks, Recreation, Fitness, and Sports" (36) that outlines six strategies:

1. Promote programs and facilities where people work, learn, live, play, and worship to provide easy access to safe and affordable physical activity opportunities.
2. Enhance the existing parks, recreation, fitness, and sports infrastructure to build capacity to disseminate policy and environmental interventions that promote physical activity.
3. Use existing professional, amateur, and college athletics and sports infrastructures and programs to enhance physical activity opportunities in communities.
4. Increase funding and resources for parks, recreation, fitness, and sports programs and facilities in areas of high need.
5. Improve physical activity monitoring and surveillance capacity to gauge program effectiveness in parks, recreation, fitness, and sports settings based on geographical population representation and physical activity levels not merely numbers served.
6. Increase social marketing efforts to maximize use of recreation programs and facilities and promote benefits with environmental and other related approaches.

Strategy 1 recommends promoting programs by reducing cost for participation, increasing operating hours, making childcare available, or establishing new parks and trails. Thus, many of the barriers that people encounter when being physically active would be proactively planned for with the use of this strategy. Strategy 6 focuses on communication channels with an emphasis on social marketing. Why might this matter to fitness professionals? First, the United States is in the middle of a health crisis because of diseases and conditions of which many are related to physical inactivity. Second, the more people who realize they need to get moving, the more opportunities there are for fitness professionals.

Advocating to state and local government representatives can initiate policy change that is called for in the National Physical Activity Plan. Policy change has targeted many unhealthy behaviors in the past.

Take tobacco use, for example. Smoke-free workplaces, restaurants, trains, and creating designated outdoor smoking areas have made it more difficult for smoking to be accepted as a cultural norm. An increase in cigarette taxes has also made it more expensive, thus creating economic barriers to smoke cigarettes. These factors, along with education about health-related risks of smoking, have contributed to a decrease in smoker prevalence (2).

Policies can also increase opportunities for physical activity or increase the likelihood that populations will choose to be more active. For example, charging a fee for parking near a business or other destination, although free parking is available within a short walking distance.

The "Transportation, Land Use, and Community Design" section of the National Physical Activity Plan outlines four strategies that include promoting active transportation, improving infrastructure such as networks of greenways, trails, and multiuse pathways (36). Fitness professionals can partner with urban and community designers to bring fitness knowledge to the design of neighborhoods and pathways. Fitness professionals in a workplace could also collect data on the users of their services to better support giving time and resources to physical activity during the workday. Many companies have decided to not only offer heavily subsidized gym fees, fitness trainers, and nutrition specialists but have also realized the need to change the social culture of their workplace to allow employees to be physically active. For example, managers at Dow Chemical Company allow employees to exercise during the day, have 5-K Fridays, and have color coded the cafeteria's utensils at the salad bar so that green handles signify "healthy foods," yellow handles signify "eat with caution," and red handles signify "temptation foods." Dow reports that since launching their efforts, the rates of obesity within the company has remained stable rather than increasing (8).

Tax incentives or medical insurance reductions are new ways to incorporate regulations and policies to impact behavior. Private health care systems are starting to use health-based incentives that track adherence to medical checkups, maintaining a healthy body mass index (BMI) or weight, not smoking, and obtaining certain amounts of physical activity (e.g., reported steps from a step counter) as ways for policy holders to qualify for reduced premiums (13). Some workplaces incorporate the amount of times associates visit an enrolled exercise facility, whereas others rely on self-report, such as pedometer steps and not smoking. Although there are limitations in some of the strategies companies use, the concept of rewarding healthy behaviors and their associated markers are ways to incentivize adoption of a healthy lifestyle. Fitness professionals in a workplace setting can use many of these strategies when developing their communication channels to advocate health programs such as publicizing rewards when using pedometers, attending physical activity classes, offering incentives for hitting body composition targets, or participating in health screenings. More examples of policy-related programs for the community setting can be found in *Chapter 48*.

SOCIAL MARKETING

Social marketing applies commercial marketing technologies to the analysis, planning, execution, and evaluation of programs designed to influence a target audience's behavior with the aim of improving personal welfare and society (16). Similar to a marketing agency who desires to sell a product to consumers to earn a profit, social marketing can use approaches such as mass media, small group interactions, and message boards while including various communication media like television, radio, print materials, billboards, and events to influence behavior change (27). Social marketing is a framework that is used during the process planning phase when developing behavior change strategies. It also provides structure during the evaluation and implementation phases of a program or campaign. It uses marketing concepts (see *Table 47-2*) to communicate specific messages to its target audience by identifying and delivering specific tailored needs (10).

The CDC has developed a free online course that walks a user through the concepts of social marketing (9), which fitness professionals can use to target participants and potential clients. Care should be taken when choosing appropriate communication channels because socially disadvantaged groups may not have the necessary means to gain access to the information and therefore, reach into specific populations may not be accomplished (*e.g.*, language barriers, lack of Internet access).

To use social marketing, it is important to understand the current behaviors of the target audience; the behavior you want them to start, limit, or stop; and the steps to move the audience to the new behavior. Examples could include reducing the time watching television, increasing the number of walks per week, or starting strength training. Another strategy that makes social marketing unique from other health promotion strategies is the use of the *marketing mix*. The marketing mix uses the "4 P's" — Product, Price, Place, and Promotion (22). The first "P" is *Product*, or what the target audience receives from the program. The important part of the product is the adopted behavior but could also consist of other benefits that are part of the program, such as receiving physical activity monitors or memberships to exercise centers. The second "P" is the *Price*. The Price addresses the cost or barriers when adopting the healthy behavior. For example, if a client

---

TABLE 47-2. Conceptual Considerations from Social Marketing for Application in Campaign Development (10)

✓ Market segmentation
✓ Market research
✓ Competitive assessment
✓ Use of product, price, promotion, and placement (distribution) tactics
✓ Pretesting and ongoing evaluation of campaign strategies
✓ Models of consumer behavior adapted from psychological and communications literature

substitutes going to the gym for watching a regular lineup of television programming, the price would be a potential loss in pleasure because of missing television shows that he or she enjoys. The Price can also include actual monetary costs, as well as other perceived "prices" such as embarrassment and inconveniences. Social marketing tries to identify and minimize these costs or, on the flipside, increase the costs of the undesirable behavior. The third "P" is *Place*. The marketing mix uses the Place to identify where the audience gathers or performs the undesirable behavior, accesses other products or behaviors, or is thinking about the health issue in question. This could lead to using television commercials to communicate the risks for sedentary behavior, information flyers at elevators to increase stair use, or workplace e-mail directed at employees at places of business. The last "P" is *Promotion*. This is the message of the program and includes the channels of communication to reach the target audience. Promotion incorporates all the other P's to deliver the message with the intent to change the behavior as well as to deliver the benefits, incentives, and activities of the program (21).

When starting the process to target a specific population, it is important to incorporate formative research principles. This will not only help you better understand your target audience's needs but also helps develop strategies with an audience-focused direction. Formative research uses a representative sample of the audience you have selected for the behavior change. In this sample, you can investigate the needs, identify common barriers, identify gaps in their knowledge about the desired behavior change, refine the message, and develop the marketing mix (the 4 "P's"). Focus groups are commonly used to gather much of this information.

Evaluation is another key part of social marketing. To establish the effectiveness of a campaign or program, professionals must use measurable outcomes to assess the targeted behavior. Usually, measures are taken before and after an intervention or program, with possible frequent measurement points along the way. Program evaluations deliver important feedback to the program designers to examine if the outcome is being affected and to identify if any program elements need modification. If a program is designed to increase physical activity, tracking activity with a monitor or diary can be used. Other methods include polling a random sample of the population to see if the target population knows about the program or campaign.

An example of a research-based, effective, social marketing campaign is the VERB campaign (38). This was a multiethnic national media campaign to increase physical activity in children ages 9–12 yr (*i.e.*, the "tween" years). Starting in 2002, the campaign delivered tailored messages using various channels to deliver their message. The planning phase used formative research to create focus groups consisting of different ethnicities and subgroups across the country to gain insight into their target audiences' needs. The tagline was "VERB: It's what you do." The 4 P's were used to develop their campaign, using enjoyment as the Product. Messaging was directed at parents and tweens to communicate that physical activity had the "right Price" and the benefits outweighed the costs (16). VERB promoted backyards, schools, churches, and parks for their year-round sponsored activities. They also placed posters in schools, radio ads, Web sites, trading cards, and television commercials to advertise the campaign. For the Promotion of VERB, messages were tailored to activities tweens like doing and included culturally relevant dancing and sports. This was accomplished through the campaign messages and targeting different ethnic groups (38).

The evaluation of VERB's effectiveness spanned multiple years. It consisted of surveys that measured awareness of VERB and gathered estimates of free-time and organized physical activity sessions during non–school hours (18). Overall, VERB is a successful model illustrating how to use social marketing concepts in a physical activity campaign. However, in a review of 18 other mass media campaigns for physical activity promotion, there have been mixed results (24) indicating that the way the campaign is implemented is an important factor.

SOCIAL MOVEMENTS

Strategies that can produce significant behavioral changes to the populations can be successful, but such endeavors can be very expensive and may have only localized effects. Another way to get more people to become physically active is through a social movement. A definition of social movement for the purposes of this chapter could be a large informal grouping of individuals and/or organizations that use political and social forces to create social change in which physical activity becomes a social and cultural norm (34). Many mass media campaigns for health promotion try to inspire a social movement in the population in order for the campaign to take on meaning and traction for sustained change. The National Physical Activity Plan and VERB, mentioned previously, are two campaigns that attempted to influence culture on a national level by making it clear why physical activity was important and highlighting that it can be fun and rewarding. Entities such as the U.S. Surgeon General's call to action on obesity (33) cannot maintain a presence in today's media, so true societal change must take place to make a lasting difference.

Creating social change uses political, social, and economic incentives to support healthy behavioral choices, but this can take a long time (17). Hill and colleagues stated that for a society to change, they need to perceive a crisis that is clearly visible and threatening to the average citizen. For example, the childhood obesity problem has activated many individuals, organizations, and institutions to take actions to promote healthy eating and active living. Similarly, the current health crisis has the potential to spur populations to become more engaged in creating a healthy change. Economics, especially economic injustices, have played a role in previous social movements (12). A strong emotional connection through a crisis or "shock" from a situation can also drive individuals to become involved into a social movement. This could include a catastrophic economic event, disease associated with childhood obesity, or premature death of family or friends. At an individual level, this causes people to feel threatened by their current surroundings and provides the motivation to adopt healthy behaviors (20). In order for this to grow into a social movement, enough people in a society or community need to personalize the crisis and start to protest the status quo. This is beginning to happen throughout the country. Take for example, Greenville, South Carolina. Through a partnership of public and private organizations, the community is working to make it a healthier place to live. The "LiveWell Greenville" social movement is creating policies, systems, and environmental changes that support making the healthy choice the easy choice (http://www.livewellgreenville.org).

There are many ways that fitness professionals can extend their expertise beyond the traditional one-on-one or group intervention and expand their reach in physical activity promotion. Fitness professionals can get involved in implementing aspects of the National Physical Activity Plan. For example, fitness professionals could create or support a social marketing campaign that encourages a target population (children, the elderly, the economically disadvantaged, etc.) to get moving more. Or, they could work in their local community to overcome injustices such as unsafe playgrounds that prevent people from being active or improve the environment or resources to make it easier for people to exercise. All of these population-based approaches could enhance a fitness professional's status and increase his or her visibility in the community, which in turn, may increase clientele. At the very least, it could help a health professional feel good to know he or she is doing something to give back to the community.

CASE STUDIES

To illustrate how various delivery channels can be used, consider the case studies in *Boxes 47-2* and *47-3*, which involve a personal trainer working with an individual at a fitness facility and a wellness director working at a company, respectively.

BOX 47-2   Case Study: A Personal Trainer Working with an Individual at a Fitness Facility

Setting: Fitness facility

Practitioner: Personal trainer

Client: 44 yr old, married, mother of two children, ages 6 and 8. She works part time as an office administrator for about 25 hr · wk^{-1}.

Scenario: You have been working with Sandra for 3 mo on resistance training and some cardio as well. She has made substantial improvements in strength and endurance. However, her work schedule has changed and instead of seeing you twice per week, she now needs to see you once per week on Fridays. Together, you work on a plan for her to increase her walking program.

To do this, you decide to implement the following mediated interventions:

1. You send her to the American Heart Association Web site to learn more about the overall benefits of physical activity and to join their "Start! Walking program" (31). This walking program contains a walking path app download, a "My Start!" online tracker to track walking frequency and time, walking paths, and diet, and provides a personalized walking plan.
2. You decide that you will also check in with her every Monday so that you can find out how the weekend went and plan for the week until you see her again on Friday. You ask her if she prefers a phone call,

text message, or e-mail session. She indicated that she would like to set up a specific time and conduct a "chat" session every Monday. Before your chat with her, she e-mails you her tracking sheet before the session. During your chat session, you are sure to check in on her progress, comment on her tracking and praise her for progress, problem solve barriers, and set new goals. You arrange for these sessions to last 10 min every Monday at 4 p.m. and agree upon a fee.

This process seems to work well and Sandra goes from walking 15 min several times per week to walking 4 d · wk^{-1} for about 36 min. She also sees a campaign for Heart Health on the American Heart Association Web site and notices that they have Heart Walks. She signs up to do a walk and uses their toolkit to take posters into work to drum up support for a walking team. She successfully recruits five coworkers who start walking with her on occasion during lunch breaks, thereby influencing the office culture to some extent. She also uses materials on the Web site to organize a GoRed for Women's Heart Health day at her workplace when it is held in February. Sandra becomes very eager to help others benefit from healthy lifestyles. You tell her about the safe routes to school campaign that the local schools and township are starting. She joins the planning group and becomes a community advocate for creating a healthy environment.

BOX 47-3	Case Study: A Wellness Director Working at a Company

Setting: A manufacturing plant that has a mix of office, administrative, and assembly line workers

Practitioner: Wellness director

Clients: The workforce of this company

Scenario: In your new role as wellness director of a medium-sized company among other responsibilities, you have been charged with increasing physical activity in the workplace.

To do this, you decide on a multipronged approach:

1. You decide to enroll in the social marketing class on the CDC Web site so that you can bring a physical activity program to your workers. You hold some focus groups with the administrative staff, line workers, and management to determine how best to approach the campaign. Using this information, you design a program that includes posting signs to promote use of stairs, encourages walking breaks and walking meetings, advertises health fairs, and walking programs.
2. You get permission and funding to conduct health fairs. At these fairs, for which the workers are allowed time away from the job, screenings are done for blood pressure, cholesterol, weight, and BMI and include a table where results are reviewed with the worker and different programs are presented. Some of these programs will be for physical activity such as exercise group classes, walking programs, or to sign up to receive contact from a wellness coach.

3. The wellness coaches can be someone on staff or be outsourced to a company providing this service. The wellness coach will continue the assessment of the behaviors and provide counseling to support change. These sessions will be mediated through phone calls and/or e-mails.
4. You received funding to incentivize participation in physical activity and set up a program where workers who wear pedometers and upload their data are eligible for prizes if they reach a daily step total of 10,000 steps per day and are also entered to win a larger prize every time they upload their steps 12 wk in a row. This program blossoms and walking teams and competitions are formed.
5. You send out weekly e-mails with tips and strategies for wellness (how to avoid the flu, the benefits of drinking water, heart health, etc.) that also contain updates on programs you are offering.

Through the process, you collect data on participation rates and also on employee satisfaction with the programs so that you are able to support the impact of the work you do. After collaborating with human resource (HR) and payroll, you also are able to access some data showing that employee attendance rates are higher. Over time, the culture of the organization shifts such that employees and managers believe that physical activity becomes a "need to do" rather than a "nice to do." You encourage the organization to join forces with others in the local community to build more sidewalks, bike lanes, parks, and trails so that physical activity is easier for all.

CONCLUSION

This chapter has outlined communication options for reaching beyond individual clients to larger groups of people. As we have shown, communications can be used for multiple purposes, including motivating and educating individuals, promoting other physical activity interventions, and encouraging individuals to advocate for policy and environmental changes. Channel selection is guided by consideration of the target audience's preferred format and context, as well as characteristics of the message or program to be delivered. With the dramatic increases in communication technology, a wide variety of delivery channels is available. To maximize the reach of behavioral programs, the use of multiple channels is encouraged. In addition, supplementing communications with other intervention strategies and advocating for policy and environmental changes are important adjuncts

for you to consider. For example, getting involved in social movement and social marketing may be of personal interest to you in your workplace or community.

In working with clients, we recommend that professionals evaluate communication delivery channels for mutual fit. Not all clients will be open to the use of the Internet or to using their cell phones to receive text messages. Working together, professionals and clients can develop a communication and intervention plan best tailored to their needs and preferences. A number of new and emerging technologies may also provide ways to promote physical activity. Interactive technologies (39) that have not been extensively studied include "exergaming" such as Dance Revolution, the Wii, and Xbox Kinect as well as social networking options such as Facebook. Such technologies may help provide variety and fun to a behavior that can be difficult for people to adopt and maintain. Fitness professionals should consider integrating mediated interventions to augment and expand their work of promoting physical activity and fitness at the individual level and beyond. In summary, although working with clients in one-to-one and small group formats is important, to increase physical activity in large populations, it will be necessary to use various communication channels to deliver an array of messages to multiple target audiences.

REFERENCES

1. *2008 Physical Activity Guidelines for Americans* [Internet]. Washington (DC): U.S. Department of Health and Human Services; [cited 2011 Sep 2]. Available from: http://www.health.gov/paguidelines/pdf/paguide.pdf

2. Achievements in Public Health, 1900–1999: Tobacco Use—Center of Disease Control, United States, 1900–1999. *MMWR Morb Mortal Wkly Rep.* 1999;48(43):986–993.

3. Andreasen AR. *Marketing Social Change: Changing Behavior to Promote Health, Social Development, and the Environment.* San Francisco (CA): Jossey-Bass; 1995. 348 p.

4. Artinian NT, Fletcher GF, Mozaffarian D, et al. Interventions to promote physical activity and dietary lifestyle changes for cardiovascular risk factor reduction in adults: a scientific statement from the American Heart Association. *Circulation.* 2010;122(4):406–41.

5. Barry VW, McClain AC, Shuger S, et al. Using a technology-based intervention to promote weight loss in sedentary overweight or obese adults: a randomized controlled trial study design. *Diabetes Metab Syndr Obes.* 2011;4:67–77.

6. Castro CM, King AC. Telephone-assisted counseling for physical activity. *Exerc Sport Sci Rev.* 2002;30(2):64–8.

7. Cole-Lewis H, Kershaw T. Text messaging as a tool for behavior change in disease prevention and management. *Epidemiol Rev.* 2010;32(1):56–69.

8. *Corporations Offer Help in Trimming the Waist* [Internet]. Washington (DC): National Public Radio; [cited 2011 Nov 4]. Available from: http://www.npr.org/2011/10/28/141768942/corporations-offer-help-in-trimming-the-waist11/4/11

9. *Division of Nutrition, Physical Activity, and Obesity: Social Marketing Resources* [Internet]. Atlanta (GA): Centers for Disease Control and Prevention; 2011 [cited 2011 Nov 22]. Available from: http://www.cdc.gov/nccdphp/dnpao/socialmarketing/index.html

10. Donovan RJ, Owen N. Social marketing and population interventions. In: Dishman RK, editor. *Advances in Exercise Adherence.* Champaign:Human Kinetics; 1994. p. 249–290.

11. Eakin EG, Lawler SP, Vandelanotte C, Owen N. Telephone interventions for physical activity and dietary behavior change: a systematic review. *Am J Prev Med.* 2007;32(5):419–34.

12. Economos CD, Brownson RC, DeAngelis MA, et al. What lessons have been learned from other attempts to guide social change? *Nutr Rev.* 2001;59(3 Pt 2):S40–56; discussion S57–65.

13. *Employers' Stock in Wellness Rise with No End in Site* [Internet]. MediMedia USA: Managed Care; [cited 2011 Nov 4]. Available from: http://www.managedcaremag.com/archives/0607/0607.wellness.html

14. *Exercising with Type 2 Diabetes: Your Prescription for Health Series* [Internet]: Exercise is Medicine; [cited 2012 Mar 12]. Available from: http://exerciseismedicine.org/documents/YPH_DiabetesType2.pdf

15. *Formative research* [Internet]. California (CA): California Department of Public Health; [cited 2011 Nov 10]. Available from: http://www.cdph.ca.gov/programs/cpns/Pages/FormativeResearch.aspx

16. Graham JL. Marketing social change: changing behavior to promote health, social development, and the environment. *J Marketing Res.* 1997;34(2):294–6.

17. Hill JO, Wyatt HR, Reed GW, Peters JC. Obesity and the environment: where do we go from here? *Science.* 2003;299(5608):853–5.

18. Huhman M, Potter LD, Wong FL, Banspach SW, Duke JC, Heitzler CD. Effects of a mass media campaign to increase physical activity among children: year-1 results of the VERB campaign. *Pediatrics.* 2005;116(2):e277–84.

19. Hurling R, Catt M, Boni MD, et al. Using internet and mobile phone technology to deliver an automated physical activity program: randomized controlled trial. *J Med Internet Res.* 2007;9(2):e7.

20. Jasper JM. The emotions of protest: affective and reactive emotions in and around social movements. *Sociological Forum.* 1998;13(3):397–424.

21. Kotler P, Lee NR. *Social Marketing: Influencing Behaviors for Good.* 3rd ed. Thousand Oaks (CA): Sage Publications; 2007. 456 p.

22. Kotler P, Zaltman G. Social marketing: an approach to planned social change. *J Mark.* 1971;35(3):3–12.

23. Kreuter MW, Strecher VJ, Glassman B. One size does not fit all: the case for tailoring print materials. *Ann Behav Med.* 1999;21(4):276–83.

24. Leavy JE, Bull FC, Rosenberg M, Bauman A. Physical activity mass media campaigns and their evaluation: a systematic review of the literature 2003–2010. *Health Educ Res.* 2011;26(6):1060–85.

25. Marcus BH, Emmons KM, Simkin-Silverman LR, et al. Evaluation of motivationally tailored vs. standard self-help physical activity interventions at the workplace. *Am J Health Promot.* 1998;12(4):246–53.

26. Marcus BH, Napolitano MA, King AC, et al. Telephone versus print delivery of an individualized motivationally tailored physical activity intervention: project STRIDE. *Health Psychol.* 2007;26(4):401–9.

27. Marcus BH, Owen N, Forsyth LH, Cavill NA, Fridinger F. Physical activity interventions using mass media, print media, and information technology. *Am J Prev Med.* 1998;15(4):362–78.

28. Napolitano MA, Marcus BH. Targeting and tailoring physical activity information using print and information technologies. *Exerc Sport Sci Rev.* 2002;30(3):122–8.

29. Neve M, Morgan PJ, Jones PR, Collins CE. Effectiveness of web-based interventions in achieving weight loss and weight loss maintenance in overweight and obese adults: a systematic review with meta-analysis. *Obes Rev.* 2010;11(4):306–21.

30. *Review of Physical Activity Promotion Policy Development and Legislation in European Union Member States.* EUR/10/EUDHP1003693/ 8.1/10 [Internet]. Copenhagen (Denmark): World Health Organization Regional Office for Europe; [cited 2011 Nov 10]. Available from: http://www.euro.who.int/__data/assets/pdf_file/0015/146220/e95150.pdf

31. *Start Walking Now* [Internet]. Dallas (TX): American Heart Association; [cited 2011 Nov 4]. Available from: http://www.startwalkingnow.org/home.jsp

32. Strecher V. Internet methods for delivering behavioral and health-related interventions (eHealth). *Annu Rev Clin Psychol.* 2007;3:53–76.

33. *The Surgeon General's Call to Action to Prevent and Decrease Overweight and Obesity* [Internet]. Rockville (MD): Office of the Surgeon General, U.S. Department of Health and Human Services; [cited 2011 Nov 4]. Available from: http://www.surgeongeneral.gov/topics/obesity/

34. Tilly C. *Social Movements, 1768–2004.* Boulder (CO): Paradigm Publishers; 2004. 262 p.

35. Tudor-Locke C, Bassett DR,Jr. How many steps/day are enough? Preliminary pedometer indices for public health. *Sports Med.* 2004;34(1):1–8.

36. *The U.S. National Physical Activity Plan* [Internet]. Columbia (SC): National Physical Activity Plan; [cited 2011 Nov 4]. Available from: http://www.physicalactivityplan.org/faq.php

37. van der Bij AK, Laurant MG, Wensing M. Effectiveness of physical activity interventions for older adults: a review. *Am J Prev Med.* 2002;22(2):120–33.

38. Wong F, Huhman M, Heitzler C, et al. VERB™—A social marketing campaign to increase physical activity among youth. *Prev Chronic Dis*. 2004 July; 1(3): A10. Available from: http://www.ncbi.nlm.nih.gov/pmc/articles/PMC1253475/

39. Zhu W. Promoting physical activity using technology. *President's Council on Physical Fitness and Sports Research Digest*. 2008; 9(3): 1–7.

SELECTED REFERENCES FOR FURTHER READING

Heath GW, Brownson RC, Kruger J, et al. The effectiveness of urban design and land use and transport policies and practices to increase physical activity: a systematic review. *J Phys Activity Health*. 2006;3(suppl 1):S55–76.

Heath GW, Martin SL, editors. *Promoting Physical Activity: A Guide to Community Action*. 2nd ed. Champaign (IL): Human Kinetics; 2008.

Hillsdon M, Foster C, Thorogood M. Interventions for promoting physical activity. *Cochrane Database Syst Rev*. 2005;25(1):CD003180.

Kroeze W, Werkman A, Brug J. A systematic review of randomized trials on the effectiveness of computer-tailored education on physical activity and dietary behaviors. *Ann Behav Med*. 2006;31:205–23.

Marcus BH, Williams DM, Dubbert PM, et al. Physical activity intervention studies: what we know and what we need to know. *Circulation*. 2006;114:2739–52.

Sallis JF, Owen N. Interventions to promote physical activity in communities and populations. In: *Physical Activity & Behavioral Medicine*. Thousand Oaks: Sage Publications; 1999. p. 153–74.

Weinreich NK. *Hands-On Social Marketing: A Step-by-Step Guide*. Thousand Oaks (CA): Sage Publications; 1999. 255 p.

INTERNET RESOURCES

- Active Living by Design: http://www.activelivingbydesign.org
- Active Living Network: Communications Toolkit: http://www.activeliving.org/index.php/Communications_Toolkit/80
- *Agita Mundo* (meaning "shake or move the world"): http://www.agitasp.com.br
- Centers for Disease Control and Prevention Community Guide (Task force recommendations on increasing physical activity with links to sample evidence-based programs focused on informational approaches, behavioral and social approaches, and environmental and policy approaches): http://www.thecommunityguide.org/pa/default.htm
- National Coalition for Promoting Physical Activity (Resource Guide): http://www.ncppa.org/resources.asp
- Smart Growth America: http://www.smartgrowthamerica.org
- Surface Transportation Policy Project: http://www.stpp.org
- VERB Campaign, Centers for Disease Control and Prevention: http://www.cdc.gov/youthcampaign

CHAPTER
48
Promoting Physical Activity in the Community

FOUNDATIONS OF COMMUNITY PHYSICAL ACTIVITY INTERVENTIONS

The relationship between physical activity and public health has been well established (1). Unfortunately, most people in the United States do not engage in recommended levels of physical activity (16). Furthermore, physical inactivity has been identified as one of the leading causes of death in the United States (63). Thus, increasing physical inactivity is becoming a compelling public health crisis, and significant attention must be devoted to reversing current trends. Communities can positively impact public health by promoting the adoption and maintenance of physical activity for all ages. As understandings of physical activity behaviors deepen, contemporary programs increasingly apply multilevel and multistrategy approaches to program design and implementation. In fact, the literature suggests that physical activity interventions that are organized within an ecologic framework emerge as the preferable method to enhance community-wide physical activity (9). Therefore, the purpose of this chapter is to identify and discuss the community-wide promotion of increased physical activity with a particular focus on multilevel intervention approaches represented in an ecologic model.

The *Guide to Community Preventives Services* ("the *Guide*") provides a systematic review of the literature

The Guide to Community Preventive Services Recommended Approaches to Increase Physical Activity

- Point-of-decision prompts
- Community-wide campaigns
- School-based physical education
- Social support interventions in community settings
- Individually adapted health behavior change programs
- Creation of or enhanced access to places for physical activity combined with informational outreach activities

and recommendations for community intervention across various behaviors including physical activity (49). The *Guide* provides insights and recommendations related to effective physical activity interventions ranging from placing signs that promote stair use to providing individually tailored interventions (*Box 48-1*) (49). Although the content and reports from the *Guide* suggest a range of strategies that can be used, it does not clarify the question of the boundaries of what should be considered as a "community" intervention. Unfortunately, the *Guide* does not clearly define community or community intervention nor does it distinguish community interventions from similar interventions that may be more limited in reach.

COMMUNITY INTERVENTIONS DEFINED

In order to fully explore community physical activity interventions, it is first important to understand what is meant by community (93). A *community* can be defined as an aggregate of people who share a common identity, set of values, or institution (6). This could include among others, communities based on racial background (*e.g.*, the Latino community), sexual preference (*e.g.*, the gay community), educational status (*e.g.*, the academic community), professional affiliations (*e.g.*, the built environment professionals community), or religious preference (*e.g.*, faith-based community). Communities may also be defined to include a spatial component that refers to the location of groups of people or institutions, such as neighborhoods, schools, or work sites. Finally, communities may be linked based on social norms, belief structures, and personal attachments (72). A second issue is that community physical activity interventions may be operationalized and implemented in several different ways within and across community settings. For example, the Stanford Five-City Project, with a multilevel intervention

approach, included policy, program, and environmental intervention strategies across several boroughs (35), whereas the Rockford Coronary Health Improvement Project (CHIP) adopted primarily intrapersonal and interpersonal strategies such as an intensive educational curriculum presented to employees and community residents 5 d · wk⁻¹ for a month (27). Furthermore, the Partnership for Active Community Environments (PACE) project (61,62) adopted a community-based participatory approach to develop and implement initiatives identified and promoted by the built environment professional community (planners, engineers, builders, etc.) to encourage the promotion of activity-friendly communities in metropolitan and suburban areas.

It is clear then that the term *community* is used to represent different groups that share common factors. It is also clear that community programs may target, develop, and implement intervention strategies at different levels of influence. Although each has a distinctly different focus and applies to specific communities, the programs share the overall goal of facilitating and maintaining behavior change across an identified group of people through various population-specific strategies such as point-of-decision prompts, community-wide campaigns, school-based and work-based interventions, policy changes, increased access to physical activity resources, and even individually adapted behavior change programs.

FACILITATING COMMUNITY CHANGE

Becoming a physically active community is likely the result of a series of well-developed projects or programs that are informed by stakeholder and professional expertise, embraced by the priority population, and sustained by the community through an intrinsic commitment to the program purpose, intent, and practices. Transforming a sedentary population into an active population may require significant changes in awareness, attitudes, beliefs, actions, and policy. Ayre et al. (4) recommend the use of community participation as a way to empower sometimes diverse groups to work together toward the development of an action agenda responsive to a shared vision of a physically active community. It is well recognized that initiatives tailored to the specific needs of stakeholders and decision makers are essential to successful change efforts, and including them as active partners in the change process enhances the likelihood of success. This participatory approach is particularly important for interventions based on ecologic models, which include strategies across multiple levels of influence. The *Community Health Assessment and Group Evaluation* (CHANGE) guide provides recommendations for the development of a community action plan for improving policies, systems, and the environment to support healthy lifestyles and assist with prioritizing community needs and allocating available resources (15). It offers the following eight actions to guide community change:

1. Identify and assemble a diverse team.
2. Develop a strategy team.
3. Review the five CHANGE sectors (community at large, institution/organizations, health care, school, work site).
4. Gather data from individual sites or locations within each sector.
5. Review data with community team.
6. Enter data.
7. Review data to determine areas of improvement.
8. Build community action plan.

The challenge in community-wide change, then, is to identify and implement strategies, which promote sustainable engagement of all stakeholder groups, and to direct the combined creativity and resources to bring about change, which results in an active community. It is also important to identify methods to sustain the shared commitment and focus necessary to realize a measurable return on time and resource investment.

If true transformation in thought and practice are to be realized, significant changes in processes must be embraced. Successful and sustainable initiatives are dependent, in large part, on expanding influences on decision making and design. Unfortunately, community change efforts are often hampered by the failure of community members to recognize and own the problem, skepticism of proposed strategies, and distrust of motives and intent of the change champions. Therefore, the establishment of focused and committed collaboratives dedicated to creating new understandings and shared agendas is essential to successful outcomes. Application of community-based participatory practices and interdisciplinary, collaborative teamwork may be a preferred method to bring about desired results. There is much to be gained from interdisciplinary work; however, it requires a significant investment of time, attention, and energy. Team purpose and potential outcomes must be highly valued by all collaborating members, with an implicit commitment to seeing the initiative through to completion with strategies in place for sustainability and eventual institutionalization of successful efforts. Changes then to existing practices are dependent on challenging existing paradigms and establishing new paradigms, which promote increased participation by everyone in the efforts to promote physical activity and improved community health.

Leading communities to adopt healthy lifestyles is a formidable challenge. Increased public interest in the adoption and maintenance of healthy lifestyles has heightened the need for qualified professionals to lead individuals and communities toward increased participation in physical activity. Because behaviors are influenced by multiple sources, professionals from various disciplines (e.g., physical education, health promotion, exercise science, behavioral psychology) may offer physical activity guidance and programming. These professionals seek to prevent and treat illnesses by promoting the adoption of physical activity and by providing individual and population-specific recommendations, programs, initiatives, and activities. Physical activity professionals are found in multiple settings (e.g., schools, hospitals, community centers, corporations) and may also serve as personal trainers and independent consultants. Physical activity specialists assess needs, plan, develop, implement, supervise, evaluate, and report outcomes of activity programs for individuals, groups, and populations. Recognizing the relationship between physical inactivity and lifestyle-related diseases and conditions, many physicians now refer patients to physical activity specialists for individual activity counseling or to community-wide classes or initiatives. The ultimate goal of the physical activity professionals is to help participants understand the importance of being physically active and equip them with the skills and abilities needed to achieve and maintain a healthy lifestyle. Physical activity professionals, then, play a critical role in community health as they encourage increased participation in physical activity at all levels of potential influence in order to move people toward improved health and well-being.

COMMUNITY PHYSICAL ACTIVITY INTERVENTIONS

Recognizing the important interrelationships that exist among individuals, groups, and the environment, the socioecologic model provides an attractive framework for the development, implementation, and evaluation of community physical activity interventions. This model proposes that actions are the result of five levels of influence: intrapersonal, interpersonal, organizational, community, and policy. The model can be appropriately applied to individuals, organizations in specific settings such as schools, clinics, work sites, or faith-based groups, as well as to a larger community-wide initiatives and policy changes (23,24,30,37,60,73,76,82,90, 91,96,99). An ecologic approach encourages the selection of population-specific strategies, which will influence behaviors through multiple levels of influences. Simultaneous implementation of intervention strategies at multiple levels of influence will intensify the intervention and increase the likelihood of desirable outcomes.

SITE-BASED INTERVENTIONS

Many programs are developed for specific sites within the community that serve large groups of people such as educational, workplace, clinical, and community settings. Recently, a small number of programs have employed a more comprehensive approach by including environmental and policy strategies to promote physical activity. Strategies targeting individual behavior change may be used in combination with environmental and policy approaches to intensify the intervention and increase the likelihood of successful outcomes.

School-Based Physical Activity Interventions

Schools offer multiple avenues for promoting physical activity through physical education classes, recess, after-school programs, classroom activities, and by taking part in active transportation to and from school (110). Children spend most of their waking hours at school. Therefore, schools play a pivotal role in adoption and maintenance of physical activity behaviors (110). Unfortunately, despite a wide range of bodies providing recommendations for increased promotion of physical activity in schools (19,44,71), several factors present significant barriers and challenges to the realization of these goals. For example, an increased focus on instructional time devoted to traditional academic subjects such as science and math in many cases have led to the unintended consequence of reduced time spent in physical education and recess, and time once devoted to physical activity has been replaced with increased time spent on academics and other sedentary activities. Some schools have also increased instructional time into the after-school hours, further compromising the time available for children and youth to be physically active. Unfortunately, a reduction in physical activity classes has been documented as demands for competitive priorities has increased.

The National Association for Sport and Physical Education's *Shape of the Nation Report* (92) documented the reduction in the percentage of students attending physical education classes on a daily basis between 1991 and 2003 — from 42% to 28%. The report also highlights that approximately 30% of states do not mandate physical education for elementary and middle school students, and almost a quarter of states allow physical education to be completed using online course work (92). In addition, the proportion of schools that provide daily physical education or the recommended amount of time per week of physical education is only approximately 8% for elementary and 6% for middle and high schools (12). When physical education is required, it is also important to consider the amount of time spent in moderate-to-vigorous activity. It has been reported that in many classes, less than 40% of the class time is used for moderate-to-vigorous physical activity (64,94).

Fortunately, there is some evidence to support education settings as the ideal setting for interventions to increase student participation in physical activity (57,65,66,68,76,89,103). An early and seminal example is the Sports, Play, and Active Recreation for Kids

(SPARK) program (89). SPARK was a randomized control trial, which included two general intervention components: changes to the physical education environment and student self-management. These components highlight the interrelationship between enhancing student perceptions of and confidence in their ability to be active, along with modifications of the physical education class to include a greater opportunity for participation in moderate-to-vigorous activity. SPARK intervention strategies were designed to enhance the physical education class by training teachers and after-school leaders in methods to promote high levels of physical activity, teaching movement skills, and including fun activities for the students. In addition to the physical education component, SPARK designed and implemented strategies for self-management of physical activity behaviors. These strategies sought to equip children with general behavior change skills (*e.g.*, self-monitoring, goal setting, and problem solving) to increase physical activity outside of school time (89).

Outcomes of the initial SPARK trial demonstrated that the program was successful at increasing participation in moderate-to-vigorous physical activity during physical education classes and improved some fitness indices (66,89). Follow-up to this trial provided evidence that teachers who were trained in the SPARK curriculum were able to sustain the delivery 18 mo after the training occurred (66). Increased student physical activity during classes was also sustained (66). Although SPARK did not significantly increase physical activity (PA) outside of school time, another trial, Child and Adolescent Trial for Cardiovascular Health (CATCH) (76), which used a more comprehensive approach but had similar curricular principles, was able to influence both in class and outside of school PA (96). These effects were sustained at 2-yr follow-up (68).

The Middle School Physical Activity and Nutrition (M-SPAN) project (90), the Healthy Youth Places project (24), and the Lifestyle Education for Activity Program (LEAP) (73) all used comprehensive multicomponent strategies and were successful in increasing physical activity. In M-SPAN and Healthy Youth Places, the students were the primary drivers of activities and were provided with ideas for policy and environmental changes that could facilitate increased participation in physical activity. These interventions also used social marketing and communications strategies to promote increased participation in physical activity at multiple levels of influence. In the Healthy Youth Places project, students were provided with computers, software, and cameras, which they used to develop public service videos played over the school announcement and multimedia systems. Policies such as required physical education classes and recess time play an important role in school settings. In a summary of literature, Pate et al. (71) provide recommendations for physical activity policy and practice (*Box 48-2*). Schools often seem to be an ideal setting to

---

BOX 48-2	**School-Based Policy and Practice Recommendations to Increase Physical Activity**

- All children participate in a minimum of 30 min of moderate-to-vigorous physical activity during each school day.
- Evidence-based physical education programs should be used.
- Physical education should be taught by certified physical education teachers.
- State policy should hold schools accountable for meeting national physical education standards.
- Schools should expand physical activity opportunities beyond physical education.
- Schools should promote active transportation to and from school.
- Child development and elementary schools should provide 30 min of recess every day.
- Schools should provide evidence-based health education that emphasizes behavioral skills to increase physical activity and decrease sedentary behavior.
- University training programs should provide professional preparation so that qualified teachers are available to deliver evidence-based physical and health education.

Adapted from Pate RR, Davis MG, Robinson TN, et al. Promoting physical activity in children and youth: a leadership role for schools: a scientific statement from the American Heart Association Council on Nutrition, Physical Activity, and Metabolism (Physical Activity Committee) in collaboration with the Councils on Cardiovascular Disease in the Young and Cardiovascular Nursing. *Circulation.* 2006;114(11):1214–24..

---

promote positive behaviors; however, they unfortunately often emerge as a barrier to participation in physical activity because children are required to sit quietly for most of the day to focus on academic work. With this in mind, the International Life Sciences Institute Center for Health Promotion (ILSICHP) developed the TAKE 10! program, which integrates activity into the elementary classroom. Using objective measures of physical activity (*e.g.*, accelerometers, pedometers), Stewart et al. (102) examined the influence of the program on exercise level and energy expenditure and reported the program to be useful in promoting meaningful physical activity among school children.

Donnelly et al. (21) partnered with TAKE 10! and classroom teachers to develop Physical Activity across the Curriculum (PAAC). Through this partnership, they designed and implemented a low cost, minimal intervention mode aimed at increasing physical activity in the classroom. They found that children who received PAAC were more physically active than those

who were not exposed to the program. Furthermore, they found that the program was well received by both teachers and administrators, and the teachers were able to sustain the curriculum without any further contact by the investigators (21).

It is also important to recognize the influence of district and state policies on activity behaviors. Schools should become strong advocates for the development and adoption of activity-friendly district and state policies such as implementing and enforcing policy that requires certified and highly qualified professionals to lead physical education classes including physical education in core educational accountability systems, directing schools to deliver 150 min of physical education per week for children in kindergarten through eighth grade or for $225 \text{ min} \cdot \text{wk}^{-1}$ for grades 9 through 12 while ensuring that training institutions (*i.e.*, colleges and universities) provide appropriate preparation so that teachers are highly qualified and prepared to deliver evidence-based health and physical education curriculum. The adoption and maintenance of such policies will positively influence both physical education instruction and opportunities for self-selected participation in physical activity.

Work Site Physical Activity Interventions

Work sites also emerge as optimal settings for physical activity interventions because adults spend a large proportion of their waking hours at work (31). However, like schools, the work site environment often revolves around sedentary activities with minimal opportunities for participation in physical activity. Therefore, work sites may also present an ideal setting to develop and implement strategies at multiple levels of influence, intensifying the intervention and producing a more powerful influence than any one type of strategy in isolation (39,97). Furthermore, the opportunities for cooperation, communication, and friendly competition among employees provide a strong foundation for various forms of social support strategies such as group rewards, participatory employee wellness teams, and incentive programs. Also, work site programs can reach a broader population and encourage many persons to take advantage of physical activity programs who may not otherwise participate (40). Finally, comprehensive work site wellness programs can be of benefit to employers by increasing employee recruitment and retention, reducing health care costs and absenteeism, and enhancing employee morale and productivity (75,86).

Although work sites often seem to be ideal settings for intervention, it is important for physical activity professionals to be aware of complexities associated with work site physical activity interventions. Even if support from top management (98) is obtained, gatekeepers such as midlevel supervisors may not be supportive or provide workers with the time necessary to participate, which can result in barriers to participation and challenges to program success. To overcome some of these challenges, it may be beneficial to strategically place physical activity programming as a critical part of an overall comprehensive wellness plan offered or promoted by the workplace. This approach may be more likely to achieve buy-in from administrators when compared with, for example, a simple physical activity program such as 12-wk pedometer program (98). Finally, competing demands, availability of appropriate space for program implementation, and the logistics of including part-time and night shift employees highlight reasons why interventions that focus on class-based corporate fitness or health education programs do not effectively reach a large proportion of employees or result in sustained behavior change (59).

Dishman et al. (20) completed a systematic review of the literature examining work site PA promotion. The review documented that the mean effect size across the 26 studies included in the analysis was small (*i.e.*, average $r = 0.11$). It is of note that three of the studies included a more ecological approach to physical activity promotion by making work site environmental changes (*e.g.*, public signage documenting participant success, employee contests, and awards or providing on-site exercise facilities) *in addition* to providing behavioral skills training (50,54,69). In comparison to the small overall effect reported in the review, these studies demonstrated a medium-sized effect (*i.e.*, average $r = 0.41$), suggesting the importance of addressing both individual and environmental strategies. Similarly, an American Heart Association scientific statement provides a similar summary of the current state of work site PA intervention research that suggests that work site physical activity promotion should be based on a multilevel approach that includes individually and environmentally tailored strategies (58). Improving diet and physical activity with A Lifestyle Intervention Via E-mail (ALIVE) (101) was a work site randomized trial that offered individually tailored small-step goals, personal electronic messages with tips, educational materials, and tracking simulation tools to 787 administrative employees. The 16-wk program, delivered by e-mail, led to significant improvements in physical activity (101).

Research on the effectiveness of comprehensive work site health promotion (*i.e.*, target multiple behavior change) programs that include physical activity provides additional findings that are important for a physical activity professional attempting to intervene at the work site. This literature demonstrated that behavior modification and incentives were used regularly, whereas competitions and capitalizing on the work site organizational characteristics were used less frequently (46,67). Yet, strategies such as promoting friendly competition increased healthy eating, physical activity, and work site smoking cessation rates (53,74). Interactive computer technologies, such as automated telephone support, Internet and e-mail support, and tailored print strategies

to develop lifestyle behavior skills are becoming more and more common in work site programs and may be as effective as time-intensive and costly individual face-to-face sessions (45). Finally, social support is an important strategy in many health promotion programs. Studies that used employee wellness teams demonstrated improved delivery of health programs on-site, and an increased number of employees found the programs appealing (47). Using the body of research on work site health promotion and the tacit knowledge of work site health professionals, the Wellness Councils of America (WELCOA) developed a set of seven benchmarks necessary for the successful implementation, effectiveness, and sustainability of work site wellness initiatives (*Box 48-3*) (105). The first benchmark is to **obtain senior level support** by matching the wellness policy to (a) the organizations' short- and long-term priorities, (b) expectations from a wellness initiative (and level of value placed on health promotion), and (c) pressures and demands on leadership that could influence support. Once senior level support is achieved, a **cohesive wellness team should be developed** to include employees from all sectors of the organization (about 8–15 members in total). Volunteer members are likely to be more energetic about the initiative, but it is necessary to work the wellness team responsibilities into the performance goals of the employees involved to reduce the likelihood of burnout.

The wellness team becomes integral in carrying out the remaining benchmarks for success. First, a brief needs assessment is conducted, which includes determining what the business needs to get out of the wellness efforts and, equally as important, what the employees want. Second, the team should develop a work site wellness **operating plan** that includes a vision for the health of employees, goals and objectives, strategies (intervention components), specific timelines, marketing strategies, budget needs, and methods to evaluate whether the goals and objectives are being achieved. Third, the wellness team should identify and select **appropriate intervention**

BOX 48-3 | **The Wellness Councils of America Benchmarks to Work Site Intervention Success**

- Obtain senior level support.
- Create cohesive wellness teams.
- Collect data to drive health efforts.
- Craft an operating plan.
- Choose appropriate interventions.
- Create a supportive environment.
- Consistently evaluate outcomes.

components. The selection of specific strategies should be informed by the needs assessment and vision of the organization for its wellness initiative. The wellness team is directed to use evidence-based interventions when available or to base the strategies on the best evidence that is available. Fourth, the team should identify and implement strategies to develop an **environment that supports healthy lifestyle behaviors**. Recommended strategies to develop a supportive environment include creating proactive policies that make the healthy decision the easy decision (*e.g.*, implement "walk-and-talk" meetings), creating incentive programs, increasing manager role modeling of healthy behaviors, and integrating healthy messages into company communications. Fifth, the team should **evaluate outcomes** that are important to the organization and employees — and that can demonstrate success or the need to modify the wellness plan (105).

Clinical Setting

In addition to programs at school sites and work sites, there is a strong rationale for promoting PA during medical visits. First, community health clinics and family physician offices are geographically distributed across the United States and have contact with a large proportion of the population (17,79,112). Physicians are also considered by patients to be experts in health-related information (79). The credibility that physicians bring to a patient visit is highlighted by a study that found as many as 90% of patients would consider registering for a physical activity intervention through a medical office (48). Based on this rationale, several physician-delivered physical activity counseling interventions have been developed (26,78,81,104,107,109). However, a review of that literature by the United States Preventive Services Task Force (USPSTF) documented that the findings of efficacy were inconsistent (26). What is clear from the USPSTF findings is that it is difficult to document consistent effects of clinical physical activity interventions when they rely primarily on interactions between the physician and the patient. That is, simply asking about patients' physical activity and advising them to do more will not lead to sustained behavior change (38,77,80). Similar to other site-specific community interventions, clinic-based physical activity promotions may be enhanced through the use of an ecological approach that uses the entire social and physical environment of a clinic (and, optimally, the surrounding community) (30). The literature supports that when the role of the physician is reduced to a short period of time to provide brief advice (*e.g.*, 3 min) and is coupled with intervention strategies delivered by other clinical staff (particularly an exercise professional) or community organizations, significant increases in patients' physical activity can be achieved (2,80). Personnel that can be used to deliver other intervention components include health educators, exercise professionals, community personnel (*e.g.*, YMCA staff), or other clinical staff (*e.g.*, nurses, front desk staff) (2,25,56,80). Finally, a promising path to improve the maintenance of clinical physical activity intervention effects is to integrate physical activity counseling with the identification of community opportunities for physical activity support (2,11,49,80,91).

Opportunities for individual health counseling presented in the physician's office may benefit from the use of the five A's of behavior change as a guide to promoting physical activity. Programs using this health counseling approach have been successful at influencing positive behavior changes in several settings and may also be of benefit in clinical settings (32,42,80,81). The five A elements are as follows: (a) **Assessing** patient physical activity level, ability, and readiness to change; (b) **Advising** physical activity relative to personalized benefits and recommended guidelines; (3) **Agreeing** with a patient on a collaboratively developed plan of action; (4) **Assisting** patients with barrier resolution and problem solving to aid in the successful completion of the action plan; and (5) **Arranging** for a positive feedback loop through designated follow-up periods and links to environmental resources for active living (32,100,111). *Figure 48-1* provides a pictorial representation of the five A's process as it may be delivered in a primary care setting.

Faith-Based Setting

Reported ethnic disparities in cancer-related morbidity and mortality and the associated risk factors (*e.g.*, poor diet quality and low activity levels) underlie a recent scientific movement to target culturally tailored interventions for African Americans within faith organizations (6). Churches serve several social, organizational, and religious functions and offer unique opportunities for promoting healthy behaviors (84). Of particular interest for physical activity professionals wishing to engage churches as a local for health promotion is the National Cancer Institute and American Cancer Society program, Body & Soul, which includes several free resources and practical instructions for implementing church-based healthy eating and, more recently, physical activity promotion (7). The genesis of Body & Soul began with two efficacy trials: Black Churches United for Better Health (13) and Eat for Life (85). Taking the information and content from the interventions tested in these trials, representatives from the National Cancer Institute, the American Cancer Society, and the respective intervention development groups identified the core behavioral principles that lead to efficacy and adapted them to a program that could be widely disseminated. Both the Black Churches United for Better Health and Eat for Life targeted nutrition rather than physical activity behaviors. However, in 2004, the Healthy Body/Healthy

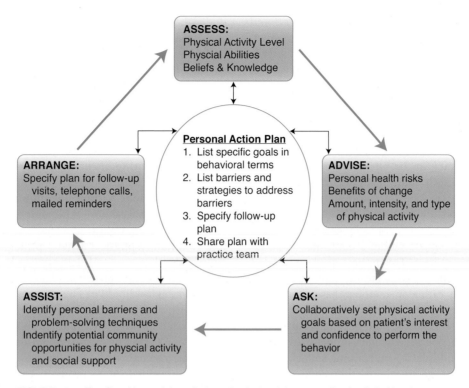

FIGURE 48-1. The five A's model applied to physical activity promotion in clinical settings.

Spirit trial (83,84) was completed based on the same underlying principles, and it targeted both nutrition and physical activity behavior. Healthy Body/Healthy Spirit demonstrated that churches could focus on both behaviors simultaneously and achieve significant dietary and physical activity changes (83). More recently, the Faith, Activity, and Nutrition (FAN) program recognized the importance of intervening on multiple levels of influence and successfully applied a participatory approach to develop a program to increase physical activity and improve dietary habits in African American churches. After engaging key stakeholders form the priority population in the process, the social, cultural, and policy environment was modified to promote healthy lifestyles (108). The principles and content of these faith-based interventions were adapted for dissemination by operationalizing the four pillars of faith-based lifestyle behavior change programs (see *Box 48-4*) (7). As with the other site-specific interventions reviewed, an ecologic approach was used to guide the selection and implementation of comprehensive strategies for a given locale.

COMMUNITY-WIDE INTERVENTIONS

In contrast to site-specific interventions, community-wide interventions typically include a multilevel and multisector approach. Community-wide interventions can include several site-specific interventions that may or may not be interwoven into a broad community action plan that attempts to increase the physical activity (or other health behaviors) across the entire population rather than singularly focusing on students, employees, patients, or congregation members. Community-wide interventions are also often inherently based on ecological models and include a range of policy, environmental, and program components (35,55,60). The Stanford Five-City Project is a well-known example of a successful community-wide intervention (35). Briefly, the project used mass media, which included television public service announcements, news stories, and newspaper articles (in Spanish and English) to promote cardiovascular risk reduction via lifestyle behavior changes. Community and scientific representation was used to determine the

---

BOX 48-4

The Four Pillars of Church-Based Lifestyle Behavior Change Programs

- A pastor who is committed to and involved with physical activity and healthy eating
- Church activities that promote healthy eating and active living
- A church environment that promotes healthy eating and active living
- Peer counseling to motivate healthy lifestyle behavior change

range of interpersonal contacts, classes, seminars, and other group interventions that would be implemented. Ultimately, each of the community programs were offered in several settings and delivered through various community agencies (*e.g.*, the health department, colleges, hospitals, nonprofit organizations). Assessments of physical activity indicated that there was a positive treatment effect for men in estimated daily energy expenditure and percent participation in vigorous activities. Similarly, women in the intervention communities engaged in significantly more moderate physical activities than those in the control community. The Naval Community Project in California (55) is worthy of note to provide some practical examples of community changes that can be made within a controlled community, such as a naval base. This project used an array of environmental and policy strategies to improve physical activity and healthy eating on a military base. During the project, the intervention community constructed bicycle paths along preexisting roads, purchased new equipment for the gymnasium, opened a women-only fitness center, and marked out multiple 1.5-mi running routes around the base. In addition, social environmental changes were implemented, including the development of jogging clubs and other athletic events. Policy approaches included extending the hours the base recreation center was open and integrating, into structured communications between superiors and subordinates, the expectation that all personnel on the base should participate in regular exercise (55).The Naval Community Project resulted in significant improvements in fitness and body composition for personnel on the intervention base when compared with a control base and the population of navy personnel (55). The benefits of the intervention demonstrated the value of comprehensive community-wide strategies in that the improvements in fitness occurred in both men and women, officers and enlisted personnel, and within each age category. That is, all segments of the population on the base benefited from the project, highlighting the value of integrating physical and social environmental changes with policy approaches to increasing PA (51). Building on these and other community-health promotion studies, Agita Sao Paulo developed an elegant yet comprehensive strategy for community-wide PA promotion for a Brazilian state of 645 municipalities with 40 million residents (60). Agita is arguably the first community-wide intervention to be developed on a specified ecological model with linked strategies across intrapersonal, social environment, and physical environment categories while being implemented with the active participation and sponsorship of the region's highest government health authority (the state health secretariat). The program has a simply stated goal: to change the physical activity of the population (60). The driving strategic principle of Agita Sao Paulo is a "mobile management" approach to strategies that fall under the umbrella of intrapersonal, social environment, and physical environment (*Table 48-1*). Specifically, "the multi-level components of the ecological model are distributed three-dimensionally in a dynamic balance as in a mobile" (60). The mobile management approach recommends that strategies across the ecological model be addressed concurrently to facilitate a balanced approach. Thus, Agita Sao Paulo engaged with several partnership institutions and a coalition of more than 300 members. To ensure a sharing of the workload as strategies were identified, the central organizing committee also identified the appropriate partner institution to lead the planning and implementation. Although Agita Sao Paulo is clearly a Herculean effort and may seem overwhelming to a community physical activity professional, the principle of development and delivery can be generalized to small or large community-wide initiatives. That principle is that strategies should be balanced across the ecological framework and matched to the appropriate partner for implementation. Also, it is clearly seen from the model that no one person or organization can plan, implement, and sustain a community-wide initiative.

Community efforts to promote improved health and well-being through increased participation in physical activity may also be seen in initiatives such as Exercise Is Medicine (EIM). This initiative promotes physical activity as a standard part of disease prevention and treatment plans. It encourages physicians to assess and review every patient's physical activity levels at each visit, and it encourages individuals to assume responsibility for their own health and adopt positive health behaviors such as regular participation in physical activity. The initiative also encourages open dialog among multiple community sectors and promotes an increased emphasis on the health benefits of being physically active. In addition to having a presence in the health care setting, EIM also has a college presence through "EIM on Campus" where opportunities for participation in physical activity are promoted campus wide and where the benefits of being active are an integral part of the college curriculum (see http://exerciseismedicine.org/campus.htm).

POLICY AND ENVIRONMENTAL APPROACHES

Pinpointing the specific reasons people choose to be active or inactive and quantifying the proportional contribution of these causes to the inactivity crisis is a tough challenge. Recent literature suggest that the built environment, structures that are made by humans for humans (buildings, roads, sidewalks, land development patterns, and other structures that are built to enhance some aspect of human life) exert powerful influences on physical activity behaviors. It has been proposed that physical activity participation may be encouraged

TABLE 48-1. The Ecological Categories and Example Community-wide Intervention Strategies Used in Agita Sao Paulo

Primary Ecological Category	Ecological Subcategory	Intervention Strategy
Intrapersonal	Demographic	Physical activity promotion materials tailored for specific age and socioeconomic groups
	Cognitive/affective	Behavioral skills–based activities that will lead to the initiation of an active lifestyle: courses, print materials, talks
	Biological	Adapt physical activity materials to address men and women and other special groups (handicapped, chronic disease)
	Behavioral	Stage-based messages to encourage sedentary people to become a little more active, insufficiently active people to become regularly active, and regularly active people to maintain their behavior
Social environment	Culture	Incentives for local executive committees to form within each municipality; allow local adaptation of logo, mascot, and icons to be culturally relevant
	Social climate	Developed executive committee that unites the representatives of government, private, and social spheres to discuss permanent intervention actions
	Supportive behaviors	Engage employers, government entities, school leaders, and health care providers to implement incentives for physical activity
	Policies governing resources	Define human, material, structural, logistic, and financial resources necessary to execute physical activity promotion; use unpaid media to promote action and results of the program
	Policies governing incentives	The establishment of policies, statutes, and laws to provide incentives and practice of physical activity promotion; health care discounts for the regularly active
Physical environment	Natural environment: geography	Establish practices that use the naturally occurring environment as much as possible
	Natural environment: weather	Adapt intervention strategies specific to the seasons
	Constructed environment: architectural	Construct new sidewalks, tracks, trails where necessary; use school grounds and resources for weekend activities and increase maintenance efforts for existing parks
	Constructed environment: entertainment	Create specific physical activity groups for diverse social groups, including children, adolescents, and the elderly
	Constructed environment: transport	Improve storage and parking of bikes; develop or improve private and public policies to support active transportation to work or school

or discouraged through both land and building design, and it seems that in many places, physical activity has been inadvertently engineered out of daily life. The culmination of zoning regulations (single use vs. mixed use, sidewalk and street design requirements, and traffic flow regulations), land development practices (density, mix, street connectivity, structure placement, pedestrian systems), and limited access to green space recreation areas encourages people to drive instead of walk or bike (34,36). Patterns of land design, development, and use have been proposed as possible explanations for shifts away from pedestrian or nonmotorized destination trips. Researchers suggest that utilitarian walking relies on design practices such as high density, a mix of residential and commercial zoning, and grid-like street design. These practices have been replaced in many areas with the familiar "sprawl" designs of low density, separated residential and commercial zoning, and cul-de-sacs (18).

One design strategy that may encourage residents in sprawling neighborhoods to be more physically active is the presence of walking trails or other amenities within newly constructed subdivisions. Several authors have reported an association between increased access to recreational facilities and higher levels of participation in physical activity (5,10,88,106). Brownson et al. (10) found trail use to be associated with increased physical activity. Similarly, others have uncovered an association between the addition of community walking/biking trails and improvements in physical activity (10,43,70). Ducan and Mummery (22) also found the distance to a foot path (walking trail, sidewalk, etc.) to be positively linked to recreational walking.

Founded in 2001 by the Robert Wood Johnson Foundation, Active Living By Design (ALBD) encourages participatory practices and community-led change to build an active community culture. ALBD provides support through funding and expertise to promote the development of active communities. Process evaluations documenting the feasibility and effectiveness of specific strategies and approaches are an important part of ALBD projects. Outcomes of these demonstration projects offer valuable insights and lessons for other communities as they strive to adopt an active community culture. In order to promote community change, ALBD offers a community action model to guide intervention development and implementation. This model is grounded in a socio-ecological approach to change encouraging targeted intervention at multiple levels of influence and begins with establishing strong support from key stakeholders and gatekeepers. Using this approach, an interdisciplinary team engages key stakeholders and gatekeepers in participatory practices aimed at developing population-specific strategies aimed that will lead to optimal outcomes (3). The selection of specific strategies will be informed by preparation, promotion, programs, policy, and physical projects. Small changes are then encouraged through increased awareness, social support, and policy changes. Then broader changes are observed as increases in community engagement are realized. As the larger population embraces a physical activity

and healthy lifestyles, decreases in chronic conditions such as obesity, diabetes, and hypertension may be realized.

ALBD supported 25 diverse communities (2003–2008) across the nation with funds to be used to facilitate the development of communities that support active lifestyles. Although outcomes will continue to evolve, current results support the importance of multidisciplinary partnerships and passionate, engaged leaders (8). Specific strategies adopted and implemented by some cities are highlighted in *Box 48-5* (8).

PRINCIPLES FOR PLANNING AND EVALUATING COMMUNITY PHYSICAL ACTIVITY INTERVENTIONS

THE RE-AIM FRAMEWORK

Consider this scenario: A local physical activity professional is interested in helping every child in her state to become active at the recommended levels. She picks up the current issue of *Medicine and Science in Sports and Exercise* and reads about a fantastic new intervention that takes only 15 min · wk^{-1}, is offered during an after-school program, and helped half of the sedentary and insufficiently active children who received it to meet the recommended guidelines within a month. Further, when the researchers went back and checked on the children 6 mo later, half of those who saw the original benefit were still meeting recommended guidelines. When she reads further, she finds that the intervention needs to be delivered by a trained and certified physical education teacher. The physical activity professional takes the information with her and successfully lobbies her state's governor to strongly recommend that all schools implement the new intervention.

The earlier scenario would be exciting for all involved. The researchers would be excited about the large effect size. The physical activity professional would be excited because the intervention will be implemented. The governor would be excited because of all of the good press. But take the scenario a little further using *Figure 48-2*. At the top of the figure, a group of clip art people represent the total population of students within the school system of the state in question. Following the governor's strong recommendation, 50% of the schools adopt the program and these schools reflect 50% of the student population (see *Fig. 48-2*: Adoption). However, only half of the schools have a certified teacher who can lead the program, so they have to use volunteers. Unfortunately, the volunteers can't implement the program with the same fidelity as certified teachers, and the intervention doesn't work in those sites. Now, 25% of the student population receives the intervention (see *Fig. 48-2*: Implementation). In the schools that are offering the program, only half of the students in their school attend the after-school program, which decreases full participation to 12.5% of

BOX 48-5	**Active Living by Design Project Focus Areas**
Partnerships	Initiated interdisciplinary partnerships
	Worked with government leaders (planners, engineers, etc.) regarding zoning, transportation, prioritize improvement projects, etc.
	Leveraged with other sources to secure additional funding
Infrastructure	Promoted, prioritized, and/or implemented infrastructure improvements
	Promoted nonmotorized travel (bikes, pedestrian systems)
Environmental	Provided environmental cues to be active (stairs, signage, etc.)
Trails	Developed and/or promoted the use of trails (biking and walking)
	Developed active living neighborhood map
School	School-based initiatives such as Safe Routes to School
Community/ neighborhood	Completed assessments (neighborhood, activity, etc.)
	Launched new programs (dance, sports, challenge programs, etc.)
	Developed social marketing plan to encourage active living

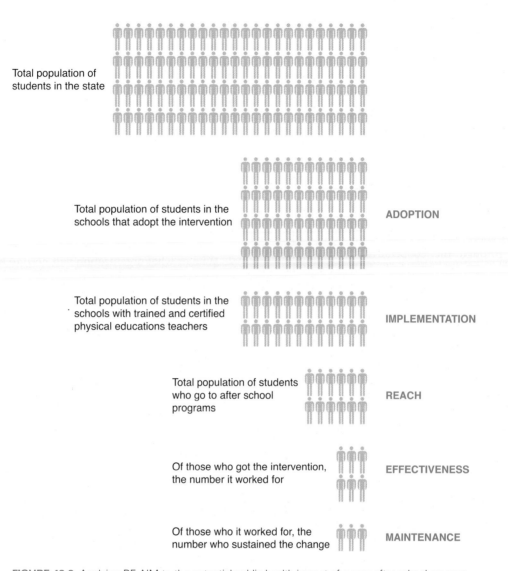

Total population of students in the state

Total population of students in the schools that adopt the intervention — **ADOPTION**

Total population of students in the schools with trained and certified physical educations teachers — **IMPLEMENTATION**

Total population of students who go to after school programs — **REACH**

Of those who got the intervention, the number it worked for — **EFFECTIVENESS**

Of those who it worked for, the number who sustained the change — **MAINTENANCE**

FIGURE 48-2. Applying RE-AIM to the potential public health impact of a new after-school program physical activity intervention.

the student population (see *Fig. 48-2*: Reach). Based on the efficacy data, half of the children increased activity to recommended guidelines, or 6.25% of the state population of students (see *Fig. 48-2*: Effectiveness), and half of those (about 3% of the total population) sustain that level of activity (see *Fig. 48-2*: Maintenance).

This scenario highlights the need for evaluation and planning efforts that address several different issues beyond simply determining if an intervention "works." Each step of the described scenario relates to a dimension of the RE-AIM planning and evaluation framework (http://www.re-aim.org) (33,41). One purpose of the RE-AIM framework is to increase attention to both individual and organizational level indicators with an effort to either predict or document the public health impact of a given intervention.

RE-AIM is an acronym that stands for *Reach, Effectiveness, Adoption, Implementation,* and *Maintenance.*

Reach is defined as the participation rate and representativeness of participants who engage in an intervention. *Effectiveness* is defined as the extent to which the intervention achieves targeted outcomes in real-world contexts and also includes assessing for potential negative consequences. *Adoption* can be defined as the participation rate of organizations that will ultimately implement the intervention and the representativeness of those organizations to the population that could implement the intervention. *Implementation* is defined as the degree to which an intervention is implemented as intended. Finally, maintenance is defined at both the individual and organizational level. For individuals, *maintenance* is defined as sustained behavior change for more than 6 mo; at the organizational level, maintenance is defined as the sustained delivery of a given intervention or the institutionalization of an intervention within typical community settings (see http://cancer control.cancer.gov/is/reaim/).

An example of a community physical activity intervention that used the RE-AIM framework for evaluation is Walk Kansas (28,29). Walk Kansas was developed by a team that was organized to respond to the need to increase the rates of physical activity in rural Kansas. The conceptual model, developed by Carron and Spink (14), uses group dynamic principles and was applied within the physical activity promotion program. Walk Kansas aimed to develop a sense of group distinctiveness, target norms through group goal setting, form groups of individuals within geographic proximity, and foster ongoing group interactions and communication to provide feedback, information sharing, and collective problem solving. In addition, the program was developed to be delivered through the cooperative extension system, which included representatives in each of the 105 counties in Kansas (28). *Table 48-2* describes the metrics used to assess each dimension of the RE-AIM framework.

RE-AIM IMPLICATIONS FOR PLANNING

One of the broad appeals of community interventions is the potential to improve the physical activity of a large proportion of the population. Schools, work sites, clinics, churches, and community-wide interventions and changes to the built environment share the commonality that by intervening through them, a large proportion of the population can be influenced. Using RE-AIM in the planning process for community physical activity programs begins with a series of questions related to each dimension that will help physical activity professionals realize the positive potential for community change (52). By addressing the questions, physical activity professionals can prepare an initiative to reach a broad cross-section of the target population, increase and sustain physical activity for those reached, and successfully adapt physical activity interventions to different settings. Four primary questions are helpful when beginning to plan a community physical activity intervention.

1. For which individuals or groups do you intend to increase physical activity as a result of the intervention?
2. Who or what organization will need to be involved in decision making and planning?
3. Who will be responsible for delivering or implementing the strategies?
4. What organization or institution will be needed to ensure sustainability?

By answering these questions, a physical activity professional can determine who else needs to be involved before comprehensive planning begins (37). Answering these questions and getting the appropriate partners at the table is the first step in the planning process. Once a partnership is formed, careful planning around

TABLE 48-2. Operationalizing the RE-AIM Framework: Walk Kansas

RE-AIM Dimension	Indicator	Outcome
Reach	Number of participants	Ranged from approximately 6,000 participants in 2002 to 20,000 in 2006
	Percent of county population that participated	Ranged from approximately 3% in 2002 to 5% in 2006
	Representativeness of participants to county populations based on sex, ethnicity, age	Walk Kansas participants were more likely to be female and older than the general population but representative on ethnicity
Effectiveness	Preevaluation/postevaluation on subsample of 1,400 program participants divided by baseline activity level (active, inactive, insufficiently active)	Active participants maintained activity levels over the course of the program; inactive and insufficiently active increased moderate-intensity physical activity by approximately 150 min · wk^{-1}
Adoption	Number of counties that participated out of 105 eligible	Ranged from 48 in 2002 to 97 in 2006
	Percent of counties that participated	Ranged from 46% in 2002 to 92% in 2006
	Representativeness of counties within the state based on population, proportion female, proportion minority	Counties were representative of the state across variables until 2006, when counties with small populations were less likely to participate (*i.e.*, 8% of the counties)
Implementation	Proportion that delivered core components (*i.e.*, used teams, goal setting, and feedback)	100% of the counties reported delivering the core components
	Proportion that used task force	Approximately 50% used a task force to market and implement the program; the remaining used their own office staff
Maintenance: individual	Random selection of 225 participants surveyed on physical activity 6 mo postintervention completion	On average, participants sustained 150 min of moderate physical activity each week
Maintenance: organizational	Percentage of counties that sustained delivery for 2, 3, 4, or 5 yr	Approximately 42% of counties delivered the program for all 5 yr, 35% for 4 yr, 10% for 3 yr, and 5% each delivered the program for 2, 1, or 0 yr.

each RE-AIM dimension will enhance the impact of the community initiative.

When planning to improve the reach of a community physical activity intervention, it is important to define a target population and have a clear understanding of its denominator. For example, if a community program attracted 500 participants, one might consider this a success. However, if the denominator of the target population was a community of 50,000, then 500 participants is not a success. Conversely, if the program targeted a small rural community of 1,000 people, then 500 participants would be exceptional. Once the denominator is clarified, building relationships with members of the target population and those who provide services to them can help to determine strategies that will be the most salient in that community. The partnership with community members can also aid in the development of population-specific recruitment materials and strategies. Finally, to ensure a broad reach into the population, go to where the target population is to deliver the intervention and distribute recruitment materials.

As suggested by WELCOA, planning for effectiveness and individual maintenance of behavior begins by understanding the evidence base (105). However, for many community contexts, there are few evidence-based interventions or specific recommendations. In these cases, development of community physical activity programs should be based on the best available evidence or developed to match the underlying principles of an efficacious intervention (87).

Planning to enhance the adoption of a community intervention begins with the same process that is used when planning for reach — by determining the denominator and characteristics of the settings that will ultimately deliver the intervention (52). As highlighted in the recommendations and processes reviewed for school, work site, clinic, church, and community-wide strategies, using a participatory model of development can enhance the perceived community ownership of a program and help ensure that the end product is consistent with the needs of the potential participants and delivery sites. It is critical to understand the system that you anticipate will use the program or implement a policy. The organizational mission, flow of day-to-day operations, and available resources are all factors that can either facilitate or impede adoption. Finally, when meeting with a new organization, have data that demonstrate the program's reach, effectiveness, ease of implementation (including cost), and relative advantage (87).

Inevitably, community physical activity interventions will be adapted over time by those who deliver them (87). This can either be a positive or negative outcome. A positive adaptation would be to make the program easier to deliver while adhering to the principles that made it effective (95). A negative adaptation would be to drop the intervention components that are most difficult but integral to intervention success and deliver only those that are easy to implement. To avoid negative adaptation, program developers should identify and market the functioning principles of the intervention or core components of policy and allow for local adaptation. Manualized programs are also more likely to facilitate fidelity to the intervention program, as are training and technical support during early stages of implementation (52).

Organizational sustainability of community physical activity programs can be challenging. Issues of program cost and organizational climate can result in the abandonment of new and effective programs. To optimize the chances for a sustained program, it is important to collect information on the effectiveness of the program including reach, implementation, and impact on both physical activity behavior as well as other things, such as participant satisfaction and program costs. Foster *program champions* at multiple levels who can advocate for the program and provide resources. Program champions are people who really believe in the program and its positive outcomes. Previous participants can be excellent advocates for both the future reach of the program and for sustained funding. It is also important to identify a program sponsor within the organization that is delivering the program. An organizational level program sponsor will be most effective if the organization holds some decision-making authority. Also, programs that have the perception of broad-based local ownership are much more likely to be sustained than those that are considered to be from a research shop that has little understanding of local needs and barriers. Finally, integrate the program into the regular service of the organization that is delivering the program.

COMMUNITY PHYSICAL ACTIVITY INTERVENTIONS: RECOMMENDATIONS AND CONSIDERATIONS

Many resources and case studies are available to assist community efforts to promote increased participation in physical activity by thorough programming and environmental strategies (see *Table 48-1*). This chapter has reviewed various community physical activity interventions and provided suggestions on how to assess the potential or actual impact of those interventions. Through this review, several commonalities arose that can be used to provide some recommendations for physical activity professionals who are interested in developing and delivering community interventions.

First, interventionists should use a broad ecological model as the basis of strategy development. This includes understanding the characteristics of potential participants and the social and physical environmental contexts of the places they reside, work, and spend leisure time. Defining the target population and completing assessments of the target population's perception of need for a physical activity program and preferences for format and content should improve the chances that the program will reach a broad audience and have intended positive effects. Addressing

TABLE 48-3. Resources: Creating Active Environments

Physical Activity Guidelines	• Physical Activity Guidelines for Americans: http://www.health.gov/paguidelines/ • Youth Physical Activity Guidelines Toolkit: http://www.cdc.gov/Healthyyouth/physicalactivity/guidelines.htm#1 • Compendium of Physical Activities: http://sites.google.com/site/compendiumofphysicalactivities/
Environmental Influences on Physical Activity	• Does the Built Environment Influence Physical Activity? Examining the Evidence: http://gulliver.trb.org/news/blurb_detail.asp?id=4536 • Designing for Active Recreation: http://www.activelivingresearch.org/alr/files/recreationrevised021105.pdf • Physical Activity and the Built Environment: http://www.fitness.gov/digests/December2006Digest.pdf • Does the Built Environment Influence Physical Activity?: http://onlinepubs.trb.org/onlinepubs/sr/sr282.pdf
Building Activity-Friendly Environments	• National Trails Training Partnership: http://www.americantrails.org/resources/index.html • Robert Wood Johnson Active Living by Design: http://www.activelivingbydesign.org/ • National Center for Bicycling & Walking: Increasing Physical Activity through Community Design, a Guide for Public Health Practitioners, May 2002: http://www.bikewalk.org/pdfs/IPA_full.pdf • Pedestrian and Bicycling Information Center: http://www.pedbikeinfo.org/ • North Carolina's Active Community Environments (ACEs) Page: http://www.eatsmartmovemorenc.com/programs_tools/community/aces.html • Active Community Environments Virtual Backpack: http://www.doh.wa.gov/CFH/NutritionPA/our_communities/active_community_environments/toolkit/default.htm
Data Collection/Survey Tools	• Surface Transportation Policy Project — State-Specific Statistics: http://www.transact.org/states/default.asp • Pedestrian and Bicycle Information Center: http://www.bicyclinginfo.org/ • Environmental Supports for Physical Activity Questionnaire: http://prevention.sph.sc.edu/tools/environmental.htm • The Path Environment Audit Tool (PEAT): http://www.activelivingresearch.org/node/10652 • Tools and Measures: http://www.activelivingresearch.org/resourcesearch/toolsandmeasures • County Health Rankings: http://www.countyhealthrankings.org/health-factors/built-environment • Exercise Is Medicine: http://exerciseismedicine.org/index.htm
Implementation	• Models for Change: Lessons for Creating Active Living Communities: http://www.activelivingresearch.org/files/ALR%20Planning%20Magazine_Case%20Studies_0.pdf • Active Living by Design-Community Partnership Profiles: http://www.activelivingbydesign.org/index.php?id=6#CPPages • Fix It First: http://www.nga.org/Files/pdf/0408FIXINGFIRST.pdf • Pedestrian and Bicycle Information Center's Sample Pedestrian Plans: http://www.walkinginfo.org/develop/sample-plans.cfm • From the Field: Four Communities Implement Active Aging Programs: http://www.prevent.org/images/stories/Files/publications/CCFAA_case_studies.pdf

TABLE 48-3. Resources: Creating Active Environments (*Continued*)

Creating A Healthy Culture	• Promoting Active Living Communities: http://www.activelivingbydesign.org/fileadmin/template/documents/rwjf_toolkit.pdf • Developing Effective Coalitions — An Eight Step Guide: http://xnet.kp.org/communitybenefit/chi/tools/docs/other_resources/EffectiveCoalitions.pdf • Local Physical Activity and Nutrition (LPAN) Coalition Manual, Guide for Community Action: http://www.eatsmartmovemorenc.com/programs_tools/community/docs/lpans/070317_lpan_manual.pdf • Getting to Smart Growth: http://www.smartgrowth.org/pdf/gettosg.pdf • Healthy Community Design, Success Stories from State and Local Leaders: http://www.activeliving.org/files/HealthyCommunityDesign_ALL.pdf • Working with Elected Officials to Promote Healthy Land Use Planning & Community Design: http://www.planning.org/research/pdf/healthycommfactsheet2.pdf • CDC's Nutrition, Physical Activity, and Obesity Legislative Database: http://apps.nccd.cdc.gov/DNPALeg • CDC's Physical Activity Policy Research Network: http://prc.slu.edu/paprn.htm
Organizations	• National Organizations: Pedestrian and Bicycle Information Center: http://www.pedbikeinfo.org • International City/County Management Association: http://www.icma.org • Local Government Commission: http://www.lgc.org • Congress for New Urbanism: http://www.cnu.org • National Association for County and City Health Officials: http://www.naccho.org/topics/hpdp/land_use_planning/LUP_Toolbox.cfm • American Planning Association: http://www.planning.org/

the social environment in terms of policy, group activities, and social marketing can provide a foundation for successful programming. Finally, ensuring that the physical environment is supportive of regular physical activity or highlighting existing community resources are promising directions for strategy development.

Second, and related to the first point, use a balanced approach to ensure that all domains in an ecological approach are addressed. The Agita Sao Paulo's mobile management system is an excellent method to ensure that there is a balanced approach to individual, social, and physical environment components. Also, implicitly balanced in the Agita approach were the components of the intervention that were based on programs and policies. This balance has applicability regardless of the type of community intervention being completed. That is, even for an intervention that targets a single school, workplace, church, or clinic, the intervention should include strategies that affect individual, social, and environmental factors to optimize the likelihood of success.

Third, to be successful, community physical activity interventions should be conceptualized, developed, delivered, and monitored by a partnership that includes representatives of those intended to benefit from the intervention, those intended to deliver it, and those intended to

provide support for it. This crosscutting of issues is critical to improve the reach, implementation, and sustainability of community physical activity interventions. Working with a group that includes all the key stakeholders within a community setting will facilitate the identification of individual, organizational, and contextual barriers that could arise over the course of the program. More importantly, such a group can aid in resolving barriers before they arise.

Fourth, evaluation of community physical activity interventions should include various outcomes in addition to assessing the potential effectiveness of the program. As demonstrated in *Figure 48-2*, there are several points in the life course of a behavioral intervention when, without careful planning, large proportions of the target population can be lost. By assessing the outcomes across the RE-AIM framework, one can identify and market individual and organizational success.

REFERENCES

1. *2008 Physical Activity Guidelines for Americans* [Internet]. Washington (DC): U.S. Department of Health and Human Services; 2008 [cited 2011 Sep 2]. 76 p. Available from: http://www.health.gov/paguidelines/pdf/paguide.pdf

2. Ackermann RT, Deyo RA, LoGerfo JP. Prompting primary providers to increase community exercise referrals for older adults: a randomized trial. *J Am Geriatr Soc.* 2005;53(2):283–9.

3. Active Living by Design Web site [Internet]. Chapel Hill (NC): North Carolina Institute for Public Policy; [cited 2011 Nov 21]. Available from: http://www.activelivingbydesign.org/

4. Ayre D, Clough G, Norris T. *Facilitating Community Change.* San Francisco (CA): Community Initiatives, Grove Consultants International; 2000. 6 p.

5. Baker EA, Brennan LK, Brownson R, Houseman RA. Measuring the determinants of physical activity in the community: current and future directions. *Res Q Exerc Sport.* 2000;71(2 Suppl):S146–58.

6. Baskin ML, Resnicow K, Campbell MK. Conducting health interventions in black churches: a model for building effective partnerships. *Ethn Dis.* 2001;11(4):823–33.

7. *Body & Soul: A Celebration of Healthy Eating & Living* [Internet]. Bethesda (MD): National Cancer Institute; [cited 2008 Nov 25]. Available from: http://www.bodyandsoul.nih.gov/

8. Bors P, Dessauer M, Bell R, Wilkerson R, Lee J, Strunk SL. The Active Living by Design national program: community initiatives and lessons learned. *Am J Prev Med.* 2009;37(6 Suppl 2):S313–21.

9. Brownson RC, Baker EA, Boyd RL, et al. A community-based approach to promoting walking in rural areas. *Am J Prev Med.* 2004;27(1):28–34.

10. Brownson RC, Baker EA, Housemann RA, Brennan LK, Bacak SJ. Environmental and policy determinants of physical activity in the United States. *Am J Public Health.* 2001;91(12):1995–2003.

11. Brownson RC, Housemann RA, Brown DR, et al. Promoting physical activity in rural communities: walking trail access, use, and effects. *Am J Prev Med.* 2000;18(3):235–41.

12. Burgeson CR, Wechsler H, Brener ND, Young JC, Spain CG. Physical education and activity: results from the School Health Policies and Programs Study 2000. *J Sch Health.* 2001;71(7): 279–93.

13. Campbell MK, Motsinger BM, Ingram A, et al. The North Carolina Black Churches United for Better Health Project: intervention and process evaluation. *Health Educ Behav.* 2000;27(2):241–53.

14. Carron AV, Spink KS. Team building in an exercise setting. *Sport Psychol.* 1993;7:8–18.

15. *CDC's Healthy Communities Program: Community Health Assessment and Group Evaluation (CHANGE): Building a Foundation of Knowledge to Prioritize Community Needs* [Internet]. Atlanta (GA): Centers for Disease Control and Prevention; [cited 2011 Nov 21]. Available from: http://www.cdc.gov/healthycommunitiesprogram/tools/change.htm

16. Centers for Disease Control and Prevention. Prevalence of regular physical activity among adults—United States, 2001 and 2005. *MMWR Morb Mortal Wkly Rep.* 2007;56(46):1209–12.

17. Chin MH, Cook S, Jin L, et al. Barriers to providing diabetes care in community health centers. *Diabetes Care.* 2001;24(2):268–74.

18. Coogan PF, Coogan MA. When worlds collide: observations on the integration of epidemiology and transportation behavioral analysis in the study of walking. *Am J Health Promot.* 2004;19(1):39–44.

19. Council on Sports Medicine and Fitness, Council on School Health. Active healthy living: prevention of childhood obesity through increased physical activity. *Pediatrics.* 2006;117(5):1834–42.

20. Dishman RK, Oldenburg B, O'Neal H, Shephard RJ. Worksite physical activity interventions. *Am J Prev Med.* 1998;15(4):344–61.

21. Donnelly JE, Greene JL, Gibson CA, et al. Physical Activity Across the Curriculum (PAAC): a randomized controlled trial to promote physical activity and diminish overweight and obesity in elementary school children. *Prev Med.* 2009;49(4):336–41.

22. Duncan M, Mummery K. Psychosocial and environmental factors associated with physical activity among city dwellers in regional Queensland. *Prev Med.* 2005;40(4):363–72.

23. Dzewaltowski DA. The ecology of physical activity and sport: merging science and practice. *J Appl Sport Psychol.* 1997;9(2):254–76.

24. Dzewaltowski DA, Estabrooks PA, Johnston JA. Healthy youth places promoting nutrition and physical activity. *Health Educ Res.* 2002;17(5):541–51.

25. Eakin EG, Glasgow RE, Riley KM. Review of primary care-based physical activity intervention studies: effectiveness and implications for practice and future research. *J Fam Pract.* 2000;49(2):158–68.

26. Eden KB, Orleans CT, Mulrow CD, Pender NJ, Teutsch SM. Does counseling by clinicians improve physical activity? A summary of the evidence for the U.S. Preventive Services Task Force. *Ann Intern Med.* 2002;137(3):208–15.

27. Englert HS, Diehl HA, Greenlaw RL, Willich SN, Aldana S. The effect of a community-based coronary risk reduction: the Rockford CHIP. *Prev Med.* 2007;44(6):513–9.

28. Estabrooks PA, Bradshaw M, Dzewaltowski DA, Smith-Ray RL. Determining the impact of Walk Kansas: applying a team-building approach to community physical activity promotion. *Ann Behav Med.* 2008;36(1):1–12.

29. Estabrooks P, Bradshaw M, Fox E, Berg J, Dzewaltowski DA. The relationships between delivery agents' physical activity level and the likelihood of implementing a physical activity program. *Am J Health Promot.* 2004;18(5):350–3.

30. Estabrooks PA, Glasgow RE. Translating effective clinic-based physical activity interventions into practice. *Am J Prev Med.* 2006;31(4 Suppl):S45–56.

31. Estabrooks PA, Glasgow RE. Worksite interventions. In: Ayers S, editor. *Cambridge Handbook of Psychology, Health and Medicine.* 2nd ed. New York: Cambridge University Press; 2007. p. 407–416.

32. Estabrooks PA, Glasgow RE, Dzewaltowski DA. Physical activity promotion through primary care. *JAMA.* 2003;289(22):2913–6.

33. Estabrooks PA, Gyurcsik NC. Evaluating the impact of behavioral interventions that target physical activity: issues of generalizability and public health. *Psychol Sport Exerc.* 2003;4(1):41–55.

34. Ewing R, Schmid T, Killingsworth R, Zlot A, Raudenbush S. Relationship between urban sprawl and physical activity, obesity, and morbidity. *Am J Health Promot.* 2003;18(1):47–57.

35. Farquhar JW, Fortmann SP, Maccoby N, et al. The Stanford Five-City Project: design and methods. *Am J Epidemiol.* 1985;122(2):323–34.

36. Frank LD. Land use and transportation interaction: implications on public health and quality of life. *J Plan Educ Res.* 2000;20(1):6–22.

37. Glasgow RE, Bayliss EA, Estabrooks PA. Translation research in diabetes: asking broader questions. In: Montori VM, editor. *Evidence-Based Endocrinology.* Totowa: Humana Press; 2006. p. 241–256.

38. Glasgow RE, Eakin EG. Medical office-based interventions. In: Snoek FJ, Skinner TC, editors. *Psychol Diabetes Care.* Chichester: Wiley; 2000. p. 141–168.

39. Glasgow RE, Hollis JF, Ary DV, Lando HA. Employee and organizational factors associated with participation in an incentive-based worksite smoking cessation program. *J Behav Med.* 1990;13(4):403–18.

40. Glasgow RE, McCaul KD, Fisher KJ. Participation in worksite health promotion: a critique of the literature and recommendations for future practice. *Health Educ Q.* 1993;20(3):391–408.

41. Glasgow RE, Vogt TM, Boles SM. Evaluating the public health impact of health promotion interventions: the RE-AIM framework. *Am J Public Health.* 1999;89(9):1322–7.

42. Goldstein MG, Whitlock EP, DePue J, Planning Committee of the Addressing Multiple Behavioral Risk Factors in Primary Care Project. Multiple behavioral risk factor interventions in primary care. Summary of research evidence. *Am J Prev Med.* 2004;27(2 Suppl):61–79.

43. Gordon PM, Zizzi SJ, Pauline J. Use of a community trail among new and habitual exercisers: a preliminary assessment. *Prev Chronic Dis.* 2004;1(4):A11.

44. Guidelines for school health programs to promote lifelong healthy eating. Centers for Disease Control and Prevention. *MMWR Recomm Rep.* 1996;45(RR–9):1–41.

45. Harvey-Berino J, Pintauro S, Buzzell P, Gold EC. Effect of internet support on the long-term maintenance of weight loss. *Obes Res.* 2004;12(2):320–9.

46. Hennrikus DJ, Jeffery RW. Worksite intervention for weight control: a review of the literature. *Am J Health Promot.* 1996;10(6):471–98.

47. Hunt MK, Lederman R, Potter S, Stoddard A, Sorensen G. Results of employee involvement in planning and implementing the Treatwell 5-a-Day work-site study. *Health Educ Behav.* 2000;27(2):223–31.

48. Jimmy G, Martin BW. Implementation and effectiveness of a primary care based physical activity counselling scheme. *Patient Educ Couns.* 2005;56(3):323–31.

49. Kahn EB, Ramsey LT, Brownson RC, et al. The effectiveness of interventions to increase physical activity. A systematic review. *Am J Prev Med.* 2002;22(4 Suppl):73–107.

50. King AC, Carl F, Birkel L, Haskell WL. Increasing exercise among blue-collar employees: the tailoring of worksite programs to meet specific needs. *Prev Med.* 1988;17(3):357–65.

51. King AC, Jeffery RW, Fridinger F, et al. Environmental and policy approaches to cardiovascular disease prevention through physical activity: issues and opportunities. *Health Educ Q.* 1995;22(4):499–511.

52. Klesges LM, Estabrooks PA, Dzewaltowski DA, Bull SS, Glasgow RE. Beginning with the application in mind: designing and planning health behavior change interventions to enhance dissemination. *Ann Behav Med.* 2005;29 Suppl:66–75.

53. Klesges RC, Vasey MM, Glasgow RE. A worksite smoking modification competition: potential for public health impact. *Am J Public Health.* 1986;76(2):198–200.

54. Larsen P, Simons N. Evaluating a federal health and fitness program: indicators of improving health. *AAOHN J.* 1993;41(3):143–8.

55. Linenger JM, Chesson CV,2nd, Nice DS. Physical fitness gains following simple environmental change. *Am J Prev Med.* 1991;7(5):298–310.

56. Lobo CM, Frijling BD, Hulscher ME, et al. Improving quality of organizing cardiovascular preventive care in general practice by outreach visitors: a randomized controlled trial. *Prev Med.* 2002;35(5):422–9.

57. Luepker RV, Perry CL, McKinlay SM, et al. Outcomes of a field trial to improve children's dietary patterns and physical activity. The child and adolescent trial for cardiovascular health. CATCH collaborative group. *JAMA.* 1996;275(10):768–76.

58. Marcus BH, Williams DM, Dubbert PM, et al. Physical activity intervention studies: what we know and what we need to know: a scientific statement from the American Heart Association Council on Nutrition, Physical Activity, and Metabolism (Subcommittee on Physical Activity); Council on Cardiovascular Disease in the Young; and the Interdisciplinary Working Group on Quality of Care and Outcomes Research. *Circulation.* 2006;114(24):2739–52.

59. Marshall AL. Challenges and opportunities for promoting physical activity in the workplace. *J Sci Med Sport.* 2004;7(1 Suppl):60–6.

60. Matsudo SM, Matsudo VKR, Andrade DR, Araújo TL, Pratt M. Evaluation of a physical activity promotion program: the example of Agita São Paulo. *Eval Program Plann.* 2006;29(3):301–11.

61. McClanahan BS, Stockton MB. Engaged Scholarship: Participatory practices enhance outcomes. In: *21st Annual Art and Science of Health Promotion Conference*; 2011 Mar 21-25: Colorado Springs (CO). Health Promotion; 1992.

62. McClanahan B, Stockton M, McClanahan R, Clark S. Interdisciplinary stakeholders identify supports and barriers to building activity friendly environments. In: *American College of Sports Medicine 59th Annual Meeting*; 2012 May 29-Jun 2: San Francisco (CA). ACSM; 2012.

63. McGinnis JM, Foege WH. Actual causes of death in the United States. *JAMA.* 1993;270(18):2207–12.

64. McKenzie TL, Feldman H, Woods SE, et al. Children's activity levels and lesson context during third-grade physical education. *Res Q Exerc Sport.* 1995;66(3):184–93.

65. McKenzie TL, Nader PR, Strikmiller PK, et al. School physical education: effect of the Child and Adolescent Trial for Cardiovascular Health. *Prev Med.* 1996;25(4):423–31.

66. McKenzie TL, Sallis JF, Kolody B, Faucette FN. Long-term effects of a physical education curriculum and staff development program: SPARK. *Res Q Exerc Sport.* 1997;68(4):280–91.

67. McTigue KM, Harris R, Hemphill B, et al. Screening and interventions for obesity in adults: summary of the evidence for the U.S. Preventive Services Task Force. *Ann Intern Med.* 2003;139(11):933–49.

68. Nader PR, Stone EJ, Lytle LA, et al. Three-year maintenance of improved diet and physical activity: the CATCH cohort. Child and adolescent trial for cardiovascular health. *Arch Pediatr Adolesc Med.* 1999;153(7):695–704.

69. Oden G, Crouse SF, Reynolds C. Worker productivity, job satisfaction, and work-related stress: the influence of an employee fitness program. *Fitness Business.* 1989;4(198):204.

70. Owen N, Humpel N, Leslie E, Bauman A, Sallis JF. Understanding environmental influences on walking: review and research agenda. *Am J Prev Med.* 2004;27(1):67–76.

71. Pate RR, Davis MG, Robinson TN, et al. Promoting physical activity in children and youth: a leadership role for schools: a scientific statement from the American Heart Association Council on Nutrition, Physical Activity, and Metabolism (Physical Activity Committee) in collaboration with the Councils on Cardiovascular Disease in the Young and Cardiovascular Nursing. *Circulation.* 2006;114(11):1214–24.

72. Pate RR, Trost SG, Mullis R, Sallis JF, Wechsler H, Brown DR. Community interventions to promote proper nutrition and physical activity among youth. *Prev Med.* 2000;31(2):S138–49.

73. Pate RR, Ward DS, Saunders RP, Felton G, Dishman RK, Dowda M. Promotion of physical activity among high-school girls: a randomized controlled trial. *Am J Public Health.* 2005;95(9):1582–7.

74. Patterson RE, Kristal AR, Glanz K, et al. Components of the working well trial intervention associated with adoption of healthful diets. *Am J Prev Med.* 1997;13(4):271–6.

75. Pelletier KR. A review and analysis of the clinical- and cost-effectiveness studies of comprehensive health promotion and disease management programs at the worksite: 1998–2000 update. *Am J Health Promot.* 2001;16(2):107–16.

76. Perry CL, Stone EJ, Parcel GS, et al. School-based cardiovascular health promotion: the child and adolescent trial for cardiovascular health (CATCH). *J Sch Health.* 1990;60(8):406–13.

77. Petrella RJ, Koval JJ, Cunningham DA, Paterson DH. Can primary care doctors prescribe exercise to improve fitness? The Step Test Exercise Prescription (STEP) project. *Am J Prev Med.* 2003;24(4):316–22.

78. Pfeiffer BA, Clay SW, Conatser RR,Jr. A green prescription study: does written exercise prescribed by a physician result in increased physical activity among older adults? *J Aging Health.* 2001;13(4):527–38.

79. *Physician Workforce of the United States: A Family Medicine Perspective* [Internet]. Washington (DC): Robert Graham Center; [cited 2011 Feb 6]. Available from: http://www.graham-center.org/PreBuilt/physician_workforce.pdf

80. Pinto BM, Goldstein MG, Ashba J, Sciamanna CN, Jette A. Randomized controlled trial of physical activity counseling for older primary care patients. *Am J Prev Med.* 2005;29(4):247–55.

81. Pinto BM, Lynn H, Marcus BH, DePue J, Goldstein MG. Physician-based activity counseling: intervention effects on mediators of motivational readiness for physical activity. *Ann Behav Med.* 2001;23(1):2–10.

82. Resnicow K, Campbell MK, Carr C, et al. Body and soul. A dietary intervention conducted through African-American churches. *Am J Prev Med.* 2004;27(2):97–105.

83. Resnicow K, Jackson A, Blissett D, et al. Results of the healthy body healthy spirit trial. *Health Psychol.* 2005;24(4):339–48.

84. Resnicow K, Jackson A, Braithwaite R, et al. Healthy Body/Healthy Spirit: a church-based nutrition and physical activity intervention. *Health Educ Res.* 2002;17(5):562–73.

85. Resnicow K, Jackson A, Wang T, et al. A motivational interviewing intervention to increase fruit and vegetable intake through Black churches: results of the Eat for Life trial. *Am J Public Health.* 2001;91(10):1686–93.

86. Riedel JE, Lynch W, Baase C, Hymel P, Peterson KW. The effect of disease prevention and health promotion on workplace productivity: a literature review. *Am J Health Promot.* 2001;15(3):167–91.

87. Rogers EM. *Diffusion of Innovations.* 5th ed. New York (NY): Free Press; 2003. 551 p.

88. Sallis JF, Hovell MF, Hofstetter CR, et al. Distance between homes and exercise facilities related to the frequency of exercise among San Diego residents. *Public Health Reports.* 105:179–185. Reprinted. In: Shephard RJ, editor. *Year Book of Sports Medicine.* Chicago: Mosby-Year Book; 1990. 470 p.

89. Sallis JF, McKenzie TL, Alcaraz JE, Kolody B, Faucette N, Hovell MF. The effects of a 2-year physical education program (SPARK) on physical activity and fitness in elementary school students. Sports, Play and Active Recreation for Kids. *Am J Public Health.* 1997;87(8):1328–34.

90. Sallis JF, McKenzie TL, Conway TL, et al. Environmental interventions for eating and physical activity: a randomized controlled trial in middle schools. *Am J Prev Med.* 2003;24(3):209–17.

91. Sallis JF, Owen N. *Physical Activity & Behavioral Medicine.* Thousand Oaks (CA): Sage Publications; 1999. 210 p.

92. *Shape of the Nation Report: Status of Physical Education in the USA: 2006* [Internet]. Reston (VA): National Association for Sport and Physical Education; 2006 [cited 2011 Feb 6]. 53 p. Available from: http://www.heartland.org/policybot/results/21578/2006 _Shape_of_The_Nation_Report_Status_of_Physical_Education _in_the_USA.html

93. Sharpe PA. Community-based physical activity intervention. *Arthritis Rheum.* 2003;49(3):455–62.

94. Simons-Morton BG, Taylor WC, Snider SA, Huang IW, Fulton JE. Observed levels of elementary and middle school children's physical activity during physical education classes. *Prev Med.* 1994;23(4):437–41.

95. Smith-Ray RL, Almeida FA, Bajaj J, et al. Translating efficacious behavioral principles for diabetes prevention into practice. *Health Promot Pract.* 2009;10(1):58–66.

96. Sorensen G, Barbeau E, Hunt MK, Emmons K. Reducing social disparities in tobacco use: a social-contextual model for reducing tobacco use among blue-collar workers. *Am J Public Health.* 2004;94(2):230–9.

97. Sorensen G, Stoddard AM, LaMontagne AD, et al. A comprehensive worksite cancer prevention intervention: behavior change results from a randomized controlled trial (United States). *J Public Health Policy.* 2003;24(1):5–25.

98. Sorensen G, Thompson B, Glanz K, et al. Work site-based cancer prevention: primary results from the Working Well Trial. *Am J Public Health.* 1996;86(7):939–47.

99. Spence JC, Lee RE. Toward a comprehensive model of physical activity. *Psychol Sport Exerc.* 2003;4(1):7–24.

100. Stange KC, Woolf SH, Gjeltema K. One minute for prevention: the power of leveraging to fulfill the promise of health behavior counseling. *Am J Prev Med.* 2002;22(4):320–3.

101. Sternfeld B, Block C, Quesenberry CP,Jr, et al. Improving diet and physical activity with ALIVE: a worksite randomized trial. *Am J Prev Med.* 2009;36(6):475–83.

102. Stewart JA, Dennison DA, Kohl HW, Doyle JA. Exercise level and energy expenditure in the TAKE 10! in-class physical activity program. *J Sch Health.* 2004;74(10):397–400.

103. Stone EJ, McKenzie TL, Welk GJ, Booth ML. Effects of physical activity interventions in youth. Review and synthesis. *Am J Prev Med.* 1998;15(4):298–315.

104. Swinburn BA, Walter LG, Arroll B, Tilyard MW, Russell DG. The green prescription study: a randomized controlled trial of written exercise advice provided by general practitioners. *Am J Public Health.* 1998;88(2):288–91.

105. *WELCOA's Seven Benchmarks of Success* [Internet]. Omaha (NE): WELCOA: Wellness Council of America; [cited 2007 May 15]. Available from: http://www.welcoa.org/wellworkplace/index.php ?category=16

106. Wendel-Vos GC, Schuit AJ, de Niet R, Boshuizen HC, Saris WH, Kromhout D. Factors of the physical environment associated with walking and bicycling. *Med Sci Sports Exerc.* 2004;36(4):725–30.

107. Whitlock EP, Orleans CT, Pender N, Allan J. Evaluating primary care behavioral counseling interventions: an evidence-based approach. *Am J Prev Med.* 2002;22(4):267–84.

108. Wilcox S, Laken M, Parrott AW, et al. The faith, activity, and nutrition (FAN) program: design of a participatory research intervention to increase physical activity and improve dietary habits in African American churches. *Contemp Clin Trials.* 2010;31(4):323–35.

109. Writing Group for the Activity Counseling Trial Research Group. Effects of physical activity counseling in primary care: the activity counseling trial: a randomized controlled trial. *JAMA.* 2001;286(6):677–87.

110. Wuest DA, Bucher CA. Historical foundations of physical education and sport. In: Wuest DA, Bucher CA, editors. *Foundations of Physical Education and Sport.* 13th ed. Boston: WCB/McGraw-Hill; 1999. p. 146–193.

111. Yarnall KS, Pollak KI, Ostbye T, Krause KM, Michener JL. Primary care: is there enough time for prevention? *Am J Public Health.* 2003;93(4):635–41.

112. Zuvekas A. Health centers and the healthcare system. *J Ambul Care Manage.* 2005;28(4):331–9.

SELECTED REFERENCES FOR FURTHER READING

Anderson LM, Quinn TA, Glanz K, et al. The effectiveness of worksite nutrition and physical activity interventions for controlling employee overweight and obesity: a systematic review. *Am J Prev Med.* 2009;37(4):340–57.

Bors P, Dessauer M, Bell R, Wilkerson R, Lee J, Strunk SL. The Active Living by Design national program: community initiatives and lessons learned. *Am J Prev Med.* 2009;37(6 Suppl 2):S313–21.

Brown T, Summerbell C. Systematic review of school-based interventions that focus on changing dietary intake and physical activity levels to prevent childhood obesity: an update to the obesity guidance produced by the National Institute for Health and Clinical Excellence. *Obesity Rev.* 2008;10(1):110–41.

Brownson RC, Hoehner CM, Day K, Forsyth A, Sallis JF. Measuring the built environment for physical activity: state of the science. *Am J Prev Med.* 2009;36(4):S99–123.e12.

CDC's Healthy Communities Program: Community Health Assessment and Group Evaluation (CHANGE): Building a Foundation of Knowledge to Prioritize Community Needs [Internet]. Atlanta (GA): Centers for Disease Control and Prevention; [cited 2011 Nov 21]. Available from: http://www.cdc.gov/healthycommunitiesprogram/tools/change.htm

Grandes G, Sanchez A, Sanchez-Pinilla R, et al. Effectiveness of physical activity advice and prescription by physicians in routine primary care. *Arch Intern Med.* 2009:169(7):694–701.

INTERNET RESOURCES

See *Table 48-3.*

American College of Sports Medicine Certifications

Note: This appendix is reprinted with permission from *ACSM's Guidelines for Exercise Testing and Prescription.* 9th ed. Baltimore (MD): Lippincott Williams and Wilkins; 2014.

Exercise practitioners are becoming increasingly aware of the advantages of maintaining professional credentials. In efforts to ensure quality, reduce liability, and remain competitive, more and more employers are requiring professional certification of their exercise staff. Additionally, in efforts to improve public safety, mandates for certification by state and/or regulatory agencies (*e.g.*, licensure) as well as third party payers now exist. The American College of Sports Medicine (ACSM) offers five primary and three specialty certifications for exercise professionals. These include the following:

Primary Certifications:
- ACSM Certified Group Exercise Instructor^{SM} (GEI)
- ACSM Certified Personal Trainer® (CPT)
- ACSM Certified Health Fitness Specialist^{SM} (HFS)
- ACSM Certified Clinical Exercise Specialist^{SM} (CES)
- ACSM Registered Clinical Exercise Physiologist® (RCEP)*

Specialty Certifications:
- ACSM/NCPAD Certified Inclusive Fitness Trainer^{SM}
  - NCPAD = National Center on Physical Activity and Disability
- ACSM/ACS Certified Cancer Exercise Trainer^{SM}
  - ACS = American Cancer Society
- ACSM/NPAS Physical Activity in Public Health Specialist^{SM}
  - NPAS = National Physical Activity Society

Advances in the exercise profession have been substantial over the past decade. Specific conditions that are considered essential for a formalized profession to exist are now in place (1). These include:

- A standardized system to develop skills.
- A standardized system to validate skills.
- An organized community to advocate for the profession.

The Committee on Accreditation for the Exercise Sciences (CoAES) under the auspices of the Commission on Accreditation of Allied Health Education Programs (CAAHEP) now validates and accredits university curriculum in the exercise sciences (*i.e.*, standardized skills development). The National Commission for Certifying Agencies (NCCA) provides a standardized, independent, and objective third party evaluation of examination design, development, and performance to ensure certification integrity (*i.e.*, skills validation). ACSM and other organizations such as Clinical Exercise Physiology Association (CEPA), a member of the ACSM affiliate societies, have created professional communities that advocate specifically for the interests of exercise and fitness practitioners.

ACSM CERTIFICATION DEVELOPMENT

The process of developing a certification examination begins with a job task analysis (JTA) (2). The purpose of the JTA is to define the major areas of professional practice (*i.e.*, domains), delineate the tasks performed "on-the-job," and identify the knowledge and skills required for safe and competent practice. The domains are subsequently weighted according to the importance and frequency of performance of their respective tasks. The number of examination test items is then determined based on the domain weight. Each examination reflects the content and weights defined by the JTA. By linking the content of the examination to the JTA (*e.g.*, what professionals do), it is possible to ensure that the examination is practice related.

Examination development continues with question writing. Content experts representing academia and practice are selected and trained on examination item writing. This examination writing team is charged with the task of creating test items that are representative of and consistent with the JTA. Each test item is evaluated psychometrically, undergoing extensive testing, editing, and retesting before being included as a scored item on the examination. Finally, passing scores are determined using a criterion-referenced methodology. Passing scores for each examination are associated with a minimum level of mastery necessary for safe and competent practice. Setting passing scores in this manner ensures that qualified candidates will become certified regardless of how other candidates perform on the examination.

The job definition, domains, and tasks from the JTA for ACSM's five primary certifications are listed in the following sections, and the primary population served, the eligibility criteria, and the competencies for these certifications are found in *Table D.1*. The complete

TABLE D.1. American College of Sports Medicine's Certifications at a Glance

Certification	Primary Population Served	Eligibility Criteria	Competencies
ACSM Certified Group Exercise Instructor^{SM}	Apparently healthy individuals and those with health challenges who are able to exercise independently	• ≥18 yr • High school diploma or equivalent • Current CPR and AED certifications (must contain a live skills component) — AED not required for those practicing outside of the United States and Canada	• Develops and implements a variety of exercises in group settings and modifies exercise according to need • Leads safe and effective exercise using a variety of leadership techniques to enhance the motor skills related to the domains of physical fitness
ACSM Certified Personal Trainer®	Apparently healthy individuals and those with health challenges who are able to exercise independently	• ≥18 yr • High school diploma or equivalent • Current CPR and AED certifications (must contain a live skills component such as the American Heart Association [AHA] or the American Red Cross) — AED not required for those practicing outside of the United States and Canada	• Identifies health risk factors, performs fitness appraisals and preparticipation health screenings, and develops exercise programs that promote lasting behavior change • Incorporates suitable and innovative activities to improve functional capacity and manages health risk to promote lasting behavior change
ACSM Certified Health Fitness Specialist^{SM}	Apparently healthy individuals and those with medically controlled diseases	• Bachelor's degree in an exercise science, exercise physiology, kinesiology, or exercise science based degree (one is eligible to sit for the examination if the candidate is in the last term of their degree program) • Current CPR and AED certifications (must contain a live skills component such as the AHA or the American Red Cross) — AED not required for those practicing outside of the United States and Canada	• Applies knowledge of exercise science including kinesiology, functional anatomy, exercise physiology, nutrition, program administration, psychology, and injury prevention in the health fitness setting • Performs preparticipation health screenings and fitness assessments • Interprets assessment results and develops exercise prescriptions • Performs duties related to fitness management, administration, and program supervision • Incorporates suitable physical activities to improve functional capacity • Applies appropriate behavioral change techniques to effectively educate and counsel on lifestyle modification
ACSM Certified Clinical Exercise Specialist^{SM}	Apparently healthy individuals and those with cardiovascular, pulmonary, and metabolic disease	• Bachelor's degree in an exercise science, exercise physiology, kinesiology, or exercise science based degree (one is eligible to sit for the exam if the candidate is in the last term of their degree program) • Minimum of 400 h of clinical experience for graduates from a CAAHEP accredited program or 500 h of clinical experience for graduates from a non-CAAHEP accredited program • Current certification for the AHA BLS for Healthcare Provider or American Red Cross CPR/AED for the Professional Rescuer or equivalent (must contain live skills component) — AED not required for those practicing outside of the United States and Canada	• Applies extensive knowledge of functional anatomy, exercise physiology, pathophysiology, electrocardiography, human behavior/psychology, gerontology, and graded exercise testing in the clinical setting • Provides exercise supervision/leadership and counsels patients on lifestyle modification • Conducts emergency procedures in exercise testing and training settings

TABLE D.1. American College of Sports Medicine's Certifications at a Glance (*Continued*)

Certification	Primary Population Served	Eligibility Criteria	Competencies
ACSM Registered Clinical Exercise Physiologist®	Apparently healthy individuals and those with cardiovascular, pulmonary, metabolic, orthopedic/musculoskeletal, neuromuscular, neoplastic, immunologic, and hematologic disorders	• Graduate degree in clinical exercise physiology with coursework in clinical assessment, exercise testing, exercise prescription, and exercise training (one is eligible to sit for the exam if the candidate is in the last term of their degree program) • Minimum of 600 h of clinical experience (external to classroom/laboratory) working with individuals with chronic disease • Current certification for the AHA BLS for Healthcare Provider or American Red Cross CPR/AED for the Professional Rescuer or equivalent (must contain live skills component) — AED not required for those practicing outside of the United States and Canada	• Performs exercise screening and exercise and fitness testing • Develops exercise prescriptions and supervises exercise programs • Conducts exercise and physical activity education counseling • Conducts measurement and evaluation of exercise and physical activity-related outcomes

CPR, cardiopulmonary resuscitation; AED, automated external defibrillators; BLS, basic life support.

JTA including knowledge and skill statements for all eight ACSM certifications can be found online at http://certification.acsm.org/exam-content-outlines. Because every question on each of the certification examinations must refer to a specific knowledge or skill statement within the associated JTA, these documents provide a resource to guide exam preparation.

ACSM'S FIVE PRIMARY CERTIFICATIONS

ACSM CERTIFIED GROUP EXERCISE INSTRUCTOR^{SM} JOB TASK ANALYSIS

The JTA is intended to serve as a blueprint of the job of a GEI. As one prepares for the examination, it is important to remember that all questions are based on the following outline.

Job Definition

The GEI (a) possesses a minimum of a high school diploma; and (b) works in a group exercise setting with apparently healthy individuals and those with health challenges who are able to exercise independently to enhance quality of life, improve health-related physical fitness, manage health risk, and promote lasting health behavior change. The GEI leads safe and effective exercise programs using a variety of leadership techniques to foster group camaraderie, support, and motivation to enhance muscular strength and endurance, flexibility, cardiorespiratory fitness, body composition, and any of the motor skills related to the domains of health-related physical fitness.

Performance Domains and Associated Job Tasks

The JTA for the GEI certification describes what the professional does on a day-to-day basis. The JTA is divided into domains and associated tasks performed on the job. The percentages listed in this section indicate the number of questions representing each domain on the 100 question GEI examination.

The performance domains are the following:

- Domain I: Participant and Program Assessment — 10%.
- Domain II: Class Design — 25%.
- Domain III: Leadership and Instruction — 55%.
- Domain IV: Legal and Professional Responsibilities — 10%.

Domain I: Participant and Program Assessment

Associated Job Tasks

A. Evaluate and establish participant screening procedures to optimize safety and minimize risk by reviewing assessment protocols based on ACSM standards and guidelines.

B. Administer and review as necessary participants' health risk to determine if preparticipation assessment is needed prior to exercise using Physical Activity Readiness Questionnaire (PAR-Q), ACSM preparticipation health screening, or other appropriate tools.

C. Screen participants as needed for known acute or chronic health conditions to provide recommendations and/or modifications.

Domain II: Class Design

Associated Job Tasks

A. Establish the purpose and determine the objectives of the class based on the needs of participants and facility.
B. Determine class content (*i.e.,* warm-up, stimulus, cool-down) in order to create an effective workout based on the objectives of the class.
C. Select and sequence appropriate exercises in order to provide a safe workout based on the objectives of the class.
D. Rehearse class content, exercise selection, and sequencing and revise as needed in order to provide a safe and effective workout based on the purpose and objectives of the class.

Domain III: Leadership and Instruction

Associated Job Tasks

A. Prepare to teach by implementing preclass procedures including screening new participants and organizing equipment, music, and room setup.
B. Create a positive exercise environment in order to optimize participant adherence by incorporating effective motivational skills, communication techniques, and behavioral strategies.
C. Demonstrate all exercises using proper form and technique to ensure safe execution in accordance with ACSM standards and guidelines.
D. Incorporate verbal and nonverbal instructional cues in order to optimize communication, safety, and motivation based on industry guidelines.
E. Monitor participants' performance to ensure safe and effective exercise execution using observation and participant feedback techniques in accordance with ACSM standards and guidelines.
F. Modify exercises based on individual and group needs to ensure safety and effectiveness in accordance with ACSM standards and guidelines.
G. Monitor sound levels of vocal and/or audio equipment following industry guidelines.
H. Respond to participants' concerns in order to maintain a professional, equitable, and safe environment by using appropriate conflict management or customer service strategies set forth by facility policy and procedures and industry guidelines.
I. Educate participants in order to enhance knowledge, enjoyment, and adherence by providing health/fitness-related information and resources.

Domain IV: Legal and Professional Responsibilities

Associated Job Tasks

A. Evaluate the class environment (*e.g.,* outdoor, indoor, capacity, flooring, temperature, ventilation, lighting, equipment, and acoustics) to minimize risk and optimize safety by following preclass inspection procedures based on established facility and industry standards and guidelines.
B. Promote participants' awareness and accountability by informing them of classroom safety procedures and exercise and intensity options in order to minimize risk.
C. Follow industry accepted professional, ethical, and business standards in order to optimize safety and reduce liability.
D. Respond to emergencies in order to minimize untoward events by following procedures consistent with established standards of care and facility policies.
E. Respect copyrights to protect original and creative work, media, etc., by legally securing copyright material and other intellectual property based on national and international copyright laws.
F. Engage in healthy lifestyle practices in order to be a positive role model for class participants.
G. Select and participate in continuing education programs that enhance knowledge and skills on a continuing basis, maximize effectiveness, and increase professionalism in the field.

ACSM CERTIFIED PERSONAL TRAINER® (CPT) JOB TASK ANALYSIS

The JTA is intended to serve as a blueprint of the job of a CPT. As you prepare for the examination, it is important to remember that all examination questions are based on the following outline.

Job Definition

The CPT (a) possesses a minimum of a high school diploma; and (b) works with apparently healthy individuals and those with health challenges who are able to exercise independently to enhance quality of life, improve health-related physical fitness, performance, manage health risk, and promote lasting health behavior change. The CPT conducts basic preparticipation health screening assessments, submaximal aerobic exercise tests, and muscular strength/endurance, flexibility, and body composition tests. The CPT facilitates motivation and adherence as well as develops and administers programs designed to enhance muscular strength/endurance, flexibility, cardiorespiratory fitness, body composition, and/or any of the motor skill-related components of physical fitness (*i.e.,* balance, coordination, power, agility, speed, reaction time).

Performance Domains and Associated Job Tasks

The JTA for the CPT certification describes what the professional does on a day-to-day basis. The JTA is divided into domains and associated tasks performed on the job. The percentages listed in this section indicate the number of questions representing each domain on the 150 question CPT examination.

The performance domains are the following:

- Domain I: Initial Client Consultation and Assessment — 26%.
- Domain II: Exercise Programming and Implementation — 27%.
- Domain III: Exercise Leadership and Client Education — 27%.
- Domain IV: Legal, Professional, Business, and Marketing — 20%.

Domain I: Initial Client Consultation and Assessment

Associated Job Tasks

A. Provide instructions and initial documents to the client in order to proceed to the interview.
B. Interview client in order to gather and provide pertinent information to proceed to the fitness testing and program design.
C. Review and analyze client data (*i.e.*, classify risk) to formulate a plan of action and/or conduct physical assessments.
D. Evaluate behavioral readiness to optimize exercise adherence.
E. Assess physical fitness including cardiorespiratory fitness, muscular strength, muscular endurance, flexibility, and anthropometric measures in order to set goals and establish a baseline for program development.
F. Develop a comprehensive (*i.e.*, physical fitness, goals, behavior) reassessment plan/timeline.

Domain II: Exercise Programming and Implementation

Associated Job Tasks

A. Review assessment results, medical history, and goals to determine appropriate training program.
B. Select exercise modalities to achieve desired adaptations based on goals, medical history, and assessment results.
C. Determine initial frequency, intensity, time (duration), and type (*i.e.*, the FITT principle of exercise prescription [Ex R$_x$]) of exercise based on goals, medical history, and assessment results.
D. Review proposed program with client; demonstrate and instruct the client to perform exercises safely and effectively.
E. Monitor client technique and response to exercise modifying as necessary.
F. Modify FITT to improve or maintain the client's physical fitness level.

G. Seek client feedback to ensure satisfaction and enjoyment of the program.

Domain III: Leadership and Education Implementation

Associated Job Tasks

A. Create a positive exercise experience in order to optimize participant adherence by applying effective communication techniques, motivation techniques, and behavioral strategies.
B. Educate clients using scientifically sound health/fitness information and resources to enhance client's knowledge base, program enjoyment, adherence, and overall awareness of health/fitness related information.

Domain IV: Legal, Professional, Business, and Marketing

Associated Job Tasks

A. Obtain medical clearance for clients based on ACSM guidelines prior to starting an exercise program.
B. Collaborate with various health care professionals and organizations in order to provide clients with a network of providers that minimizes liability and maximizes program effectiveness.
C. Develop a comprehensive risk management program (including emergency action plan and injury prevention program) to enhance the standard of care and reflect a client-focused mission.
D. Participate in approved continuing education programs on a regular basis to maximize effectiveness, increase professionalism, and enhance knowledge and skills in the field of health/fitness.
E. Adhere to ACSM's Code of Ethics by practicing in a professional manner within the Scope of Practice of a CPT (see ACSM's Code of Ethics for Certified and Registered Professionals at http://certification.acsm.org/faq28-codeofethics).
F. Develop a business plan to establish mission, business, budgetary, and sales objectives.
G. Develop marketing materials and engage in networking/business exchanges to build client base, promote services, and increase resources.
H. Obtain appropriate personal training and liability insurance and follow industry accepted professional, ethical, and business standards in order to optimize safety and to reduce liability.
I. Engage in healthy lifestyle practices in order to be a positive role model for all clients.
J. Respect copyrights to protect original and creative work, media, etc., by legally securing copyright material and other intellectual property based on national and international copyright laws.

K. Safeguard client confidentiality and privacy rights unless formally waived or in emergency situations.

ACSM CERTIFIED HEALTH FITNESS SPECIALIST[SM] JOB TASK ANALYSIS

The JTA is intended to serve as a blueprint of the job of an HFS. As one prepares for the examination, it is important to remember that all examination questions are based on the following outline.

Job Definition

The HFS is a health fitness professional with a minimum of a bachelor's degree in exercise science. The HFS performs preparticipation health screenings, conducts physical fitness assessments, interprets results, develops exercise prescriptions, and applies behavioral and motivational strategies to apparently healthy individuals and individuals with medically controlled diseases and health conditions to support clients in adopting and maintaining healthy lifestyle behaviors. The academic preparation of the HFS also includes fitness management, administration, and supervision. The HFS is typically employed or self-employed in commercial, community, studio, corporate, university, and hospital settings.

Performance Domains and Associated Job Tasks

The JTA for the HFS describes what the professional does on a day-to-day basis. The JTA is divided into domains and associated tasks performed on the job. The following percentages listed in this section indicate the number of questions representing each domain on the 150 question HFS examination.

The performance domains are the following:

- Domain I: Health and Fitness Assessment — 30%.
- Domain II: Exercise Prescription and Implementation (and Ongoing Support) — 30%.
- Domain III: Exercise Counseling and Behavioral Strategies — 15%.
- Domain IV: Legal/Professional — 10%.
- Domain V: Management — 15%.

Domain I: Health and Fitness Assessment

Associated Job Tasks

A. Implement assessment protocols and preparticipation health screening procedures to maximize participant safety and minimize risk.
B. Determine participant's readiness to take part in a health-related physical fitness assessment and exercise program.
C. Select and prepare physical fitness assessments for healthy participants and those with controlled disease.
D. Conduct and interpret cardiorespiratory fitness assessments.
E. Conduct assessments of muscular strength, muscular endurance, and flexibility.
F. Conduct anthropometric and body composition assessments.

Domain II: Exercise Prescription and Implementation

Associated Job Tasks

A. Review preparticipation health screening including self-guided health questionnaires and appraisals, exercise history, and physical fitness assessments.
B. Determine safe and effective exercise programs to achieve desired outcomes and goals.
C. Implement cardiorespiratory Ex R_x using the FITT principle (*i.e.*, frequency, intensity, time, and type) for apparently healthy participants based on current health status, fitness goals, and availability of time.
D. Implement Ex R_x using the FITT principle for flexibility, muscular strength, and muscular endurance for apparently healthy participants based on current health status, fitness goals, and availability of time.
E. Establish exercise progression guidelines for resistance, aerobic, and flexibility activity to achieve the goals of apparently healthy participants.
F. Implement a weight management program as indicated by personal goals that are supported by preparticipation health screening, health history, and body composition/anthropometrics.
G. Prescribe and implement exercise programs for participants with controlled cardiovascular, pulmonary, and metabolic diseases and other clinical populations.
H. Prescribe and implement exercise programs for healthy and special populations (*i.e.*, older adults, youth, pregnant women).
I. Modify Ex R_x based on environmental conditions.

Domain III: Exercise Counseling and Behavioral Strategies

Associated Job Tasks

A. Optimize adoption and adherence to exercise programs and other healthy behaviors by applying effective communication techniques.
B. Optimize adoption of and adherence to exercise programs and other healthy behaviors by applying effective behavioral and motivational strategies.
C. Provide educational resources to support clients in the adoption and maintenance of healthy lifestyle behaviors.
D. Provide support within the scope of practice of an HFS and refer to other health professionals as indicated.

Domain IV: Legal/Professional

Associated Job Tasks

A. Create and disseminate risk management guidelines for a health/fitness facility, department, or organization to reduce member, employee, and business risk.
B. Create an effective injury prevention program and ensure that emergency policies and procedures are in place.

Domain V: Management

Associated Job Tasks

A. Manage human resources in accordance with leadership, organization, and management techniques.
B. Manage fiscal resources in accordance with leadership, organization, and management techniques.
C. Establish policies and procedures for the management of health/fitness facilities based on accepted safety and legal guidelines, standards, and regulations.
D. Develop and execute a marketing plan to promote programs, services, and facilities.
E. Use effective communication techniques to develop professional relationships with other allied health professionals (*e.g.*, nutritionists, physical therapists, physicians, and nurses).

ACSM CERTIFIED CLINICAL EXERCISE SPECIALIST^SM (CES) JOB TASK ANALYSIS

The JTA is intended to serve as a blueprint of the job of the CES. As one prepares for the examination, it is important to remember that all examination questions are based on the following outline.

Job Definition

The CES is an allied health professional with a minimum of a bachelor's degree in exercise science. The CES works with patients and clients challenged with cardiovascular, pulmonary, and metabolic diseases and disorders, as well as with apparently healthy populations in cooperation with other health care professionals to enhance quality of life, manage health risk, and promote lasting health behavior change. The CES conducts preparticipation health screening, maximal and submaximal graded exercise tests, and performs strength, flexibility, and body composition tests. The CES develops and administers programs designed to enhance cardiorespiratory fitness, muscular strength and endurance, balance, and range of motion. The CES educates their clients about testing, exercise program components, and clinical and lifestyle self-care for control of chronic disease and health conditions.

Performance Domains and Associated Job Tasks

The JTA for the CES describes what the professional does on a day-to-day basis. The JTA is divided into domains and associated tasks performed on the job. The percentages listed in this section indicate the number of questions representing each domain on the 100 question CES examination.

The performance domains are the following:

- Domain I: Patient/Client Assessment — 30%.
- Domain II: Exercise Prescription — 30%.
- Domain III: Program Implementation and Ongoing Support — 20%.
- Domain IV: Leadership and Counseling — 15%.
- Domain V: Legal and Professional Considerations — 5%.

Domain I: Patient/Client Assessment

Associated Job Tasks

A. Determine and obtain the necessary physician referral and medical records to assess the potential participant.
B. Perform a preparticipation health screening including review of the participant's medical history and knowledge, their needs and goals, the program's potential benefits, and additional required testing and data.
C. Evaluate the participant's risk to ensure safe participation and determine level of monitoring/supervision in a preventive or rehabilitative exercise program.

Domain II: Exercise Prescription

Associated Job Tasks

A. Develop a clinically appropriate Ex R_x using all available information (*e.g.*, clinical and physiological status, goals, and behavioral assessment).
B. Review the Ex R_x and exercise program with the participant including home exercise, compliance, and participant's expectations and goals.
C. Instruct the participant in the safe and effective use of exercise modalities, exercise plan, reporting symptoms, and class organization.

Domain III: Program Implementation and Ongoing Support

Associated Job Tasks

A. Implement the program (*e.g.*, Ex R_x, education, counseling, and goals).
B. Continually assess participant feedback, clinical signs and symptoms, and exercise tolerance, and provide feedback to the participant about their exercise, general program participation, and clinical progress.

C. Reassess and update the program (*e.g.*, exercise, education, and client goals) based on the participant's progress and feedback.

D. Maintain participant records to document progress and clinical status.

Domain IV: Leadership & Counseling

Associated Job Tasks

A. Educate the participant about performance and progression of aerobic, strength, and flexibility exercise programs.

B. Provide disease management and risk factor reduction education based on the participant's medical history, needs, and goals.

C. Create a positive environment for participant adherence and outcomes by incorporating effective motivational skills, communication techniques, and behavioral strategies.

D. Collaborate and consult with health care professionals to address clinical issues and provide referrals to optimize participant outcomes.

Domain V: Legal and Professional Considerations

Associated Job Tasks

A. Evaluate the exercise environment to minimize risk and optimize safety by following routine inspection procedures based on established facility and industry standards and guidelines.

B. Perform regular inspections of emergency equipment and practice emergency procedures (*e.g.*, crash cart, advanced cardiac life support procedures, and activation of emergency medical system).

C. Promote awareness and accountability and minimize risk by informing participants of safety procedures and self-monitoring of exercise and related symptoms.

D. Comply with Health Insurance Portability and Accountability Act (HIPAA) laws and industry accepted professional, ethical, and business standards in order to maintain confidentiality, optimize safety, and reduce liability.

E. Promote a positive image of the program by engaging in healthy lifestyle practices.

F. Select and participate in continuing education programs that enhance knowledge and skills on a continuing basis, maximize effectiveness, and increase professionalism in the field.

ACSM REGISTERED CLINICAL EXERCISE PHYSIOLOGIST® (RCEP) JOB TASK ANALYSIS

The JTA is intended to serve as a blueprint of the job of a RCEP. As one prepares for the examination, it is important to remember that all examination questions are based on the following outline.

Job Definition

The RCEP (a) is an allied health professional with a minimum of a master's degree in exercise science; and (b) works in the application of physical activity and behavioral interventions for those clinical diseases and health conditions that have been shown to provide therapeutic and/or functional benefit. Persons that RCEP services are appropriate for may include, but are not limited to, individuals with cardiovascular, pulmonary, metabolic, orthopedic, musculoskeletal, neuromuscular, neoplastic, immunologic, and hematologic disease. The RCEP provides primary and secondary prevention and rehabilitative strategies designed to improve physical fitness and health in populations ranging across the lifespan.

The RCEP provides exercise screening, exercise and physical fitness testing, exercise prescriptions, exercise and physical activity counseling, exercise supervision, exercise and health education/promotion, and measurement and evaluation of exercise and physical activity-related outcome measures. The RCEP works individually or as part of an interdisciplinary team in a clinical, community, or public health setting. The practice and supervision of the RCEP is guided by published professional guidelines, standards, and applicable state and federal laws and regulations.

Performance Domains and Associated Job Tasks

The JTA for the RCEP describes what the professional does on a day-to-day basis. The JTA is divided into domains and associated tasks performed on the job. The percentages listed in this section indicate the number of questions representing each domain on the 125 question RCEP examination.

The performance domains are the following:

- Domain I: Clinical Assessment — 20%.
- Domain II: Exercise Testing — 20%.
- Domain III: Exercise Prescription — 20%.
- Domain IV: Exercise Training — 20%.
- Domain V: Education and Behavior Change — 10%.
- Domain VI: Program Administration — 5%.
- Domain VII: Legal and Professional Considerations — 5%.

Domain I: Clinical Assessment

Associated Job Tasks

In this domain, chronic disease(s) includes cardiovascular, pulmonary, metabolic, orthopedic/musculoskeletal, neuromuscular, neoplastic, immunologic, and hematologic disorders.

A. Review patient's medical record for information pertinent to the reason for their visit.

B. Interview patient for medical history pertinent to the reason for their visit and reconcile medications.
C. Assess resting vital signs and symptoms.
D. Collect and evaluate clinical and health measurements including, but not limited to ECG, spirometry, or blood glucose.

Domain II: Exercise Testing

Associated Job Tasks

In this domain, chronic disease(s) includes cardiovascular, pulmonary, metabolic, orthopedic/musculoskeletal, neuromuscular, neoplastic, immunologic, and hematologic disorders.

A. Assess appropriateness of and contraindications to symptom-limited, maximal exercise testing and/or other health assessments.
B. Select, administer, and interpret tests to assess muscular strength and/or endurance.
C. Select, administer, and interpret tests to assess flexibility and/or body composition.
D. Select, administer, and interpret submaximal aerobic exercise tests.
E. Select, administer, and interpret functional and balance tests (*e.g.,* Get Up and Go, Berg Balance).
F. Prepare patient for a symptom-limited, maximal exercise test by providing an informed consent and prepping the patient for electrocardiogram (ECG) monitoring.
G. Administer a symptom-limited, maximal exercise test using appropriate protocol and monitoring.
H. Evaluate results from a symptom-limited, maximal exercise test and report in the medical record and to health care providers.
I. Calibrate, troubleshoot, operate, and maintain testing equipment.

Domain III: Exercise Prescription

Associated Job Tasks

In this domain, chronic disease(s) includes cardiovascular, pulmonary, metabolic, orthopedic/musculoskeletal, neuromuscular, neoplastic, immunologic, and hematologic disorders.

A. Evaluate and document exercise goals and motivations of the patient to design an individualized Ex R_x.
B. Determine and document the Ex R_x for exercise training based on the patient's history, available data, and goals and discuss with the patient.
C. Determine the appropriate level of supervision and monitoring needed to provide a safe exercise environment based on risk classification guidelines.
D. Explain exercise intensity and measures to guide exercise intensity (*e.g.,* target heart rate, ratings of perceived exertion, signs/symptoms, and ability to carry on a conversation) to the patient.

E. Design a home component for an exercise program to help transition a patient to more independent exercise using appropriate behavioral strategies.
F. Discuss the importance of, barriers to, and strategies to optimize adherence.
G. Regularly evaluate the appropriateness of and modify, as needed, the Ex R_x based on the patient's compliance, signs/symptoms, and physiologic response to the exercise program.

Domain IV: Exercise Training

Associated Job Tasks

In this domain, chronic disease(s) includes cardiovascular, pulmonary, metabolic, orthopedic/musculoskeletal, neuromuscular, neoplastic, immunologic, and hematologic disorders.

A. Meet with patient to discuss exercise training plan, expectations, and goals.
B. Identify, adapt, and instruct patient in appropriate exercise modes in order to reduce risk and maximize the development of cardiorespiratory fitness, strength, and flexibility.
C. Monitor and/or supervise patient during exercise based on their level of risk (*e.g.,* cardiopulmonary risk and fall risk) in order to provide a safe exercise environment.
D. Evaluate patient's contraindications to exercise training to make a risk/reward assessment.
E. Evaluate, document, and report patient's clinical status and response to exercise training in the medical record and to their health care provider.
F. Discuss clinical status and response to exercise training with patients and adapt and/or modify the exercise program as needed in order to prevent injury, maximize adherence, and progress toward desired outcomes.
G. Report new or worsening symptoms and adverse events in the patient's medical record and consult with the health care provider.

Domain V: Education and Behavior Strategies

Associated Job Tasks

In this domain, chronic disease(s) includes cardiovascular, pulmonary, metabolic, orthopedic/musculoskeletal, neuromuscular, neoplastic, immunologic, and hematologic disorders.

A. Evaluate patients to identify those who may benefit from mental health services using industry accepted screening tools.
B. Observe and interact with patients on an ongoing basis to identify recent changes that may benefit from counseling or other mental health services.
C. Assess patient for level of understanding of their disease and/or disability, readiness to adopt behavior change, and learning needs.

D. Conduct group and individual education sessions to teach patients about their disease/disability, secondary prevention, and how to manage their condition.

E. Assess knowledge of and compliance with health behaviors and apply behavior change techniques to encourage the adoption of healthy behaviors.

F. Teach relapse prevention techniques for maintenance of healthy behaviors.

Domain VI: Program Administration

Associated Job Tasks

In this domain, chronic disease(s) includes cardiovascular, pulmonary, metabolic, orthopedic/musculoskeletal, neuromuscular, neoplastic, immunologic, and hematologic disorders.

A. Maintain patient records as an ongoing documentation device to provide continuity of care and to meet legal standards.

B. Develop and/or maintain program evaluation tools and report program outcomes.

C. Develop strategies to improve program outcomes.

D. Develop and maintain relationships with referring physicians and other health care providers to enhance patient care.

E. Recruit, hire, train, motivate, and evaluate staff, students, and volunteers in order to provide effective services within a positive work environment.

F. Manage fiscal resources to provide efficient and effective services.

G. Develop, update, and/or maintain policies and procedures for daily operations, routine care, and adverse events.

H. Develop and maintain a safe environment that promotes positive outcomes and follows current industry recommendations and facility policies.

I. Develop and maintain an atmosphere of caring and support in order to promote patient adherence.

J. Promote the program and enhance its reputation through excellent communication and customer service.

K. Regularly conduct departmental needs assessment and develop/modify programs to accommodate changing environment.

Domain VII: Legal and Professional Considerations

Associated Job Tasks

In this domain, chronic disease(s) includes cardiovascular, pulmonary, metabolic, orthopedic/musculoskeletal, neuromuscular, neoplastic, immunologic, and hematologic disorders.

A. Follow industry accepted professional, ethical, and business standards in order to optimize safety, reduce liability, and protect patient confidentiality.

B. Participate in continuing education and/or professional networks to maintain certification, enhance knowledge, and remain current in the profession.

C. Maintain an environment that promotes ongoing written and verbal communication (*e.g.*, insurance providers and patients) and provides documentation of treatment that meets legal standards.

D. Take action in emergencies consistent with current certification, institutional procedures, and industry guidelines.

E. Inform patients of personal and facility safety procedures in order to minimize risk.

THE BOTTOM LINE

Obtaining professional credentials enhances the career development of health/fitness, clinical exercise, and health care professionals conducting exercise programs and exercise testing and improves the delivery of care to the consumer, client, and patient. ACSM offers high quality professional certifications for a variety of health/fitness, exercise, and health care professionals in corporate, health/fitness, and clinical settings.

ONLINE RESOURCES

- American College of Sports Medicine Certifications: http://certification.acsm.org/get-certified
- American College of Sports Medicine Certifications Job Task Analysis: http://certification.acsm.org/exam-content-outlines
- American College of Sports Medicine Code of Ethics for Certified and Registered Professionals: http://certification.acsm.org/faq28-codeofethics
- Clinical Exercise Physiology Association: http://www.acsm-cepa.org
- Commission on Accreditation of Allied Health Education Programs: http://www.caahep.org
- Committee on Accreditation for the Exercise Sciences: http://www.coaes.org
- The National Commission for Certifying Agencies under the National Organization for Competency Assurance: http://www.noca.org

REFERENCES

1. Costanzo DG. ACSM Certification: The Evolution of the Exercise Professional. *ACSM Health Fitness J.* 2006;10(4):38–9.
2. Paternostro-Bayles M. The role of a job task analysis in the development of professional certifications. *ACSM Health Fitness J.* 2010; 14(4):41–2.

Editors for the Previous Two Editions

EDITORS FOR THE 6TH EDITION

SENIOR EDITOR

Jonathan K. Ehrman, PhD, FACSM
ACSM Program Director^{SM}
ACSM Certified Clinical Exercise Specialist®
Henry Ford Hospital
Detroit, Michigan

SECTION EDITORS

Adam deJong, MA
ACSM Certified Clinical Exercise Specialist®
William Beaumont Hospital
Royal Oak, Michigan

Bonnie Sanderson, PhD, RN
ACSM Program Director^{SM}
ACSM Certified Clinical Exercise Specialist®
University of Alabama at Birmingham
Birmingham, Alabama

David Swain, PhD, FACSM
ACSM Program Director^{SM}
ACSM Certified Clinical Exercise Specialist®
Old Dominion University
Norfolk, Virginia

Ann Swank, PhD, FACSM
ACSM Program Director^{SM}
ACSM Certified Clinical Exercise Specialist®
University of Louisville
Louisville, Kentucky

Chris Womack, PhD, FACSM
ACSM Certified Clinical Exercise Specialist®
James Madison University
Harrisonburg, Virginia

EDITORS FOR THE 5TH EDITION

SENIOR EDITOR

Leonard A. Kaminsky, PhD, FACSM
ACSM Program Director® Certified
ACSM Exercise Test Technologist® Certified
Human Performance Laboratory
Adult Fitness/Cardiac Rehabilitation Program
Ball State University
Muncie, Indiana

SECTION EDITORS

Kimberly A. Bonzheim, MS, FACSM
ACSM Program Director® Certified
Noninvasive Cardiology
William Beaumont Hospital
Royal Oak, Michigan

Carol Ewing Garber, PhD, RCEP®, FACSM
ACSM Program Director® Certified
ACSM Exercise Test Technologist® Certified
ACSM Health Fitness Instructor® Certified
Bouvé College of Health Sciences
Northeastern University
Boston, Massachusetts

Stephen C. Glass, PhD, FACSM
ACSM Exercise Specialist® Certified
Department of Movement Science
Grand Valley State University
Allendale, Michigan

Larry F. Hamm, PhD, FACSM
ACSM Program Director® Certified
ACSM Exercise Test Technologist® Certified
ACSM Exercise Specialist® Certified
Cardiac Rehabilitation Program Neuroscience Center
National Rehabilitation Hospital
Washington, DC

Harold W. Kohl III, PhD, FACSM
Centers for Disease Control and Prevention
National Center for Chronic Disease Prevention and Health Promotion
Division of Nutrition and Physical Activity
Physical Activity and Health Branch
Atlanta, Georgia

Alan Mikesky, PhD, FACSM
Department of Physical Education
Indiana University–Purdue University Indianapolis
Indianapolis, Indiana

CONTRIBUTORS TO THE 6TH EDITION

Kent J. Adams
Department of Kinesiology
California State University
Chico, California
Chapter 3

Rafael Bahamonde, PhD, FACSM
School of Physical Education
Indiana University–Purdue University Indianapolis
Indianapolis, Indiana
Chapter 1

David Bassett, PhD, FACSM
ACSM Certified Clinical Exercise Specialist®
Department of Exercise, Sports and Leisure Studies
University of Tennessee
Knoxville, Tennessee
Chapter 12

Susan Beckham, PhD, FACSM
ACSM Program Director ᔆᴹ
ACSM Registered Clinical Exercise Physiologist®
ACSM Exercise Technologist®
Dallas Veteran Affairs Medical Center
Dallas, Texas
Chapter 50

Ghazelah Bigdeli, MD
Alleghany General Hospital
Pittsburgh, Pennsylvania
Chapter 23

Clinton A. Brawner, MS
ACSM Registered Clinical Exercise Physiologist®
ACSM Certified Clinical Exercise Specialist®
Preventive Cardiology
Henry Ford Hospital
Detroit, Missouri
Chapter 30

Cedric X. Bryant, PhD, FACSM
American Council on Exercise
San Diego, California
Chapter 48

Barbara Bushman, PhD
ACSM Program Director ᔆᴹ
ACSM Certified Clinical Exercise Specialist®
ACSM Certified Fitness Specialist
ACSM Certified Personal Trainer ᔆᴹ
Department of Health, Physical Education and
    Recreation
Missouri State University
Springfield, Missouri
Chapter 26

Brian W. Carlin, MD
Alleghany General Hospital
Pittsburgh, Pennsylvania
Chapter 23

Heather O. Chambliss, PhD, FACSM
Health, Exercise Science and Recreation Arrangement
University of Memphis
Memphis, Tennessee
Chapter 42

Dawn P. Coe, PhD
ACSM Certified Clinical Exercise Specialist®
Department of Health, Physical Education and
    Recreation
University of Tennessee
Knoxville, Tennessee
Chapter 41

Sheri R. Colberg, PhD
ACSM Exercise Test Technologist®
Exercise Science, Physical Education and Recreation
Old Dominion University
Norfolk, Virginia
Chapter 13

Christopher B. Cooper, MD
ACSM Health/Fitness Director®
David Geffen School of Medicine
University of California Los Angeles Medical Center
Los Angeles, California
Chapter 36

Laura Cupper, BSW, CCRC
Minto Prevention and Rehabilitation Centre
University of Ottawa Heart Institute
Ottawa, Ontario
Chapter 25

Adam deJong, MA
ACSM Certified Clinical Exercise Specialist®
Preventive Cardiology and Rehabilitation
William Beaumont Hospital
Royal Oak, Michigan
Chapter 20

Shawn Drake, PhD, PT
ACSM Program Director℠
ACSM Certified Clinical Exercise Specialist®
Department of Physical Therapy
Arkansas State University
Jonesboro, Arizona
Chapter 18

Andrea L. Dunn, PhD, FACSM
Klein Buendel, Inc.
Golden, Colorado
Chapter 9

J. Larry Durstine, PhD
Department of Exercise Science
The University of South Carolina
Columbia, South Carolina
Chapter 38

Paul Estabrooks, PhD
Human Nutrition, Foods, and Exercise
Virginia Tech
Blacksburg, Virginia
Chapter 47

Maria A. Fiatarone-Singh, MD
School of Exercise and Sport Science
University of Sydney
Lidcombe, NSW, Australia
Chapter 41

Carl Foster, PhD
ACSM Program Director℠
Department of Exercise and Sport Science
University of Wisconsin
LaCrosse, Wisconsin
Chapter 21

Barry Franklin, PhD
ACSM Program Director℠
ACSM Certified Clinical Exercise Specialist®
Preventive Cardiology and Rehabilitation
William Beaumont Hospital
Royal Oak, Michigan
Chapter 20

Peter W. Grandjean, PhD, FACSM
ACSM Certified Clinical Exercise Specialist®
Department of Health and Human Performance
Auburn University
Auburn, Alabama
Chapter 46

B. Sue Graves, EdD, FACSM
ACSM Certified Health Fitness Specialist®
Department of Exercise Science & Health Promotion
Florida Atlantic University
Boca Raton, Florida
Chapter 5

Jennifer Guthrie, MS
StayWell Corporation
Auburn Hills, Michigan
Chapter 19

Patrick Hagerman, EdD
ACSM Certified Health Fitness Specialist®
Department of Exercise and Sport Science
University of Tulsa
Tulsa, Oklahoma
Chapter 19

Chad Harris
Department of Allied Health
Western New Mexico University
Silver City, New Mexico
Chapter 3

Jeffrey Hastings, MD
Institute for Exercise and Environmental Medicine
Presbyterian Hospital of Dallas and University of Texas
Southwestern Medical Center
Dallas, Texas
Chapter 34

David L. Herbert, JD
David L. Herbert and Associates, LLC
Canton, Ohio
Chapter 51

William G. Herbert, PhD, FACSM
ACSM Program Director^{SM}
Human Nutrition, Foods, and Exercise
Virginia Polytechnic Institute and State University
Blacksburg, Virginia
Chapter 51

Julie M. Hughes
School of Kinesiology
University of Minnesota
Minneapolis, Minnesota
Chapter 39

Megan E. Jablonski, MS
Department of Psychological and Brain Sciences
University of Louisville
Louisville, Kentucky
Chapter 16

Patrick L. Jacobs, PhD, FACSM
Department of Exercise Science & Health Promotion
Florida Atlantic University
Boca Raton, Florida
Chapter 5

Rachel A. Jarvis, MS
ACSM Registered Clinical Exercise Physiologist®
ACSM Certified Clinical Exercise Specialist®
Edward Hospital
Naperville, Illinois
Chapter 35

Lyndon Joseph, PhD
University of Maryland School of Medicine
Division of Gerontology
Baltimore, Maryland
Chapter 8

Anthony S. Kaleth, PhD
ACSM Program Director^{SM}
ACSM Registered Clinical Exercise Physiologist®
ACSM Certified Clinical Exercise Specialist®
ACSM Certified Health Fitness Specialist
School of Physical Education
Indiana University–Purdue University Indianapolis
Indianapolis, Indiana
Chapter 1

Peter Kaplan, MD
Alleghany General Hospital
Pittsburgh, Pennsylvania
Chapter 23

Carol Kennedy-Armbruster, MS
ACSM Certified Health Fitness Specialist®
Department of Kinesiology
Indiana University
Bloomington, Indiana
Chapter 32

Steven J. Keteyian, PhD, FACSM
ACSM Registered Clinical Exercise Physiologist®
Preventive Cardiology
Henry Ford Hospital
Detroit, Michigan
Chapters 30,35

Abby C. King, PhD
Stanford Prevention Research Center
Stanford University School of Medicine
Stanford, California
Chapter 42

Duane Knudson, PhD, FACSM
Department of Physical Education and Exercise Science
California State University
Chico, California
Chapter 2

William J. Kraemer, PhD, FACSM
Department of Kinesiology
University of Connecticut
Storrs, Connecticut
Chapters 29,31

William E. Kraus, MD, FACSM, FACC
Duke University Medical Center
Durham, North Carolina
Chapter 11

Diana Lahue, RN, BSN
Research Medical Center
Kansas City, Missouri
Chapter 27

John Lee, MD, FACC
Research Medical Center
Kansas City, Missouri
Chapter 27

Benjamin Levine, MD
Institute for Exercise and Environmental Medicine
Presbyterian Hospital of Dallas and University of Texas
Southwestern Medical Center
Dallas, Texas
Chapter 34

Shel Levine, MS, MSA
ACSM Certified Clinical Exercise Specialist®
School of Health Promotion and Human
    Performance
Eastern Michigan University
Ypsilanti, Missouri
Chapter 26

Beth A. Lewis, PhD
Health Partners Research Foundation
Minneapolis, Minnesota
Chapters 43,44

G. William Lyerly, MS
ACSM Certified Clinical Exercise Specialist®
ACSM Certified Health Fitness Specialist
Department of Exercise Science
The University of South Carolina
Columbia, South Carolina
Chapter 38

Bess H. Marcus, PhD
Department of Psychiatry and Human Behavior
Brown University
Providence, Rhode Island
Chapters 43,44

Bonita Marks, PhD, FACSM
ACSM Certified Clinical Exercise Specialist®
Department of Exercise and Sport Science
University of North Carolina
Chapel Hill, North Carolina
Chapter 10

Timothy Maynard, MS
ACSM Program Director ᔆᴹ
Providence Rehab and Wellness Center
Providence Hospital
Mobile, Alabama
Chapter 24

Peter A. McCullough, MD, MPH
Preventive and Nutritional Medicine
William Beaumont Hospital
Royal Oak, Michigan
Chapter 22

A. Lynn Millar, PT, PhD, FACSM
Department of Physical Therapy
Andrews University
Berrien Springs, Minnesota
Chapter 40

Nancy Houston Miller, RN, BSN
Stanford University School of Medicine
Palo Alto, California
Chapter 15

Geoffrey E. Moore, MD, FACSM
Cayuga Center for Healthy Living
Ithaca, New York
Chapter 38

Paul Nagelkirk, PhD
ACSM Certified Clinical Exercise Specialist®
School of Physical Education, Sport and
    Exercise Science
Ball State University
Muncie, Indiana
Chapter 6

Melissa A. Napolitano, PhD
Department of Kinesiology, Center for Obesity
    Research and Education
Temple University
Philadelphia, Pennsylvania
Chapters 43,44

Stefan M. Pasiakos, PhD
ACSM Certified Health Fitness Specialist
University of Connecticut
Department of Nutritional Science
Storrs, Connecticut
Chapter 4

James A. Peterson, PhD, FACSM
Healthy Learning/Coaches Choice
Monterey, California
Chapter 48

Moira A. Petit, PhD
School of Kinesiology
University of Minnesota
Minneapolis, Minnesota
Chapter 39

John P. Porcari, PhD
ACSM Program Director ᔆᴹ
ACSM Registered Clinical Exercise Physiologist®
Department of Exercise and Sport Science
University of Wisconsin
LaCrosse, Wisconsin
Chapter 21

Judith J. Prochaska, PhD, MPH
Department of Psychiatry
University of California
San Francisco, California
Chapter 45

Nicholas Ratamess, PhD
Department of Health and Exercise Science
College of New Jersey
Ewing, New Jersey
Chapter 17

Nancy R. Rodriguez, PhD, FACSM
Department of Nutritional Science
University of Connecticut
Storrs, Connecticut
Chapter 4

Jeffrey L. Roitman, EdD, FACSM
ACSM Program Director SM
Research Medical Center
Kansas City, Missouri
Chapter 27

Lee M. Romer, PhD
Centre for Sports Medicine and Human Performance
School of Sport and Education
Brunel University
Uxbridge, Middlesex, England
Chapter 7

Alice Ryan, PhD
ACSM Certified Clinical Exercise Specialist®
University of Maryland School of Medicine
Division of Gerontology
Baltimore, Maryland
Chapter 8

James F. Sallis, PhD
Department of Psychology
San Diego State University
San Diego, California
Chapter 45

Paul Salmon, PhD
ACSM Certified Health Fitness Specialist
Department of Psychological and Brain Sciences
University of Louisville
Louisville, Kentucky
Chapter 16

Bonnie K. Sanderson PhD, RN, FAACVPR
ACSM Certified Exercise Specialist®
ACSM Program Director SM
Department of Cardiovascular Services
University of Alabama at Birmingham
Birmingham, Alabama
Chapters 46,49

Patrick Savage, MS, FAACVPR
Cardiac Rehabilitation
Fletcher Allen Health Care
South Burlington, Vermont
Chapter 49

Matthew Saval, MS
ACSM Registered Clinical Exercise Physiologist®
ACSM Certified Clinical Exercise Specialist®
Preventive Cardiology
Henry Ford Hospital
Detroit, Michigan
Chapter 30

John R. Schairer, DO
Preventive Cardiology
Henry Ford Hospital
Detroit, Michigan
Chapter 35

Tom Spring, MS
ACSM Certified Clinical Exercise Specialist®
ACSM Certified Personal Trainer SM
Preventive Cardiology and Rehabilitation
William Beaumont Hospital
Royal Oak, Michigan
Chapter 20

Thomas W. Storer, MD
David Geffen School of Medicine
University of California Los Angeles Medical Center
Los Angeles, California
Chapter 36

David P. Swain, PhD, FACSM
ACSM Program Director SM
ACSM Certified Clinical Exercise Specialist®
Department of Exercise Science
Old Dominion University
Norfolk, Virginia
Chapter 28

Stephen J. Tharrett, MS
ACSM Program Director SM
Club Industry Consulting
Highland Village, Texas
Chapter 48

Larry Verity, PhD
ACSM Certified Clinical Exercise Specialist®
Department of Exercise and Nutritional Sciences
San Diego State University
San Diego, California
Chapter 37

David E. Verrill, MS, FAACVPR
ACSM Program Director SM
ACSM Registered Clinical Exercise Physiologist®
ACSM Exercise Test Technologist®
Presbyterian Hospital Pulmonary Rehabilitation
    Program
Charlotte, North Carolina
Chapter 49

Stella L. Volpe, PhD, RD, LDN, FACSM
ACSM Certified Clinical Exercise Specialist®
School of Nursing
University of Pennsylvania
Philadelphia, Pennsylvania
Chapter 33

Joseph M. Warpeha
ACSM Registered Clinical Exercise Physiologist®
ACSM Certified Clinical Exercise Specialist®
School of Kinesiology
University of Minnesota
Minneapolis, Minnesota
Chapter 39

Michael Whitehurst, EdD, FACSM
Department of Exercise Science & Health Promotion
Florida Atlantic University
Boca Raton, Florida
Chapter 5

Jessica A. Whiteley, PhD
Department of Exercise and Health Sciences
University of Massachusetts
Boston, Massachusetts
Chapters 43,44

CONTRIBUTORS TO THE 5TH EDITION

Leonard A. Kaminsky, PhD, FACSM
ACSM Program Director® Certified
ACSM Exercise Test Technologist® Certified
Human Performance Laboratory
Adult Fitness/Cardiac Rehabilitation Program
Ball State University
Muncie, Indiana

Kent Adams, PhD, FACSM
Exercise Physiology Lab
University of Louisville
Louisville, Kentucky

Simon Bacon, PhD
Department of Psychiatry
Duke University Medical Center
Durham, North Carolina

Rafael E. Bahamonde, PhD, FACSM
Department of Physical Education
Indiana University–Purdue University Indianapolis
Indianapolis, Indiana

Susan G. Beckham, PhD, FACSM, RCEP®
ACSM Program Director® Certified
ACSM Exercise Test Technologist® Certified
Noninvasive Cardiology
Dallas VA Medical Center
Dallas, Texas

Valerie Bishop, PhD, RCEP®
ACSM Health Fitness Instructor®Certified
ACSM Exercise Specialist® Certified
Independent Consultant
Ojai, California

James A. Blumenthal, PhD
Department of Psychiatry
Duke University Medical Center
Durham, North Carolina

Clinton A. Brawner, CES
ACSM Exercise Specialist® Certified
Preventive Cardiology
Henry Ford Hospital
Detroit, Michigan

Suzanne Brodney-Folse, PhD, RD
Department of Community Health
Brown University
Providence, Rhode Island

Cedric X. Bryant, PhD, FACSM
Educational Services
American Council on Exercise
Redmond, Washington

Barbara N. Campaigne, PhD, FACSM
Diabetes and Endocrine Platform Team
Eli Lilly and Company
Indianapolis, Indiana

Brian Carlin, MD
Division of Pulmonary and Critical Care Medicine
Drexel University
Philadelphia, Pennsylvania

Ruth Ann Carpenter, MS, RD, LD
Cooper Institute
Dallas, Texas

Cynthia Castro, PhD
Stanford Prevention Research Center
Stanford University School of Medicine
Stanford, California

Heather O. Chambliss, PhD
The Cooper Institute
Southaven, Mississippi

Timothy Church, MD, MPH, PhD
Center for Medical & Laboratory Research
Cooper Institute
Dallas, Texas

Christopher B. Cooper, MD, FRCP, FACSM, FCCP
ACSM Health Fitness Director® Certified
Departments of Medicine and Physiology
UCLA—David Geffen School of Medicine
Los Angeles, California

Kerry S. Courneya, PhD
Faculty of Physical Education
University of Alberta
Edmonton, Alberta

Joel T. Cramer, PhD, HFI; CSCS,*D; NSCA-CPT, *D
ACSM Health Fitness Instructor® Certified
Department of Kinesiology
The University of Texas at Arlington
Arlington, Texas

Tim L.A. Doyle, MSc, CSCS
Exercise Biomechanics
University of Notre Dame Australia
Fremantle WA Australia

Eric L. Dugan, PhD
Biomechanics Laboratory
Ball State University
Muncie, Indiana

Andrea Dunn, PhD, FACSM
Klein Buendel, Inc.
Golden, Colorado

Gregory B. Dwyer, PhD, FACSM, RCEP®
ACSM Program Director® Certified
ACSM Exercise Specialist® Certified
ACSM Exercise Test Technologist® Certified
Movement Studies and Exercise Science Department
East Stroudsburg University
East Stroudsburg, Pennsylvania

Kyle Ebersole, PhD
Department of Human Movement Science
University of Wisconsin, Milwaukee
Milwaukee, Wisconsin

Jonathan K. Ehrman, PhD, FACSM
ACSM Program Director® Certified
ACSM Exercise Specialist® Certified
Department of Preventive Cardiology
Henry Ford Heart & Vascular Institute
Detroit, Michigan

Eve V. Essery, PhD
Department of Nutrition and Food Sciences
Texas Woman's University
Denton, Texas

Tammy K. Evetovich, PhD, FACSM
ACSM Health Fitness Instructor®Certified
Department of Health, Human Performance and Sport
Wayne State College
Wayne, Nebraska

Brian W. Findley, MEd
Health Sciences Department
Palm Beach Community College
Boca Raton, Florida

Shannon J. Fitzgerald, PhD
Department of Kinesiology, Health Promotion, & Recreation
University of North Texas
Denton, Texas

Carl Foster, PhD, FACSM
ACSM Program Director® Certified
Department of Exercise and Sport Science
University of Wisconsin-LaCrosse
LaCrosse, Wisconsin

Barry A. Franklin, PhD, FACSM
ACSM Program Director® Certified
ACSM Exercise Specialist® Certified
Preventive Cardiology
Beaumont Health Center
Royal Oak, Michigan

Neil F. Gordon, MD, PhD, FACSM
Center for Heart Disease Prevention
St. Joseph's/Candler Health System
Savannah, Georgia

B. Sue Graves, EdD, FACSM
ACSM Health Fitness Instructor®Certified
Department of Exercise Science and Health Promotion
Florida Atlantic University
Davie, Florida

Suzanne L. Groah, MD, MSPH
Rehabilitation Research and Training Center on
    Secondary Conditions after Spinal Cord Injury
National Rehabilitation Hospital
Washington, DC

Larry R. Gurchiek, PhD
Department of Health, Physical Education,
    & Leisure Studies
University of South Alabama
Mobile, Alabama

Chad Harris, PhD
Department of Kinesiology
Boise State University
Boise, Idaho

David L. Herbert, JD
Herbert and Benson, Attorneys at Law
Canton, Ohio

William G. Herbert, PhD, FACSM
ACSM Program Director® Certified
Department of Human Nutrition, Foods, and Exercise
Virginia Polytechnic Institute and State University
Blacksburg, Virginia

Brendan Humphries, PhD
School of Science and Primary Industries
Charles Darwin University
Darwin, Northern Territory, Australia

Kurt Jackson, PhD, GCS
Kettering Medical Center
Kettering, Ohio

Anthony S. Kaleth, PhD, RCEP®
ACSM Program Director® Certified
ACSM Health Fitness Instructor®Certified
ACSM Exercise Specialist®Certified
Department of Physical Education
Indiana University–Purdue University Indianapolis
Indianapolis, Indiana

Peter T. Katzmarzyk, PhD, FACSM
School of Physical and Health Education
Queen's University
Kingston, Ontario

NiCole Keith, PhD
Department of Physical Education
Indiana University–Purdue University Indianapolis
Indianapolis, Indiana

Steven John Keteyian, PhD, FACSM, RCEP®
Henry Ford Heart & Vascular Institute
Detroit, Michigan

Abby King, PhD, FACSM
Training Program
Stanford University School of Medicine
Palo Alto, California

Duane V. Knudson, PhD, FACSM
Department of Kinesiology
California State University, Chico
Chico, California

John E. Kovaleski, PhD
Department of Health & Physical Education
University of South Alabama
Mobile, Alabama

Len Kravitz, PhD
ACSM Health Fitness Instructor® Certified
Department of Physical Performance & Development
University of New Mexico
Albuquerque, New Mexico

Jessica Krenkel, MS, RD, CNSD
Division of Medical Nutrition
University of Nevada School of Medicine
Reno, Nevada

Doina Kulick, MD
Division of Medical Nutrition
University of Nevada School of Medicine
Reno, Nevada

Richard Mearl Lampman, PhD, FACSM
Department of Surgery
St. Joseph Mercy Hospital
Ann Arbor, Michigan

John A. Larry, MD
Division of Cardiology
The Ohio State University Medical Center
Columbus, Ohio

Richard F. Leighton, MD
Medical College of Ohio
Toledo, Ohio

Beth Lewis, PhD
Health Partners Research Foundation
Minneapolis, Minnesota

Bess H. Marcus, PhD
Division of Behavioral Medicine
The Miriam Hospital
Providence, Rhode Island

John E. Martin, PhD
Department of Psychology
San Diego State University
San Diego, California

Sara McGlynn, MBA, CPA
Cardiology
William Beaumont Hospital
Royal Oak, Michigan

Stephen P. Messier, PhD, FACSM
Department of Health & Exercise Science
Wake Forest University
Winston-Salem, North Carolina

Aryan N. Mooss, MD
Division of Cardiology
Creighton University School of Medicine
Omaha, Nebraska

James R. Morrow, Jr., PhD, FACSM
Department of Kinesiology, Health Promotion
    & Recreation
University of North Texas
Denton, Texas

Janet A. Mulcare, PhD, FACSM
Department of Physical Therapy
Andrews University
Berrien Springs, Michigan

Melissa A. Napolitano, PhD
Centers for Behavioral and Preventive Medicine
Brown Medical School and the Miriam Hospital
Providence, Rhode Island

David L. Nichols, PhD, FACSM
Department of Kinesiology
Texas Woman's University
Denton, Texas

David C. Nieman, DrPH, FACSM
Department of Health, Leisure and Exercise Science
Appalachian State University
Boone, North Carolina

Nancy E. O'Hare, ScD, FACSM
Cardiovascular Division
Beth Israel Deaconess Medical Center
Boston, Massachusetts

Patricia Painter, PhD, FACSM
Department of Physiological Nursing
University of California at San Francisco
San Francisco, California

Albert Washington Pearsall IV, MD
Department of Orthopaedic Surgery
University of South Alabama Medical Center
Mobile, Alabama

Laura Peno-Green, MD, FCCP
Marietta Pulmonary Medicine
Marietta, Georgia

James A. Peterson, PhD, FACSM
Healthy Learning
Monterey, California

John P. Porcari, PhD, FACSM, RCEP®
ACSM Program Director® Certified
Department of Exercise and Sport Science
University of Wisconsin-La Crosse
LaCrosse, Wisconsin

Judith J. Prochaska, PhD, MPH
Department of Psychiatry
University of California, San Francisco
San Francisco, California

Jeanne E. Ruff, MS
Cardiovascular Rehab and Health Promotion
Peninsula Regional Medical Center
Salisbury, Maryland

Khaleel Salahudeen, MD
Pulmonary Laboratory
Allegheny General Hospital
Pittsburgh, Pennsylvania

James F. Sallis, PhD, FACSM
Department of Psychology
San Diego State University
San Diego, California

Robert Scales, PhD
Albuquerque, New Mexico

Stephen F. Schaal, MD
Division of Cardiology
The Ohio State University Medical Center
Columbus, Ohio

John Schairer, DO
Advanced Cardiovascular Health Specialists
Livonia, Michigan
Henry Ford Heart & Vascular Institute
Detroit, Michigan

Lois Sheldahl, PhD
Veteran's Administration Medical Center
Milwaukee, Wisconsin

Ray W. Squires, PhD, FACSM
ACSM Program Director®Certified
ACSM Exercise Specialist®Certified
Division of Cardiovascular Diseases &
   Internal Medicine
Mayo Clinic and Foundation
Rochester, Minnesota

Satchiko St. Jeor, PhD
Division of Medical Nutrition
University of Nevada School of Medicine
Reno, Nevada

Stephen J. Tharrett, MS
Club Corps of America
Dallas, Texas

Larry S. Verity, PhD, FACSM
ACSM Exercise Specialist®Certified
Department of Exercise & Nutritional Sciences
San Diego State University
San Diego, California

Stella Lucia Volpe, PhD, RD, FACSM
ACSM Exercise Specialist®Certified
Department of Nutrition
University of Massachusetts
Amherst, Massachusetts

Janet P. Wallace, PhD, FACSM
ACSM Program Director®Certified
ACSM Exercise Specialist®Certified
Adult Fitness Program
Indiana University
Bloomington, Indiana

Joe P. Weir, PhD, FACSM
Department of Physical Therapy
Des Moines University
Des Moines, Iowa

Michael Whitehurst, EdD, FACSM
Department of Exercise Science & Health Promotion
Florida Atlantic University
Davie, Florida

Jessica Whiteley, PhD
The Centers for Behavioral and Preventative Medicine
Brown Medical School/The Miriam Hospital
Providence, Rhode Island

Index

Page numbers followed by "f" denote figures, those followed by "t" denote tables, and those followed by "b" denote boxes.

coronary artery disease, 624t
heart failure, 624t
pacemakers, 624t
after percutaneous coronary intervention, 624t, 627
after percutaneous transluminal angioplasty, 624t, 627
after valve surgery, 624t
Cardiovascular disease (CVD), 110–117. *See also specific types*
atherosclerosis, 110–112, 110b, 111f
definition of, 110b
with diabetes mellitus, exercise precautions in, 673–674, 673t
diet in, 208–211
medical nutrition therapy in, 208, 209t–210t
epidemiology of, 110, 208, 248
on exercise prescription, 173
key terms in, 110b
myocardium healing in, 117, 117b
outcomes and manifestations of
coronary heart disease, 112
heart failure, 112–113, 112t
hypertension, 112
peripheral arterial disease, 113, 113t
stroke, 113
preparticipation screening and risk assessment with, 172
psychosocial interventions for, 250–251, 274–275
psychosocial status and, 248–250, 250f
anxiety in, 249, 274
depression in, 248–250, 274
social support on, 249
stress in, 248, 249, 250f, 274
resistance training with, 608
risk factors and their modification in
dyslipidemia, 115
fasting glucose, impaired, 116, 207b
hypertension, 114–115, 115t
obesity, 115–116
sedentary lifestyle, 115
smoking, 114
treatment of
pharmacologic, 116–117
surgical, 113–114, 114f
warm-up and cool-down with, 608
Cardiovascular disease (CVD), diagnosis, 382–395
chest discomfort evaluation in, 384–386, 386b
as coronary artery disease screening, 384, 385f
decision statistics in, 386–388, 387t, 388f
graded exercise testing with electro-cardiography in, 388–389, 390b
guidelines for, 382–383
history and physical examination in, 383–384, 383b
imaging methods in, 389–395
cardiac magnetic resonance imaging, 393
coronary angiography, 394, 394b
coronary computed tomography angiography, 393, 394b
echocardiography, 390–391, 391b

intravascular ultrasound, 394–395
myocardial perfusion imaging, 391–393, 392b
positron emission tomography, 393
value and use of, 389–390
key terms in, 382b
management guidance in, 386
prognosis determination in, 386
test selection in, 388, 388b, 389f
Cardiovascular disease (CVD), exercise prescription with, 250–251, 619–629
with angina and myocardial infarction, 626–630 (*See also* Angina; Myocardial infarction [MI])
cardiac rehabilitation in, 623–624
disease-specific effects in
on blood pressure, 620, 620t
on cardiac output and oxygen uptake, 620, 620t
on heart rate, 619–620, 620t
key terms in, 619b
programming in, 624–626, 624t, 625t
with coronary artery disease, 624t, 626
rationale for exercise therapy in, 620–623
autonomic nervous system in, 622
hemostatic components in, 623
HR variability in, 622
myocardial oxygen demand in, 621, 621f
myocardial oxygen supply in, 621–622, 622t
Cardiovascular drift, exercise on, 55
Cardiovascular endurance training, 578. *See also* Cardiorespiratory exercise prescription
Cardiovascular exercise, 469. *See also specific types and applications*
Cardiovascular risk factors, exercise on, 624, 625t
Cardiovascular system
aging on, 92–93
resistance training on, 513t
Carina, 12f, 13
Carotid pulse, 326, 327f
Carpal tunnel syndrome, 605b
Cartilage
articular, 17, 19f
resistance training on, 522
Cartilaginous joints, 18, 19t
Casting, deconditioning from, 97t, 98
Catecholamines, resistance training on, 519, 519t, 520
Center of gravity, 32b, 41
in weightlifting, 41
Center of mass, displacing, 588–589
Center of rotation (COR), 29, 30f
Central fatigue, 44b, 62
Central nervous system, aging on, 95
Central obesity, 685
Cerebral edema, high-altitude, 71, 614–615
Cerebrovascular disease
epidemiology and pathophysiology of, 686
exercise prescription in, 694
exercise responses and adaptations in, 691–692
medical management of, 689

Certifications, American College of Sports Medicine (ACSM), 805–814
CES. *See* American College of Sports Medicine (ACSM), Certified Clinical Exercise Specialist (CES)
Chambers, heart, 3–4, 4f, 5, 6f
enlargement of
atrial enlargement in, 462
metabolic disorders in, 462, 462t
ventricular hypertrophy, 461–462, 461t, 462f
Change
processes of, 730b, 761b, 764
stages of (*See* Stages of change [SOC] model)
Change talk, 764
Channels, 774b, 775
Chest discomfort, 384–386, 386b
Chest pain, 601b
Chest wall, 15, 16f
Chest wall deformities, 641
Chilblain, 610t
Child and Adolescent Trial for Cardiovascular Health (CATCH), 789
Children
body composition assessment in, 303
definition of, 565b
exercise assessment in, 439–444
echocardiography in, 424
exercise protocols in, 442–443
exercise testing in, 439–440, 568–569
hemodynamic and pulmonary characteristics of, 440t
indications for, 439
maximal effort criteria in, 441
muscular strength and endurance testing in, 351–352
relative risks for, 443t
stress testing in, 441–442, 443b, 443t
stress testing in, pharmacologic, 424
testing equipment in, 440–441, 440b, 441t
test termination in, 442, 443b
exercise in, 568–570
benefits of, 568
cardiovascular risk factors in, 568
exercise response in, 568
exercise prescription in, 569–570
obesity and overweight in, 568
special considerations in, 569–570
Cholesterol, 82, 83, 683, 684t
in coronary artery disease, 211–213
omega-3 fatty acids, 207b, 212
omega-6 fatty acids, 207b, 212–213
saturated and unsaturated, 82–83, 211–212
trans fatty acids and interesterified fats, 213
definition of, 206b
in diabetes, 225
high-density lipoprotein, 206b, 683, 684t
low-density lipoprotein
in atherosclerosis, 110–111
cardiovascular disease from, 115
definition of, 207b
preparticipation testing of, 329
Chondroitin, 717